AIIMS NOV

Multiple Choice Questions

ANATOMY

1. Which of following is not the branch of external carotid artery in Kiesselbach's plexus?
   a. Anterior and posterior ethmoidal
   b. Sphenopalatine artery
   c. Greater palatine artery
   d. Septal branch of superior labial artery

2. Structure passing through the central tendon of the diaphragm:
   a. Esophagus   b. Aorta
   c. IVC   d. Sympathetic chain

3. Talocalcaneonavicular joint is what type of joint?
   a. Saddle   b. Hinge
   c. Ellipsoid   d. Ball and socket

4. Marked structure in the given image connects which of the following?

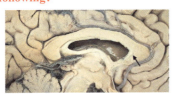

   a. Striate cortex   b. Orbital cortex
   c. Hippocampus   d. Dentate nucleus

5. Development the of heart is from which of the following marked structure?

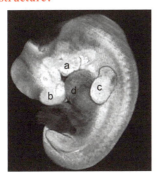

   a. a   b. b
   c. c   d. d

6. Which of the following sinus grows till early adulthood?
   a. Maxillary   b. Ethmoidal
   c. Frontal   d. Sphenoid

7. What is the shape of the trapezius muscle?
   a. Quadrangular b. Triangular
   c. Strap   d. Fusiform

8. Which of the marked muscle helps in the opening of jaw?

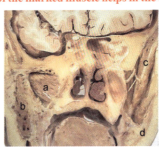

   a. a   b. b
   c. c   d. d

9. Dense irregular collagen fibres are found in which of the following?
   a. Tendon   b. Ligament
   c. Dermis   d. Lamina propria

10. Holocrine cells in the given slide are:

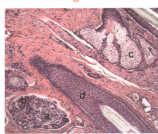

    a. a   b. b
    c. c   d. d

11. Identify the marked nerve:

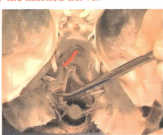

    a. Abducent nerve
    b. Spinal accessory nerve
    c. Hypoglossal nerve
    d. Labyrinthine artery

12. What is the root value of cremasteric reflex?
    a. L1-L2   b. L2-L3
    c. L4-L5   d. S1-S2

13. All of the following are true about grey communicans *except*:
    a. Unmyelinated
    b. Connects to spinal nerves
    c. Preganglionic
    d. Present medial to the white ramus communicans

14. Which of the following junctional complexes are not seen in the marked region of the given slide?

    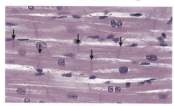

    a. Gap junction (communicating junctions)
    b. Zonula occludens (tight junction)
    c. Fascia adherens (adhering junction)
    d. Macula adherens (desmosomes)

15. Which of the following layer contains abundant desmosomes?

    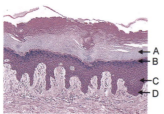

    a. A   b. B
    c. C   d. D

16. Which of the following refers to the lateral semicircular canal in the specimen of cortical mastoidectomy with posterior tympanostomy?

    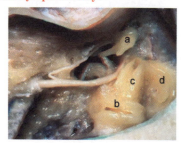

    a. a   b. b
    c. c   d. d

PHYSIOLOGY

17. Slow waves are generated by:
    a. Myenteric neurons   b. Smooth muscle
    c. Interstitial cells of Cajal   d. Parasympathetic neurons

18. Reflex responsible for tachycardia during right atrial distension is:
    a. Bezold-Jarisch reflex   b. Bainbridge reflex
    c. Cushing reflex   d. J-reflex

19. Identify the stage of sleep from the given picture:

    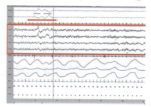

    a. Stage I NREM   b. Stage II NREM
    c. Stage III NREM d. REM

20. Identify the hormone from the picture:

    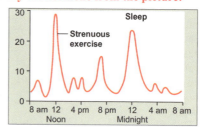

    a. Growth hormone   b. Cortisol
    c. Estrogen   d. Insulin

21. Feed forward control system is employed during the regulation of:
    a. Blood volume   b. pH
    c. Temperature   d. Blood pressure

22. Efferent arteriolar constriction causes all of the following *except*:
    a. Decrease in GFR
    b. Decreases renal blood flow
    c. Decreases oncotic pressure in peritubular capillaries
    d. Increases hydrostatic pressure in glomerular capillaries

23. Difference in trajectory between inspiratory loop and the expiratory loop in the curve is due to:

    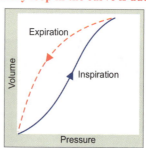

    a. Difference in alveolar pressure during inspiration and expiration
    b. Difference in concentration of surfactant during inspiration and expiration
    c. Difference in airway resistance during inspiration and expiration
    d. Inspiration is active and expiration is passive

24. Absolute refractory period is due to:
    a. Opening of calcium channels
    b. Closure of potassium channels
    c. Closure of active gates of sodium channel
    d. Closure of inactive gates of sodium channel

25. X, Y, Z are the three ions permeable. X = –50 and Y = –30. If at resting membrane potential (RMP), when there is no net electro genic transfer, what is the value of Z?
    a. +20
    b. –20
    c. +80
    d. –80

BIOCHEMISTRY

26. Which of the following amino acid does not include post-translational modification?
    a. Selenocysteine
    b. Triiodothyronine
    c. Hydroxyproline
    d. Hydroxylysine

27. Which of the following vitamin is required for glycogen phosphorylase?
    a. Pyridoxal phosphate
    b. Thiamine pyrophosphate
    c. Riboflavin
    d. Lipoic acid

28. Structure of DNA is shown. What are the bonds between 2 nitrogenous bases?

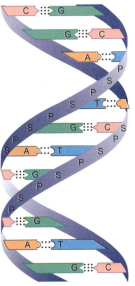

    a. 3'5' phosphodiester bonds
    b. 2'5' phosphodiester bonds
    c. Hydrogen bonds
    d. Covalent bonds

29. Following are the test done for proteins, sugar and ketones. Which of the following will be positive in starvation state in urine?

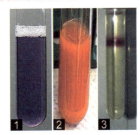

    a. 1 and 2
    b. Only 2
    c. Only 3
    d. 2 and 3

30. Which type of DNA repair is defective in severe combined immunodeficiency disease (SCID)?
    a. Homologous end joining repair
    b. Nucleotide excision repair
    c. Non-homologous end joining repair
    d. Base excision repair

31. Child presents with hypotonia and seizures. It was confirmed to be Zellweger syndrome. Which of the following is accumulated in the brain in zellweger syndrome?
    a. Glucose
    b. Lactic acid
    c. Long chain fatty acid
    d. Triglycerides

32. Dried blood drop of an infant can be used to know:
    a. Blood sugar
    b. Inborn errors of metabolism
    c. Hepatitis
    d. Cataract

PATHOLOGY

33. Storage period of 35 days for blood is seen with:
    a. CPD
    b. CPDA-1
    c. ACD
    d. CP2D

34. In Prothrombin time (PT) estimation, on addition of calcium and thromboplastin to platelet poor plasma, which of the following pathway is activated?
    a. Extrinsic
    b. Intrinsic
    c. Fibrinolysis
    d. Common

35. What is the correct order of blood sampling?
    1. Verification of patient's profile
    2. Labeling at bedside
    3. Sampling
    4. Identification of patient
    a. 1, 2, 3, 4
    b. 4, 1, 3, 2
    c. 4, 3, 1, 2
    d. 1, 4, 2, 3

36. Which of the following anticoagulant is used for electrolyte estimation?
    a. EDTA
    b. Citrate
    c. Sodium fluoride
    d. Lithium heparin

37. Patient with bilateral proptosis is being investigated. Identify the diagnosis based on given biopsy from the region:

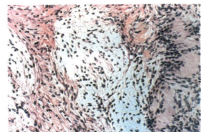

    a. Leiomyoma
    b. Schwannoma
    c. Rhabdomyosarcoma
    d. Fibromatosis

38. Which of the following will be seen on the peripheral smear of a 5 years old patient with HbA2 3% and HbF 97%?

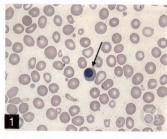
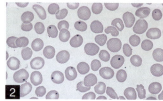
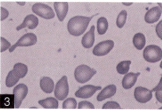

a. 1 and 2
b. 1 and 3
c. 2 and 3
d. 1, 2 and 3

39. Which of the following is not involved in iron metabolism?
    a. Transthyretin
    b. Hepcidin
    c. Ceruloplasmin
    d. Ferritin

40. All of the followings are reduced in iron deficiency anaemia *except*:
    a. Serum ferritin
    b. TIBC
    c. Hepcidin
    d. Transferrin saturation

41. In the cases of carcinoma breast with Her-2 neu immunohistochemistry staining, which of the following score needs further FISH study?
    a. 0
    b. 1+
    c. 2+
    d. 3+

42. A depressed patient came with the history of sudden onset of dyspnea. Chest X-ray shows bilateral diffuse infiltrates with predominant involvement of right middle and lower lobes. He could not be saved despite treatment and on autopsy, the lungs appeared normal grossly. Histopathology showed the following. What is your diagnosis?

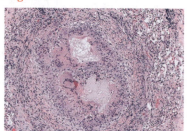

a. Necrotizing TB granuloma
b. Vegetative matter aspiration pneumonia
c. Sarcoid granuloma
d. Severe fungal pneumonia

43. Origin of CLL/SLL:
    a. Centrocytes
    b. Extranodal mature peripheral b cells
    c. Naive B cells in inter-follicular zones
    d. Bone marrow progenitors

44. In a child with bilateral proptosis. Which investigation will help you in arriving at the diagnosis of chloroma?
    a. Peripheral smear
    b. Platelets
    c. Hb concentration
    d. Leucocytic count

45. A hilly area, male patient presented with fever and splenomegaly. TLC was 21000, differential showed metamyelocytes and myelocytes (around 40%). Hb was 16, lymphocytes and platelets were normal. Next investigation will be:
    a. EPO estimation
    b. Philadelphia chromosome
    c. JAK2 mutations
    d. Bone marrow biopsy with reticulin stain

46. Endoscopic picture of a lesion in esophagus is shown below. What is the expected histopathology finding?

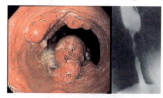

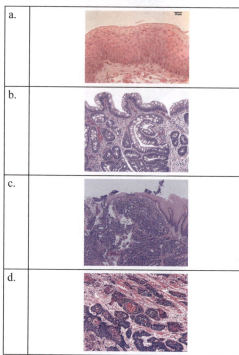

47. A 30 years old male patient presented with severe dyspnoea. Mitral stenosis with LA hypertrophy was seen. Vegetations on the mitral valve, which was excised. Image of HPE shows:

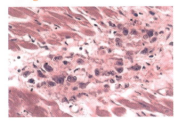

   a. Sarcoidosis
   b. Tuberculosis
   c. Aschoff nodule
   d. Fungal granuloma

48. Asymptomatic hepatitis B is common in 2-3% normal population, but there is increased risk of transmission into hepatocellular carcinoma. Why?
   a. Inability to induce inflammation to remove the organism
   b. High level of transaminases
   c. High rate of proliferation of hepatocytes
   d. Integration of viral DNA with host DNA

49. Which of the following statement is not true about glomerular basement membrane?
   a. Type III collagen is present
   b. Glomerular basement membrane is stained with PAS
   c. Glomerular basement membrane acts as filtration barrier
   d. Glomerular basement membrane is involved in charge dependent filtration

PHARMACOLOGY

50. A patient requires ceftriaxone 180 mg. You have a 2 ml syringe with 10 divisions per ml. The vial contains 500 mg/5 ml of ceftriaxone. How many divisions in the 2 ml syringe will you fill to give 180 mg ceftriaxone?
   a. 18   b. 1.8
   c. 20   d. 2

51. Mechanism of action of vancomycin is:
   a. Cell wall synthesis inhibition
   b. Protein synthesis inhibition
   c. Increase membrane permeability
   d. Inhibit folic acid metabolism

52. Atropine is indicated in all the following poisonings *except*:
   a. Baygon   b. Tik 20
   c. Parathion   d. Endrin

53. A patient of septic shock was given intravenous norepinephrine. The response to this drug is best checked by:
   a. Increase in heart rate
   b. Decrease in heart rate
   c. Increase in mean arterial pressure
   d. Decreased renal perfusion and reduced urine output

54. A diabetic and hypertensive patient taking several drugs presented with septicemia. Serum creatinine levels are 5.7 mg/dl. Which of the following drug should be stopped?
   a. Insulin   b. Metoprolol
   c. Linagliptin   d. Metformin

55. A morbidly obese diabetic woman was on failed metformin therapy. She has the history of pancreatitis and family history of bladder cancer. Patient does not want to take injections. Which of the following would be suitable to reduce her glucose levels?
   a. Liraglutide   b. Sitagliptin
   c. Canagliflozin d. Pioglitazone

56. Which of the following drug can decrease the size of prostate?
   a. Tamsulosin   b. Sildenafil
   c. Finasteride   d. Prazosin

57. A young male developed 5 episodes of loose stool 2 hours after eating in a restaurant. He is afebrile and has mild dehydration. What should be the treatment?
   a. Ciprofloxacin and tinidazole
   b. Only ciprofloxacin
   c. Only ORS
   d. Ciprofloxacin, tinidazole and ORS

58. A patient presented with pain in the right lower quadrant of abdomen. He has history of stones in the right kidney. He was prescribed an opioid, which is partial agonist at mu receptors and antagonist at kappa receptors. The likely drug given was:
   a. Pentazocine   b. Buprenorphine
   c. Tramadol   d. Fentanyl

59. A person has to go to Shimla next morning. Which of the following medication might help him to reduce his motion sickness?
   a. Scopolamine patch a night before
   b. Ranitidine one night before and then before the trip
   c. Dimenhydrinate 1 hour before journey
   d. Omeprazole half hour before trip

60. A patient on antitubercular drug therapy developed tingling sensation on lower limb. Which of the following when substituted can result in improvement of symptoms?
   a. Thiamine   b. Folic acid
   c. Pyridoxine   d. Vitamin B12

61. Which of the following is an example of placebo?
   a. Herbal medication with no known effect
   b. Physiotherapy
   c. Sham surgery
   d. Cognitive behavioral therapy

62. An unknown drug is being tested in experimental set-up. The results obtained are given in the table. From these actions, new drug is likely to be:

Parameter	Placebo treated	New drug treated
Heart rate	72	86
Systolic BP	110	150
Diastolic BP	80	68
Tremors	Absent	Present

a. Beta-1 and beta-2 agonist
b. Alpha-1 antagonist and beta-2 agonist
c. M2 and M3 agonist
d. Alpha-1 and beta-1 agonist

63. Which of the following instructions should be given to a lactating mother regarding drug usage?
   a. No advice is required as most of the drugs are secreted negligibly in the milk
   b. Take drugs with longer half-life
   c. Tell her to feed the baby just before next dose
   d. Tell mother to feed when it is least efficacious

64. Treatment of choice for anaphylactic shock is:
   a. Adrenaline 0.5 ml of 1:1000 solution by intramuscular route
   b. Adrenaline 1 ml of 1:10000 by intravenous route
   c. Atropine 3 mg intravenously
   d. Adenosine 12 mg intravenously

65. Drug of choice for scrub typhus is:
   a. Azithromycin   b. Ciprofloxacin
   c. Doxycycline   d. Chloramphenicol

66. Treatment of choice for a patient with gonococcal as well as non-gonococcal urethritis is:
   a. Ceftriaxone 250 mg IM single dose
   b. Cefixime 400 mg oral single dose
   c. Ciprofloxacin 500 mg oral single dose
   d. Azithromycin 2 gm oral single dose

67. A patient of Prinzmetal angina is started on isosorbide mononitrate. What is the mechanism of action of nitrates in this condition?
   a. Reduced cardiac contractility
   b. Increased left ventricular end diastolic volume
   c. Decreased diastolic perfusion pressure
   d. Endothelium independent coronary vasodilation

68. A patient presented with acute exacerbation of bronchial asthma. Salbutamol inhalation didn't improve the condition of the patient. So, intravenous corticosteroids and aminophylline were added and the condition improved. What is the mechanism of action of corticosteroids in this condition?
   a. They cause bronchodilatation when given with xanthines
   b. They increase bronchial responsiveness to salbutamol
   c. They increase the action of aminophylline on adenosine receptors
   d. They increase the mucociliary clearance

MICROBIOLOGY

69. Which of the following is not a dimorphic fungi?
   a. Blastomyces dermatidis   b. Histoplasma capsulatum
   c. Pneumocystis jirovecii   d. Penicillin marneffei

70. A patient with HIV develops diarrhea and fecal examination showing Isospora belli. He was given treatment with trimethoprim-sulfamethoxazole. Diarrhea subsided but fever persisted. Bone marrow examination showed the following picture with an intracellular fungi. Which of the following is the wrong statement about this fungus?

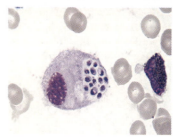

   a. It cannot be grown in Sabouraud Dextrose Agar (SDA)
   b. Spores are the infective form
   c. It is intracellular budding yeast
   d. It can cause systemic disease

71. Identify the following organism on the basis of given image:

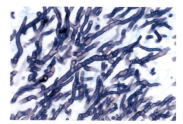

   a. Obtuse-angled mucor
   b. Acute-angled Penicillium
   c. Obtuse-angled Rhizopus
   d. Acute-angled branching Aspergillus

72. A female from Himachal Pradesh presented with history of thorn prick a year back, has verrucous lesions in the skin with following microscopic findings. Identify the agent:

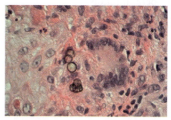

   a. Blastomycosis   b. Pheohyphomycosis
   c. Sporotrichosis   d. Chromoblastomycosis

73. 1,3-beta-D-glucan is helpful for identification of:
   a. Invasive candidiasis   b. Rhizopus
   c. Cryptococcus   d. Mucormycosis

74. Best method of the diagnosis for Clostridium difficle infection:
   a. Pure strain isolation from culture
   b. Immunofluorescence
   c. Toxin detection by ELISA
   d. Toxin gene detection by PCR

75. Viral hemorrhagic fever which have occurred in India?
   a. Marburg
   b. Yellow fever
   c. Crimean Congo hemorrhagic fever
   d. Ebola

76. Blood spills in OT is cleaned with:
    a. Phenol
    b. Alcohol
    c. Quarternary ammonium compound
    d. Chloride compounds

77. Identify the organism from the given image?

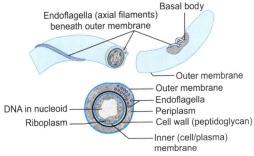

    a. Helicobacter pylori
    b. Leptospira
    c. Vibrio cholerae
    d. Salmonella typhi

78. Biofilm forming bacteria causes antimicrobial resistance by all of the following *except*:
    a. Mechanical barrier
    b. Increased excretion of antibiotics
    c. Altered metabolism
    d. Adherence

79. Identify the following organism on the basis of given image:

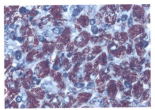

    a. Mycobacterium
    b. Nocardia
    c. Actinomyces
    d. Corynebacterium

80. Identify the virus based on the given cycle:

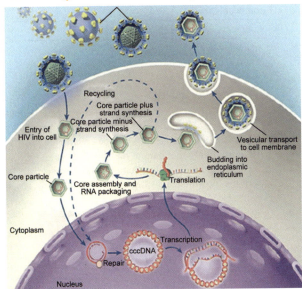

    a. HIV
    b. Hepatitis
    c. Influenza
    d. Herpes simplex

81. Fecal smear showed the following findings. Identify the organism:

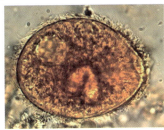

    a. Entamoeba dispar
    b. Cryptosporidium
    c. Giardia lamblia
    d. Balantidium coli

82. Identify the organism on the basis of given stool microscopy:

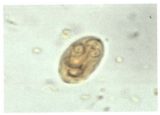

    a. Entamoeba dispar
    b. Cryptosporidium
    c. Giardia lamblia
    d. Balantidium coli

83. Urine LAM is used for the diagnosis of:
    a. Mycoplasma
    b. Mycobacterium tuberculosis
    c. Mycobacterium leprae
    d. Listeria monocytogenes

84. In which of the following malarial parasite, relapse is seen?
    a. Plasmodium vivax and falciparum
    b. Plasmodium ovale and falciparum
    c. Plasmodium vivax and ovale
    d. Plasmodium vivax and malariae

FORENSIC MEDICINE

85. Nothing is an offence, which is done by a person who, at the time of doing it, by reason of unsoundness of mind, is incapable of knowing the nature of the act, or that he is doing, what is either wrong or contrary to law?
    a. McNaughten's rule
    b. Durham's rule
    c. Curren's rule
    d. American law institute test

86. According to the Nysten's rule, order of development of rigor mortis:
    a. Orbicularis oculi, facial muscles, jaw, upper limb
    b. Orbicularis oculi, facial muscle upper limb, thorax
    c. Orbicularis oculi, neck, upper limb, thorax
    d. Orbicularis oculi, facial muscles, thorax, upper limb

87. A 14 years old rape victim with 22 weeks of gestation coming to hospital. All of the following can be done *except*:
   a. Male doctor can examine her with female attendant
   b. Gynecologist can abort the fetus upon the patient request
   c. No need to collect vaginal swab
   d. UPT not required

88. First carpal bone to ossify:
   a. Capitate   b. Lunate
   c. Scaphoid   d. Hamate

89. Blackfoot's disease is caused by:
   a. Arsenic   b. Copper
   c. Mercury   d. Lead

90. Match the following declarations:

1. Geneva	a. Torture
2. Tokya	b. Abortion
3. Oslo	c. Human experimentation
4. Helsinki	d. Ethics

   a. 1 =a, 2=b, 3=c, 4=d   b. 1 =b, 2=c, 3=d, 4=a
   c. 1 =d, 2=a, 3=b, 4=c   d. 1 =c, 2=d, 3=a, 4=b

91. Match the following:

1. Cocaine	a. Hunan hand
2. LSD	b. White lady
3. Abrus	c. Purple haze
4. Capsaicin	d. Gunchi

   a. 1 =a, 2=b, 3=c, 4=d   b. 1 =b, 2=c, 3=d, 4=a
   c. 1 =d, 2=a, 3=b, 4=c   d. 1 =c, 2=d, 3=a, 4=b

92. A middle-aged lady was found in a robbed room lying in a pool of blood. On forensic examination, there was an entry wound of size around 2 cm x 2 cm on the left temporal region with tattooing and blackening around the wound. There was also an exit wound with beveling at the right temporal region. On further examination, two bullet fragments were found inside the brain parenchyma. Which of the following could be used to determine the distance from which the weapon was fired?
   a. Hair   b. Cloth
   c. Bullet fragments d. Blood

93. Autopsy of a female brought dead to the casualty was performed. No specific signs were seen. On external examination, only a mark on the chin was seen as shown below and on internal examination, following appearance was seen. What is the likely cause of death?   *(AIIMS November 2017, May 2017)*

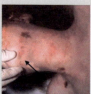
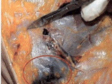

   a. Smothering   b. Throttling
   c. Hanging   d. Ligature strangulation

PSM

94. In a subcenter area with crude birth rate of 20, what would be the expected number of ANC registrations?
   a. 60   b. 80
   c. 100   d. 120

95. Pics of vials of oral polio vaccine—which one can be used dark colored or white colored?

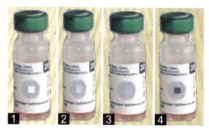

   a. 1 and 2   b. 2 and 3
   c. 3 and 4   d. 1 and 4

96. Chronic liver disease is classified into Child–Pugh class A to C, employing the added score from above. Class A: 5–6, B: 7–9, C: 10–15. This is ………… scale:
   a. Nominal   b. Ordinal
   c. Qualitative   d. Continuous

97. A clinical trail was conducted with 15225 hypertensive patients alloted in the intervention group (New drug) and control group (Old drug) respectively. Results of the research study are given in the following table. Calculate the absolute risk reduction (ARR) and relative risk (RR):

	Control group (old drug)	Intervention group (new drug)
Developed HT complications	1800	1620
Did not develop HT complications	13425	13605
Total subjects	15225	15225

   a. ARR = 10% and RR = 0.9
   b. ARR = 1% and RR = 9
   c. ARR = 1% and RR = 0.9
   d. ARR = 10% and RR = 9

98. A doctor uses a highly sensitive test on a patient and the result is positive. What does this mean?
   a. If it is a rare disease, this can be considered positive
   b. Highly likely that patient has the disease
   c. Highly unlikely that patient has the disease
   d. If the prevalence is high, then the patient has the disease

99. Annual new case detection rate of leprosy as on 31st March, 2016 is:
   a. 0.66 /10,000 population
   b. 0.66/1,00,000 population
   c. 9.7/10,000 population
   d. 9.7/1,00,000 population

100. Supplementary nutrition provided in the Mid-day meal program should satisfy:
    a. 1/3 of the total protein requirement + 1/2 of the total energy requirement
    b. 2/3 of the total protein requirement + 1/2 of the total energy requirement
    c. 1/2 of the total protein requirement + 1/3 of the total energy requirement
    d. 1/2 of the total protein requirement + 2/3 of the total energy requirement

101. In a statistical study for calculating the effect of drug on patients sugar level, the test showed significant difference, whereas in reality there was no difference. This is due to:
    a. Alpha error   b. Beta error
    c. Gamma error   d. Power of the test

MEDICINE

102. A patient comes with the history of sudden onset palpitations. ECG showed a narrow complex tachycardia without 'P' waves and with a rate of 160 BPM. His blood pressure is 96/68 mm Hg. What is the next management?
    a. Carotid body massage   b. Adenosine
    c. Beta-blocker   d. Defibrillator

103. The most sensitive index for renal tubular function is:
    a. Specific gravity of urine b. Blood urea
    c. GFR   d. Creatinine clearance

104. A 53 years old man is admitted with a history of CVA 2 days ago. Patient is drowsy with minimal response. CT picture is shown as in the figure. What will be your next line of management?

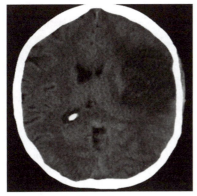

    a. Aspirin and clopidogrel
    b. Mannitol
    c. Decompressive surgery
    d. Mechanical thrombectomy

105. A patient comes to emergency with headache describing it as worst headache in his life. What is the next step?
    a. CT brain
    b. Lumbar puncture
    c. MRI brain
    d. Observation and analgesics

106. Loud S1 in mitral stenosis is lost in all except:
    a. First degree heart block b. Aortic regurgitation
    c. Calcified valve   d. Mild MS

107. During a routine follow-up of a hypertensive patient, an intern noticed that blood pressure in the right arm was 180/100 mm Hg and in the left arm was 130/90 mm Hg. Which of the following conditions would be least likely associated with these findings?
    a. Supravalvular aortic stenosis
    b. Coarctation of aorta
    c. Takayasu arteritis
    d. Aortic dissection

108. Normal anion gap metabolic acidosis seen in all *except*:
    a. Proximal RTA   b. Pancreatitis
    c. Diarrhea   d. Salicylate poisoning

109. Diagnosis of the following ECG:

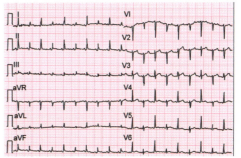

    a. Bigeminy   b. Electrical alternans
    c. 'P' pulmonale   d. Left ventricular failure

110. A patient comes to emergency with fever and headache. On examination he has neck stiffness. CSF analysis was done: Opening pressure –Increased; Proteins- Mild increased; Glucose – Normal; Lymphocytes - Increased. Most likely organism responsible is:
    a. Mycobacterium tuberculosis
    b. Neisseria meningitidis
    c. Cryptococcus
    d. Coxsackie virus

111. A patient came with ascites. Ascitic fluid analysis was done and found to have SAAG more >1.1. All of the following can be the cause *except*:
    a. Cirrhosis   b. Liver failure
    c. Metastasis to liver   d. Tubercular peritonitis

112. A young donor came to the blood bank for the first time for platelet apheresis with platelet count of 1.9L. During the course he developed paresthesias, circumoral numbness during donation. His vitals remain stable though. ECG showed tachycardia with ST-T changes. What is the reason for his symptoms?
    a. Hypovolemic shock   b. Hypocalcemia
    c. Seizures   d. Allergic reaction

113. A patient presents with unilateral ptosis and hypotonia in the same eye. He was given an IV injection, following which symptoms go away. The diagnosis is:

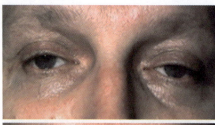
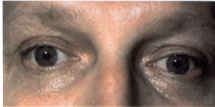

  a. Horner syndrome   b. Myasthenia gravis
  c. Third nerve palsy   d. Sixth nerve palsy

114. **All of the following drugs are used in emergency management of acute hyperkalemia *except*:**
  a. Calcium gluconate
  b. Salbutamol
  c. Glucose-Insulin
  d. Intravenous magnesium sulphate

SURGERY

115. **Best guide for the management of resuscitation is:**
  a. CVP   b. Urine output
  c. Blood pressure   d. Saturation of oxygen

116. **Modified shock index formula is:**
  a. Heart rate/Systolic BP
  b. Heart rate/Diastolic BP
  c. Heart rate/Mean arterial pressure
  d. Pulse rate/Systolic BP

117. **22 Gauge IV cannula color is:**
  a. Green   b. Grey
  c. Blue   d. Pink

118. **For the transport of traumatized and conscious patient all the following are done *except*:**
  a. On a hard board with head/spine stabilized
  b. In lateral lying position
  c. Talk to patient while he is on board
  d. Rolling without moving the spine

119. **In a school bus accident, which of the following victim you will attend first?**
  a. A child with airway obstruction
  b. A child with shock
  c. A child with flail chest
  d. A child with severe head injury

120. **Which of the following colour code and explanation is matched correctly as per the triage used in disaster management?**
  a. Red- Decreased
  b. Black- Minor injuries
  c. Yellow- Stable patients, observation
  d. Green- Need immediate intervention

121. **A patient who had traumatic head injury has spontaneous eye opening, tries to remove examiners hands on painful stimuli and irrelevant talks/stances. What is the GCS score?**
  a. 11   b. 13
  c. 3   d. 1

122. **Which of the following is the correct sequence?**
  a. Assess the patient's response, call for help, Check carotid pulse, start CPR
  b. Check carotid pulse, start CPR, call for help, defibrillate
  c. Defibrillate, assess response, check carotid pulse, maintain airway
  d. Start CPR, call for help, defibrillate, check pulse

123. **French in Foley's catheter refers to:**
  a. Outer circumference measurement
  b. Inner circumference measurement
  c. Diameter of catheter
  d. Lumen size

124. **In a preoperative patient surgical checklist, which of the following is not required?**
  a. Oral consent
  b. Doctor's signature
  c. Site marking
  d. Confirming patient's identity

125. **Balanced resuscitation in trauma management is:**
  a. Giving colloids and crystalloids ratio of 1:1
  b. Maintaining pH by ensuring acid base are balanced
  c. Maintaining permissible hypotension to avoid bleeding
  d. Maintaining airway, breathing and circulation simultaneously

126. **Identify the diagnosis of the given gross specimen:**

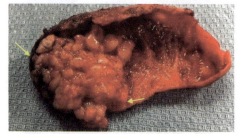

  a. Cancer gallbladder   b. Cholesterolosis
  c. Strawberry gallbladder   d. Polyps in gallbladder

127. **Most common presentation of abdominal desmoid tumor is:**
  a. Abdominal pain   b. Abdominal mass
  c. Fever   d. Rectal prolapse

128. **A 10 years old child with pain and mass in right lumbar region with no was brought to the emergency, with right hip flexed and X-ray showed spine changes. Most probable diagnosis is:**
  a. Psoas abscess
  b. Pyonephrosis
  c. Retrocecal appendicitis
  d. Torsion of right undescended testis

129. How will you check the functioning of the ICD tube?
    a. By observing for continuous air bubbles coming out of the underwater drain
    b. By observing the movement of air water column in the tube during respiration
    c. By taking X-ray chest repeatedly
    d. By auscultation
130. Following a blunt trauma abdomen, a patient had renal laceration and urinoma. Even after 12 days, urinoma persisted, but patient was stable and there was no fever. Next step in management would be:
    a. Percutaneous exploration and repair
    b. Wait and watch
    c. J-shaped urinary stent
    d. Percutaneous nephrostomy
131. Management of 4 cm size renal staghorn calculus:
    a. ESWL
    b. PCNL
    c. Intra renal repair surgery
    d. Open pyelolithotomy
132. Tumor lysis syndrome is characterized by all *except*:
    a. Hyperuricemia
    b. Hypercalcemia
    c. Hyperkalemia
    d. Hyperphosphatemia
133. A 53 years old patient was admitted complains of dyspnea. On examination he has puffy face with engorged veins over the chest. SVC obstruction is suspected. Chest X-ray shows mediastinal enlargement. What is the next step?
    a. Total blood count with peripheral smear
    b. CT thorax
    c. Start cyclophosphamide
    d. Urgent referral to RT
134. How to measure nasogastric tube length?
    a. Tip of nose to ear to xiphisternum
    b. Tip of nose to angle of ear to umbilicus
    c. Mouth to ear to umbilicus
    d. Mouth to ear to midway between xiphisternum and umbilicus
135. Which layer is involved in the blister formation in a superficial partial thickness burn?
    a. Epidermis
    b. Dermis
    c. Papillary dermis
    d. Reticular dermis

OBSTETRICS AND GYNECOLOGY

136. Identify the grip in the picture used for checking ballotability of head:

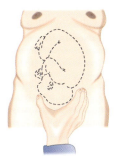

    a. Pelvic grip
    b. Pawlick grip
    c. Fundal grip
    d. Umbilical grip

137. Name the instrument seen in the picture:

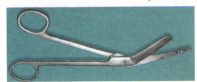

    a. Mayo scissor
    b. Episiotomy scissor
    c. Suture remover
    d. Curved scissor
138. In the partogram, first time of the initial markings are made in:
    a. Left side of the action line
    b. Right side of the action line
    c. Left side of the alert line
    d. Right side of the alert line
139. Fixative used in the PAP smear:
    a. 55% ethyl alcohol
    b. 95% formalin
    c. 95% ethyl alcohol
    d. Normal saline
140. Nanovalent vaccine offers protection against which type of HPV virus?
    a. Types 6, 8, 10, 11, 31, 33, 45, 52, 58
    b. Types 6, 11, 16, 18, 31, 33, 45, 52, 58
    c. Types 6, 11, 16, 18, 31, 35, 45, 52, 58
    d. Types 6, 11, 16, 18, 19, 31, 32, 33, 34
141. According to the Naegele's rule, calculate EDD of a patient with LMP 9/01/2017
    a. 16/10/2017
    b. 16/09/2017
    c. 16/11/2017
    d. 9/10/2017
142. A 18 years old female presents with an ovarian mass, her serum biomarker are found to be normal except for LDH, which is found to be elevated. The most likely diagnosis is:
    a. Dysgerminoma
    b. Endodermal sinus tumor
    c. Malignant teratoma
    d. Mucinous cystadenocarcinoma
143. A primigravida came with 6 cm cervical dilatation with contraction rate of 3/10 min. Which stage of labour is she in?
    a. First stage
    b. Second stage
    c. Third stage
    d. Fourth stage
144. A postmenopausal female with biopsy report as endometrial hyperplasia with atypia. Next line of management is:
    a. Type 1 hysterectomy
    b. Oral progestins
    c. Mirena
    d. Dilatation and curettage
145. For effective protection after unprotected intercourse one single tab of levonorgestrel 0.75 mg already been taken, when to take the next dose?
    a. 1 tab after 24 hours
    b. 1 tab after 12 hours
    c. 2 tabs after 12 hours
    d. 2 tabs after 24 hours
146. A female in the labour ward was administered opioid analgesic. Which of the following drugs should be kept ready for emergency?
    a. Fentanyl
    b. Naloxone
    c. Morphine
    d. Bupivacaine

147. **A patient, who is the father of 2 children, his wife is not able to conceive, is diagnosed to have hypogonadotropic hypogonadism. Which of the following is not true?**
    a. Low LH and FSH
    b. Low testosterone
    c. Oligospermia
    d. Low prolactin levels

148. **A 27 years old female presented to the OPD of infertility clinic. She was prescribed bromocriptine. What could be the possible reason?**
    a. Hyperprolactinemia
    b. Polycystic ovarian disease
    c. Hypogonadotropic hypogonadism
    d. Pelvic inflammatory disease

149. **Injury to which of the following deep part of perineal body causes cystocele, enterocele and urethral descent?**
    a. Pubococcygeus
    b. Ischiocavernosus
    c. Bulbospongiosus
    d. Sphincter of urethra and anus

150. **An 18 years old girl presents with primary amenorrhea. On evaluation, she was having a karyotype of 45XO and infantile uterus. What should be done next?**
    a. HRT to induce puberty
    b. Vaginoplasty
    c. Clitoroplasty
    d. Bilateral gonadectomy

151. **In a patient of Down's syndrome, triple test was done. Expected result is:**
    a. High HCG, low ue3, low AFP
    b. Low HCG, high ue3, high AFP
    c. High HCG, high ue3, low AFP
    d. Low HCG, low ue3, high AFP

152. **A primigravida was given dietary advice in the first trimester. What should be the extra calorie intake in pregnancy?**
    a. 200 kilocal
    b. 300 kilocal
    c. 500 kilocal
    d. No extra calories

153. **Pregnant women with following is called systemic hypertension:**
    a. Hypertension diagnosed at 10 weeks of gestation
    b. Diabetic retinopathy
    c. Diabetic nephropathy
    d. Episode of seizure

154. **A 35 years old woman comes with the history of postcoital bleeding. What is the next step?**
    a. PAP smear
    b. Conisation
    c. Cryotherapy
    d. Targeted biopsy

PEDIATRICS

155. **A 3 years old child is said to have delayed milestone, if he fails to:**
    a. Use spoon
    b. Draw square
    c. Skip
    d. Climb alternate steps downwards

156. **A 4 years old child was brought to the hospital with kinky hair and growth retardation. Most probable diagnosis is:**
    a. Menke's disease
    b. Pompe's disease
    c. Nieman-Pick disease
    d. Wilson's disease

157. **Preferred treatment option for a 4 days old baby with bilirubin of 8 mg/dL:**
    a. Stop breastfeeding and phototherapy
    b. Continue breastfeeding and phototherapy
    c. Exchange transfusion
    d. IV fluids and phototherapy

158. **APGAR expansion: (Asked twice in the exam)**
    a. Appearance, Pulse, Grimace, Activity, Respiration
    b. Alert, Pulse, Grimace, Activity, Respiration
    c. Assessment, Pulse, Grimace, Alive, Respiration
    d. Appearance, Pressure, Grimace, Activity, Respiration

159. **APGAR expansion: (Asked twice in the exam)**
    a. Appearance, Pulse, Grimace, Activity, Respiration
    b. Alert, Pulse, Grimace, Activity, Respiration
    c. Assessment, Pulse, Grimace, Alive, Respiration
    d. Appearance, Pressure, Grimace, Activity, Respiration

160. **An 18 months old baby was brought to the clinic who didn't receive immunization so far. Which of the following vaccines can be given?**
    a. Pentavalent vaccine only
    b. Pentavalent vaccine + BCG + OPV
    c. BCG + OPV + MMR
    d. OPV + DPT booster

161. **A neonate was diagnosed to have periventricular calcification on CT brain. Best method of diagnosis of this etiological agent:**
    a. Liver biopsy
    b. Urine examination
    c. CSF examination
    d. Blood

162. **A 10 years old boy rapidly develops hypoglycemia after moderate activity. Blood examination reveals raised levels of ketone bodies, lactic acid and triglycerides. On examination, liver and kidneys were enlarged. Histopathology of liver shows deposits of glycogen in excess amount. What is the diagnosis?**
    a. Von-Gierke diseases
    b. Cori's diseases
    c. McArdle's diseases
    d. Pompe's disease

ORTHOPEDICS

163. **All of the following are true about Sprengel's shoulder *except*:**
    a. Associated with diastematomyelia
    b. Most commonly associated with Klippel-Feil syndrome
    c. Usually associated with dextrocardia
    d. Associated with congenital scoliosis

164. **Glucosamine is used in the treatment of:**
    a. Arthritis
    b. Diabetes
    c. Cataract
    d. Asthma

165. **A patient came with complaints of lower limb weakness. Examiner places one hand under the patient's heel and patient is asked to raise his other leg against downward resistance. What is the name of this test?**
    a. Hoover test
    b. Waddell's test
    c. O'Donoghue test
    d. McBride test

166. A 40 years old body builder taking steroids and creatinine presented with bilateral hip pain and unable to squat. On MRI there is marrow edema, subchondral cyst, flattening of weight bearing areas of femoral head and X-ray shows crescent sign. Most probable diagnosis is:
    a. Avascular necrosis of femur
    b. Fracture femur
    c. Osteochondroma
    d. Tuberculosis of hip

167. An adult with POP cast for forearm fracture is given analgesic. Earliest way to detect development of compartment syndrome by the nurse is:
    a. Check radial pulse by displacing the cast
    b. Decreased response to analgesic
    c. Change in odor
    d. Check colour change in fingertip

168. What type of fracture is shown in the image?

    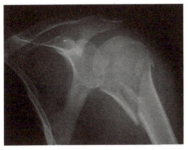

    a. Neer's type III proximal humerus
    b. Garden's type II proximal humerus
    c. Schatzker's type III proximal humerus
    d. Ideberg type III proximal humerus

169. A 40 years old male fell on the outstretched hand with radial side pain and tenderness in anatomical snuff-box and restriction of wrist movement. Following is the X-ray image. Most probable diagnosis is:

    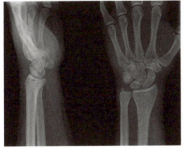

    a. Trans-scaphoid perilunate fracture
    b. Scaphoid fracture
    c. Distal radius fracture
    d. Hamate fracture

170. A patient with history of RTA presents in emergency department. Attending orthopedic surgeon writes IIIB for his both lower limbs injury fracture. According to Gustilo-Anderson classification, which of the following is correct?
    a. Bilateral limb wound of >10 cm adequate soft tissue coverage in spite of extensive laceration, flaps, avulsion injury and regardless of size of wound
    b. Bilateral limb wound of size <1 cm
    c. Bilateral limb wound of size >10 cm with extensive soft tissue damage and periosteal stripping
    d. Wound between 1 and 10 cm with extensive soft tissue damage, flaps or avulsions

171. Which of the following statement is not true about posterior cruciate ligament?
    a. Prevents posterior displacement of tibia on femur
    b. Extra-synovial
    c. Primary action is to prevent internal rotation of knee joint
    d. Attached to anterolateral aspect of medial condyle

OPHTHALMOLOGY

172. Identify the refractive error:

    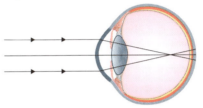

    a. Myopia
    b. Hypermetropia
    c. Compound astigmatism
    d. Mixed astigmatism

173. Following picture exhibit which cranial nerve palsy?

    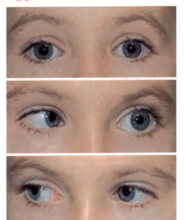

    a. Oculomotor nerve
    b. Abducent nerve
    c. Trochlear nerve
    d. Facial nerve

174. Most common tumor of lacrimal gland:
    a. Pleomorphic adenoma
    b. Adenoid cystic carcinoma
    c. Mucoepidermoid carcinoma
    d. Non-Hodgkin's lymphoma

175. A patient presented to eye OPD with glaucoma and bulging of cornea. What is the most probable diagnosis?
    a. Granular dystrophy
    b. Keratoconus
    c. Staphyloma
    d. Keratomalacia

176. A 60 years old diabetic male presented with history of decreased vision on reading. Fluorescein angiography shows:

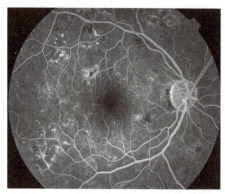

a. Mild non-proliferative diabetic retinopathy
b. Birdshot choroidopathy
c. Proliferative diabetic retinopathy
d. Severe non-proliferative diabetic retinopathy

177. A patient came to eye OPD with following clinical picture after 5 days of cataract surgery. All of the following should be done in the management of this condition *except*:

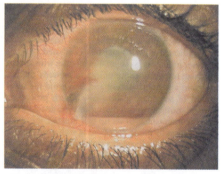

a. Pars plana vitrectomy
b. Topical antibiotics
c. Intravitreal antibiotics
d. Intravenous antibiotics

178. Identify the given condition:

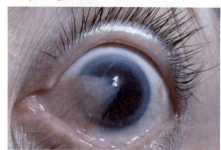

a. Thermal burn
b. Squamous cell carcinoma
c. Pinguecula
d. Pterygium

ENT

179. Noise induced hearing loss mostly affects:
    a. Inner hair cell   b. Outer hair cell
    c. Macula   d. Cupula

180. Target sign is seen in:
    a. Spontaneous CSF rhinorrhea
    b. Traumatic CSF rhinorrhea
    c. Traumatic epistaxis
    d. Petrositis

181. Hutchinson's triad is:
    a. Interstitial keratitis + Eighth nerve deafness + Hutchinson incisor
    b. Interstitial keratitis + Eighth nerve deafness + Mulberry incisor
    c. Interstitial keratitis + Eighth nerve deafness + Hutchinson molar
    d. Interstitial keratitis + Eighth nerve deafness + Mulberry molar

SKIN

182. An 18 years old male presented with pruritus over fingers. The clinical picture of the lesion and the causative agent is given below. What is the most probable diagnosis?

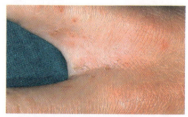

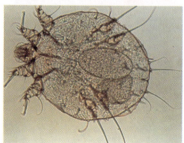

a. Scabies   b. Pediculosis
c. Contact dermatitis d. Insect bile allergy

183. What is the most probable diagnosis based on the given image?

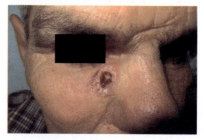

a. Basal cell carcinoma
b. Malignant melanoma
c. Squamous cell carcinoma
d. Marjolin's ulcer

184a. This condition is associated with:

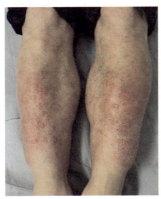

a. Diabetes mellitus　　b. Hypothyroidism
c. Hyperthyroidism　　d. Sarcoidosis

184b. This condition is associated with:

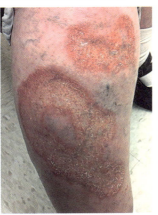

a. Diabetes mellitus　　b. Hypothyroidism
c. Hyperthyroidism　　d. Sarcoidosis

185. A 40 years old female came to OPD with the history of fever, joint pain and rash. NSAIDs were prescribed. After one week, the patient developed brownish discoloration over nose. This was due to:

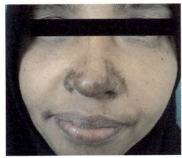

a. Melasma　　b. Dengue
c. Chikungunya　　d. Fixed drug eruption

186. Which of the following causative organism is responsible for this condition?

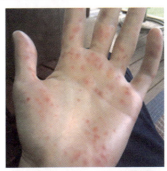

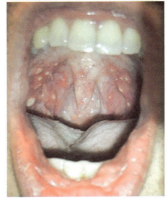

a. Coxsackie
b. Pox virus
c. Molluscus contagiosum
d. Human herpes virus 7

ANESTHESIA

187. Which group of nerve fibers is least susceptible to local anesthetics?
    a. A-alpha　　b. A-beta
    c. B　　d. C

188. Highest concentration of oxygen is delivered through:
    a. Nasal cannula
    b. Venturi mask
    c. Bag and mask
    d. Face mask with reservoir

189. What is the recommended duration of pre-oxygenation before intubation?
    a. 1 minute of tidal volume breathing
    b. 3 minutes of tidal volume breathing
    c. 3 minutes of deep breathing
    d. 5 minutes of deep breathing

190. Tracheal secretions should be suctioned for:
    a. 10–15 seconds　　b. 60 seconds
    c. 30 seconds　　d. 3 minutes

191. Which of the following drug can be used as intravenous induction agent?
    a. Bupivacaine　　b. Lorazepam
    c. Neostigmine　　d. Dexmetomidine

AIIMS ESSENCE

192. **A patient who was on ventilator and being ventilated for past few days, suddenly pulls out the endotracheal tube. What is the next step of management?**
    a. Assess the patient, give bag and mask ventilation and look for spontaneous breathing
    b. Start bag and mask ventilation and reintubate
    c. Sedate and reintubate
    d. Make him sit and do physiotherapy

RADIOLOGY

193. **The chest X-ray shows:**

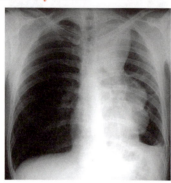

    a. Pneumothorax
    b. Hydropneumothorax
    c. Pleural effusion
    d. Consolidation

194. **Reduced uptake in FDG-PET scan is seen in:**
    a. Atypical carcinoid
    b. Typical carcinoid
    c. Small cell carcinoma
    d. Large cell neuroendocrine tumor

195. **The digital subtraction angiography in a patient with history of headache shows:**

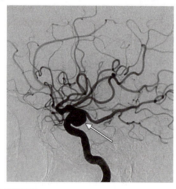

    a. Aneurysm
    b. Cavernous angioma
    c. Arteriovenous fistula
    d. None of the above

PSYCHIATRY

196. **A young male patient is on 5 mg haloperidol for many days, recently for last 4 days of duration he has inner restlessness and urge to move. Diagnosis is:**
    a. Akathisia
    b. Tardive dyskinesia
    c. Rabbit syndrome
    d. Acute dystonia

197. **A patient believes he is the most important person in the world than anyone so his neighbors and family is trying to harm him as they are jealous of him. His wife says otherwise and says he behaves like this recently only before he was working as a school-teacher peacefully and brought to OPD. He is suffering from:**
    a. Delusion of grandiosity
    b. Delusion of persecution
    c. Delusion of grandiosity and persecution
    d. Delusion of grandiosity, persecution and reference

198. **A young patient was admitted to hospital with acute psychosis. He wakes up and asks the nurse to call his wife who was there in the same room in the same area. Upon seeing her, he started beating her thinking that it was nurse who was masquerading as his wife. He also said she was the same nurse who gave her wrong medication 2 days back as well to make him ill, because she wanted to harm him but who was actually his wife. What syndrome he is suffering from?**
    a. Capgras syndrome
    b. Frégoli's syndrome
    c. Delusion of subjective doubles
    d. Othello syndrome

199. **Which of the following is the test for immediate memory?**
    a. Serial (100-7) subtraction test up to 5 steps
    b. Digit span forward up to 7 digits with 2 skips allowed
    c. Digit span backwards upto 5 digits with 2 skips allowed
    d. Serial (20-1) subtraction test up to 5 steps

200. **An IT employee after taking up the job is feeling guilty, hopeless and not able to concentrate on work. His symptoms started 3 years back when he entered college. Most likely diagnosis is:**
    a. Depressive disorder
    b. Dysthymia
    c. Adjustment disorder
    d. Cyclothymic disorder

201. **Basis of reliability of information of patient provided by informants depend on all *except*:**
    a. Biological relationship
    b. Educational status
    c. Observational skills
    d. Duration of stay with patient

Explanations

ANATOMY

1. **Ans. a. Anterior and posterior ethmoidal** *(Ref: Gray's 41/e p563, 40/e p554; Dhingra 7/e p197)*

   Anterior and posterior ethmoidal arteries are branches of ophthalmic artery, which in turn is a branch of internal carotid artery. Sphenopalatine and greater palatine arteries are branches of maxillary artery, which in turn is branch of external carotid artery. Superior labial artery is the branch of facial artery, which in turn is branch of external carotid artery.

   > *"Little's area: It is situated in the anterior inferior part of nasal septum, just above the vestibule. Four arteries, anterior ethmoidal, septal branch of superior labial, septal branch of sphenopalatine artery and the greater palatine, anastomose here to form a vascular plexus called "Kiesselbach's plexus". This area is exposed to the drying effect of inspiratory current and to finger nail trauma, and is the usual site for epistaxis in children and young adults."- Dhingra 7/e p197*

   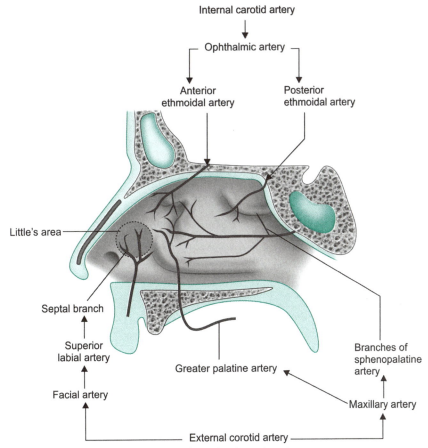

   Fig. 1: Blood supply of nasal septum

Blood Supply of Nasal Septum	
Internal Carotid System	**External Carotid System**
• Anterior & posterior ethmoidal artery[Q] (Branch of **ophthalmic artery**[Q])	• **Sphenopalatine artery**[Q] (branch of **maxillary artery**[Q]) gives **nasopalatine & posterior medial nasal branches**[Q]. • Septal branch of **greater palatine artery**[Q] (branch of **maxillary artery**[Q]) • Septal branch of **superior labial artery**[Q] (branch of **facial artery**[Q]).

2. **Ans. c. IVC** *(Ref: Gray's 41/e p899, 40/e p1008)*
Inferior vena cava (IVC) passes through central tendon of diaphragm.

> "The vena caval aperture, the highest of the three large openings, lies at about the level of the disc between the eighth and ninth thoracic vertebrae. It is quadrilateral, and located at the junction of the right leaf with the central area of the tendon, and so its margins are aponeurotic. It is traversed by the inferior vena cava, which adheres to the margin of the opening, and by some branches of the right phrenic nerve."-*Gray's 40/e p1008*

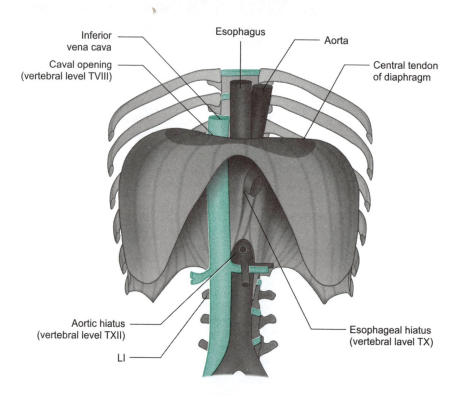

Fig. 2: Openings in diaphragm

Opening	Vertebral level	Part of diaphragm	Passing structure
Vena Caval	T_8^Q	Central tendon^Q	Inferior vena cava^Q Right phrenic nerve^Q
Esophageal	T_{10}^Q	Muscular portion derived from right crus^Q	Esophagus^Q Esophageal branch of left gastric artery Gastric or vagus nerve^Q
Aortic	T_{12}^Q	Osseoaponeurotic between right & lateral crus^Q	Aorta^Q Thoracic duct^Q Azygous vein^Q

Small Openings in the Diaphragm		
Opening	Location	Passing structure
Medial lumbocostal Arch	Behind medial arcuate ligament	Sympathetic chain^Q
Lateral lumbocostal arch	Behind arcuate ligament	Subcostal nerve & vessels^Q
Larry's space / Foramen of Morgagni	Between xiphoid & costal origin of diaphragm	Superior epigastric vessels^Q some lymphatics

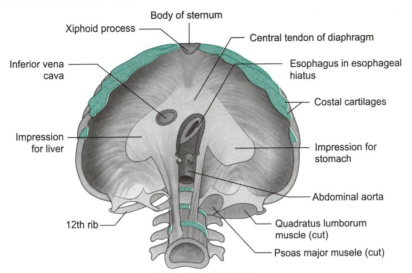

Fig. 3: Openings in diaphragm

3. **Ans. d. Ball and socket** *(Ref: Gray's 40/e p; BDC 7/e Vol-III/p164)*
Talocalcaneonavicular joint is a type of synovial joint, ball and socket joint.

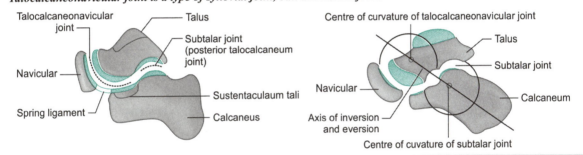

"Talocalcaneonavicular joint: The joint has some of the features of a ball and socket joint. The head of the talus fits into a socket formed partly by the navicular bone, and partly by the calcaneum. Two ligaments also take part in forming the socket: these are the spring ligament medially, and the medial limb of the bifurcate ligament laterally."- BDC 7/e Vol-III/p164

\	Classification of Joints	
Fibrous Joints	• **Suture**: Skull • **Syndesmosis**: Inferior tibiofibular joint[Q] • **Gomphosis**: Tooth socket	
Cartilaginous Joints	**Primary Cartilaginous Joint** **(Synchondrosis / hyaline cartilage)** • Costochondral joint[Q] • 1st chondrosternal joint[Q] • Spheno-occipital joint • Between epiphysis & diaphysis	**Secondary Cartilaginous Joint** **(Symphysis / fibrocartilaginous)** • Symphysis pubis[Q] • Intervertebral joint[Q] • Manubriosternal joint[Q]
Synovial Joints	Plane	1. Intercarpal & intertarsal joint 2. Between articular process of vertebra
	Hinge	1. Elbow, ankle[Q] & interphalyngeal[Q] joint
	Condylar	• Knee[Q], TM joint[Q], atlanto-occipital joint
	Pivot (trochoid)	• Radioulnar joint & atlantoaxial joint
	Ellipsoid	• Wrist[Q] & MCP joint[Q]

Contd...

Contd...

	Saddle (Sellar)	• 1st carpometacarpal[Q] joint • Sternoclavicular[Q] joint • Calcaneocuboid joint
	Ball & socket (THIS)	• Talo-calcaneo-navicular joint • Hip[Q] joint • Incudostapedial joint • Shoulder[Q] joint

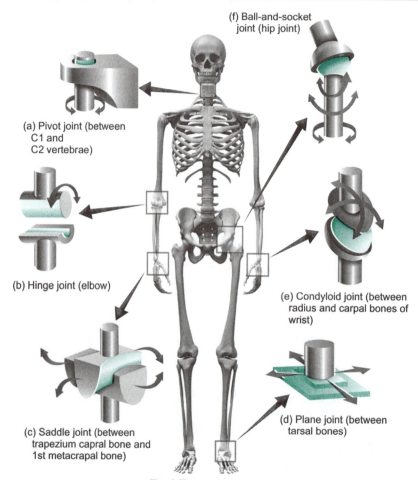

Fig. 4: Types of synovial joints

4. **Ans. b. Orbital cortex** (Ref: Gray's 41/e p393, 40/e p355)

   Marked structure in the image is rostrum. Commissural fibres forming the rostrum extend laterally, below the anterior horn of the lateral ventricle, connecting the orbital surfaces of the frontal lobes.

   "Nerve fibres of the corpus callosum radiate into the white matter core of each hemisphere, thereafter dispersing to the cerebral cortex. **Commissural fibres forming the rostrum extend laterally, below the anterior horn of the lateral ventricle, connecting the orbital surfaces of the frontal lobes.** Fibres in the genu curve forwards, as the forceps minor, to connect the lateral and medial surfaces of the frontal lobes. Fibres of the trunk pass laterally, intersecting with the projection fibres of the corona radiata to connect wide neocortical areas of the hemispheres. Fibres of the trunk and splenium, which form the roof and lateral wall of the posterior horn and the lateral wall of the inferior horn of the lateral ventricle, constitute the tapetum. The remaining fibres of the splenium curve back into the occipital lobes as the forceps major." - *Gray's 40/e p355*

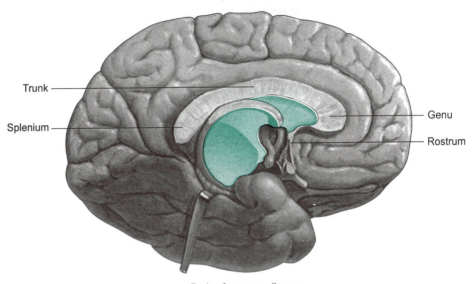

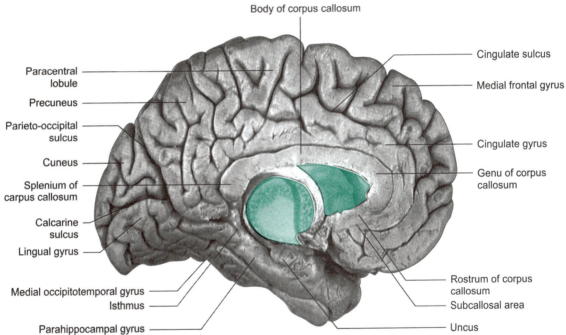

Commissure	Parts of Brain Connected
Rostrum	• Orbital surfaces of frontal lobes[Q]
Genu	• Medial & lateral surfaces of the frontal lobes[Q]
Body	• Surface of the hemisphere[Q]
Splenium	• Two occipital lobes[Q]
Anterior commissure	• Olfactory cortex[Q]
Posterior commissure	• Language processing[Q]
Hippocampal commissure (commissure of the fornix)	• Two hippocampi
Habenular commissure	• Habenular nuclei

5. **Ans. d. d**   *(Ref: Gray's 40/e p1016)*

Development of heart is from the structure labeled as 'd'.

Structures Marked in the Diagram	
a	• Pharyngeal arches
b	• Developing forebrain
c	• Upper limb bud
d	• **Developing heart**

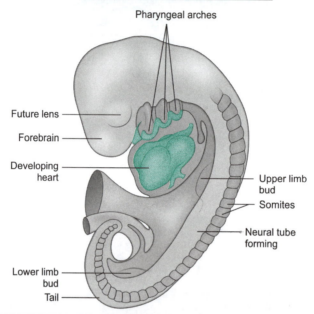

"The heart is formed from tissues derived from the midline splanchnopleuric coelomic epithelium with later contributions from neural crest mesenchyme. The splanchnopleuric coelomic epithelium gives rise to the myocardium, including the conduction system of the heart, and the endocardium, including its derived cardiac mesenchymal population, which produces the valvular tissues of the heart. Splanchnopleuric coelomic epithelium is also the source of the epicardium, coronary arteries and interstitial fibroblasts." -Gray's 40/e p1016

Development of the heart

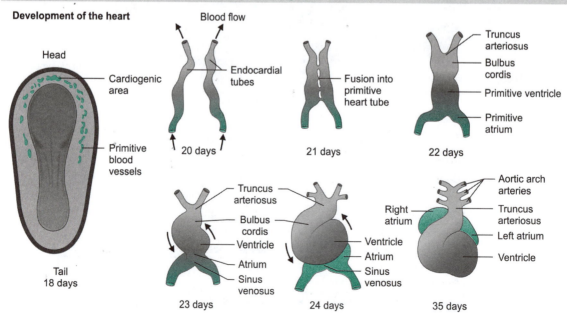

Partitioning of the heat into four chambers

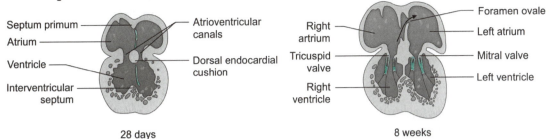

28 days   8 weeks

Development of Primitive Heart Tube

- A pair of **endocardial heart tubes (mesodermal in origin**^{Q}**)** forms within the cardiogenic region.
- As lateral folding occur, the **endocardial heart tubes fuse to form the primitive heart tube**, which **develops into the endocardium**^{Q}.
- **Mesoderm** surrounding the primitive heart tube **develops into myocardium & epicardium**^{Q}.

  - **Primitive heart tube forms five dilatations: truncus arteriosus, bulbus cordis, primitive ventricle, primitive atrium & sinus venosus**^{Q}.

Embryonic Dilatation	Adult Structure
Truncus arteriosus (T)	• Aorta^Q • Pulmonary trunk^Q
Bulbus cordis (B)	• Smooth part of right ventricle (conus arteriosus)^Q • Smooth part of left ventricle (aortic vestibule)^Q
Primitive ventricle (PV)	• Trabeculated part of right ventricle^Q • Trabeculated part of left ventricle^Q
Primitive atrium (PA)	• Trabeculated part of right atrium^Q • Trabeculated part of left atrium^Q
Sinus venosus (SV)	• Smooth part of right atrium (sinus venarum)^Q • Coronary sinus^Q • Oblique vein of left atrium^Q

6. **Ans. c. Frontal**   *(Ref: Gray's 40/e p557, 558, 478)*

The frontal sinuses are rudimentary or absent at birth, generally well developed between the seventh and eighth years, but reach full size only after puberty.

> *"The frontal sinuses are rudimentary or absent at birth, generally well developed between the seventh and eighth years, but reach full size only after puberty. They are more prominent in males, and lend the forehead an obliquity that contrasts with the vertical or convex profile typical of children and females. In the presence of a persistent metopic suture, the frontal sinuses develop separately on either side of the suture, which can be helpful in excluding frontal fractures."- Gray's 40/e p557*

> *"Sphenoid sinus: At birth the sinuses are minute cavities, and their main development occurs after puberty."- Gray's 40/e p557*

> *"Ethmoid sinus: They grow rapidly between the ages of 6 and 8 years and after puberty."- Gray's 40/e p558*

> *"The maxillary sinus appears as a shallow groove on the nasal aspect at about the fourth month in utero. Though small at birth, the sinus is identifiable radiologically. After birth it enlarges with the growing maxilla, though it is only fully developed following the eruption of the permanent dentition."-Gray's 40/e p478*

Development of Sinuses

Sinus	Gestational Month When Development Starts	Present in Clinically Significant Size	Fully Developed
Maxillary	2^Q	Birth^Q	12 years^Q
Ethmoid	3^Q	Birth^Q	12 years^Q
Frontal	4^Q	3 years^Q	18-20 years^Q
Sphenoid	3^Q	8 years^Q	12-15 years^Q

7. Ans. b. Triangular   *(Ref: Gray's 40/e p747, 809)*

Trapezius is a flat, triangular muscle, which extends over the back of the neck and upper thorax.

"Trapezius is a flat, triangular muscle that covers the back of the neck and shoulder. Together, the two trapezius muscles resemble a trapezium or quadrilateral in which two of the angles correspond to the shoulders, a third to the occipital protuberance and the fourth to the spine of the 12th thoracic vertebra." -Gray's 40/e p747

"Trapezius is a flat, triangular muscle which extends over the back of the neck and upper thorax. The paired trapezius muscles form a diamond shape, from which the name is derived: the lateral angles occur at the shoulder tips, the superior angle at the occipital protuberance and superior nuchal lines, and the inferior angle at the spine of the twelfth thoracic vertebra." - Gray's 40/e p809

Trapezius
• Trapezius is a **flat, triangular muscle**[Q] • Extends over the **back of neck & upper thorax**. • **Paired trapezius** muscles form a **diamond shape**[Q]
Origin
• Occipital bone, ligamentum nuchae, spine of 7th cervical vertebra, spines of all thoracic vertebrae[Q]
Insertion
• Upper fibers into lateral third of clavicle; middle & lower fibers into acromion & spine of scapula[Q]
Nerve Supply
• Spinal part of accessory nerve (motor) and C3 & 4 (sensory)[Q]
Action
• Upper fibers elevate the scapula[Q] • Middle fibers pull scapula medially[Q] • Lower fibers pull medial border of scapula downward[Q]

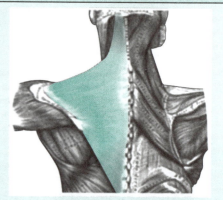

Note: Look at the muscle from one side only

8. Ans. a. a   *(Ref: Gray's 41/e p569, 40/e p539)*

Opening of jaw is carried out by the bilateral action of lateral pterygoid muscle, which is represented by 'a' in the diagram, originating by two heads from sphenoid bone and getting inserted at anterior surface of mandibular condyle.

Structures Marked in the Diagram		
a	Lateral pterygoid	Opening & Protraction
b	Masseter	Closing
c	Temporalis	Closing & retraction
d	Buccinator	Cheek inflation

"Lateral pterygoid: When left and right muscles contract together the condyle is pulled forward and slightly downward. This protrusive movement alone has little or no function except to assist opening the jaw. Digastric and geniohyoid are the main jaw opening muscles: unlike lateral pterygoid, when acting alone they rotate the jaw open, provided other muscles attached to the hyoid prevent if from being pulled forward. If only one lateral pterygoid contracts, the jaw rotates about a vertical axis passing roughly through the opposite condyle and is pulled medially toward the opposite side. This contraction together with that of the adjacent medial pterygoid (both attached to the lateral pterygoid plate) provides most of the strong medially directed component of the force used when grinding food between teeth of the same side. It is arguably the most important function of the inferior head of lateral pterygoid."- Gray's 40/e p539

Movements of Mandible				
Protrusion	**Retraction**	**Depression**	**Elevation**	**Side to side**
• Lateral pterygoid[Q] • Medial pterygoid[Q]	• Posterior fibers of temporalis	• Lateral pterygoid[Q] • Digastric[Q] • Geniohyoid[Q] • Mylohyoid[Q]	• Masseter[Q] • Medial pterygoid[Q] • Temporalis[Q]	• Lateral pterygoid[Q] • Medial pterygoid[Q]

9. **Ans. c. Dermis** *(Ref: Gray's 40/e p38, 112, 150; Rook's 8/e p8.22)*

Dense irregular connective tissue is found in the dermis of the skin, the walls of large tubular organs, such as the alimentary canal, in glandular tissue, and in organ capsules. Regular connective tissues include highly fibrous tissues in which fibres are regularly orientated, either to form sheets such as fasciae and apo- neuroses, or as thicker bundles such as ligaments or tendons.

"Dense irregular connective tissue occurs in: the reticular layer of the dermis; the superficial connective tissue sheaths of muscle and nerves and the adventitia of large blood vessels; the capsules of various glands and organs (e.g. testis, sclera of the eye, periostea and perichondria)."- Gray's 40/e p38

"Regular connective tissues include highly fibrous tissues in which fibres are regularly orientated, either to form sheets such as fasciae and aponeuroses, or as thicker bundles such as ligaments or tendons."- Gray's 40/e p38

"The dermis is an irregular, moderately dense connective tissue. It has a matrix composed of an interwoven collagenous and elastic network in an amorphous ground substance of glycosaminoglycans, glycoproteins and bound water, which accommodates nerves, blood vessels, lymphatics, epidermal appendages and a changing population of cells. Mechanically, the dermis provides considerable strength to the skin by virtue of the number and arrangement of its collagen fibres (which give it tensile strength), and its elastic fibres (which give it elastic recoil)."-Gray's 40/e p150

"Tendons take the form of cords or straps of round or oval cross-section, and consist of dense, regular connective tissue."- Gray's 40/e p112

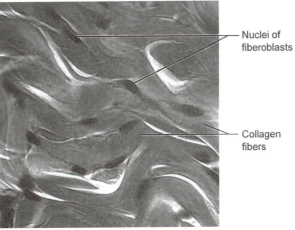

Fig. 5: Dense irregular connective tissue from the dermis of skin
(Collagen fibers are arranged in bundles without a definite orientation & form three-dimensional network)

Dense Irregular Connective Tissue (DICT)

- DICT is found in **regions** that are **under considerable mechanical stress** & where **protection is given to ensheathed organs**.
- **Collagen fibers** are **arranged in bundles without a definite orientation** & form **three-dimensional network**
- **Provide resistance to stress from all directions**

Dense Irregular Connective Tissue occurs in	
Reticular layer of dermis[Q]	Capsules of various glands & organs (e.g. testis, sclera of the eye)[Q]
Superficial connective tissue sheaths of muscle & nerves[Q]	Periosteum[Q]
Adventitia of large blood vessels[Q]	Perichondrium[Q]

Dense Regular Connective Tissue (DRCT)

- **Provides connection between different tissues in the human body.**
- The **collagen fibers** are **bundled in a parallel fashion.**
- In this kind of tissue, **elastic** & **reticular fibers** are **completely absent.**

Contd...

Contd...

Dense Regular Connective Tissue (DRCT)
• Dense regular tissue can be **divided into white fibrous connective tissue** and **yellow fibrous connective tissue**. Both of these types can be arranged in **cord or sheet arrangement**.

Dense Regular Connective Tissue	
Cord arrangement	**Sheet arrangement**
• Bundles of **collagen & matrix** are distributed in **regular alternate patterns**.	• **Collagen bundles & matrix** are **distributed in irregular patterns**, • Similar to areolar tissue

Dense Regular Connective Tissue	
Structures formed	**Functions**

• **Tendons**:
   – **Connect muscle to bone**[Q]
   – Derive their strength from the **regular, longitudinal arrangement of bundles of collagen fibers**[Q].
 • **Ligaments**:
   – **Bind bone to bone**[Q]
   – Similar in structure to tendons.
 • **Aponeurosis**
	• Has **great tensile strength**[Q] that resists pulling forces especially well in one direction.
	 • Has a **very poor blood supply**[Q] (damaged tendons & ligaments are slow to heal)

10. **Ans. c. c** *(Ref: Gray's 40/e p153; Ross Histology 6/e p147)*

Holocrine cells in the given slide are marked with the legend 'c'.

Structures Marked in the Diagram	
a	• Sweat gland
b	• Sweat gland ducts
c	• Sebaceous gland
d	• Root of hair follicle

"Sebaceous glands are small saccular structures lying in the dermis; together with the hair follicle and arrector pili muscle, they constitute the pilosebaceous unit. They are present over the whole body except the thick hairless skin of the palm, soles and flexor surfaces of digits. Typically, they consist of a cluster of secretory acini, which open by a short common duct into the dermal pilary canal of the hair follicle. They release their lipid secretory product, sebum, into the canal by a holocrine mechanism. In some areas of thin skin which lack hair follicles, their ducts open instead directly on to the skin surface, e.g. on the lips and corners of the mouth, the buccal mucosa, nipples, female breast areolae, penis, inner surface of the prepuce, clitoris and labia minora. At the margins of the eyelids, the large complex palpebral tarsal glands (Meibomian glands) are of this type. They are also present in the external auditory meatus."- Gray's 40/e p153

Sebaceous Glands
• Sebaceous glands **empty their secretory product into upper parts of hair follicles**.   • Found in **parts of the skin where hair is present (Exception: Lips, oral surfaces of cheeks & external genitalia**, sebaceous glands are present without hair)[Q]   • **Pilosebaceous unit: Hair follicle** & its **associated sebaceous gland**   • Sebaceous glands are **simple & branched**   • Secretory portion consists of **alveoli**.

- **Basal cells** in outermost layer of alveolus **are flattened. Basal cells** are **mitotically active**.
- Some of the **new cells** will **replenish the pool of basal cells**, while the remaining cells are displaced towards the centre of alveolus as more cells are generated by basal cells.
- **Secretory cells** will gradually **accumulate lipids & grow in size**[Q].
- Finally their **nuclei disintegrate & cells rupture**.
- **Resulting secretory product of lipids & constituents of the disintegrating cell** is a **holocrine secretion**.

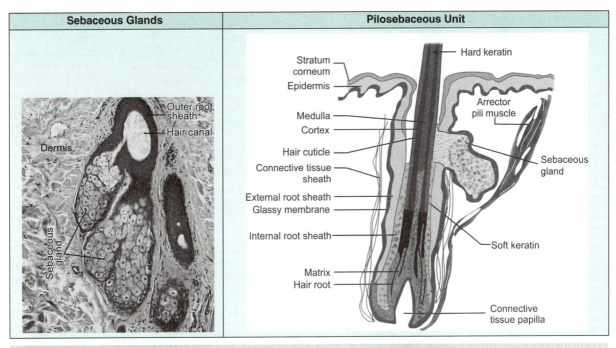

"*Exocrine glands* secrete their products through a duct onto an outer surface of the body, such as the skin or the human gastrointestinal tract. Secretion is directly onto the apical surface. The glands in this group can be divided into three groups: *Apocrine glands, holocrine glands & merocrine glands.*"

Types of Glands		
Apocrine Glands	**Holocrine Glands**	**Eccrine (Merocrine) Glands**
• Apical part of cell is shed off to discharge secretion (decapitation[Q] secretion). • Responds mainly to sympathetic adrenergic stimuli[Q] • Becomes functional at puberty[Q] • Example: Apocrine sweat glands in axilla & groin, mammary glands; external auditory canal (ceruminous gland)[Q] & eyelids (gland of Moll)[Q]	• Whole cell disintegrates[Q] discharging secretion. • Found throughout skin except palms & soles. • Sebaceous glands are usually associated with hair follicles except in following locations: • Gland of Zeis & Meibomian gland[Q] in eyelids • Montgomery tubercle[Q]: Nipple & areola • Tyson's[Q] gland: External fold of prepuce • Fordyce[Q] spot: vermillion border of lips & mucosa	• Cell is intact & secretions are thrown out by exocytosis[Q]. • Example: Sweat gland on palms & soles[Q]. • Found everywhere except clitoris, gland penis, labia minora, external auditory canal & lips[Q].

11. **Ans. a. Abducent nerve**   *(Ref: Gray's 40/e p430)*

    Marked nerve in the given picture is abducent nerve. Abducent nerve enters the subarachnoid space when it emerges from the brainstem. It runs upward between the pons and the clivus, and then pierces the dura mater to run between the dura and the skull through Dorello's canal. At the tip of the petrous temporal bone it makes a sharp turn forward to enter the cavernous sinus.

*"The **abducens nerve** is the **sixth cranial nerve** and **innervates lateral rectus exclusively**. It emerges from the brain stem between the pons and the medulla oblongata and usually **runs through** the inferior venous compartment of the **petroclival venous confluence** in a bow-shaped canal, Dorello's canal. It then bends sharply across the upper border of the petrous part of the temporal bone to enter the cavernous sinus, where it lies lateral to the internal carotid artery (unlike the oculomotor, trochlear, ophthalmic and maxillary nerves, which merely invaginate the lateral dural wall of the sinus). The abducens nerve **enters the orbit through the superior orbital fissure**, within the common tendinous ring, at first below, and then between, the two divisions of the oculomotor nerve and lateral to the nasociliary nerve. It **passes forwards to enter the medial (ocular) surface of lateral rectus**."-Gray's 40/e p430*

12. **Ans. a. L1-L2**   *(Ref: Gray's 40/e p1064; Snell's 9/e p131)*

The root value of cremasteric reflex is L1-L2. The afferent fibers of cremasteric reflex arc travel in the femoral branch of the genitofemoral nerve (L1 and 2), and the efferent motor nerve fibers travel in the genital branch of the genitofemoral nerve.

"Cremaster is innervated by the genital branch of the genitofemoral nerve, derived from the first and second lumbar spinal nerves."-Gray's 40/e p1064

"Cremaster pulls the testis up towards the superficial inguinal ring. Although its fibres are striated, it is not usually under voluntary control. Stroking the skin of the medial side of the thigh evokes a reflex contraction of the muscle, the cremasteric reflex, which is most pronounced in children. It may represent a protective reflex, and the cremaster may also have a role in testicular thermoregulation."-Gray's 40/e p1064

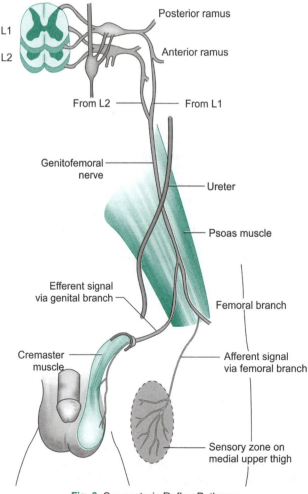

Fig. 6: Cremasteric Reflex Pathway

"The cremaster muscle is supplied by the genital branch of the genitofemoral nerve. The cremaster muscle can be made to contract by stroking the skin on the medial aspect of the thigh. This is called the cremasteric reflex. The afferent fibers of this reflex arc travel in the femoral branch of the genitofemoral nerve (L1 and 2), and the efferent motor nerve fibers travel in the genital branch of the genitofemoral nerve."- *Snell's 9/e p131*

Superficial Reflexes			
Reflex	**Stimulation**	**Clinical Result**	**Root Value**
Plantar reflex	Scratching laterally on sole of the foot	Flexion of big toe (downward movement)	L5, S1[Q]
Scapular reflex	Scratching skin in interscapular region	Contraction of scapular muscles	C5 to T1[Q]
Abdominal reflex	Scratching on abdominal wall below costal margin and in iliac fossa	Contraction of abdominal muscles	T7 to T12[Q]
Anal reflex	Scratching near anus	Contraction of anal sphincter	S3, S4[Q]
Cremasteric reflex	**Stoking skin at upper & inner thigh**	**Upward movement of testes**	L1, L2[Q]

13. **Ans. c. Preganglionic** *(Ref: Gray's 40/e p1042)*

Each spinal nerve receives a branch called a gray ramus communicans from the adjacent paravertebral ganglion of the sympathetic trunk. The gray rami communicans contain postganglionic nerve fibers of the sympathetic nervous system and are composed of largely unmyelinated neurons. This is in contrast to the white rami communicans, in which heavily myelinated neurons give the rami their white appearance.

"Anterior rami of T1 to L2 are connected to the sympathetic trunk or to a ganglion, by a white ramus communicans, which carries preganglionic sympathetic fibers and appears white because the fibers it contains are myelinated."- *Gray's Anatomy for Students (2009)/p44*

"The gray ramus communicans connects the sympathetic trunk or a ganglion to the anterior ramus and contains the postganglionic sympathetic fibers. It appears gray because postganglionic fibers are nonmyelinated. The gray ramus communicans is positioned medial to the white ramus communicans."- *Gray's Anatomy for Students (2009)/p44*

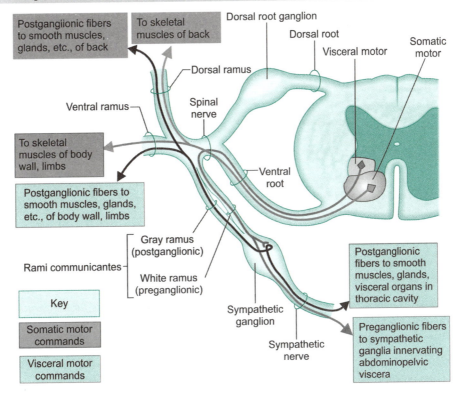

*"The cell bodies of neurones of the sympathetic supply of the abdomen and pelvis lie in the intermediolateral grey matter of the first to 12th thoracic and first two lumbar spinal segments. These neurones give rise to myelinated axons which travel in the ventral ramus of the spinal nerve of the same level, leaving it via the white ramus communicans to enter a thoracic or lumbar paravertebral ganglion. Visceral branches may exit at the same level or ascend or descend several levels before exiting but leave the ganglia without synapsing in medial (visceral) branches. These give rise to the greater, lesser and least splanchnic nerves, and the lumbar and sacral splanchnic nerves. **Axons destined for supply to somatic structures always synapse in the ganglion of the same level and post-ganglionic, unmyelinated axons leave the ganglion via the grey ramus communicans to enter the spinal nerve of the same level."*- Gray's 40/e p1042

	White Ramus Communicans	Gray Ramus Communicans
Type of fibers	**Myelinated**^Q	**Nonmyelinated**^Q
Source of origin	**Lateral horn cells of spinal cord**^Q	**Cells of sympathetic ganglion**^Q
Destination	Relay in the sympathetic ganglion (**preganglionic fibers**)^Q	Distributed to **blood vessels, hair & sweat glands** through branches of anterior & posterior rami of spinal nerves (**postganglionic fibers**)^Q

14. **Ans. b. Zonula occludens**   *(Ref: Ganong 25/e p112, 41; Gray's 40/e p7, 140)*

The arrow in the given diagram is showing intercalated discs of cardiac muscle, which contains all types of cellular junctions except occluding tight junction (Zonula occludens). Cardiac muscle cells are connected by fascia adherens (the structural analog of zonula adherens), gap junctions & macula adherens.

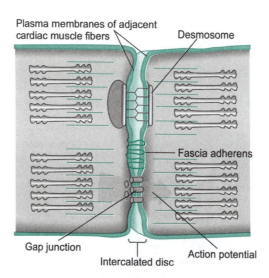

"Intercalated disc is a junctional complex between neighbouring cells in cardiac muscle cells. The interdigitating transverse parts of the intercalated disc form a fascia adherens, with numerous desmosomes; gap junctions are found in the longitudinal parts of the disc."-Gray's 40/e p140

"Three types of cell junction make up an intercalated disc- fascia adherens, desmosomes & gap junctions."

"Gap Junctions: They occur in numerous tissues including the liver, epidermis, pancreatic islet cells, connective tissues, cardiac muscle and smooth muscle, and are also common in embryonic tissues."- Gray's 40/e p7

"A fascia adherens is similar to a zonula adherens, but is more limited in extent and forms a strip or patch of adhesion, e.g. between smooth muscle cells, in the intercalated discs of cardiac muscle cells and between glial cells and neurones."- Gray's 40/e p7

"Tight junctions characteristically surround the apical margins of the cells in epithelia such as the intestinal mucosa, the walls of the renal tubules, and the choroid plexus."- Ganong 25/e p41

Intercalated discs

- Intercalated discs are unique & identifying features of cardiac muscle[Q].
- **Cardiac muscle** consists of individual heart muscle cells (**cardiomyocytes**) connected by intercalated discs to work as a **single functional organ** or syncytium[Q].
- **Skeletal muscle** consists of **multinucleated muscle fibers** and exhibit **no intercalated discs**[Q].
- Support synchronized contraction of cardiac tissue; Occur at **Z line of sarcomere**[Q]
  - Three types of cell junction make up an intercalated disc-fascia adherens, desmosomes & gap junctions. [Q]
- Light microscope: **Transverse lines crossing the tracts of cardiac cells**[Q].
- Have **transverse & lateral portions**[Q]
- **Transverse portion contain desmosomes & lateral portions contain gap junctions**[Q]

Specialized Adhesive Contacts

- Specialized adhesive contacts are **localized regions of the cell surface** with particular ultrastructural characteristics.

Major Classes of Specialized Adhesive Contacts		
Occluding junctions (tight junctions, zonula occludens)		• **Create diffusion barriers in continuous layers of cells**, including **epithelia, mesothelia & endothelia**[Q] • **Prevent the passage of materials** across the cellular layer through intercellular spaces[Q]. • They form a **continuous belt (zonula) around cell perimeter**[Q], near the apical surface in cuboidal or columnar epithelial cells.
Adhesive junctions		• Adhesive junctions include **intercellular & cell-extracellular matrix contacts**[Q] • **Cells adhere strongly** to each other or to adjacent matrix components[Q].
	Zonula adherens (intermediate junction)	• **Continuous, belt-like zone of adhesion** around **apical perimeters of epithelial, mesothelial and endothelial cells**, parallel & just basal to tight junction in epithelia[Q]. • **High concentrations of cadherins** occur in this zone[Q].
	Fascia adherens	• **Similar to a zonula adherens**, but is more limited in extent & forms a strip or patch of adhesion, e.g. **between smooth muscle cells**, in **intercalated discs of cardiac muscle cells** and between **glial cells & neurons**[Q].
	Desmosomes (maculae adherentes)	• Desmosomes are limited, **plaque-like areas** of **strong intercellular contact**[Q]. • **Located anywhere** on the cell surface • Desmosomes **form strong anchorage points**[Q], likened to spot-welds, between cells subject to mechanical stress
	Hemides-mosomes	• **Anchoring junctions** between **bases of epithelial cells & basal lamina**[Q]. • Resemble a **single-sided desmosome**, anchored on **one side to plasma membrane** & on the other to **basal lamina & adjacent collagen fibrils**[Q]. • Hemidesmosomes use **integrins** as adhesion molecules, whereas desmosomes use **cadherins**[Q].
	Focal adhesion plaques	• **Regions of local attachment** between cells & extracellular matrix. • **Situated at or near ends of actin filament bundles** • **Usually short-lived**
Gap junctions (commu-nicating junctions)		• **Resemble tight junctions** in transverse section, but **two apposed lipid bilayers** are separated by an apparent gap of 3 nm, bridged by connexons. • **Connexons** are formed by a **ring of six connexin proteins** in each membrane[Q]. • **Form limited attachment plaques, allow free passage of substances** within the adjacent intercellular space. • Occur in **liver, epidermis, pancreatic islet cells, connective tissues, cardiac muscle, smooth muscle, embryonic tissues, CNS** (in **ependyma** & between **neuroglial cells**)

15. **Ans. c. C** *(Ref: Gray's 40/e p145, 147; DeFiore's Atlas of Histology 11/e p225)*
   Stratum spinosum or prickle cell layer contains abundant desmosomes marked with the legend 'C' in the image.

Picture shows layers of epidermis	
A	Stratum corneum
B	Stratum granulosum
C	Stratum spinosum
D	Stratum basale

"The epidermis can be divided into a number of layers from deep to superficial as follows: basal layer (stratum basale), spinous or prickle cell layer (stratum spinosum), granular layer (stratum granulosum), clear layer (stratum lucidum) and cornified layer (stratum corneum)."-Gray's 40/e p145

"The prickle cell layer (stratum spinosum) consists of several layers of closely packed keratinocytes that interdigitate with each other by means of numerous cell surface projections. The cells are anchored to each other by desmosomes that provide tensile strength and cohesion to the layer. These suprabasal cells are committed to terminal differentiation and gradually move upwards towards the cornified layer as more cells are produced in the basal layer. When skin is processed for routine light microscopy, the cells tend to shrink away from each other except where they are joined by desmosomes, which gives them their characteristic spiny appearance. Prickle cell cytoplasm contains prominent bundles of keratin filaments, (mostly K1 and K10 keratin proteins) arranged concentrically around a euchromatic nucleus, and attached to the dense plaques of desmosomes. The cytoplasm also contains melanosomes, either singly or aggregated within membrane-bound organelles (compound melanosomes). Langerhans cells and the occasional associated lymphocyte are the only non-keratinocytes present in the prickle cell layer."-Gray's 40/e p147

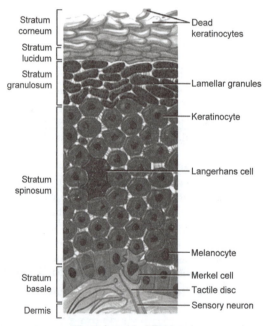

Fig. 7: Layers of Epidermis

Layers of Epidermis	
Stratum basale	• Also known as **stratum germinativum**[Q] • It contains **mitotically active keratinocytes containing house keeping organelles**[Q] (RER, golgi complex, mitochondria, lysosomes, ribosomes) • **Give rise to superficial layer**[Q]
Stratum spinosum	• **Spine like appearance**[Q] of cell margins in histological sections • These **spines are abundant desmosomes**[Q], calcium dependent cell surface modifications that promote adhesion of epidermal cells & resistance to mechanical stresses.
Stratum granulosum	• Characterized by **buildup of components necessary for the process of programmed cell death** & formation of **superficial water impermeable barrier**[Q]. • Most apparent structure within these cells is **basophilic contain keratohyaline granules**[Q]

Contd...

Contd...

Layers of Epidermis	
Stratum lucidum	• Clear layer, seen only in thick skin[Q]
Stratum corneum	• Formed of **cornified or horny cells (largest cell of epidermis)** and have **highest concentration of free amino acids**[Q]

16. **Ans. c. c** *(Ref: Gray's 40/e p632)*
    Lateral semi-circular canal in the given picture is marked as 'c'.

Structures Marked in the Diagram	
a	Incus
b	Posterior semicircular canal
c	Lateral semicircular canal
d	Superior semicircular canal

"The three semicircular canals, anterior (superior), posterior and lateral (horizontal), are located posterosuperior to the vestibule. They are compressed from side to side and each forms approximately two-thirds of a circle. They are unequal in length, but similar in diameter along their lengths, except where they bear a terminal swelling, an ampulla, which is almost twice the diameter of the canal." -Gray's 40/e p632

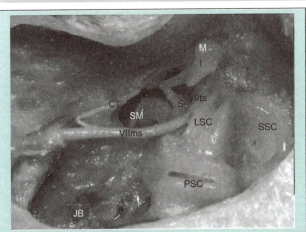 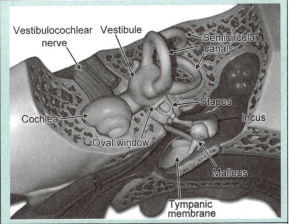

CT: Chorda tympani; I: Incus; JB: Jugular bulb; LSC: Lateral semicircular canal; M: Malleus; PSC: Posterior semicircular canal; S: Stapes; SM: Stapedius muscle; SSC: Superior semicircular canal; VIIms: Mastoid segment of VII cranial nerve; VIIts: Tympanic segment of VII cranial nerve

Semicircular Canal		
Anterior Semicircular Canal	**Posterior Semicircular Canal**	**Lateral Semicircular Canal**
Length: 15–20 mm	Length: 18–22 mm	Length: 12–15 mm
Vertical in orientation & lies **transverse to the long axis of the petrous temporal bone** under the anterior surface of its arcuate eminence. **Ampulla at anterior end of the canal opens into upper & lateral part of vestibule**[Q]. Its other end unites with the upper end of posterior canal to form crus commune, opens into the medial part of vestibule.	Vertical but curves backwards almost parallel with the posterior surface of petrous bone. **Ampulla opens low in the vestibule**[Q], below the cochlear recess where the macula cribrosa inferior transmits nerves to it. Its **upper end joins the crus commune**[Q].	Its arch runs horizontally backwards & laterally. Its **anterior ampulla opens into upper & lateral angle of vestibule**[Q], above the oval window & just below the ampulla of superior canal; its posterior end opens below the opening of crus commune.

PHYSIOLOGY

17. **Ans. c. Interstitial cells of Cajal** *(Ref: Ganong 25/e p496; Guyton 13/e p797, 798)*
    Slow waves are generated by complex interactions among the smooth muscle cells and specialized cells, called the interstitial cells of Cajal.

"Most gastrointestinal contractions occur rhythmically, and this rhythm is determined mainly by the frequency of so-called "slow waves" of smooth muscle membrane potential."- Guyton 13/e p797

"The precise cause of the slow waves is not completely understood, although they appear to be caused by complex interactions among the smooth muscle cells and specialized cells, called the interstitial cells of Cajal, which are believed to act as electrical pacemakers for smooth muscle cells. These interstitial cells form a network with each other and are interposed between the smooth muscle layers, with synaptic-like contacts to smooth muscle cells. The interstitial cells of Cajal undergo cyclic changes in membrane potential due to unique ion channels that periodically open and produce inward (pacemaker) currents that may generate slow wave activity."-Guyton 13/e p798

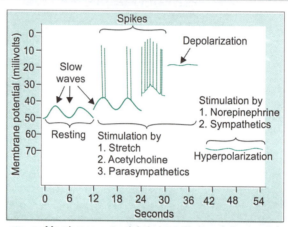

Fig. 8: Membrane potentials in intestinal smooth muscle
Note the slow waves, the spike potentials, total depolarization, and hyperpolarization, all of which occur under different physiological conditions of the intestine

Slow Waves

• **Most gastrointestinal contractions occur rhythmically**, and this rhythm is determined mainly by the frequency of so-called "slow waves" of smooth muscle membrane potential[Q].
• **Slow waves** are slow, undulating changes in the resting membrane potential[Q].
• **Intensity: 5-15 millivolts**[Q]
• **Frequency: 3-12/minute**[Q] (Body of stomach-3/minute, duodenum-12/minute, terminal ileum-8 or 9/minute)[Q]
• **Precise cause of slow waves** is not completely understood.
    • **Slow waves** appear to be **caused by complex interactions among smooth muscle cells & interstitial cells of Cajal**[Q] (electrical pacemakers for smooth muscle cells).
    • **Interstitial cells of Cajal** undergoes **cyclic changes in membrane potential** due to **unique ion channels that periodically open & produce inward (pacemaker) currents** that may **generate slow wave activity**.
• **Slow waves** usually do not by themselves cause muscle contraction in most parts of GIT, **except** perhaps in the **stomach**[Q].
• **Slow waves** mainly excite the appearance of intermittent spike potentials & spike potentials in turn actually excite the muscle contraction[Q].

18. Ans. b. Bainbridge reflex *(Ref: Ganong 25/e p591; Guyton 13/e p223)*
Bainbridge reflex is responsible for tachycardia during right atrial distension.

"Atrial Reflex Control of Heart Rate (the Bainbridge Reflex): An increase in atrial pressure also causes an increase in heart rate, sometimes increasing the heart rate as much as 75 percent. A small part of this increase is caused by a direct effect of the increased atrial volume to stretch the sinus node; such direct stretch can increase the heart rate as much as 15 percent.

An additional 40 to 60 percent increase in rate is caused by a nervous reflex called the Bainbridge reflex. The stretch receptors of the atria that elicit the Bainbridge reflex transmit their afferent signals through the vagus nerves to the medulla of the brain. Then efferent signals are transmitted back through vagal and sympathetic nerves to increase heart rate and strength of heart contraction. Thus, this reflex helps prevent damming of blood in the veins, atria, and pulmonary circulation."-Guyton 13/e p223

"Another important factor is that stretching the heart causes the heart to pump faster, resulting in an increased heart rate. That is, stretch of the sinus node in the wall of the right atrium has a direct effect on the rhythmicity of the node to increase the heart rate as much as 10 to 15 percent. In addition, the stretched right atrium initiates a nervous reflex called the Bainbridge reflex, passing first to the vasomotor center of the brain and then back to the heart by way of the sympathetic nerves and vagi, also to increase the heart rate."- Guyton 13/e p246

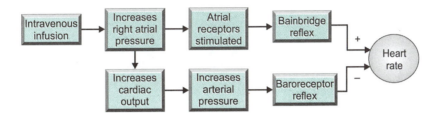

Bezold-Jarisch reflex	• In experimental animals, **injections of serotonin, veratridine, capsaicin, phenyldiguanide,** and **some other drugs into the coronary arteries supplying the left ventricle cause apnea followed by rapid breathing, hypotension, and bradycardia** (the **coronary chemoreflex** or **Bezold-Jarisch reflex[Q]**). • The **receptors are probably C fiber endings**, and the **afferents are vagal[Q]**. • The response is **not produced by injections into the blood supply of the atria or the right ventricle[Q]**.
Hering-Bruer reflex	• The **Hering-Breuer inflation reflex is an increase in the duration of expiration produced by steady lung inflation**, and the **Hering-Breuer deflation reflex is a decrease in the duration of expiration produced by marked deflation of the lung[Q]**.
Bainbridge's reflex	• **Rapid infusion of blood or saline in anesthetized animals** sometimes produces a **rise in heart rate if the initial heart rate is low[Q]**. • This effect was described by Bainbridge in 1915, and since then it has been known as the **Bainbridge reflex**.
Cushing reflex	• **Cushing reflex** (also referred to as the **vasopressor response**), is a **physiological nervous system response to increased intracranial pressure** (ICP) that results in **Cushing's triad of increased blood pressure, irregular breathing, and a reduction of the heart rate[Q]**. • It is usually seen in the **terminal stages of acute head injury** and **may indicate imminent brain herniation[Q]**. • These symptoms can be **indicative of insufficient blood flow** to the **brain (ischemia)** as well as **compression of arterioles[Q]**.
J-reflex (Pulmonary chemoreflex)	• **J or Juxtacapillary/juxtapulmonary receptors** are **C fibre endings located close to pulmonary capillaries** (These were **discovered by Dr Paintal** in 1970). • They are **stimulated by hyperinflation of the lungs[Q]**, but they also respond to intravenous and intracardiac administration of chemicals such as capsaicin, phenyldiguanide. • The reflex that is produced is known as the **pulmonary chemoreflex** and consists of: **Apnea followed by rapid, shallow breathing, bradycardia & hypotension[Q]**. • The physiologic role of this reflex is uncertain, but it probably occurs in pathologic states such as **pulmonary congestion, pulmonary embolism or pulmonary edema[Q]**. • They may play a role in dyspnea associated with left heart failure, interstitial lung disease, pneumonia & microembolism[Q].

19. Ans. d. REM *(Ref: Ganong 25/e p273, 275; Guyton 13/e p762, 763)*

Saw tooth waves (as mentioned in the picture) corresponding to eye movements are seen during REM sleep.

"REM sleep, also known as dream sleep, is characterized by EEG pattern similar to that of stage 1 sleep with superimposed sawtooth waves."-Textbook of Psychiatry By Sethi (2008)/p115

"REM sleep is marked by low-voltage activity, alpha waves, "sawtooth waves," and artifact consistent with horizontal eye movements."- Neurology Examination and Board Review by Nizar Souayah 3/e p198

REM Sleep: Low voltage, random, fast with sawtooth waves

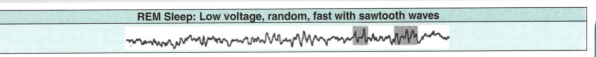

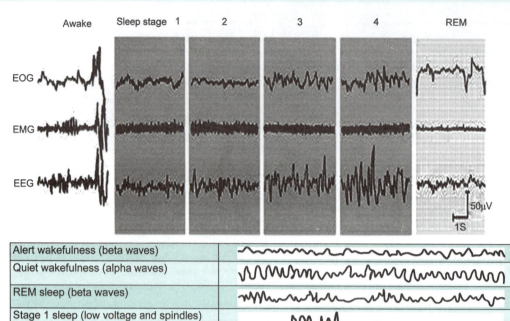

	EEG Patterns In Sleep			
	Beta (β) Wave	**Alpha (α) Wave**	**Theta Wave**	**Delta Wave**
Seen in	• Parietal & frontal[Q] region • Patients awake, at rest with eyes open[Q]	• Recorded from parieto occipital region[Q]. • Related to decreased level of attention • Seen in awake patient at rest with eyes closed[Q] & mind wandering	• Seen in hippocampus[Q] in children[Q] & drowsiness • Found over parietal & temporal areas.	• Seen in deep NREM sleep[Q] & infant[Q]
Frequency	>14 Hz[Q]	8-13 Hz	4-7 Hz	3-5 Hz (minimum)[Q]
Amplitude	Low amplitude	High amplitude	High amplitude[Q]	Large amplitude (Maximum)[Q]
Characteristic Feature	• Low-voltage, high frequency desynchronized electrical activity • Can be produced by any form of sensory stimulation or mental concentration, such as solving arithmetic problems alpha rhythm gets replaced by beta, therefore beta rhythm known as alpha block • Beta rhythm is also known as arousal or alerting response, because it is correlated with the aroused, alert state	Frequency of alpha rhythm is decreased by: • Old age • Low blood glucose • Low body temperature • Low levels of adrenal glucocorticoids • High arterial $PaCO_2$ • Sleep	Recorded in: • Newborn infants • Stage 1 of NREM sleep • Emotional stress in adults particularly disappointment & frustration • Many brain disorders • Accentuated in children when they are crying	• High-voltage, low frequency synchronized electrical activity. • Evoked by overbreathing • Seen in pathological states in which thalamocortical transmission is blocked, such as coma. • Presence of intracranial tumor act as a source of delta wave activity. • In metabolic encephalopathy, Delta waves are seen predominantly due to a decrease in the consciousness.

EEG Pattern In Sleep	
Non Rapid Eye Movement (NREM) Sleep	**Rapid Eye Movement (REM) Sleep**
• Also known as **Slow wave sleep or Orthodox sleep**[Q] (70-80% of total sleep[Q])	• Also known as **Paradoxical sleep**[Q] (20-30% of total sleep)
Stage I: • First & lightest stage of sleep. • Predominantly **theta waves**[Q] **Stage II:** Characterized by- • **Sleep spindles**[Q] • **K-complex (easily evoked)**[Q] **Stage III:** (deep sleep transition) • **Delta wave first appear**[Q] • **K-complex** (with strong stimuli only) **Stage IV:** (Cerebral sleep) • Predominant **delta activity**[Q]	• Light phase of sleep, but **arousal is difficult**[Q] • Mixed frequency, **low amplitude**[Q] waves on EEG. Predominantly β-like activity. • Also known as **Desynchronized**[Q] or paradoxical sleep (because EEG is rapid) • **Dreaming is seen**[Q] • Active sleep
Sleep disorder during NREM IV	**Sleep disorder of REM (3N)**
1. Sleep walking (**Somnambulism**)[Q] 2. Sleep talking (**Somniloquy**)[Q] 3. **Night terror**[Q] (Pavor nocturnes) 4. **Bruxism**[Q] (tooth grinding) 5. **Nocturnal enuresis**[Q] (bed wetting)	6. Night mares[Q] 7. **Narcolepsy**[Q]: The hallmark of this disorder being decreased sleep latency. 8. **Nocturnal penile tumescene**[Q]

20. **Ans. a. Growth hormone** *(Ref: Ganong 25/e p328; Guyton 13/e p945)*

Release of growth hormone is stimulated by strenuous exercise. During sleep, large pulsatile bursts of growth hormone secretion occur.

"Growth hormone is found at relatively low levels during the day, unless specific triggers for its release are present. During sleep, on the other hand, large pulsatile bursts of growth hormone secretion occur."- Ganong 25/e p328

"Growth hormone is secreted in a pulsatile pattern, increasing and decreasing. The precise mechanisms that control secretion of growth hormone are not fully understood, but several factors related to a person's state of nutrition or stress are known to stimulate secretion: (1) starvation, especially with severe protein deficiency; (2) hypoglycemia or low concentration of fatty acids in the blood; (3) exercise; (4) excitement; (5) trauma; and (6) ghrelin, a hormone secreted by the stomach before meals. Growth hormone also characteristically increases during the first 2 hours of deep sleep."- Guyton 13/e p945

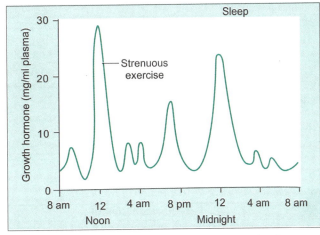

Fig. 9: Typical variations in growth hormone secretion throughout the day, demonstrating the powerful effect of strenuous exercise & high rate of GH secretion that occurs during the first few hours of deep sleep

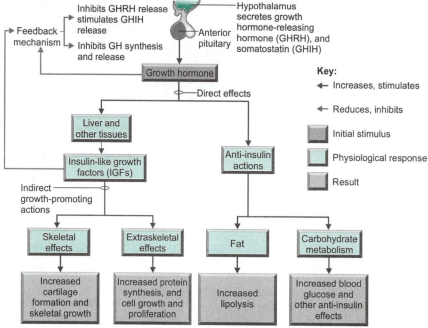

Fig. 10: Metabolic actions of growth hormone

Growth Hormone
• GH is **most abundant anterior pituitary hormone**[Q]
• **GH-secreting somatotrophs** cells constitute **upto 50% of total anterior cell population**[Q]
• **GH is released in pulsatile fashion**[Q]

Factors Stimulating GH Secretion	Factors Inhibiting GH Secretion
• **Hypoglycemia**[Q] • **Decreased blood free fatty acids**[Q] • Increased blood amino acids (arginine) • Other conditions causing hypoglycemia: **Stress, fasting & exercise**[Q] • **Deep sleep (NREM stage II & IV)**[Q] • **Glucagon**[Q] • **Ghrelin**[Q] • **Hormones:** Vasopressin, Androgen, Estrogen, Dopamine agonists, Thyroid hormones, α adrenergic agonists[Q]	• **Increased blood glucose**[Q] • **Increased blood free fatty acids**[Q] • Obesity[Q] • Somatostatin[Q] • Insulin like growth factor-1 (**IGF-1**) • Cortisol[Q] • β adrenergic agonists[Q] • REM sleep[Q]

Actions of Growth Hormone	
Direct Actions of GH	Actions of GH via IGF
• **Decreased glucose uptake into cells**[Q] • **Increased lipolysis**[Q] • **Increased protein synthesis**[Q] • **Epiphyseal growth**[Q] • **GH promotes Na⁺, K⁺ & water retention** and elevates serum levels of inorganic phosphate[Q]	• **Increased protein synthesis in chondrocytes**[Q] • **Increased linear growth**[Q] (pubertal growth spurt) • Increased protein synthesis in most organs • Increased organ size • **Antilipolytic**[Q]

21. **Ans. c. Temperature** *(Ref: Guyton 13/e p10; Understanding Medical Physiology by RL Bijlani 4/e p12)*
Feed forward control system is employed during the regulation of temperature.

Feed Forward Control
• There is a control system in our body when **no stimulus is required** but still the **system anticipates** and **makes corrective changes**. Such a system is called **feed forward** or **anticipatory** or **adaptive control**.

Contd...

Contd...

Examples of Feed Forward Control
• **Temperature control**[Q]: Thermoregulatory responses are initiated by hypothalamus before the changes in **environmental temperature** have succeeded in changing the body's core body temperature • **Cephalic phase of gastric secretion**[Q]: Just thinking about food increases gastric acid production • **Thinking about exercise** itself increases heart rate & respiratory rate[Q] • **Role of cerebellum in motor coordination**[Q]

22. **Ans. c. Decreases oncotic pressure in peritubular capillaries**   *(Ref: Ganong 25/e p678, 679; Guyton 13/e p339; Harrison 19/e p332e-3, p332e-11)*

Constriction of efferent arteriole leads to increase in proteins that escape filtration in glomerular capillaries leading to rise in oncotic pressure (not the decrease in oncotic pressure) in the glomerular capillaries & peritubular capillaries.

"Constriction of the efferent glomerular arteriole by angiotensin II indirectly increases the filtration fraction and raises peritubular capillary oncotic pressure to promote tubular Na^+ reabsorption. Finally, angiotensin II inhibits renin secretion through a negative feedback loop."-Harrison 19/e p332e-11

"Angiotensin II evokes vasoconstriction of the efferent arteriole, and the resulting increased glomerular hydrostatic pressure elevates filtration to normal levels."-Harrison 19/e p332e-3

"Constriction of the efferent arterioles increases the resistance to outflow from the glomerular capillaries. This mechanism raises glomerular hydrostatic pressure, and as long as the increase in efferent resistance does not reduce renal blood flow too much, GFR increases slightly. However, because efferent arteriolar constriction also reduces renal blood flow, filtration fraction and glomerular colloid osmotic pressure increase as efferent arteriolar resistance increases. Therefore, if constriction of efferent arterioles is severe (more than about a threefold increase in efferent arteriolar resistance), the rise in colloid osmotic pressure exceeds the increase in glomerular capillary hydrostatic pressure caused by efferent arteriolar constriction. When this situation occurs, the net force for filtration actually decreases, causing a reduction in GFR."-Guyton 13/e p339

"Thus, efferent arteriolar constriction has a biphasic effect on GFR. At moderate levels of constriction, there is a slight increase in GFR, but with severe constriction, there is a decrease in GFR. The primary cause of the eventual decrease in GFR is as follows: As efferent constriction becomes severe and as plasma protein concentration increases, there is a rapid, nonlinear increase in colloid osmotic pressure caused by the Donnan effect; the higher the protein concentration, the more rapidly the colloid osmotic pressure rises because of the interaction of ions bound to the plasma proteins, which also exert an osmotic effect."-Guyton 13/e p339

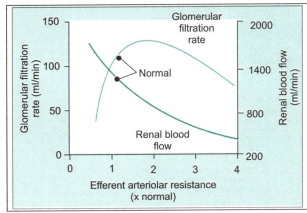 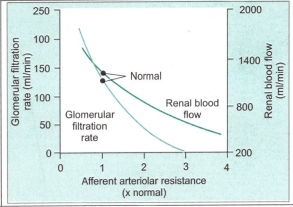

Fig. 11: Effect of change in afferent arteriolar resistance or efferent arteriolar resistance on glomerular filtration rate and renal blood flow

Effects of Constriction of Efferent Arteriole
• If there is **more than threefold increase in resistance, GFR decreases** because of **decrease in renal blood flow & increase in colloid osmotic pressure**[Q]

Contd...

Contd...

- **Efferent arteriolar constriction reduces peritubular capillary hydrostatic pressure**, which **increases net tubular reabsorption**[Q]
- **Increase in the filtration fraction & raises peritubular capillary oncotic pressure to promote tubular Na⁺ reabsorption**[Q]

23. **Ans. b. Difference in concentration of surfactant during inspiration and expiration** *(Ref: Ganong 25/e p629, 631; Guyton 13/e p500)*

    Difference in trajectory between inspiratory loop and the expiratory loop in the curve is due to difference in concentration of surfactant during inspiration and expiration.

    *"Differences are also obvious in the curves generated during inflation and deflation. This difference is termed **hysteresis**, and notably is not present in the saline generated curves. The alveolar environment, and specifically the secreted factors that help reduce surface tension and keep alveoli from collapsing, contribute to hysteresis. **The low surface tension when the alveoli are small is due to the presence of surfactant in the fluid lining the alveoli. Surfactant is a mixture of dipalmitoylphosphatidylcholine (DPPC), other lipids, and proteins. If the surface tension is not kept low when the alveoli become smaller during expiration, they collapse in accordance with the law of Laplace.**"*- Ganong 25/e p631

    ### Compliance Curve
    - The curve has inspiratory & expiratory components
    - **Inspiratory & expiratory compliance curves do not coincide. This difference** is called **hysteresis**[Q].
        - The difference between inflation & deflation paths—**hysteresis**—exists because a **greater trans-pulmonary pressure is required to open a previously closed airway, owing to a deficit of surfactant at the air-water interface, than to keep an open airway from closing, reflecting abundant surfactant**[Q].
    - Lung volume at any given pressure is greater during expiration than during inspiration
    - **Compliance** is **greatest at mid pressure range**[Q]
        - Pulmonary compliance = $\Delta V / \Delta P$
        - ΔV is the **change in volume** or amount of air inhaled in mL or L
        - ΔP is the **change in intrapleural pressure in cm H_2O**

24. **Ans. d. Closure of inactive gates of sodium channel** *(Ref: Ganong 25/e p91, 93; Guyton 13/e p73)*

    Absolute refractory period is due to closure of inactive gates of sodium channel.

    *"**Absolute Refractory Period**: The Na⁺ channels rapidly enter a closed state called the inactivated state and remain in this state for a few milliseconds before returning to the resting state, when they again can be activated."-Ganong 25/e p91*

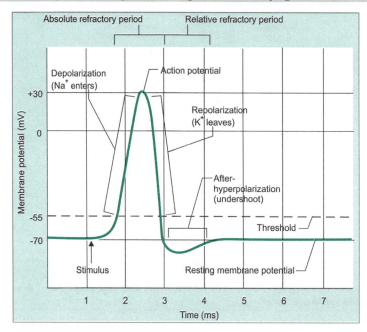

Refractory Period

- During the rising and much of the falling phases of the spike potential, the neuron is refractory to stimulation.
- This refractory period is divided into:
- **Absolute refractory period: Period from the time the firing level is reached until repolarization is about one-third complete**[Q]
- **Relative refractory period:** Lasting from this point to the **start of after-depolarization**[Q].

  - During the **absolute refractory period, no stimulus, no matter how strong, will excite the nerve;** but during the **relative refractory period, stronger than normal stimuli** can cause **excitation**[Q].

Refractory Period	
Absolute Refractory Period	**Relative refractory period**
• **Period from the time firing level is reached until repolarization is about 1/3rd complete**[Q]. • **No stimulus, no matter how strong, will not excite the nerve during absolute refractory period**[Q] • **Cause: Inactivation gates of the Na+ channel are closed when the membrane potential is depolarized. They remain closed until repolarization occurs. No action potential can occur until the inactivation gates open**[Q].	• Begins from the remaining part of repolarization to the end of action potential • **Stronger than normal stimulus** (suprathreshold stimulus) **produces action potential in relative refractory period**[Q] • **Cause: K+ conductance is higher than at rest, and the membrane potential is closer to the K+ equilibrium potential**[Q] and, therefore, farther from threshold; more inward current is required to bring the membrane to threshold

25. **Ans. c. +80**   *(Ref: Ganong 25/e p90)*

Resting membrane potential (RMP) is the static state of a membrane, where the net transmembrane electric flux is zero. Non-electrogenic transfer at RMP means X+Y+Z = 0 . Since X = −50 and Y = −30, then Z must be +80 since (-80 +80 = 0)

BIOCHEMISTRY

26. **Ans. a. Selenocysteine**   *(Ref: Harper 30/e p16, 18, 286)*

Selenocysteine is not the product of post-translational modification. Unlike hydroxyproline or hydroxylysine, selenocysteine arises co-translationally during its incorporation into peptides.

	Name	Codon	Modification
21st amino acid	**Selenocysteine**[Q]	**UGA** (STOP codon)[Q]	**Co-translational**[Q]
22nd amino acid	**Pyrrolysine**[Q]	**UAG** (STOP codon)[Q]	**Co-translational**[Q]

"Selenocysteine is an L-alpha-amino acid found in proteins from every domain of life. Humans contain approximately two dozen selenoproteins that include certain peroxidases and reductases, selenoproteins P, which circulates in the plasma, and the iodothyronine deiodinases responsible for converting the prohormone thyroxine (T4) to the thyroid hormone 3,3'5-triiodothyronine (T3). As its name implies, a selenium atom replaces the sulphur atom of its element analog, cysteine. Selenocysteine is not the product of a posttranslational modification, but is inserted directly into a growing polypeptide during translation. Selenocysteine thus is commonly termed the '21st amino acid'. However, unlike the other 20 amino acids, incorporation of selenocysteine is specified by a large and complex genetic element for he unusual tRNA called tRNASec which utilizes the UGA anticodon that normally signals STOP. However, the protein synthetic apparatus can identify a selenocysteine-specific UGA codon by the presence of an accompanying stem-loop structure, the selenocysteine insertion element, in the untranslated region of the mRNA."-Harper 30/e p16

Selenocysteine (the 21st Amino Acid)

- While its occurrence in proteins is uncommon, **selenocysteine** is **present at the active site of several human enzymes** that **catalyze redox reactions**[Q]. **Examples: thioredoxin reductase, glutathione peroxidase, & deiodinase** (that converts thyroxine to triiodothyronine)
- Significantly, **replacement of selenocysteine by cysteine** can significantly **decrease catalytic activity**[Q].

  - **Impairments in human selenoproteins** have been implicated in tumorigenesis & atherosclerosis, and are associated with **selenium deficiency cardiomyopathy** (**Keshan disease**[Q]).

Contd...

Contd...

Selenocysteine (the 21st Amino Acid)

- **Biosynthesis of selenocysteine requires cysteine, selenate, ATP, a specific tRNA** & several enzymes.
- **Serine provides the carbon skeleton of selenocysteine.** Selenophosphate, formed from ATP & selenate, serves as the selenium donor.

  - Unlike hydroxyproline or hydroxylysine, selenocysteine arises co-translationally during its incorporation into peptides.
  - UGA anticodon of the unusual tRNA designated tRNA^{Sec} normally signals STOP^Q.

- The ability of the protein synthetic apparatus to identify a **selenocysteine-specific UGA codon** involves the **selenocysteine insertion element, a stem-loop structure in the untranslated region of the mRNA**^{Q}.
- **Selenocysteine- tRNA^{Sec} is first charged with serine** by the ligase that charges tRNA^{Ser}. Subsequent replacement of the serine oxygen by selenium involves selenophosphate formed by selenophosphate synthase.
- Successive enzyme-catalyzed reactions convert cysteyl- tRNA^{Sec} to aminoacryl- tRNA^{Sec} and then to selenocysteyl- tRNA^{Sec}.
- In the presence of a specific elongation factor that recognizes selenocysteyl- tRNA^{Sec}, selenocysteine can then be incorporated into proteins.

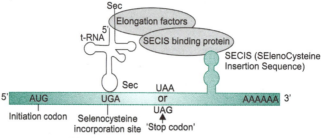

Fig. 12: Mechanism of incorporation of selenocysteine

27. Ans. a. Pyridoxal phosphate   *(Ref: Harper 30/e p557)*

Pyridoxal phosphate is the cofactor of glycogen phosphorylase, where the phosphate group is catalytically important.

> "Pyridoxal phosphate is a coenzyme for many enzymes involved in amino acid metabolism, especially transamination and decarboxylation. It is also the cofactor of glycogen phosphorylase, where the phosphate group is catalytically important. In addition, B_6 is important in steroid hormone action. Pyridoxal phosphate removes the hormone-receptor complex from DNA binding, terminating the action of the hormones. In vitamin B_6 deficiency, there is increased sensitivity to the actions of low concentrations of estrogens, androgens, cortisol, and vitamin D." -*Harper 30/e p557*

Pyridoxine (Vitamin B_6)

- **Vitamin B_6** is involved in **heme & neurotransmitter synthesis**; metabolism of glycogen, lipids, steroids, sphingoid bases, conversion of tryptophan to niacin^Q.
- **Active form** of Pyridoxine: Pyridoxal phosphate (Mainly used for amino acid metabolism^Q)
- Approx. 80% of the body's total vitamin B_6 is pyridoxal phosphate in muscle, mostly **associated with glycogen phosphorylase**^{Q}.

  - RDA of Pyridoxine: 1-2 mg/day^Q
  - Dietary Sources: Rich food sources are legumes, nuts, wheat bran & meat^Q

Coenzyme Roles of Pyridoxal Phosphate		
Decarboxylation of Amino Acids	**Results in the formation of Biogenic Amines**	
	• 5-Hydroxy Tryptophan → Serotonin^Q • Cysteine → Taurine^Q • DOPA → Dopamine^Q	• Glutamate → GABA^Q • Histidine → Histamine^Q • Serine → Ethanolamine^Q
Glycogenolysis	• Glycogen phosphorylase^Q	
Heme Synthesis	• ALA synthase that catalyze condensation of succinyl Co-A & glycine.	

Contd...

Contd...

Pyridoxine (Vitamin B$_6$)	
Coenzyme Roles of Pyridoxal Phosphate	
Transamination	• Alanine aminotransferase (**ALT**), Aspartate aminotransferase (**AST**) • **Alanine glyoxylate aminotransferase**[Q]
Transulfuration	• Involved in metabolism of sulfur containing amino acids. • **Synthesis of cysteine from methionine**[Q]
Tryptophan Metabolism	• Coenzyme of **kynureninase** involved in **synthesis of niacin from tryptophan**[Q]

Deficiency Diseases:

- Epithelial changes, **peripheral neuropathy (generalized axonal sensorimotor polyneuropathy)**, abnormal EEG & **personality changes** (depression & confusion)[Q]
- **Convulsions:** Due to decreased synthesis of GABA[Q]; **Pellagra:** Due defective niacin synthesis[Q].
- **Microcytic hypochromic Anemia:** Due to decreased heme synthesis[Q]

   - **Hyperhomocysteinemia** & increased risk of cardiovascular disease[Q]
   - **Infants: Diarrhea, seizures & anemia**[Q]

Clinical Applications:

- **Vitamin B$_6$ deficiency** is most commonly seen in **patients treated with isoniazid or hydralazine**[Q].
- **Pyridoxine** is of proven benefit in **correcting the sideroblastic anemias** associated with **ATT (isoniazid & pyrazinamide), which act as vitamin B$_6$ antagonists**[Q].

   - **Prophylactic administration of pyridoxine prevents** the **development of ATT induced peripheral neuritis & CNS disorders**[Q]

- **Pyridoxine deficiency**, an important cause of **neonatal seizures** can be effectively **treated with pyridoxine replacement**[Q].
- **High-dose of Pyridoxine** is given in: **Carpal Tunnel syndrome, premenstrual syndrome, schizophrenia & diabetic neuropathy**[Q].
- Drugs that interact with carbonyl group & cause pyridoxal phosphate deficiencies: **Levodopa, penicillamine & cycloserine**[Q]
- **Vitamin B$_6$ should not be given with levodopa**[Q]

   Pyridoxine dependency syndromes needing Pharmacological Dose of Pyridoxal Phosphate
   - **Classic homocystinuria:** Due to cystathionine beta-synthase deficiency[Q]
   - **Sideroblastic anemia:** Due to ALA synthase deficiency[Q]
   - **Gyrate atrophy of retina & choroid** in ornithine delta-amino transferase mutation[Q]

Assessment of Vitamin B$_6$ status:

- **Most widely used method: Activation of erythrocyte aminotransferases by pyridoxal phosphate added in vitro,** expressed as the activation coefficient[Q].

Vitamin B$_6$ Toxicity:

- **Vitamin B$_6$** toxicity causes **severe sensory neuropathy, photosensitivity & dermatitis**[Q].

28. **Ans. c. Hydrogen bonds**   *(Ref: Harper 30/e p361)*

Nitrogenous bases are held together by hydrogen bonds. Three hydrogen bonds, formed by hydrogen bonded to electronegative N or O atoms, hold the deoxyguanosine nucleotide to the deoxycytidine nucleotide, whereas the other pair, the A–T pair, is held together by two hydrogen bonds.

"The two strands, in which opposing bases are held together by interstrand hydrogen bonds, wind around a central axis in the form of a double helix. In the test tube double stranded DNA can exist in at least six forms (A–E and Z). The B form is usually found under physiologic conditions (low salt, high degree of hydration). A single turn of B- DNA about the long axis of the molecule contains ten base pairs. The distance spanned by one turn of B-DNA is 3.4 nm (34 A°). The width (helical diameter) of the double helix in B-DNA is 2 nm (20 A°). Three hydrogen bonds, formed by hydrogen bonded to electronegative N or O atoms, hold the deoxyguanosine nucleotide to the deoxycytidine nucleotide, whereas the other pair, the A–T pair, is held together by two hydrogen bonds. Thus, the G–C bonds are more resistant to denaturation, or strand separation, termed "melting," than A–T-rich regions of DNA."- Harper 30/e p361

Diagrammatic representation of Watson & Crick model of double-helical structure of B form of DNA

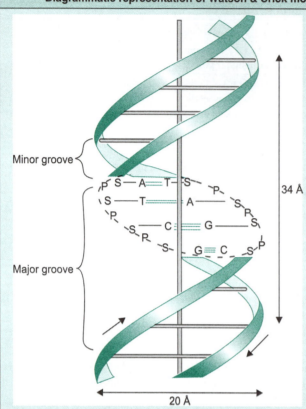

- Horizontal arrow indicates the **width of double helix (20 A°)**
- Vertical arrow indicates the **distance spanned by one complete turn of the double helix (34 A°).**
- **One turn of B-DNA includes 10 base pairs (bp), so the rise is 3.4 per bp.**
- Central axis of double helix is indicated by vertical rod.
- Short arrows designate the polarity of the antiparallel strands.
- Major & minor grooves are depicted.
- (A, adenine; C, cytosine; G, guanine; T, thymine; P, phosphate; S, sugar [deoxyribose].)
- **Hydrogen bonds between A/T and G/C bases indicated by short, horizontal lines.**

DNA Base Pairing

- **DNA base pairing between adenosine & thymidine** involves the formation of **2 hydrogen bonds**[Q].
- **DNA base pairing between cytidine & guanosine** involves the formation of **3 hydrogen bonds**[Q].
- The broken lines represent hydrogen bonds.

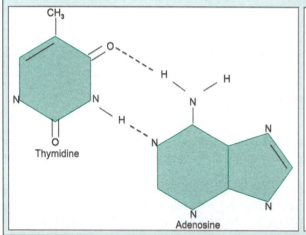
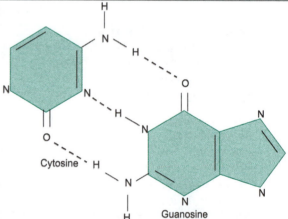

DNA Structure

- **Watson, Crick & Wilkins** proposed the DNA model in 1953 based on **X-ray diffraction** photographs of DNA taken **by Rosalind Franklin**[Q].

Contd...

Contd...

DNA Structure
Salient Features of Watson-Crick Model of DNA
• **Right handed double-stranded** DNA helix[Q]
• **Base Pairing Rule: Adenine** always pairs **with thymine** by **2 hydrogen bonds; Guanine** pairs **with cytosine** by **3 hydrogen bonds**[Q]
• **Two strands are antiparallel;** one strand in 5' to 3' direction & second in 3' to 5' direction[Q].
• **Grooves of the DNA: Major groove & Minor groove; Grooves** often acts **as sites of DNA-Protein interaction** needed for **regulation of gene expression. DNA-Protein interaction** is via **hydrophobic interaction & ionic bond**[Q].

Types of DNA:
- 6 types of DNA: A, B, C, D & E are right handed; Z is left handed[Q]

Characteristics	A-DNA	B-DNA	Z-DNA
Base pairs per turn	11[Q]	10.5[Q]	12[Q]
Morphology	Broad & short[Q]	Longer & thinner[Q]	Elongated & thin[Q]
Base pair tilts the axis of helix	20° tilt[Q]	Base pair perpendicular to helix[Q]	9° tilt[Q]
Screw sense	Right-handed[Q]	Right-handed[Q]	Left-handed[Q]

- Physiologically MC DNA: **B-DNA**[Q]
- Distance spanned by one turn of B-DNA: **3.4 nm (34 A°)**[Q]
- Width of double helix in B-DNA: **2 nm (20 A°)**[Q]
- Under **low salt & high degree of hydration, B-DNA** is usually found[Q]
- Under **high salt concentration & low degree of hydration, A-DNA** is usually found[Q].

29. Ans. c. Only 3 *(Ref: Harper 30/e p231, 148-149; Textbook of Biochemistry by DM Vasudevan 7/e p365)*

Higher than normal quantities of ketone bodies present in the blood or urine constitutes hyperketonemia or ketonuria, respectively. The overall condition is called ketosis. The basic form of ketosis occurs in starvation. Ketone bodies will be positive in starvation in the patient's urine.

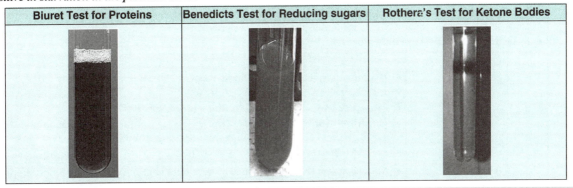

"Higher than normal quantities of ketone bodies present in the blood or urine constitutes ketonemia (hyperketonemia) or ketonuria, respectively. The overall condition is called ketosis. The basic form of ketosis occurs in starvation and involves depletion of available carbohydrate coupled with mobilization of free fatty acids." -Harper 30/e p231

Tests for Ketonuria (Ketone bodies in urine)
• **Ketone bodies** are **products of incomplete fat metabolism**[Q].
• **Three ketone bodies excreted in urine: Acetoacetic acid (20%), acetone (2%) & beta-hydroxybutyric acid (78%)**[Q].

Tests for Ketonuria	
Rothera's test	• **Ketone bodies** (acetone & Acetoacetic acid) combine with **alkaline solution of Sodium nitroprusside** forms **purple coloured ring**[Q]
Gerhardt's test	• Addition of **ferric chloride to urine** leads to formation of **brownish-red colour**[Q]
Reagent strip test	• **Stripes** coated with **alkaline sodium nitroprusside** dipped in urine & it **turns purple**

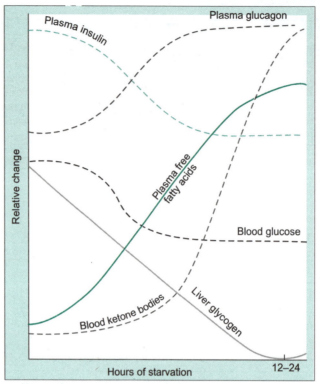

Fig. 13: Relative changes in metabolic parameters during the onset of starvation

Fasting & Starvation
• Priorities are to supply sufficient glucose to brain & RBCs and to preserve protein[Q].
• In starvation, activity of key gluconeogenic enzymes (pyruvate carboxylase, phosphoenol pyruvate carboxykinase, fructose 1, 6-bisphosphatase & glucose 6-phosphatase) is increased[Q].
• In fasting state, RBCs use only glucose[Q].

Day 1-3	• Blood glucose level is maintained by: • Hepatic glycogenolysis & glucose release[Q] • Adipose release of free fatty acids (FFA)[Q] • Muscle & liver shifting fuel use from glucose to FFA[Q] • Hepatic gluconeogenesis from peripheral tissue lactate & alanine and from adipose tissue glycerol & propionyl co-A from odd chain free fatty acid metabolism[Q] • By 12-16 hours, glycogen stores are depleted[Q].
After day 3	• Muscle protein loss is maintained by hepatic formation of ketone bodies, supplying the brain & heart[Q].
After several days	• Ketone bodies become main source of energy for brain, so less muscle protein is degraded than during days 1-3[Q].

Organ	Fed	Fasting	Starvation
Brain	Glucose	Glucose	Ketone bodies[Q]
Heart	Fatty acids[Q]	Fatty acids[Q]	Ketone bodies[Q]
Liver	Glucose	Fatty acids[Q]	Amino acids[Q]
Muscles	Glucose	Fatty acids[Q]	Fatty acids & ketone bodies
Adipose tissue	Glucose	Fatty acids[Q]	Fatty acids & ketone bodies
RBCs	Glucose	Glucose	

Contd...

Contd...

Colour Reactions of Amino Acids

Biuret Test	Ninhydrin Test
• General test **for proteins**[Q] • **Cupric ions** in alkaline medium forms violet colour with **peptide bond nitrogen**[Q] • **Dipeptides & individual amino acid do not answer biuret test** because this **test needs a minimum of two peptide bonds**[Q].	• General test **for all alpha-amino acids**[Q] • Amino acid + 2 mols of Ninhydrin →Aldehyde with 1 carbon atom less+ CO_2 + Purple Complex (**Ruhemann's Purple**[Q]) • Amino acid which do not give purple colour are: • **Proline & hydroxyproline**[Q] (Yellow colour) • **Glutamine & asparagine**[Q] (Brown colour)

Colour Reactions	Test Answered By
Aldehyde Tests: • **Acree-Rosenheim Test** (Formaldehyde & Mercuric Sulphate is used) • **Hopkins-Cole Test**[Q] (Glyoxylic acid is used)	• Tryptophan (Indole group)[Q]
Cyanide Nitroprusside Test	• **Homocysteine**[Q]
Milton's test	• Tyrosine (Phenol)[Q]
Sakaguchi's test	• Arginine (**Guanidinium** group)[Q]
Sulphur test	• Cysteine[Q] • **Methionine does not answer sulphur test** because **sulphur in methionine is in thioether linkage**, which is **difficult to break.**
Pauly's Test	• Histidine (Imidazole) & tyrosine (Phenol)[Q]
Xanthoproteic Test (Reagent: **Conc. HNO_3**)	• Aromatic amino acid: Phenylalanine, tyrosine & tryptophan[Q]

Tests for Carbohydrates

General test for all carbohydrates	• **Molisch** test[Q]
Test for reducing substances	• **Benedict's** test[Q]
Test to differentiate monosaccharides & disaccharides	• **Barfoed's** test[Q] • **Moore's** test[Q] • **Fehling's** test[Q]
Test to differentiate aldoses & ketoses	• **Seliwanoff's** test[Q] • **Rapid furfural** test[Q] • **Foulger's** test[Q]
Test to detect deoxy sugar	• **Feulgen staining**[Q]
Test for Pentoses (to differentiate pentoses from hexoses)	• **Bial's** test[Q]
Test for galactose	• **Mucic acid test**[Q]

30. **Ans. c. Non-homologous end joining repair** *(Ref: Harper 30/e p390)*

Non-homologous end joining repair is defective in severe combined immunodeficiency disease (SCID).

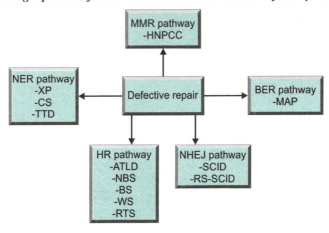

Human Diseases of DNA Damage Repair			
Defective Nonhomologous End Joining Repair (NHEJ)	**Defective Homologous Repair (HR)**	**Defective DNA Nucleotide Excision Repair (BER)**	**Defective DNA Mismatch Repair (MMR)**
• Severe combined immunodeficiency disease (SCID)[Q] • **Radiation sensitive severe combined immunodeficiency disease (RS-SCID)**[Q]	• At-like disorder (ATLD) • Nijmegen breakage syndrome (NBS) • **Bloom syndrome**[Q] **(BS)** • **Werner syndrome**[Q] **(WS)** • **Rothmund-Thomson syndrome**[Q] **(RTS)** • Breast cancer susceptibility 1 & 2 (**BRCA1, BRCA2**)[Q]	• **Xeroderma pigmentosum**[Q]**(XP)** • **Cockayne syndrome**[Q] **(CS)** • Trichothiodystrophy (TTD)	• Hereditary nonpolyposis colorectal cancer (**HNPCC**)[Q]

31. **Ans. c. Long chain fatty acid** *(Ref: Harper 30/e p231, 614)*

    Zellweger's (cerebrohepatorenal) syndrome is characterized by accumulation of very-long-chain fatty acids, abnormalities of the synthesis of bile acids, and a marked reduction of plasmalogens.

    "Zellweger's (cerebrohepatorenal) syndrome occurs in individuals with a rare inherited absence of peroxisomes in all tissues. They accumulate C_{26}–C_{38} polyenoic acids in brain tissue and also exhibit a generalized loss of peroxisomal functions. The disease causes severe neurological symptoms, and most patients die in the first year of life."-Harper 30/e p231

    "Interest in import of proteins into peroxisomes has been stimulated by studies on Zellweger syndrome. This condition is apparent at birth and is characterized by profound neurologic impairment, victims often dying within a year. The number of peroxisomes can vary from being almost normal to being virtually absent in some patients. Biochemical findings include an accumulation of very-long-chain fatty acids, abnormalities of the synthesis of bile acids, and a marked reduction of plasmalogens. The condition is believed to be due to mutations in genes encoding certain proteins—so called peroxins—involved in various steps of peroxisome biogenesis (such as the import of proteins described above), or in genes encoding certain peroxisomal enzymes themselves."- Harper 30/e p614

32. **Ans. b. Inborn errors of metabolism** *(Ref: Harper 30/e p33, 296, 297)*

    Dried blood drop of an infant can be used to know inborn errors of metabolism with the help of tandem mass spectrometry.

    *"Inborn errors of metabolism: Left untreated, these disorders can result in irreversible brain damage and early mortality. Prenatal or early postnatal detection and timely initiation of treatment thus are essential. Many of the enzymes concerned can be detected in cultured amniotic fluid cells, which facilitate prenatal diagnosis by amniocentesis. Almost all states conduct screening tests for up to as many as 30 metabolic diseases. These tests include, but are not limited to, disorders that result from defects in the catabolism of amino acids. **The best screening tests use tandem mass spectrometry to detect, in a few drops of neonate blood, catabolites suggestive of a metabolic defect.**"-Harper 30/e p297*

    "Tandem mass spectrometry can be used to screen blood samples from newborns for the presence and concentrations of amino acids, fatty acids, and other metabolites. Abnormalities in metabolite levels can serve as diagnostic indicators for a variety of genetic disorders, such as phenylketonuria, ethylmalonic encephalopathy, and glutaric acidemia type 1."-Harper 30/e p33

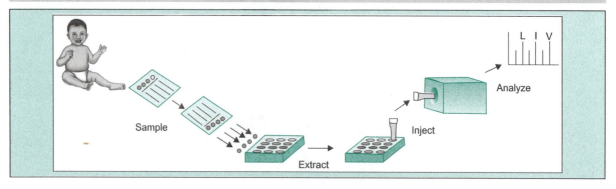

- Figure: From droplet to diagnosis by Tandem Mass Spectrometry
- A drop of blood is blotted onto a sample card, and an aliquot is extracted for analysis by mass spectrometry. The peak profile is used to diagnose metabolic errors.

- Tandem Mass Spectrometry (MS)

- **Complex peptide mixtures** can now be **analyzed, without prior purification, by tandem mass spectrometry**, which employs the equivalent of two mass spectrometers linked in series[Q].
- **First spectrometer separates individual peptides based upon their differences in mass**. By adjusting the field strength of the first magnet, a single peptide can be directed into the **second mass spectrometer**, where **fragments are generated & their masses determined**[Q].
  - **Tandem MS** can be used to **screen blood samples from newborns** for **presence & concentrations of amino acids, fatty acids, and other metabolites**[Q].
  - **Abnormalities in metabolite levels** can serve as **diagnostic indicators for** a variety of genetic disorders, such as **phenylketonuria, ethylmalonic encephalopathy, and glutaric acidemia type 1**[Q].

PATHOLOGY

33. Ans. b. CPDA-1 *(Ref: Wintrobe's 13/e p1278)*

CPDA-1 is a common anticoagulant-preservative and allows storage of RBC concentrates for 35 days.

"CPDA-1, which is CPD fortified with adenine, became available in the United States in 1978. It had been used extensively in Europe for several years before then. Initial concerns about potential toxicity of adenine proved to be unfounded. CPDA-1 is now a common anticoagulant-preservative and allows storage of RBC concentrates for 35 days."-Wintrobe's 13/e p1278

Additive Solutions Used for Storage of Blood Products		
Name	**Full Form**	**Shelf-life**
ACD	Acid Citrate Dextrose	**21** days[Q]
CPD	Citrate Phosphate Dextrose	**21** days[Q]
CPDA-1	Citrate Phosphate Dextrose with Adenine	**35** days[Q]
SAGM	**Sodium Adenine Glucose Mannitol** (also contains CPD as anticoagulant)	**42** days[Q]

Action of Ingredients of Additive Solution	
Ingredient	**Action**
Glucose	• **ATP generation by glycolysis**[Q]
Adenine	• **Synthesis of ATP, increases shelf-life of RBCs to 42 days**[Q]
Citrate	• **Prevents coagulation by chelating calcium**[Q]
Sodium diphosphate	• **Prevents fall in pH**[Q]

34. Ans. a. Extrinsic *(Ref: Robbins 9/e p119, 656; Harrison 19/e p405)*

In Prothrombin time (PT) estimation, addition of calcium and thromboplastin to platelet poor plasma activates extrinsic pathway.

"The prothrombin time (PT) assay assesses the function of the proteins in the extrinsic pathway (factors VII, X, V, II, and fibrinogen). In brief, tissue factor, phospholipids, and calcium are added to plasma and the time for a fibrin clot to form is recorded."-Robbins 9/e p119

"The partial thromboplastin time (PTT) assay screens the function of the proteins in the intrinsic pathway (factors XII, XI, IX, VIII, X, V, II, and fibrinogen). In this assay, clotting of plasma is initiated by addition of negative- charged particles (e.g., ground glass) that activate factor XII (Hageman factor) together with phospholipids and calcium, and the time to fibrin clot formation is recorded."-Robbins 9/e p119

"Prothrombin time (PT): This test assesses the extrinsic and common coagulation pathways. The clotting of plasma after addition of an exogenous source of tissue thromboplastin (e.g., brain extract) and Ca^{2+} ions is measured in seconds. A prolonged PT can result from deficiency or dysfunction of factor V, factor VII, factor X, prothrombin, or fibrinogen."- Robbins 9/e p656

"Partial thromboplastin time (PTT): This test assesses the intrinsic and common clotting pathways. The clotting of plasma after addition of kaolin, cephalin, and Ca^{2+} ions is measured in seconds. Kaolin activates the contact-dependent factor XII, and cephalin substitutes for platelet phospholipids. Prolongation of the PTT can be due to deficiency or dysfunction of factors V, VIII, IX, X, XI, or XII, prothrombin, or fibrinogen, or to interfering antibodies to phospholipid."- Robbins 9/e p656

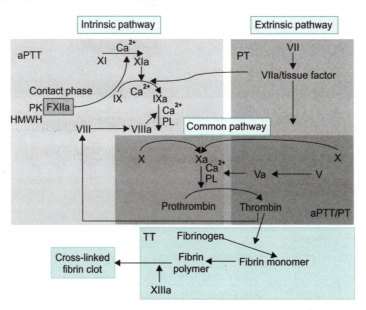

Fig. 14: Coagulation cascade and laboratory assessment of clotting factor deficiency by aPTT, PT & thrombin time (TT)

Prothrombin Time
For Prothrombin Time estimation

• **Platelet poor plasma** is used
• Sample should be kept at **room temperature**[Q] (if stored at room temperature, PT is shortened due to VII activation in cold)
• **Activation is done with thromboplastin** (derived from rabbit brain or lung)
• **Activation with kaolin is done for PTT not for PT**
• PT, APTT are **carried out on fresh samples**
    • The test done **within 2 hours**[Q]
    • **Normal value** is **11-16 seconds**[Q]

Interpretation of increased Prothrombin Time
• **Administration of oral anticoagulants (vitamin K antagonists)**[Q] • **Liver disease** particularly **obstructive type**[Q] • **Vitamin K deficiency**[Q]   • **DIC**[Q]   • Rarely, previously undiagnosed **factor VII, X, V or prothrombin deficiency or defect**[Q]

Contd...

Contd...

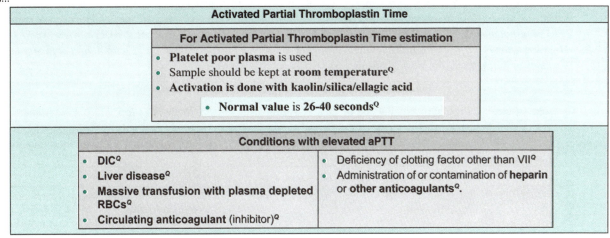

35. Ans. b. 4, 1, 3, 2 *(Ref: Practical Medical Procedures at a Glance By Rachel K. Thomas (2015)/p29)*
Correct order of blood sampling: Identification of patient; Verification of patient's profile; Sampling; Labeling at bedside.

Procedure for drawing blood (WHO)	
Step	**Procedure**
1	**Assemble equipment**, include **needle & syringe or vacuum tube**, depending on which is to be used.
2	Perform **hand hygiene** (if using soap & water, dry hands with single-use towels).
3	**Identify & prepare the patient**.
4	**Select the site**, preferably at the **antecubital area**. Warming the arm with a hot pack, or hanging the hand down may make it easier to see the veins. Palpate the area to locate the anatomic landmarks. **Do not touch the site once alcohol or other antiseptic has been applied.**
5	**Apply a tourniquet**, about 4–5 finger widths **above the selected venepuncture site**.
6	Ask the **patient to form a fist** so that the veins are more prominent.
7	Put on well-fitting, non-sterile gloves.
8	**Disinfect the site using 70% isopropyl alcohol for 30 seconds** & allow to dry completely (30 sec).
9	**Anchor the vein by holding the patient's arm & placing a thumb below the venepuncture site.**
10	**Enter the vein** swiftly at a **30 degree angle**.
11	Once sufficient blood has been collected, **release the tourniquet before withdrawing the needle.**
12	Withdraw the needle gently and then give the patient a clean gauze or dry cotton-wool ball to apply to the site with gentle pressure.
13	Discard the used needle & syringe or blood-sampling device into a puncture-resistant container.
14	Check the label & forms for accuracy.
15	Discard sharps & broken glass into the sharps container. Place items that can drip blood or body fluids into the infectious waste.
16	Remove gloves & place them in the general waste. Perform hand hygiene. If using soap & water, dry hands with single-use towels.

36. Ans. d. Lithium heparin *(Ref: Wintrobe's 13/e pB-7; Textbook of Biochemistry for Medical Students By D M Vasudevan 8/e p441)*
Lithium heparin is the anticoagulant used for electrolyte estimation.

"Lithium-heparin is the preferred anticoagulant for hematology in nonmammalians because EDTA causes in vitro hemolysis in some amphibian, reptile, and fish species; moreover, plasma harvested from blood anticoagulated with lithium-heparin can be used for routine chemistry/electrolyte analysis, which is especially advantageous with small sample volumes."-Wintrobe's 13/e pB-7

AIIMS ESSENCE

"Commonly used anticoagulants are heparin, EDTA, oxalates, citrate and fluoride. Of these, lithium heparin is best suited for most of the biochemical estimations. All other anticoagulants chelate calcium and hence unsuitable for calcium estimation. The possibility of enzyme inhibition especially creatine kinase, ALP, ACP, amylase and LDH are observed with several of these anticoagulants. Oxalates are unsuitable for estimation of sodium and potassium also."- Textbook of Biochemistry for Medical Students By D M Vasudevan 8/e p441

Recommended Order of Draw for Plastic Vacuum Tubes (WHO)				
Order of use	**Type of tube/usual colour**	**Additive**	**Mode of action**	**Uses**
1	**Blood culture bottle (yellow-black striped tubes)**	**Broth mixture[Q]**	**Preserves viability of microorganisms[Q]**	Microbiology – aerobes, anaerobes, fungi[Q]
2	Non-additive tube	–	–	–
3	**Coagulation tube (light blue top)**	**Sodium citrate[Q]**	**Forms calcium salts to remove calcium[Q]**	Coagulation tests (protime & prothrombin time), requires full draw
4	**Clot activator (red top)**	**Clot activator[Q]**	Blood clots & serum is separated by centrifugation	Chemistries, immunology & serology, blood bank (cross-match)
5	**Serum separator tube (red-grey tiger top or gold)**	None	Contains a gel at the bottom to separate blood from serum on centrifugation	Chemistries, immunology and serology
6	**Sodium heparin (dark green top)**	**Sodium heparin or lithium heparin[Q]**	Inactivates thrombin & thromboplastin	For lithium level use sodium heparin, for ammonia level use either
7	**PST (light green top)**	**Lithium heparin anticoagulant and a gel separator[Q]**	Anticoagulants with lithium, separates plasma with PST gel at bottom of tube	Chemistries
8	**EDTA (purple top)**	**EDTA[Q]**	**Forms calcium salts to remove calcium[Q]**	**Haematology, Blood Bank[Q]** (cross-match) requires full draw
9	**Blood tube (pale yellow top)**	**Acid-citrate-dextrose[Q] (ACD, ACDA or ACDB)**	**Complement inactivation[Q]**	**HLA tissue typing, paternity testing, DNA studies[Q]**
10	**Oxalate/fluoride (light grey top)**	**Sodium fluoride & potassium oxalate[Q]**	**Antiglycolytic agent preserves glucose up to five days[Q]**	**Glucoses, requires full draw[Q]** (may cause haemolysis if short draw)

37. **Ans. b. Schwannoma** *(Ref: Robbins 9/e p257, 854; Harrison 19/e p207)*

Schwannoma is the rare cause of proptosis. Schwannomas often abut orbital apertures, and patients present with nonspecific symptoms such as progressive painless proptosis.

"Tumors of the orbit cause painless, progressive proptosis. The most common primary tumors are cavernous hemangioma, lymph- angioma, neurofibroma, schwannoma, dermoid cyst, adenoid cystic carcinoma, optic nerve glioma, optic nerve meningioma, and benign mixed tumor of the lacrimal gland. Metastatic tumor to the orbit occurs frequently in breast carcinoma, lung carcinoma, and lymphoma."-Harrison 19/e p207

"Schwannomas often abut orbital apertures, and patients present with nonspecific symptoms such as progressive painless proptosis." - Nerves and Nerve Injuries by R. Shane Tubbs (2015)/p287

> *"Schwannoma: In the Antoni A^Q pattern of growth, elongated cells with cytoplasmic processes are arranged in fascicles in areas of moderate to high cellularity and scant stromal matrix; the "nuclear-free zones" of processes that lie between the regions of nuclear palisading are termed Verocay bodies^Q. In the Antoni B^Q pattern of growth, the tumor is less densely cellular and consists of a loose meshwork of cells, microcysts and myxoid stroma."- Robbins 9/e p854*

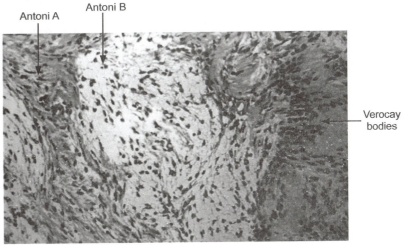

Fig. 15: Tumor showing cellular areas (Antoni A), including Verocay bodies (far right), as well as looser, myxoid regions (Antoni B, center).

Schwannoma
Benign tumor <ul><li>Arise from the **neural crest–derived Schwann cell**[Q]</li><li>Cause **symptoms by local compression** of involved nerve or adjacent structures (brainstem or spinal cord).</li><li>Schwannomas are a **component of NF2**[Q]</li><li>**Loss of expression of the *NF2* gene product, merlin**[Q], is a **consistent finding in all schwannomas.**</li></ul>
Morphology. <ul><li>**Well-circumscribed, encapsulated masses** that are attached to the nerve but can be separated from it</li><li>On microscopic examination tumors show a **mixture of two growth patterns**<ul><li>In the **Antoni A**[Q] pattern of growth, **elongated cells with cytoplasmic processes** are **arranged in fascicles in areas of moderate to high cellularity & scant stromal matrix**; the **"nuclear-free zones"** of processes that lie between the regions of nuclear palisading are termed **Verocay bodies**[Q].</li><li>In the **Antoni B**[Q] pattern of growth, **tumor is less densely cellular & consists of a loose meshwork of cells, microcysts & myxoid stroma.**</li></ul></li><li>**Schwann cell origin** of these tumors is borne out by their **S-100 immunoreactivity**[Q].</li><li>**Malignant change is extremely rare**[Q], but **local recurrence can follow incomplete resection.**</li></ul>
Clinical Features: <ul><li>Within the cranial vault **most schwannomas occur at cerebellopontine angle**, where they are **attached to the vestibular branch of eighth nerve**[Q].</li><li>Affected individuals often present with **tinnitus & hearing loss**; tumor is often referred to as an **"acoustic neuroma,"** although it actually is a **vestibular Schwannoma**.<ul><li>Elsewhere within dura, sensory nerves are preferentially involved, including **branches of the trigeminal nerve & dorsal roots**[Q].</li><li>When extradural, schwannomas are most commonly found in association with **large nerve trunks**[Q], where motor & sensory modalities are intermixed.</li></ul></li></ul>

38. Ans. d. 1, 2 and 3 (*Ref: Harrison 19/e p81e-1, 638; Henry's Clinical Diagnosis and Management by Laboratory Methods 23/e p588; Robbins 9/e p640*)

Presence of 3% of HbA2 and 97% of HbF in a child is highly suggestive of thalassemia major. In thalassemia major, nucleated RBCs with target cells, Howell-Jolly bodies and teardrop cells (Dacrocytes) are seen.

"*β-thalassemia major: Unlike most hemolytic diseases, the anemia is hypochromic and microcytic. Extreme Poikilocytosis with bizarre shapes, target cells, ovalocytosis, Cabot rings, Howell-Jolly bodies, nuclear fragments, siderocytes, aniosochromia, anisocytosis, and often extreme normoblastosis are present.*"-*Henry's Clinical Diagnosis and Management by Laboratory Methods 23/e p588*

"*The diagnosis of β-thalassemia major is readily made during child-hood on the basis of severe anemia accompanied by the characteristic signs of massive ineffective erythropoiesis: hepatosplenomegaly, profound microcytosis, a characteristic blood smear, and elevated levels of HbF, HbA_2, or both.*"-*Harrison 19/e p638*

"*Dacrocytes are teardrop-shaped cells that can be seen in hemolytic anemias, severe iron deficiency, thalassemias, myelofibrosis, and myelodysplastic syndromes.*"-*Harrison 19/e p81e-1*

"*Elliptocytes are elliptical-shaped red cells that can reflect an inherited defect in the red cell membrane, but they also are seen in iron deficiency, myelodysplastic syndromes, megaloblastic anemia, and thalassemias.*"-*Harrison 19/e p81e-1*

"*Target cells have an area of central pallor that contains a dense center, or bull's-eye. These cells are seen classically in thalassemia, but they are also present in iron deficiency, cholestatic liver disease, and some hemoglobinopathies.*"-*Harrison 19/e p81e-1*

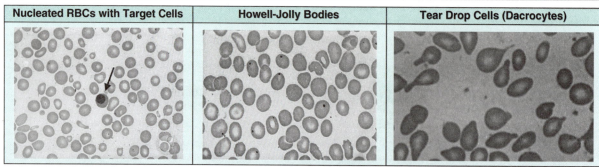

Pathologic Red Cells in Blood Smears in β-thalassemia major	
• Anisocytosis[Q]	• Cabot rings[Q]
• Poikilocytosis[Q]	• Howell-Jolly bodies[Q]
• Target cells (codocytes[Q])	• Nuclear fragments[Q]
• Tear drop cells (Dacrocytes[Q])	• Siderocytes[Q]
• Nucleated RBCs[Q]	• Aniosochromia[Q]
• Basophilic stippling[Q]	• Extreme normoblastosis[Q]
• Ovalocytosis[Q]	

Pathologic Red Cells in Blood Smears			
Red Cell Type	**Description**	**Underlying Change**	**Disease State Associations**
Acanthocyte (spur cell)	**Irregularly spiculated red cells with projections of varying length & dense center[Q]**	Altered cell membrane lipids	**Abetalipoproteinemia, parenchymal liver disease, post-splenectomy[Q]**
Basophilic stippling	**Punctuate basophilic inclusions[Q]**	**Precipitated ribosomes (RNA)[Q]**	**Coarse stippling**: Lead intoxication, thalassemia[Q] **Fine stippling**: A variety of anemias
Bite cell (degmacyte)	Smooth semicircle taken from one edge	**Heinz body pitting by spleen[Q]**	**G-6-PD deficiency, drug-induced oxidant hemolysis[Q]**
Burr cell (echinocyte) or crenated red cell	**Red cells with short evenly spaced spicules & preserved central pallor[Q]**	May be associated with altered membrane lipids	Usually artifactual; seen in **uremia, bleeding ulcers, gastric carcinoma[Q]**
Cabot rings	**Circular, blue, threadlike inclusion with dots**	**Nuclear remnant[Q]**	**Postsplenectomy, hemolytic anemia, megaloblastic anemia[Q]**
Ovalocyte (elliptocyte)	Elliptically shaped cell	Abnormal cytoskeletal proteins	**Hereditary elliptocytosis[Q]**
Howell-Jolly bodies	**Small, discrete, basophilic, dense inclusions; usually single**	Nuclear remnant (DNA)	**Postsplenectomy, hemolytic anemia, megaloblastic anemia[Q]**
Hypochromic red cell	Prominent central pallor	Diminished hemoglobin synthesis	**Iron deficiency anemia, thalassemia, sideroblastic anemia[Q]**
Leptocyte	**Flat, wafer like, thin, hypochromic cell**	—	**Obstructive liver disease, thalassemia[Q]**
Macrocyte	Red cells larger than normal (>8.5 μm), well filled with hemoglobin	Young red cells, abnormal red cell maturation	Increased erythropoiesis; oval macrocytes in megaloblastic anemia; round macrocytes in liver disease
Microcyte	Red cells smaller than normal (<7.0 μm)	—	Hypochromic red cell
Pappenheimer bodies	Small, dense, basophilic granules	**Iron-containing siderosome or mitochondrial remnant[Q]**	**Sideroblastic anemia, post-splenectomy[Q]**
Poly-chromatophilia	Grayish or blue hue often seen in macrocytes	**Ribosomal material[Q]**	**Reticulocytosis**, premature marrow release of red cells[Q]
Rouleaux	Red cell aggregates resembling stack of coins	Red cell clumping by circulating paraprotein	**Paraproteinemia[Q]**
Schistocyte (helmet cell)	Distorted, fragmented cell; two or three pointed ends	Mechanical distortion in microvasculature by fibrin strands, disruption by prosthetic heart valve	**Microangiopathic hemolytic anemia (DIC, TTP, prosthetic heart valves, severe burns)[Q]**
Sickle cell (drepanocyte)	**Bipolar, spiculated forms, sickle shaped, pointed at both ends[Q]**	Molecular aggregation of HbS	**Sickle cell disorders**, not including S trait[Q]

Contd...

Contd...

Red Cell Type	Description	Underlying Change	Disease State Associations
Spherocyte	Spherical cell with dense appearance & absent central pallor, usually decreased diameter[Q]	Decreased membrane surface area	Hereditary spherocytosis, immunohemolytic anemia[Q]
Stomatocyte	Mouth or cuplike deformity[Q]	Membrane defect with abnormal cation permeability	Hereditary stomatocytosis, immunohemolytic anemia[Q]
Target cell (codocyte)	Target like appearance, often hypochromic[Q]	Increased redundancy of cell membrane	Liver disease, post-splenectomy, thalassemia, hemoglobin C disease[Q]
Teardrop cell (dacryocyte)	Distorted, drop-shaped cell[Q]	—	Myelofibrosis, myelophthisic anemia[Q]

Clinical spectrum of Thalassemia (β thalassemia)			
Syndrome	Thalassemia major	Thalassemia intermedia	Thalassemia minor
General characteristic	Presentation in **early infancy** with: • **Progressive pallor**[Q] • **Hepatosplenomegaly**[Q] • **Bony changes**[Q] • **Invariably fatal during first few years of life** if left untreated[Q] • Require **repeated blood transfusions**[Q]	Patient present somewhere between the two extremes with variable clinical manifestations of: • **Progressive pallor**[Q] • **Hepatosplenomegaly**[Q] • **Bony changes**[Q] • These patients maintain **hemoglobin levels** between **6-10 g/dl** and lead their life fairly comfortably. • **May need occasional transfusions**[Q] but are not dependent on blood transfusions for their survival.	• **Presents late** and patient can lead a practically **normal life** except for **mild persistent anemia**[Q] • **Not dependent on blood transfusions**[Q]
Clinical Features			
Severity of disease	++++[Q]	++	±
Growth and development	Impaired[Q]	-	-
Splenomegaly	++++[Q]	++	-
Jaundice	++[Q]	+/-	-
Skeletal changes	+++[Q]	+	-
Thalassemia facies	+++[Q]	+	-
Hematological findings			
Hb gm/dl (Anemia)	< 7 (severe)[Q]	7-10 (moderate)	>10
Microcytosis	+++[Q]	++	+
Hypochromia	+++[Q]	++	+
Basophilic stippling	++[Q]	+	+
Anisopoikilocytosis	+++[Q]	++	±
Target cells	+++[Q]	++	+
Nucleated red cells	+++[Q]	+/- occasional	-
Reticulocytes	2-15[Q]	2-10	< 5
HbF	30-90%[Q]	20-100%	0-5%
HbA2	<3.5%[Q]	<3.5%	3.5-8%
Bone marrow iron	++++[Q]	++	±
Iron overload	+	-	-
Life expectancy	20-28 years	Normal	Normal

39. Ans. a. Transthyretin *(Ref: Harper 30/e p672; Robbins 9/e p572, 848, 64; Ganong 25/e p341)*

Transthyretin is a normal serum protein synthesized in the liver that transports thyroxine and retinol-binding protein. Transthyretin is not involved in iron metabolism.

"Transthyretin is a normal serum protein synthesized in the liver that transports thyroxine and retinol-binding protein."- Robbins 9/e p572

Proteins Involved in Iron Metabolism		
• Ceruloplasmin[Q] (ferrioxidase activity) • DMT1[Q] • Ferrireductase[Q] (cytochrome *b* reductase I) • Ferritin[Q]	• Ferroportin[Q] • Heme transporter • Hemojuvelin • Hepcidin[Q] • Hephaestin[Q]	• HFE[Q] • Iron-responsive element-binding protein[Q] • Transferrin[Q] • Transferrin receptors 1 & 2

"Ceruloplasmin, a copper-containing plasma protein synthesized by liver, is a ferrioxidase required for the oxidation of Fe^{2+} to Fe^{3+}. Fe^{3+} is then bound to transferrin in blood. The iron released from macrophages in this way (about 25 mg/d) is recycled and forms the major source of iron for the body. In comparison, intestinal iron absorption contributes only 1 to 2 mg of the body's daily iron needs."-Harper 30/e p672

"The main regulator of iron absorption is the protein hepcidin, encoded by the HAMP gene and secreted by the liver. Hepcidin is named for its originally elucidated properties as a hepatocellular protein with bactericidal activities. Transcription of hepcidin is increased by inflammatory cytokines and iron, and decreased by iron deficiency, hypoxia, and ineffective erythropoiesis. Hepcidin binds to the cellular iron efflux channel ferroportin, causing its internalization and proteolysis, thereby inhibiting the release of iron from intestinal cells and macrophages. Therefore, hepcidin lowers plasma iron levels. Conversely, a deficiency in hepcidin causes iron overload."- Robbins 9/e p848

"Ferritin is a constituent of most cell types. When there is a local or systemic excess of iron, ferritin forms hemosiderin granules, which are easily seen with the light microscope. Hemosiderin pigment represents aggregates of ferritin micelles. Under normal conditions small amounts of hemosiderin can be seen in the mononuclear phagocytes of the bone marrow, spleen, and liver, which are actively engaged in red cell breakdown."- Robbins 9/e p64

Duodenal epithelial cell uptake of heme and nonheme iron is depicted. *When the storage sites of the body are replete with iron and erythropoietic activity is normal, plasma hepcidin levels are high. This leads to down-regulation of ferroportin and trapping of most of the absorbed iron, which is lost when duodenal epithelial cells are shed into the gut. Conversely, when body iron stores decrease or when erythropoiesis is stimulated, hepcidin levels fall and ferroportin activity increases, allowing a greater fraction of the absorbed iron to be transferred to plasma transferrin. DMT1,* Divalent metal transporter 1.

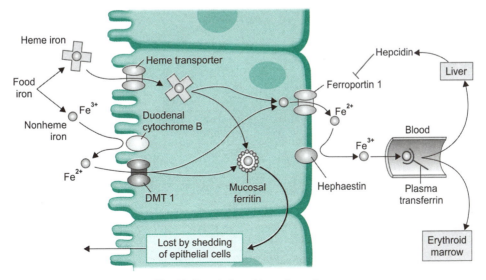

Fig. 16: Regulation of iron absorption

40. **Ans. b. TIBC** *(Ref: Robbins 9/e p652)*
Total iron binding capacity (TIBC) is decreased in iron deficiency anemia and increased in anemia of chronic disease.

> "The diagnosis of iron deficiency anemia ultimately rests on laboratory studies. Both the hemoglobin and hematocrit are depressed, usually to a moderate degree, in association with hypochromia, microcytosis, and modest poikilocytosis. The serum iron and ferritin are low, and the total plasma iron-binding capacity (reflecting elevated transferrin levels) is high. Low serum iron with increased iron-binding capacity results in a reduction of transferrin saturation to below 15%. Reduced iron stores inhibit hepcidin synthesis, and its serum levels fall. In uncomplicated iron deficiency, oral iron supplementation produces an increase in reticulocytes in about 5 to 7 days that is followed by a steady increase in blood counts and the normalization of red cell indices."-Robbins 9/e p652

> "Iron Deficiency Anemia: When iron stores become depleted, the serum iron begins to fall. Gradually, the TIBC increases, as do red cell protoporphyrin levels."-Harrison 19/e p626

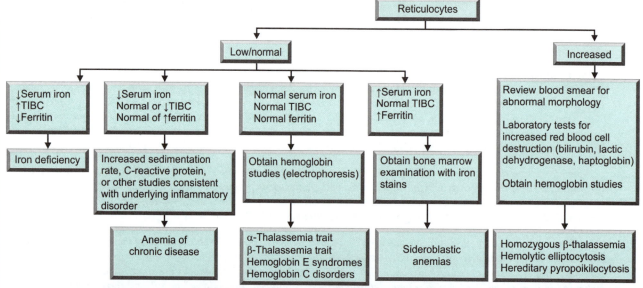

Test (normal values)	Iron deficiency	Thalassemia	Sideroblastic anemia	Anemia of chronic disease
Smear	Microcytic hypochromic[Q]	Microcytic hypochromic[Q]	Microcytic hypochromic[Q]	Normocytic normochromic[Q] > Micro/ hypochromic
Serum iron (50-150 mg/dl)	Low[Q] (<30)	Normal	Normal	↓[Q] (<50)
TIBC (300-360 mg/dl)	High[Q] (>360)	Normal	Normal	↓[Q] (<300)
% Saturation (30-50%)	< 10 (↓ed)[Q]	N or ↑ed (30-80)	N or ↑ (30-80)	↓[Q] (10-20)
Ferritin (mg/l) (50-200 mg/L)	< 15 (↓ed)[Q]	↑ (50-300)[Q]	↑ (50-300)[Q]	Normal or ↑[Q] (30-200)
Hemoglobin pattern	Normal	Abnormal[Q]	Normal	Normal
Free Erythrocyte Protporphrin	↑ed[Q]	Normal	↑ed[Q]	↑ed[Q]
RDW	↑ed[Q]	Normal	Normal	Normal

Low serum iron with **increased TIBC**	Iron deficiency anemia[Q]
Low serum iron with **decreased TIBC**	Anemia of chronic disease[Q]

41. Ans. c. 2+ *(Ref: Sabiston 20/e p840, 857; Diagnostic Histopathology of Tumors By Christopher D. M. Fletcher 4/e p1117)*

Even though FISH is a more complex and expensive procedure, it should be considered the method of choice for assessment of Her-2/neu gene status especially for equivocal cases (2+) by IHC that are not accompanied by true gene amplification in the majority of breast carcinoma cases.

"HER-2 protein overexpression is measured clinically by immunohistochemistry and scored on a scale from 0 to 3+. Alternatively, fluorescent in situ hybridization, which directly detects the number of HER-2 gene copies, can be used to detect gene amplification."-Sabiston 20/e p840

"Trastuzumab is a humanized monoclonal antibody developed to target the extracellular domain of the HER-2 receptor. HER-2 gene amplification or protein overexpression occurs in approximately 20% to 25% of breast cancers. Amplification leads to protein overexpression, measured clinically by immunohistochemistry and scored on a scale from 0 to 3+. Alternatively, fluorescent in situ hybridization directly detects the quantity of HER-2 gene copies; the normal copy number is two."-Sabiston 20/e p857

"Scoring of HER-2 Immunohistochemistry Assays: Only membrane staining of the invasive tumor should be considered when scoring IHC tests. If a commercial kit assay system is used, it is recommended that laboratories adhere strictly to the kit assay protocol and scoring methodology. Local modifications of techniques can lead to false-positive and false-negative assay results. The scoring method recommended is a semi quantitative system based on the intensity of reaction product and percentage of membrane positive cells, giving a score of 0 to 3+. Samples scoring 3+ are regarded as positive and those scoring 0/1+ as negative. Borderline scores of 2+ require confirmation with use of another analysis system, ideally FISH."-Diagnostic Histopathology of Tumors By Christopher D. M. Fletcher 4/e p1117

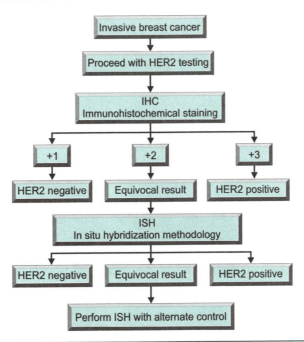

Scoring of HER-2 Immunohistochemistry Assays		
Score	**HER-2 Status**	**Staining Pattern**
0	Negative	• **No staining** or membrane staining in **<10%** of tumor cells[Q]
1+	Negative	• A **faint barely perceptible membrane staining** is detected **in >10%** of tumor cells. The cells are only stained in part of the membrane[Q].
2+	Equivocal	• **Weak to moderate complete membrane staining** is seen in **>10%** of tumor cells or **<30% with strong staining**[Q]
3+	Positive	• **Strong complete membrane staining** is seen in **>30%** of tumor cells[Q]

42. **Ans. b. Vegetative matter aspiration pneumonia** *(Ref: Robbins 9/e p708)*
The given histopathological slide shows granuloma with multinucleated giant cell reaction to acellular debris suggestive of aspirated foreign material, seen in vegetative matter aspiration pneumonia. Points which favor the diagnosis of aspiration of pneumonia are depressed patient, history of sudden onset of dyspnea and Chest X-ray showing bilateral diffuse infiltrates with predominant involvement of right middle and lower lobes.

Aspiration Pneumonia (Vegetative matter)	Necrotizing Tubercular Granuloma
• **Aspirated foreign material.** There is a **multinucleated giant cell reaction to acellular debris**	• Characteristic **tubercle** with central **caseation surrounded** by **epithelioid & multinucleated giant cells.**

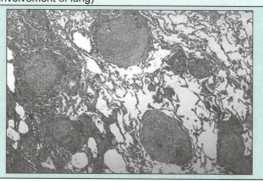

Sarcoid Granuloma	Severe fungal pneumonia
• **Noncaseating granuloma associated with sarcoidosis** involving the lung. **Circular scars** represent a form of **inflammation & scarring** (characteristic of sarcoidosis involvement of lung)	• Severe fungal pneumonia showing **septate hyphae with acute-angle branching**, consistent with **Aspergillus.**

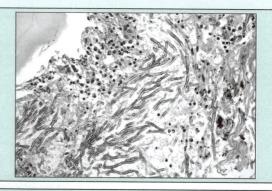

Aspiration Pneumonia

- Aspiration pneumonia occurs in **markedly debilitated patients** or those who **aspirate gastric contents** either while **unconscious** (e.g., after a stroke) or **during repeated vomiting**[Q].
- These patients have **abnormal gag & swallowing reflexes** that predispose to aspiration.
- **Resultant pneumonia is partly chemical**[Q] due to **irritating effects of gastric acid & partly bacterial**[Q] (from the **oral flora**).
- Typically, **more than one organism is recovered on culture**, **aerobes**[Q] being **more common** than anaerobes.
- This type of pneumonia is **often necrotizing**, pursues a **fulminant clinical course**[Q], and is a **frequent cause of death**. In those who survive, **lung abscess** is a **common complication**[Q].

Microaspiration

- **Microaspiration**, in contrast, **occurs frequently in almost all people**, especially those with **gastroesophageal reflux disease**[Q].
- It usually results in **small, poorly formed non-necrotizing granulomas with multinucleated foreign body giant cell reaction**[Q].
- It is **usually inconsequential**, but **may exacerbate** other preexisting lung diseases such as **asthma, interstitial fibrosis & lung rejection**[Q].

AIIMS November 2017

43. **Ans. c. Naive B cells in inter-follicular zones**   *(Ref: Robbins 9/e p593; Wintrobes 13/e p4304, 4308)*
    Cell of origin of chronic lymphocytic leukemia (CLL)/small lymphocytic lymphoma (SLL) is naive B-cells in inter-follicular zones.

    "DNA sequencing has revealed that the Ig genes of some CLL/SLL are somatically hypermutated, whereas others are not, suggesting that the cell of origin may be either a postgerminal center memory B cell or a naive B cell."- Ref: Robbins 9/e p593

    "Chronic lymphocytic leukemia (CLL) is characterized by the accumulation of mature-appearing lymphocytes in the blood, marrow, lymph nodes, and spleen. Small lymphocytic lymphoma (SLL) is the same disease, but primarily there is involvement of lymph nodes and spleen. Both CLL and SLL are antedated by monoclonal B-cell lymphocytosis (MBL) in which small numbers of CLL cells can be detected in the blood of asymptomatic individuals. The CLL cells are monoclonal B lymphocytes that express CD19, CD5, and CD23 with weak or no expression of surface immunoglobulin (Ig), CD20, CD79b, and FMC7."-Wintrobes 13/e p4304

    "Cell of Origin: CLL cell is antigen-experienced, suggesting that the expressions of CD5 and CD23 on these cells are secondary changes, perhaps representing cell activation or nonspecific changes secondary to the malignancy. Thus, the cell of origin of the CLL cell may be the memory B-cell, regardless of whether there are mutations of the IgVH gene. This would explain why all CLL cells are CD27+, which is typically a marker of the memory B-cell. Although most normal CD27+ B-cells have IgVH gene mutations, a small fraction does not. Altered DNA methylation is observed in CLL and the methylation pattern in the unmutated IgVH form of CLL is similar to a CD5+ naive B-cell form, whereas the mutated form is most similar to a memory B-cell."-Wintrobes 13/e p4308

	Chronic Lymphocytic Leukemia
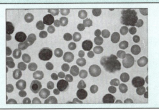	• **Peripheral blood smear** is flooded with **small lymphocytes with condensed chromatin** & scant cytoplasm. • A characteristic finding: **Presence of disrupted tumor cells (smudge cells).** • **Smudge cells or basket cells**[Q] are disintegrated lymphocytes & represent the spread out nuclear material observed in the peripheral blood film. They are **due to rupture of the neoplastic lymphoid cells** while making the peripheral smear due to its fragile nature.

Chronic Lymphocytic Leukemia (CLL)

- CLL is tumor composed of **monomorphic small B lymphocytes** in the **peripheral blood, bone marrow & lymphoid organs**[Q] (spleen & lymph nodes).
- Age: **50-60 years**; More common in **males**
- MC leukemia of adults in western world: **CLL**[Q]
    - **Cell of Origin:** Postgerminal center **memory B cell** or **a naive B cell**[Q]

	Pripheral Blood Picture
Peripheral smear	• RBCs: Show **normocytic normochromic anemia**[Q] or rarely hemolytic blood picture. • WBCs: Total leukocyte count is increased and varies from **20-50 x 10⁹/L**.
	Differential Leukocyte Count • **Lymphocytosis** is the **characteristic feature**[Q] • **Absolute lymphocyte count** should be **>5 x 10⁹/L**. • Usually **absolute lymphocyte count >10 x 10⁹/L** is common at **the time of diagnosis**[Q]. • **Lymphocytes** constitute **>50% of the white cells** and may reach up to 90-98% with **resultant neutropenia**[Q] (lymphocytes 70-98% & polymorphs 2-30%). • **Smudge cells** or **basket cells**[Q]
Platelet count	• Initially the platelet count is normal. • **Decreased platelet count** due to **bone marrow infiltration & autoimmune destruction of platelets associated with hypersplenism** • **Platelet count <100 x 10⁹/L** is associated with **worse prognosis**[Q].
Hemoglobin	• Hb <13 gm/dL (as the disease progresses, it may decrease <10 gm/dL) • Due to **marrow failure & associated autoimmune hemolysis**[Q]

Contd...

Contd...

Chronic Lymphocytic Leukemia (CLL)

Bone marrow:
- **Cellularity: hypercellular marrow[Q]**
- **Erythropoiesis: Erythropoiesis is normal[Q].** Patients are **prone to develop autoimmune diseases**, most commonly directed against red cells or platelets. Such cases which result in hemotytic anemia show normoblasticerythroid hyperplasia.
- **Myelopoiesis:Myelopoiesis is normal** in the **initial stages** of the disease.
- **Megakaryopoiesis:**Megakaryopoiesis is **within normal limits**.

> - **Neoplastic lymphocytes replace** the **normal cells of erythroid, myeloid** & **megakaryocytic series** in the **bone marrow[Q]**.
> - This **results in anemia, neutropenia** & **thrombocytopenia** indicates that the **disease is advancing[Q]**.

Special Tests:
- **Antiglobulin (Coombs) Test:** About **15-20%** of patients **manifest autoimmune hemolytic anemia** & have **positive direct Coombs test[Q]**.
- **Immunophenotype:** Tumor cells in **CLL** express the **pan-B cell markers CD19 & CD20[Q]**.
- **B cell CLL** is characterized by **aberrant expression of T cell antigen CD5** (found only in a small subset of normal B cells). There is also weak expression of monoclonal surface immunoglobulin with κ or λ light chains.

Cytogenetic Abnormalities

- **Chromosomal translocations** are **rarely observed** in CLL.
- **MC genetic anomalies: Deletions of l3q14.3, 11q22-23 & 17p13[Q]**
- About **20% of CLL** show **trisomy 12[Q]**

Clinical Features:
- **Asymptomatic:** About **25% of patients** are often asymptomatic and are detected either because of nonspecific symptoms or routine blood examination for some other disease
- **Non specific symptoms**: Fatigue, malaise, weight loss & anorexia
- **Symptoms from splenomegaly**
- **Generalized lymphadenopathy:** Initially the cervical lymph nodes are enlarged and in later stages there may be generalized lymphadenopathy. **Involved nodes** are **rubbery, discrete, non-tender, small** & **mobile[Q]**
- **Hypogammaglobulinemia[Q]** is common and is responsible for **increased risk of opportunistic infections**.

Prognostic Factors of CLL

- **Plasma beta-2 microglobulin level[Q]: High levels** are associated with a **poor prognosis**.
- Presence of **deletions of 11q** & **l7p[Q]: Worse prognosis**
- **Bone marrow trephine biopsy[Q]**: Pattern of marrow infiltration.
- **Nodular & interstitial pattern of infiltration** has **better prognosis** than mixed and diffuse types.
- **Lack of somatic hypermutation[Q]: Worse prognosis**

44. **Ans. a. Peripheral smear**   *(Ref: Wintrobes 13/e p3760, 3602, 3603; Hurwitz Clinical Pediatric Dermatology 5/e p239)*
Although biopsies of lesions of chloroma may suggest the diagnosis, the findings may mimic a variety of inflammatory or neoplastic diseases. Therefore immunophenotyping and examination of peripheral blood smears and bone marrow aspirates are often required in an effort to confirm the diagnosis. Platelet count and Hb concentration are not useful in making the diagnosis of chloroma. Leucocyte count might not raised in chloroma as it is caused by extramedullary blast proliferation.

> *"Chloroma: The diagnosis is suggested by presence of eosinophilic myelocytes in hematoxylin and eosin-stained biopsy sections. Imprint preparations can be helpful. The diagnosis can be made if Auer rods are detected or if myeloid origin is confirmed by cytochemical or immunohistochemical methods."- Wintrobes 13/e p3603*

> *"Cutaneous leukemic infiltrates may be known by a variety of names, including leukemia cutis, granulocytic sarcoma, and chloroma. Although biopsies of lesions of leukemia cutis may suggest the diagnosis, the findings may mimic a variety of inflammatory or neoplastic diseases. Therefore immunophenotyping and examination of peripheral blood smears and bone marrow aspirates are often required in an effort to confirm the diagnosis."- Hurwitz Clinical Pediatric Dermatology 5/e p239*

Chloroma (Myeloid sarcoma or Extramedullary AML or Granulocytic sarcoma)
• Type of **AML** presenting as a **solid tumor from the localized proliferation of malignant myeloblasts[Q]**. • Occur in 2-14% cases of AML
Pathology: • Term **chloroma** derives from a **green appearance** due to **expression of MPO[Q]**. • **Most frequently associated with AML** with **t(8;21) translocation[Q]**
Clinical Features: • Tumors are **usually localized**, frequently in **bone, periosteum, soft tissues, lymph nodes, or skin[Q]**. • **Common sites: Orbit & paranasal sinuses[Q]** • Other sites: GIT, genitourinary tract, breast, cervix, salivary glands, mediastinum, pleura, peritoneum & bile duct.
Diagnosis: • Diagnosis is suggested by **presence of eosinophilic myelocytes in hematoxylin & eosin-stained biopsy sections**. • Diagnosis can be made if **Auer rods are detected** or if **myeloid origin is confirmed by cytochemical or immunohistochemical methods[Q]**. • **Biopsy of a chloroma** with **special immunohistochemical staining for myeloid markers, FISH & cytogenetics** for AML-related alterations as well as **flow immunophenotyping** should be done[Q].
Treatment: • **Similar to AML (intensive AML-directed chemotherapy[Q])** • **Radiation therapy** may be **reserved** for **non-responsive cases to intensive AML-directed chemotherapy[Q]**.

45. **Ans. a. EPO estimation**   *(Ref: Robbins 9/e p656; Harrison 19/e p400)*

In this patient, who is staying in hilly area, with raised hemoglobin, erythropoietin estimation should be done first to find out whether the patients is having is having primary polycythemia (EPO is normal or decreased) or secondary polycythemia (EPO is increased).

"Polycythemia can be spurious (related to a decrease in plasma volume; Gaisbock's syndrome), primary, or secondary in origin. The secondary causes are all associated with increases in EPO levels: either a physiologically adapted appropriate elevation based on tissue hypoxia (lung disease, high altitude, CO poisoning, high-affinity hemoglobinopathy) or an abnormal overproduction (renal cysts, renal artery stenosis, tumors with ectopic EPO production). A rare familial form of polycythemia is associated with normal EPO levels but hyper-responsive EPO receptors due to mutations."-Harrison 19/e p400

"Polycythemia, Approach to the Patient: The first step is to document the presence of an increased red cell mass using the principle of isotope dilution by administering ^{51}Cr-labeled autologous red blood cells to the patient and sampling blood radioactivity over a 2-h period. If the red cell mass is normal (<36 mL/kg in men, <32 mL/kg in women), the patient has spurious or relative polycythemia. If the red cell mass is increased (>36 mL/kg in men, >32 mL/kg in women), serum EPO levels should be measured."-Harrison 19/e p400

Polycythemia: Approach to the Patient

• **First step: Document the presence of an increased red cell mass** using the principle of isotope dilution by administering ^{51}Cr-labeled autologous red blood cells to the patient and sampling blood radioactivity over a 2-h period.
• If the **red cell mass is normal**, the patient has **spurious or relative polycythemia[Q]**.
• If the **red cell mass is increased**, serum EPO levels should be measured[Q].
    • **If EPO levels are low or unmeasurable, the patient most likely has polycythemia vera[Q]**.
    • **A mutation in JAK2 (Val617Phe), a key member of the cytokine intracellular signaling pathway, can be found in 90–95% of patients with polycythemia vera[Q]**.
    • Short workup is to **measure EPO levels, check for JAK2 mutation & perform an abdominal ultrasound to assess spleen size[Q]**.
    • Polycythemia vera is associated with **elevated WBC count, increased absolute basophil count & thrombocytosis[Q]**.
• If serum **EPO levels** are **elevated,** one needs to **distinguish** whether the elevation is a **physiologic response to hypoxia** or related to **autonomous EPO production[Q]**.
• Patients with **low arterial O$_2$ saturation** (<92%) should be further evaluated for the presence of **heart or lung disease**, if they are **not living at high altitude[Q]**.

Contd...

Polycythemia: Approach to the Patient
• Patients with **normal O₂ saturation** who are **smokers** may have **elevated EPO levels because of CO displacement of O₂**. • If **carboxyhemoglobin (COHb) levels are high**, the diagnosis is **"smoker's polycythemia"**[Q]

- Patients with **normal O₂ saturation who do not smoke** either have an **abnormal hemoglobin that does not deliver O₂ to the tissues** or have a **source of EPO production** that is **not responding to the normal feedback inhibition**[Q].
- Further workup is dictated by the **differential diagnosis of EPO-producing neoplasms**.

  - **Hepatoma, uterine leiomyoma & renal cancer or cysts** are diagnosed with abdominopelvic CT scans[Q].
  - **Cerebellar hemangiomas may produce EPO**, but they present with **localizing neurologic signs & symptoms** rather than polycythemia-related symptoms[Q].

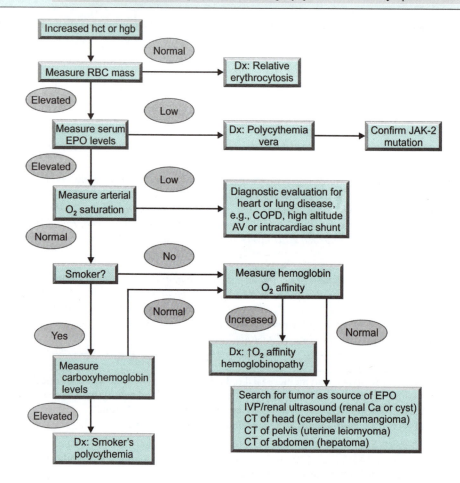

46. **Ans. d. Squamous cell carcinoma**   *(Ref: Robbins 9/e p759; Bailey 27/e p1081-1083, 26/e p1004-1013)*
    Endoscopic image shows exophytic lesion and stricture is present in the middle-third of esophagus. Most common malignancy seen in the middle-third of esophagus is squamous cell carcinoma, given in option 'd'.

    *"In contrast to adenocarcinoma, half of squamous cell carcinomas occur in the middle third of the esophagus. Squamous cell carcinoma begins as an in situ lesion termed **squamous dysplasia**. Early lesions appear as small, gray-white, plaque-like thickenings. **Over months to years they grow into tumor masses that may be polypoid, or exophytic, and protrude into and obstruct the lumen.**"-Robbins 9/e p759*

Contd...

Normal Stratified Squamous Epithelium (Squamous epithelial cells arranged in layers upon a basal membrane)	Barrett's Esophagus: (Intestinal metaplasia with goblet cells; Columnar or glandular epithelium)
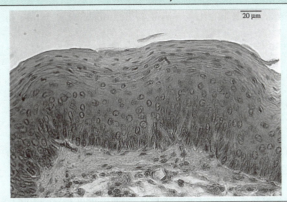	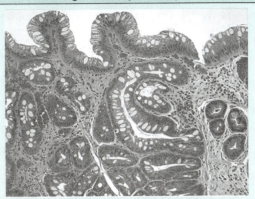
Adenocarcinoma Esophagus (Irregular infiltrative glands are seen)	Squamous Cell Carcinoma Esophagus (Keratinization & Keratin pearls are seen)
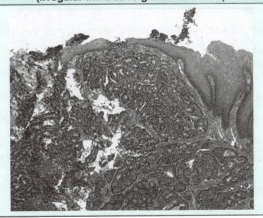	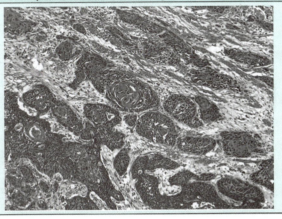

Carcinoma Esophagus

- MC esophageal cancer worldwide: **Squamous cell carcinoma**[Q]
- MC esophageal cancer in United States (Western countries): **Adenocarcinoma**[Q]
- More common in **males**[Q]
- MC site of CA esophagus: Middle 1/3rd (Overall)[Q]
- Chemotherapy regimen: **E**pirubicin + **C**isplatin[Q] + 5-**F**U (ECF)

Squamous cell carcinoma	Adenocarcinoma
• Rarely seen before the age of 30 years	• Seen infrequently before the age of 40 years
• **Highest mortality rates** seen in **men** between **60-70 years**[Q] of age.	• **Increases in incidence** with age[Q]
• Predominantly affects **African American men**[Q]	• Disease affecting **white men**[Q]
• **MC site: Middle 1/3**rd[Q]	• **Barrett's esophagus: 40-fold**[Q] increased risk for adenocarcinoma
• Obesity is protective	• MC site: Lower 1/3rd[Q]
• **H. pylori** CAG-A strain is a **risk factor**[Q]	• **Obesity** is a **risk factor**
• Usually appears as an **exophytic lesion** with a **large fungating mass**[Q]	• **H. pylori CAG-A strain** is a **protective**
• More sensitive to **chemoradiotherapy**	• Polypoid (5-10%), flat (10-15%), fungating (20-25%), or infiltrative (40-50%)[Q]
• Treated aggressively with **nonsurgical therapy**[Q]	• Not as sensitive to chemoradiotherapy
	• Treated by a more **aggressive surgical approach**[Q]

Contd...

Contd...

Carcinoma Esophagus
Pathology:
• Esophageal cancer asserts **aggressive biologic behavior**.
• With **only two layers** to the **esophageal wall**, tumors **rapidly infiltrate through** the **muscular wall into surrounding structures**[Q].
• **Rich vascular** & **lymphatic supply facilitates spread** to **regional LNs**[Q].
Clinical Features:
• **Early-stage cancers**: Asymptomatic or mimic symptoms of **GERD**.
• **MC symptom**: Dysphagia >Weight loss[Q]
• **Most patients** with esophageal cancer **present with dysphagia** & **weight loss**, symptoms that usually indicate advanced disease.
• **Choking, coughing**, and **aspiration** from a **tracheoesophageal fistula** (In advanced cases)[Q]
• **Hoarseness** & **vocal cord paralysis** from **direct invasion** into **recurrent laryngeal nerve** (In **advanced cases**)[Q]
• **MC site of metastasis: Liver**[Q] >lung >bone
Diagnosis:
• **Barium swallow: First investigation done**[Q] in suspected case of **CA esophagus** (classic finding of an **apple core lesion**[Q])
• **Endoscopy** with **biopsy: Investigation of choice** for **diagnosis of CA esophagus**[Q].
• **Endoscopic Ultrasound: Investigation of choice** for **staging of CA esophagus, best** for **T staging** & **LN metastasis**[Q].
• **CECT (abdomen & chest):** Assess the length of the tumor, thickness of the esophagus and stomach, **regional LN status** and **metastasis to liver** & **lungs**[Q].

Treatment of CA Esophagus	
High grade dysplasia (Tis) or T1a	• Endoscopic Mucosal Resection[Q]
Localized Esophageal Cancer	• **T1**: Vagal sparing or transhiatal or **minimal invasive esophagectomy** with limited LN dissection[Q]
	• **T2 & T3: Neo-adjuvant chemoradiation + Surgery**[Q]
	• **Cervical SCC** or **Non-ideal candidate** for resection: **Definitive chemoradiation**[Q]
Locally Advanced Cancer	• **Chemoradiation**[Q] (± Surgical resection in T4a)
Metastatic Disease	• **Definitive chemoradiation**[Q] (for involved distant LN or metastatic disease)
Malignant TEF	• **Coated SEMS**[Q] (self expanding metallic stents)

• **Post-operative chemoradiation** is reserved for **GE junction tumors**[Q]
• **Extent of Resection:** An in-situ **margin of 10 cm**[Q] should be the goal
Prognosis:

Long-term survival following esophagectomy depends on
• **Depth** of **tumor invasion** (T)[Q]
• **Number** of **involved lymph nodes** (N)[Q]
• **Location**[Q] of the tumor in the esophagus

• **Prognosis is better** for **tumors of cervical esophagus** & tumors **located at GE junction**[Q], in comparison to tumors located in thoracic esophagus.

47. **Ans. c. Aschoff nodule** *(Ref: Robbins 9/e p558)*

   The given image shows circumscribed nodule of mixed mononuclear inflammatory cells with associated necrosis; within the inflammation, large activated macrophages show prominent nucleoli, as well as chromatin condensed into long, wavy ribbons (caterpillar cells). The findings are suggestive of Aschoff body.

   "During acute RF, focal inflammatory lesions are found in various tissues. Distinctive lesions occur in the heart, called Aschoff bodies, consisting of foci of T lymphocytes, occasional plasma cells, and plump activated macrophages called Anitschkow cells (pathognomonic for RF). These macrophages have abundant cytoplasm and central round-to-ovoid nuclei (occasionally binucleate) in which the chromatin condenses into a central, slender, wavy ribbon (hence the designation "caterpillar cells")."-Robbins 9/e p558

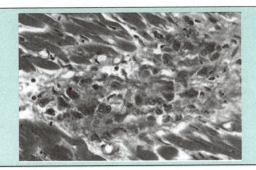

Microscopic appearance of an Aschoff body
- Myocardium exhibits a **circumscribed nodule of mixed mononuclear inflammatory cells with associated necrosis**; within the inflammation, **large activated macrophages show prominent nucleoli, as well as chromatin condensed into long, wavy ribbons (caterpillar cells)**.

Rheumatic Fever (RF) & Rheumatic Heart Disease (RHD)

- **RHD** is **characterized principally by deforming fibrotic valvular disease**, particularly **mitral stenosis**, of which **RHD** is **virtually the only cause**[Q].

Pathogenesis:
- **Acute rheumatic fever results from host immune responses to group A streptococcal antigens that cross-react**[Q] **with host proteins.**
- **Antibodies & CD4+ T cells directed against streptococcal M proteins can also in some cases recognize cardiac self-antigens**[Q].
- Antibody binding can activate complement, as well as recruit Fc-receptor bearing cells (neutrophils & macrophages); **cytokine production by the stimulated T cells leads to macrophage activation (e.g., within Aschoff bodies)**[Q].
- **Damage to heart tissue** caused by a combination of **antibody- & T cell–mediated reactions**.

Morphology:
- During **acute RF**, focal inflammatory lesions are found in various tissues.
- **Distinctive lesions** occur in the **heart,** called **Aschoff bodies**[Q], which **consist of foci of lymphocytes (primarily T cells)**, occasional plasma cells & **plump activated macrophages** called **Anitschkow cells**[Q] **(pathognomonic for RF)**.
   - These **macrophages** have **abundant cytoplasm** & **central round to ovoid nuclei** in which the **chromatin is disposed in a central, slender, wavy ribbon ("caterpillar cells")**[Q], and may become **multinucleated**[Q].
- During acute RF, **diffuse inflammation & Aschoff bodies** may be found in **any of the three layers of the heart,** causing **pericarditis, myocarditis,** or **endocarditis (pancarditis)**[Q].
- Inflammation of endocardium & left-sided valves typically results in **fibrinoid necrosis** within the cusps or along tendinous cords.
- Overlying these necrotic foci are **small (1-2 mm) vegetations**, called **verrucae, along the lines of closure**[Q].
- **Subendocardial lesions**, perhaps exacerbated by regurgitant jets, may **induce irregular thickenings** called **MacCallum plaques**, usually in the **left atrium**[Q].
   - Cardinal anatomic changes of the mitral valve in chronic RHD are **leaflet thickening, commissural fusion & shortening, and thickening & fusion of tendinous cords**[Q].
   - Fibrous bridging across the valvular commissures & calcification create "fish mouth" or "buttonhole" stenoses[Q].

48. **Ans. d. Integration of viral DNA with host DNA** *(Ref: Sabiston 20/e p696; Blumgart 5/e p148; Robbins 9/e p328)*
The DNA of the HBV integrates randomly into hepatocyte chromosomes and acts as a nonselective insertional mutagenic agent. Integration of HBV DNA into the host genome occurs in 90% of HBV-related HCC and has been postulated as an early event in chronic viral infection.

"Integration of HBV DNA into the host genome occurs in 90% of HBV-related HCC and has been postulated as an early event in chronic viral infection. Thus far, no specific genes have been identified to be the preferential target for HBV insertion. However, the insertion itself may induce general genomic instability."-Sabiston 20/e p696

"The DNA of the HBV integrates randomly into hepatocyte chromosomes and acts as a nonselective insertional mutagenic agent. Secondary chromosomal rearrangements involving duplications, translocations, and deletions reveal that the major oncogenic effect of HBV integration may be increased genomic instability of the host's cellular DNA. In greater than 90% of patients with HBV-related HCC, fragments of viral DNA have been found integrated into the host genome."-Blumgart 5/e p148

Hepatitis B virus

- **Development of HCC after HBV infection** involves a combination of **indirect & direct mechanisms**.
- **Chronic liver injury secondary to persistent viral infection** leads to necrosis, inflammation & hepatocyte regeneration.
- **Constitutive induction of liver cell progression into cell cycle** overwhelms DNA repair mechanisms in the presence of **mutational events**. This may induce **fixed DNA mutations & chromosomal rearrangements**, which are major determinants of cell transformation; **fibrosis disrupts the normal lobular structure & modifies cell-cell & cell-ECM interactions,** with further **loss of control over cell growth**[Q].
  - **Integration of HBV DNA into host genome** occurs in **90% of HBV-related HCC** & an **early event in chronic viral infection; insertion** may **induce general genomic instability**[Q].

- Dysregulation of cellular genes controlling immortalization (hTERT), proliferation (MAPK1, cyclin A), and viability (TNF receptor–associated protein 1) has been observed.
- **HBV cell surface proteins** have been shown to **increase hepatocyte proliferation** & may contribute to **carcinogenesis by accumulating in the endoplasmic reticulum**, inducing endoplasmic reticulum stress.
  - **HBV X protein (HBx)** may also act as a **potential viral oncoprotein**. It is a **potent transcriptional activator**, acting on a number of viral & cellular promoters[Q].
  - **HBx binds p53 and inhibits several critical p53-mediated processes**, including **DNA sequence-specific binding, transcriptional transactivation & apoptosis**[Q].

49. **Ans. a. Type III collagen is present** *(Ref: Robbins 9/e p20-23; Guyton 13/e p335, 336)*

Type IV collagens (not the type III collagen) are the main components of the basement membrane, together with laminin.

"The basement membrane is synthesized by contributions from the overlying epithelium and underlying mesenchymal cells, forming a flat lamellar "chicken wire" mesh (although labeled as a membrane, it is quite porous). The major constituents are amorphous nonfibrillar type IV collagen and laminin."-Robbins 9/e p21

"Type IV collagens have long but interrupted triple-helical domains and form sheets instead of fibrils; they are the main components of the basement membrane, together with laminin."-Robbins 9/e p23

"In the PAS reaction, the mesangial matrix and basement membranes are stained purple, and this allows a good assessment of the amount of matric and the thickness of the GBM. PAS also stains the tubular basement membranes and hyaline deposits."-Brenner and Rector's The Kidney (2015)/p 920

"The glomerular capillary membrane is similar to that of other capillaries, except that it has three (instead of the usual two) major layers: (1) the endothelium of the capillary, (2) a basement membrane, and (3) a layer of epithelial cells (podocytes) surrounding the outer surface of the capillary basement membrane. Together, these layers make up the filtration barrier, which, despite the three layers, filters several hundred times as much water and solutes as the usual capillary membrane. Even with this high rate of filtration, the glomerular capillary membrane normally prevents filtration of plasma proteins."-Guyton 13/e p335

"Note that for any given molecular radius, positively charged molecules are filtered much more readily than are negatively charged molecules. Neutral dextrans are also filtered more readily than are negatively charged dextrans of equal molecular weight. The reason for these differences in filterability is that the negative charges of the basement membrane and the podocytes provide an important means for restricting large negatively charged molecules, including the plasma proteins."-Guyton 13/e p336

Main Types of Collagens, Tissue Distribution, and Genetic Disorders		
Collagen Type	**Tissue Distribution**	**Genetic Disorders**
Fibrillar Collagens		
I	Ubiquitous in hard & soft tissues (**Bone, cornea & myofibrils**[Q])	**Osteogenesis imperfecta; Ehlers-Danlos syndrome-**arthrochalasias type I
II	Cartilage, **intervertebral disc**[Q], **vitreous**[Q]	Achondrogenesis type II, spondyloepiphysea dysplasia syndrome
III	Hollow organs, soft tissues, **granulation tissue**[Q]	**Vascular Ehlers-Danlos syndrome**[Q]

Contd...

Contd...

Collagen Type	Tissue Distribution	Genetic Disorders
V	Soft tissues, blood vessels[Q]	Classical Ehlers-Danlos syndrome[Q]
IX	Cartilage, vitreous[Q]	Stickler syndrome
Basement Membrane Collagens		
IV	Basement membranes, eye lens[Q]	Alport syndrome[Q]
Other Collagens		
VI	Ubiquitous in microfibrils	Bethlem myopathy
VII	Anchoring fibrils at dermal-epidermal junctions[Q]	Dystrophic epidermolysis bullosa[Q]
IX	Cartilage, intervertebral discs[Q]	Multiple epiphyseal dysplasias
XVII	Transmembrane collagen in epidermal cells[Q]	Benign atrophic generalized epidermolysis bullosa[Q]
XV & XVIII	Endostatin-forming collagens, endothelial cells[Q]	Knobloch syndrome[Q] (type XVIII collagen)

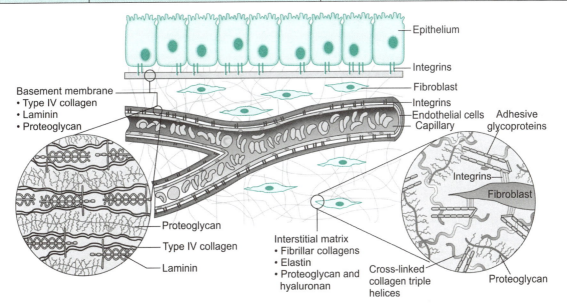

PHARMACOLOGY

50. **Ans. a. 18**

    18 divisions in the 2 ml syringe should be filled to give 180 mg ceftriaxone.

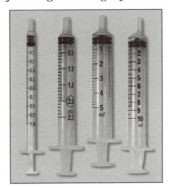

- 5 mL contains 500 mg drug
- So, 1 mL will contain 100 mg
- 1.8 mL will contain 180 mg.
- So 1.8 mL of drug solution is required to give 180 mg drug to the patient. That is to be taken in a 2 mL syringe.
- In 2 mL syringe, 1 mL contains 10 divisions. So 1.8 mL would come up to 18 divisions.

51. Ans. a. Cell wall synthesis inhibition   *(Ref: Goodman Gilman 12/e p1540; Katzung 13/e p781-782, 12/e p802)*
Vancomycin inhibits cell wall synthesis by binding firmly to the D-Ala-D-Ala terminus of nascent peptidoglycan pentapeptide

"Vancomycin and teicoplanin inhibit the synthesis of the cell wall in sensitive bacteria by binding with high affinity to the D-alanyl-D-alanine terminus of cell wall precursor units. Because of their large molecular size, they are unable to penetrate the outer membrane of gram-negative bacteria."-Goodman Gilman 12/e p1540

"Vancomycin inhibits cell wall synthesis by binding firmly to the D-Ala-D-Ala terminus of nascent peptidoglycan pentapeptide. This inhibits the transglycosylase, preventing further elongation of peptidoglycan and cross-linking. The peptidoglycan is thus weakened, and the cell becomes susceptible to lysis. The cell membrane is also damaged, which contributes to the antibacterial effect."-Katzung 13/e p781

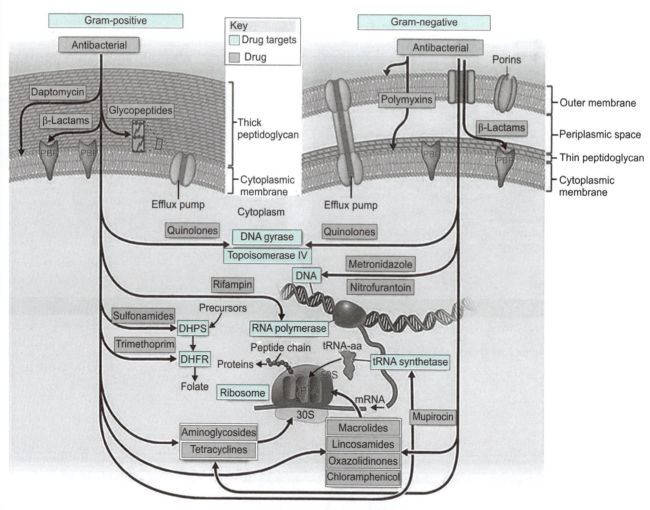

Fig. 17: Antibacterial targets (A: Aminoacyl site; DHFR: Dihydrofolate reductase; DHPS: Dihydropteroate synthetase; P: Peptidyl site; PBP: Penicillin-binding protein: tRNA-aa: Aminoacyl tRNA)

AIIMS November 2017

Classification of antibiotics according to the type of action	
Bacteriostatic	**Bactericidal**
Protein synthesis inhibitors: • **Tetracyclines**[Q] • **Tigecycline**[Q] • **Chloramphenicol**[Q] • **Macrolides**[Q] • **Lincosamide**[Q] • **Linezolid**[Q]	**Protein synthesis inhibitors:** • **Aminoglycosides**[Q] • **Streptogramins**[Q]
Drugs affecting DNA: • **Nitrofurantoin**[Q] • **Novobiocin**[Q]	**Drugs affecting DNA:** • **Quinolones**[Q] • **Metronidazole**[Q]
Drugs affecting metabolism: • **Sulfonamides**[Q] • **Dapsone**[Q] • **PAS** • **Trimethoprim**[Q] • **Ethambutol**[Q]	**Cell wall synthesis inhibitors:** • **Fosfomycin** • **Cycloserine**[Q] • **Bacitracin**[Q] • **Vancomycin**[Q] • **Penicillins**[Q] • **Cephalosporins**[Q]

Vancomycin
• **Glycopeptide antibiotic**[Q] produced by **Streptococcus orientalis & Amycolatopsis orientalis**. • With the **exception of Flavobacterium**, it is **active only against gram-positive bacteria**. • **Effective against MRSA**[Q], Strep. viridans, Enterococcus and **Cl. difficile**[Q]
Mechanism of Action: • Acts by **inhibiting bacterial cell wall synthesis**[Q] (binds terminal "D-ala-D-ala" sequence)
Uses: • **Oral**: Antibiotic associated pseudonembranous colitis [Q] • **Intravenous**: Serious MRSA infection, Enterococcal endocarditis , Empirical therapy of bacterial meningitis, Pneumococcal infections[Q]
Side-Effects: • **High systemic toxicity**[Q] • Causes plasma **conc. dependent nerve deafness**[Q] which may be permanent • **Dose related kidney damage**[Q] • **Histamine release : Skin allergy , fall in BP & Red man syndrome**[Q]   • **Rapid IV injection** has caused chills, fever, urticaria & **intense flushing** called **'Red man' or 'red neck' syndrome'**[Q]

52. Ans. d. Endrin *(Ref: Goodman Gilman 12/e p248; Katzung 13/e p118, 979-980, 12/e p122, 123, 1033)*

Atropine is drug of choice in organophosphate and carbamate poisoning. Atropine is drug of choice in poisoning of Baygon (contains carbamates & organophosphorus), Tik-20 (contains organophosphorus) and Parathion (organophosphate) but not endrin (organochlorine). No specific antidote is available for organochlorine poisoning.

Anticholinesterases			
Reversible		**Irreversible**	
Carbamates	**Acridine**	**Organophosphate**	**Carbamates**
• **Physostigmine**[Q] • **Neostigmine**[Q] • **Pyridostigmine**[Q] • **Edrophonium**[Q] • **Rivastigmine**[Q] • **Donepezil**[Q] • **Galantamine**[Q]	• Tacrine	• **Dyflos**[Q] **(DFP)** • **Echothiophate**[Q] • **Parathion**[Q] • **Malathion**[Q] • **Diazinon**[Q] **(TIK -20)** • **Tabun**[Q] • **Sarin**[Q] • **Soman**[Q]	• **Carbaryl**[Q] • **Propoxur**[Q]

AIIMS ESSENCE

Drug of Choice in Poisoning

• Organophosphate, carbamate, early mushroom poisoning	• Atropine[Q]
• Atropine, belladona & dhatura poisoning	• Physostigmine[Q]
• Acetaminophen poisoning	• Acetylcystine[Q]
• Benzodiazepine poisoning	• Flumazenil[Q]
• Opioid poisoning	• Naloxone[Q]
• Acute iron poisoning	• Desferrioxamine[Q]
• Chronic iron poisoning	• Deferiprone[Q]
• Cyanide poisoning	• Amyl nitrate[Q]
• Beta-blocker poisoning	• Glucagon[Q]
• TCA (Amitriptyline, clomipramine & imipramine) poisoning	• IV sodium bicarbonate[Q]

"To reverse the muscarinic effects, a tertiary (not quaternary) amine drug must be used (preferably atropine) to treat the CNS effects as well as the peripheral effects of the organophosphate inhibitors. Large doses of atropine may be needed to oppose the muscarinic effects of extremely potent agents like parathion and chemical warfare nerve gases: 1–2 mg of atropine sulfate may be given intravenously every 5–15 minutes until signs of effect (dry mouth, reversal of miosis) appear."- Katzung 13/e p128

"Anticholinesterases (organophosphate & carbamate) Poisoning: Atropine in sufficient dosage effectively antagonizes the actions at muscarinic receptor sites, including increased tracheobronchial and salivary secretion, bronchoconstriction, bradycardia, and to a moderate extent, peripheral ganglionic and central actions. Larger doses are required to get appreciable concentrations of atropine into the CNS. Atropine is virtually without effect against the peripheral neuromuscular compromise, which can be reversed by pralidoxime (2-PAM), a cholinesterase reactivator."- Goodman Gilman 12/e p248

Common Antidotes & Their Indications

Antidote	Poisoning Indication
Acetylcysteine	• Acetaminophen[Q]
Atropine sulfate	• Organophosphorus[Q] & carbamate[Q] pesticides
Benztropine	• Drug-induced dystonia[Q]
Sodium Bicarbonate	• Na[+] channel blocking drugs
Bromocriptine	• Neuroleptic malignant syndrome[Q]
Calcium gluconate or chloride	• Ca[2+] channel blocking drugs, Fluoride
Carnitine	• Valproate[Q], hyperammonemia[Q]
Crotalidae polyvalent immune Fab	• North American crotaline snake envenomation
Dantrolene	• Malignant hyperthermia[Q]
Deferoxamine	• Iron[Q]
Digoxin immune Fab	• Cardiac glycosides[Q]
Diphenhydramine	• Drug-induced dystonia[Q]
Dimercaprol (BAL)	• Lead[Q], mercury[Q], arsenic[Q]
EDTA, CaNa$_2$	• Lead[Q]
Ethanol	• Methanol[Q], ethylene glycol[Q]
Fomepizole	• Methanol[Q], ethylene glycol[Q]
Flumazenil	• Benzodiazepines [Q]
Glucagon	• β adrenergic antagonists[Q]
Hydroxocobalamin hydrochloride	• Cyanide[Q]
Insulin (high dose)	• Ca[2+] channel blockers[Q]
Leucovorin	• Methotrexate[Q]
Methylene blue	• Methemoglobinemia[Q]
Naloxone	• Opioids[Q]

Contd...

Contd...

Antidote	Poisoning Indication
Octreotide	• Sulfonylurea-induced hypoglycemia [Q]
Oxygen (hyperbaric)	• Carbon monoxide[Q]
Penicillamine	• Lead[Q], mercury[Q], copper[Q]
Physostigmine salicylate	• Anticholinergic syndrome[Q]
Pralidoxime chloride (2-PAM)	• Organophosphorus pesticides[Q]
Pyridoxine hydrochloride	• Isoniazid seizures[Q]
Succimer (DMSA)	• Lead[Q], mercury[Q], arsenic[Q]
Sodium Thiosulfate	• Cyanide[Q]
Vitamin K$_1$ (phytonadione)	• Coumarin[Q], indanedione[Q]

53. Ans. c. Increase in mean arterial pressure *(Ref: Katzung 13/e p97-99, 12/e p89-91; Miller 7/e p473)*

Noradrenaline is a powerful peripheral vasoconstrictor and inotrope and used in patients of septic shock and cardiogenic shock. Noradrenaline causes peripheral vasoconstriction thereby increasing diastolic blood pressure as well as venous return. The increase in diastolic blood pressure and systolic blood pressure can increase mean arterial pressure (MAP) which is the therapeutic outcome expected in any septic shock patient as a response to vasopressor.

"Autonomic reflexes are particularly important in understanding cardiovascular responses to autonomic drugs. The primary controlled variable in cardiovascular function is mean arterial pressure. Changes in any variable contributing to mean arterial pressure (eg, a drug-induced increase in peripheral vascular resistance) evoke powerful homeostatic secondary responses that tend to compensate for the directly evoked change. The homeostatic response may be sufficient to reduce the change in mean arterial pressure and to reverse the drug's effects on heart rate. A slow infusion of norepinephrine provides a useful example. This agent produces direct effects on both vascular and cardiac muscle. It is a powerful vasoconstrictor and, by increasing peripheral vascular resistance, increases mean arterial pressure."- Katzung 13/e p97

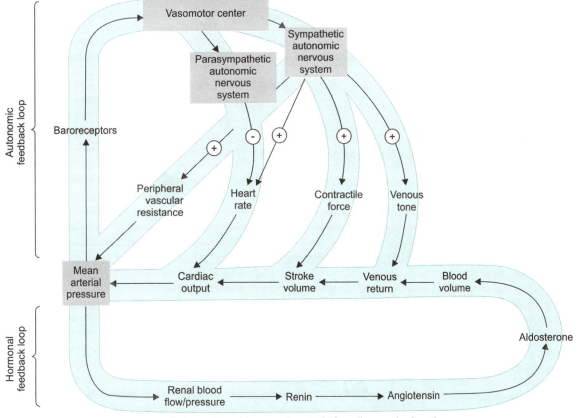

Fig. 18: Autonomic and hormonal control of cardiovascular function

"In patients with septic shock, profound hypotension, and oliguria, vasopressor therapy with norepinephrine may actually improve renal function by enhancing renal perfusion pressure. Desjars and coworkers evaluated a group of septic patients who remained oliguric despite volume resuscitation and the use of dopamine up to doses of 15 µg/kg/ min. The addition of norepinephrine and reduction of dopamine to a low-dose level resulted in an improvement in mean arterial pressure from 50 to 70 mm Hg, a tripling of urine flow, and a doubling of creatinine clearance. Norepinephrine increased the systemic vascular resistance (SVR) with little change in cardiac index or Do₂. Subsequent studies have confirmed that the **use of norepinephrine to keep mean arterial pressure greater than 60 mm Hg results in improved cardiac function (increase in stroke volume and decrease in heart rate) and GFR without deleterious effects on cardiac index, Vo₂, or oxygen extraction.** *Large doses of norepinephrine may be required to achieve these goals, because in septic shock, the peripheral vasculature is notoriously refractory to norepinephrine-induced vasoconstriction. This occurs because of massive inducible nitric oxide release as well as vasopressin deficiency. Nonetheless, these findings strongly support the concept that renal autoregulation is impaired in sepsis and that maintenance of adequate renal perfusion pressure is an important component of renal protection."-Miller 7/e p473*

---

54. **Ans. d. Metformin** *(Ref: Goodman Gilman 12/e p1259; Katzung 13/e p736-737, 12/e p757)*

Serum creatinine >1.5 mg/dL (men) >1.4 mg/dL (women), CHF, radiographic contrast studies, hospitalized patients and acidosis are contraindications for the use of metformin in diabetes mellitus.

"Metformin should not be used in patients with renal insufficiency (glomerular filtration rate [GFR] <60 mL/min), any form of acidosis, unstable congestive heart failure (CHF), liver disease, or severe hypoxemia."-Harrison 19/e p2413

"Metformin should be withheld when radiographic contrast media will be given or if unstable CHF, acidosis, or declining renal function is present."-Harrison 19/e p2413

Insulin	• Insulin is preferred in hospitalized patients, patients with sepsis and unstable patients admitted to ICU
Metoprolol	• Metoprolol are **extensively metabolized in liver**, with little unchanged drug appearing in urine. • **Metoprolol is safe in renal failure**
Linagliptin	• **Predominantly excreted via enterohepatic system (84.7%** of drug is eliminated in **feces & 5% eliminated via urine)** • Appears to be **safe in renal failure**^{Q} • **Approved for use as monotherapy** & in **combination with metformin, glimepiride & pioglitazone.**

"Many cases of lactic acidosis associated with the use of metformin have been reported in patients with concurrent conditions that can cause poor tissue perfusion such as sepsis, myocardial infarction, and congestive heart failure. Renal failure is another common comorbidity reported in patients having lactic acidosis associated with metformin use, and decreased glomerular filtration rates are thought to increase plasma metformin levels by reducing clearance of drug from the circulation. Metformin should not be used in severe pulmonary disease, decompensated heart failure, severe liver disease, or chronic alcohol abuse."-Goodman Gilman 12/e p1259

"Biguanides (metformin) are contraindicated in patients with renal disease, alcoholism, hepatic disease, or conditions predisposing to tissue anoxia (eg, chronic cardiopulmonary dysfunction) because of the increased risk of lactic acidosis induced by these drugs."-Katzung 12/e p757

Metformin
• **Biguanide class of oral hypoglycemic drugs,** available for use today

• Mechanism of Action:
 • **Metformin increases** the activity of **AMP-dependent protein kinase (AMPK)**^{Q}
 • **Activated AMPK stimulates fatty acid oxidation, glucose uptake & monoxidative metabolism**, and it **reduces lipogenesis & gluconeogenesis. Net result** is **increased glycogen storage** in skeletal muscle, **lower rates** of **hepatic glucose production, increased insulin sensitivity & lower blood glucose levels**^{Q}.
 	
      • **Metformin lowers blood glucose by reducing hepatic glucose production & increasing peripheral glucose uptake** in persons with **hyperglycemia**^{Q},
      • **Hepatic effect** is **dominant mode of action & involves suppression of gluconeogenesis**^{Q}.

Contd...

Contd...

Metformin
Pharmacokinetics:
• **Absorbed** primarily **from small intestine, does not bind to plasma proteins, excreted unchanged in urine**[Q].
• **Organic cation transporter 1 (OCT-1) carry drug into cells** (hepatocytes & myocytes) where it is pharmacologically active.
• **Organic cation transporter 2 (OCT-2) transports metformin into renal tubules** for excretion.

Therapeutic Uses:
• **Metformin** is currently the **most commonly used oral agent to treat type 2 DM**[Q]
• **Accepted as the 1st-line treatment for type 2 DM**[Q]
• **Metformin** is **not effective in the treatment of type 1 DM**[Q]
• **Metformin** has been used as a **treatment for infertility in women with polycystic ovarian syndrome**[Q].

Adverse Effects:
- **MC side-effects: Gastrointestinal**[Q] (anorexia, nausea, vomiting, abdominal discomfort & diarrhea)
- Use of metformin is associated with **lower blood levels of vitamin B_{12}**[Q]
- Associated with **lactic acidosis** [Q]

Contraindications of Metformin	
• **Serum creatinine >1.5 mg/dL in men**[Q] **& >1.4 mg/dL in women**[Q]	• **Radiographic contrast studies**[Q]
	• **Hospitalized patients**[Q]
• **CHF**[Q]	• **Lactic acidosis**[Q]

55. Ans. c. Canagliflozin   *(Ref: Harrison 19/e p2414, 2415; Katzung 13/e p256, 740, 12/e p760)*

Canagliflozin is a Sodium-Glucose Co-Transporter 2 Inhibitor, given orally and reduces body weight. For the given clinical scenario, Canagliflozin is the preferred drug, as Sitagliptin increases the risk of acute pancreatitis, use of pioglitazone is associated with a small increased risk of bladder cancer and Liraglutide is given subcutaneously.

*"**Sodium-Glucose Co-Transporter 2 Inhibitors (SLGT2):** These agents lower the blood glucose by selectively inhibiting this co-transporter, which is expressed almost exclusively in the proximal, convoluted tubule in the kidney. This inhibits glucose reabsorption, lowers the renal threshold for glucose, and leads to increased urinary glucose excretion. **Thus, the glucose-lowering effect is insulin independent and not related to changes in insulin sensitivity or secretion.** Because these agents are the newest class to treat type 2 DM, clinical experience is limited. **Due to the increased urinary glucose, urinary or vaginal infections are more common, and the diuretic effect can lead to reduced intravascular volume. As part of the FDA approval of canagliflozin in 2013, postmarketing studies for cardiovascular outcomes and for monitoring bladder and urinary cancer risk are under way.**"-Harrison 19/e p2415*

*"**The SGLT-2 inhibitors have been found to reduce systolic blood pressure, uric acid and weight and are lipid neutral. The SGLT-2 inhibitors put to clinical use include canagliflozin.**"-API Textbook of Medicine 10/e p495*

*"**Sitagliptin is contraindicated in patient with a history of a serious hypersensitivity reaction to sitagliptin, including anaphylaxis and angioedema. There have been postmarketing reports of acute pancreatitis, including fatal and nonfatal hemorrhagic or necrotizing pancreatitis, in patients taking sitagliptin. If pancreatitis is suspected, sitagliptin should be discontinued promptly.**"-Diagnosis and Management of Type 2 Diabetes By Steven V. Edelman (2011)/p113*

*"**The use of pioglitazone is associated with a small increased risk of bladder cancer it is therefore not recommended in patients with history of bladder cancer or uninvestigated hematuria and should be used with caution in the elderly, given that the risk of bladder cancer rises with age.**"-Clinical Biochemistry: Metabolic and Clinical Aspects By William J. Marshall, (2014)/P316*

*"**Liraglutide, another GLP-1 receptor agonist, is almost identical to native GLP-1 except for an amino acid substitution and addition of a fatty acyl group (coupled with a γ-glutamic acid spacer) that promote binding to albumin and plasma proteins and pro- long its half-life. GLP-1 receptor agonists increase glucose-stimulated insulin secretion, suppress glucagon, and slow gastric emptying. These agents do not promote weight gain; in fact, most patients experience modest weight loss and appetite suppression. Treatment with these agents should start at a low dose to minimize initial side effects (nausea being the limiting one). GLP-1 receptor agonists, available in twice daily, daily, and weekly injectable formulations, can be used as combination therapy with metformin, sulfonylureas, and thiazolidinediones.**"-Harrison 19/e p2414*

AIIMS ESSENCE

"Liraglutide is approved for the treatment of type 2 diabetes as an injectable therapy in patients who achieve inadequate control with diet and exercise, and are receiving concurrent treatment with metformin, sulfonylureas, or Tzds. It is not recommended as a first-line therapy or for use with insulin."-Katzung 12/e p760

Anti-hyperglycemic Drugs

Oral	Parenteral

Oral

Insulin Secretagogues (Increase Insulin Secretion)

Sulfonylureas	1st Generation: • Tolbutamide, Chlorpropamide 2nd Generation: • Glibenclamide, Glipizide • Gliclazide, Glimepiride
Meglitinides	• Repaglinide, Nateglinide^Q
Dipeptidyl Peptidase-4 inhibitors	• Sitagliptin, Vildagliptin^Q • Saxagliptin, Alogliptin^Q • Linagliptin^Q

Other Mechanisms

Overcome insulin resistance	• Biguanides: Metformin^Q • Thiazolidinediones
Alpha-glucosidase inhibitors	• Acarbose, Miglitol^Q • Vaglibose^Q
Sodium glucose Contransporter-2 (SGLT-2) inhibitors	• Dapagliflozin • Sergliflozin • Remogliflozin • Canagliflozin

Parenteral

Insulin

Ultra short acting	• Lispro, Aspart, Glulisine
Short acting	• Regular (Crystalline zinc) • Semi lente
Intermediate Acting	• NPH, Lente
Long Acting	• Glargine, Detemir
Newer generation	• Albulin, Inhaled insulin

GLP-1analogs: Exenatide^Q, Liraglutide^Q

Amylin analogues: Pramlintide^Q

Liver — Glycogenolysis — Gluconeogenesis — *Increased hepatic glucose production*

② Glucose — Metformin (−)

Adipose tissue and muscle — Storage — Oxidation

① Glucose — Rosiglitazone Pioglitazone (+)

Hyperglycemia

Decreased response to insulin (Insulin resistance)

③ Insulin — Beta cells — Insulin secretion — *Decreased response to glucose*

Tolbutamide, Glyburide, Glipizide, Glimepiride, Repaglinide, Nateglinide (+)

④ Glucose — Acarbose Miglitol (−)

Gut — Diet — *Excess or rapid ingestion of carbohydrate*

Primary drug action
+ Stimulation
− Inhibition

56. **Ans. c. Finasteride** *(Ref: Goodman Gilman 12/e p308, 1205; Katzung 13/e p720, 12/e p738)*
Finasteride inhibit conversion of testosterone to dihydrotestosterone and can reduce the prostate volume.

> *"Finasteride has been reported to be moderately effective in reducing prostate size in men with benign prostatic hyperplasia and is approved for this use in the USA."-Katzung 13/e p720*

> *"Finasteride and dutasteride, two drugs that inhibit conversion of testosterone to dihydrotestosterone and can reduce prostate volume in some patients, are approved as monotherapy and in combination with α receptor antagonists."-Goodman Gilman 12/e p308*

> *"Finasteride is an antagonist of 5α-reductase, especially the type II; dutasteride is an antagonist of both type I and type II. Both agents block the conversion of testosterone to dihydrotestosterone, especially in the male external genitalia. These drugs were developed to treat benign prostatic hyperplasia, and they are approved in the U.S. and many other countries for this purpose. When they are administered to men with moderately severe symptoms due to obstruction of urinary tract outflow, serum and prostatic concentrations of dihydrotestosterone decrease, prostatic volume decreases, and urine flow rate increases."- Goodman Gilman 12/e p1205*

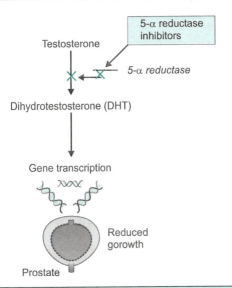

Finasteride
• Finasteride **inhibits type II isozyme of 5α-reductase**, the enzyme that converts testosterone to DHT[Q]
Mechanism of Action: • Inhibition of type II isozyme of 5α-reductase[Q] (enzyme that converts testosterone to dihydrotestosterone)
Therapeutic Uses: • **Reduces prostate size in BPH & increase urine flow rate**[Q]   • **Androgenic alopecia**: Promotes hair growth and prevents further hair loss[Q]   • **Hirsutism**[Q]
Adverse Effects: • **Decreased libido, erectile dysfunction, ejaculation disorder & decreased ejaculate volume**[Q].   • **Increased risk of hypospadias** in the male fetus if given to pregnant women[Q]

57. **Ans. c. Only ORS** *(Ref: Harrison 19/e p267)*
In the given clinical scenario, patient is having diarrhea with mild dehydration. Fluid and electrolyte replacement are of central importance to all forms of acute diarrhea. Fluid replacement alone with ORS is sufficient.

> *"Fluid and electrolyte replacement are of central importance to all forms of acute diarrhea. Fluid replacement alone may suffice for mild cases. Oral sugar-electrolyte solutions (iso-osmolar sport drinks or designed formulations) should be instituted promptly with severe diarrhea to limit dehydration, which is the major cause of death. Profoundly dehydrated patients, especially infants and the elderly, require IV rehydration."-Harrison 19/e p267*

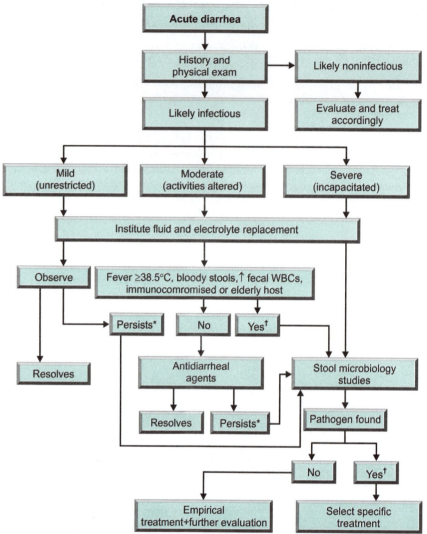

Fig. 19: Algorithm for the management of acute diarrhea
Consider empirical treatment before evaluation with (∗) metronidazole and with (†) quinolone

Management of Acute Diarrhea

- **Fluid & electrolyte replacement** are of **central importance to all forms of acute diarrhea**ᵉ.
- **Fluid replacement alone** may suffice for **mild cases**ᵉ.
- **Oral sugar-electrolyte solutions (ORS)** should be **instituted promptly with severe diarrhea to limit dehydration**, which is the major cause of deathᵉ.
- **Profoundly dehydrated patients, especially infants & elderly, require IV rehydration**ᵉ.
    - In **moderately severe non-febrile & non-bloody diarrhea, anti-motility & anti-secretory agents** such as **loperamide** can be useful adjuncts to control symptoms. Such agents should be **avoided with febrile dysentery**, which **may be exacerbated or prolonged by them**ᵉ.
- **Bismuth subsalicylate** may reduce symptoms of **vomiting & diarrhea** but **should not be used to treat immunocompromised patients** or those **with renal impairment** because of **risk of bismuth encephalopathy**ᵉ.
- **Judicious use of antibiotics** is appropriate in selected instances of acute diarrhea and may **reduce its severity & duration**ᵉ.
- Many physicians treat **moderately to severely ill patients with febrile dysentery** empirically without diagnostic evaluation using a quinolone, such as **ciprofloxacin**ᵉ.

Contd...

AIIMS November 2017

Contd...

Management of Acute Diarrhea
• **Empirical treatment** can also be considered for **suspected giardiasis with metronidazole**. • **Bismuth subsalicylate** may **reduce the frequency of traveler's diarrhea**[Q].
• **Antibiotic prophylaxis** is only indicated for certain **patients traveling to high-risk countries** in whom the likelihood or **seriousness of acquired diarrhea** would be especially **high (immunocompromised, IBD, hemochromatosis, or gastric achlorhydria)**[Q] • Use of **ciprofloxacin, azithromycin, or rifaximin** may **reduce bacterial diarrhea in such travelers by 90%**[Q].

58. Ans. a. Pentazocine *(Ref: Goodman Gilman 12/e p510; Katzung 13/e p547, 544, 548, 12/e p552, 558)*

Pentazocine can be given as analgesic and it is a κ (kappa) agonist with weak μ-antagonist or partial agonist properties. It is the oldest mixed agent available. It may be used orally or parenterally.

"Pentazocine is a κ (kappa) agonist with weak μ-antagonist or partial agonist properties. It is the oldest mixed agent available. It may be used orally or parenterally. However, because of its irritant properties, the injection of pentazocine subcutaneously is not recommended."-Katzung 13/e p547

"Buprenorphine is a potent and long-acting phenanthrene derivative that is a partial μ-receptor agonist and a κ–receptor antagonist."- Katzung 13/e p546

"Buprenorphine is an opioid agonist that displays high binding affinity but low intrinsic activity at the μ receptor. Its slow rate of dissociation from the μ receptor has also made it an attractive alternative to methadone for the management of opioid withdrawal. It functions as an antagonist at the δ and κ receptors and for this reason is referred to as a "mixed agonist-antagonist." Although buprenorphine is used as an analgesic, it can antagonize the action of more potent μ agonists such as morphine."- Katzung 13/e p546

"Tramadol is a centrally acting analgesic whose mechanism of action is predominantly based on blockade of serotonin reuptake. Tramadol has also been found to inhibit norepinephrine transporter function."-Katzung 13/e p547

"Fentanyl is a synthetic opioid related to the phenylpiperidines. The actions of fentanyl and its congeners, sufentanil, remifentanil, and alfentanil, are similar to those of other mu-opioid receptor (MOR) agonists."-Goodman Gilman 12/e p505

Opioid Receptor	Agonist	Partial Agonist	Antagonist
μ (mu)	• **Morphine**[Q] • **Methadone**[Q] • **Codeine**[Q] • **Endogenous opioids**[Q] (enkephalin, endorphin, dynorphin)	• Pentazocine[Q] • Butorphanol[Q] • **Buprenorphine**[Q]	• **Pentazocine**[Q] • **Naloxone**[Q] • **Naltrexone**[Q]
κ (kappa)	• **Morphine**[Q] • **Nalorphine**[Q] • **Pentazocine**[Q]	• –	• **Pentazocine**[Q] • **Naloxone**[Q] • **Naltrexone**[Q]
δ (delta)	• **Morphine**[Q] • **Endogenous opioids**[Q] (enkephalin, endorphin, dynorphin)	• –	• **Naloxone**[Q] • **Naltrexone**[Q]

Actions ascribed to Opioid Receptors		
μ (mu)	**κ (kappa)**	**δ (delta)**
• **Physical dependence**[Q] (morphine type) • **Miosis**[Q] • **Constipation**[Q] (μ2) • **Analgesia**[Q] (supraspinalμ1 + spinal μ2) • **Respiratory depression**[Q] (μ2) • **Euphoria**[Q] • **Sedation**[Q] • (PM CARES)	• **Dysphoria**[Q], pscychomimetic • **Miosis**[Q] (lower ceiling) • **Analgesia**[Q] (Spinal k1, supraspinal k3) • **Respiratory depression**[Q] (lower ceiling) • **Diuresis**[Q] • **Sedation**[Q] • **Physical dependence**[Q] (nalorphine type) • **Reduced GI motility**[Q] • (DMARDS)	• **Analgesia**[Q] (Spinal + affective component of supraspinal) • **Respiratory depression**[Q] • Affective behavior • **Reinforcing actions**[Q] • **Reduced GI motility**[Q]

Buprenorphine
• **Buprenorphine** is a **potent & long-acting phenanthrene derivative** that is a **partial mu-receptor agonist & a kappa–receptor antagonist**[Q].   • 25-50 times more potent than morphine
Mechanism of Action   • **Partial mu-receptor agonist & a kappa–receptor antagonist**[Q]   • Produces **analgesia** & other **CNS effects similar to morphine**[Q].
Clinical Applications: • Used as an **analgesic for moderate pain**[Q]   • Used for the **treatment of opioid addiction**[Q]   • **Reduces craving for alcohol**[Q]
Adverse-effects   • May precipitate **abstinence syndrome**[Q]   • Sedation, nausea, vomiting, dizziness, sweating & headache

59. Ans. a. Scopolamine patch a night before *(Ref: Goodman Gilman 12/e p233; Katzung 13/e p131, 12/e p121)*

Scopolamine, the muscarinic antagonist, given orally, parenterally, or transdermally, is the most effective drug for the prophylaxis and treatment of motion sickness. A transdermal preparation of scopolamine (TRANSDERM SCOP) has been shown to be highly effective when used prophylactically for the prevention of motion sickness.

"The belladonna alkaloids were among the first drugs to be used in the prevention of motion sickness. Scopolamine is the most effective prophylactic agent for short (4-6 hour) exposures to severe motion, and probably for exposures of up to several days. All agents used to combat motion sickness should be given prophylactically; they are much less effective after severe nausea or vomiting has developed. A transdermal preparation of scopolamine (TRANSDERM SCOP) has been shown to be highly effective when used prophylactically for the prevention of motion sickness. The drug, incorporated into a multilayered adhesive unit, is applied to the postauricular mastoid region, an area where transdermal absorption of the drug is especially efficient, resulting in the delivery of ~ 0.5 mg of scopolamine over 72 hours."-Goodman Gilman 12/e p233

"Motion sickness: Certain vestibular disorders respond to antimuscarinic drugs (and to antihistaminic agents with antimuscarinic effects). Scopolamine is one of the oldest remedies for seasickness and is as effective as any more recently introduced agent. It can be given by injection or by mouth or as a transdermal patch. The patch formulation produces significant blood levels over 48–72 hours. Useful doses by any route usually cause significant sedation and dry mouth."-Katzung 13/e p131

Scopolamine
• **Scopolamine (l-hyoscine)** is **muscarinic receptor antagonists**, found chiefly in **Hyoscyamus niger** (henbane).

      • **Most effective drug for prophylaxis & treatment of motion sickness**[Q]
      • **Transdermal patch used for motion sickness**[Q]

Mechanism of Action: • **Muscarinic antagonists prevent the effects of ACh by blocking its binding to muscarinic receptors on effector cells** at **parasympathetic** (and sympathetic cholinergic) **neuro-effector junctions, in peripheral ganglia, & in CNS**[Q].
Effect: • **Reduces vertigo, postoperative nausea**[Q]
Clinical Applications: • **Prevention & treatment of motion sickness**[Q]   • **Prevention postoperative nausea & vomiting**[Q]
Adverse Effects: • **Tachycardia, blurred vision, xerostomia, delirium**[Q]

60. Ans. c. Pyridoxine *(Ref: Harrison 19/e p2689; Goodman Gilman 12/e p1557, 1558, 1562, 1565; Katzung 13/e p817, 12/e p841)*

Prophylactic administration of pyridoxine can prevent the ATT induced neuropathy. If pyridoxine is not given concurrently, peripheral neuritis (most commonly paresthesias of feet and hands) is encountered in ~2% of patients receiving isoniazid 5 mg/kg of the drug daily.

"INH inhibits pyridoxal phosphokinase, resulting in pyridoxine deficiency and the neuropathy. Prophylactic administration of pyridoxine 100 mg/d can prevent the neuropathy from developing."-Harrison 19/e p2689

"Isoniazid is often given together with 25–50 mg of pyridoxine daily to prevent drug-related peripheral neuropathy."-Harrison 19/e p205e-3

"Ethionamide should be taken with food to reduce gastrointestinal effects and with pyridoxine (50–100 mg/d) to limit neuropathic side effects."-Harrison 19/e p205e-6

"If pyridoxine is not given concurrently, peripheral neuritis (most commonly paresthesias of feet and hands) is encountered in ~2% of patients receiving isoniazid 5 mg/kg of the drug daily."-Goodman Gilman 12/e p1557

"Isoniazid: The prophylactic administration of pyridoxine prevents the development not only of peripheral neuritis, as well as most other nervous system disorders in practically all instances, even when therapy lasts as long as 2 years."-Goodman Gilman 12/e p1558

61. **Ans. c. Sham surgery**   *(Ref: Pediatric Surgery and Urology: Long-Term Outcomes by Mark D. Stringer (2006)/p22)*

Sham surgery is a faked surgical intervention that omits the step thought to be therapeutically necessary. In clinical trials of surgical intervention, sham surgery is an important scientific control. This is because it isolates the specific effects of the treatment as opposed to the incidental effects caused by anesthesia, the incisional trauma, pre- and post-operative care, and the patients perception of having had a regular operation. Thus, sham surgery serves an analogous purpose to placebo drugs, neutralizing biases such as the placebo effect.

"The placebo effect, therefore, is the measurable, observable, or felt improvement in health not attributable to treatment. In place of a placebo, in surgery we could consider a sham operation. The risks here are great, however. In drug trials, the risk of placebo is that active treatment is not being pursued. In sham surgery, the added risk of the surgery itself must be considered. This is ethically thin ice – performing sham surgery for the sole purpose of blinding and controlling for the placebo effect. Hence, these trials are rare in surgery."- Pediatric Surgery and Urology: Long-Term Outcomes by Mark D. Stringer (2006)/p22

62. **Ans. a. Beta-1 and beta-2 agonist**   *(Ref: Goodman Gilman 12/e p283; Katzung 13/e p141, 12/e p137)*

Beta-1 stimulation increases heart rate and systolic blood pressure. Beta-2 stimulation cause vasodilation and thus decreases diastolic blood pressure and tremors. Hence, the drug appears to be beta-1 and beta-2 agonist.

"Alpha-1 receptors are widely expressed in vascular beds, and their activation leads to arterial and venous vasoconstriction. Their direct effect on cardiac function is of relatively less importance. A relatively pure alpha-agonist such as phenylephrine increases peripheral arterial resistance and decreases venous capacitance. The enhanced arterial resistance usually leads to a dose-dependent rise in blood pressure. In the presence of normal cardiovascular reflexes, the rise in blood pressure elicits a baroreceptor-mediated increase in vagal tone with slowing of the heart rate, which may be quite marked."-Katzung 13/e p141

"Alpha-2 adrenoceptors are present in the vasculature, and their activation leads to vasoconstriction. This effect, however, is observed only when alpha-2 agonists are given locally, by rapid intravenous injection or in very high oral doses. When given systemically, these vascular effects are obscured by the central effects of alpha-2 receptors, which lead to inhibition of sympathetic tone and blood pressure. Hence, alpha-2 agonists are used as sympatholytics in the treatment of hypertension."-Katzung 13/e p141

"The blood pressure response to a beta-adrenoceptor agonist depends on its contrasting effects on the heart and the vasculature. Stimulation of beta-receptors in the heart increases cardiac output by increasing contractility and by direct activation of the sinus node to increase heart rate. Beta agonists also decrease peripheral resistance by activating beta-2 receptors, leading to vasodilation in certain vascular beds. Isoproterenol is a nonselective beta-agonist; it activates both beta-1 and beta-2 receptors. The net effect is to maintain or slightly increase systolic pressure and to lower diastolic pressure, so that mean blood pressure is decreased."- Katzung 13/e p141

\multicolumn{3}{c}{**Distribution of Adrenoceptor Subtypes**}
Type	**Tissue**	**Actions**
α_1	**Most vascular smooth muscle[Q] (innervated)**	**Contraction[Q]**
	Pupillary dilator muscle[Q]	Contraction[Q] (dilates pupil[Q])
	Pilomotor smooth muscle[Q]	Erects hair[Q]
	Prostate[Q]	Contraction[Q]
	Heart[Q]	**Increases force of contraction[Q]**
α_2	Postsynaptic CNS neurons[Q]	Probably multiple[Q]
	Platelets[Q]	Aggregation[Q]
	Adrenergic & cholinergic nerve terminals[Q]	Inhibits transmitter release[Q]
	Some vascular smooth muscle[Q]	Contraction[Q]
	Fat cells[Q]	Inhibits lipolysis[Q]
β_1	**Heart, juxtaglomerular cells[Q]**	**Increases force & rate of contraction[Q]; increases renin release[Q]**
β_2	**Respiratory, uterine & vascular smooth muscle[Q]**	**Promotes smooth muscle relaxation[Q]**
	Skeletal muscle[Q]	Promotes potassium uptake[Q]
	Human liver[Q]	Activates glycogenolysis[Q]
β_3	Fat cells[Q]	Activates lipolysis[Q]
D_1	Smooth muscle[Q]	Dilates renal blood vessels[Q]
D_2	Nerve endings[Q]	Modulates transmitter release[Q]

Effector Organs	**Parasympathetic Nervous System**	\multicolumn{2}{c}{**Sympathetic Nervous System**}	
		Receptor Type	**Response**
Heart			
SA node	**Decreased heart rate[Q]**	β_1	**Increased heart rate[Q]**
Atria & ventricle	**Decreased atrial contractility[Q]**	β_1, β_2	**Increased contractility[Q] In-**
AV node & Purkinje	**Decreased conduction velocity[Q]**	β_1	**creased conduction velocity**
Arterioles			
Skin, splanchnic vessels	—	α_1	**Constriction[Q] Constriction/Dila-**
Skeletal muscle	—	α_1 / β_2, M	**tion[Q]**
Systemic veins	—	$\alpha_1, \alpha_2 / \beta_2$	**Constriction/Dilation[Q]**

63. Ans. c. Tell her to feed the baby just before next dose *(Ref: Understanding Pharmacology: Essentials for Medication Safety By M. Linda Workman 2/e p22; Obstetrics: Normal and Problem Pregnancies By Steven G. Gabbe, 6/e p158)*

Regarding drug usage, lactating mother should be advised to feed the baby just before next dose because least plasma concentration of the drug will just before the next loading dose.

"Feeding the baby just before the mother takes a drug results in the baby receiving the lowest possible drug concentration."- https://www.ncbi.nlm.nih.gov/pmc/articles/PMC4657301/

"For drugs requiring daily dosing during lactation, knowledge of pharmacokinetics may minimize the dose to the infant. For example, dosing immediately after nursing decreases the neonatal exposure because the blood level will be at its nadir just before the next dose."-Obstetrics: Normal and Problem Pregnancies By Steven G. Gabbe, 6/e p158

\multicolumn{2}{c}{**Recommended Methods of Reducing Infant Exposure to Drugs During Breastfeeding**}
For drugs that should not be given to infants	**For Drugs that do not have to be avoided but should have levels reduced**
• **Switch the infant to formula feeding temporarily** or to **breast milk obtained when you were not taking the drug.** • Maintain your milk supply by pumping your breasts on a regular schedule, and discard the pumped milk • When you are **no longer taking the drug** and it has been **eliminated, resume breastfeeding.**	• Nurse your baby right before taking the next dose of the drug. • Drink plenty of liquids to dilute the amount of the drug in the breast milk. • Take the drug just before the baby's longest sleep.

AIIMS November 2017

64. Ans. a. Adrenaline 0.5 ml of 1:1000 solution by intramuscular route *(Ref: Harrison 19/e p2117; Goodman Gilman 12/e p; Katzung 13/e p148, 12/e p145)*

In anaphylactic shock, the syndrome of bronchospasm, mucous membrane congestion, angioedema, and severe hypotension usually responds rapidly to the parenteral administration of epinephrine, 0.3–0.5 mg (0.3–0.5 mL of a 1:1000 epinephrine solution). Intramuscular injection may be the preferred route of administration, since skin blood flow (and hence systemic drug absorption from subcutaneous injection) is unpredictable in hypotensive patients.

"Early recognition of an anaphylactic reaction is mandatory, since death can occur within minutes to hours after the first symptoms. Mild symptoms such as pruritus and urticaria can be controlled by administration of 0.3–0.5 mL of 1:1000 (1 mg/mL) epinephrine SC or IM, with repeated doses as required at 5- to 20-min intervals for a severe reaction."- Harrison 19/e p2117

"Anaphylactic shock and related immediate (type I) IgE-mediated reactions affect both the respiratory and the cardiovascular systems. The syndrome of bronchospasm, mucous membrane congestion, angioedema, and severe hypotension usually responds rapidly to the parenteral administration of epinephrine, 0.3–0.5 mg (0.3–0.5 mL of a 1:1000 epinephrine solution). Intramuscular injection may be the preferred route of administration, since skin blood flow (and hence systemic drug absorption from subcutaneous injection) is unpredictable in hypotensive patients"- Katzung 13/e p148

Drug of Choice in Shock	
Anaphylactic shock	• Adrenaline[Q]
Cardiogenic shock	• Noradrenaline or dopamine[Q]
Distributive shock	• Noradrenaline or phenylephrine[Q]
Hypovolemic shock	• Fluids[Q] (crystalloids)
Secondary shock	• Prazosin[Q] (alpha blockers)
Shock with oliguria	• Dopamine[Q]
Shock due to adrenal insufficiency	• Corticosteroids[Q]
Septic shock	• Broad spectrum antibiotics[Q]

Treatment of Anaphylaxis (Anaphylactic Shock)

- **Early recognition of an anaphylactic reaction is mandatory,** since **death occurs within minutes to hours** after first symptoms[Q].
- **Mild symptoms** (pruritus & urticaria) can be **controlled by** administration of 0.3 to 0.5 mL of 1:1000 (1 mg/mL) **epinephrine SC or IM,** with repeated doses as required at 5- to 20-min intervals for a severe reaction[Q].
- **If antigenic material was injected into an extremity,** rate of absorption may be reduced by **prompt application of a tourniquet proximal to reaction site**, administration of 0.2 mL of 1:1000 **epinephrine into the site**[Q] & removal without compression of an insect stinger, if present.
  - An **IV infusion** should be initiated to provide a **route for administration of 2.5 mL epinephrine,** diluted 1:10,000, at 5- to 10-min intervals, **volume expanders such as normal saline & vasopressor agents** such as **dopamine if intractable hypotension occurs**[Q].
- Replacement of intravascular volume due to post-capillary venular leakage may require several liters of saline.
  - **Epinephrine provides both alpha & beta-adrenergic effects,** resulting in **vasoconstriction, bronchial smooth-muscle relaxation & attenuation of enhanced venular permeability**[Q].
- When epinephrine fails to control the anaphylactic reaction, hypoxia due to airway obstruction or related to a cardiac arrhythmia, or both, must be considered.
  - **Oxygen alone via a nasal catheter** or **with nebulized albuterol** may be helpful, but either **endotracheal intubation** or a **tracheostomy is mandatory for oxygen delivery if progressive hypoxia develops**[Q].
- Ancillary agents such as **diphenhydramine,** 50-100 mg IM or IV & **aminophylline,** 0.25-0.5 g IV, are appropriate **for urticaria-angioedema & bronchospasm, respectively**[Q].
  - **Intravenous glucocorticoids,** 0.5-1 mg/kg of medrol, are **not effective for acute event** but **may alleviate later recurrence of bronchospasm, hypotension, or urticaria**[Q].

Direct Sympathomimetics		
Drug	**Selectivity**	**Indications**
Epinephrine	$\alpha_1, \alpha_2, \beta_1, \beta_2, \beta_3$	• Anaphylactic shock^Q, open angle glaucoma^Q, bronchodilator in acute asthma^Q, hypotension, complete heart block^Q • With **local anesthetics to prolong action**^{Q}
Norepinephrine	$\alpha_1, \alpha_2 > \beta_1$	• **Hypotension**^{Q}
Isoproterenol	$\beta_1 = \beta_2$	• **Bronchodilator in asthma, complete heart block**, **shock**^{Q}
Dopamine	$D_1 = D_2 > \beta > \alpha$	• **Inotropic & chronotropic**^{Q}; used in shock
Dobutamine	$\beta_1 > \beta_2$	• **Inotropic but not chronotropic**^{Q} • **Short term treatment** of **cardiac decompensation** after surgery, or patients with **CHF** or **MI**
Phenylephrine	$\alpha_1 > \alpha_2$	• Used as **pure mydriatic**^{Q} when cycloplegia is not required (fundus examination), **nasal decongestion, vasoconstriction, antagonizes hypotension of spinal anesthesia**^{Q}
Albuterol, terbutaline	$\beta_2 > \beta_1$	• **Albuterol for acute attack of asthma**^{Q} • **Terbutaline as tocolytic**^{Q}
Ritodrine	β_2	• **To stop premature labour (Tocolytic)**^{Q}

65. Ans. c. Doxycycline   *(Ref: Harrison 19/e p782; Goodman Gilman 12/e p1525)*

Scrub typhus is caused by Orientia tsutsugamushi, transmitted by larval mites or chiggers. Drug of choice for scrub typhus is doxycycline.

> *"Scrub typhus, caused by Orientia tsutsugamushi (a separate genus in the family Rickettsiaceae), is transmitted by larval mites or chiggers and is one of the most common infections in southeastern Asia and the western Pacific. The organism is found in areas of heavy scrub vegetation (e.g., along riverbanks). Patients may have an inoculation eschar and may develop a maculopapular rash. Severe cases progress to pneumonia, meningoencephalitis, DIC, and renal failure. Mortality rates range from 1% to 35%. If recognized in a timely fashion, rickettsial disease is very responsive to treatment. Doxycycline (100 mg twice daily for 3–14 days) is the treatment of choice for both adults and children."-Harrison 19/e p782*

66. Ans. d. Azithromycin 2 gm oral single dose   *(Ref: Harrison 19/e p1008)*

Treatment of choice for a patient with gonococcal as well as non-gonococcal urethritis is Azithromycin 2 gm oral single dose.

> *"Gonococcal Infections: Because co-infection with C. trachomatis occurs frequently, initial treatment regimens must also incorporate an agent (e.g., azithromycin or doxycycline) that is effective against chlamydial infection. Pregnant women with gonorrhea, who should not take doxycycline, should receive concurrent treatment with a macrolide antibiotic for possible chlamydial infection. A single 1-g dose of azithromycin, which is effective therapy for uncomplicated chlamydial infections, results in an unacceptably low cure rate (93%) for gonococcal infections and should not be used alone. A single 2-g dose of azithromycin, particularly in the extended-release microsphere formulation, delivers azithromycin to the lower gastrointestinal tract, thereby improving tolerability." - Harrison 19/e p1008*

Azithromycin
• **Azithromycin** is a 15-atom lactone **macrolide ring** compound   • It **penetrates into most tissues (except CSF) & phagocytic cells**^{Q}
• **Elimination half-life: 3 days**^{Q} (permit **once-daily dosing & shortening of duration of treatment**)   • **Does not inhibit cytochrome P450 enzymes**^{Q}
Mechanism of Action: • **Prevents bacterial protein synthesis by binding to the 50S ribosomal subunit**^{Q}
Antimicrobial Activity: • Highly active against **Chlamydia species**^{Q} • Enhanced activity against **M. avium-intracellulare** & protozoa^Q (e.g., **Toxoplasma gondii, Cryptosporidium & Plasmodium spp.**).   • Good activity against **M. catarrhalis, L. pneumophila, B. burgdorferi, Mycoplasma pneumoniae & H. pylori**.   • Active against **H. influenzae & Campylobacter spp**^{Q}

Contd...

Contd...

Azithromycin
Clinical Applications: • **Community-acquired pneumonia** can be treated with azithromycin given as a 500-mg loading dose, followed by a 250-mg single daily dose for the next 4 days[Q]. • **A single 2-gm dose** of extended-release microspheres is an **alternative regimen for treatment of community-acquired pneumonia or acute exacerbations of chronic bronchitis**[Q]. <blockquote>• Treatment or prophylaxis of M. avium-intracellulare infection in AIDS patients[Q] • STDs, especially during pregnancy when tetracyclines are contraindicated[Q].</blockquote>• **Treatment of uncomplicated non-gonococcal urethritis,** presumed to be caused by **C. trachomatis** consists of a **single 1-gm dose of azithromycin**. This dose also is **effective for chancroid**[Q]. • A **single 1-gm dose** is recommended for **uncomplicated urethral, endocervical, rectal, or epididymal infections**[Q].

Gonococcal Infections
• A **single 1-g dose of azithromycin**, which is effective therapy for uncomplicated chlamydial infections, results in an **unacceptably low cure rate (93%) for gonococcal infections** and should not be used alone. • A **single 2-g dose of azithromycin**, particularly in the extended-release microsphere formulation, **delivers azithromycin to the lower gastrointestinal tract, thereby improving tolerability.**

67. Ans. d. Endothelium independent coronary vasodilation *(Ref: Harrison 19/e p1588; Goodman Gilman 12/e p; Katzung 13/e p195, 12/e p200)*

Mechanism of action of nitrates in Prinzmetal's angina is endothelium independent coronary vasodilation. When metabolized, organic nitrates release nitric oxide (NO) that binds to guanylyl cyclase in vascular smooth muscle cells, leading to an increase in cyclic guanosine monophosphate, which causes relaxation of vascular smooth muscle.

> *"Nitrates benefit patients with variant (also known as Prinzmetal) angina by relaxing the smooth muscle of the epicardial coronary arteries and relieving coronary artery spasm."-Katzung 13/e p195*

> *"The organic nitrates are a valuable class of drugs in the management of angina pectoris. Their major mechanisms of action include systemic venodilation with concomitant reduction in left ventricular end-diastolic volume and pressure, thereby reducing myocardial wall tension and oxygen requirements; dilation of epicardial coronary vessels; and increased blood flow in collateral vessels. When metabolized, organic nitrates release nitric oxide (NO) that binds to guanylyl cyclase in vascular smooth muscle cells, leading to an increase in cyclic guanosine monophosphate, which causes relaxation of vascular smooth muscle. Nitrates also exert antithrombotic activity by NO-dependent activation of platelet guanylyl cyclase, impairment of intraplatelet calcium flux, and platelet activation."-Harrison 19/e p1588*

> *"Nitrates improve exercise tolerance in patients with chronic angina and relieve ischemia in patients with unstable angina as well as patients with Prinzmetal's variant angina."- Harrison 19/e p1588*

Prinzmetal's Variant Angina (PVA)
• Syndrome of **severe ischemic pain** that usually **occurs at rest** and is associated with **transient ST-segment elevation**[Q]. • **Caused by focal spasm of an epicardial coronary artery,** leading **to severe transient myocardial ischemia & occasionally infarction**[Q]. • **Atherosclerotic plaques** in **at least one proximal coronary artery** occur in about **half** of patients • **Spasm** usually occurs **within 1 cm of plaque; Focal spasm** is **most common in right coronary artery**[Q].
Clinical Manifestations: • Patients are **relatively younger with fewer coronary risk factors** (with the exception of cigarette smoking)[Q] • Clinical diagnosis is made by **detection of transient ST-segment elevation with rest pain**[Q]. • Many patients also exhibit **multiple episodes of asymptomatic ST-segment elevation**[Q] (silent ischemia). • **Small elevations of troponin** may occur in patients **with prolonged attacks**[Q].
Diagnosis: • **Coronary angiography: Transient coronary spasm** is the **diagnostic hallmark of PVA**[Q].
Treatment: • **Main therapeutic agents: Nitrates & calcium channel blockers**[Q] • **Coronary revascularization** may be helpful in patients who also have discrete, flow-limiting, proximal fixed obstructive lesions.

Contd...

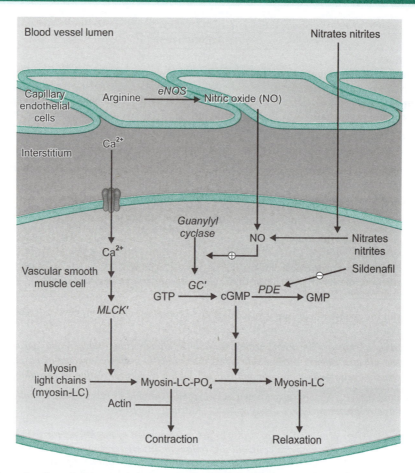

Fig. 20: Mechanism of action of nitrates, nitrites, and other substances that increase the concentration of nitric oxide (NO) in vascular smooth muscle cells. (MLCK: Activated myosin light-chain kinase; GC: Activated guanylyl cyclase: PDE, Phosphodiesterase; eNOS: Endothelial nitric oxide synthase)

68. **Ans. b. They increase bronchial responsiveness to salbutamol** *(Ref: Goodman Gilman 12/e p1049; Katzung 13/e p344, 12/e p347; Harrison 19/e p1677)*

Corticosteroids has a dual effect in acute asthma with an early facilitator effect on airway beta-2 adrenoreceptor sensitivity and a later effect on airway inflammation, which further emphasizes the need for corticosteroids to be administered as early as possible during an acute asthma attack.

"Corticosteroids have been used to treat asthma since 1950 and are presumed to act by their broad anti-inflammatory efficacy, mediated in part by inhibition of production of inflammatory cytokines. They do not relax airway smooth muscle directly but reduce bronchial reactivity and reduce the frequency of asthma exacerbations if taken regularly. Their effect on airway obstruction may be due in part to their contraction of engorged vessels in the bronchial mucosa and their potentiation of the effects of β-receptor agonists, but their most important action is inhibition of the infiltration of asthmatic airways by lymphocytes, eosinophils, and mast cells."- Katzung 13/e p344

"Effect on beta-2 Adrenergic Responsiveness: Corticosteroids increase beta adrenergic responsiveness, but whether this is relevant to their effect in asthma is uncertain. Steroids potentiate the effects of beta agonists on bronchial smooth muscle and prevent and reverse beta-receptor desensitization in airways in vitro and in vivo. At a molecular level, corticosteroids increase the transcription of the beta-2 receptor gene in human lung in vitro and in the respiratory mucosa in vivo and also increase the stability of its messenger RNA. They also prevent or reverse uncoupling of beta-2 receptors to Gs. In animal systems, corticosteroids prevent down-regulation of beta-2 receptors."-Goodman Gilman 12/e p1049

"The molecular mechanism of action of corticosteroids involves several effects on the inflammatory process. The major effect of corticosteroids is to switch off the transcription of multiple activated genes that encode inflammatory proteins such as cytokines, chemokines, adhesion molecules, and inflammatory enzymes. This effect involves several mechanisms, including inhibition of the transcription factor NF-κB, but an important mechanism is recruitment of HDAC2 to the inflammatory gene complex, which reverses the histone acetylation associated with increased gene transcription. Corticosteroids also activate anti-inflammatory genes, such as mitogen-activated protein (MAP) kinase phosphatase-1, and increase the expression of β2-receptors. Most of the metabolic and endocrine side effects of corticosteroids are also mediated through transcriptional activation."-Harrison 19/e p1677

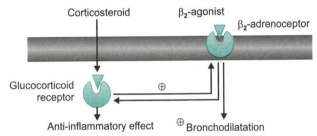

Drug of Choice in Bronchial Asthma	
• Acute attack of bronchial asthma • Acute attack of bronchial asthma in pregnancy • Exercise & aspirin induced acute attack of bronchial asthma	• Salbutamol[Q]
• Acute attack of bronchial asthma during labour • Acute attack of bronchial asthma on beta blockers therapy	• Ipratropium[Q]
• Prophylaxis of bronchial asthma, Exercise induced, aspirin induced bronchial asthma	• Corticosteroids[Q]

MICROBIOLOGY

69. Ans. c. Pneumocystis jirovecii   *(Ref: Ananthanarayan 10/e p609, 618; Jawetz 27/e p678, 691)*

Dimorphic fungi have two growth forms, such as a mold and a yeast, which develop under different growth conditions. Pneumocystis jirovecii is not a dimorphic fungi, it is a fungus with a close relationship to ascomycetes.

"Systemic mycoses refer to disseminated or deep fungal infection not restricted to the superficial areas. They are caused by fungi that are mostly soil saprophytes. Systemic mycoses occur in varying degrees of severity, ranging from asymptomatic infection to fatal disease. The fungi causing systemic mycoses are dimorphic (they are in the yeast from at 37° C and mold at 25° C) and include: Histoplasma capsulatum, Blastomyces dermatitidis, Paracoccidioides brasiliensis & Coccidioides immitis."-Ananthanarayan 10/e p609

"Opportunistic mycoses occur in patients who are immunosuppressed, those with haematological malignancies or diabetes, those on immunosuppressive drugs, corticosteroids, X-rays or broad-spectrum antibiotics. Opportunistic mycoses are caused by fungi that are of low virulence and found as contaminants in the environment, such as Mucor, Penicillium, Aspergillus species, etc."- Ananthanarayan 10/e p609

"Only one of the numerous and ubiquitous environmental species of Penicillium is dimorphic, Penicillium marneffei, and this species has emerged as an endemic, opportunistic pathogen."- Jawetz 27/e p692

Dimorphic Fungi	
• Blastomyces dermatitidis[Q] • Coccidioides immitis[Q] • Coccidioides posadasii[Q] • Histoplasma capsulatum[Q]	• Paracoccidioides brasiliensis[Q] • Penicillium marneffei[Q] • Sporothrix schenckii[Q]

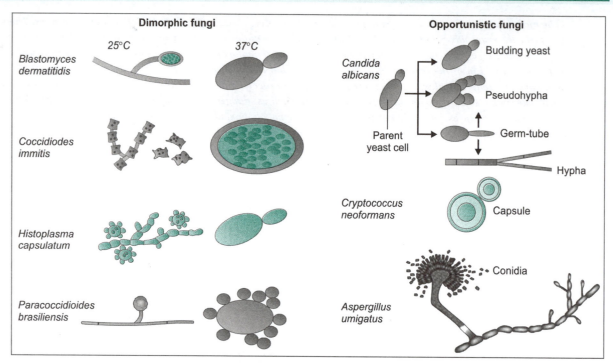

70. **Ans. a. It cannot be grown in Sabouraud Dextrose Agar (SDA)** *(Ref: Ananthanarayan 10/e p610; Jawetz 27/e p678, 679; Harrison 19/e p1332, 1333)*

Presence of intracellular fungi on Bone marrow examination (in tissues) in an HIV positive patient is highly suggestive of Disseminated histoplasmosis caused by Histoplasma capsulatum. Specimens are cultured in rich media, such as glucose-cysteine blood agar at 37°C and on SDA (Sabouraud Dextrose Agar) or IMA Inhibitory Mold Agar) at 25–30°C.

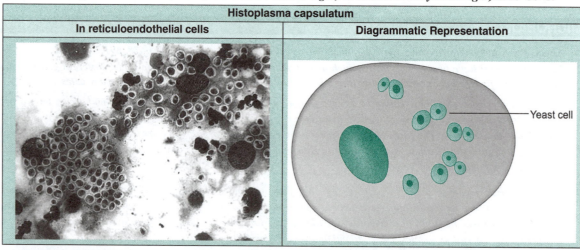

"*Histoplasma capsulatum is a dimorphic soil saprophyte that causes histoplasmosis, the most prevalent pulmonary fungal infection in humans and animals. In nature, H capsulatum grows as a mold in association with soil and avian habitats, being enriched by alkaline nitrogenous substrates in guano. H capsulatum and histoplasmosis, which is initiated by inhalation of the conidia, occur worldwide. However, the incidence varies considerably, and most cases occur in the United States. H capsulatum received its name from the appearance of the yeast cells in histopathologic sections; however, it is neither a protozoan nor does it have a capsule.*"-*Jawetz 27/e p678*

"*Histoplasma capsulatum: Specimens are cultured in rich media, such as glucose-cysteine blood agar at 37°C and on SDA (Sabouraud Dextrose Agar) or IMA (Inhibitory Mold Agar) at 25–30°C.*"-*Jawetz 27/e p679*

"In patients with impaired cellular immunity, the infection is not contained and can disseminate. Progressive disseminated histoplasmosis (PDH) can involve multiple organs, most commonly the bone marrow, spleen, liver, adrenal glands, and mucocutaneous membranes."-Harrison 19/e p1332

"Progressive disseminated histoplasmosis (PDH) is typically seen in immunocompromised individuals, who account for ~70% of cases. Common risk factors include AIDS (CD4+ T cell count, <200/μL), extremes of age, immunosuppressive medications administered for prevention or treatment of rejection following transplantation (e.g., prednisone, mycophenolate, calcineurin inhibitors, and biologic response modifiers), and methotrexate, anti-TNF-α agents, or other biologic response modifiers given for inflammatory arthritis or Crohn's disease."- Harrison 19/e p1333

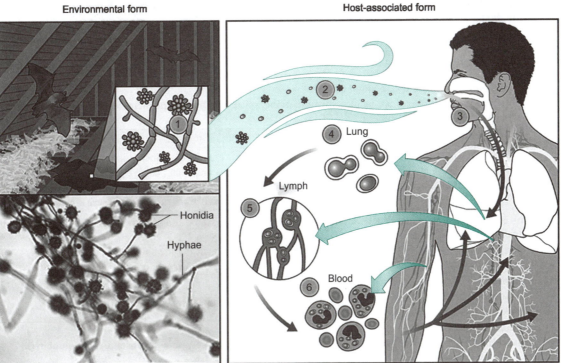

Fig. 21: Life-cycle of histoplasma capsulatum

Histoplasma capsulatum
• **Dimorphic soil saprophyte**, causes histoplasmosis[Q] • **Most prevalent pulmonary fungal infection** in **humans & animals**[Q]. • **Grows as a mold** in soil mixed with bird feces (e.g., starling roosts, chicken houses) or **bat guano (caves)**[Q]. • Appearance of yeast cells in histopathologic sections; does not have a capsule[Q].

Morphology & Identification:
• Primary isolates develop **brown mold colonies** at temperatures <37°C.
• **Hyaline, septate hyphae** produce **microconidia** & **large, spherical thick-walled macroconidia** with peripheral projections of cell wall material[Q].
    • In tissue or in vitro on rich medium at 37°C, hyphae & conidia convert to small, oval yeast cells[Q].
    • In tissue, yeasts are typically seen within macrophages, as **Histoplasma capsulatum** is a **facultative intracellular parasite**[Q].

Epidemiology • **Highest incidence in the United States**; also found in Africa & Far East
Mode of Transmission: • **Inhalation of airborne environmental conidia by wind & dust**[Q] • Histoplasmosis is **not communicable from person to person**[Q]

Contd...

Contd...

Histoplasma capsulatum
Pathogenesis:
• **Clinical Incubation Period:** 3–17 days for acute manifestations; chronic manifestations over months to years
• After inhalation, **conidia develop into yeast cells** & engulfed by alveolar macrophages & replicate[Q].
• Within macrophages, yeasts may disseminate to reticuloendothelial tissues (liver, spleen, bone marrow & LNs)[Q]
• **Initial inflammatory reaction** becomes **granulomatous**[Q].
Clinical Features:
• Chronic, systemic disease with **fever, weight loss, fatigue, cytopenias, hepatosplenomegaly**[Q]
• **Chronic pulmonary disease** similar to tuberculosis. **Granulomatous nodules in the lungs** or other sites **heal with calcification**[Q].
• **Severe disseminated histoplasmosis** particularly in **infants, elderly & immunosuppressed**, including **AIDS patients**[Q].
Diagnosis
• **Gold-standard diagnostic test: Fungal culture**[Q]
• **Specimens:** Specimens for culture include **sputum, urine, scrapings from superficial lesions, bone marrow aspirates & buffy coat blood cells**[Q].
Microscopic Examination
• Blood films, bone marrow slides & biopsy specimens may be examined microscopically.
• In disseminated histoplasmosis, **bone marrow cultures** are often **positive**[Q].
• **Small ovoid cells may be observed within macrophages in histologic sections** stained with **fungal stains,** such as **GMS or PAS,** or in **Giemsa-stained smears** of **bone marrow or blood**[Q].
• **Culture:** Specimens are cultured in **rich media,** such as **glucose-cysteine blood agar at 37°C & on SDA (Sabouraud Dextrose Agar) or IMA (Inhibitory Mold Agar) at 25–30°C**[Q].
• **Serology: Radioassay** or **enzyme immunoassay** for circulating polysaccharide antigen of H. capsulatum[Q].
• **Radiographic examination:** **Hilar lymphadenopathy & pulmonary infiltrates** or nodules[Q].
Treatment:
• **Itraconazole:** For the treatment of **mild to moderate infection**[Q]
• **Amphotericin B:** For the treatment of **disseminated disease**[Q]
Prevention & Control:
• **Personal protective measures** in selected high-risk environments **(caves, pigeon roosts & chicken houses)**
• **Spraying formaldehyde on infected soil** may destroy H. capsulatum.

71. **Ans. d. Acute angle branching Aspergillus** *(Ref: Harrison 19/e p1348; Robbins 9/e p389; Ananthanarayan 10/e p613; Jawetz 27/e p690)*

The given shows septate hyphae, with acute angle branching suggestive of Aspergillus. Aspergillus hyphae are hyaline, narrow, and septate, with branching at 45° (acute angle branching).

"Aspergillus forms fruiting bodies (usually in lung cavities) and septate filaments, 5 to 10 µm thick, branching at acute angles (40 degrees). Aspergillus hyphae cannot be distinguished from Pseudallescheria boydii and Fusarium species by morphology alone. Aspergillus has a tendency to invade blood vessels, therefore areas of hemorrhage and infarction are usually superimposed on the necrotizing, inflammatory tissue reactions."-Robbins 9/e p389

"Aspergillus hyphae are hyaline, narrow, and septate, with branching at 45°; no yeast forms are present in infected tissue. Hyphae can be seen in cytology or microscopy preparations, which therefore provide a rapid means of presumptive diagnosis."-Harrison 19/e p1348

"Mucormycetes form non-septate hyphae of variable width (6-50 µm) with frequent right angle branching, distinct from Aspergillus hyphae, that are readily demonstrated by hematoxylin and eosin or special fungal stains."-Robbins 9/e p389

"Penicillium organisms have uniformly cylindrical septate hyphae 2–5 mm in width that branch at an angle of 25°–45°. Characteristics helpful in distinguishing them from Aspergillus are the presence of their hyphae of clear vacuoles alternating with basophilic zones, and the occurenece of chlamydospores. Penicillium, like aspergillus, may have a radiating growth and invade vessels."- The Pathologic Anatomy of Mycoses: By Roger Denio Baker (2012)/p774

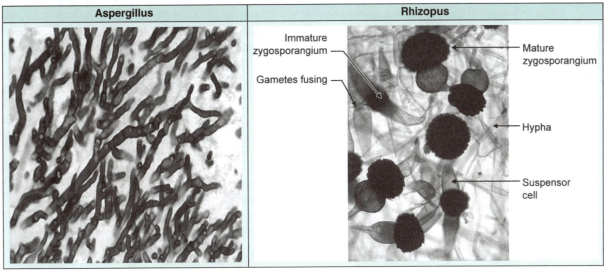

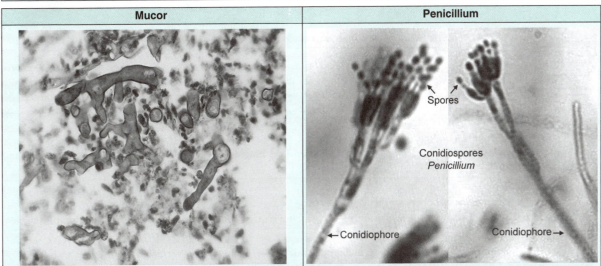

Hyphae Features	Aspergillus	Zygomycetes (Mucormycosis)	Fusarium	Pseudoallescheria	Penicillium
Width	3-6 mm	6-50 mm	3-8 mm	2-5 mm	2-5 mm
Outline appearance	**Parallel lines**[Q]	**Irregular lines**[Q]	Parallel lines	**Parallel lines**[Q]	**Parallel lines**[Q]
Branching pattern	**Dichotomous** (daughter branch has same width as parent branch) **branching at acute angles**[Q]	**Haphazard branching: Frequent right angle & >90° angle branching**[Q]	Frequently **right angle branching**, sometimes 45° branching[Q]	**Haphazard** branching[Q]	**Branch** at **an angle** of **25-45°**[Q]
Septation	**Septate**[Q]	**Aseptate or pauciseptate**[Q]	**Septate**[Q]	**Septate**[Q]	**Septate**[Q]

72. **Ans. d. Chromoblastomycosis**   (Ref: Ananthanarayan 10/e p605; Jawetz 27/e p671, 672, 674; Harrison 19/e p1355)

History of thorn prick and the image showing sclerotic bodies (medlar bodies or copper penny bodies) is highly suggestive of chromoblastomycosis.

> "*Chromoblastomycosis occurs mainly in the tropics. The fungi are saprophytic in nature, probably occurring on vegetation and in soil. The disease occurs chiefly on the legs of barefoot agrarian workers following traumatic introduction of the fungus.*"-*Jawetz 27/e p672*

"The diagnostic feature of chromoblastomycosis is the microscopic observation of brownish (melanized), spherical sclerotic bodies within the lesions."- Jawetz 27/e p674

Chromoblastomycosis showing Sclerotic bodies
(Rounded cells surrounded by thick walls known as Medlar bodies or copper pennies)

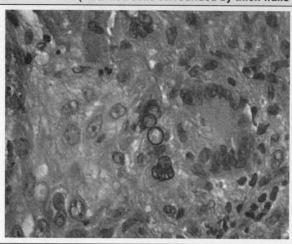 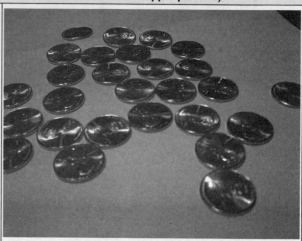

"The agents of chromoblastomycosis are identified by their modes of conidiation. In tissue they appear the same, producing spherical brown cells (4–12 μm in diameter) termed muriform or sclerotic bodies that divide by transverse septation. Septation in different planes with delayed separation may give rise to a cluster of four to eight cells."-Jawetz 27/e p671

Chromoblastomycosis (Verrucous Dermatitis)

- **MC form of chromomycosis**[Q]
- **Subcutaneous mycotic infection** caused by **traumatic inoculation** of causative fungal agents **residing in soil & vegetation**[Q].

Epidemiology:
- Chromoblastomycosis occurs **mainly in the tropics**[Q].
- Disease occurs chiefly on the **legs of barefoot agrarian workers following traumatic introduction** of fungus[Q].

Causative Agents:
- All are **dematiaceous fungi**, having **melanized cell walls**: **Phialophora** verrucosa, **Fonsecaea** pedrosoi, Fonsecaea compacta, **Rhinocladiella** aquaspersa & **Cladophialophora** carrionii[Q].

Pathogenesis:
- Fungi are **introduced into the skin by trauma**[Q].
- Over months to years, **primary lesion becomes verrucous & wart-like** with **extension along the draining lymphatics. Cauliflower-like nodules with crusting abscesses** eventually cover the area[Q].
  - Small ulcerations or "black dots" of hemopurulent material are present on the warty surface[Q].
  - **Histology**: Lesions are **granulomatous & dark sclerotic bodies (medlar bodies or copper penny bodies**[Q]) seen within leukocytes or giant cells.

Clinical Features:
- Indolent subcutaneous infection characterized by **nodular, verrucous, or plaque-like painless lesions** that occur predominantly on the **lower extremities** & grow slowly over months to years.

Diagnosis:
- **Specimens from lesions** are examined microscopically **in KOH for dark, spherical cells**[Q].
- **Detection of the sclerotic bodies** is **diagnostic of chromoblastomycosis** regardless of the etiologic agent[Q].

Treatment:
- **Small lesions**: Surgical excision with wide margins is the **therapy of choice**[Q]
- **Larger lesions**: Antifungal agents of choice are **itraconazole, voriconazole & posaconazole**[Q]

AIIMS November 2017

Body/Figures	Feature	Seen in
Alder Reilly bodies[Q]	Deeply **basophilic granules** seen within **neutrophils**[Q]	**Hunter's & Hurler's syndrome**[Q]
Antoni A bodies[Q]	Densely cellular areas with palisaded nuclei, fascicles & **Verocay bodies**[Q]	**Schwannoma**[Q]
Antoni B bodies[Q]	Loose, gelatinous stroma, fewer cells microcystic changes	**Schwannoma**[Q]
Arao-Perkins bodies[Q]	Small fibrous bodies in dermal papilla	Androgenic alopecia[Q]
Aschoff body[Q]	**Small granulomatous lesion composed of macrophages, lymphocytes & giant cells**[Q]	**Rheumatic fever**[Q]
Asteroid body[Q]	Star-like cytoplasmic inclusions in giant cells	**Sarcoidosis**[Q] & other **granulomatous disease** (TB, Botryomycosis, sporotrichosis, actinomycosis, leprosy, Berylliosis)[Q]
Bamboo bodies[Q]	Cylindrical, high density foreign bodies in lung.	**Asbestosis**[Q]
Banana bodies[Q]	**Crescentic shaped bodies within Schwann cells**[Q]	**Disseminated lipogranulomatosis**[Q] Farber disease, Ochronosis[Q]
Birbeck granules[Q]	**Tennis racket structures on EM**[Q]	**Langerhans cells**[Q]
Bodies of Arantius[Q]	**Small nodules located at cusps of aortic & pulmonary valves**[Q]	**Aortic valve nodules**[Q]
Body of Highmore[Q]	Mass of fibrous tissue continuous with tunica albuginea that project into testis.	**Mediastinum testis**[Q]
Bollinger bodies[Q]	**Intracytoplasmic, eosinophilic inclusions in epithelial cells of birds**[Q].	**Fowlpox**[Q]
Brassy body[Q]	**Dark shrunken blood corpuscles**[Q]	**Malaria**[Q]
Bunina bodies[Q]	Small eosinophilic intraneuronal inclusions in **lower motor neurons**[Q]	**Amyotrophic lateral sclerosis**[Q]
Call-Exner bodies[Q]	**Small eosinophilic, fluid-filled spaces found in ovary between granulosa cells**[Q]	**Granulosa cell tumor**[Q]
Caterpillar bodies[Q]	**Elongated epidermal eosinophilic bodies**[Q]	**Porphyria cutanea tarda**[Q]
Chromatid bodies[Q]	**Cytoplasmic elongated cigar-shaped bars with bluntly rounded ends**[Q]	**Entamoeba histolytica precyst**[Q]
Cigar bodies[Q]	**Elongated, cigar like**[Q]	**Sporotrichosis**[Q]
Citron bodies[Q]	**Boat or leaf shaped pleomorphic bacteria**[Q]	**Clostridium septicum**[Q]
Civatte bodies (colloid bodies)[Q]	**Spherical, eosinophilic hyaline bodies seen in or below the epidermis**[Q]	**Lichen planus**[Q]
Councilman bodies[Q]	**Cytoplasmic inclusion**[Q]	**Viral hepatitis**[Q] yellow fever[Q]
Cowdry type A bodies[Q]	**Lipschutz inclusions, intranuclear eosinophilic inclusions surrounded by clear halo**[Q]	**Herpes simples, Varicella Zoster lesions**[Q]
Cowdry type B bodies[Q]	Droplet like masses of acidophilic material surrounded by clear halo within nuclei	**Polio & adenovirus**[Q]
Coccoid X bodies[Q]	**Minute bodies (elementary & reticulate) found in the blood**[Q]	**Psittacosis**[Q]
Comma shaped bodies[Q]	**Two electron dense membranes within histiocytes**[Q]	**Juvenile Xanthogranuloma, histiocytosis**[Q]
Creola bodies[Q]	**Clumps of benign respiratory epithelium in sputum indicative of asthma**[Q]	**Asthma**[Q]
Cystoid bodies[Q]	Heterogeneous round, oval, or polygonal deposit, usually in dermis	**Collective form for colloid bodies, Russell bodies amyloid, elastic globes**[Q]

Contd...

Contd...

Body/Figures	Feature	Seen in
Davidson bodies[Q]	**Nuclear chromatin buds**[Q]	**Female's neutrophils**[Q]
Donovan bodies[Q]	Single or clustered rod safety pin like bacteria in macrophages	**Granuloma inguinale**[Q]
Dutcher bodies[Q]	Intranuclear, eosinophilic globules found in plasma cells.	**B-cell lymphoma, multiple myeloma, Farber disease**[Q]
Farber bodies[Q]	Comma-shaped tubular structures in cytoplasm of fibroblasts	**Farber disease**[Q]
Ferruginous bodies (Asbestos bodies)[Q]	**Thin, curved or drumstick appearance; stain positively with Perl's Prussian blue**[Q]**.**	**Asbestosis, silicosis**[Q]
Flame Figures[Q]	Poorly circumscribed, small areas of amorphous eosinophilic material adherent to dermal collagen	Eosinophilic cellulitis + flame figures was syndrome > arthropod bites, parasites, BP, of eosinophilic panniculi
Floret cells[Q]	Multinucleated giant cells with marginally placed nuclei	**Pleomorphic (spindle cell) lipoma**[Q]
Flower cells[Q]	Atypical CD4+ T cells, prominent nuclear lobation	**HTLV-1, ATL**[Q]
Gamma Gandy bodies[Q]	Nodules secondary to accumulation of hemosiderin	**CML, sickle cell anemia, cirrhosis of liver**[Q]
Guarnieri bodies (Paschen bodies)[Q]	Cytoplasmic, eosinophilic inclusion in keratinocytes	**Smallpox, Vaccinia**[Q]
Heinz bodies (Ehrlich or Heinz-Ehrlich bodies)[Q]	Small rounded distensions that deform RBCs. Ehrlich or Heinz-Ehrlich bodies	**G-6-PD deficiency**[Q]
Henderson-Patterson bodies[Q]	Large, cytoplasmic eosinophilic inclusions in keratinocytes	**Molluscum contagiosum**[Q]
Herring bodies[Q]	Large eosinophilic masses of neurosecretary granules located in posterior lobe of pituitary at dilatations along the axons & their endings.	**Neurohypophysis**[Q]
Hirano bodies[Q]	Intracellular, eosinophilic rod-shaped structures in nerve cells.	**Alzheimer's disease**, Creutzfeldt-Jacob disease[Q]
Homer-Wright Rosettes	Central nerve fibrils, peripheral small tumor cells	**Cutaneous neuroblastoma**[Q]
Kamino bodies[Q]	Eosinophilic globoid bodies, probably apoptotic lesional cells.	**Spindle cell naevi**[Q]
Lafora bodies[Q]	Concentric amyloid deposits (**polyglucosan bodies**)[Q]	**Lafora disease**[Q]
Levinthal-Coles-Lillie bodies[Q]	Cytoplasmic inclusion bodies in macrophages of lung	**Psittacosis**[Q]
Lewy bodies[Q]	**Round eosinophilic structures found in cytoplasm of neurons**[Q]**.**	**Parkinsonism,** Alzheimer's disease[Q]
Lipofuscin-like granules	Yellow-brown granules in dermal macrophages	**Amiodarone hyperpigmentation**[Q]
Marquee sign[Q]	Organisms at the periphery of macrophages	**Leishmania**[Q]
Medlar (sclerotic) bodies[Q]	Muriform cells, "copper pennies, "round thick-walled brown fungi	**Chromoblastomycosis**[Q]
Michaelis-Gutmann bodies[Q]	Calcified, degraded bacteria in macrophages, lamellated	**Malakoplakia**[Q]
Mikulicz cells[Q]	**Large macrophages containing Klebsiella rhinoscleromatis**[Q]	**Rhinoscleroma**[Q]
Morulae[Q]	**Leukocyte intracytoplasmic inclusions, Ehrlichia multiplying in cell vacuoles**[Q]	**Ehrlichiosis**[Q]

Contd...

Contd...

Body/Figures	Feature	Seen in
Mooser bodies[Q]	Large mononuclear cells filled with Rickettsia typhi in patients with endemic typhus fever	Endemic typhus[Q]
Mott bodies (Mott cells)[Q]	Plasma cells with spherical inclusions (Russell bodies) packed in their cytoplasm.	Multiple myeloma[Q]
Negri bodies[Q]	Eosinophilic, cytoplasmic inclusions in neutrons	Rabies[Q]
Odland bodies[Q]	Small, granular, membrane-bound vacuoles found in cytoplasm of skin keratinocytes	Derived from the Golgi apparatus Shows synthesis of epidermal lipids
Psammoma bodies[Q]	Concentrically laminated, round calcified bodies	Papillary carcinoma thyroid, Serous cyst-adenoma of ovary, Meningioma, Malignant Mesothelioma[Q]
Pustule-ovoid bodies of Milian[Q]	Large eosinophilic granules with clear halo	Granular cell tumor[Q]
Reilly bodies[Q]	Granular inclusions found in WBCs in Alder-Reilly anomaly[Q]	Hurler's syndrome[Q]
Rokitansky bodies[Q]	Yellowish appearance of adipose tissue on CT	Benign cystic teratomas[Q]
Ross's bodies[Q]	Spherical copper-coloured bodies[Q]	Syphilis[Q]
Rushton bodies[Q]	Intraepithelial, curvilinear & eosinophilic lamellar structures	Odontogenic cyst[Q]
Russell bodies[Q]	Immunoglobulin deposits in plasma cells	Rhinoscleroma, plasmacytosis[Q]
Sandstorm bodies[Q]	Synonymous with parathyroid glands	Parathyroid glands[Q]
Schaumann bodies[Q]	Shell-like, lamellated, basophilic, calcified protein complexes in giant cells[Q]	Sarcoidosis[Q]
Schiller-Duval bodies[Q]	Perivascular structures consisting of tumour cells arranged around a blood vessel[Q].	Yolk sac tumor[Q]
Sclerotic bodies[Q]	Rounded cells surrounded by thick walls often known as Medlar bodies or copper pennies[Q].	Chromoblastomycosis[Q]
Spiderweb cells[Q]	Globular, striated, vacuolated cells	Adult rhabdomyoma[Q]
Verocay bodies[Q]	Palisading nuclei in rows around eosinophilic cytoplasm[Q]	Schwannoma[Q]
Winkler bodies[Q]	Spherical structures in lesions in syphilis	Syphilis[Q]
Weibel-Palade bodies[Q]	Dense rod or oval organelles on EM[Q]	Endothelial cells[Q]
Zebra bodies[Q]	Vacuoles with transverse membrane with endothelial cells[Q]	Metachromatic leukodystrophy[Q]

73. **Ans. a. Invasive candidiasis** *(Ref: Nelson 19/e p881e-1; Jawetz 27/e p665; Harrison 19/e p489, 1360; J. Clin. Microbiol, July 2014, vol. 52 no. 7 2328)*

1,3-beta-D-glucan is helpful for identification of invasive candidiasis. (1-3)-β-D-glucan (BG) is a component of the cell walls of most fungi. The main exceptions are Mucorales (Rhizopus, Mucor & Absidia) and cryptococci, which release no or little BG to be detected in human serum.

"Mannan antigen and (1,3)β-d-glucan have utility in rapid detection of invasive candidiasis."-Nelson 19/e p881e-1

"Another serum marker for the presence of invasive fungal infections is (1-3)-β-D-glucan (BG), which has been included in the relevant European Organization for Research and Treatment of Cancer (EORTC)/Mycoses Study Group diagnostic criteria. BG is a component of the cell walls of most fungi. The main exceptions are Mucorales and cryptococci, which release no or little BG to be detected in human serum."-J. Clin. Microbiol, July 2014, vol. 52 no. 7 2328

"β-(1,3)-d-glucan levels of ≥80 pg/mL are positive and associated with invasive candidiasis, aspergillosis, dimorphic pathogens, and other mycoses."-Jawetz 27/e p665

74. Ans. c. Toxin detection by ELISA *(Ref: Ananthanarayan 10/e p270; Jawetz 27/e p187; Harrison 19/e p859: Sabiston 20/e p312)*

ELISA that detects toxin A or B in stool is highly sensitive and specific for diagnosis of Clostridium difficile colitis.

"Cell cytotoxin assay in tissue culture is a highly sensitive and specific test for the detection of toxin B (rounding effect) and is the gold standard diagnostic test for Clostridium difficile colitis. ELISA that detects toxin A or B in stool is highly sensitive and specific. In contrast to the stool cytotoxic test, which requires 24 to 48 hours, results of ELISA are obtained within hours, the test is less expensive, and it does not require specific training. "-Sabiston 20/e p312

Pseudomembranous Colitis
• **PMC** is caused by **C. difficile**, a **gram-positive**[Q] bacillus. • **C. difficile colitis** is the **leading cause** of **nosocomially acquired diarrhea**[Q].

Pathogenesis:
• Colitis is thought to result from **overgrowth** of this **organism after depletion of** the **normal commensal flora** of the gut **with** the use of **antibiotics**[Q].
     • **Clindamycin**[Q] was the **first antimicrobial agent** associated with **C. difficile colitis,** almost **any antibiotic** may **cause this disease.**
     • Toxins produced: **Toxin A** (an **enterotoxin**) & **toxin B** (a **cytotoxin**)[Q].
• **Immunosuppression, medical comorbidities, prolonged hospitalization** or **nursing home residence**, and **bowel surgery increase** the **risk**[Q].

Clinical Features: • The **spectrum of disease** ranges from **watery diarrhea** to **fulminant, life-threatening** colitis
Diagnosis: • Diagnosis is made after **detection of one** or **both toxins by:** • **Stool cytotoxin assay**[Q] (Gold standard diagnostic test) • **ELISA: ELISA that detects toxin A or B in stool is highly sensitive & specific**[Q] • **Colonoscopy**: Characteristic **ulcers, plaques**, and **pseudomembranes**[Q]
Treatment: • **Immediate cessation** of the **offending antimicrobial agent**[Q]. • **Mild disease:** • **Oral metronidazole** (10-day course): **Drug of choice**[Q] • **Oral vancomycin: Second-line agent,** used in **metronidazole allergy** or in **recurrent disease**[Q] • **Severe disease: Bowel rest, IV hydration**, and **IV metronidazole** or oral **vancomycin**[Q].   • **Fidoxamicin (specific RNA polymerase inhibitor against C. difficile)**

Fecal Microbiota Transplantation (FMT)

• Also known as **stool transplant**[Q]
• Process of **transplantation of fecal bacteria from a healthy individual into a recipient**[Q].
• **FMT Hypothesis: Bacterial interference (using harmless bacteria to displace pathogenic bacteria)**
     • **FMT restores the colonic microbiota** to its natural state by **replacing missing Bacteroidetes & Firmicutes species**[Q].
     • Used successfully as a **treatment for patients suffering from C. difficile infection**[Q].

75. Ans. c. Crimean Congo hemorrhagic fever *(Ref: Harrison 19/e p782, 1321; https://www.nhp.gov.in/disease/blood-lymphatic/crimean-congo-haemorrhagic-fever-cchf)*

Viral hemorrhagic fevers are zoonotic illnesses caused by viruses that reside in either animal reservoirs or arthropod vectors. These diseases occur worldwide and are restricted to areas where the host species live; examples are- Ebola and Marburg virus infections in Africa; yellow fever in Africa and South America. Crimean-Congo hemorrhagic fever has an extensive geographic distribution. In India, first confirmed case of CCHF was reported during a nosocomial outbreak in Ahmadabad, Gujarat, in January 2011.

AIIMS November 2017

"Viral hemorrhagic fevers are zoonotic illnesses caused by viruses that reside in either animal reservoirs or arthropod vectors. These diseases occur worldwide and are restricted to areas where the host species live. They are caused by four major groups of viruses: Arenaviridae (e.g., Lassa fever in Africa), Bunyaviridae (e.g., Rift Valley fever in Africa; hantavirus hemorrhagic fever with renal syndrome in Asia; or Crimean-Congo hemorrhagic fever, which has an extensive geographic distribution), Filoviridae (e.g., Ebola and Marburg virus infections in Africa), and Flaviviridae (e.g., yellow fever in Africa and South America and dengue in Asia, Africa, and the Americas). Lassa fever and Ebola and Marburg virus infections are also transmitted from person to person. The vectors for most viral fevers are found in rural areas; dengue and yellow fever are important exceptions. After a prodrome of fever, myalgias, and malaise, patients develop evidence of vascular damage, petechiae, and local hemorrhage. Shock, multifocal hemorrhaging, and neurologic signs (e.g., seizures or coma) predict a poor prognosis. Dengue is the most common arboviral disease worldwide."-Harrison 19/e p782

"Crimean-Congo haemorrhagic fever (CCHF): The disease was first described in the Crimea (former USSR) in 1944 and given the name Crimean haemorrhagic fever. In 1969, it was recognized that the pathogen causing Crimean haemorrhagic fever was the same as that responsible for an illness identified in 1956 in the Congo and linkage of the both place names resulted in the current name for the disease and the virus. The disease is widespread in many countries in Africa, Europe, Middle East and Central Asia with sporadic outbreaks recorded in Kosovo, Albania, Iran, and Turkey. In India the first confirmed case of CCHF was reported during a nosocomial (Infections caught in hospitals) outbreak in Ahmadabad, Gujarat, in January 2011. Subsquently outbreaks were reported from different districts of Gujarat every year. During 2012–2015, several outbreaks and cases of CCHF transmitted by ticks via livestock and several nosocomial infections were reported in the states of Gujarat and Rajasthan. Cases were documented from 6 districts of Gujarat (Ahmadabad, Amreli, Patan, Surendranagar, Kutch, and Aravalli) and 3 districts of Rajasthan (Sirohi, Jodhpur, and Jaisalmer). A CCHF case was also reported from Uttar Pradesh state. Pakistan reports 50-60 cases annually."- https://www.nhp.gov.in/disease/blood-lymphatic/crimean-congo-haemorrhagic-fever-cchf

Crimean-Congo Hemorrhagic Fever (CCHF)

- Caused by **tick-borne virus (Nairovirus)**[Q]
- This **severe VHF** has a **wide geographic distribution**[Q]
- **Zoonotic** (could be transmitted from animals to humans) **vector-borne disease**[Q].
- CCHF causes **severe illness in humans** and has a **case-fatality rate of up to 40%.**

> - **In India, first confirmed case of CCHF** was reported during a **nosocomial outbreak in Ahmadabad, Gujarat, in January 2011**[Q].

Route of Infection:
- **Human infections are acquired via tick bites** or during the **crushing of infected ticks**[Q].
- **Risk of acquiring CCHF during sheep shearing, slaughter** & contact with **infected hides or carcasses**[Q]
- **Nosocomial epidemics** are usually related to **extensive blood exposure or needle sticks**[Q].

Clinical Features:
- Generally similar to other VHFs, **CCHF causes extensive liver damage**, resulting in **jaundice** in some patients.
- Clinical laboratory values indicate **DIC** & elevations of **AST, creatine phosphokinase & bilirubin**[Q].
- **Thrombocytopenia** is **more marked** & **develops earlier in patients who do not survive** than in survivors.

Treatment:
- **No human** or **veterinary vaccines are recommended**.
- **Oral ribavirin** has been recommended **for the treatment & prophylaxis**[Q]

---

76. **Ans. d. Chloride compounds** *(Ref: Infection Control in Clinical Practice By Jennie Wilson (2006)/p173)*

Blood spills in OT is cleaned with chloride compounds. High-concentration chlorine-releasing compounds provide the most economical and effective method of treating many spills, especially large spills of blood.

"High-concentration chlorine-releasing compounds provide the most economical and effective method of treating many spills, especially large spills of blood. Chlorine-releasing granules have the advantage of containing the spill rather than adding to it; they have a longer shelf-life than hypochlorite solutions and are more portable."-Infection Control in Clinical Practice By Jennie Wilson (2006)/p173

"Blood and body fluid spillage is a daily occurrence in the operation theatre, and each hospital policy on the management of such occurrences should clearly state the solutions and strengths to be used. Sodium hypochlorite, a chlorine based solution, is the established one of choice; however, chlorine solutions need to be accurately diluted to be effective (1:1000 for cleaning floors; 1:10000 for dealing with blood and body fluid splashes)."-A Textbook of Perioperative Care By Kate Woodhead (2005)/p94

Disinfectant	Effective against			Susceptible to organic matter
	Bacteria	Spores	Virus	
Formaldehyde	+++	+++	+++	-
Glutaraldehyde	+++	+++	+++	-
Chlorine (hypochlorite)	+++	+/-	+++	+++
Phenols	++(+)	-	+	+/-

Techniques of Sterilization	
Steam (121°C for 15 minutes)	• Surgical instruments[Q]
Ethylene oxide	• **Heart lung machine**[Q], respirators, dental labs
Hot air oven	• **Glass syringe**[Q], **test tubes, flasks**[Q], cutting instruments
Irradiation (**gamma rays**)	• Industrial packaging[Q]
Paracetic acid (STERIS)	• Flexible endoscopes[Q]
Isopropyl alcohol	• Clinical thermometer[Q]
Beta propiolactone >Formaldehyde	• Fumigation of OT, labs, wards[Q]
2% Glutaraldehyde	• **Endoscope (cystoscope, bronchoscope)**[Q]
Autoclaving	• Culture media, suture materials except catgut[Q]
Sodium hypochlorite	• **Blood & body fluid spillage** in the **operation theatre**

77. **Ans. b. Leptospira**   *(Ref: Ananthanarayan 10/e p377; Jawetz 27/e p330)*

All members of spirochetes (Treponema, Borrelia & Leptospira) have the characteristic presence of endoflagellum (axial filament).

"The spirochetes have many structural characteristics in common, as typified by Treponema pallidum. They are long, slender, helically coiled, spiral, or corkscrew-shaped bacilli. T pallidum has an outer sheath or glycosaminoglycan coating. Inside the sheath is the outer membrane, which contains peptidoglycan and maintains the structural integrity of the organisms. Endoflagella (axial filaments) are the flagella-like organelles in the periplasmic space encased by the outer membrane. The endoflagella begin at each end of the organism and wind around it, extending to and overlap- ping at the midpoint. Inside the endoflagella is the inner membrane (cytoplasmic membrane) that provides osmotic stability and covers the protoplasmic cylinder. A series of cytoplasmic tubules (body fibrils) are inside the cell near the inner membrane. Treponemes reproduce by transverse fission."- *Jawetz 27/e p323*

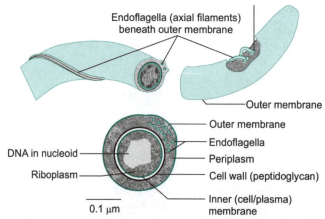

Fig. 22: Endoflagella of a spirochete (Treponema, Borrelia & Leptospira)

AIIMS November 2017

"Elongated, motile, flexible bacteria twisted spirally along the long axis are termed spirochetes (from speira, meaning coil and chaite, meaning hair). They are structurally more complex than other bacteria. A characteristic feature is the presence of varying numbers of endoflagella (axial filament), which are polar flagella wound along the helical protoplasmic cylinder, and situated between the outer membrane and the cell wall."-Ananthanarayan 10/e p377

"Leptospirae are tightly coiled, thin, flexible spirochetes 5–15 μm long, with very fine spirals 0.1–0.2 μm wide; one end is often bent, forming a hook. They are actively motile, which is best seen using a dark-field microscope. Electron micrographs show a thin axial filament and a delicate membrane. The spirochete is so delicate that in the dark-field view, it may appear only as a chain of minute cocci. It does not stain readily but can be impregnated with silver."-Jawetz 27/e p330

78. Ans. d. Adherence   *(Ref: Ananthanarayan 10/e p77, 208; Jawetz 27/e p58, 165; Harrison 19/e p145e-4; Goodman Gilman 12/e p1367)*

Biofilm in the bacteria leads antimicrobial resistance by acting as mechanical barrier, increased excretion of antibiotics and altered metabolism inside the biofilms.

*"A topic of major interest is the ability of many bacterial, fungal, and protozoal species to grow in multicellular masses referred to as **biofilms**. These masses are biochemically and morphologically quite distinct from the free-living individual cells referred to as planktonic cells. Growth in biofilms leads to altered microbial metabolism, production of extracellular virulence factors, and decreased susceptibility to biocides, antimicrobial agents, and host defense molecules and cells. P. aeruginosa growing on the bronchial mucosa during chronic infection, staphylococci and other pathogens growing on implanted medical devices, and dental pathogens growing on tooth surfaces to form plaque are several examples of microbial biofilm growth associated with human disease. Many other pathogens can form biofilms during in vitro growth. It is increasingly accepted that this mode of growth contributes to microbial virulence and induction of disease and that biofilm formation can also be an important factor in microbial survival outside the host, promoting transmission to additional susceptible individuals."-Harrison 19/e p145e-4*

"Similarly, biofilms are associated with Streptococcus viridians on heart valves, Pseudomonas aeruginosa lung infections, Staphylococcus aureus on catheters, or Legionella pneumophila colonization of hospital water systems, among many others."- Jawetz 27/e p58

"Bacterial and fungal biofilms are colonies of slowly growing cells that are enclosed within an exopolymer matrix. The exopolysaccharide is negatively charged, which restricts positively charged antibiotics from reaching their target. This physical barrier restricts the diffusion of antimicrobial molecules and sometimes binds them. To be effective against infections in these compartments, antibiotics have to be able to penetrate the biofilm and endothelial barriers."-Goodman Gilman 12/e p1367

79. Ans. a. Mycobacterium   *(Ref: Ananthanarayan 10/e p; Jawetz 27/e p309, 199, 295, 192)*

The image shows acid-fast staining with blue background and clumps of pink bacilli. Bacilli are clustered together and single at some places. Acid fastness rules out Actinomyces and Corynebacterium. Nocardia appears as branching filaments, long and slender. Hence from the above scenario, the image should be the culture smear of Mycobacterium, showing many bacilli.

"In tissue, tubercle bacilli are thin, straight rods measuring about 0.4×3 μm. On artificial media, coccoid and filamentous forms are seen with variable morphology from one species to another. Mycobacteria cannot be classified as either gram positive or gram negative. When stained by basic dyes, they cannot be decolorized by alcohol, regardless of treatment with iodine. True tubercle bacilli are characterized by "acid fastness"—that is, 95% ethyl alcohol containing 3% hydrochloric acid (acid-alcohol) quickly decolorizes all bacteria except the mycobacteria. Acid fastness depends on the integrity of the waxy envelope. The Ziehl-Neelsen technique of staining is used for identification of acid-fast bacteria."-Jawetz 27/e p309

"Nocardiae: These bacteria are gram positive and catalase positive, and they produce urease. Nocardiae form extensive branching substrates and aerial filaments that fragment, breaking into coccobacillary cells. The cell walls contain mycolic acids that are shorter chained than those of Mycobacteria. They are considered to be weakly acid fast, that is, they stain with the routine acid-fast reagent (carbol fuchsin) and retain this dye when decolorized with 1–4% sulfuric acid instead of the stronger acid-alcohol decolorant."-Jawetz 27/e p199

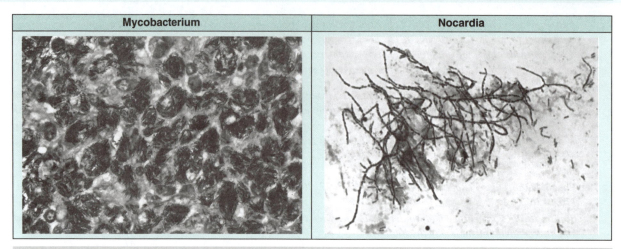

"Actinomyces: On Gram stain, they vary considerably in length; they may be short and club shaped or long, thin, beaded filaments. They may be branched or unbranched. Because they often grow slowly, prolonged incubation of the culture may be necessary before laboratory confirmation of the clinical diagnosis of actinomycosis can be made."-Jawetz 27/e p295

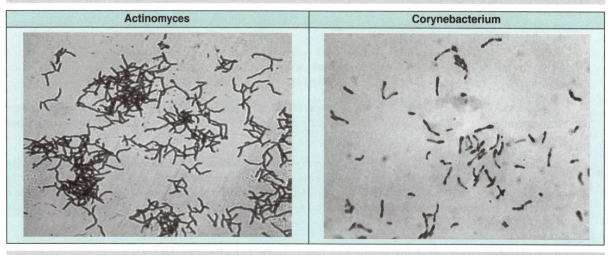

"Corynebacteria are 0.5–1 µm in diameter and several micrometers long. Characteristically, they possess irregular swellings at one end that give them the "club-shaped" appearance. Irregularly distributed within the rod (often near the poles) are granules staining deeply with aniline dyes (metachromatic granules) that give the rod a beaded appearance. Individual corynebacteria in stained smears tend to lie parallel or at acute angles to one another. True branching is rarely observed in cultures."- Jawetz 27/e p192

80. **Ans. b. Hepatitis** *(Ref: Ananthanarayan 10/e p548; Harrison 19/e p2005; Robbins 9/e p831-832; Jawetz 27/e p500)*
The given lifecycle is of hepatitis B virus.

"HBV attachment to a receptor on the surface of hepatocytes occurs via a portion of the pre-S region of hepatitis B surface antigen (HBsAg). After uncoating of the virus, unidentified cellular enzymes convert the partially double-stranded DNA to covalent closed circular (ccc) DNA that can be detected in the nucleus. The cccDNA serves as the template for the production of HBV mRNAs and the 3.5-kb RNA pre-genome. The pre-genome is encapsidated by a packaging signal located near the 5' end of the RNA into newly synthesized core particles, where it serves as template for the HBV reverse transcriptase encoded within the polymerase gene. An RNase H activity of the polymerase removes the RNA template as the negative-strand DNA is being synthesized. Positive-strand DNA synthesis does not proceed to completion within the core, resulting in replicative intermediates consisting of full-length minus-strand DNA plus variable-length (20–80%) positive-strand DNA. Core particles containing these DNA replicative intermediates bud from pre-Golgi membranes (acquiring HBsAg in the process) and may either exit the cell or reenter the intracellular infection cycle."-Jawetz 27/e p500

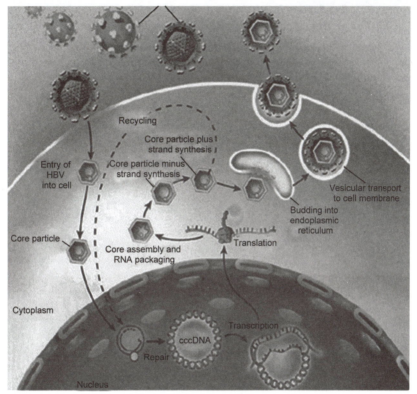

Fig. 23: Hepatitis B virus (HBV) replication cycle

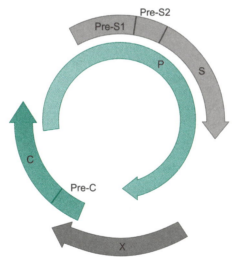

Fig. 24: Compact genomic structure of HBV

Hepatitis B virus Genes & Antigens	
Gene	Antigen Produced
C gene	HBcAg (Hepatitis B core antigen)[Q]
C & Pre C genes	HBeAg (Hepatitis B e antigen)[Q]
S gene	HBsAg (Hepatitis B surface antigen): large, middle & small HBsAg[Q]
P gene	DNA polymerase (pol) & reverse transcriptase[Q]
X gene	HBxAg: virus replication & transcriptional transactivator[Q]

81. **Ans. d. Balantidium coli**   *(Ref: Paniker 7/e p107, 109; Jawetz 27/e p705)*
In the given image, cilia are present all over the trophozoite. Balantidium coli is the only ciliate known to infect humans.

> *"Balantidium coli: Trophozoite is oval shaped with a slightly pointed anterior end with a grove, peristome leading to the mouth, cystostome. Rounded posterior end has a small anal pore, cytopyge and has a large kidney shaped macronucleus and small micronucleus."* -Paniker 7/e p109

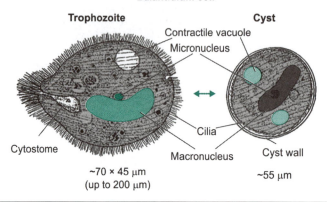

Balantidium coli
• Balantidium coli is a **large ciliated protozoal parasite**[Q] that can produce a spectrum of large-intestinal disease analogous to amebiasis. • **Only ciliate parasite of humans; Largest protozoan** parasite in **large intestine**[Q]

Life-cycle:
• **Balantidium coli** passes its **life cycle in one host only (monoxenous)**[Q].
• **Natural host: Pig**[Q]; **Accidental host: Man**[Q]; **Reservoirs: Pig, monkey & rat**[Q]
• **Infective form: Cyst**[Q]
  • **Mode of transmission:** Ingestion of **food & water contaminated with** feces containing the **cyst of B. coli**[Q].
  • **Ingested cysts liberate trophozoites**, which **reside & replicate in large bowel**[Q].

Pathogenesis: • In symptomatic patients, pathology in the bowel is **similar to amebiasis**, with varying degrees of **mucosal invasion, focal necrosis & ulceration**[Q].
Clinical Features: • Many patients remain **asymptomatic**, but some have **persisting intermittent diarrhea** & a few develop more **fulminant dysentery**[Q].
Diagnosis: • Diagnosis is made by detection of **trophozoite** stage in **stool or sampled colonic tissue**[Q].
Treatment: • **DOC: Tetracycline**[Q] (500 mg four times daily for 10 days)

82. **Ans. c. Giardia lamblia**   *(Ref: Paniker 7/e p31; Jawetz 27/e p710)*
In the given stool microscopy, quadrinucleate cyst of Giardia lamblia is seen.

> *"Giardia lamblia cyst: It is the infective form of the parasite. The cyst is small and oval, measuring 12mm x 8mm and is surrounded by a hyaline cyst wall. Its internal structure includes 2 pairs of nuclei grouped at one end. A young cyst contains 1 pair of nuclei. The axostyle lies diagonally, forming a dividing line within cyst wall. Remnants of the flagella and the sucking disc may be seen in the young cyst."* - Paniker 7/e p31

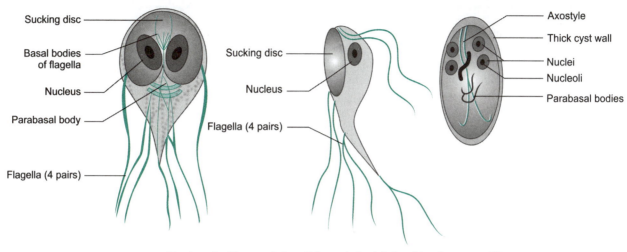

Fig. 25: Trophozoite (A-ventral view; B-Lateral view) & Quadrinucleate cyst (C)

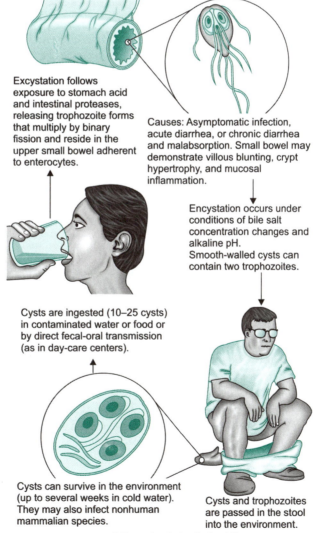

Fig. 26: Life cycle of giardia lamblia

Giardiasis

• Caused by **Giardia lamblia**[Q] (also known as **G. duodenalis** or **G. intestinalis**)
• **MC parasitic pathogen in humans**[Q]
• **Only common pathogenic protozoan** found in **duodenum & jejunum** of humans[Q]
• Infection may occur after **ingestion of as few as 10 cysts**[Q].
    • **Cysts** are **resistant to chlorine** (Giardia are **endemic in unfiltered public water supplies**)[Q].
    • Causes **decreased expression of brush-border enzymes** & cause **microvillous damage & apoptosis of small intestinal epithelial cells**[Q].

Pathology: • **Mode of Transmission:** Spread by **fecally contaminated water or food**[Q] • **Site of Infection: Small intestine**[Q] (Duodenum & jejunum) • **Clinical Incubation Period: 7–10 days**[Q]

Morphology:
• Two forms: Trophozoite & cyst
• **Giardia trophozoites:** Characteristic **pear shape** with **two equally sized nuclei & four pairs of flagella**[Q]
• **Cyst: Ellipsoid, thick-walled** with **four nuclei**[Q]
    • **Trophozoites** are **tightly bound to brush border of villous enterocytes without invasion**[Q]
    • **Villous blunting** with **increased numbers of intraepithelial lymphocytes** & mixed lamina propria inflammatory infiltrates in patients with **heavy infections**[Q].

Clinical Features: • Giardiasis may be subclinical or accompanied by **acute or chronic diarrhea**, **malabsorption, weight loss** & flatus due to **post-infectious irritable bowel syndrome** or **protein losing enteropathy**[Q]

Diagnosis:
• Diagnosed by **detection of parasite antigens in feces**, by **identification of cysts in feces** or **of trophozoites in feces or small intestines**, or by **nucleic acid amplification tests**[Q].
    • **Stool examination: Pear shaped & binucleate trophozoites**[Q]
    • **Small intestinal biopsy: Identification of organisms**[Q]

Treatment: • **DOC** for Giardiasis: **Metronidazole**[Q]
Prevention: • Prevented by **consumption of uncontaminated food & water**[Q]

83. Ans. b. Mycobacterium tuberculosis *(Ref: Clinical Tuberculosis, by Peter D.O. Davies 5/e p198; Infectious Diseases By Jonathan Cohen (2016)/p870)*

Urine lipoarabinomannan (LAM) is used for the diagnosis of Mycobacterium tuberculosis.

*"A recent innovative approach that has been explored is the **urinary detection of Lipoarabinomannan (LAM). LAM is a 17.5 kD glycolipid component of the outer cell wall of mycobacteria. LAM is heat stable, cleared by the kidney and detectable in urine. As a bacterial product, it has the theoretical potential to discriminate active TB from latent infection, the former having higher quantities of bacteria.** The sensitivity of urinary LAM in adults varies widely (44%-67%)."- Clinical Tuberculosis, by Peter D.O. Davies 5/e p198*

*"Thus, this is a major breakthrough for diagnosis **of HIV-associated TB and is now being widely implemented around the world. Another development is a simple, low-cost, lateral flow assay that detects the mycobacterial cell wall glycolipid antigen, lipoarabinomannan(LAM), in urine samples, permitting a diagnosis of TB to be made with high specificity within 30 minutes.**"-Infectious Diseases By Jonathan Cohen (2016)/p870*

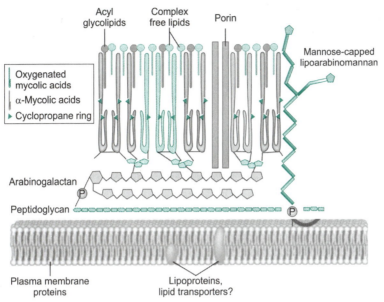

Fig. 27: Constituents of mycobacterium cell wall

84. **Ans. c. Plasmodium vivax and ovale** *(Ref: Harrison 19/e p1369; Paniker 7/e p66; Jawetz 27/e p718)*
    In *Plasmodium vivax* and *Plasmodium ovale* infections, a proportion of the intrahepatic forms remain inert for a period ranging from 3 weeks to ≥1 year before reproduction begins. These dormant forms, or hypnozoites, are the cause of the relapses that characterize infection with these two species.

> "In *P. vivax* and *P. ovale* infections, a proportion of the intrahepatic forms do not divide immediately but remain inert for a period ranging from 3 weeks to ≥1 year before reproduction begins. These dormant forms, or hypnozoites, are the cause of the relapses that characterize infection with these two species."- *Harrison 19/e p1369*

> "*P. vivax* and *P. ovale* may persist as dormant forms, or hypnozoites, after the parasites have disappeared from the peripheral blood. Resurgence of an erythrocytic infection (relapse) occurs when merozoites from hypnozoites in the liver break out, are not phagocytosed in the bloodstream, and succeed in reestablishing a red cell infection. Without treatment, *P. vivax* and *P. ovale* infections may persist as periodic relapses for up to 5 years."-*Jawetz 27/e p718*

\multicolumn{5}{c}{Characteristics of plasmodium species infecting Humans}				
Characteristic	**P. falciparum**	**P. vivax**	**P. ovale**	**P. malariae**
Incubation period	12 days (shortest)[Q]	14 days	14 days	30 days (longest)[Q]
Duration of erythrocytic cycle (hours)	48 (malignant tertian malaria)[Q]	48 (benign tertian malaria)	50 (ovale tertian malaria)	72 (Quatran malaria)[Q]
Red cell preference	Younger cells[Q] (but can invade cells of all ages), >2% of RBC infected[Q]	Red cells upto 14 days old[Q], <1% of RBC infected	Reticulocytes[Q]	Older cells[Q]
Morphology	Usually only **ring forms, banana shaped gametocytes**[Q]	Irregularly shaped **large rings and trophozoites; enlarged erythrocytes; Schuffner's dots**[Q]	Infected erythrocytes **enlarged and oval with tufted ends**[Q]; **Schuffner's dots**	**Band of rectangular forms** of trophozoites common
Pigment	Black[Q]	Yellow-brown[Q]	Dark brown[Q]	Brown-black[Q]
Relapse (hypnozoits or exo-erythrocytic schizogony)	No	Yes[Q]	Yes[Q]	No

Stages	Parasites			
	Plasmodium vivax	*Plasmodium ovale*	*Plasmodium malariae*	*Plasmodium falciparum*
Ring stage				
Developing trophozoite				
Developing schizont				
Schizont				
Microgametocyte				
Macrogametocyte				

Blood Smears of Plasmodium				
Features	**P. falciparum**	**P. vivax**	**P. malariae**	**P. ovale**
Features of red cells				
Size	All sizes/ normal	Large (young) pale	Small (Old), normal	Large (young)
Shape	Round, may be crenated	Round or oval	Round	Round or pear-shaped fimbriated
Stippling	**Maurer's clefts**[Q] Large; red up to 20 Basophilic stippling ±	**Schuffner's dots**[Q]; numerous small red	None, Occasionally **Zieman's dots**[Q]	**Schuffner's dots, James dot**[Q]
Features of Parasite				
Ring (early trophozoite)	**Threadlike, multiple infections, double chromatin dots form accole**[Q]	**Thicker**[Q]	**Compact**[Q]	**Compact**[Q]
Mature/Late trophozoites (amoeboid form)	**Absent**/ occasionally seen	**Ameboid** may fill cell	More regular, smaller, **Band form**[Q]	**Less ameboid** & smaller than those of P vivax
Diagnostic keys				
	Gametocyte, multiple rings, double chromatin dots, accole forms, heavy infection[Q]	**Schizont, large RBCs, amoeboid forms**[Q]	**Schizont, small RBCs, band forms**[Q]	**Schizont and large RBCs; pear-shaped, fimbriated RBCs**[Q]

| AIIMS November 2017 | 483 |

FORENSIC MEDICINE

85. Ans. a. McNaughten's rule   *(Ref: Reddy 34/e p459, 460, 33/e p493)*

In the question, description of McNaughten's rule is given.

> *"McNaughten's Rule: An accused person is not legally responsible, if it is clearly proved, that at the time of committing the crime, he was suffering from such a defect of reason from abnormality of mid, that he did not know the nature and quality of the act he was doing, or that what he was doing was wrong."-Reddy 34/e p459*

> *"Durham rule (1954): An accused person is not criminally responsible, if his unlawful act is the mental disease or mental defect."-Reddy 34/e p460*

> *"Curren's rule (1961): An accused person is not criminally responsible, if at the time of committing the act, he did not have the capacity to regulate his conduct to the requirements of the law, as a result of mental disease or defect."-Reddy 34/e p460*

> *"American Law Institute Test (1972): A person is not responsible for criminal conduct, if at the time of such conduct, as the result of mental disease or defect, he lacks adequate capacity either to appreciate the criminality of his conduct or to the requirements of the law."- Reddy 34/e p460*

McNaughten's Rule (Legal test or right or Wrong Test)

- Deals with **responsibilities of mentally ill persons in criminal cases.**
- An **accused person is not legally responsible**, if it is clearly proved, that **at the time of committing the crime**, he was **suffering from such a defect of reason from abnormality of mid, that he did not know the nature and quality of the act he was doing, or that what he was doing was wrong.**
  - **Section 84 IPC** states that: **Nothing is an offence** which is **done by a person, who at the time of doing it, by reason of unsoundness of mind, is incapable of knowing the nature of the act, or that he is doing what is either wrong or contrary to the law."**

It must be clearly proved that:

- The **offence is directly related to the insanity**
- The **offence could not have occurred if there was no mental abnormality**
- Insanity subsequent to the act is not a defence.

86. Ans. d. Orbicularis oculi, facial muscles, thorax, upper limb   *(Ref: Reddy 34/e p152, 33/e p161)*

According to Nysten's rule, order of development of rigor mortis is orbicularis oculi, facial muscles, thorax, upper limb.

> *"Order of appearance of Rigor: All muscles of the body, both voluntary and involuntary are affected. It does not start in all muscles simultaneously (Nysten's rule). It first appears in the involuntary muscles; the myocardium becomes rigid in hour. It begins in the eyelids, neck and lower jaw and passes upwards to the muscles of the face, and downwards to the muscles of the chest, upper limbs, abdomen and lower limbs and lastly in the fingers and toes."-Reddy 34/e p152*

Rigor Mortis

- In **India, Rigor mortis commences in 2-3 hours**, takes about **12 hours to develop from head to foot, persist for another 12 hours** and **takes about 12 hours to pass off[Q].**
- So if **rigor mortis is not set in**, the **time since death** would be **within 2 hours** & if it has **affected the whole body**, the **time since death would be 12-24 hours[Q].**
- It does not start in all muscles simultaneously (**Nysten's rule[Q]**).

Order of Appearance & Disappearance

- **Heart (Left chamber in 1 hour)** → **Eyelids (3-4 hours)** → Face muscles → Neck & trunk → Upper extremities → Legs → Small muscles of **fingers & toes (Last to be affected, 11-12 hours)[Q].**
- **It passes off in same order of appearance.**
- It takes about **12 hours to develop from head to foot, persist for another 12 hours** & takes about **12 hours to pass off[Q].**
- It usually **lasts for 18-36 hours in summer** & **24-48 hours in winter[Q].**

- **Rigor mortis may not be perceivable in many infant & child corpses due to their smaller muscle mass[Q]**

87. Ans. b. Gynecologist can abort the fetus upon the patient request *(Ref: Reddy 34/e p388, 33/e p416; Shaw 15/e p244-245, Williams 24/e p368)*

Consent of woman is required before conducting abortion. Written consent of guardian is required if the woman is a minor (<18 years) or mentally ill person. In the question, age of patient is 14 years only, so the consent of the guardian is required for termination. Termination is permitted upto 20 weeks of pregnancy only. So, gynecologist cannot abort the fetus upon the patient request.

"The (rape) victim is examined in the presence of a third person, preferably a female nurse or a female relative of the woman whose name should be recorded."- Reddy 34/e p388

Medical termination of pregnancy Act, 1971

- **MTP act** was **passed** in **August 1971 in India** & came into **effect from April 1972**[Q]
- Extends to whole of India **except Jammu & Kashmir**[Q]

Indications of MTP	
Therapeutic	• Continuation of pregnancy **endangers the life of woman** or may cause **serious injury to physical or mental health**[Q].
Eugenic	• When there is risk of the child being born with serious physical or mental abnormalities. This may occur: • If the pregnant woman in **first three months suffers from: German measles, smallpox or chicken pox, toxoplasmosis, viral hepatitis** or any severe viral infection[Q] • **Drug treatment: Thalidomide, cortisone, antimitotic drugs, hallucinogens** or **antidepressants**[Q]. • Mother is treated by **X-rays or radioisotopes**[Q] • **Insanity of parents**[Q]
Humanitarian	• **Pregnancy caused by rape**[Q]
Social	• Pregnancy due to **failure of contraceptive methods,** likely to cause serious injury to mental health[Q]. • When **social or economic environment,** actual or reasonably expected **can injure the mother's health**[Q].

Rules for MTP

- **Only a qualified registered medical practitioner**[Q] possessing prescribed experience **can terminate pregnancy**[Q]. Chief medical officer (CMO) of district is empowered to certify that a doctor has the **necessary training** to do abortions. A medical practitioner can qualify if has **assisted in performance of 25 cases of MTP in a recognized hospital**[Q].
- Pregnancy should be terminated in **government hospitals**[Q] or in the **hospitals recognized by government** for this purpose[Q]

  - **Non-governmental institutions** may take up abortion if they obtain a **license form CMO of the district**[Q].
  - **Consent of woman**[Q] is required before conducting abortion. **Written consent of guardian** is required if the woman is a **minor (<18 years)**[Q] or **mentally ill person**[Q] **(consent of husband is not necessary)**
  - **Abortion cannot be performed on the request of husband,** if the **woman** herself is **not willing**[Q].

- **Woman need not produce proof of her age**[Q]: Statement of woman that she is >18 years of age is accepted
- It is **enough for the woman to state that she was raped**[Q]: It is not necessary to lodge a complaint with the police
- **Professional secrecy has to be maintained: Admission register** for MTP is secret document & information should not be disclosed to any person.
- If the **period of pregnancy** is between **12 & 20 weeks, two doctors must agree that there is an indication** once the opinion is formed, the **termination can be done by any one doctor**[Q].
- **Termination is permitted up to 20 weeks of pregnancy**[Q]

  - **In an emergency, pregnancy can be terminated by a single doctor, even without required training (even after 20 weeks), without consulting a second doctor, in a private hospital, which is not recognized**[Q].
  - **Termination of pregnancy** by a person who is **not registered medical practitioner** (person concerned), or in an **unrecognised hospital** (the administrative head) shall be **punished with rigorous imprisonment** for a term which **shall not be <2 years, but which may extend to seven years**[Q].

AIIMS November 2017

88. Ans. a. Capitate *(Ref: Reddy 34/e p73, 33/e p72)*

Capitate is the first carpal bone to ossify. Sequence of ossification in carpal bones: <u>C</u>apitate→<u>H</u>amate →<u>T</u>riquetral →<u>Lu</u>nate →<u>S</u>caphoid →<u>T</u>rapezoid →<u>T</u>rapezium →<u>P</u>isiform (CHaT LuST TraP).

> "As a rule, ossification begins centrally in an epiphysis and spreads peripherally as it gets bigger. At first, it is entirely amorphous, rounded and pinhead sized. As it grows, bones are ossified from a single centre, e.g., carpus and tarsus. **The ossification centres in carpal bones appear as follows: capitate 2 to 3 months, hamate first year; triquetral 3, lunate 4, scaphoid and trapezoid 5, trapezium 6, pisiform 11 years. At the end of one year, two carpal bones are seen in X-ray of the wrist. Between 2 to 6 years, the number of carpal bones present on X-ray indicates the approximate age in years."**- *Reddy 33/e p72*

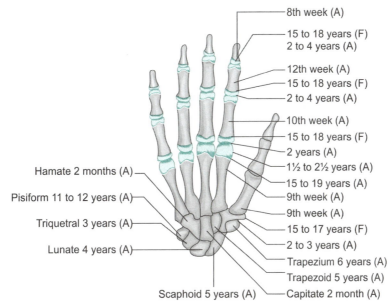

Fig. 28: Appearance and fusion of epiphysis in bones of hand

Ossification of Carpal Bones

- Ossification of carpal bones occurs in a predictable sequence, **starting with capitate & ending with pisiform.**
- **At birth**, there is **no calcification in carpal bones**.

Ossification of Carpal Bones (CHaT LuST TraP)				
Bone	**Ossification time**	**Bone**	**Ossification time**
<u>C</u>apitate	1-3 months[Q]	<u>S</u>caphoid	4-6 years[Q]
<u>H</u>amate	2-4 months[Q]	<u>T</u>rapezium	4-6 years[Q]
<u>T</u>riquetral	2-3 years[Q]	<u>T</u>rapezoid	4-6 years[Q]
<u>Lu</u>nate	2-4 years[Q]	<u>P</u>isiform	8-12 years[Q]

- **Ossification centers of distal radius & ulna (Distal radius: 1 year & Distal ulna: 5-6 years)[Q]**

Appearance of Centres of Ossification & Union of Bones & Epiphysis		
Age	**Appearance of Centres of Ossification**	**Union of Bones & Epiphysis**
5th year	Head of radius, trapezoid, scaphoid[Q]	Greater tubercle fuses with head of humerus[Q]
6th year	Lower end of ulna, trapezium[Q]	Rami of pubis & ischium unite[Q]
6th to 7th year	Medial epicondyle of humerus[Q]	–
9th year	Olecranon[Q]	–

Contd...

Contd...

Age	Appearance of Centres of Ossification	Union of Bones & Epiphysis
9th to 11th year	Trochlea of humerus[Q]	–
10th to 11th year	Pisiform[Q]	–
11th year	Lateral epicondyle of humerus[Q]	–
13th year	Separate centres in triradiate cartilage of acetabulum[Q]	–
12th to 14th year	Lesser trochanter of femur[Q]	–
14th year	Crest of ilium; head & tubercles of ribs[Q]	Medial epicondyle of humerus; lateral epicondyle with trochlea; patella complete[Q]
15th year	Acromian[Q]	Coracoid with scapula; triradiate cartilage of acetabulum[Q]
16th year	Ischial tuberosity[Q]	Lower end of humerus; olecranon to ulna; upper end of radius; metacarpals; proximal phalanges[Q]
17th to 18th year	–	Head of femur; lesser 7 greater trochanter of femur; acromian; lower end of ulna[Q]
18th to 19th year	Inner end of clavicle[Q]	Lower end of femur; upper end of tibia & fibula; head of humerus; lower end of radius[Q]
20th to 21st year	–	Iliac crest; inner head of clavicle; ischial tuberosity, head of ribs[Q]

First primary center of ossification First bone to ossify	• Clavicle[Q]
First secondary center of ossification	• Lower end of femur[Q]
First bone to completely ossify	• Ossicles[Q]
First tarsal bone to ossify	• Calcaneum[Q]

89. Ans. a. Arsenic *(Rerf: Reddy 34/e p482, 33/e p540; Lippincott's Manual of Toxicology edited by Joshua J. Lynch (2012)/ p1970)*

Blackfoot's disease, a form of arsenic-induced peripheral vascular disease resulting in gangrene, is caused by arsenic poisoning.

"Subacute or chronic symptoms from arsenic poisoning include anemia, leukopenia, aplastic anemia, and sensory motor neuropathy. Arsenic-induced skin changes may include hyperpigmentation, hypopigmentation, hyperkeratosis, Bowen's disease, squamous cell cancers, basal cell cancers, or Blackfoot's disease (a form of arsenic-induced peripheral vascular disease resulting in gangrene). Mees lines (transverse white lines in the nails) occur in a minority of arsenic toxic patients."– Lippincott's Manual of Toxicology edited by Joshua J. Lynch (2012)/p197

Arsenic Poisoning		
Black Foot	Aldrich-Mees lines	Raindrop pigmentation

Poisoning	Characteristic Features
Arsenic (As)	• **Blackfoot's disease**[Q] (a form of arsenic-induced peripheral vascular disease resulting in gangrene) • **Yellow colour of skin, hair & mucous membrane**[Q] • **Raindrop type of pigmentation**[Q] • **Aldrich-Mees lines**[Q] (transverse white lines in the nails) • **Milk rose (Brownish pigmentation)**[Q]

Contd...

Copper (Cu)	• **Jaundiced skin**^{Q} • **Green-Blue skin, hair & perspiration**^{Q} • **Green-Purple line of gums**^{Q}
Mercury (Hg)	• **Brown/Black-Blue line on gums**^{Q} with **loosening of tooth & necrosis of jaw** • **Brown deposits on anterior lens capsule**^{Q} **(Mercuria lentis)** • **Acrodynia (Pink disease)**^{Q}
Lead (Pb)	• **Blue stippled burtonian line on gums**^{Q}, especially on **upper jaw near dirty & infected teeth**

90. **Ans. c. 1 =d, 2=a, 3=b, 4=c** *(Ref: Reddy 34/e p25, 278, 600, 33/e p26, 400, 647; Parikh 6/e p1.26)*

1. Geneva	Ethics
2. Tokyo	Torture
3. Oslo	Abortion
4. Helsinki	Human experimentation

Declaration of **Geneva (1948)**	**Modernized version of Hippocratic oath**^{Q}
Declaration of **London (1949)**	International code of **medical ethics**
Declaration of **Helsinki (1964)**	**Human experimentation & clinical trials**^{Q}
Declaration of **Sydney (1968)**	Definition of **death & recovery of organs**
Declaration of **Oslo (1970)**	**Therapeutic (legalized) abortion**^{Q}
Declaration of **Munich (1973)**	**Discrimination in medicine**
Declaration of **Tokyo (1975)**	**Torture & medicine**^{Q}
Declaration of **Lisbon (1981)**	**Rights of patients**
Declaration of **Venice (1983)**	**Terminal illness**
Declaration of **Malta (1992)**	**Role of doctors in hunger strikes**
Declaration of **Istanbul (2008)**	**Organ trafficking & transplant tourism**

91. **Ans. b. 1 =b, 2=c, 3=d, 4=a** *(Ref: Reddy 34/e p559, 554, 516, 33/e p602, 596, 555; Modern Medical Toxicology By Pillay (2012)/p 285; APC Essentials of Forensic Medicine and Toxicology/p509, 536)*

1. Cocaine	White lady
2. LSD	Purple haze
3. Abrus	Gunchi
4. Capsaicin	Human hand

*"**Cocaine:** It is obtained from the **leaves of Erythroxylum coca,** which grows wild in South America, India, Java, etc. **The leaves contain about 0.5 to 1% cocaine.** It is a colourless, odourless, crystalline substance with bitter taste. **It contains alkaloids ecgonine, hygrine, and cinnamyl cocaine. It is used as local anaesthetic. It is also known as coke, snow, Cadillac and white lady. Crack is prepared by combining cocaine with baking soda and water, which is suitable for smoking.**"-Reddy 34/e p559*

*"**LSD Post-hallucinogen Perception Disorder:** A persistent perceptual disorder often described by the person as if he is residing in a bubble under water in a "**purple haze**" with trailing of lights and images. Associated anxiety, panic and depression are common."- Modern Medical Toxicology By Pillay (2012)/p 285*

*"**Abrus precatorius (Ratti, Gunchi, Jequirity, Crab's eye, Rosary pea) is a slender, perennial climber found all over India that twins around trees, shrubs and hedges.**"-APC Essentials of Forensic Medicine and Toxicology/p509*

*"**Hunan Hand: Intense burning pain, hyperalgesia, erythema and dermatitis, after handling chili (Capsicum annuum) powder with bare hands.** Common in cooks, who prepare food with chilies without using gloves. **Hunan hand is so named because it was common in Hunan province of China. Capsaicin releases Substance P, an undecapeptide from afferent sensory neurons causing pain. The symptoms are due to nerve receptor stimulation and not local injury to the skin.**"-APC Forensic Medicine and Toxicology/p536*

92. Ans. a. Hair *(Ref: Reddy 34/e p206-208, 33/e p217-219)*

To calculate range, required findings are presence of burning or singeing (due to flame), blacking (due to smoke) & tattooing (due to gun powder). Given finding is tattooing which is seen upto intermediate range. To check if the gun was fired from near, then hair should be analyzed for presence of any singeing or smoke deposits. The same can be done with clothes, however, the injury here is on the skull, and hence the better answer is hair.

"The hair of the trunk and limbs may be completely burnt around the wound. If the distance is greater, the keratin of the hair may melt with the flame, and then solidify on cooling, producing clubbed appearance of the hair because of rounded bulges at the tips." - Reddy 34/e p206

Feature	Contact Shot	Close Shot	Near Shot	Distant Shot
Definition, Range and Discharge reaching victim	**In firm (hard or actual) contact**, muzzle end is pushed hard against the skin & all **discharge from muzzle are blown into the track taken by bullet**[Q], producing severe disruption of deeper tissues	When victim is **within the range of flame. Point blank** is used when range is very close to or in near contact with skin & is with in range of all discharge from muzzle.	When victim is **within the range of gun-powder** but outside the range of flame.	When victim is **outside the range of all** discharges of muzzle **except bullet.**
Rifled firearm (Revolver, Pistol) range Shot gun range (~)	In touch with skin	5-8 cm (2.5-7.5 cm) Short range (1-2 meter)	Up to 50 cm (60cm) Intermediate range (2-4 metres)	>50 cm (or 60cm) Long (distant) range (>4 metres)
Discharge	**Bullet, gun powder, soot,** (smoke, carbon particles), **gases, flame** (fire, burn, heat) with **imprinted barrel marks & tearing in actual contact**[Q]	Bullet, gun powder, soot, gases and burn	Bullet, gun powder, and ± soot	**Only bullet** (± coarse particles of gun powder)
Blast effect	**Muzzle end imprint, eversion of edges, back spatter, soiling** of internal structures & pocket formation, **burst (comminution) fracture of skull and crazy paving fracture of base of skull**[Q] are all seen	**Absent**	**Absent**	**Absent**
Heat Effect on surface & cloths	Absent	**Scorching of skin, singeing of hair & burning melting – ironing of cloths present**	**Absent**	**Absent**
Blackening (smudging)	**Absent outside present inside the track**[Q]	**Present outside**[Q] the wound	Absent (±)	Absent
Tattooing	Absent outside present inside	**Present outside**	**Present outside**	Absent (±)
Abrasion / Grease collar	Absent outside present inside	**Present**	**Present**	Present (skin adjacent to hole shows two zones inner grease & outer abrasion collar)
Lead snow storm	**Absent**	**Absent**	**Absent**	Present (on x-ray) in shotgun injury
Carboxy Hb, Cherry red discoloration	Present **in wound track**	Present in surrounding tissue	+	±
Surrounding skin around entrance wound shows	**No** burning, blackening (soot), tattooing, abrasion/grease collar	**Burning, blackening (soot), tattooing, abrasion / grease collar** present	**Tattooing & abrasion / grease collar** present	**Abrasion** (grease / dirt) **collar & lead storm** present
Entrance Wound Size	**Largest**	Bullet size	Smaller	**Smallest** due to initial stretching of skin

Contd...

Contd...

Feature	Contact Shot	Close Shot	Near Shot	Distant Shot
Shape	Stellate (star shaped[Q]), triangular, cruciform (cruciate[Q]) or raged (irregular with crenated & scalloped edges)	Circular (or rat hole[Q])	Circular (central big wound with smaller wounds around)	Circular (wide spread[Q])
Number	Single	Single	Multiple	Multiple
Edges (Margin)	Scorched, contused, undermined or everted margins from which tears (lacerations) over skin radiating outwards from entrance hole because of expansion of gases (between scalp & skull)	Inverted & well defined	Inverted	Inverted

93. Ans. b. Throttling *(Ref: Reddy 34/e p329, 33/e p352; Knight's Forensic Pathology 4/e p374)*

On external examination, a single abrasion is seen, likely due to assailant's fingers grasping the neck. Bruising of the neck is seen as well. On internal examination, we can see contused tissues of the neck with bleeding from strap muscles. All these features are suggestive of throttling. Hanging can be ruled out in absence of ligature mark. Absence of ligature mark rules out ligature strangulation.

"Throttling or Manual Strangulation: Asphyxia produced by compression of the neck by human hands is called throttling. Death occurs due to occlusion of carotid arteries. Occlusion of airway plays minor role."- Reddy 34/e p329

"Postmortem Appearances: External-Bruises on the neck: The situation and extent of the bruised area on the neck will depend upon the relative positions of assailant and victim, the manner of grasping neck, and the degree of pressure exerted upon the throat. The bruises are produced by the tips or the pads of the fingers."- Reddy 34/e p329

Smothering: If the orifices are closed by the hand, there may be scratches, distinct nail marks, or laceration of the soft parts of the victim face. The lips, gum and tongue may show bruising or laceration. Slight bruising may be found in the mouth and nose, which should be confirmed by microscopy. The asphyxial signs and symptoms are severe, because death usually results due to slow asphyxia and often the fatal period is three to five minutes."- Reddy 34/e p329

Throttling or Manual Strangulation
• **Asphyxia produced by compression of the neck by human hands** is called **throttling[Q]**.
• **Death** occurs due to **occlusion of carotid arteries. Occlusion of airway** plays **minor role.**
• **Vagal inhibition** is much **more common in manual strangulation** than with a ligature[Q].

Usual Diagnostic Signs of Death due to Manual Strangulation	
• **Cutaneous bruising & abrasions[Q]**	• Fracture of **larynx, thyroid cartilage & hyoid bone[Q]**
• **Extensive bruising** with or without **rupture of neck muscles[Q]**	• **Cricoid cartilage** is almost **exclusively fractured in throttling[Q]**
• **Engorgement of the tissues at & above the level of compression[Q]**	• General signs of **asphyxia[Q]**

PSM

94. Ans. a. 60 *(Ref: Park 24/e p559)*

In a subcenter area with crude birth rate of 20, the expected number of ANC registrations should be approximately 55.

Number of Expected Pregnancies per Year
• Expected no. of live-births (Y)/year = Birth rate (per 1000 population) x Population of the area/1000

• As some pregnancies may not result in a live birth (i.e., **abortions & stillbirth may occur**), the expected number of live births would be an under-estimation of the total number of pregnancies. Hence, a correction factor of 10% is required, i.e., add 10% to the figure obtained above.

• **Total number of Expected Pregnancies Z = Y + 10% of Y**
• **Population under the subcentre = 5000**
• **Birth rate = 20**

Contd...

Contd...

Number of Expected Pregnancies per Year
• **Expected no. of live-births (Y)/year = 20 x 5000/1000 = 100** • Total number of Expected Pregnancies **Z** = Y + 10% of Y = 100 + 10% of 100 = 110 • **Expected number of ANC registrations will be half of yearly calculation = 55**

95. Ans. a. 1 and 2 *(Ref: Park 24/e p118)*

If the colour of inner square is the same colour or darker than the outer circle, the vaccine has been exposed to too much heat and should be discarded. Vaccine 1 and 2 can be used.

"Monitoring heat exposure using vaccine vial monitor: Vaccine vial monitors (VVMs) are the only temperature monitoring devices that routinely accompany vaccines throughout the entire supply chain. A VVM is a chemical indicator label attached to the vaccine container (vial, ampoule or dropper) by the vaccine manufacturer. As the container moves through the supply chain, the VVM records its cumulative heat exposure through a gradual change in colour. If the colour of inner square is the same colour or darker than the outer circle, the vaccine has been exposed to too much heat and should be discarded."- Park 24/e p118

Symbol	Explanation	Stage
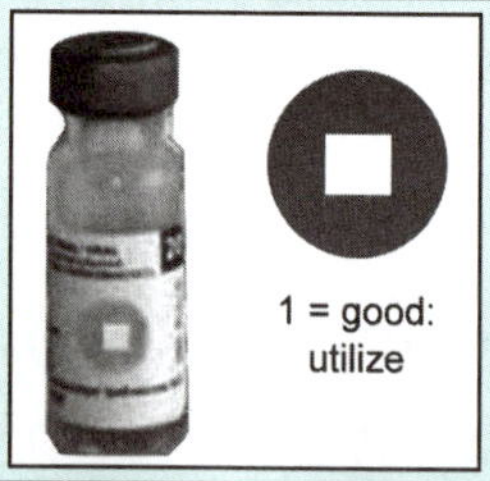 1 = good: utilize	• The **inner square is lighter than the outer circle** • If the expiry date has not passed, **use the vaccine**	I
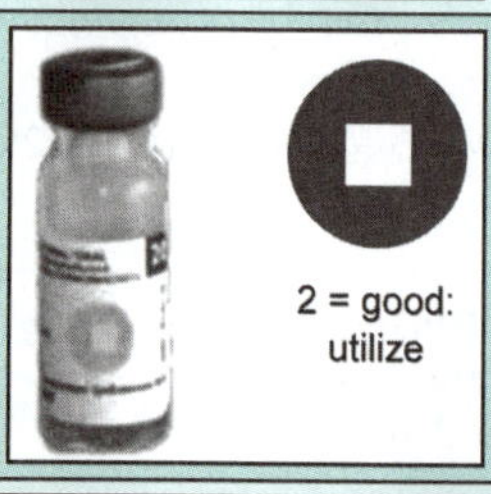 2 = good: utilize	• As the time passes, the **inner square is still lighter than the outer circle** • If the expiry date has not passed, **use the vaccine**	II
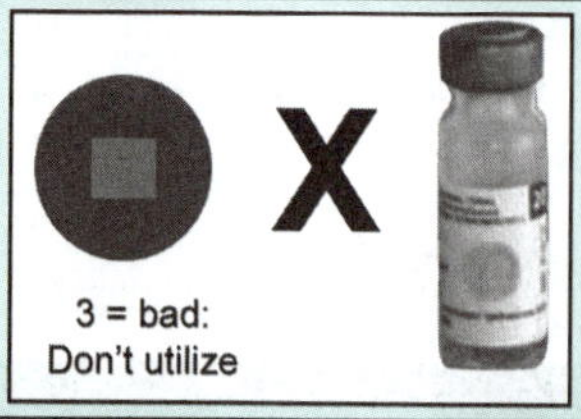 3 = bad: Don't utilize	• **Discard point:** The **colour of inner square matches that of the outer circle** • **Do not use the vaccine**	III
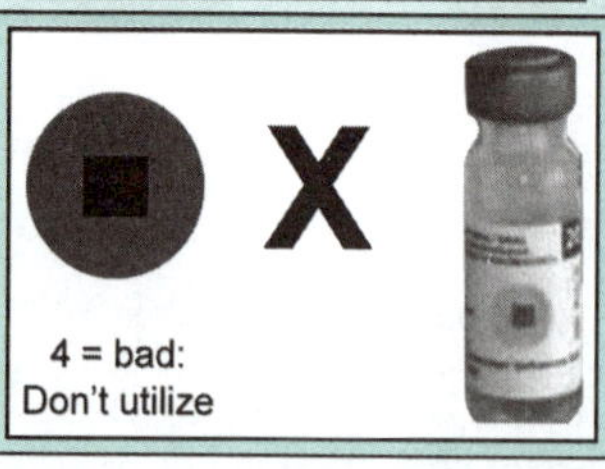 4 = bad: Don't utilize	• **Beyond the discard point: Inner square is darker than the outer circle** • **Do not use the vaccine**	IV

Vaccine Vial Monitors (VVMs)
• **VVMs** are the only **temperature monitoring devices** that **routinely accompany vaccines throughout the entire supply chain.** • A **VVM** is a **chemical indicator label attached to vaccine container** (vial, ampoule or dropper) by the vaccine manufacturer.

Contd...

AIIMS November 2017

- As the container moves through the supply chain, the **VVM records its cumulative heat exposure through a gradual change in colour.**
    - If the **colour of inner square** is the **same** colour or **darker than the outer circle, vaccine has been exposed to too much heat & should be discarded.**

Types of VVM
• Four types of **VVM** to **match the heat sensitivity** of vaccine: **VVM2, VVM7, VVM14, VVM30** • **VVM number**: **Time in days** that it takes for the **inner square to reach the colour indicating the discard point**, if the vial is exposed to a constant temperature of **37°C.**

VVM Locations	
On the Vaccine Label	**Other than Vaccine Label**
• **Vaccine vial, once opened** can be **kept for subsequent immunization sessions upto 28 days**, regardless of the formulation of product (liquid or freeze dried)	• **Vaccine vial, once opened** must be **discarded at the end of the immunization session** or **within six hours** whichever comes first regardless of the product (liquid or freeze dried)

Advantages of VVM
• Main purpose of VVM: To ensure that heat-damaged vaccines are nor administered • To decide, which vaccines can be safely be kept after a cold chain break occurs, minimizing unnecessary vaccine wastage. • VVM status helps to decide which vaccine should be used first   • VVMs do not measure exposure to the freezing temperature.

96. Ans. b. Ordinal   *(Ref: High yield Biostatistics 2/e p4; BK Mahajan 6/e p11-13, 36-48, 58-76)*

Chronic liver disease is classified into Child–Pugh class A to C, employing the added score from above. Class A: 5–6, B: 7–9, C: 10–15. This is ordinal scale as the data can be arranged in a meaningful order but there is no information about the size of the interval between them.

Types of Statistical data			
Qualitative Data		**Quantitative data**	
No notion of magnitude or **size of variables**[Q] (as they cannot be measured) **Variables** can be **categorized according to** some **characteristics or quality** **Example:** Sex, marital status, education level, vaccinated or not vaccinated, grades in the class. **Qualitative data** can be placed on 2 scales: **Nominal & Ordinal**		**Quantitative data have a magnitude**[Q], i.e. they can be measured. **Example:** Height, weight, blood pressure, serum cholesterol level, temperature, number of children in a family etc. **Quantitative data** can be measured on 2 scales: **Interval & Ratio scales**	
Nominal Scale	• **Data cannot be placed in a meaningful order**[Q] • Nominal scale data are **divided into qualitative categories or groups**, such as **male/female, black/white, died/cured, attacked/not attacked, vaccinated/not vaccinate, urban/sub urban/rural.** • There is **no implication of order or ratio**, means that the **data cannot be placed in a meaningful order**[Q].	**Interval scale**	• Interval scale data can be **placed in a meaningful order with meaningful intervals** between items, **which can be measured**[Q]. • **Example: Temperature on the Celsius scale** (the difference between 80° and 70° is the same as between 40° and 30°) • Interval scale data **do not have an absolute zero, ratios of the scores are not meaningful**, i.e. 80 °C of Celsius temperature is not twice as hot as 40 °C because 0 °C does not indicated a complete absence of heat.
Ordinal Scale	• **Data** can be **placed into categories that can be rank ordered** (e.g. students may be ranked 1st/2nd/3rd/4th etc.) • **No information about the size of interval**[Q], i.e. no conclusion can be drawn about whether the difference between the 1st & 2nd students is the same as the difference between 2nd & 3rd.	**Ratio Scale**	• Ratio scale **has an absolute zero, meaningful ratio do exist**[Q].

AIIMS ESSENCE

Contd...

	Qualitative Data		Quantitative data
	• Variables in the form of **mild, moderate & severe** (or **very satisfied, satisfied & dissatisfied**) are analyzed by ordinal scale as they can be **arranged in a meaningful order** but there is **no information about the size of interval between them**[Q].	**Ratio Scale**	• **Example: weights, time, blood pressure, temperature on the Kelvin scale** (not Celsius scale), on the Kelvin scale, zero degrees indicate an absolute absence of heat, just as a zero pulse indicates an absolute absence of heartbeat. Thus we can say that 400 K is twice as hot as 200 K.

97. **Ans. c. ARR = 1% and RR = 0.9** *(Ref: Park 24/e p83)*

In the given situation, absolute risk reduction (ARR) is 1% and relative risk (RR) is 0.9.

Relative Risk (RR)	Attributable Risk (AR)	Population Attributable Risk (PAR)
$RR = I_{Exp} / I_{Non\text{-}exp}$	$AR = (I_{Exp} - I_{Non\text{-}exp})/ I_{Non\text{-}exp} \times 100$	$AR = (I_{Total} - I_{Non\text{-}exp})/ I_{Total} \times 100$
• **RR** is the **ratio of the risk in the exposed divided by the risk in the unexposed.**	• **AR** indicates the **number of cases of a disease among exposed individuals that can be attributed to that exposure** • It is **excess risk** or **risk difference** • **Useful measure of extent of public health problem caused by an exposure**	• PAR indicates the number (or proportion) of cases that would not occur in a population if the factor were eliminated.

	Control group (old drug)	Intervention group (New drug)
Developed HT complications	1800	1620
Did not develop HT complications	13425	13605
Total subjects	15225	15225

- **IC** = Incidence of events (hypertensive complications) in the control group = **1800/15225 = 0.118 = 11.8%**
- **IT** = Incidence of events (hypertensive complications) in the treatment group = **1620/15225 = 0.106 = 10.6%**
- **Absolute risk reduction (ARR) is also known as risk difference.**
- **ARR = IC–IT = 11.8 –10.6 = 1.2%**
- **Relative risk (RR) = IT/IC = 0.106/0.118 = 0.9**

98. **Ans. b. Highly likely that patient has the disease** *(Ref: Park 24/e p149, 23/e p141)*

If the result of highly sensitive test is positive, it is highly likely that patient has the disease.

"Sensitivity: The term sensitivity was introduced by Yerushalmy in 1940s as a statistical index of diagnostic accuracy. It has been defined as the ability of a test to identify correctly all those who have the disease, that is true positive."- Park 24/e p149

Sensitivity	• Proportion of persons with the condition who test positive: True positive /(True positive + False negative)[Q]
Specificity	• Proportion of persons without the condition who test negative: True negative /(False positive + True negative)[Q]

Assessment & Value of A Diagnostic Test		
	Condition Present	Condition Absent
Positive Test	a (True positive)	b (False positive)
Negative Test	c (False negative)	d (True negative)

Sensitivity	Proportion of persons with the condition who test positive: $a /(a + c)$[Q]
Specificity	Proportion of persons without the condition who test negative: $d /(b + d)$[Q]
Positive predictive value (PPV)	Proportion of persons with a positive test who have the condition: $a /(a + b)$[Q]
Negative predictive value (NPV)	Proportion of persons with a negative test who do not have the condition: $d /(c + d)$[Q]

Predictive Value
• Prevalence, sensitivity, and specificity determine predictive value[Q] • PPV = Prevalence × Sensitivity /(Prevalence × Sensitivity) + (1 − Prevalence)(1 − Specificity)[Q] • NPV = (1 − Prevalence)(Specificity) /(1 − Prevalence)(Specificity) + (1 − Sensitivity)(Prevalence)[Q]

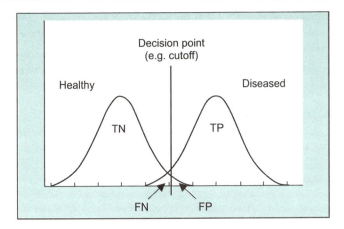

99. **Ans. d. 9.7/1,00,000 population** *(Ref: NLEP-Annual Report for the year 2015-16, Central Leprosy Division, DGHS, MOHFW, GOI*

Annual new case detection rate of leprosy as on 31ˢᵗ March, 2016 is 9.7/1,00,000 population.

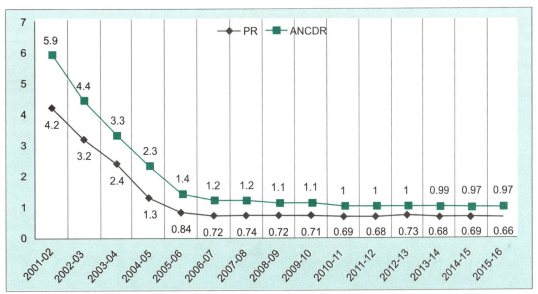

Fig. 29: The trend of prevallence and Annual New Case Detection Rate per 10,000 population since 2001-02 to 2015-16 (provisional) is shown in the Graph-source: NLEP operational guidelines 2016

NLEP – Annual Report for the year 2015-16
• Based on the reports received from all the States and UTs for the year of 2015 -16 (Annexure –I), current leprosy situation in the country is as below:
• A total of **127334 new cases** were **detected during the year 2015-16,** which gives **Annual New Case Detection Rate (ANCDR) of 9.71 per 100,000 population**, as against 125785 cases in 2014-15.
• A total of 86028 leprosy cases are on record as on 1st April 2016, giving a **Prevalence Rate (PR) of 0.66 per 10,000 population**, as against 88833 cases in 1ˢᵗ April 2015.
• Detailed information on new leprosy cases detected during 2015-16 indicates the proportion of MB (51.27%), Female (38.33%), Child (8.94%), Grade II Deformity (4.60%), ST cases (18.79%) and SC cases (18.57%).
• A total of 5851 Gr. II disability detected amongst the New Leprosy Cases during 2015-16, indicating the Gr. II Disability Rate of 4.46 / million population (Annexure-II)
• A total of 11389 child cases were recorded, indicating the **Child Case rate of 8.94%** (Annexure-III).

100. **Ans. c. 1/2 of the total protein requirement + 1/3 of the total energy requirement** *(Ref: Park 24/e p698)*
Supplementary nutrition provided in the Mid-day meal program should satisfy 1/2 of the total protein requirement and 1/3 of the total energy requirement.

> "Mid-day meal programme Meal should supply at least one third of the total energy requirement & half of the protein need."- Park 24/e p698

101. **Ans. a. Alpha error** *(Ref: High Yield Biostatistics/p46)*
In a statistical study for calculating the effect of drug on patients sugar level, the test showed significant difference, whereas in reality there was no difference. This is due to alpha error or type I error.

> "Type I error, also known as an **error of the first kind**, occurs **when the null hypothesis (H_0) is true, but is rejected**. It is **asserting something that is absent**, a **false hit**. A type I error may be compared with a so-called false positive (a result that indicates that a given condition is present when it actually is not present) in tests where a single condition is tested for. **The type I error rate or significance level is the probability of rejecting the null hypothesis, given that it is true. It is denoted by the Greek letter α (alpha) and is also called the alpha level.** Often, the significance level is set to 0.05 (5%), implying that it is acceptable to have a 5% probability of incorrectly rejecting the null hypothesis.

> Type I errors are philosophically a focus of skepticism and Occam's razor. A type I error occurs when we believe in falsehood ("believing in a lie"). In terms of folk tales, an investigator may be "crying wolf" without a wolf in sight (raising a false alarm) (H_0: no wolf)."

> "A type II error, also known as an **error of the second kind**, occurs when the null hypothesis is false, but erroneously fails to be rejected. It is failing to assert what is present, a miss. A type II error may be compared with a so-called false negative (where an actual 'hit' was disregarded by the test and seen as a 'miss') in a test checking for a single condition with a definitive result of true or false. A type II error is committed when we fail to believe a truth. In terms of folk tales, an investigator may fail to see the wolf ("failing to raise an alarm"). Again, H_0: no wolf. **The rate of the type II error is denoted by the Greek letter β (beta) and related to the power of a test (which equals 1−β)."**

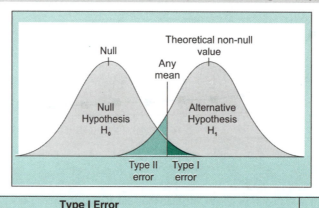

Type I Error	Type II Error
• The **null hypothesis is true but rejected (False positive)**[Q] • **Probability of type I error is given by p value**[Q] • **Significance (alpha) level is the maximum tolerable probability of type I errors**[Q] • **Keep type I error to be minimum;** then results are declared to be statistically significant[Q] • **Type I error is more serious than type II error**[Q]	• **Null hypothesis is not false but is not rejected/accepted (false negative)**[Q] • **Probability of type II error is given by beta**[Q]

MEDICINE

102. **Ans. a. Carotid body massage** *(Ref: Harrison 19/e p1483-1484, 1479)*
Narrow complex tachycardia without visible P waves and sudden nature of the palpitations clinically suggest the likelihood of Atrioventricular Nodal Reentry Tachycardia (AVNRT), most common form of PSVT. Patient is clinically stable (Systolic BP > 90 mm Hg). So there is no need for defibrillation or cardioversion. Carotid sinus massage (or any other vagal maneuver) will be the best next step in management as vagal maneuvers can terminate an approximate 10-20% of AVNRT's. The drug of choice would still be adenosine > Beta-blockers, which can be used in cases of failed vagal maneuvers in hemodynamically stable patients.

*"Acute management of narrow QRS PSVT is guided by the clinical presentation. Continuous ECG monitoring should be implemented and a 12-lead ECG should always be obtained when possible. **In the presence of hypotension with unconsciousness or respiratory distress, QRS-synchronous direct current cardioversion is warranted, but this is rarely needed, because intravenous adenosine works promptly in most situations**. For stable individuals, initial therapy takes advantage of the fact that most PSVTs are dependent on AV nodal conduction (AV nodal reentry or orthodromic AV reentry) and therefore likely to respond to sympatholytic and vagotonic maneuvers and drugs."* - Harrison 19/e p1483

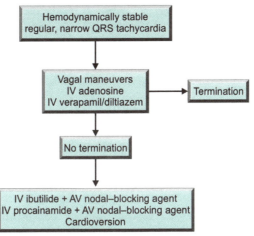

Fig. 30: Treatment algorithm of PSVT in hemodynamically stable patient

Atrioventricular Nodal Reentry Tachycardia (AVNRT)
- **AVNRT is MC form of PSVT**[Q]   - Most commonly manifests in **2nd to 4th decades**.
Mechanism: - **Reentry involving AV node**[Q]   - **MC form**: A slowly conducting AV nodal pathway extends from compact AV node near the bundle of His, **inferiorly along tricuspid annulus**, adjacent to coronary sinus os. **Reentry wave-front propagates up this slow pathway to compact AV node** & then **exits from fast pathway at the top of AV node**[Q].
Clinical Features: - It is **often well tolerated**, but **rapid tachycardia**, particularly in the elderly, may **cause angina, pulmonary edema, hypotension, or syncope**[Q].   - **Usually not associated with structural heart disease**[Q].
ECG Findings: - **Long PR interval, narrow QRS complex tachycardia**[Q]   - **P-wave buried inside QRS complex**[Q] (**not visible** or **distort initial** or **terminal portion of QRS complex**)

Acute Treatment:
 - Treatment is directed at **altering conduction within the AV node**[Q].
 - **Vagal stimulation (Valsalva maneuver or carotid sinus massage)** can **slow conduction in AV node sufficiently to terminate AVNRT**[Q].
   - If physical maneuvers do not terminate tachyarrhythmia, **1st-line treatment: Adenosine**[Q]
   - **2nd-line treatment: IV beta blockade or calcium channel therapy**[Q]
   - In hemodynamically unstable patients, R-wave synchronous DC cardioversion using 100–200 J can terminate the tachyarrhythmia[Q].

Catheter Ablation
- **Catheter ablation** of **slow AV nodal pathway** is recommended for **recurrent or severe episodes** or when **drug therapy is ineffective, not tolerated, or not desired** by the patient[Q].   - **Catheter ablation is curative in over 95% of patients**[Q].   - Major risk: Heart block requiring permanent pacemaker implantation

496 AIIMS ESSENCE

Adenosine
• **Adenosine** is administered as a **rapid IV bolus for acute termination of re-entrant supraventricular arrhythmias**^{Q}.   • **Used to produce controlled hypotension**^{Q} during some surgical procedures & in diagnosis of coronary artery disease.

Pharmacologic Effects:
 • Effects of adenosine are **mediated by interaction with specific G protein-coupled adenosine receptors**^{Q}.
 • **Adenosine activates acetylcholine-sensitive K$^+$ current in the atrium, sinus & AV nodes**, resulting in **shortening of APD, hyperpolarization, & slowing of normal automaticity**^{Q}.
 	
    • **Adenosine reduces Ca^{2+} currents**, it can be **anti-arrhythmic by increasing AV nodal refractoriness** and by **inhibiting DADs elicited by sympathetic stimulation**^{Q}.
    • **IV bolus of adenosine** transiently **slows sinus rate & AV nodal conduction velocity & increases AV nodal refractoriness**^{Q}.

Clinical uses: • Treatment of **reentrant supraventricular tachycardias**^{Q} • **IV adenosine terminates majority of PSVT by transiently blocking conduction in AV node**^{Q}.

103. Ans. a. Specific gravity of urine   *(Ref: Miller 7/e p2108, 2109, 2110)*

Urinary specific gravity is an index of the kidney›s concentrating ability, specifically, renal tubular function. The serum creatinine concentration and clearance are better indicators of general kidney function and GFR. The GFR is the best measure of glomerular function.

"Urinary specific gravity is an index of the kidney›s concentrating ability, specifically, renal tubular function. Determination of urinaryosmolality (i.e., measurement of the number of moles of solute [osmoles] per kilogram of solvent) is a similar, more specific test. Excretion of concentrated urine (specific gravity, 1.030; 1050 mOsm/kg) is indicative of excellent tubular function, whereas a urinaryosmolality fixed at that of plasma (specific gravity 1.010; 290 mOsm/Kg) indicates renal disease. The urinary dilution mechanism persists after concentrating defects are present, so a urinary osmolality of 50 to 100 mOsm/Kg still may be consistent with adavanced renal disease."-Miller 7/e p2110

"The GFR is the best measure of glomerular function. Normal GFR is approximately 125 mL/min. Manifestations of reduced GFR are not seen, however, until the GFR has decreased to 50% of normal. When GFR decreases to 30% of normal, a stage of moderate renal insufficiency sets in. Patients remain asymptomatic with only biochemical evidence of a decline in GFR (i.e., an increase in serum concentrations of urea and creatinine). Further workup usually reveals other abnormalities, such as nocturia, anemia, loss of energy, decreasing appetite, and abnormalities in calcium and phosphorus metabolism."-Miller 7/e p2108

"The blood urea nitrogen (BUN) concentration is not a direct correlate of reduced GFR. BUN is influenced by non-renal variables, such as exercise, bleeding, steroids, and massive tissue breakdown. The more important factor is that BUN is not elevated in kidney disease until the GFR is reduced to almost 75% of normal."-Miller 7/e p2109

"The serum creatinine concentration and clearance are better indicators of general kidney function and GFR than similar measurements of urea nitrogen. There are disease states, however, in which even the serum creatinine may be affected independent of the GFR."-Miller 7/e p2109

104. Ans. c. Decompressive surgery   *(Ref: Harrison 19/e p1735)*

The patient is having a low GCS with CT showing significant edema in the MCA territory (at least >50%). In such cases brain herniation is impending and need to be referred for decompressive neurosurgery.

"Stroke is a common cause of neurologic critical illness. Hypertension must be managed carefully, since abrupt reductions in blood pressure may be associated with further brain ischemia and injury. Acute ischemic stroke treated with tissue plasminogen activator (tPA) has an improved neurologic outcome when treatment is given within 3 h of onset of symptoms. The mortality rate is not reduced when tPA is compared with placebo, despite the improved neurologic outcome. The risk of cerebral hemorrhage is significantly higher in patients given tPA. No benefit is seen when tPA therapy is given beyond 3 h after symptom onset. Heparin has not been convincingly shown to improve outcomes in patients with acute ischemic stroke. Decompressive craniectomy is a surgical procedure that relieves increased intracranial pressure in the setting of space-occupying brain lesions or brain swelling from stroke; available evidence suggests that this procedure may improve survival among select patients (≤55 years or age), albeit at a cost of increased disability for some."-Harrison 19/e p1735

AIIMS November 2017

105. Ans. a. CT brain *(Ref: Harrison 19/e p1785, 1786)*

Worst headache of the life is a typical feature of a subarachnoid hemorrhage. More than 95% of cases have enough blood to be visualized on a high-quality noncontrast CT scan obtained within 72 h. If the scan fails to establish the diagnosis of SAH and no mass lesion or obstructive hydrocephalus is found, a lumbar puncture should be performed to establish the presence of subarachnoid blood.

*"**Most unruptured intracranial aneurysms are completely asymptomatic. Symptoms are usually due to rupture and resultant SAH**, although some unruptured aneurysms present with mass effect on cranial nerves or brain parenchyma. At the moment of aneurysmal rupture with major SAH, the ICP suddenly rises. This may account for the sudden transient loss of consciousness that occurs in nearly half of patients. **Sudden loss of consciousness may be preceded by a brief moment of excruciating headache, but most patients first complain of headache upon regaining consciousness**. In 10% of cases, aneurysmal bleeding is severe enough to cause loss of consciousness for several days. In ~45% of cases, severe headache associated with exertion is the presenting complaint. **The patient often calls the headache "the worst headache of my life"; however, the most important characteristic is sudden onset**. Occasionally, these ruptures may present as headache of only moderate intensity or as a change in the patient's usual headache pattern. The headache is usually generalized, often with neck stiffness, and vomiting is common."- Harrison 19/e p1785*

*"**The hallmark of aneurysmal rupture is blood in the CSF. More than 95% of cases have enough blood to be visualized on a high-quality noncontrast CT scan obtained within 72 h. If the scan fails to establish the diagnosis of SAH and no mass lesion or obstructive hydrocephalus is found, a lumbar puncture should be performed to establish the presence of subarachnoid blood.** Lysis of the red blood cells and subsequent conversion of hemoglobin to bilirubin stains the spinal fluid yellow within 6–12 h. This xanthochromic spinal fluid peaks in intensity at 48 h and lasts for 1–4 weeks, depending on the amount of subarachnoid blood."- Harrison 19/e p1786*

Subarachnoid Hemorrhage
• **MC cause: Trauma** >Spontaneous rupture of **Berry aneurysm**[Q]
Clinical Features: • **Sudden transient loss of consciousness**[Q] (occurs in nearly half of the patients) • **Excruciating severe headache**[Q]: presenting complaint in 45% of cases (worst headache of patients life) more common upon regaining consciousness when loss of consciousness is associated <ul><li>**Neck stiffness & vomiting**[Q]: are common associations</li><li>**Focal neurological deficit: uncommon.**</li><li>**Sudden headache** in the **absence of focal neurological deficit** is the **hallmark of aneurysmal rupture**[Q]</li></ul>
• Associated prodromal symptoms (suggest **location** of progressively enlarging unruptured aneurysm): – Third cranial nerve palsy[Q]: Aneurysm at junction of PCA & ICA – Sixth nerve palsy[Q]: Aneurysm in cavernous sinus – Occipital and posterior cervical pain: Inferior cerebellar artery aneurysm – Pain in or behind the eye[Q]: MCA aneurysm
Diagnosis: • **Non contrast CT scan: Investigation of choice**[Q] (Lumbar puncture is not indicated prior to an imaging procedure) • **CSF picture: Hallmark** of aneurysmal rupture is **blood in CSF (Xanthochromic spinal fluid**[Q]**)** <ul><li>**Lumbar puncture** should be performed **if the CT scan fails to establish the diagnosis of SAH** and **no mass lesion** or **obstructive hydrocephalus** is found to establish the presence of subarachnoid blood[Q]</li></ul>
Treatment: • **Traumatic subarachnoid hemorrhage** is **managed conservatively**[Q].
Prognosis assessed by: • **Hunt and Hess scale**[Q] • **WFNS** (World Federal of Neurological Scale).

106. Ans. d. Mild MS *(Ref: Harrison 19/e p1447)*

The first heart sound (S1) is usually accentuated in the early stages of the disease. Loud S1 in MS does not depend upon severity of MS. The intensity of S1 is determined by the distance over which the anterior leaflet of the mitral valve must travel to return to its annular plane, leaflet mobility, left ventricular contractility, and the PR interval.

"The first heart sound (S1) includes mitral and tricuspid valve closure. Normal splitting can be appreciated in young patients and those with right bundle branch block, in whom tricuspid valve closure is relatively delayed. The intensity of S1 is determined by the distance over which the anterior leaflet of the mitral valve must travel to return to its annular plane, leaflet mobility, left ventricular contractility, and the PR interval. S1 is classically loud in the early phases of rheumatic mitral stenosis (MS) and in patients with hyperkinetic circulatory states or short PR intervals. S1 becomes softer in the later stages of MS when the leaflets are rigid and calcified, after exposure to β-adrenergic receptor blockers, with long PR intervals, and with left ventricular contractile dysfunction. The intensity of heart sounds, however, can be reduced by any process that increases the distance between the stethoscope and the responsible cardiac event, including mechanical ventilation, obstructive lung disease, obesity, pneumothorax, and a pericardial effusion."-Harrison 19/e p1447

First Heart Sound (S1)

Cause of Soft S1	Causes of Loud S1
• **Poor conductance of sound through chest wall:** Obesity, emphysema, pleural effusion & pericardial effusion[Q] • **Decrease in rate of LV pressure development:** Myxedema, cardiomyopathy, acute **MI & MR**[Q] • **PR interval & velocity of valve closure:** Prolonged PR interval[Q] (1st degree heart block) • **Mobility of valve:** Severe calcification of valve or reduced mobility of valve is associated with **soft S1. Long standing MS** is associated with **severe calcification of mitral valve & soft S1**[Q].	• **Tachycardia:** S1 is louder if diastole is shortened due to tachycardia especially in **anemia, anxiety & fever**[Q] • **Increased AV Flow:** Due to high cardiac output (**Thyrotoxicosis & AV fistula**) or due to **left to right shunting (ASD, PDA)**[Q] • **Prolonged AV Flow:** Due to stenosis in **MS & TS**[Q] • **Short PR interval**[Q]

"Auscultatory Findings in MS: The first heart sound (S1) is usually accentuated in the early stages of the disease and slightly delayed. The pulmonic component of the second heart sound (P2) also is often accentuated with elevated PA pressures, and the two components of the second heart sound (S2) are closely split. The opening snap (OS) of the mitral valve is most readily audible in expiration at, or just medial to, the cardiac apex. This sound generally follows the sound of aortic valve closure (A2) by 0.05–0.12 s. The time interval between A2 and OS varies inversely with the severity of the MS. The OS is followed by a low-pitched, rumbling, diastolic murmur, heard best at the apex with the patient in the left lateral recumbent position; it is accentuated by mild exercise (e.g., a few rapid sit-ups) carried out just before auscultation."-Harrison 19/e p1540

Mitral stenosis

Auscultatory findings	X-Ray findings
• **S1:** Accentuated[Q] • **S2:** Normally split S2[Q] with accentuated P2[Q] • **Murmur:** Low-pitched[Q], rumbling diastolic murmur with 'Pre-systolic accentuation', heard best at the **apex in left lateral recumbent position**[Q]. • **Opening snap:** Brief, high pitched[Q], early diastolic[Q] sound, best heard at the **lower left sternal border**[Q].	• **Straightening of left border of cardiac silhouette**[Q] • **Prominence** of main pulmonary artery[Q] • **Dilation of upper lobe pulmonary veins**[Q] • **Kerley B lines**[Q] • **Backward displacement of esophagus**[Q]

Features suggesting severe MS
• Proximity of S2-OS gap[Q] • Longer duration of mid-diastolic murmur[Q]

107. Ans. a. Supravalvular aortic stenosis *(Ref: Harrison 19/e p1525, 1531, 2190, 1641)*

Coarctation of aorta, Takayasu arteritis and aortic dissection can cause mid-diastolic murmur but aortic stenosis causes systolic murmur.

"The murmur of aortic stenosis (AS) is characteristically an ejection (mid) systolic murmur that commences shortly after the S_1, increases in intensity to reach a peak toward the middle of ejection, and ends just before aortic valve closure. It is characteristically low-pitched, rough and rasping in character, and loudest at the base of the heart, most commonly in the second right intercostal space. It is transmitted upward along the carotid arteries. Occasionally it is transmitted downward and to the apex, where it may be confused with the systolic murmur of mitral regurgitation (MR) (Gallavardin effect)."- Harrison 19/e p1531

*"**Coarctation of aorta:** Most children and young adults with isolated, discrete coarctation are asymptomatic. **Headache, epistaxis, chest pressure, and claudication with exercise may occur, and attention is usually directed to the cardiovascular system when a heart murmur or hypertension in the upper extremities and absence, marked diminution, or delayed pulsations in the femoral arteries are detected on physical examination.** Enlarged and pulsatile collateral vessels may be palpated in the intercostal spaces anteriorly, in the axillae, or posteriorly in the interscapular area. **The upper extremities and thorax may be more developed than the lower extremities. A mid-systolic murmur over the left interscapular space may become continuous if the lumen is narrowed sufficiently to result in a high-velocity jet across the lesion throughout the cardiac cycle.**"- Harrison 19/e p1525*

*"**The diagnosis of Takayasu's arteritis should be suspected strongly in a young woman who develops a decrease or absence of peripheral pulses, discrepancies in blood pressure, and arterial bruits.** The diagnosis is confirmed by the characteristic pattern on arteriography, which includes irregular vessel walls, stenosis, post-stenotic dilation, aneurysm formation, occlusion, and evidence of increased collateral circulation."- Harrison 19/e p2190*

*"The peak incidence of aortic dissection is in the sixth and seventh decades. Men are more affected than women by a ratio of 2:1. **The presentations of aortic dissection and its variants are the consequences of intimal tear, dissecting hematoma, occlusion of involved arteries, and compression of adjacent tissues.** Acute aortic dissection presents with the sudden onset of pain, which often is described as very severe and tearing and is associated with diaphoresis. The pain may be localized to the front or back of the chest, often the interscapular region, and typically migrates with propagation of the dissection. Other symptoms include syncope, dyspnea, and weakness. **Physical findings may include hypertension or hypotension, loss of pulses, aortic regurgitation, pulmonary edema, and neurologic findings due to carotid artery obstruction (hemiplegia, hemianesthesia) or spinal cord ischemia (paraplegia).**"- Harrison 19/e p1641*

Principal Causes of Heart Murmurs			
Systolic Murmurs	**Early systolic**	• **Mitral: Acute MR**[Q] • **VSD**[Q]**:** Muscular, nonrestrictive with pulmonary hypertension • **Tricuspid: TR** with normal pulmonary artery pressure[Q]	
	Mid-systolic	**Aortic**	**Pulmonary**

		• Obstructive:
		   – **Supravalvular: Supravalvular aortic stenosis, coarctation of aorta**
		   – **Valvular: AS & aortic sclerosis** [Q]
		   – **Subvalvular: Discrete, tunnel or HOCM**[Q]
		 • **Increased flow, hyperkinetic states, AR, complete heart block**[Q]
		 • **Dilation of ascending aorta**, atheroma, aortitis
			• **Obstructive :**
			 • **Supravalvular:** Pulmonary artery stenosis
			 • **Valvular:** Pulmonic valve stenosis
			 • **Subvalvular:** Infundibular stenosis (dynamic)
			 • **Increased flow, hyperkinetic states, left-to-right shunt** (e.g., **ASD**)
			 • Dilation of pulmonary artery

	Late systolic	• **Mitral : MVP**, acute myocardial ischemia[Q] • **Tricuspid:** Tricuspid valve prolapse (**TVP**)[Q]	
	Holosystolic	• Atrioventricular valve regurgitation (**MR, TR**)[Q] • Left-to-right shunt at ventricular level (**VSD**)[Q]	
Diastolic Murmurs	**Early Diastolic Murmurs**	**Aortic regurgitation (AR)** [Q] **Pulmonic regurgitation (PR)**[Q]	
	Mid-Diastolic Murmurs	• Mitral: • **Mitral stenosis** [Q] • **Carey-Coombs murmur**[Q] (mid-diastolic apical murmur in acute rheumatic fever) • **Increased flow across non-stenotic mitral valve** (e.g., **MR, VSD, PDA**, high-output states, & complete heart block)[Q] • Tricuspid: • **Tricuspid stenosis** [Q] • Increased flow across non-stenotic tricuspid valve (e.g., **TR, ASD** & anomalous pulmonary venous return) • **Left & right atrial tumors (myxoma)**[Q] • **Severe AR (Austin Flint murmur)**[Q]	

Principal Causes of Heart Murmurs		
Continuous Murmurs	• **PDA**[Q] • **Coronary AV fistula**[Q] • **Ruptured sinus of Valsalva aneurysm**[Q] • **ASD** [Q] • Cervical venous hum • Anomalous left coronary artery	• Proximal coronary artery stenosis • **Mammary souffle of pregnancy**[Q] • **Pulmonary artery branch stenosis**[Q] • **Bronchial collateral circulation**[Q] • **Small (restrictive) ASD with MS**[Q] • **Intercostal AV fistula**[Q]

108. Ans. d. Salicylate poisoning *(Ref: Harrison 19/e p319, 320)*

Salicylate poisoning leads to high anion-gap metabolic acidosis. Proximal renal tubular acidosis (RTA), pancreatitis and diarrhea lead to normal anion gap metabolic acidosis.

> *"Salicylate intoxication in adults usually causes respiratory alkalosis or a mixture of high-AG metabolic acidosis and respiratory alkalosis. Only a portion of the AG is due to salicylates. Lactic acid production is also often increased."*-*Harrison 19/e p319*

> *"Alkali can be lost from the gastrointestinal tract from diarrhea or from the kidneys (renal tubular acidosis, RTA). In these disorders, reciprocal changes in [Cl⁻] and [HCO₃⁻] result in a normal AG. In pure non–AG acidosis, therefore, the increase in [Cl⁻] above the normal value approximates the decrease in [HCO₃⁻]. The absence of such a relationship suggests a mixed disturbance."*-*Harrison 19/e p320*

Causes of Non-Anion-Gap Acidosis			
Gastrointestinal bicarbonate loss	**Renal Acidosis**	**Drug-induced Hyperkalemia (with renal insufficiency)**	**Others**
Diarrhea[Q] External pancreatic or small-bowel drainage **Uretero-sigmoidostomy**[Q], jejunal loop, ileal loop **Drugs:** Calcium chloride (acidifying agent), magnesium sulphate (diarrhea), **cholestyramine (bile acid diarrhea)**[Q]	**Hypokalemia: Proximal RTA** (type 2) & **Distal (classic) RTA** (type 1)[Q] **Hyperkalemia:** Generalized distal nephron dysfunction (**type 4 RTA**)[Q] **Mineralocorticoid deficiency**[Q] **Mineralocorticoid resistance**[Q] Voltage defect Tubulointerstitial disease **Normokalemia :** Chronic progressive kidney disease	**Potassium sparing diuretics**[Q] (**amiloride, triamterene, spirono-lactone**) **Trimethoprim**[Q] **Pentamidine**[Q] **ACE inhibitors & AT-II receptor blockers**[Q] **NSAIDs**[Q] **Cyclosporine**[Q]	**Acid loads** (ammonium chloride, hyper-alimenta-tion) **Loss of potential bicar-bonate:** ketosis with ke-tone excretion **Expansion acidosis** (rap-id saline administration) Hippurate **Cation exchange resins**[Q]

109. Ans. b. Electrical alternans *(Ref: Harrison 19/e p1457)*

This is a classical ECG showing electrical alternans where there is alternate high and low amplitude QRS.

> *"Electrical alternans—a beat-to-beat alternation in one or more components of the ECG signal—is a common type of nonlinear cardiovascular response to a variety of hemodynamic and electrophysiologic perturbations. Total electrical alternans (P-QRS-T) with sinus tachycardia is a relatively specific sign of pericardial effusion, usually with cardiac tamponade. The mechanism relates to a periodic swinging motion of the heart in the effusion at a frequency exactly one-half the heart rate. In contrast, pure repolarization (ST-T or U wave) alternans is a sign of electrical instability and may precede ventricular tachyarrhythmias."*-*Harrison 19/e p1457*

110. Ans. d. Coxsackie virus *(Ref: Harrison 19/e p1289, 1291)*

History of fever and headache with neck stiffness suggest the diagnosis of meningitis. CSF analysis findings of increased opening pressure, mildly increased proteins, normal glucose, increased lymphocytes are highly suggestive of viral (Coxsackie virus) meningitis. Meningitis with normal glucose is highly suggestive of viral meningitis.

> *"Enteroviruses encompass more than 100 human serotypes: 3 serotypes of poliovirus, 21 serotypes of coxsackievirus A, 6 serotypes of coxsackievirus B, 28 serotypes of echovirus, enteroviruses 68–71, and multiple new enteroviruses (beginning with enterovirus 73) that have been identified by molecular techniques."*-*Harrison 19/e p1289*

"In children and young adults, enteroviruses are the cause of up to 90% of cases of aseptic meningitis in which an etiologic agent can be identified. Patients with aseptic meningitis typically present with an acute onset of fever, chills, headache, photophobia, and pain on eye movement. Nausea and vomiting also are common. Examination reveals meningismus without localizing neurologic signs; drowsiness or irritability may also be apparent. In some cases, a febrile illness may be reported that remits but returns several days later in conjunction with signs of meningitis. Other systemic manifestations may provide clues to an enteroviral cause, including diarrhea, myalgias, rash, pleurodynia, myocarditis, and herpangina. Examination of the CSF invariably reveals pleocytosis; the CSF cell count shows a shift from neutrophil to lymphocyte predominance within 1 day of presentation, and the total cell count does not exceed 1000/µL. The CSF glucose level is usually normal (in contrast to the low CSF glucose level in mumps), with a normal or slightly elevated protein concentration."-Harrison 19/e p1291

Typical CSF Profiles for Meningitis

	Normal	Bacterial Meningitis	Viral Meningitis	Fungal Meningitis	Parasitic Meningitis	Tuberculous Meningitis
WBC count (per µL)	<5	>1000[Q]	25–500[Q]	40–600	150–2000	25–100
Differential of WBC	60–70% lympho-cytes, ≤30% monocytes / macrophages	↑↑**PMNs**[Q] (≥80%)	Predominantly **lymphocytes**[Q]	Lymphocytes or PMNs, depending on specific organism	↑↑ Eosinophils (≥50%)	Predominantly **lymphocytes**[Q]
Gram's stain	Negative	**Positive**[Q] (in >60% of cases)	**Negative**[Q]	Rarely positive	Negative	**Occasionally positive**[Q]
Glucose (mg/dL)	40–85	<40[Q]	**Normal**[Q]	↓ to normal	Normal	<50 in 75% of cases[Q]
Protein (mg/dL)	15–45	>100[Q]	20–80[Q]	150–300	50–200	100–200[Q]
Opening pressure (mm H$_2$O)	50–180	>300[Q]	100–350[Q]	160–340	Normal	150–280[Q]

111. Ans. d. Tubercular peritonitis   *(Ref: Harrison 19/e p287)*

In tubercular peritonitis, Serum-Ascites Albumin Gradient (SAAG) is <1.1 gm/dL.

"The SAAG is useful for distinguishing ascites caused by portal hypertension from non-portal hypertensive ascites. The SAAG reflects the pressure within the hepatic sinusoids and correlates with the hepatic venous pressure gradient. The SAAG is calculated by subtracting the ascitic albumin concentration from the serum albumin level and does not change with diuresis. A SAAG ≥1.1 g/dL reflects the presence of portal hypertension and indicates that the ascites is due to increased pressure in the hepatic sinusoids. According to Starling's law, a high SAAG reflects the oncotic pressure that counterbalances the portal pressure. Possible causes include cirrhosis, cardiac ascites, hepatic vein thrombosis (Budd-Chiari syndrome), sinusoidal obstruction syndrome (veno-occlusive disease), or massive liver metastases. A SAAG <1.1 g/dL indicates that the ascites is not related to portal hypertension, as in tuberculous peritonitis, peritoneal carcinomatosis, or pancreatic ascites."-Harrison 19/e p287

Classification of Ascites by Serum-Ascites Albumin Gradient (SAAG)

High Gradient (>1.1 gm/dL) or Transudate	Low Gradient (<1.1 gm/dL) or Exudate
• **Cirrhosis (MC)**[Q] • **Alcoholic hepatitis**[Q] • **Cardiac ascites**[Q] • Mixed ascites • Massive liver metastases • **Fulminant hepatic failure**[Q] • **Budd-Chiari syndrome**[Q] • **Portal vein thrombosis**[Q] • Sinusoidal obstruction syndrome • **Myxedema**[Q] • Fatty liver of pregnancy	• **Peritoneal carcinomatosis (MC)**[Q] • **Tubercular peritonitis**[Q] • Pancreatic ascites • **Bowel obstruction** or **infarction**[Q] • Biliary ascites • **Nephrotic syndrome**[Q] • Post-operative lymphatic leak • **Serositis** in connective tissue disease

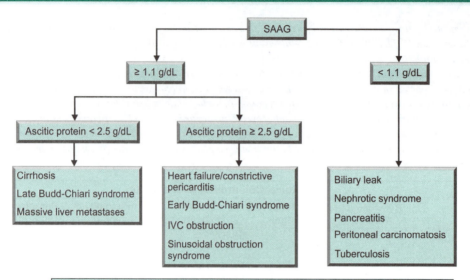

- MC cause of low-albumin gradient ascites: Peritoneal carcinomatosis[Q]
- MC cause of high-albumin gradient ascites: Cirrhosis[Q]

112. **Ans. b. Hypocalcemia** *(Ref: Harrison 19/e p315, 2482, 138e-5)*
Clinical findings of paresthesias, circumoral numbness and ECG showing tachycardia with ST-T changes are highly suggestive of hypocalcemia, which has been caused by extensive transfusion of citrated blood.

"Citrate, commonly used to anticoagulate blood components, chelates calcium and thereby inhibits the coagulation cascade. Hypocalcemia, manifested by circumoral numbness and/or tingling sensation of the fingers and toes, may result from multiple rapid transfusions."-Harrison 19/e p 138e-5

"Transient hypocalcemia is seen with severe sepsis, burns, acute kidney injury, and extensive transfusions with citrated blood."-Harrison 19/e p2482

"Patients with hypocalcemia may be asymptomatic if the decreases in serum calcium are relatively mild and chronic, or they may present with life-threatening complications. Moderate to severe hypocalcemia is associated with paresthesias, usually of the fingers, toes, and circumoral regions, and is caused by increased neuromuscular irritability. On physical examination, a Chvostek's sign (twitching of the circumoral muscles in response to gentle tapping of the facial nerve just anterior to the ear) may be elicited, although it is also present in ~10% of nor- mal individuals. Carpal spasm may be induced by inflation of a blood pressure cuff to 20 mmHg above the patient's systolic blood pressure for 3 min (Trousseau's sign). Severe hypocalcemia can induce seizures, carpopedal spasm, bronchospasm, laryngospasm, and prolongation of the QT interval."-Harrison 19/e p315

Clinical Manifestations of Hypocalcemia	
Neuro-psychiatric manifestations	- Seizures, increased ICT & papilledema[Q] - **Dementia** in adults & **mental retardation** in children[Q] - Irritability, depression & psychosis[Q] - Calcification of basal ganglia[Q]
Increased Neuromuscular irritability	- Mild: Numbness of perioral region & finger tips[Q] - Severe: - Carpopedal spasm, laryngeal spasm & convulsions[Q] - Chvostek's sign: Twitching of circumoral muscles in response to gentle tapping of facial nerve just anterior to ear[Q] - Trousseau's sign: Carpal spasm may be induced by inflation of a BP cuff to 20 mmHg above the patient's systolic blood pressure for 3 min[Q]
CVS symptoms	- Prolongation of QT interval, CHF & hypotension[Q]
Autonomic	- Biliary colic, bronchospasm & diaphoresis[Q]
Others	- Cataract, dry coarse skin, steatorrhea & achlorhydria[Q]

113. Ans. b. Myasthenia gravis *(Ref: Harrison 19/e p2701-2702; Goodman Gilman 12/e p251)*
Clinical findings of unilateral ptosis and hypotonia in the eye with improvement after an IV injection (most probably edrophonium) suggest the diagnosis of Myasthenia gravis.

"*Although the diagnosis of autoimmune myasthenia gravis usually can be made from the history, signs, and symptoms, its differentiation from certain neurasthenic, infectious, endocrine, congenital, neoplastic, and degenerative neuromuscular diseases can be challenging. However, myasthenia gravis is the only condition in which the aforementioned deficiencies can be improved dramatically by anti-ChE medication. The edrophonium test for evaluation of possible myasthenia gravis is performed by rapid intravenous injection of 2 mg of edrophonium chloride, followed 45 seconds later by an additional 8 mg if the first dose is without effect; a positive response consists of brief improvement in strength, unaccompanied by lingual fasciculation (which generally occurs in non-myasthenic patients).*"-Goodman Gilman 12/e p251

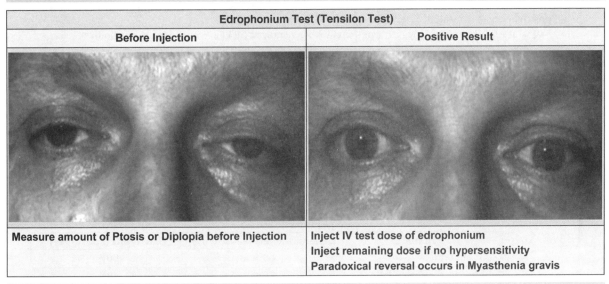

"*The edrophonium (Tensilon) test is sometimes of value in distinguishing botulism (usually a negative result) from myasthenia gravis (usually a positive result).*"- Harrison 19/e p989

Myasthenia Gravis (MG)
• MG is a **neuromuscular disorder** characterized by **weakness & fatigability of skeletal muscles**[Q].   • Associated with **thymomas**[Q] & certain **autoimmune diseases**[Q]   • More common in women[Q]   • Peaks of incidence: Women in **twenties & thirties**; men in **fifties & sixties**[Q].
Pathophysiology: • **Decrease in number of available acetylcholine receptors (AChRs) at NM junctions** due to an **antibody-mediated autoimmune attack** resulting in **decreased efficiency of NM transmission**[Q].

Clinical features:
 • **Cardinal features**: Weakness & fatigability of muscles[Q].
 • **Weakness increases during repeated use** (fatigue) or late in the day and may **improve following rest or sleep**.
 • **Distribution of muscle weakness** has a **characteristic pattern**[Q].
     • **Cranial muscles (lids & extraocular muscles)** are typically involved early in the course of MG
     • **Diplopia & ptosis** are **common initial complaints**[Q].
 • **Facial weakness** produces a **"snarling" expression** when the **patient attempts to smile**[Q].
 • **Weakness in chewing** is most noticeable after prolonged effort, as in chewing meat.
 • **Speech**: **Nasal timbre** (due to weakness of palate) & **dysarthric "mushy" quality**[Q] (due to tongue weakness)
 • **Difficulty in swallowing** as a result of **weakness of palate, tongue, or pharynx**, giving rise to **nasal regurgitation or aspiration**[Q].

Contd...

Myasthenia Gravis (MG)

- **Bulbar weakness** is especially prominent in **MuSK antibody–positive MG[Q]**.

  - In ~85% of patients, **weakness becomes generalized**, affecting the **limb muscles as well**.
  - **Limb weakness in MG is often proximal** and may be **asymmetric[Q]**.
  - **Despite the muscle weakness, deep tendon reflexes are preserved[Q]**.

- If **weakness of respiration** becomes so severe as to **require respiratory assistance,** the patient is said to be in **crisis.**
- **Ocular MG:** Weakness restricted to extraocular muscles[Q]

Diagnosis:

- **Anti-AChR radioimmunoassay:** ~85% positive in generalized MG; 50% in ocular MG; **definite diagnosis if positive;** negative result does not exclude MG[Q]
- **~40% of AChR antibody–negative patients** with generalized MG have **anti-MuSK antibodies[Q]**

  - **Repetitive nerve stimulation: Decrement of >15% at 3 Hz:** highly probable[Q]
  - **Single-fiber electromyography: Blocking & jitter, with normal fiber density; confirmatory,** but not specific[Q]

- **Edrophonium chloride** 2 mg + 8 mg IV; **highly probable diagnosis** if unequivocally positive[Q]
- **For ocular or cranial MG:** exclude **intracranial lesions** by CT or MRI

Single most sensitive test for diagnosis of MG	Single muscle electromyography[Q]
Single most specific test for diagnosis of MG	AChR antibodies[Q]

Treatment:

- **Most useful treatments** for MG: **Anticholinesterase medications, immunosuppressive agents, thymectomy & plasmapheresis** or intravenous immunoglobulin **(IVIg)[Q]**

Test	Generalized MG (sensitivity)	Ocular MG (sensitivity)
AChR antibodies	80%	60%
Repetitive nerve stimulation	75%	48%
Single fiber EMG	99%	97%
Edrophonium (Tensilon) test	95%	85%

114. Ans. d. Intravenous magnesium sulphate *(Ref: Harrison 19/e p312, 463e-4, 18/e p359)*

Intravenous magnesium sulphate is not used in emergency management of acute hyperkalemia.

"Hyperkalemia is defined as a serum potassium level >5.5 mmol/L (>5.5 meq/L) and can neurologically present as muscle weakness with or without paresthesias. Hyperkalemia becomes life threatening when it produces electrocardiographic abnormalities such as peaked T waves or a widened QRS complex. In these cases, prompt treatment is essential and consists of strategies that protect the heart against arrhythmias (calcium gluconate administration); promote potassium redistribution into cells (with glucose, insulin, and β2-agonist medications); and increase potassium removal (through sodium polystyrene sulfonate, loop diuretics, or hemodialysis)."- Harrison 19/e p312

"Intravenous calcium serves to protect the heart, whereas other measures are taken to correct hyperkalemia. Calcium raises the action potential threshold and reduces excitability, without changing the resting membrane potential. By restoring the difference between resting and threshold potentials, calcium reverses the depolarization blockade due to hyperkalemia."- Harrison 19/e p312

Hyperkalemia

- **Hyperkalemia** is defined as **plasma K$^+$ >5.0 mmol/L,** but **every case of hyperkalemia doesn't require treatment.**
- **Management strategy of hyperkalemia depends upon:** Plasma K$^+$ concentration, associated muscular weakness & changes on ECG

- Treatment of Hyperkalemia is required in following cases:
- Serum K$^+$ >5 along with ECG manifestation of hyperkalemia
- Serum K$^+$ >6 (even when ECG manifestation are not present)

Contd...

Contd...

Hyperkalemia		
In Hyperkalemia the treatment is directed at		
Minimizing membrane depolarization	**Redistribution of potassium (shifting of K+ back into cells)**	**Increased excretion of potassium**
Administration of calcium in the form of **calcium gluconate, decreases membrane excitability**[Q] **Calcium directly reverses** the effect of potassium on the **cardiac conduction system**[Q]	Administering **insulin & glucose**[Q] Alkali therapy with **I.V. NaHCO$_3$.**[Q] **Beta$_2$ adrenergic agonist**[Q] (When administered parenterally or in nebulized form, **beta$_2$ adrenergic agonist** promote cellular uptake of K+)[Q]	**Cation exchange resin**[Q] (Sodium polystyrene sulfonate) **Diuretics (Enhance K+ excretion)**[Q] **Hemodialysis (Most effective and rapid way of lowering plasma K+ conc.)**[Q]

SURGERY

115. Ans. b. Urine output *(Ref: Sabiston 20/e p520; Schwartz 10/e p169; Bailey 27/e p17, 26/e p18)*

Best guide for the management of resuscitation is urine output.

> *"Ultimately, the goal of treatment is to restore cellular and organ perfusion. Ideally, therefore, monitoring of organ perfusion should guide the management of shock. The best measures of organ perfusion and the best monitor of the adequacy of shock therapy remains the urine output."- Bailey 27/e p17*

> *"Patients who have a good response to fluid infusion (i.e., normalization of vital signs, clearing of the sensorium) and evidence of good peripheral perfusion (warm fingers and toes with normal capillary refill) are presumed to have adequate overall perfusion. Urine output is a quantitative, reliable indicator of organ per- fusion. Adequate urine output is 0.5 mL/kg per hour in an adult, 1 mL/kg per hour in a child, and 2 mL/kg per hour in an infant <1 year of age."- Schwartz 10/e p169*

> *"Urine output of more than 1 mL/kg is an adequate measure of renal perfusion in the absence of underlying renal disease."- Sabiston 20/e p520*

116. Ans. c. Heart rate/Mean arterial pressure *(Ref: Sabiston 20/e p52)*

Modified shock index (MSI) is defined as heart rate divided by mean arterial pressure.

> *"Modified shock index (MSI) is defined as heart rate divided by mean arterial pressure. High MSI indicates a value of stroke volume and low systemic vascular resistance, a sign of hypodynamic circulation. In contrast, low MSI indicates a hyperdynamic state. MSI has been considered a better marker than shock index (SI) for mortality rate prediction. Although SI or MSI is better than heart rate and systolic BP alone, the combination of these variables will undoubtedly be more useful."-Sabiston 20/e p52*

Shock Index (SI)	Modified Shock Index (MSI)
• SI is defined as **heart rate divided by systolic BP**[Q]. • **Better marker for assessing severity of shock than heart rate & BP alone**[Q]. • Utility in **trauma patients, sepsis, obstetrics, myocardial infarction, stroke & other acute critical illnesses**[Q]. • **Correlated with need for interventions** such as blood transfusion & invasive procedures including operations. • SI is known as a **hemodynamic stability indicator**[Q]. • SI does **not take into account** the **diastolic BP**	• MSI is defined as **heart rate divided by mean arterial pressure**[Q]. • **High MSI** indicates a **value of stroke volume & low systemic vascular resistance**, a sign of hypodynamic circulation[Q]. • **Low MSI** indicates a hyperdynamic state[Q]. • **MSI** has been considered a **better marker than SI for mortality rate prediction**[Q].

117. Ans. c. Blue *(Ref: Manual of ICU Procedures By Mohan Gurjar (2015)/p240)*

The 22 Gauge IV cannula color is blue.

"Present day IV cannulae are available from sizes 14 gauge to 26 gauge with universal color coding for easy recognition of IV cannula. Commonly used adult size is 20 gauze. In cases of rapid fluid transfusion, even large gauge 18 (green) or 16 (gray) can be used in adult patient. Cannula size 22 (blue) is preferred in pediatric age group and size 24 (yellow) in infants and neonates."- Manual of ICU Procedures By Mohan Gurjar (2015)/p240

Gauge	Color code	External Diameter	Length	Flow Rate
14G	OrangeQ	2.1 mm	45 mm	240 ml/min
16G	GreyQ	1.8 mm	45 mm	180 ml/min
18G	GreenQ	1.3 mm	32/45 mm	90 ml/min
20G	PinkQ	1.1 mm	32 mm	60 ml/min
22G	BlueQ	0.9 mm	25 mm	36 ml/min
24G	YellowQ	0.7 mm	19 mm	20 ml/min
26G	VioletQ	0.6 mm	19 mm	13 ml/min

118. **Ans. b. In lateral lying position**   *(Ref: Sabiston 20/e p414, 420, 473; Schwartz 10/e p161)*

In patients of trauma, maintaining the patient in a supine flat position at all times protects the thoracic, lumbar, and sacral segments of the spine. That's why patient should not be put in lateral lying down position.

"Cervical spine protection includes the use of a hard cervical collar and the maintenance of the log roll technique for all movement of the patient."- Sabiston 20/e p414

"Spinal immobilization with a rigid cervical collar and a long spine board is an immediate priority for pre-hospital personnel as a scene is approached."-Sabiston 20/e p420

"The trauma team must always take steps to protect the patient from self-inflicted or iatrogenic spinal cord injury. Therefore, full spine precautions must be observed until it is confirmed that the patient's vertebral column is intact, either by physical examination and clinical findings or by radiologic confirmation, when warranted. Fitting the patient with a hard cervical collar stabilizes the cervical spine. Maintaining the patient in a supine flat position at all times protects the thoracic, lumbar, and sacral segments of the spine. If the patient is to be moved, a strict log roll technique is used. At times, a patient may have to be physically restrained to prevent potential self-inflicted injury by head or lower extremity movements that could impart rotational, translational, or bending moments to the vertebral column. Special care must be taken with combative patients or those with altered mental status who may have lost the ability to protect themselves from further injury. On examination of the back, the examiner notes the presence of deformity, edema, or ecchymosis. Tenderness elicited on palpation of the spine is recorded for each level at which the patient complains of pain. Distinction is made regarding whether the pain is midline or paraspinal. Perianal sensation and rectal sphincter tone should be evaluated to test sacral nerve root function. Deep tendon reflexes and pathologic reflexes, such as the bulbocavernosus and Babinski reflexes, are tested."- Sabiston 20/e p473

119. **Ans. a. airway obstruction**   *(Ref: Sabiston 20/e p413; Schwartz 10/e p161; Advanced Trauma Life Support (ATLS) Manual 7/e p33-34; CSDT 11/e p205)*

The first priority in management of a case trauma is airway maintenance. Ensuring an adequate airway is the first priority in the primary survey of trauma.

"Following a defined order of assessment, life-threatening conditions are immediately addressed at the time of identification. This initial assessment, also termed the primary survey, follows the mnemonic ABCDE: Airway and cervical spine protection, Breathing, Circulation, Disability or neurologic condition, Exposure and environmental control."- Sabiston 20/e p413

"Ensuring a patent airway is the first priority in the primary survey. This is essential, because efforts to restore cardiovascular integrity will be futile unless the oxygen content of the blood is adequate. Simultaneously, all patients with blunt trauma require cervical spine immobilization until injury is excluded. This is typically accomplished by applying a hard collar or placing sandbags on both sides of the head with the patient's forehead taped across the bags to the backboard. Soft collars do not effectively immobilize the cervical spine. For penetrating neck wounds, however, cervical collars are not believed useful because they provide no benefit, but may interfere with assessment and treatment."- Schwartz 10/e p161

Primary Survey - ATLS Protocol

A: Airway with Cervical Spine Protection

- **Assess Airway Patency**[Q]

If Not Patent (Management):
- Chin lift / Jaw thrust[Q]
- Clear airway[Q] of Foreign body
- Insert oropharyngeal /Nasopharyngeal airway[Q]
- Establish definitive airway[Q]

B: Breathing (Ventilation and Oxygenation)

- **Assess Breathing**
  - **Rate and depth**
  - **Percuss chest**
  - **Auscultate chest**
- **Administer Oxygen**[Q]
- Attach patient to **pulse oximeter**[Q]

Abnormal Breathing detected: **Management**
- **Ventilate if required**[Q]
- **Alleviate tension pneumothorax**[Q]
- **Seal open pneumothorax**[Q]

C: Circulation with Hemorrhage Control

- **Assess circulation** –
- Identify **external hemorrhage**[Q]
- **Pulse**
- **BP** (time permitting)
- Skin colour
- Identify potential **internal hemorrhage**[Q]

If Abnormality detected
- Apply direct pressure to external bleeding[Q]
- Insert **2 large bore IV catheters**[Q]
- Simultaneously obtain **blood** for **hematological chemical analysis**, **type & cross match**[Q]
- Initiate **IV fluid therapy**[Q]

Consider potential need for **operative intervention**, if suspected internal hemorrhage.

D: Disability (Brief Neurological Examination)

- **Assess Consciousness**
  GCS score

Assess Pupils
Size / Equality / Reaction[Q]

E: Exposure / Environment

Completely undress the patient but **prevent hypothermia**

---

120. **Ans. c. Yellow- Stable patients, observation** *(Ref: Pediatric Emergency Medicine By Jill M. Baren (2008)/p1087)*

Triage consists of classifying the injured rapidly on the basis of illness severity and survival likelihood. Yellow color represents second priority in which, if the patient is stable, observation is required.

"Triage is the prioritization of patient care (or victims during a disaster) based on illness/injury, severity, prognosis, and resource availability. The disaster triage categories are red (most urgent, first priority), yellow (urgent, second priority), green (nonurgent, walking wounded, third priority), and black (dead or catastrophic)."-Pediatric Emergency Medicine By Jill M. Baren (2008)/p1087

Triage
- **Triage means "to sort,"** involves **prioritizing victims into categories based on** their **severity of injury, likelihood of survival,** and **urgency of care**[Q].
- The method of triage widely used by **municipalities** is the **START triage scheme**, which stands for **simple triage** and **rapid treatment**[Q]. This is accomplished by color tagging of patients.

Red color	• **First priority** and signifies a **critical patient**[Q]
Yellow color	• **Urgent, second priority**[Q]
Green color	• Minor injuries, **ambulatory** patient, **third-priority**[Q]
Black color	• **Expectant** or **dead** patients[Q]

121. Ans. b. 13 *(Ref: Harrison 19/e p1730; Sabiston 20/e p411; Schwartz 10/e p1712; Bailey 27/e p325, 26/e p312)*

Here, E = 4 (spontaneous eye opening); V= 4 (confused and irrelevant talks); M = 5 (Localizes pain). Hence, GCS = E4V4M5 = 13.

Glasgow Coma Scale (GCS)					
Eye Opening		**Verbal response**		**Best Motor response**	
Spontaneous	4	Oriented	5	Obeys commands	6
To loud voice	3	Confused, disoriented	4	Localizes pain	5
To pain	2	Inappropriate words	3	Flexion (withdrawal) to pain)	4
No response	1	Incomprehensible sounds	2	Abnormal flexion posturing	3
		No response	1	Extension posturing	2
				No response	1

- **Maximum score-15^Q, minimum score-3^Q.**
- **Best predictor of outcome: Motor response^Q**
- Patients scoring **3 or 4** have an **85% chance of dying** or **remaining vegetative**, while scores above **11** indicate only a **5-10% likelihood of death^Q.**

122. Ans. a. Assess the patient's response, Call for help, Check carotid pulse, Start CPR *(Ref: BLS/ACLS Guidelines: https:// www.resus.org.uk/resuscitation guidelines /adult- advanced-life-support; Harrison 19/e p1768; Braunwald's 10/e p844-845)*

According to Adult Basic Life Support (BLS) algorithm, steps followed are: Assess the patient's response, Call for help, check carotid pulse, Start CPR.

Adult Basic Life Support (BLS) Algorithm	
Safety	• Make sure you, the victim and any bystanders are safe
Response	• Check the victim for a response
Airway	• Open the airway
Breathing	• **Look, listen and feel for normal breathing for no more than 10 seconds^Q**
Dial 999	• Call an ambulance (999)
Send For AED	• Send someone to get an AED if available
Circulation	• **Start chest compressions** • Place **heel of one hand in lower half of victim's sternum** ^{Q} • Place **heel of your other hand on top of first hand**^{Q} • Interlock the fingers of your hands & ensure that pressure is not applied over the victim's ribs • Keep your arms straight; Position your shoulders vertically above the victim's chest • **Press down on sternum to a depth of 5–6 cm^Q** • After each compression, release all the pressure on chest without losing contact between your hands & sternum • **Repeat at a rate of 100–120/min^Q**
Give Rescue Breaths	• **After 30 compressions open the airway again using head tilt & chin lift & give 2 rescue breaths^Q** • **Do not interrupt compressions by more than 10 seconds to deliver two breaths. Then return your hands without delay to correct position on sternum & give a further 30 chest compressions ^{Q}** • **Continue with chest compressions & rescue breaths in a ratio of 30:2^Q** • If you are untrained or unable to do rescue breaths, give chest compression only CPR (i.e. continuous compressions at a rate of at least 100–120/min^Q)
If an AED Arrives	• **Switch on the AED** & follow the spoken/visual directions • Ensure that nobody is touching the victim while AED is analyzing the rhythm • **If a shock is indicated, deliver shock** & ensure that nobody is touching the victim • **Immediately restart CPR at a ratio of 30:2^Q** • **If no shock is indicated, continue CPR^Q**

Contd...

Contd...

	Adult Basic Life Support (BLS) Algorithm
Continue CPR	• Do not interrupt resuscitation until: • A health professional tells you to stop ; You become exhausted • The victim is definitely waking up, moving, opening eyes and breathing normally • It is rare for CPR alone to restart the heart. Unless you are certain the person has recovered continue CPR
Recovery Position	• If you are certain the victim is breathing normally but is still unresponsive, place in the recovery position[q]

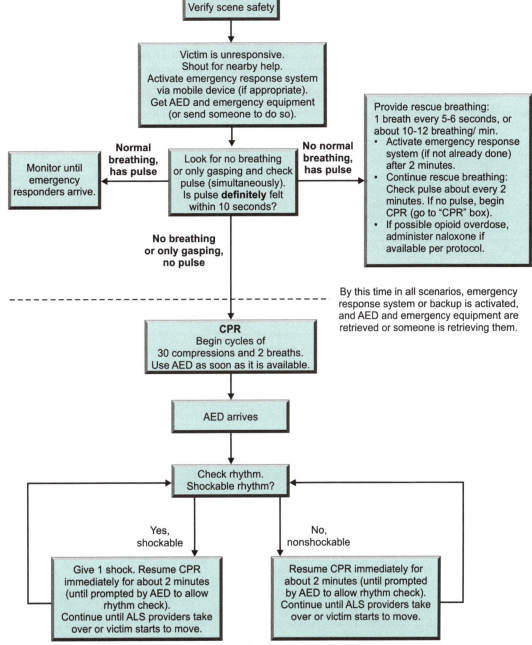

Fig. 31: Adult BLS cardiac arrest algorithm 2015 update

AIIMS ESSENCE

Cardiopulmonary Resuscitation (AHA 2015 Guidelines)

- **"CAB"[Q]** is followed (**not ABC**): **Circulation, Airway, Breathing**[Q] (**Immediately start chest compressions rather than airway opening**[Q])
- To allow **full chest wall recoil** after each compression, **rescuer must avoid leaning on the chest** between compressions[Q].

  - **Rescuer should not interrupt compressions for >10 seconds**[Q].
  - For patients with **ongoing CPR and an advanced airway in place**, a simplified **ventilation rate of 1 breath every 6 seconds**[Q] (**10 breaths per minute**[Q]) is recommended.

- **Routine use of impedance threshold device** (ITD) as an adjunct to conventional CPR is **not recommended**[Q].
- In **ACLS** (Advanced Cardiac Life Support), **vasopressin does not offer an advantage over the use of epinephrine alone**[Q]. Therefore, **vasopressin has been removed from the Adult Cardiac Arrest Algorithm-2015 Update. In 2010 update, atropine was removed**[Q] (earlier vasopressin was recommended as an alternative to epinephrine).
- Low end-tidal carbon dioxide (ETCO$_2$) in intubated patients **after 20 minutes of CPR** is associated with a **very low likelihood of resuscitation**[Q].
- **Emergency coronary angiography** is recommended for **all patients with ST elevation** and for **hemodynamically or electrically unstable patients without ST elevation** for whom a **cardiovascular lesion is suspected**[Q].

  - During **adult CPR tidal volume of 600 ml (6-7 ml/kg)** should be **adequate to cause the chest to rise**[Q].

- During airway management in an **unconscious trauma patient with possible cervical injury, neck hyperextension** should be **avoided.**
- The **most widely used waveform** in the automated electrical defibrillators (AEDs) now is the **biphasic truncated exponential (BTE) waveform.**

  - The following **drugs** may be **given through the endotracheal tube during CPR**: **L**ignocaine[Q], **E**pinephrine[Q], **V**asopressin[Q], **A**tropine[Q], **N**aloxone[Q] (**LEVAN**); (Amiodarone & sodium bicarbonate are not given endotracheally[Q])
  - **Atropine is not recommended for routine use** in the management of **Pulseless Electrical Activity/asystole** and has been **removed from the ACLS Cardiac Arrest Algorithm**[Q] (Epinephrine, vasopressin & amiodarone are used[Q])

	Adult (>12 years)	Child (1-12 years)	Infant (<1 year)
Compression Depth	At least **2 inches**[Q] (**5 cm, but not >2.4 inches/6 cm**[Q])	About **2 inches**[Q] (**5 cm; 1/3rd of chest depth**[Q])	About **1.5 inches**[Q] (**4 cm; 1/3rd of chest depth**[Q])
Compression: Ventilation ratio	**30:2**[Q] (one or two rescuer CPR)	**30:2**[Q] (single rescuer) or **15:2**[Q] (two rescuer)	
Compression rate	**100-120/min**[Q]		

123. Ans. c. Diameter of catheter *(Ref: The ICU Book By Paul L. Marino 3/e p108)*

French in Foley's catheter refers to diameter of catheter.

"The size of vascular catheters is expressed in terms of outside diameter of the catheter. Two units of measurements are used to describe catheter size: a metric-based French size and a wire-based gauge size. The French size is a series of whole numbers that increases from zero in increments of 0.33 millimeters (e.g., a size 5 French catheter will have an outside diameter of 5 x 0.33 = 1.65 mm). The gauge size was introduced for solid wires and is an expression of how many wires can be placed side-by-side in a given space. The gauge size varies inversely with the diameter of the wire (or catheter)."- The ICU Book By Paul L. Marino 3/e p108

124. Ans. b. Doctor's signature *(Ref: Sabiston 20/e p232; Schwartz 10/e p1969)*

In a pre-operative patient surgical checklist, doctor's signature is not required.

Elements of the Surgical Safety Checklist		
Sign In	**Time-Out**	**Sign Out**
Before induction of anesthesia, members of the team (at least the nurse and an anesthesia professional) state that the following have been done:	Before skin incision, the entire team (nurses, surgeons, anesthesia professionals, and any others participating in the care of the patient) or specific members state aloud the following:	Before the patient leaves the operating room, the following are done:
Patient has verified his or her identity, surgical site & procedure and consent.	Team confirms that all team members have been introduced by name & role.	Nurse reviews the following aloud with the team:
		Name of procedure, as recorded

Contd...

Contd...

Sign In	Time-Out	Sign Out
The **surgical site is marked** or site marking is not applicable. **Pulse oximeter** is on the patient & functioning. All members of the team are aware of whether the patient has a **known allergy**. **Patient's airway & risk of aspiration** have been evaluated, and appropriate equipment & assistance are available. If there is a risk of blood loss of at least 500 mL (or 7 mL/kg body weight in children), appropriate access and fluids are available.	Team confirms the patient's identity, surgical site & procedure. Team reviews the anticipated critical events. Surgeon reviews critical and unexpected steps, operative duration & anticipated blood loss. Anesthesia professionals review concerns specific to patient. Nurses review confirmation of sterility, equipment availability, and other concerns. **Team confirms that prophylactic antibiotics have been administered ≤60 minutes before incision is made or that antibiotics are not indicated.** Team confirms that all **essential imaging results for correct patient are displayed in operating room.**	That **needle, sponge, & instrument counts are complete** (or not applicable) That specimen (if any) is correctly labeled, including patient's name Whether there are any issues with equipment that need to be addressed The surgeon, nurse & anesthesia professional review aloud the key concerns for the recovery and care of the patient.

Surgical Safety checklist

Before induction of anaesthesia
(with at least nurse and anaesthetist)

Has the patient confirmed his/her identity, site, procedure, and consent?
□ Yes

Is the site marked?
□ Yes
□ Not applicable

□ Is the anaesthesia machine and medication check complete?
□ Yes

Is the pulse oximeter on the patient and functioning?
□ Yes

Does the patient have a:
Known allergy?
□ No
□ Yes
Difficult airway or aspiration risk?
□ No
□ Yes, and equipment/assistance available
Risk of > 500 ml blood loss (7ml/kg in children)?
□ No
□ Yes, and two IVs/central access and fluids planned

Before skin incision
(with nurse, anaesthetist and surgeon)

□ Confirm all team members have introduced themselves by name and role,

□ Confirm the patient's name, procedure, and where the incision will be made.

Has antibiotic prophylaxis been given within the last 60 minutes?
□ Yes
□ Not applicable

Anticipated Critical Events
To Surgeon:
□ What are the critical or non-routine steps?
□ How long will the case take?
□ What is the anticipated blood loss?
□ To Anaesthetist:
□ Are there any patient-specific concerns?
□ To Nursing Team:
□ Has sterility (inducing indicator results) been confirmed?
□ Are there equipment issues or any concerns?
Is essential imaging displayed?
□ Yes
□ Not applicable

Before patient leaves
operating room
(with nurse, anaesthetist and surgeon)

Nurse Verbally Confirms:
□ The name of the procedure
□ Completion of instrument, sponge and needle counts
□ Specimen labelling (read specimen labels aloud, including patient name)

To Surgeon, Anaesthetist and Nurse:
□ What are the key concerns for recovery and management of this patient?

Fig. 32: Surgical safety checklist (WHO surgical safety checklist 2009)

125. Ans. c. Maintaining permissible hypotension to avoid bleeding *(Ref: Schwartz 10/e p98; Current Therapy of Trauma and Surgical Critical Care By Juan A. Asensio 2/e p602)*

Balanced resuscitation in trauma management is maintaining permissible hypotension to avoid bleeding.

*"One of the most widely lauded and discussed advances in combat trauma care over the past decade has been a radical change in resuscitation strategy, now known as **damage control resuscitation (DCR)**. The core principle of this strategy is to replace blood loss with a balanced resuscitation of red blood cells, plasma, platelets, and clotting factors. This is achieved by either the use of fresh whole blood or with component therapy including PRBCs, fresh frozen or thawed plasma, and platelets. The optimal ratio of administration of each type of product remains a matter of debate, with the current practice being to aim for 1:1:1 ratio starting with the initial administration and continuing through the early resuscitation period."-Current Therapy of Trauma and Surgical Critical Care By Juan A. Asensio 2/e p602*

512   AIIMS ESSENCE

"Damage Control Resuscitation: Standard advanced trauma life support guidelines start resuscitation with crystalloid, followed by packed red blood cells. Only after several liters of crystalloid have been transfused does transfusion of units of plasma or platelets begin. This conventional massive transfusion practice was based on a several small uncontrolled retrospective studies that used blood products containing increased amounts of plasma, which are no longer available. Because of the known early coagulopathy of trauma, the current approach to managing the exsanguinating patient involves early implementation of damage control resuscitation (DCR). Although most of the attention to hemorrhagic shock resuscitation has centered on higher ratios of plasma and platelets, DCR is actually composed of three basic components: permissive hypotension, minimizing crystalloid-based resuscitation, and the immediate release and administration of pre-defined blood products (red blood cells, plasma, and platelets) in ratios similar to those of whole blood."- Schwartz 10/e p98

Components of Damage Control Resuscitation
• **Permissive hypotension**[Q]   • **Minimizing crystalloid-based resuscitation**[Q]   • **Immediate release & administration of pre-defined blood products** (red blood cells, plasma & platelets) **in ratios similar to those of whole blood**[Q].

126. **Ans. d. Polyps in gallbladder**   *(Ref: Sabiston 20/e p1511; Bailey 27/e p1210, 26/e p1109; Blumgart 5/e p751; Shackelford 7/e p1364)*

The diagnosis of the given gross specimen is gallbladder polyp.

Polypoid Lesions of the Gallbladder	
Cholesterol polyps	**Adenomatous polyp**
• **Cholesterol polyps (MC**[Q]**)** • Usually **<10 mm** in size[Q] • Have a characteristic echogenic **pedunculated**[Q] appearance on USG • **Multiple (30%** of cases)[Q]	• **Malignant potential**[Q]. • **Difficult to distinguish from adenocarcinoma** of GB • Main differentiating feature is a **lack of transmural invasion** on USG[Q] **Risk factors associated with malignancy** • **Age >60 years**[Q] • Coexistence of **gall stones**[Q] • Documented **increase in size**[Q] • **Size >10 mm**[Q]

127. **Ans. b. Abdominal mass**   *(Ref: Sabiston 20/e p765, 1073, 1085; Schwartz 10/e p1454; Bailey 27/e p1045, 26/e p969; Schackelford 7/e p974, 2035)*

Most common presentation of abdominal desmoid tumor is abdominal mass.

"Clinically, the most common areas of origin include the extremity, intraperitoneal, abdominal wall, and chest wall. Affected patients may present with a painful versus asymptomatic firm mass, bowel obstruction, or bowel ischemia."- Sabiston 20/e p765

"Patients with a desmoid tumor present with an asymptomatic mass or with symptoms related to mass effect from the tumor."-Sabiston 20/e p1073

Desmoid Tumour

• **MC primary malignant neoplasm of the mesentery**: Desmoid tumor
 • Arises from **musculoaponeurotic structures** of abdominal wall, especially **below** the **level of umbilicus**[Q].
 • It is a **completely unencapsulated fibroma**[Q] and is **so hard** that it **creaks when** it is **cut**[Q].
 • **Distribution: Extra-abdominal (60%), abdominal wall (25%), intra-abdominal (15%)**.
 • About **80% of cases** occur **in women**[Q], many of whom have borne children
 	
      • Occurs **occasionally in scars**[Q] of old hernial or other abdominal **operation wounds**.
      • **Surgical trauma**[Q]: Important etiological factor
      • **Estrogens stimulate**[Q] desmoid growth
      • Occur in cases of **FAP**[Q] (Gardener's syndrome)

Contd...

Contd...

Desmoid Tumour
Pathology: • Tumour is composed of **fibrous tissue** containing **multinucleated plasmodial masses** resembling **foreign body giant cells**[Q]. • Usually of **very slow growth**, it tends to **infiltrate muscle** in the **immediate area**[Q]. • Eventually it **undergoes a myxomatous change** and it then **increases in size more rapidly**. • **Metastasis does not occur**[Q], **no sarcomatous change**[Q]
Clinical Features: • **Desmoids classically arise in pregnancy** as an **abdominal mass independent of uterus**. • **MC presentation: Abdominal mass** • Affected patients may present with a **painful versus asymptomatic firm mass, bowel obstruction, or bowel ischemia.**
Diagnosis: • **MRI** is **investigation of choice** for **extremity & abdominal wall desmoids**[Q]. • **Biopsy** is required to **establish the diagnosis**.
Treatment: • **Wide local excision** (with **2 cm margin**) is **treatment of choice**[Q]. • **Surgery + Radiotherapy:** For **recurrent desmoid tumors**[Q] • Doxorubicin, dacarbazine, or carboplatin can produce remission in up to 50% of patients.
Prognosis: • Involvement of margins is associated with **recurrence rates** as high as **80%.**

128. **Ans. a. Psoas abscess** *(Ref: Harrison 19/e p852, 1110; Bailey 27/e p1065, 26/e p1204, 1380; Campbell 10/e p303)*

History of abdominal pain and mass in right lumbar region with no fever, with right hip flexed and X-ray showing spine changes suggest the diagnosis of psoas abscess of tubercular origin. Flexion deformity is not seen in undescended testis. Fever is the characteristic feature of pyonephrosis. Spine changes on X-ray are not seen in acute appendicitis.

"Psoas Abscesses: The psoas muscle is another location in which abscesses are encountered. Psoas abscesses may arise from a hematogenous source, by contiguous spread from an intra-abdominal or pelvic process, or by contiguous spread from nearby bony structures (e.g., vertebral bodies). Associated osteomyelitis due to spread from bone to muscle or from muscle to bone is common in psoas abscesses. When Pott's disease was common, Mycobacterium tuberculosis was a frequent cause of psoas abscess. Currently, either S. aureus or a mixture of enteric organisms including aerobic and anaerobic gram-negative bacilli is usually isolated from psoas abscesses in the United States. S. aureus is most likely to be isolated when a psoas abscess arises from hematogenous spread or a contiguous focus of osteomyelitis; a mixed enteric flora is the most likely etiology when the abscess has an intra- abdominal or pelvic source. Patients with psoas abscesses frequently present with fever, lower abdominal or back pain, or pain referred to the hip or knee. CT is the most useful diagnostic technique."-Harrison 19/e p852

"Spinal TB (Pott's disease or tuberculous spondylitis) often involves two or more adjacent vertebral bodies. Whereas the upper thoracic spine is the most common site of spinal TB in children, the lower thoracic and upper lumbar vertebrae are usually affected in adults. From the anterior superior or inferior angle of the vertebral body, the lesion slowly reaches the adjacent body, later affecting the intervertebral disk. With advanced disease, collapse of vertebral bodies results in kyphosis (gibbus). A paravertebral "cold" abscess may also form. In the upper spine, this abscess may track to and penetrate the chest wall, presenting as a soft tissue mass; in the lower spine, it may reach the inguinal ligaments or present as a psoas abscess."-Harrison 19/e p1110

"The term pyonephrosis refers to infected hydronephrosis associated with suppurative destruction of the parenchyma of the kidney, in which there is total or nearly total loss of renal function. The patient is usually very ill, with high fever, chills, flank pain, and tenderness."-Campbell 10/e p303

"Retrocecal appendicitis: Rigidity is often absent, and even application of deep pressure may fail to elicit tenderness (silent appendix), the reason being that the caecum, distended with gas, prevents the pressure exerted by the hand from reaching the inflamed structure. However, deep tenderness is often present in the loin, and rigidity of the quadratus lumborum may be in evidence. Psoas spasm, due to the inflamed appendix being in contact with that muscle, may be sufficient to cause flexion of the hip joint. Hyperextension of the hip joint may induce abdominal pain when the degree of psoas spasm is insufficient to cause flexion of the hip."-Bailey 27/e p1304

"*Testicular torsion is most common between 10 and 25 years of age, although a few cases occur in infancy. Typically, there is sudden agonizing pain in the groin and the lower abdomen. The patient feels nauseated and may vomit. Torsion of a fully descended testis is usually easily recognized. The testis seems high and the tender twisted cord can be palpated above it. The cremasteric reflex is lost.*"- Bailey 27/e p1500

129. **Ans. b. By observing the movement of air water column in the tube during respiration** *(Ref: Pleural Diseases By Richard W. Light 5/e p400)*

Functioning of the ICD tube is assessed by observing the movement of air water column in the tube during respiration.

"*When the patient is not receiving suction, the patency of the chest tube can be assessed by observing the oscillations in the water seal chamber with respiratory movements.*"-Pleural Diseases By Richard W. Light 5/e p400

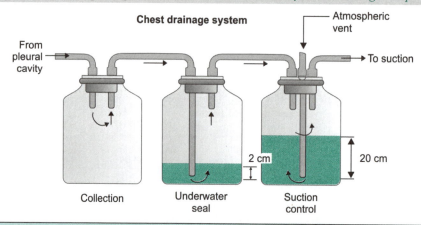

Intercostal Drain (Chest Tube) Insertion

- Chest tube insertion is used to provide **evacuation of abnormal collections of air** or **fluid from pleural space**.
- Tube thoracostomy may be indicated for **pleural effusions associated with malignancy, infection, or hemothorax** in the post-surgical setting (drainage is imperative **to allow for lung re-expansion**)

Underwater Seal Chamber

- **Underwater seal chamber** is the **most important element** in pleural drainage. It acts as a **low-resistance, one-way valve for the evacuation of pleural contents**[Q].
- When **intrapleural pressure rises** (eg, expiration, coughing), the **free contents of the pleural space are forced out through the chest tube and into the underwater seal drainage chamber**[Q].
  - **Reentry of air into pleural space** when intrapleural pressures become negative (eg, inspiration) is **blocked by underwater seal.** The **water in this tube is referred to as the "column" of water;** its **movements reflect the changes in intrathoracic pressure with each inspiration and expiration**[Q].
- **End of tube in the underwater seal chamber must remain covered with water at all times**[Q].
- Standard recommendation: Keep the **tip of tube 2-3 cm below the surface of water**[Q].

Indications of Chest Tube Insertion

• **Pneumothorax**[Q] (if it is **large or progressive**, or if the patient is **symptomatic**)	• **Chylothorax**[Q]
• **Tension pneumothorax**[Q]	• **Empyema**[Q]
• **Penetrating chest trauma**[Q]	• **Drainage of pleural effusions**[Q]
• **Hemothorax**[Q]	• Prevention of hydrothorax after cardiothoracic surgery
	• **Bronchopleural fistula**[Q]

Contraindications of Chest Tube Insertion

• Anticoagulation of a **bleeding dyscrasia**	• **Small, stable pneumothorax** (may spontaneously resolve)
• **Systemic anticoagulation**	
• **Loculated fluid accumulations**	• **Empyema** caused by **acid-fast organisms**

Contd...

AIIMS November 2017

Contd...

Intercostal Drain (Chest Tube) Insertion
Follow-up:
• **Patency of chest tube** is assessed by observing the **oscillations in water seal chamber with respiratory movements**[Q].
• **Position of chest tube** & **resolution of intrapleural air or liquid** is checked by x-ray (**AP & cross table lateral**). Tube should be **pulled back if it crosses the mediastium**[Q].
Removal:
• Chest tubes are generally removed when there has been **air or fluid drainage of <200 ml in 24 hours for >24 hours**[Q].

Complications of Chest Tube Insertion	
• Injury to heart, great vessels, or lung	• Recurrent pneumothorax
• Diaphragmatic perforation	• Empyema
• Subdiaphragmatic placement of the tube	• Lung parenchyma perforation
• Open or tension pneumothorax	• Subcutaneous placement
• Subcutaneous emphysema	• Cardiogenic shock (from chest tube compression of the right ventricle)
• Unexplained or persistent air leakage	
• Hemorrhage (especially from intercostal artery injury)	• Infection

130. Ans. c. J-shaped urinary stent *(Ref: Campbell 10/e p3736)*

Management of urinoma is by endoscopic intervention, with cystoscopy, retrograde pyelography, placement of a ureteral stent, urethral catheter drainage, and intravenous antibiotics.

"Although most post-traumatic urinomas are asymptomatic and have a spontaneous resolution rate approaching 85%, urinomas will occasionally persist. Symptomatic urinomas will develop a classic triad of findings: ipsilateral flank pain, adynamic ileus, and a low-grade temperature. Management of these patients is by endoscopic intervention, with cystoscopy, retrograde pyelography, placement of a ureteral stent, urethral catheter drainage, and intravenous antibiotics. When a ureteral stent is placed in conjunction with temporary placement of a urethral catheter, greater than 90% of the symptomatic urinomas will resolve. Classically, the urethral catheter is removed 3 to 5 days after the patient's clinical symptoms have abated. Intravenous antibiotics are discontinued and prophylactic antibiotics initiated at the time of urethral catheter removal. The author removes the ureteral stent 4 to 6 weeks post-injury and will maintain oral prophylactic antibiotic coverage for 48 hours after stent removal. It should be noted that both percutaneous nephrostomy drainage and internal stenting are equally efficacious for the treatment of symptomatic urinomas. The advantage of an internal stent is that it prevents possible dislodgment of the drainage tube and the need for external drainage devices. The two major disadvantages of internal drainage are that both stent placement and removal, in the pediatric patient population, require general anesthesia. In addition, the small-size ureteral stents (4 to 5 Fr) placed in young children may become blocked with blood clots from the dissolving hematoma, resulting in persistence of the urinoma."- Campbell 10/e p3736

131. Ans. b. PCNL *(Ref: Campbell 10/e p1364, 1374, 1380-1381, 1399-1405; Bailey 27/e p1409, 26/e p1294)*

Management of 4 cm size renal stag horn calculus is PCNL.

"The procedure of choice for patients with staghorn calculi is PNL. When they are left untreated, staghorn calculi are associated with the loss of renal function and increased mortality."-Campbell 10/e p1374

"The management of patients with staghorn stones by a combined approach must be viewed as primarily percutaneous in nature, with SWL being used only as an adjunct to minimize the number of access points required. Improved PNL techniques, incorporating the increasing use of flexible nephroscopy and providing complete or nearly complete clearance of stone material at the time of the primary procedure, may have decreased or eliminated the need for additional SWL treatment."-Campbell 10/e p1364

"PNL followed by either SWL or repeated PNL, should be used for most patients with struvite staghorn calculi, with PNL being the initial element of the combination therapy."-Campbell 10/e p1364

Renal Stones Treatment decisions by stone burden	
Stone size/ Composition	**Treatment of Choice**
Stone ≤2 cm	• **ESWL**[Q] • Unless factors of stone composition, location, location or renal anatomy shift the balance towards more invasive modalities (PCNL/URS).

AIIMS ESSENCE

Contd...

Renal Stones Treatment decisions by stone burden	
Stone >2 cm	• PCNL[Q]
Stag horn calculi	• PCNL + ESWL is TOC[Q] • Initial approach is **PCNL, followed by ESWL,** as an adjunct to minimize the number of repeat PCNL accesses.

PCNL (Percutaneous nephrolithotomy)

- Removal of kidney stone via a **'track'** developed **between surface of skin & collecting system** of kidney.
- **Posterior approach[Q]** is most commonly used, **through the posterior calyx** rather than into the renal pelvis, as it **avoids damage** to **posterior branches of renal artery[Q],** which are closely associated with renal pelvis.

Indications of PCNL	
• **Obstructive uropathy[Q]** (contraindication for ESWL) • **Large volume stone (>2 cm)** • **Stag horn calculi[Q]** • **Lower pole calyceal stone[Q]**	• Other modalities failure (**Ureteroscopic failure or ESWL failure**)[Q] • **Difficult (hard) stones for ESWL: Brushite, Hydroxyapatite, Cystine, Calcium oxalate monohydrate (BHC-2)[Q]**

Complications of PCNL	
• **Bleeding: MC complication** • **Injury** to other viscera like **pleura (MC)[Q], colon, spleen**	• Urinary extravasation • Retained fragments • Sepsis

132. Ans. b. Hypercalcemia *(Ref: Harrison 19/e p1795; Sabiston 20/e p90; Schwartz 10/e p81)*

Tumor lysis syndrome is characterized by hyperuricemia, hypocalcemia, hyperkalemia and hyperphosphatemia, not the hypercalcemia.

"Tumor lysis syndrome (TLS) is characterized by hyperuricemia, hyperkalemia, hyperphosphatemia, and hypocalcemia and is caused by the destruction of a large number of rapidly proliferating neoplastic cells. Acidosis may also develop. Acute renal failure occurs frequently."-Harrison 19/e p1795

"Tumor lysis syndrome is a constellation of electrolyte abnormalities that include hypocalcemia, hyperphosphatemia, hyperuricemia, and hyperkalemia. Such abnormalities occur when antineoplastic therapy causes a sudden surge in tumor cell death and a release of cytosolic contents. Solid tumors and lymphomas have been implicated."-Sabiston 20/e p90

Tumor Lysis Syndrome

- Caused by **destruction of** large number of **rapidly proliferating neoplastic cells[Q]**
- Frequently, **acute renal failure** develops as a result of the syndrome[Q].
- **Most frequently associated with** the treatment of **Burkitt's lymphoma, ALL** and other **high-grade lymphomas[Q], chronic leukemias** & rarely with solid tumors.

Pathophysiology:
- **Hyperuricemia**: Due to destruction of malignant cells & rapid turnover of nucleic acid
- **Hyperkalemia**: Due to release of intracellular K⁺ leading to arrhythmia.
- **Hyperphosphatemia & Hypocalcemia:** Due to **release of intracellular phosphate,** which combines with calcium into bone, **calcium phosphate** gets **deposited in renal tubules** causing **renal failure[Q].**
- **Lactic acidosis**: Due to **deranged oxidative metabolism[Q]**

Characteristic Abnormalities of Tumor Lysis Syndrome	
• Hyperuricemia[Q] • Hyperkalemia[Q] • Hyperphosphatemia[Q]	• Lactic acidosis[Q] • Hypocalcemia[Q]

Treatment:
- **Hydration, NaHCO₃, allopurinol, rasburicase** (recombinant urate oxidase), **hemodialysis[Q]**

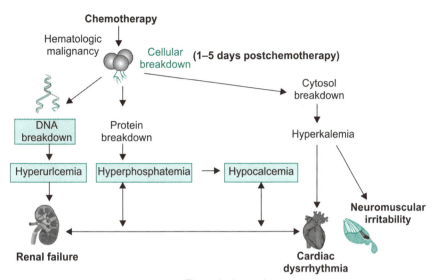

Fig. 32: Tumor lysis syndrome

133. **Ans. b. CT thorax** *(Ref: Harrison 19/e p1787-1788)*

The investigation of choice for diagnosis of SVC obstruction is CT scan. CT provides the most reliable view of the mediastinal anatomy. The diagnosis of SVCS requires diminished or absent opacification of central venous structures with prominent collateral venous circulation.

> *"The diagnosis of superior vena cava (SVC) syndrome (SVCS) is a clinical one. The most significant chest radiographic finding is widening of the superior mediastinum, most commonly on the right side. Pleural effusion occurs in only 25% of patients, often on the right side. The majority of these effusions are exudative and occasionally chylous.* However, a normal chest radiograph is still compatible with the diagnosis if other characteristic findings are present. **Computed tomography (CT) provides the most reliable view of the mediastinal anatomy. The diagnosis of SVCS requires diminished or absent opacification of central venous structures with prominent collateral venous circulation.** *Magnetic resonance imaging (MRI) has no advantages over CT."- Harrison 19/e p1788*

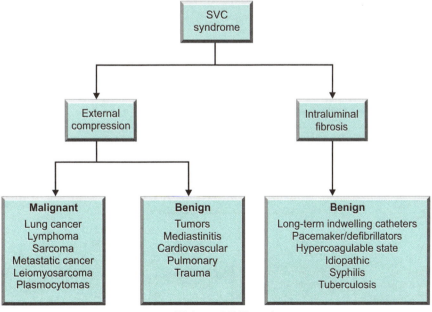

Fig. 33: Etiology of SVC syndrome

Superior Vena Cava (SVC) Syndrome

- **Clinical manifestation of SVC obstruction**, with **severe reduction in venous return from head, neck & upper extremities**[Q].
- MC cause is **Lung cancer (small cell & squamous cell carcinoma)**[Q], along with **lymphoma** & **metastatic tumors** responsible for **>90% of all SVC syndrome**[Q].
- In young adults, **malignant lymphoma** is the **leading cause** of SVC syndrome[Q].

Clinical Features:
- Patients present with **neck & facial swelling** (especially around the eyes), **dyspnoea & cough**[Q].
- Other symptoms include hoarseness, tongue swelling, headache, nasal congestion, epistaxis, dysphagia, pain, dizziness, syncope.
  - **Characteristic Physical Findings: Dilated neck veins, increased number of collateral veins** covering the **anterior chest wall, cyanosis & edema** of **face, arms & chest**[Q].

Diagnosis:
- Most significant chest radiographic finding is **widening of the superior mediastinum (MC right side)**[Q]
- **CT scan: Investigation of choice**[Q].

Treatment:
- Potentially life threatening complication of **superior mediastinal mass** is **tracheal obstruction**[Q].
- Diuretics with low salt diet, head elevation and oxygen may produce temporary symptomatic relief.

Treatment	Underlying cause
Radiation Therapy[Q]	Non-small cell lung cancer, metastatic solid tumors
Chemotherapy[Q]	Small cell carcinoma or lymphoma
Surgery[Q]	All other cases

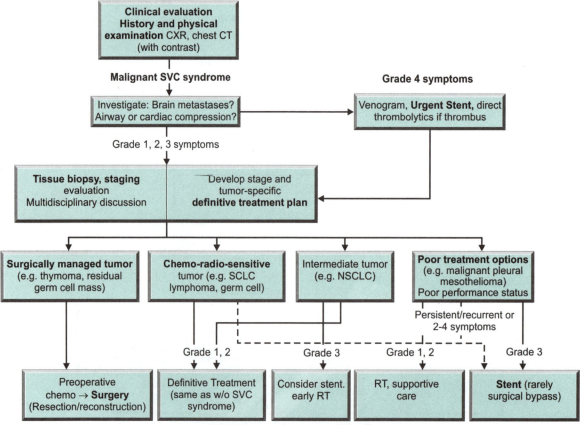

Fig. 34: Management algorithm of SVC syndrome

134. **Ans. a. Tip of nose to ear to xiphisternum** *(Ref: Practical Medical Procedures at a Glance By Rachel K. Thomas (2015)/p70)*

The commonly used method to measure nasogastric tube length is the NEX method. NEX: Nose–Ear–Xiphisternum.

> *"To measure the required length of tube, measure from the tip of the patient's nose, to their ear, and then down to the xiphisternum."*-Practical Medical Procedures at a Glance By Rachel K. Thomas (2015)/p70

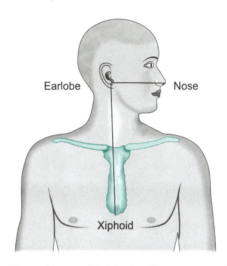

Fig. 35: Nasogastric tube length measurement

135. **Ans. c. Papillary dermis** *(Ref: Sabiston 20/e p506; Schwartz 10/e p229; Bailey 27/e p622, 26/e p390)*

Papillary dermis is involved in blister formation in a superficial partial thickness burn.

> *"Superficial partial-thickness burns: The damage in these burns goes no deeper than the papillary dermis. The clinical features are blistering and/or loss of the epidermis. The underlying dermis is pink and moist. The capillary return is clearly visible when blanched. There is little or no fixed capillary staining. Pinprick sensation is normal. Superficial partial-thickness burns heal without residual scarring in 2 weeks. The treatment is non-surgical."*-Bailey 27/e p622

Burns Depth

First Degree
- Epidermal burn[Q]
- Involve **only epidermis**[Q]
- **Do not blister**[Q]
- **Erythematous**[Q] because of dermal vasodilatation
- **Painful**[Q]
- **Heal without scarring** in **5-10 days**[Q]

Second Degree
- **Partial thickness**[Q] burn
- Involve **epidermis** & some **part of dermis**[Q]
- **Divided into: Superficial & Deep** second degree

Third Degree
- **Full thickness burn**[Q]
- Involve **all layers of dermis**[Q]
- Characterized by **hard leathery eschar**, that is **painless & black, white** or **cherry red**[Q]
- **No capillary refilling** or **pin-prick sensation**[Q]
- All dermal & epidermal components are **lost**[Q]
- **Heals** only **by wound contracture**[Q]
- Require **excision with skin grafting** to heal[Q]

Fourth Degree
- Involve **other organs** beneath the skin, such as **muscle, bone & brain**[Q].

Superficial Second Degree
- Involve **upper layer** of **dermis (papillary dermis)**[Q]
- **Erythematous**[Q]
- **Blisters** are **seen**[Q]
- **Blanch to touch**[Q]
- **Painful**[Q]
- **Heals without scarring** in **7-14 days**[Q]

Deep Second Degree
- Also known as **deep partial thickness burn**[Q]
- **Injury extends** to **reticular layer** of **dermis**[Q]
- **Don't blanch**[Q]
- **Mottled pink & white color** of wound surface[Q]
- **Capillary refilling** is **absent** or occurs slowly[Q]
- **Pain** is **absent**[Q]
- **Pin-prick sensation** is **preserved**[Q]
- **Heals in 3-9 weeks** with **scar formation**[Q]

OBSTETRICS AND GYNECOLOGY

136. Ans. b. Pawlick grip *(Ref: Williams 24/e p437, 438; Mudaliar and Menon's Clinical Obstetrics 12/e p76)*
The grip shown in the picture used for checking ballotability of head is known as Pawlick grip.

> *"First pelvic grip (Third Leopold) or Pawlick grip: The third maneuver is performed by grasping with the thumb and fingers of one hand the lower portion of the maternal abdomen just above the symphysis pubis. If the presenting part is not engaged, a movable mass will be felt, usually the head. The differentiation between head and breech is made as in the first maneuver. If the presenting part is deeply engaged, however, the findings from this maneuver are simply indicative that the lower fetal pole is in the pelvis, and details are then defined by the fourth maneuver."* - Williams 24/e p437

Importance of Pawlick grip
• To determine which part of fetus occupies the lower part of uterus: • **Head (independently ballotable)**^{Q} • **Breech (not independently ballotable)**^{Q} • **Empty lower pole (transverse lie)**^{Q}

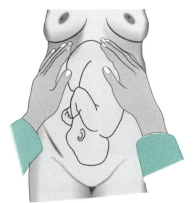
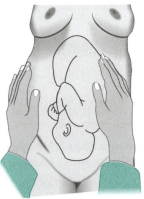
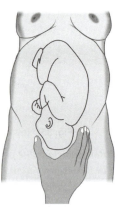
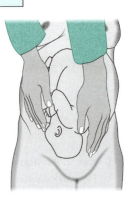

First maneuver   Second maneuver   Third maneuver   Fourth maneuver

Fig. 36: Abdominal palpation—leopold maneuvers

Abdominal Palpation—Leopold Maneuvers
• **Abdominal examination** can be conducted systematically employing the **four maneuvers described by Leopold**. • Mother lies **supine & comfortably positioned** with her **abdomen bared**.   • These maneuvers may be **difficult if not impossible to perform & interpret if the patient is obese**, if there is **excessive amnionic fluid**, or if the **placenta is anteriorly implanted**^{Q}. • Abdominal palpation can be **performed throughout the latter months of pregnancy** and **during & between the contractions of labor**^{Q}. • With experience, **it is possible to estimate the size of fetus**^{Q}. • For identification of fetal malpresentation, Leopold maneuvers have **sensitivity of 88%, specificity of 94%, positive-predictive value of 74% & negative-predictive value of 97%.**

Obstetric Grips (Leopold Maneuvers)	
1st Leopold (Fundal grip)	• Permits identification of **which fetal pole (cephalic or podalic) occupies the uterine fundus**^{Q}. • The **breech** gives the sensation of a **large, nodular mass**, whereas the **head feels hard & round** and is **more mobile & ballotable**^{Q}.
2nd Leopold (Lateral/ umbilical grip)	• Palms are placed on either side of maternal abdomen & gentle but deep pressure is exerted. • On one side, a **hard, resistant structure** is felt—the **back**. On the other, **numerous small, irregular, mobile parts** are felt—the **fetal extremities**^{Q}.

Contd...

Contd...

Abdominal Palpation—Leopold Maneuvers

Obstetric Grips (Leopold Maneuvers)	
	• By noting whether the **back is directed anteriorly, transversely, or posteriorly, fetal orientation** can be determined[Q].
3rd Leopold (First pelvic grip or Pawlick grip[Q])	• Performed by **grasping with the thumb & fingers of one hand the lower portion of maternal abdomen just above the symphysis pubis**[Q]. • If the **presenting part is not engaged, a movable mass will be felt**, usually the head. Differentiation between head & breech is made as in the first maneuver[Q]. • If the **presenting part is deeply engaged**, the findings are simply indicative that the **lower fetal pole is in the pelvis**[Q].
4th Leopold (Second pelvic grip)	• Examiner faces the mother's feet & with the tips of the first three fingers of each hand, exerts deep pressure in the direction of axis of the pelvic inlet. • In many instances, when the **head has descended into the pelvis**, the **anterior shoulder may be differentiated** readily by the third maneuver[Q].

137. Ans. b. Episiotomy scissor   *(Ref: Williams 24/e p551)*

Name of the instrument seen in the picture is episiotomy scissor, identified easily by the presence of angulation in the scissor.

Episiotomy Scissor
• Episiotomy scissor has **angulation in the scissor**[Q] • Angulation in the scissor **prevents extension of pelvic tears in to the anal margins**, obstetric anal sphincter injuries & complete perineal tear[Q].

138. Ans. c. Left side of the alert line   *(Ref: Williams 24/e p 452, Mudaliar and Menon's Clinical obstetrics 12/e p401)*

In partogram, first time of the initial markings are made in left side of the alert line.

> "A partograph was designed by the World Health Organization (WHO) for use in developing countries. According to Orji (2008), the partograph is similar for nulliparas and multiparas. **Labor is divided into a latent phase, which should last no longer than 8 hours, and an active phase. The active phase starts at 3 cm dilatation, and progress should be no slower than 1 cm/hr. A 4-hour wait is recommended before intervention when the active phase is slow. Labor is graphed, and analysis includes use of alert and action lines.**" - *Williams 24/e p452*

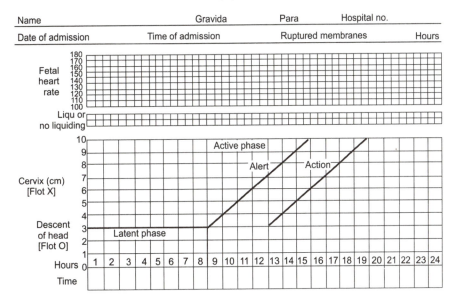

Partograph
• Partograph is a **composite graphical record of cervical dilatation in centimeters & descent of head against duration of labor in hours**[Q].
• **Introduce as an early warning system** to detect labour that was progressing normally, **for timely transfer to a referral center**[Q].

In a partograph the labor process is divided into
• **Latent phase** that **ends** when the **cervix is 3 cm dilated**[Q]
• **Active phase starts with cervical dilation of 3 cm. Cervix** should **dilate at least 1cm/hour in this active phase**[Q]

• **Cervical dilation rate (cervicograph)** is plotted in relation to alert line & action line[Q].
• Concept of Alert line & Action line **given by Philpott**[Q]

Alert line	Action line
• Alert line **starts at the end of latent phase (3 cm cervical dilation)** & ends with full dilation of the cervix (10cm) in 7 hours (1cm/hour dilation rate)[Q]	• Action line is **drawn four hours to the right of the alert line. An interval of 4 hours is allowed to diagnose delay in active phase** and then **appropriate intervention is done**[Q].

Labor is considered **abnormal when cervicograph crosses the alert line & falls on zone 2**[Q].
Intervention is required when it **crosses the action line & falls on zone 3**[Q].

139. Ans. c. 95% ethyl alcohol   *(Ref: Shaw's 16/e p343; Novak's 15/e p987; DC Dutta's Gynecology 7/e p89)*
Fixative used in PAP smear is 95% ethyl alcohol.

"Pap's smear: The principle of the staining is to achieve clear nuclear definition and to define cytoplasmic coloration. The material so collected should be immediately spread over a microscopic slide and at once put into the fixative ethyl alcohol (95%) before drying. After fixing for about 30 minutes, the slide is taken out, air-dried and sent to the laboratory with proper identification. The slide so sent is stained either with Papanicolaou's or Sorr's method and examined by a trained cytologist. Indeed, trained cytopathologist and cytotechnologist are vital for the success of any screening program."-DC Dutta's Gynecology 7/e p89

"Pap's smear: The scrapings are evenly spread onto a glass slide and immediately fixed by dipping the slide in the jar containing equal parts of 95% ethyl alcohol and ether. After fixing it for 30 minutes, the slide is air-dried and stained with Pap or short stain."- Shaw's 14/e p87

Screening Recommendations for Asymptomatic Subjects		
Cancer Type	**Test or Procedure**	**ACS: American Cancer Society**
Cervical	Pap test (cytology)	• Women **21–29 years**: Screen **every 3 years**[Q] • Women **30–65 years**: Acceptable approach to screen with cytology **every 3 years**[Q] • Women **<21 years**: **No screening**[Q] • Women **>65 years**: **No screening following adequate negative prior screening**[Q]
	HPV test	• Women **30–65 years**: Preferred approach to screen with **HPV & cytology co-testing every 5 years**[Q] • Women **<30 years**: **Do not use HPV testing** [Q] • Women **>65 years**: **No screening following adequate**[Q] **negative prior screening** • Women **after total hysterectomy** for noncancerous causes: **Do not screen**[Q]

140. Ans. b. Types 6, 11, 16, 18, 31, 33, 45, 52, 58   *(Ref: Shaw's 16/e p623; Novak's 15/e p1203; William's Gynecology/p1002)*
Nanovalent vaccine offers protection against HPV virus types 6, 11, 16, 18, 31, 33, 45, 52, 58.

*"The development of HPV-related vaccines has opened a new avenue in HPV-related cancer prevention. **The three existing HPV vaccines are Gardasil, a tetravalent vaccine that includes 4 types, HPVs 6, 11, 16, and 18; Gardasil 9 a nanovalent vaccine that includes nine types, HPV_s 6, 11, 16, 18, 31, 33, 45, 52, and 58; and Cervarix, a bivalent vaccine against HPV_s 16 and 18.** They have been licensed by several regulatory agencies such as the European Agency for the Evaluation of Medical Products (EMEA) or the US FDA. HPV vaccines have been approved in over 100 countries and have been introduced in some national immunization Programs, mainly in developed countries. **The result from randomized controlled trials have demonstrated high immunogenicity, safety, and efficacy against cervical preneoplastic lesions (CIN 2/3) and vaginal, vulvar, and anal-related lesions to the HPV types included in these vaccines. Moreover, the quadrivalent vaccine has shown high efficacy against genital warts related to HPV6 and 11.**"-Tropical Hemato-Oncology by Jean-Pierre Droz (2015)/p153*

HPV Vaccines
• HPV vaccines are **highly effective in preventing infection with the types of HPV they target when given before initial exposure to the virus**—which means **before individuals begin to engage in sexual activity.**

Types of HPV Vaccines		
Bivalent Vaccine (Cervarix)	**Quadrivalent Vaccine (Gardasil)**	**Nanovalent Vaccine (Gardasil 9)**
• Prevention against HPV types **16 & 18**[Q] • Only used for **girls**[Q] • Age **9-26 years**[Q]	• Prevention against HPV types **6, 11, 16, 18**[Q] • Used for both for **boys & girls**[Q] • Age **9-26 years**[Q]	• Prevention against HPV types **6, 11, 16, 18, 31, 33, 45, 52, 58**[Q] • Used for both **boys & girls**[Q] • **3 doses** given at 0, 2 & 6 months • 0.5 ml given IM

141. **Ans. a. 16/10/2017** *(Ref: William's 24/e p127)*

According to Naegele's rule, EDD of a patient with LMP 9/01/2017 is 16/10/2017 [9 + 7/01 (January)–3 months/2017= 16/10/2017].

"Clinicians customarily calculate gestational age as menstrual age. Approximately 280 days, or 40 weeks, elapse on average between the first day of the last menstrual period and the birth. This corresponds to 9 and 1/3 calendar months. A quick estimate of a pregnancy due date based on menstrual data can be made as follows: add 7 days to the first day of the last period and subtract 3 months. For example, if the first day of the last menses was July 5, the due date is 07–05 minus 3 (months) plus 7 (days) = 04–12, or April 12 of the following year. This calculation has been termed Naegele rule."-William's 24/e p127

Naegele's Rule

• **EDD is calculated by Naegele's rule**
 • **Add 7 days to the first day of the last period and subtract 3 months**
 • Naegele's rule is **based on 28 days regular cycle**.
 • If the **cycle is shorter or longer than 28 days**, EDD will be corrected and written as **corrected EDD**.
 • Examples:
   – **40 days** cycle regularly, to get corrected EDD, **add 12 days** (40-28) with the EDD calculated from LMP.
   – **21 days** cycle regularly, to get corrected EDD, **subtract 7 days** (28-21) with the EDD calculated from LMP.

142. **Ans. a. Dysgerminoma** *(Ref: Shaw's 16/e p821, 15/e p378; Novak's 15/e p1506-1508; Robbins 9/e p1031)*

Ovarian mass in a young female (18 years) with raised LDH suggests the diagnosis of dysgerminoma.

"Dysgerminoma is the most common malignant germ cell tumor, accounting for about 30% to 40% of all ovarian cancers of germ cell origin. The tumors represent only 1% to 3% of all ovarian cancers, but they represent as many as 5% to 10% of ovarian cancers in patients younger than 20 years."-Novak's

"Placental alkaline phosphatase (PLAP) and lactate dehydrogenase (LDH) are commonly produced by dysgerminomas and may be useful for monitoring the disease."-Novak's

Histology	AFP	hCG	LDH	PLAP	CA-125
Choriocarcinoma	–	+	–	+	–
Dysgerminoma	–	+	+	+	+
Embryonal carcinoma	+	+	–	+	–
Endodermal sinus tumor	+	–	+	–	+
Immature teratoma	+	–	–	–	–

Tumor	Tumor Marker
Dysgerminoma	• b-hCG, PLAP, LDH[Q]
Endodermal sinus tumor **Immature teratoma** **Mixed germ cell tumor**	• AFP[Q]
Granulosa cell tumor	• Inhibin[Q]
Stromal tumors (including granulosa cell tumors)	• **Estradiol**[Q]

Dysgerminoma
• MC malignant tumor of ovary[Q]
• MC ovarian malignancy detected during pregnancy[Q]
• **Usually unilateral,** but they are the **only germ cell malignancy with a significant rate of bilateral ovarian involvement (15-20%)**[Q]   • Can be found at **gonadal as well as extra-gonadal sites**[Q]
Genetics: • Express **OCT-3, OCT-4 & NANOG**[Q]   • **Activating mutations** in the **Kit gene** in one third[Q]
Pathology: • **Solid neoplasm** with areas of **softening due to degeneration, consistency is fleshy**[Q]   • Mimics the pattern of primitive gonad, lymphocytic infiltration is seen (good prognostic sign)
Clinical Features: • Primarily affects **young women**; **Average age: 20 years**   • Clinically as with all germ cell tumors, most dysgerminoma are **diagnosed at an early stage**   • **MC route of spread: Lymphatic**[Q]   • **Metastasize to opposite ovary**[Q]
Diagnosis: • **Does not secrete AFP, rarely secrete beta-HCG**[Q]   • **Secretes LDH & PLAP**[Q] (Placental alkaline phosphatase)
Treatment: • **Early Dysgerminoma (Stage IA): Unilateral oophorectomy**[Q]   • **Rest cases: Unilateral oophorectomy followed by chemotherapy**[Q]

Histopathological Features of Ovarian Tumors

Tumor	Type	Histopathological Feature
Epithelial Tumors	**Brenner tumor**	**Urothelial cells**[Q]
	Clear cell tumors	**Clear, glycogen filled cells**[Q]
	Mucinous tumors	**Adenomatous glandular cells**[Q]
	Serous tumors	**Psammoma bodies**[Q]
Sex Cord Stromal Tumors	**Granulosa cell tumor**	**Inhibin staining**[Q] **Call-Exner bodies**[Q]
	Hilus cell tumor (Pure Leydig cell tumor)	**Large lipid laden cells with distinct borders**[Q]
	Sertoli-Leydig tumors (Androblastomas)	**Stain with inhibin**[Q]
	Thecomas	**Spindle shaped cells with vacuolated cells**[Q] **Oil red 'O' stain positive**[Q]
Germ Cell Tumors	**Benign teratoma**	**Rokitansky protuberances**[Q] **Multiple cell lines**[Q]
	Monodermal teratoma	**Struma/carcinoid like with mature thyroid tissue**[Q]
	Dysgerminoma	**Large vesicular cells with clear cytoplasm & centrally placed regular nuclei**[Q]
	Yolk sac tumor	**Schiller Duval (glomeruloid bodies)**[Q]

143. **Ans. a. First stage** *(Ref: Williams 24/e p446)*

Cervical dilatation of 6 cm with contraction rate of 3/10 min in a primigravida is suggestive of first stage of labor.

"The progress of labor in nulliparas has particular significance because these curves all reveal a rapid change in the slope of cervical dilatation rates between 3 and 5 cm. Thus, cervical dilatation of 3 to 5 cm or more, in the presence of uterine contractions, can be taken to reliably represent the threshold for active labor."-Williams 24/e p446

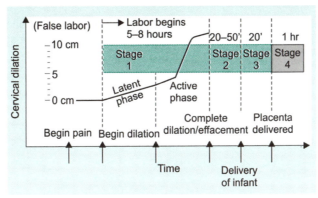

Fig. 37: Stages of normal labor

Stage of Labor			
First Stage	**Second Stage**	**Third Stage**	**Fourth Stage**
• **Initiation of labor** through **10-cm cervical dilation** • **Longest stage**, with **three phases** (**early or latent, active & transition**). • Physiologically, the uterus contracts & relaxes at frequent intervals as a response to maternal hormones. • **Estrogens stimulate uterine contractions; prostaglandins soften the cervix** and play a role in the rising level of estrogen. • **Decreasing progesterone levels** allow the body to **initiate & continue contractions** & efface (thin, 0% to 100%) and **dilate** (open, 0 to 10 cm) **the cervix.**	• **Begins with complete cervical dilatation & ends with fetal delivery.** • Once fully dilated, **involuntary contractions** (primary force of labor) & **maternal pushing** (secondary force of labor) **augment the expulsive effort** culminating in birth. • **Fetus changes position during the birth process** (cardinal movements of labor) **to accommodate maternal pelvis; positions include:** • Descent • Flexion • Internal rotation • Extension • Restitution • External rotation • Expulsion	• **Begins immediately after fetal birth & ends with placental delivery** • Contractions continue, resulting in expulsion of the placenta.	• **Delivery of placenta through the first 2 to 4 hours** postpartum. • Physiologically, the **first 2 to 4 hours after delivery** begins the **physical & emotional readjustment** to the non-pregnant state with **a rapid change in hormones** after placental delivery.

Stage 1: Dilation

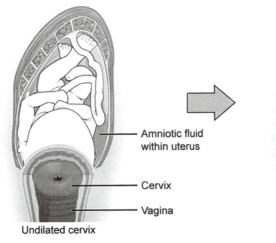
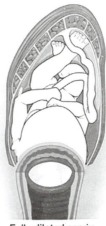

Undiluted cervix   Fully dilated cervix (> 10 cm in diameter)

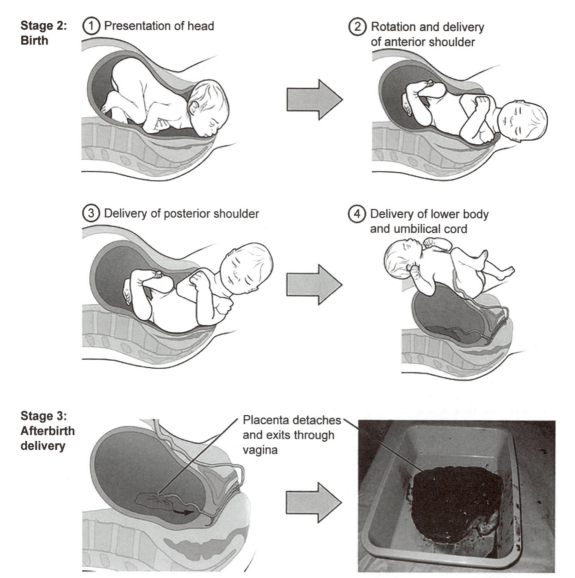

Fig. 38: Stages of normal labor

144. **Ans. a. Type 1 hysterectomy** *(Ref: Shaw's 16/e p826; Novak's 15/e p1121)*

A postmenopausal female with biopsy report as endometrial hyperplasia with atypia is having increased risk of malignancy. So the next line of management is type 1 hysterectomy.

> *"Endometrial hyperplasia carries a resonably high risk of progresssion to endometrial cancer if not adequately treated. Simple hyperplasia without cytologic atypia carries aless than 1% chance of progression to cancer, whereas complex hyperplasia without atypia has 2% to 3% chance of progression to cancer. Thus these two entities are usually treated medically using progesterone therapy.With cytologic atypia, simple hyperplasia and complex hyperplasia carry an 8% and 27% to 28% chance of progression to cancer, respectively. With cytologic atypia, hysterectomy is usually the treatment of choice unless future fertility is still desired."-Advances in Surgical Pathology: Endometrial Carcinoma by Anna Sienko (2012)/p130*

> *"Endometrial hyperplasia with atypia is less likely to respond to hormonal therapy, and for that reason, peri- and postmenopausal women with complex atypical hyperplasia (CAH) are usually treated with hysterectomy."- Gynecologic Pathology by Marisa R. Nucci (2009)/p240*

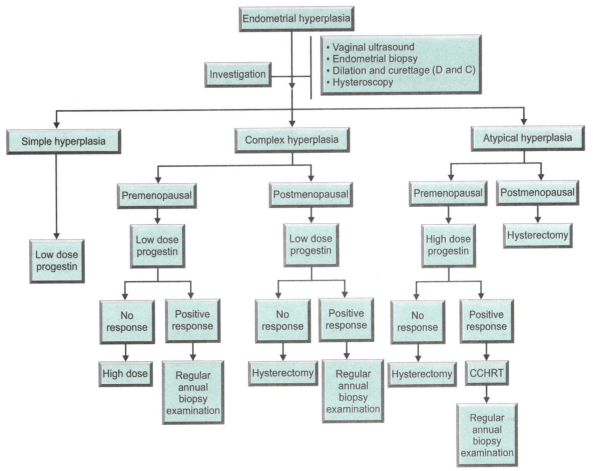

Fig. 39: Management of endometrial hyperplasia

Endometrial Hyperplasia
• **Endometrial hyperplasia** represents a spectrum of **morphologic & biologic alterations of endometrial glands** & stroma.
• Endometrial hyperplasia may cause **abnormal bleeding**, be **associated with estrogen-producing ovarian tumors**, result from **hormonal therapy** & precede or occur simultaneously with endometrial cancer.
• Risk of endometrial hyperplasia progressing to carcinoma is related to presence & severity of cytologic atypia.

Type of Hyperplasia	Progression to Cancer
Simple hyperplasia without atypia	1%[Q]
Complex hyperplasia without atypia	3%[Q]
Simple hyperplasia with atypia	8%[Q]
Complex hyperplasia with atypia	29%[Q]

Management of Endometrial Hyperplasia	
Hyperplasia without Atypia (All ages)	**Hyperplasia with Atypia**
• **Progestin therapy** is **very effective in reversing endometrial hyperplasia without atypia**[Q]. • **First line: Levonorgestrel intrauterine system (LNG-IUS)**[Q] • **Progesterone only pills (POP)** or **depot medroxyprogesterone acetate (DMPA)**[Q] • If fails **endometrial ablation**[Q]	• **Postmenopausal women or women completed family: Simple or type-1 hysterectomy**[Q] • **Young women/ not completed family: LNG-IUS/POP/DMPA**[Q] (Duration 9-12 months)

528 AIIMS ESSENCE

145. **Ans. b. 1 tab after 12 hours** *(Ref: Shaw's 16/e p609; William's 24/e p714)*

For emergency contraception levonorgestrel is used, 0.75 mg initially, followed by another 0.75 mg 12 hours later.

"With progestin-only regimens, 1.5 mg of levonorgestrel is taken, either as a single, one-time 1.5-mg dose or as two tablets, each containing 0.75 mg levonorgestrel. With these regimens, the first dose is ideally taken within 72 hours of unprotected coitus but may be given up to 120 hours. With the two-pill regimen, the second dose follows 12 hours later, although a 24-hour interval between the doses is also effective."- William's 24/e p714

"A new and better alternative for emergency contraception is using levonorgestrel alone, 0.75 mg initially, followed by another 0.75 mg 12 hours later."-Novak's

"Finally, levonorgestrel is used as so-called emergency contraception after known or suspected unprotected intercourse. The medication is given orally within 72 hours after intercourse as either a single 1.5-mg dose (PLAN B ONE STEP) or as two 0.75-mg doses (PLAN B) separated by 12 hours. The mechanism of action may involve several factors, including the prevention of ovulation, fertilization, and implantation."-Goodman Gilman 12/e p1184

146. **Ans. b. Naloxone** *(Ref: William's 24/e p507, 517; Goodman Gilman 12/e p512; Katzung 13/e p548, 12/e p560)*

Low-dose naloxone has an increasing role in the treatment of adverse effects that are commonly associated with intravenous or epidural opioids. Careful titration of the naloxone dosage can often eliminate the itching, nausea, and vomiting while sparing the analgesia.

"The major application of naloxone is in the treatment of acute opioid overdose. It is very important that the relatively short duration of action of naloxone be borne in mind, because a severely depressed patient may recover after a single dose of naloxone and appear normal, only to relapse into coma after 1–2 hours."- Katzung 13/e p548

"Low-dose naloxone (0.04 mg) has an increasing role in the treatment of adverse effects that are commonly associated with intravenous or epidural opioids. Careful titration of the naloxone dosage can often eliminate the itching, nausea, and vomiting while sparing the analgesia."- Katzung 13/e p548

"The opioid antagonist naloxone may be given in a dose of 0.4–2 mg intravenously. Naloxone reverses respiratory and CNS depression due to all varieties of opioid drugs."- Katzung 12/e p1029

"Opioid antagonists, particularly naloxone, have an established use in the treatment of opioid-induced toxicity, especially respiratory depression. Its specificity is such that reversal by this agent is virtually diagnostic for the contribution of an opiate to the depression. Naloxone acts rapidly to reverse the respiratory depression associated with high doses of opioids."- Goodman Gilman 12/e p512

Naloxone
• **Naloxone** is an **opioid antagonist; promptly reverses the respiratory depressant property of opioids**[Q].
• **Other agnostic effects of opioids** such as **effects on CNS & BP** is **also reversed**[Q].
Mechanism of Action:
• **Nonselective antagonist of opioid receptors**[Q]
• Clinical Applications:
• **Opioid overdose:** Effect much shorter than morphine (1–2 h); several injections required
Adverse Effects:
• **Antagonism of opioid** effects by **naloxone** is often accompanied by **"overshoot" phenomenon** i.e., while reversing the effect produced by the opioids it **tends to overcorrect it**[Q].
• **Precipitate seizures only in** patients who are **addicted** to or **dependent** on opioids[Q].
• **Rebound release of catecholamine** may cause **arrhythmia, hypertension & pulmonary edema** when **naloxone is administered in normal individual** to reverse the effect of opioids[Q].

147. **Ans. d. Low prolactin levels** *(Ref: Shaw's 16/e p431; Novak's 15/e p782; Harrison 19/e p2365)*

In hypogonadotropic hypogonadism LH, FSH and testosterone are low but prolactin levels are high.

AIIMS November 2017

"Pre-testicular azoospermia represents those conditions in which the hypothalamic–pituitary axis fails to stimulate spermatogenesis within the testis. Congenital, acquired, and idiopathic etiologies of hypogonadotropic hypogonadism are included in this category. A full endocrine history, including information on puberty and growth and a review of endocrine systems, should guide the physician in the evaluation of the hypogonadotropic hypogonadal patient. Laboratory investigations of particular benefit in this population include measurement of serum LH, FSH, testosterone, and prolactin levels and imaging of the pituitary gland. Low levels of gonadotropins (LH and FSH) and low serum levels of testosterone are characteristic."- Novak's 14/e p1198

"Hyperprolactinemia: Elevated prolactin (PRL) levels are associated with hypogonadotropic hypogonadism. PRL inhibits hypothalamic GnRH secretion either directly or through modulation of tuberoinfundibular dopaminergic pathways. A PRL-secreting tumor may also destroy the surrounding gonadotropes by invasion or compression of the pituitary stalk. Treatment with dopamine agonists reverses gonadotropin deficiency, although there may be a delay relative to PRL suppression."-Harrison 19/e p2365

Hypogonadism			
	Hypogonadotropic Hypogonadism	Hypergonadotropic Hypogonadism	Normogonadotropic Hypogonadism
LH & FSH	Low[Q]	High[Q]	Normal[Q]
Testosterone	Low[Q]	Low[Q]	Normal[Q]
Testicular volume	Low[Q] (oligospermia)	Low[Q] (oligospermia)	Normal[Q]

148. Ans. a. Hyperprolactinemia   *(Ref: Novaks 15/e p1107; Goodman Gilman 12/e p1114; Katzung 13/e p289, 655, 12/e p672, 290)*

Hyperprolactinemia produces a syndrome of amenorrhea and galactorrhea in women. Because of its greater track record, bromocriptine generally is recommended for fertility induction in patients with hyperprolactinemia.

"Hyperprolactinemia: Hyperprolactinemia can be associated with ovulatory factor infertility. After exclusion of a pituitary macroadenoma or other intracranial pathology, correction of the hyperprolactinemic state with bromocriptine is followed by restoration of ovulation in 90% of patients."- Novaks 15/e p1107

"Hyperprolactinemia produces a syndrome of amenorrhea and galactorrhea in women, and loss of libido and infertility in men."-Katzung 13/e p655

"Because of negative feedback effects, hyperprolactinemia is associated with amenorrhea and infertility in women as well as galactorrhea in both sexes. Rarely, the prolactin surge that occurs around the end of term pregnancy may be associated with heart failure; cabergoline has been used to treat this cardiac condition successfully.

Bromocriptine is extremely effective in reducing the high levels of prolactin that result from pituitary tumors and has even been associated with regression of the tumor in some cases."-Katzung 13/e p289

"Patients with prolactinomas who wish to become pregnant comprise a special subset of hyperprolactinemic patients because drug safety during pregnancy becomes an important consideration. The dopamine agonists described here relieve the inhibitory effect of prolactin on ovulation and permit most patients with prolactinomas to become pregnant. Clinical experience also indicates that many patients can discontinue the dopaminergic agonist during pregnancy without clinically significant tumor growth. Although drug therapy ideally is discontinued before pregnancy to avoid any fetal exposure, most experts discontinue therapy after pregnancy is confirmed and carefully follow for symptoms or signs of pituitary mass effect throughout gestation. Because of its greater track record, bromocriptine generally is recommended for fertility induction in patients with hyperprolactinemia."-Goodman Gilman 12/e p1114

Dopamine Agonists	
Ergot Derivatives	**Non-ergot Dopamine Agonists**
• Associated with **ergot-related side effects**, including **cardiac valvular damage**[Q]	• Non-ergot dopamine agonists replaced ergot derivatives
• Example:	• Example:
• **Bromocriptine**[Q]	• **Pramipexole**[Q]
• **Pergolide**[Q]	• **Ropinirole**[Q]
• **Cabergoline**[Q]	• **Rotigotine**[Q]

Bromocriptine
• Bromocriptine is the **semisynthetic ergot alkaloid** & **dopamine receptor agonist**
Mechanism of Action: • **Activates dopamine D_2 receptors** to **inhibit spontaneous & TRH-induced release of prolactin**[Q] • **Activates D_1 receptors**[Q] (to a lesser extent)
Effects: • **Suppresses pituitary secretion of prolactin** & less effectively, **GH**[Q] • **Dopaminergic effects** on CNS motor control & behavior[Q]
Therapeutic Uses: • Treatment of **hyperprolactinemia, acromegaly & Parkinson's disease**[Q]   • Bromocriptine normalizes serum prolactin levels in **70-80%** of patients with prolactinomas & decreases tumor size in **>50%**. It **does not cure** the underlying **adenoma; hyperprolactinemia & tumor growth recur upon cessation of therapy**[Q].

Bromocriptine	
Adverse effects	**Contraindications**
• Nausea, vomiting, **abdominal pain** • Muscle cramps, weakness, paresthesias • **Digital vasospasm**[Q] • **Coronary & other vascular spasm**[Q] • **Chest pain** (due to **coronary vasoconstriction**)[Q]	• Sepsis[Q] • Ischemic heart disease[Q] • Peripheral vascular disease[Q] • Hypertension[Q] • Pregnancy[Q] • Live & kidney disease[Q]

149. Ans. a. Pubococcygeus *(Ref: Shaw's 16/e p493; Novak's 15/e p861; Gray's 41/e p1223; Williams 24/e p22)*

When the pubococcygeus muscle contracts, it pulls the rectum, vagina, and urethra anteriorly toward the pubic bone and constricts the lumens of these pelvic organs. It is this contractile property that is so important in maintaining urinary and fecal continence and in providing support for the genital organs (vagina, cervix, uterus) that lie upon and are supported by the levator plate. Injury to pubococcygeus can lead to rectocele, cystocele and urinary incontinence.

"Pelvic Diaphragm: Found deep to the anterior and posterior triangles, this broad muscular sling provides substantial support to the pelvic viscera. The pelvic diaphragm is composed of the levator ani and the coccygeus muscle. The levator ani is composed of the pubococcygeus, puborectalis, and iliococcygeus muscles. The pubococcygeus muscle is also termed the pubovisceral muscle and is subdivided based on points of insertion and function. These include the pubovaginalis, puboperinealis, and puboanalis muscles, which insert into the vaginal, perineal body, and anus, respectively. Vaginal birth conveys significant risk for damage to the levator ani or to its innervation. Of these muscles, the pubovisceral muscle is more commonly damaged. Evidence supports that these injuries may predispose women to greater risk of pelvic organ prolapse or urinary incontinence. For this reason, current research efforts are aimed at minimizing these injuries."-Williams 24/e p22

"The pubovisceral (pubococcygeus) portion of the levator ani muscle consists of a thick U-shaped band of muscle arising from the pubic bone and attaching to the lateral walls of the vagina and rectum. Therefore, the rectum is supported by a muscular sling that pulls it toward the pubic bones when these muscles contract. This muscular band is often called the puborectalis or the pubococcygeus muscle, but a more accurate term is the pubovisceral muscle because these muscles arise from the pubic bone and insert directly onto pelvic viscera or provide a supporting sling for them. When the pubovisceral muscle contracts, it pulls the rectum, vagina, and urethra anteriorly toward the pubic bone and constricts the lumens of these pelvic organs. It is this contractile property that is so important in maintaining urinary and fecal continence and in providing support for the genital organs (vagina, cervix, uterus) that lie upon and are supported by the levator plate."-Novak's 13/e p271

Levator Ani Muscle	
Origin	• **Linear origin** from back of the **body of pubis**, a **tendinous arch** formed by **thickening of fascia covering obturator internus & spine of ischium**[Q].

Contd...

Contd...

	Levator Ani Muscle
Insertion	• Groups of fibers sweep downward & medially to their insertion as follows: • **Anterior fibers: Levator prostatae** or **sphincter vaginae** form a sling around the prostate or vagina and are **inserted into perineal body**^{Q}. • **Intermediate fibers: Puborectalis** forms a sling around the junction of rectum & anal canal. **Pubococcygeus** passes posteriorly to be inserted into **anococcygeal body**^{Q}. • **Posterior fibers: Iliococcygeus** is inserted into the **anococcygeal body & coccyx**^{Q}.
Action	• Levatores ani of two sides forms an **efficient muscular sling** that **supports & maintains the pelvic viscera** in position^Q. • **Resist the rise in intrapelvic pressure** during straining & expulsive efforts of abdominal muscles^Q • **Important sphincter action on anorectal junction** & serves as a **sphincter of vagina**^{Q}. • **Contractile property of pubococcygeus** helps in **maintaining urinary & fecal continence** and in **providing support for genital organs (vagina, cervix, uterus).**
Nerve supply	• **Perineal branch of 4th sacral nerve** & from perineal branch of **pudendal nerve**^{Q}

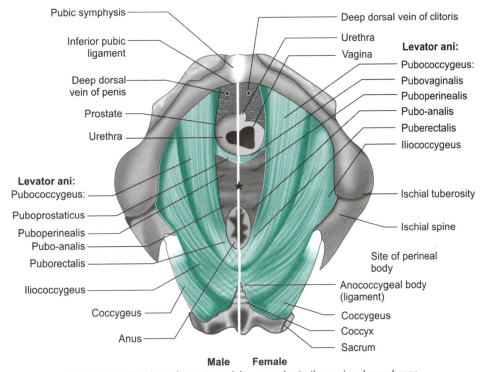

Fig. 40: Inferior view of structures lying superior to the perineal membrane

150. **Ans. d. Bilateral gonadectomy** *(Ref: Leon-Speroff 8/e p461; Novaks 15/e p1040; Harrison 19/e p2352; Nelson 20/e p2745, 19/e p1953)*

History of primary amenorrhea, karyotype of 45XO & infantile uterus is suggestive of Turner's syndrome. Approximately 5% of women with Turner's syndrome have a karyotype with Y chromosome (45X/46XY). It is important to identify a Y chromosome because affected individuals are at significant risk of gonadoblastoma (20 to 30%). Therefore, prophylactic gonadectomy should be performed.

"Turner's syndrome: Mosaicism involving the Y chromosome occurs in 5%. Gonadoblastoma among Y-positive patients occurred in 7-10%. Therefore, the current recommendation is that prophylactic gonadectomy should be performed even in the absence of MRI or CT evidence of tumors." -Nelson 20/e p2745

532   AIIMS ESSENCE

> *"Even in the presence of typical Turner stigmata, a karyotype is indicated to eliminate the possibility of any portion of a Y chromosome. If a Y chromosome is identified, with exogenous estrogen should be based mainly on circulating FSH levels because FSH levels in the normal range for the patient's age imply the presence of surgical extirpation of the gonads is warranted to eliminate any possibility of a germ cell neoplasm (estimated 20% to 30% prevalence). In individuals in whom there is no evidence of neoplastic dissemination, the uterus may be left in situ for donor in vitro fertilization and embryo transfer. The evaluation of other commonly involved organ systems should include a careful physical examination, with special attention to the cardiovascular system, and thyroid function tests (including antibody assessment), fasting blood glucose, renal function tests, and intravenous pyelography or a renal ultrasonography."-Novaks 15/e p1040*

> *"The phenotype of individuals with 45,X/46,XY mosaicism (sometimes called mixed gonadal dysgenesis) can vary considerably. Some have a predominantly female phenotype with somatic features of Turner's syndrome (TS), streak gonads, and müllerian structures, and are managed as TS with a Y chromosome. Most 45,X/46,XY individuals have a male phenotype and testes, and the diagnosis is made incidentally after amniocentesis or during investigation of infertility. In practice, most newborns referred for assessment have atypical genitalia and variable somatic features. Management is complex and needs to be individualized. A female sex-of-rearing is often assigned if uterine structures are present, gonads are intra-abdominal, and phallic development is incomplete. In such situations, gonadectomy usually is considered to prevent further androgen secretion at puberty and prevent risk of gonadoblastoma (up to 25%)."-Harrison 19/e p2352*

151. Ans. a. High HCG, low ue3, low AFP   *(Ref: Williams 24/e p289-291; Nelson 20/e p613; Pediatric Endocrinology By M. Sperling 3/e p618)*

The average hCG is higher than normal and the AFP and uE3 (unconjugated estriol) are lower than normal in the presence of fetal trisomy 21 (Down's syndrome).

> *"The measurement of concentrations of human chorionic gonadotropin (hCG), alpha-fetoprotein (AFP), and unconjugated estriol (uE3) in maternal serum in conjunction with maternal age has been used as a prenatal screen for Down syndrome and trisomy 18. The basis for the utility of this screen is that in fetal trisomy 21 the average hCG is higher than normal and the AFP and uE3 are lower than normal in the presence of fetal trisomy 21."-Pediatric Endocrinology By M. Sperling 3/e p618*

Conditions Associated with Abnormal Maternal Screening Results			
Condition	**AFP**	**hCG**	**uE3**
Neural Tube Defects (NTD)	High[Q]	−	−
Trisomy 21 (Down's syndrome)	Low[Q]	High[Q]	Low[Q]
Trisomy 18 (Edward's syndrome)	Low[Q]	Low[Q]	Low[Q]

152. Ans. d. No extra calories   *(Ref: William's 24 /e p178)*

The Institute of Medicine (2006) recommends adding 0, 340, and 452 kcal/day to the estimated non-pregnant energy requirements in the first, second, and third trimesters, respectively. So, no extra-calories are recommended in first trimester of pregnancy.

> *"Pregnancy requires an additional 80,000 kcal, mostly during the last 20 weeks. To meet this demand, a caloric increase of 100 to 300 kcal per day is recommended during pregnancy (American Academy of Pediatrics and the American College of Obstetricians and Gynecologists, 2012). This intake increase, however, should not be divided equally during the course of pregnancy. The Institute of Medicine (2006) recommends adding 0, 340, and 452 kcal/day to the estimated non-pregnant energy requirements in the first, second, and third trimesters, respectively. Calories are necessary for energy. Whenever caloric intake is inadequate, protein is metabolized rather than being spared for its vital role in fetal growth and development."- William's 24 /e p178*

153. Ans. a. Hypertension diagnosed at 10 weeks of gestation   *(Ref: Williams 24/e p730)*

Chronic underlying hypertension or systemic hypertension is diagnosed in women with documented blood pressures ≥ 140/90 mm Hg before pregnancy or before 20 weeks' gestation, or both.

> *"Chronic underlying hypertension is diagnosed in women with documented blood pressures ≥ 140/90 mm Hg before pregnancy or before 20 weeks' gestation, or both."-Williams 24/e p730*

154. Ans. a. PAP smear   *(Ref: Novaks 15/e p1305, 597-605)*

Postcoital bleeding in a 35 years old woman requires clinical examination and next step is PAP smear, and if a cancer is suspected, a targeted wedge biopsy should be performed to establish the diagnosis of invasive disease.

AIIMS November 2017

```
┌─────────────────────┐
│  Postcoital bleeding │
└─────────────────────┘
           │
           ▼
┌─────────────────────┐
│ History and physical │
│     examination      │
└─────────────────────┘
       │         │
   ┌───┘         └────┐
   ▼                  ▼
┌────────────┐  ┌──────────────────┐
│ Pap testing│  │ Identifiable lesion│
│            │  │    on cervix      │
└────────────┘  └──────────────────┘
   │                  │
   ▼                  ▼
┌────────────┐     ┌──────────────────┐
│  Abnormal  │     │ Colposcopy and   │
│  cytology  │→Yes→│    biopsy        │
└────────────┘     └──────────────────┘
```

"Symptomatic disease (e.g. postcoital bleeding) requires clinical examination, and if a cancer is suspected, a targeted wedge biopsy rather than a punch biopsy taken as this has a greater chance of establishing invasive disease."-Histopathology Reporting: Guidelines for Surgical Cancer By Derek C Allen (2013)/p273

"As cervical cytology may miss cases with cervical atypical squamous intraepithelial lesions (SIL) or cervical carcinoma, a thorough colposcopic examination and directed biopsy is essential when there is a positive risk factors like post-coital bleeding."-Gynaecology For Postgraduate And Practitioners By Sengupta (2010)/p158

PAP smear	• **False negative rate of Pap smear** in the **presence of invasive cancer is 50%** and a **negative Pap test should never be relied on in a symptomatic patient.**
Conisation	• **Conisation** is an **invasive procedure** where the cervix is cut in a cone shaped manner. It is both **diagnostic & therapeutic**.
	• **Conisation is indicated for diagnosis in women with HSIL or adenocarcinoma-in-situ** and may be considered under the following conditions:
	• **Limits of the lesion cannot be visualized with colposcopy**.
	• **SCJ is not seen at colposcopy.**
	• ECC histologic findings are positive for **CIN 2 or CIN 3.**
	• **Lack of correlation** between cytology, biopsy & colposcopy results.
	• **Microinvasion** is suspected based on biopsy, colposcopy, or cytology results.
	• Colposcopist is **unable to rule out invasive cancer**.
	• **Conisation is not indicated for all symptomatic women** and it should be **done following either a PAP, colposcopy or a biopsy with abnormal or inconclusive result.**
Cryotherapy	• **Cryotherapy destroys the surface epithelium of cervix by crystallizing the intracellular water using nitrous oxide or carbon dioxide.**
	• Cryotherapy is ideal only for small superficial lesions.
	• **Cryotherapy should be considered acceptable therapy when the following criteria are met: CIN, grade 1 to 2; Small lesion ; Ectocervical location only ; Negative ECC findings; No endocervical gland involvement on biopsy**
	• **Cryotherapy** is **indicated only for biopsy proven cases of abnormal epithelium.**

PEDIATRICS

155. Ans. a. Can't use spoon *(Ref: Nelson 20/e p75)*

Child starts self-feeding with spoon at 15 months. Failure of self-feeding with spoon in a 3 years old child is suggestive of delayed milestones. Child can draw square at the age of 4 years. Child can skip at the age of 5 years. Child can climb alternate steps downwrads at the age of 4 years.

Development Milestones in a 3 Years Old Child	
Motor	• **Rides tricycle; stands momentarily on one foot**
Adaptive	• **Makes tower of 10 cubes**; imitates construction of "bridge" of 3 cubes; **copies circle; imitates cross**
Language	• Knows age & sex; counts 3 objects correctly; repeats 3 numbers or a sentence of 6 syllables; most of speech intelligible to strangers
Social	• **Plays simple games** (in "parallel" with other children); **helps in dressing** (unbuttons clothing & puts on shoes); **washes hands**

156. Ans. a. Menke's disease *(Ref: Harrison 19/e p96e-10; Nelson 20/e p3196, 2916)*

Most probable diagnosis of A 4 years old child having kinky hair & growth retardation is Menke's disease.

> *"Menkes kinky hair syndrome is an X-linked metabolic disturbance of copper metabolism characterized by mental retardation, hypocupremia, and decreased circulating ceruloplasmin. This syndrome is caused by mutations in the copper-transporting ATP7A gene. Children with this disease often die within 5 years because of dissecting aneurysms or cardiac rupture."* -Harrison 19/e p96e-10

> *"Menkes Kinky Hair Syndrome (Trichopoliodystrophy): Males with Menkes kinky hair syndrome, an X-linked recessive trait, are born to an unaffected mother after a normal pregnancy. Neonatal problems include hypothermia, hypotonia, poor feeding, seizures, and failure to thrive. Hair is normal to sparse at birth but is replaced by short, fine, brittle, light-colored hair that may have features of trichorrhexis nodosa, pili torti, or monilethrix. The skin is hypopigmented and thin, cheeks typically appear plump, and the nasal bridge is depressed. Progressive psychomotor retardation is noted in early infancy. Mutations in the ATP7A gene, encoding a copper-transporting adenosine triphosphatase protein, cause Menkes kinky hair syndrome. It is due to maldistribution of the copper in the body."* - Nelson 20/e p3196

Menkes disease (Kinky Hair Disease or Trichopoliodystrophy)

- **Progressive neurodegenerative condition**; Inherited as a **X-linked recessive trait**[Q].
- **Mutations in ATP7A gene**, encoding a **copper-transporting adenosine triphosphatase protein**, cause Menkes kinky hair syndrome[Q].
- It is due to **maldistribution of copper in the body**[Q].

Pathology:
- **Copper uptake across the brush border of small intestine is increased**, but **copper transport from these cells into the plasma is defective**, resulting in **low total body copper stores**[Q].
    - **Neuropathologic changes**: Tortuous degeneration of gray matter & marked changes in cerebellum with **loss of internal granule cell layer & necrosis of Purkinje cells**[Q].

Clinical Features:
- Symptoms begin in **1st few months of life**
- **Symptoms: Hypothermia, hypotonia & generalized myoclonic seizures**[Q].
- **Facies: Distinctive, with chubby, rosy cheeks & kinky, colorless, friable hair**[Q].
- **Feeding difficulties** lead to **failure to thrive**[Q].
- **Severe mental retardation** & **optic atrophy** are constant features of the disease[Q].

Treatment:
- **Copper-histidine therapy** may be **effective in preventing neurologic deterioration**, particularly **when treatment is begun in the neonatal period** or, preferably, with the fetus[Q].

Prognosis:
- **Death** occurs **within 5 years** because of **dissecting aneurysms or cardiac rupture**[Q].

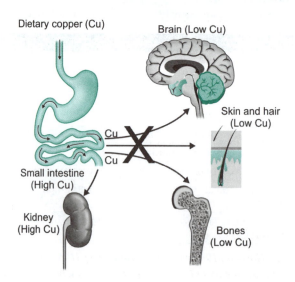

Contd...

AIIMS November 2017

157. Ans. b. Continue breastfeeding and phototherapy *(Ref: Nelson 20/e p288, 873-874, 879; Ghai 8/e p173)*

Preferred treatment option for a 4 days old baby with bilirubin of 8 mg/dL is to continue breastfeeding and phototherapy.

"Breast milk jaundice is a different disorder that causes persistently high indirect bilirubin in a thriving healthy baby that become evident later than breastfeeding jaundice, but which generally declines in the 2nd to 3rd week of life. Infants with severe or persistent jaundice should be evaluated for problems such as galactosemia, hypothyroidism, urinary tract infection, and hemolysis before ascribing the jaundice to breast milk that might contain inhibitors of glucuronyl transferase or enhanced absorption of bilirubin from the gut. Persistently high bilirubin can require changing from breast milk to infant formula for 24-48 hr and/or phototherapy without cessation of breastfeeding. Breastfeeding should resume after the decline in serum bilirubin. Parents should be reassured and encouraged to continue collecting breast milk during the period when the infant is taking formula."-Nelson 20/e p288

Phototherapy

- **Phototherapy** has been found to be **effective in treating jaundice in neonates**[Q].
- **Unconjugated bilirubin in skin converted into water-soluble photoproducts on exposure to light** of a particular wavelength (**425-475 mm**)[Q].

  - These **photoproducts** are **water soluble, nontoxic** and **excreted in intestine & urine**[Q].

- For **phototherapy to be effective, bilirubin needs to be present in skin** so there is **no role for prophylactic phototherapy**[Q].

Phototherapy Acts by		
Configurational isomerization	**Structural Isomerization**	**Photo oxidation**
• The **Z-isomers of bilirubin** are **converted into E-isomers**[Q]. • The **reaction is instantaneous** upon exposure to light but **reversible** as bilirubin reaches into the bile duct. • After exposure of 8-12 hours of phototherapy, this constitutes about **25% of STB**, which is **non-toxic**. • Since this is **excreted slowly** from body, this is **not a major mechanism for decrease of STB**[Q].	• This is an **irreversible reaction** where the **bilirubin is converted into lumirubin**. • The reaction is **directly proportional to dose of phototherapy**[Q]. • These products forms **2-6% of STB, which is rapidly excrete from body, mainly responsible for phototherapy induced decline in STB**[Q].	• This is a **minor reaction,** where **photo products are excreted in urine**[Q].

Types of Light:
- **Most effective lights** are those with **high energy output near the maximum adsorption peak of bilirubin (450-460 nm)**[Q].

  - **Special blue lamps** with a **peak output at 425-475 nm are the most efficient**[Q].

- **Cool daylight lamps** with a **principal peak at 550 to 600 nm are most commonly used but not very effective phototherapy units** in our country[Q].
- The **lamps should be changed every 3 months** or **earlier if irradiance is monitored**[Q].

  - **Double surface phototherapy is more effective** than the single surface[Q].

- **Double surface phototherapy** can be provided either by **double surface special blue lights** or by **conventional blue light & undersurface fiberoptic phototherapy**.

Factors affecting efficacy of phototherapy	
• Irradiance[Q] • Surface area exposed[Q] • Distance from phototherapy unit[Q]	• Initial serum total bilirubin[Q] • Adequacy of breast feeding[Q]

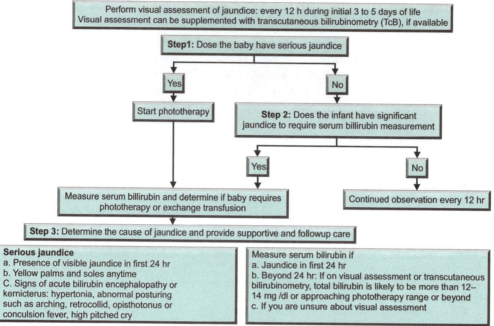

Fig. 41: Approach to an Infant with Jaundice

158. Ans. a. Appearance, Pulse, Grimace, Activity, Respiration *(Ref: Williams 24/e p627; Child development by Diane E. Papaplia (2003)/p116)*

Apgar score assesses appearance, pulse, grimace, activity, and respiration. (Asked twice in the exam)

> "Apgar scale: It assesses appearance, pulse, grimace, activity, and respiration. Its name, after its developer, Dr. Virginia Apgar (1953), helps us remember its five subtests: appearance (color), pulse (heart rate), grimace (reflex irritability), activity (muscle tone), respiration (breathing)."-Child development by Diane E. Papaplia (2003)/p116

APGAR score (Appearance, Pulse, Grimace, Activity, Respiration)
• Useful clinical tool to **identify those neonates who require resuscitation** & to assess the effectiveness of any resuscitative measures.
• Practical method of **systematically assessing newborn infants immediately after birth**.
• A **low score** may be **due to fetal distress**, prematurity & drugs given to the mother during labor.

- **1-minute Apgar score:** Reflects the **need for immediate resuscitation**[Q].
- **5-minute score** (particularly the **change in score between 1 & 5 minutes**): Useful index of the effectiveness of resuscitative efforts[Q].
- **5-minute Apgar score** also has **prognostic significance for neonatal survival** because survival is related closely to the condition of the neonate in the delivery room[Q].

- **MC cause of low APGAR score: Birth Asphyxia**[Q]
- **APGAR score at 7-10 minutes**, if low, may indicate cerebral palsy but not mortality[Q].
- Apgar score alone cannot establish hypoxia as the cause of cerebral palsy[Q].

Criteria of APGAR score				
	Score of 0	**Score of 1**	**Score of 2**	**Component of Acronym**
Skin colour/ complexion	Blue or pale all over	Blue at extremities, body pink (acrocyanosis)	No cyanosis, body & extremities pink	**A**ppearance
Pulse rate	Absent	<100	≥ 100	**P**ulse
Reflex irritability	No response to stimulation	Grimace/ feeble cry when stimulated	Cry or pull away when stimulated	**G**rimace
Muscle tone	None	Some flexion	Flexed arms & legs that resist extension	**A**ctivity
Breathing	Absent	Weak, irregular, gasping	Strong, lusty cry	**R**espiration
Apgar score interpretation: 0–3 severely depressed, 4–6 moderately depressed, 7–10 excellent condition[Q]				

AIIMS November 2017

159. Ans. a. Appearance, Pulse, Grimace, Activity, Respiration *(Ref: Williams 24/e p627; Child development by Diane E. Papaplia (2003)/p116)*

Apgar score assesses appearance, pulse, grimace, activity, and respiration. (Asked twice in the exam)

160. Ans. b. Pentavalent vaccine + BCG + OPV *(Ref: Park 24/e p132)*

Vaccines which can be given to an 18 months old unimmunized baby brought to the clinic for the first time are pentavalent vaccine (combination of DPT, Hepatitis B & Hib), BCG and OPV.

National Immunization Schedule (NIS) for Infants, Children and Pregnant Women (India)						
Vaccine	When to give	Max. Age	Dose	Diluent	Route	Site
For Pregnant Women						
TT-1	Early in pregnancy	-	0.5 ml	NO	Intramuscular	Upper arm
TT-2#	4 weeks after TT-1	-	0.5 ml	NO	Intramuscular	Upper arm
TT-Booster#	If received TT doses in a pregnancy within the last 3 years	-	0.5 ml	NO	Intramuscular	Upper arm
Vaccine	When to give	Max. Age	Dose	Diluent	Route	Site
For Infants						
BCG##	At **birth** or **as early as possible**	Till **one year** of age	**0.1 ml** (0.05 ml until 1 month age)	Sodium chloride	Intradermal	Left upper arm
Hepatitis B Birth Dose###	At **birth** or **as early as possible**	Within **24 hours**	0.5 ml	NO	Intramuscular	**Anterolateral side of mid-thigh** (Left)
OPV-0*#	At **birth** or **as early as possible**	Within the first **15 days**	2 drops	NO	Oral	-
OPV 1,2&3	At **6, 10 & 14 weeks**	Till **5 years** of age	2 drops	NO	Oral	-
Rotavirus vaccine*	At **6, 10 & 14 weeks**	Till **1 year** of age	5 drops	NO	Oral	-
IPV (Inactivated Polio Vaccine)	At **14 weeks**	Up to **1 year** of age	0.5 ml	NO	Intramuscular	**Anterolateral side of mid-thigh** (Right)
Pentavalent** 1,2 & 3	At **6, 10 & 14 weeks**	Till **1 year** of age	0.5 ml	NO	Intramuscular	**Anterolateral side of mid-thigh** (Left)
Measles- 1st dose	**9-12** completed months	Given till **5 years** of age	0.5 ml	Sterile water	Subcutaneous	Right upper arm
Japanese Encephalitis*** 1st dose	**9-12** completed months	Till **15 years**	0.5 ml	Phosphate buffer	Subcutaneous	Left upper arm
Vitamin A (1st dose)	At **9** completed months with measles	Till **5 years** of age	**1 ml** (I lakh IU)	NO	Oral	-
For Children						
DPT booster-I	**16-24** months	7 years	0.5 ml	NO	Intramuscular	**Anterolateral side of mid-thigh** (Left)
Measles 2nd dose	**16-24** months	Till **5 years** of age	0.5 ml	Sterile water	Subcutaneous	Right upper arm
OPV booster	**16-24** months	Till **5 years** of age	2 drops	NO	Oral	-
Japanese Encephalitis*** 2nd dose	**16-24** months	-	0.5 ml	Phosphate buffer	Subcutaneous	Left upper arm
Vitamin A (2nd to 9th dose)	16 months. Then, one dose every 6 months	Till **5 years** of age	**2 ml** (2 lakh IU)	NO	Oral	-
DPT Booster-2	5-6 years	7 years	0.5 ml	NO	Intramuscular	**Upper arm** (Left)
TT	10 years & 16 years	-	0.5 ml	NO	Intramuscular	Upper arm

Contd...

AIIMS ESSENCE

Contd...

Vaccine	When to give	Max. Age	Dose	Diluent	Route	Site

 # Give TT-2 or booster doses before 36 weeks of pregnancy. However, give these even if more than 36 weeks have passed. Give TT to a woman in labour, If she has not previously received TT.

BCG: There is no need to revaccinate the child if scar is not formed after BCG vaccination.

HepB: Birth dose is given only within 24 hours after birth **as** it helps to **prevent** perinatal transmission of **Hepatitis B.**

*# OPV-0 dose is given within 15 days after birth. OPV can be given till 5 years of age.

* In selected states.

** Pentavalent vaccines contain a combination of DPT, Hepatitis B & Hib. Hepatitis B birth dose and booster doses of DPT will continue as before.

*** JE Vaccine is introduced after the campaign in selected endemic districts of Uttar Pradesh, West Bengal, Karnataka, Assam & Bihar.

Children, **who have not received a single vaccine coming after 1 year, will be given 3 doses of DPT at an interval of 4 weeks. Measles-1st dose & JE 1st dose (wherever applicable) upto 2 years of age.**

- *Interval between 2 doses of Pentavalent, OPV & hepatitis B should not be <1 month.*
- *Minor cough, cold & mild fever are not a contraindication to vaccination.*
- *If the child has diarrhoea, give a dose of OPV, but do not count the dose and ask the mother to return in 4 weeks for the missing dose.*

161. Ans. b. Urine examination   *(Ref: Nelson 20/e p1592, 3074; Ghai 8/e p272)*

Periventricular calcification is caused by Cytomegalovirus (CMV) infection. For diagnosis of congenital CMV infection, urine and saliva are the best specimens for culture and saliva and cord blood is best for PCR. Among the given options, best option would be urine.

"The definitive method for diagnosis of congenital CMV infection is virus isolation or demonstration of CMV DNA by PCR, which must be performed during the 1st 2 weeks of life because viral excretion afterwards may represent infection acquired at birth or shortly thereafter. Urine and saliva are the best specimens for culture and saliva, and cord blood is best for PCR." -Nelson 20/e p1592

Congenital CMV Infection

- **Symptomatic congenital CMV infection** was originally termed **cytomegalic inclusion disease**[Q].
- **Severe** cytomegalic inclusion disease-**5%**; **Mild** involvement-**5%**; **Subclinical** chronic infection-**90%**

Cause:

- Congenital infections that are **symptomatic & most severe** & resulting in sequelae are **more likely to be caused by primary rather than reactivated infections in pregnant women**[Q].
- **Re-infection with a different strain** of CMV can lead to **symptomatic congenital infection**[Q].

Clinical Features:

- **Characteristic signs & symptoms** of clinically manifested infections: **IUGR, prematurity, hepatosplenomegaly & jaundice, blueberry muffin–like rash, thrombocytopenia & purpura, microcephaly & intracranial calcifications**[Q].
- **Other neurologic problems: Chorioretinitis, sensorineural hearing loss** & mild increases in CSF protein[Q].

  - **Asymptomatic congenital CMV infection** is likely a **leading cause of SNHL,** which occurs in **7-10% of** all infants with congenital CMV infection, **whether symptomatic at birth or not**[Q].

Diagnosis:

- **Definitive diagnosis**: **By virus isolation** or **demonstration of CMV DNA by PCR** (performed **during 1st 2 weeks of life**)[Q]
- **Urine & saliva** are **best specimens for culture; saliva & cord blood** is **best for PCR**[Q].

  - **IgG antibody test**: Little diagnostic value (positive result also reflects maternal antibodies); Negative result excludes the diagnosis of congenital CMV infection[Q].
  - **IgM tests** lack sensitivity & specificity; unreliable for diagnosis of congenital CMV infection[Q].

Treatment:

- **Ganciclovir prevents hearing deterioration & improves or maintains normal hearing function** at 6 months of age & **may prevent hearing deterioration** that occurs after 1 year of age[Q].

AIIMS November 2017

162. Ans. a. Von-Gierke's diseases *(Ref: Harrison 19/e p433e-3; Robbins 9/e p; Harper 30/e p355)*

History of hypoglycemia after moderate activity and raised levels of ketone bodies, lactic acid & triglycerides on blood examination with enlarged liver & kidneys, excess glycogen deposits in the liver is highly suggestive of Von-Gierke's diseases.

> *"Von-Gierke's Disease: Persons with type I GSD (Glycogen storage disease) may develop hypoglycemia and lactic acidosis during the neonatal period; however, more commonly, they exhibit hepatomegaly at 3–4 months of age. Hypoglycemia, hypoglycemic seizures, and lactic acidosis can develop after a short fast. These children usually have doll-like faces with fat cheeks, relatively thin extremities, short stature, and a protuberant abdomen that is due to massive hepatomegaly."-* Harrison 19/e p433e-3

> *"In the hepatic form (von Gierke disease), liver cells store glycogen because of a lack of hepatic glucose-6- phosphatase."-* Robbins 9/e p157

ORTHOPEDICS

163. Ans. c. Usually associated with dextrocardia *(Ref: Apley's 9/e p181, 361, 443; Review of Orthopaedics By Mark D. Miller, 6/e p255)*

"Sprengel's Deformity: Increased association with Klippel–Feil syndrome, kidney disease, scoliosis and diastematomyelia"- Review of Orthopaedics By Mark D. Miller, 6/e p255

> *"Sprengel's deformity may be associated with other defects of the cervical spine (e.g. Klippel–Feil syndrome), and high thoracic kyphosis or scoliosis is quite common."-* Apley's 9/e p181

> *"About 1 in 3 children with Klippel–Feil syndrome also has Sprengel's deformity of the scapula."-* Apley's 9/e p443

> *"Sprengel's deformity: Deformity is the only symptom and it may be noticed at birth. The shoulder on the affected side is elevated; the scapula looks and feels abnormally high, smaller than usual and somewhat prominent; occasionally both scapulae are affected. The neck appears shorter than usual and there may be kyphosis or scoliosis of the upper thoracic spine."-* Apley's 9/e p361

Sprengel's Deformity (Elevation of the Scapula)
• MC congenital shoulder abnormality[Q]
• Complex deformity of shoulder, characterized by congenital elevation of the scapula[Q]
• Represents a failure of scapular descent from the cervical spine. **An omovertebral bar (fibrous, cartilaginous and/or osseous connection between scapula & cervical spine) is often present.**

Clinical Features:
- **Sprengel's deformity is usually noticed at birth**
- **Asymmetry of shoulders**, with **elevation & underdevelopment** of affected side.
- **Scapula is abnormally small & too high**; associated with hypoplasia or atrophy of regional muscles[Q]
- **Elevated scapula is visually noticeable with restriction in the motion of scapula & glenohumeral joint[Q]**.
- Occasionally both sides are involved.

Associations of Sprengel's Deformity	
• **Klippel-Feil syndrome[Q]**	• **Torticollis[Q]**
• **Spina bifida & diastemetomyelia[Q]**	• Underdevelopment of clavicle or humerus
• **Kyphosis or scoliosis[Q]**	

Treatment:
- **Treatment** is required only **if shoulder movements are severely limited** or if the **deformity is particularly unsightly**.
- **Best age of operation**: **Before 6 years** of age.
- **Vertebroscapular muscles** are **released from spine, supraspinous part of scapula is excised with omovertebral bar** & scapula is repositioned by tightening the lower muscles.

164. Ans. a. Arthritis *(Ref: Apley's 9/e p572; Katzung 13/e p1104, 12/e p1135)*

Glucosamine is primarily used for pain associated with knee osteoarthritis.

> *"Osteoarthritis: New forms of medication have been introduced in recent years, particularly the oral administration of glucosamine and intra-articular injection of hyalourans. There is, as yet, no agreement about the long-term efficacy of these products."-* Apley's 9/e p572

"*As a dietary supplement, glucosamine is primarily used for pain associated with knee osteoarthritis.*"- *Katzung 13/e p1104*

"*Endogenous glucosamine is used for the production of glycosaminoglycans and other proteoglycans in articular cartilage. In osteoarthritis, the rate of production of new cartilage is exceeded by the rate of degradation of existing cartilage. Supplementation with glucosamine is thought to increase the supply of the necessary glycosaminoglycan building blocks, leading to better maintenance and strengthening of existing cartilage.*"- *Katzung 13/e p1104*

Glucosamine
• **Glucosamine** is a **substrate for the production of articular cartilage** & serves as a **cartilage nutrient**. • Commercially derived from **crabs & other crustaceans**. • As a dietary supplement, glucosamine is **primarily used for pain associated with knee osteoarthritis**.
Pharmacologic Effects & Clinical Uses: • **Endogenous glucosamine** is **used for production of glycosaminoglycans** & other proteoglycans **in articular cartilage**. • In **osteoarthritis**, the **rate of production of new cartilage is exceeded by the rate of degradation of existing cartilage**. • **Supplementation with glucosamine** is thought to **increase the supply of necessary glycosaminoglycan building blocks**, leading to **better maintenance & strengthening of existing cartilage**.
Efficacy & Results: • **No benefit for glucosamine therapy in mild to moderate disease** in osteoarthritis.

165. **Ans. a. Hoover test** (Ref: Orthopedic Physical Assessment By David J. Magee 5/e p577)
In Hoover test, the subject relaxes in a supine position on the table while the examiner places both of the subject's heels into the palm of the examiners hands.

Waddell's test	• **Waddell's test** indicate nonorganic pathology for back pain • **Tests:** • **Tenderness:** Subcutaneous pressure reproduces symptoms • **Stimulation tests: Axial loading & pain on simulated rotation** • **Distracted straight leg raise:** If a patient complains of pain on straight leg raise, but not if the examiner extends the knee with the patient seated at another time during the initial evaluation • **Non-anatomic sensory changes:** Regional sensory changes & regional weakness • **Overreaction: Exaggerated painful response to a stimulus**, that is not reproduced when the same stimulus is given later • If there are **more than 3 of 5 present** then there is high probability that patient has **non-organic pain.**
O'Donoghue test	• **Method: Examiner flexes the supine subject's knee to 90°** & then **rotates the leg inward & outward a few times.** The examiner then **fully flexes the subject's knee & again rotates it in both directions.** • **Results: Increased pain on rotation with the knee fully flexed as compared with 90° flexion indicates a meniscal tear or capsule irritation**
McBride Test	• **Ask the patient to stand on one leg while raising the opposite knee to the chest**. This should **lessen low back pain.** • A reported **increase in pain**, or a **refusal to do the test**, is a **positive behavioural sign.**

Hoover test	
• **Test positioning:** The subject relaxes in a supine position on the table while the examiner places both of the subject's heels into the palm of the examiners hands. • **Action:** The subject is asked to perform a unilateral straight leg raise • **Positive finding: Inability to lift the leg may reflect a neuromuscular weakness.** A positive finding is also noted when the examiner does not feel increased pressure in the palm that underlies the resting leg.	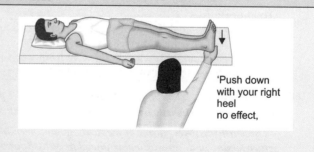 'Push down with your right heel no effect,

Contd...

Contd...

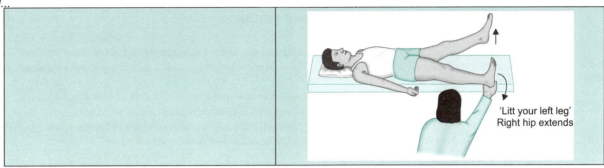

166. **Ans. a. Avascular necrosis of femur** *(Ref: Apley's 9/e p528)*

History of bilateral hip pain and unable to squat in a 40 years old body builder taking steroids and creatinine with MRI showing marrow edema, subchondral cyst, flattening of weight bearing areas of femoral head & X-ray showing crescent sign is highly suggestive of avascular necrosis (Osteonecrosis) of femur.

"Non-traumatic osteonecrosis is seen in association with infiltrative disorders of the marrow, Gaucher's disease, sickle-cell disease, coagulopathies, caisson disease, systemic lupus erythematosus and – commonest of all – high-dosage corticosteroid administration and alcohol abuse."-Apley's 9/e p528

"Osteonecrosis: The presenting complaint is usually pain in the hip (or, in over 50 per cent of cases, both hips), which progresses over a period of 2–3 years to become quite severe. However, in over 10 per cent of cases the condition is asymptomatic and discovered incidentally after x-ray or MRI during investigation of a systemic disorder or longstanding symptoms in the other hip."-Apley's 9/e p528

*"X-rays: During the early stages of osteonecrosis plain x-rays are normal. The first signs appear only 6–9 months after the occurrence of bone death and are due mainly to reactive changes in the surrounding (live) bone. **Thus, the classic feature of increased density (interpreted as sclerosis) is a sign of repair rather than necrosis.** With time, destructive changes do appear in the necrotic segment: a thin subchondral fracture line (the 'crescent sign'), slight flattening of the weight bearing zone and then increasing distortion, with eventual collapse, of the articular surface of the femoral head."- Apley's 9/e p528*

"MRI shows characteristic changes in the marrow long before the appearance of x-ray signs – a mean of 3.6 months after the initiation of steroid treatment in one published study. The diagnostic feature is a band of altered signal intensity running through the femoral head (diminished intensity in the T1 weighted SE image and increased intensity in the STIR image). This 'band' represents the reactive zone between living and dead bone and thus demarcates the ischaemic segment, the extent and location of which are important in staging the lesion."- Apley's 9/e p528

Avascular Necrosis (Osteonecrosis)

- **MC site of symptomatic osteonecrosis: Femoral head**[Q] (mainly due to its **peculiar blood supply**)

Etiology of Avascular Necrosis	
Post-traumatic	**Non-traumatic**
• Usually follows a **displaced fracture of femoral neck** or **dislocation of hip**[Q]. • **Main cause: Interruption of arterial blood supply**[Q], other contributory factors are **venous stasis & thrombosis of intramedullary arterioles & capillaries.**	• Non-traumatic osteonecrosis is seen in association with: • **High-dose corticosteroid administration & alcohol abuse**[Q] **(MC)** • Infiltrative disorders of the marrow • **Gaucher's disease**[Q] • **Sickle-cell disease**[Q] • **Coagulopathies**[Q] • **Caisson disease**[Q] • **Systemic lupus erythematosus**[Q] • **Perthes' disease**[Q]

Contd...

Avascular Necrosis (Osteonecrosis)

Clinical features:

- **Post-traumatic osteonecrosis** develops **soon after injury to the hip**, but symptoms & signs may take months to appear.
- **Non-traumatic osteonecrosis** is **more insidious**. **Children** are affected in conditions such as **Perthes' disease, sickle-cell disease & Gaucher's disease**[Q].
- **Presenting complaint: Pain in the hip**, which **progresses over a period of 2–3 years** to become quite severe.
- In **10% of cases** the **condition is asymptomatic** & discovered incidentally after X-ray or MRI[Q].
- **On examination**: Patient walks with a **limp** and may have a **positive Trendelenburg sign**; **Thigh is wasted** & **limb** may be **1 or 2 cm short**. **Movements are restricted**, particularly **abduction & internal rotation**[Q].

- A **characteristic sign** is a **tendency for the hip to twist into external rotation during passive flexion**; this corresponds to the **'sectoral sign'** in which, with the **hip extended, internal rotation is almost full**, but with the **hip flexed it is grossly restricted**[Q].

- **History of treatment with corticosteroids** or **high usage of alcohol**[Q]

Diagnosis:

- **X-rays**: Classic feature of **increased density** (interpreted as **sclerosis**) is a **sign of repair** rather than necrosis. With time, **destructive changes do appear in the necrotic segment**: a **thin subchondral fracture line** (the **'crescent sign'**[Q]), **slight flattening of weight bearing zone** & **increasing distortion**, with eventual **collapse**, of the **articular surface of femoral head**[Q].
- **MRI**: Characteristic changes in marrow; **diagnostic feature** is a **band of altered signal intensity running** through the femoral head (This **'band'** represents the **reactive zone between living & dead bone**)[Q]

Treatment	
Post-traumatic osteonecrosis	• **Young patients <40 years: Realignment osteotomy**, with or without bone grafting of the necrotic segment • **Older patients: Partial or total joint replacement.**
Non-traumatic osteonecrosis	• **Grade I lesions** (restricted to medial part of femoral head): Symptomatic treatment & reassurance • **Grade II lesions** (occupying up to one-half of femoral head & between one and two-thirds of weight bearing surface): **Conservative surgery** (core decompression or decompression and bone grafting of the femoral head). • **Grade III lesions** (occupying a large part of femoral head & more than 2/3rd of weight bearing surface): • For **younger patients**, realignment osteotomy is the **treatment of choice**. • **Older patients: Partial or total joint replacement.** • **Advanced osteonecrosis & bone collapse: Reconstructive surgery** (osteotomy, with or without bone grafting, or joint replacement)

167. **Ans. b. Decreased response to analgesic**   *(Ref: Apley's 9/e p713, 714)*

Earliest way to detect development of compartment syndrome by the nurse is decreased response to analgesic. In compartment syndrome, the ischemia occurs at the capillary level, so pulses may still be felt and the skin may not be pale.

"However in compartment syndrome the ischaemia occurs at the capillary level, so pulses may still be felt and the skin may not be pale! The earliest of the 'classic' features are pain (or a 'bursting' sensation), altered sensibility and paresis (or, more usually, weak- ness in active muscle contraction). Skin sensation should be carefully and repeatedly checked. Ischaemic muscle is highly sensitive to stretch. If the limb is unduly painful, swollen or tense, the muscles (which may be tender) should be tested by stretching them. When the toes or fingers are passively hyperextended, there is increased pain in the calf or forearm."- Apley's 9/e p714

Compartment Syndrome

- In **fractures of arm or leg, severe ischemia** can occur even if there is **no damage to a major vessel**.

- **Bleeding, edema or inflammation** may **increase the pressure within one of the osseofascial compartments**; there is **reduced capillary flow**, which results in **muscle ischemia**, further edema, still greater pressure and yet more **profound ischaemia** – a vicious circle that ends, after 12 hours or less, in **necrosis of nerve & muscle** within the compartment.

Contd...

Contd...

Compartment Syndrome
• **Nerve is capable of regeneration** but **muscle, once infarcted, can never recover** and is **replaced by inelastic fibrous tissue (Volkmann's ischemic contracture)**. • A similar cascade of events may be **caused by swelling of a limb inside a tight plaster cast**.

Clinical features:
• **High-risk injuries**: Fractures of elbow, forearm bones, proximal third of tibia & multiple fractures of hand or foot, **crush injuries & circumferential burns**.
• **Other precipitating factors**: Operation (usually for internal fixation) or **infection**.
• **Classic features of ischaemia**: Pain , Paraesthesia, Pallor , Paralysis , Pulselessness (5 Ps)
    • **In compartment syndrome, ischemia** occurs **at capillary level**, so **pulses may still be felt & skin may not be pale**.
    • **Earliest of the 'classic' features** are **pain (or a 'bursting' sensation), altered sensibility & paresis** (or, more usually, **weakness in active muscle contraction**).
    • **Skin sensation** should be **carefully & repeatedly checked**.

• **Ischemic muscle** is **highly sensitive to stretch**. If the **limb is unduly painful**, swollen or tense, the **muscles should be tested by stretching them**. • When the **toes or fingers** are **passively hyperextended**, there is **increased pain in the calf or forearm**.

Diagnosis:
• **Confirmation of diagnosis** can be made by **measuring the intracompartmental pressures**.
• **For early diagnosis, use of continuous compartment pressure monitoring for high-risk injuries** (e.g. **fractures of the tibia & fibula**) & for **forearm or leg fractures** in patients who are **unconscious**.
    • A **split catheter** is **introduced into the compartment** & pressure is measured **close to the level of fracture**.
    • A **differential pressure (ΔP)** –difference between **diastolic pressure & compartment pressure** – of **<30 mmHg** (4.00 kilopascals) is an **indication for immediate compartment decompression**.

Treatment:
• **Threatened compartment** must be **promptly decompressed**.
• **Casts, bandages & dressings** must be **completely removed** – merely splitting the plaster is utterly useless – & **limb should be nursed flat**.
• The ΔP should be carefully moni**tored**; if it **falls below 30 mmHg, immediate open fasciotomy is performed**.
    • In leg, **'fasciotomy' means opening all four compartments** through **medial & lateral incisions**.
    • **Wounds should be left open & inspected 2 days later**: debridement for **muscle necrosis**; if the **tissues are healthy, wounds** can be **sutured** (without tension) or **skin-grafted**.

168. **Ans. a. Neer's type III proximal humerus**   *(Ref: Apley's 9/e p744-746)*

    In the given X-ray of proximal humerus fracture, there is three-part fracture, which fits it into Neer's type III.

Neer Classification for Shoulder Fractures	
Type	• Description
I	• **Minimally displaced, one-part fracture**, fracture lines involve 1-4 parts • Account for ~**70-80%** of all proximal humeral fractures
II	• **Two-part fracture**, fracture lines involve 2-4 parts, **one part is displaced (Anatomical neck)**
III	• **Three-part fracture**, fracture lines involve 3-4 parts, **two parts are displaced (Surgical neck)**
IV	• **Four-part fracture**, fracture lines involve more than 4 parts & **three parts are displaced (Greater tuberosity)**
V	• Lesser tuberosity fractures
VI	• Fracture dislocations

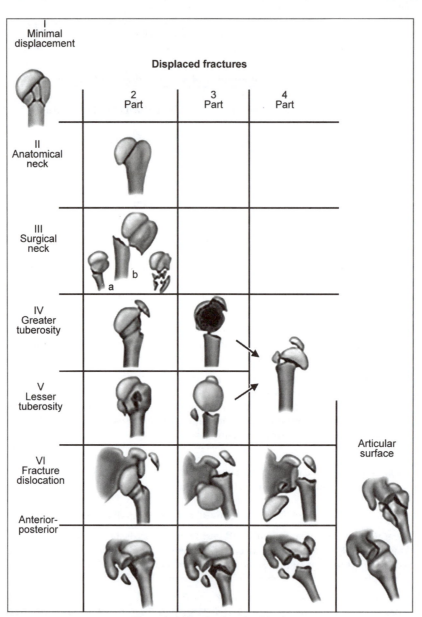

Fig. 42: Neer classification for shoulder fractures

Fractures of Proximal Humerus
• Usually occur **after middle age** & most of the patients are **osteoporotic, postmenopausal women.** • **Fracture displacement** is usually **not marked**; considerable displacement & significant risk of complications due to bone fragility, damage to rotator cuff & prevailing co-morbidities in 20% of cases.
Mechanism of Injury: • **Fall on the outstretched arm**
Classification & Pathological anatomy: • Most widely accepted classification: **Neer's classification**[Q] • **Four major segments involved: Head** of humerus, **lesser tuberosity, greater tuberosity & shaft**[Q]. • **Neer's classification** distinguishes between **number of displaced fragments**, with **displacement** defined as **>45°** of **angulation** or **1 cm of separation**[Q].

Contd...

Contd...

Fractures of Proximal Humerus

Clinical features:
- Because the **fracture is often firmly impacted, pain may not be severe.** However, the **appearance of a large bruise** on the upper part of the arm is suspicious.
- Signs of **axillary nerve or brachial plexus injury**

Diagnosis:
- **X-ray: In elderly patients: single, impacted fracture** extending across the surgical neck; **In younger patients: fragments** are usually **more clearly separated**.

Treatment of Fractures of Proximal Humerus		
Minimally displaced fractures	• **Rest for 1-2 weeks** with **arm in a sling** until the pain subsides & then gentle passive movements of shoulder. • Once the **fracture has united** (usually after 6 weeks), **active exercises** are encouraged.	
Two-part fractures	**Surgical neck fractures**	• **Fragments** are gently **manipulated into alignment & arm is immobilized in a sling for 4 weeks** or until the fracture feels stable & x-ray shows some signs of healing. • **Elbow & hand exercises** are encouraged; shoulder exercises are commenced at about 4 weeks. • If the **fracture cannot be reduced, closed** or **very unstable** after closed reduction, then **fixation is required**.
	Greater tuberosity fractures	• Often **associated with anterior dislocation** • Reduces to a good position when the shoulder is relocated. If it does not reduce, the fragment can be re-attached through a small incision with interosseous sutures or, in young hard bone, cancellous screws.
	Anatomical neck fractures	• **Young patients:** Fracture should be **fixed with a screw**. • **Older patients: Prosthetic replacement** (hemiarthroplasty) is **preferable** because of high risk of avascular necrosis of humeral head.
Three-part fractures	• Usually involve **displacement of surgical neck & greater tuberosity** • **In active individuals: Open reduction & internal fixation**	
Four-part fractures	• **In young patients: Reconstruction** • **In older patients: Closed treatment** & attempts at **open reduction & fixation**; If the fracture pattern is such that the **blood-supply is likely to be compromised**, or that **reconstruction & internal fixation will be extremely difficult**, then the **treatment of choice is prosthetic replacement of proximal humerus**.	

Named Fracture Classification Systems	
Named Classification	**Used for**
Allman[Q]	• **Clavicle fractures**
Neer[Q]	• **Proximal humerus fractures**
Rockwood[Q]	• **Acromioclavicular joint injuries**
Ideberg[Q]	• **Scapula fractures**
Gartland[Q]	• **Supracondylar fracture humerus**
Riseborough & Radin[Q]	• **Intercondylar fracture**
O'Driscoll[Q]	• **Coronoid process fracture**
Mason[Q]	• **Radial head fracture**
Bado[Q]	• **Monteggia fracture**
Frykman's[Q]	• **Distal radius fracture**
Tile[Q] **Young & Burgess**[Q]	• **Pelvic fractures**

Contd...

Contd...

Named Classification	Used for
Garden[Q] Pauwel[Q]	• Fracture neck of femur
Pipkin[Q]	• Fracture head of femur
Evan's[Q] Boyd & Griffin[Q]	• Intertrochanteric fractures
Russel-Taylor[Q]	• Subtrochanteric fractures
Winquist & Hansen[Q]	• Fracture shaft of femur
Lauge-Hansen[Q] Danis-Weber[Q]	• Bimalleolar fracture
Essex-Lopresti[Q] Sanders[Q]	• Fracture calcaneum
Hawkin's[Q]	• Fracture talus

169. Ans. b. Scaphoid fracture *(Ref: Apley's 9/e p781)*

History of fall on an outstretched hand with radial side pain and tenderness in anatomical snuff-box and restriction of wrist movement and given X-ray showing transverse line in scaphoid bone is suggestive of scaphoid fracture.

"Scaphoid Fracture: The appearance may be deceptively normal, but the astute observer can usually detect fullness in the anatomical snuffbox; precisely localized tenderness in the same place is an important diagnostic sign; the scaphoid can of course also be palpated from the front and back of the wrist and it may be tender there as well. Proximal pressure along the axis of the thumb may be painful."- Apley's 9/e p781

"X-ray in Scaphoid Fracture: Anteroposterior, lateral and oblique views are all essential; often a recent fracture shows only in the oblique view. Usually the fracture line is transverse, and through the narrowest part of the bone (waist), but it may be more proximally situated (proximal pole fracture). Sometimes only the tubercle of the scaphoid is fractured." -Apley's 9/e p781

Scaphoid Fracture

- Scaphoid fractures account for **75% of all carpal fractures**[Q]
- Rare in elderly & children.

> **Pathological Anatomy**
> - **Blood supply of scaphoid diminishes proximally**[Q]
> - **1% of distal third fractures, 20% of middle third fractures & 40% of proximal fractures** result in **non-union or avascular necrosis of proximal fragment**[Q].

Mechanism of Injury:
- Combination of **forced carpal movement & compression**, as in a **fall on the dorsiflexed hand**[Q]
- **Most scaphoid fractures** are **stable**[Q]; with unstable fractures the fragments may become displaced.
- Distal fragment, unrestrained by the scapho-lunate ligament, flexes & proximal fragment tilts dorsally with the lunate; the **hump-backed deformity of the scaphoid is permanent**[Q].

Clinical Features:
- **Fullness in anatomical snuffbox** with **precisely localized tenderness** is an **important diagnostic sign**[Q]
- **Proximal pressure** along the **axis of thumb may be painful**[Q].

Diagnosis:
- **X-ray:** Anteroposterior, lateral & oblique views are all **essential**; often a **recent fracture shows only in the oblique view**. **Fracture line** is transverse, through the **narrowest part of bone (waist)**, but it may be more proximally situated (proximal pole fracture)[Q].

> - A few weeks after the injury the fracture may be more obvious; **if union is delayed, cavitation appears on either side of the break**[Q].
> - **Old, un-united fractures** have **'hard' borders**[Q].
> - **Relative sclerosis of proximal fragment is pathognomonic of avascular necrosis**[Q].

Treatment of Scaphoid Fracture	
Fracture scaphoid tubercle	• No splintage is required[Q] • Treated as a wrist sprain (crepe bandage & encouraged movement)[Q]
Undisplaced fractures	• Reduction is not required; treated in plaster[Q] • 90% of waist fractures should heal[Q] • Wrist is held dorsiflexed & thumb forwards in 'glass-holding' position[Q]
Displaced fractures	• Open reduction & fixation with a compression screw[Q] increase the likelihood of union & reduce the time of immobilization.

Complications:
- Avascular necrosis, non-union, osteoarthritis[Q]

170. Ans. c. Bilateral limb wound of size >10 cm with extensive soft tissue damage and periosteal stripping *(Ref: Apley's 9/e p706, 897)*
Type IIIB Gustilo's Classification of Open Fractures: Wound- Usually >10 cm long; Soft-tissue injury- Severe loss of soft-tissue cover; Bone injury- Require soft-tissue reconstruction for cover.

"In type III B there is extensive periosteal stripping and fracture cover is not possible without use of local or distant flaps."-Apley's 9/e p706

Gustilo's Classification of Open Fractures			
Grade	Wound	Soft-tissue injury	Bone injury
I	<1 cm long[Q]	Minimal[Q]	Simple low-energy fractures[Q]
II	>1 cm long[Q]	Moderate, some muscle damage[Q]	Moderate comminution[Q]
IIIA	Usually >1 cm long[Q]	Severe deep contusion + compartment syndrome[Q]	High-energy fracture patterns; comminuted but soft-tissue cover possible[Q]
IIIB	Usually >10 cm long[Q]	Severe loss of soft-tissue cover[Q]	Requires soft-tissue reconstruction for cover[Q]
IIIC	Usually >10 cm long[Q]	As IIIB, with need for vascular repair[Q]	Requires soft-tissue reconstruction for cover[Q]

171. Ans. c. Primary action is to prevent internal rotation of knee joint *(Ref: Gray's 40/e p1400; Snell's 9/e p500)*
Lateral collateral ligament (LCL) not the posterior cruciate ligament (PCL) prevents internal rotation of the tibia on the femur when varus (towards the midline) stress is placed on the knee.

"The posterior cruciate ligament (PCL) is attached to the posterior intercondylar area of the tibia and passes upward, forward, and medially to be attached to the anterior part of the lateral surface of the medial femoral condyle. The PCL prevents anterior displacement of the femur on the tibia. With the knee joint flexed, the PCL prevents the tibia from being pulled posteriorly."-Snell's 9/e p500

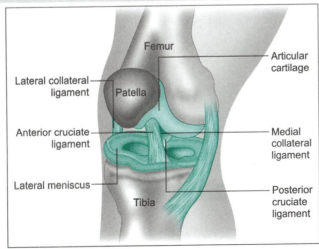

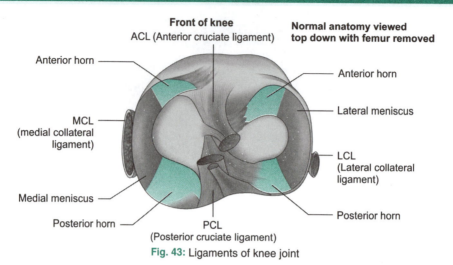

Fig. 43: Ligaments of knee joint

Ligaments of Knee Joint	
Extracapsular Ligaments	**Intracapsular Ligaments**
• **Ligamentum patellae** is attached above to lower border of patella & below to the tuberosity of tibia. It is a **continuation of central portion of common tendon of quadriceps femoris** muscle[Q]. • **Lateral collateral ligament** is cordlike and is **attached above to lateral condyle of femur & below to head of fibula. Tendon of popliteus muscle intervenes between the ligament & lateral meniscus**[Q]. • **Medial collateral ligament** is a flat band and is **attached above to medial condyle of femur & below to medial surface of shaft of tibia. It is firmly attached to the edge of medial meniscus**[Q]. • **Oblique popliteal ligament** is a **tendinous expansion** derived from **semimembranosus muscle**. It **strengthens the posterior aspect of capsule**[Q].	• **Cruciate ligaments** are two strong intracapsular ligaments that cross each other within the joint cavity. They are named **anterior & posterior**, according to their tibial attachments. • Cruciate ligaments are the **main bond between femur & tibia** throughout the joint's range of movement.

Anterior Cruciate Ligament	Posterior Cruciate Ligament
ACL is attached to anterior intercondylar area of tibia and passes upward, backward & laterally to be attached to posterior part of medial surface of lateral femoral condyle[Q]. ACL prevents posterior displacement of the femur on the tibia[Q]. With the knee joint flexed, the ACL prevents the tibia from being pulled anteriorly[Q].	PCL is attached to posterior intercondylar area of tibia & passes upward, forward & medially to be attached to anterior part of lateral surface of medial femoral condyle[Q]. PCL prevents anterior displacement of femur on tibia[Q]. With the knee joint flexed, PCL prevents the tibia from being pulled posteriorly[Q].

• **Menisci:**
  – Menisci are C-shaped sheets of fibrocartilage[Q].
  – Peripheral border is thick & attached to the capsule & inner border is thin & concave and forms a free edge[Q].
  – Upper surfaces are in contact with femoral condyles[Q].
  – Lower surfaces are in contact with tibial condyles[Q].
  – Function: To deepen the articular surfaces of tibial condyles to receive the convex femoral condyles; Serve as cushions between the two bones[Q].
  – Each meniscus is attached to the upper surface of the tibia by anterior & posterior horns.
  – Medial meniscus is also attached to medial collateral ligament, & is relatively immobile[Q].

OPHTHALMOLOGY

172. Ans. a. Myopia *(Ref: Parson 22/e p71, 51)*
In the given image, incident parallel rays come to a focus anterior to the light-sensitive layer of the retina, seen in myopia.

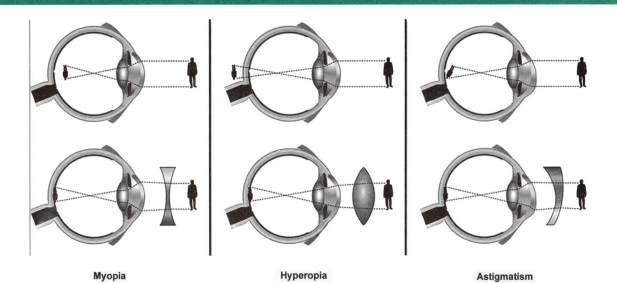

| Myopia | Hyperopia | Astigmatism |

"Myopia, also known as 'short sight', is that dioptric condition of the eye in which, with the accommodation at rest, incident parallel rays come to a focus anterior to the light-sensitive layer of the retina. The majority of cases merely result as variants in the frequency curve of axial length and curvature, the former being the more important, although curvature myopia occurs commonly as a factor in astigmatism."-Parson 22/e p71

"Hypermetropia (hyperopia) is also known as 'far sight'. In this dioptric condition of the eye, with the accommodation at rest, incident parallel rays come to a focus posterior to the light-sensitive layer of the retina. As in myopia, the chief factor in clinical hypermetropia is axial—an abnormal shortness in the length of the eye."-Parson 22/e p75

"Astigmatism: In this condition of refraction a point of light cannot be made to produce a punctate image upon the retina by any spherical correcting lens."-Parson 22/e p76

173. **Ans. b. Abducent nerve**   *(Ref: Parson 22/e p440, 441, 442; Gray's 40/e p430)*

In the given picture, abduction limitation is there on left side. Lateral gaze palsy is due to paralysis of lateral rectus, which is supplied by the abducens nerve. So, the given picture shows left (abducent) sixth nerve palsy.

"Paralysis of the lateral rectus: There is an esotropia or convergent squint with limitation of movement out wards, and the face is turned towards the paralysed side, flomonymous diplopia occurs on looking to the paralysed side; the images are on the same level and erect, becoming more separated on looking more towards the paralysed side. The false image is slightly tilted on looking up or down towards the paralysed side because of the imbalanced effect of the oblique muscles in these positions."-Parson 22/e p440

"Paralysis of the superior oblique: There is hypertropia of the affected eye with limitation of movement downwards and towards the sound side; the face is turned downwards and towards the sound side with a slight tilt of the head towards the shoulder of the sound or the normal side. Homonymous diplopia occurs on looking down; the false image is lower and its upper end is tilted towards the true image (the image is intorted because the eye is extorted when the superior oblique is paralysed). The distance between the images increases on looking down and towards the sound side and the inclination of the false image increases on looking down to the paralysed side. The patient has great difficulty in going downstairs, and vertigo is usually a particularly prominent symptom"- Parson 22/e p441

"Paralysis of the third nerve: In complete paralysis of the third nerve there is ptosis, which prevents diplopia. On raising the lid with the finger the eye is seen to be deflected outwards (divergent squint or exotropia) and rotated internally (intorted), owing to the tone of the two unparalysed muscles. The pupil is semidilated and immobile, and accommodation is paralysed. There is a slight degree of proptosis, owing to loss of tone of the paralysed muscles. There is limitation of movements upwards and inwards; to a lesser degree, downwards. With the lid raised there is diplopia, which is crossed, the false image being higher, with its upper end tilted towards the paralysed side (the eye is intorted and the image extorted)."-Parson 22/e p442

Functions of Extraocular Muscles		
Muscle	Nerve Supply	Action
Superior rectus	Oculomotor (Superior division)[Q]	Elevation, Adduction, Intortion[Q]
Inferior rectus	Oculomotor (Inferior division)[Q]	Depression, Adduction, Extortion[Q]
Medial rectus	Oculomotor (Inferior division)[Q]	Abduction[Q]
Muscle	Nerve Supply	Action
Lateral rectus	Abducens[Q]	Adduction[Q]
Superior oblique	Trochlear[Q]	Depression, Abduction, Intortion[Q]
Inferior oblique	Oculomotor (Inferior division)[Q]	Elevation, Abduction, Extortion[Q]

174. Ans. d. Non-Hodgkin's lymphoma *(Ref: Orbital Imaging By F. Allan Midyett (2014)/p192; Ocular pathology 6/e p564; Rosai and Ackerman's Surgical Pathology 10/e p2011; Sternberg's Diagnostic Surgical Pathology 5/e p1101)*

Most common tumor of lacrimal gland is Non-Hodgkin's lymphoma (37%) > Pleomorphic adenoma (25%). Most common malignant epithelial tumor of the lacrimal gland is adenoid cystic carcinoma.

"Adenoid cystic carcinoma (ACC) is the most common malignant epithelial tumor of the lacrimal gland." - Orbital Imaging By F. Allan Midyett (2014)/p192

"Benign mixed tumor (Pleomorphic adenoma): Benign mixed tumor (BMT) is the most common tumor of the lacrimal gland comprising more than 50% of all epithelial tumors. BMT accounts for 25% of lacrimal gland tumors."-Orbital Imaging By F. Allan Midyett (2014)/p192

"Lacrimal gland lymphoma: Lacrimal gland lymphoma (LGL) is usually bilateral. 75% of patients with orbital lymphoma have systemic disease. Primary orbital lymphoma is one of the most common orbital tumors found in half of orbital malignancies. Non-Hodgkin's lymphoma (NHL) is the most common primary tumor occurring in ocular adnexa. LGL comprises 37% of lacrimal gland malignancies. LGL comprises 50% of primary orbital malignancies."- Orbital Imaging By F. Allan Midyett (2014)/p192

Lacrimal Gland Tumor	
MC tumor of lacrimal gland	**Non-Hodgkin's lymphoma**[Q]
MC epithelial tumor of lacrimal gland	**Pleomorphic adenoma**[Q]
MC malignant epithelial tumor of lacrimal gland	**Adenoid cystic carcinoma**[Q]

175. Ans. c. Staphyloma *(Ref: Parson 22/e p229)*

Corneal bulging with glaucoma (raised IOP) is seen in the cases of anterior staphyloma. Intraocular pressure is lesser in keratoconus and keratomalacia because of thin corneas.

"Anterior staphyloma: This can be partial or total, depending on whether part or whole of the cornea is affected. The most common cause is a sloughing corneal ulcer, which perforates and heals with the formation of a pseudocornea by the organization of exudates and laying down of fibrous tissue. It is lined internally by the iris and externally by newly formed epithelium. The anterior chamber is flat and later secondary glaucoma may supervene. Gradually the weak anterior surface of the eye protrudes outward leading to an anterior staphyloma."-Parson 22/e p229

"Keratoconus (conical cornea): This is frequently due to a congenital weakness of the cornea, though it only manifests itself after puberty. However, it can also occur secondarily following trauma in which case it is unilateral, or in patients with vernal keratoconjunctivitis or Down syndrome due to repeated rubbing of the eye. The cornea thins near the centre and progressively bulges forwards, with the apex of the cone always being slightly below the centre of the cornea. The cornea is at first transparent and the vision is impaired due to myopic astigmatism. If the condition is marked, the conical shape is easily recognized in profile, particularly by the acute bulge given to the lower lid when the patient looks down (Munsen sign)."- Parson 22/e p216

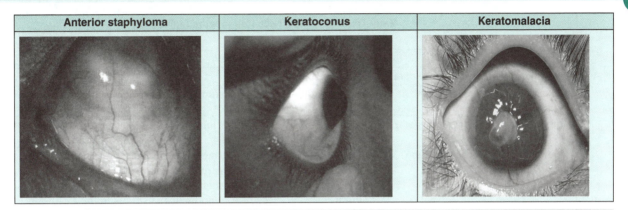

"Keratomalacia: This is common in developing countries and affects poorly nourished children who are deficient in vitamin A, often early in the first year of life; the condition is usually bilateral. The cornea becomes dull and insensitive, hazy and yellow infiltrates form until finally the whole tissue undergoes necrosis and seems to melt away (keratomalacia) within a few hours. A characteristic feature is the absence of inflammatory reaction. Keratomalacia is often precipitated by an acute systemic illness such as measles, pneumonia or severe diarrhoea. The children are usually extremely ill and very frequently die of other systemic diseases. Owing to their apathetic condition they do not close the lids, the cornea is continually exposed, and secondary bacterial infection can occur and complicate the clinical picture."-Parson 22/e p218

"In granular corneal dystrophy (nodular or granular dystrophy of Groenouw), in which the heredity is autosomal dominant, the opacities formed due to the abnormal accumulation of hyaline protein assume a discrete granular form and subsequently coalesce into various irregular shapes. The intervening cornea between the opacities and peripheral cornea remain clear."- Parson 22/e p213

176. **Ans. d. Severe non-proliferative diabetic retinopathy** *(Ref: Neema Textbook of Ophthalmology 6/e p304)*

    In the given fluorescein angiography of a diabetic patient, multiple microaneurysms are seen in all the quadrants suggesting the diagnosis of severe nonproliferative retinopathy.

    "Nonproliferative Diabetic Retinopathy (NPDR) is the most common type of diabetic retinopathy wherein the lesions are intraretinal and confined to the posterior pole. It is characterized by multiple microaneurysms, venous dilatation, hard exudates, dot and blot and flame-shaped hemorrhages, and retinal edema. The earliest sign of NPDR is a capillary microaneurysms. The microaneurysms appear as multiple, minute, round, red dots occasionally arranged like cluster of grapes at the ends of paramacular vessels. They are usually associated with yellow-white waxy-looking exudates with crenated margins."- Neema Textbook of Ophthalmology 6/e p304

    "Severity of NPDR is expressed by 4:2:1 rule, which is characterized by retinal hemorrhages and microaneurysms in 4 quadrants, venous beading in 2 quadrants and intraretinal microvascular abnormalities (IRMA), which represents shunt vessels that run from retinal arterioles to venules bypassing the capillary bed, in 1 quadrant. The presence of any one of these features represents severe NPDR while any two features indicate very severe NPDR and risk for progression to proliferative diabetic retinopathy."- Neema Textbook of Ophthalmology 6/e p304

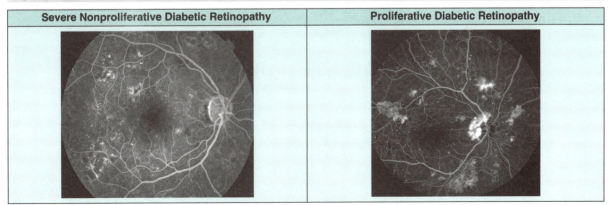

AIIMS ESSENCE

Early Treatment of Diabetic Retinopathy Scale	
Severity	**Definition**
No retinopathy	Diabetic retinopathy absent[Q]
Very mild nonproliferative retinopathy	Microaneurysm only[Q]
Mild nonproliferative retinopathy	Microaneurysm plus hard exudates, **cotton wool spots**, and/or **mild retinal hemorrhage**[Q]
Moderate nonproliferative retinopathy	Microaneurysm plus **mild intraretinal microvascular abnormalities** or moderate retinal hemorrhage[Q]
Severe nonproliferative retinopathy	Presence of **anyone** of the following (**4:2:1 rule**[Q]): Retinal hemorrhages and microaneurysms in 4 quadrants[Q] Venous beading in 2 quadrants[Q] Intraretinal microvascular abnormalities in 1 quadrant[Q]
Very severe nonproliferative retinopathy	Presence of **at least two** of the following (**4:2:1 rule**): Retinal hemorrhages and microaneurysms in 4 quadrants[Q] Venous beading in 2 quadrants[Q] Intraretinal microvascular abnormalities in 1 quadrant[Q]
Proliferative retinopathy	**Neovascularization** and/or **vitreous/pre-retinal hemorrhage**[Q]

177. Ans. d. Intravenous antibiotics   *(Ref: Parson 22/e p243)*

The given picture suggests the diagnosis of endophthalmitis. Intravenous antibiotics have no role in the management of enophthalmitis.

"Topical antibiotics: Commonly used topical antibiotics are fortified cefazolin (5%) or vancomycin (5%) with gentamicin or amikacin (1.3%) 1 hourly, alternating every half hour. Cycloplegia is achieved initially with topical atropine 1 % twice a day substituted by short-acting agents after 3-4 days."- Parson 22/e p243

"Intravitreal antibiotics are the treatment of choice and are injected after taking a 0.2-0.3 ml vitreous aspirate for preparing smears and obtaining cultures. A combination of amikacin (0.4 mg in 0.1 ml) or gentamicin (0.4 mg in 0.1 ml) and ceftriaxone (2 mg in 0.1 ml) or vancomycin (1.0 mg in 0.1ml) is generally recommended."-Parson 22/e p243

"Vitrectomy: Recovery from bacterial and fungal endophthalmitis is hastened by the removal of infected vitreous (vitrectomy) and the introduction of intravitreal antibiotics."-Parson 22/e p243

Approach to Management of Endophthalmitis

1st Step

Check the visual acuity and then plan treatment accordingly

If vision is >= HMCF*, proceed for vitreous sampling by tap for microbiology and intracanthal injection of antibiotics

If vision is only PL+**, then patient should be taken up for vitrectomy with IV antibiotics

If no light perception then no surgical intervention or evisceration if developing panophthalmitis

2nd step

After 48 hours check the vision and if there is no improvement, proceed for repeat vitreous tap for infection

If there is no improvement after 2 intravitreal injections, proceed for vitrectomy

*HMCF-hand movement close to face
**perception of light present

AIIMS November 2017

Endophthalmitis
• **Endophthalmitis** is defined as an **intraocular inflammation**, which predominantly **affects the inner spaces of eye & their contents** (**vitreous** and/or **anterior chamber**)

Etiology:
- **Organisms responsible:** Pneumococci, staphylococci, streptococci, Escherichia coli, Pseudomonas pyocyanea, Bacillus cereus & subtilis, Clostridium welchii

Fungal Endophthalmitis
• Occur **after intraocular surgery** or **injury with vegetable matter**[Q] **(thorn or wooden stick)**   • **Incubation period** of **several weeks**[Q]   • Predominantly affects **anterior vitreous & anterior uvea** with formation of a **hypopyon**[Q]   • **Granulomatous vitreous & pupils** become **occluded with inflammatory material**[Q].

- **Delayed onset exogenous endophthalmitis** can occur **after cataract surgery** or **glaucoma-filtering surgery** with thin filtering blebs following use of antifibroblastic agents. **Fungal infection & Propionibacterium acnes** are **most likely organisms in endophthalmitis** occurring several weeks or months **after cataract surgery**[Q].

Endogenous Endophthalmitis
• **Endogenous form** of purulent uveitis is **metastatic in origin**[Q].   • Seen as a **complication of exanthematous illnesses** such as **meningococcal septicemia** & in **immunosuppressed patients**[Q]   • Infection may be bacterial, fungal or viral.   • **Mucormycosis** extends **directly from nasopharynx** in debilitated individuals with **diabetic ketoacidosis**.

Clinical Features:
- **Cardinal features**: **Pain, swelling of lid & decrease in vision**[Q]
- Rise in temperature, headache & sometimes vomiting; fever is more common with endogenous infection.

> - **Edges of wound** become **yellow & necrotic, hypopyon appears** in **exogenous form**[Q]
> - **Severe chemosis** with **intense ciliary & conjunctival congestion, swollen & red lids; severe pain** in eye.
> - **Purulent vitreous** as shown by a **yellow reflex with oblique illumination**[Q].

- **Anterior chamber** becomes **full of pus** with **cloudy & yellow cornea; ring infiltration & corneal melting**[Q]
- **Proptosis & painful limitation of movement of globe** due to **extension of inflammation to Tenon's capsule**
- **Metastatic cases**: On ophthalmoscopic examination **hazy media, yellow edematous retina** & **yellow reflex**; Formation of a **hypopyon & rapid failure of vision**[Q].

Diagnosis:
- **Detailed history, ocular examination & ultrasonography** are required to **confirm the clinical diagnosis**
- **Vitreous tap or biopsy** for **Gram & Giemsa staining**, bacterial & fungal cultures

Treatment of Endophthalmitis	
Topical antibiotics	• **Commonly used topical antibiotics:** Fortified **cefazolin (5%)** or **vancomycin (5%)** with **gentamicin** or **amikacin (1.3%) 1 hourly,** alternating every half hour[Q].
Intravitreal antibiotics	• **Intravitreal antibiotics are the treatment of choice**[Q] • Injected after taking a 0.2-0.3 ml vitreous aspirate for preparing smears & obtaining cultures. • **Combination** of **amikacin or gentamicin & ceftriaxone** or **vancomycin is recommended**[Q].
Vitrectomy	• **Recovery** from bacterial & fungal endophthalmitis is **hastened by removal of infected vitreous (vitrectomy) & introduction of intravitreal antibiotics**[Q]. • **Immediate pars plana vitrectomy** if **visual acuity** on presentation is **light perception** or **worse,** or patient **does not respond to intravitreal antibiotics within 48 hours**[Q]

178. **Ans. d. Pterygium**   *(Ref: Parson 22/e p184)*

In the given picture, there is wing shaped extension of conjunctiva over cornea known as pterygium.

> *"Pterygium: This is a degenerative condition of the subconjunctival tissues which proliferate as vascularized granulation tissue to invade the cornea, destroying the superficial layers of the stroma and Bowman's membrane, the whole being covered by conjunctival epithelium. The lesion thus appears as a triangular encroachment of the conjunctiva upon the cornea with numerous small opacities lying deeply in the neighbouring part of the cornea in front of its blunt apex."- Parson 22/e p184*

Pterygium	Pinguecula
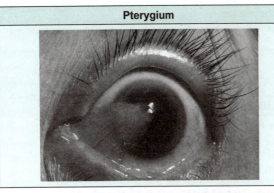	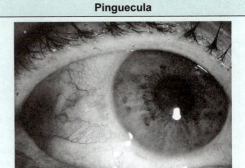

*"**Pinguecula**: This is a triangular patch on the conjunctiva, usually found in elderly people, especially those exposed to strong sunlight, dust, wind, etc. It occurs near the limbus in the palpebral aperture, the apex of the triangle being away from the cornea and affects the nasal side first, then the temporal. It is yellow in colour and looks like fat, hence the name (pinguis, fat), but is due to hyaline infiltration and elastotic degeneration of the sub-mucous tissue. Since the pinguecula remains relatively free from congestion it is particularly conspicuous when the eye is inflamed; mistakes in diagnosis may then occur. **It requires no treatment**."-Parson 22/e p184*

Pterygium

- **Degenerative condition of subconjunctival tissues** which proliferate as **vascularized granulation tissue to invade the cornea** destroying the superficial layers of stroma & Bowman's membrane[Q]
- Wing shaped triangular fold of degenerative bulbar conjunctiva encroaching upon the cornea[Q]

Etiology:
- Prolonged exposure to UV rays, dust, wind, dry heat[Q].

Pathology:
- **Degenerative:** Hyperplastic condition affecting the subconjunctival tissue
- Elastotic collagenous degeneration with proliferation of vascularized granulation tissue, which invades cornea[Q]
- Corneal epithelium, Bowman's layer & superficial stroma are destroyed by invading tissue[Q]

Features:
- Vascularized conjunctiva encroaching the cornea from canthus
- **Stocker's line:** Iron deposition anterior to advancing head[Q]
- **Visual impairment** due to pupillary involvement, **astigmatism** due to fibrosis, **diplopia** due to restriction of ocular movement & cosmetic blemish[Q].

Treatment:
- **Asymptomatic cases type 1** i.e., <2 mm corneal involvement are **best left alone**[Q].

Surgical Options in Pterygium
- **Excision with simple closure** of the wound.
- **Mc Gavics bare sclera method:** Pterygium is excised and the conjunctival defect is left as it is. High rates of recurrence **(30-80%)** and granuloma formation
- **Transplantation of the pterygium**: Pterygium excision with **auto-conjunctival graft / amniotic membrane graft**. Done in **recurrent pterygium / large pterygium**.
- **Mac Reynold's operation:** Head is sutured to the **body itself**
- **Kehr's operation:** Head is sutured **to the inferior fornix**.

ENT

179. Ans. b. Outer hair cell *(Ref: Dhingra 7/e p37; Otorhinolaryngology, Head and Neck Surgery by Matti Anniko (2010)/p128)*
Noise induced hearing loss mostly affects outer hair cell.

"Noise induced hearing loss (NIHL) causes damage to hair cells, starting in the basal turn of cochlea. Outer hair cells are affected before the inner hair cells."- Dhingra 7/e p37

"Noise-induced hearing loss damages hair cells, which begin at the basal turn of cochlea. Outer hair cells are affected earlier than the inner hair cells."-Diseases of Ear, Nose and Throat By Mohan Bansal (2012)/p161

"Chronic noise exposure causes metabolic as well as mechanic ultrastructural visible damage at the level of the organ of Corti, initially causing a loss of outer hair cells, leading finally to neuronal degeneration." Otorhinolaryngology, Head and Neck Surgery by Matti Anniko (2010)/p128

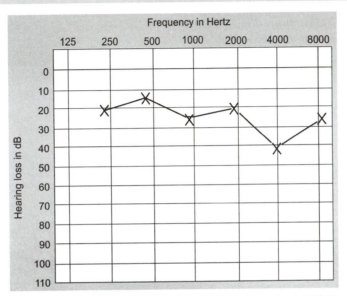

Fig. 44: Early case of noise-induced hearing loss. Note dip at 4000 Hz

	Noise-Induced Hearing Loss (NIHL)
\multicolumn{2}{l}{• **Hearing loss follows chronic exposure to less intense sounds** than seen in acoustic trauma}
\multicolumn{2}{l}{• Mainly a **hazard of noisy occupations**}
Temporary threshold shift (TTS)	• **Hearing is impaired immediately after exposure to noise** but **recovers** after an interval of a few minutes to a few hours even up to 2 weeks. • Amount of TTS depends on the noise—its **intensity, frequency & duration**[Q].
Permanent threshold shift (PTS)	• **Hearing impairment** is **permanent** and **does not recover at all.** • Damage caused by noise trauma depends on several factors: • **Frequency** of noise: A frequency of **2000–3000 Hz** causes **more damage than lower or higher frequencies**[Q] • **Intensity & duration** of noise: As the intensity increases, permissible time for exposure is reduced[Q] • **Continuous vs interrupted noise: Continuous noise** is **more harmful.** • **Susceptibility** of the individual • **Pre-existing ear disease**

Pathology:
- **Chronic noise exposure** causes **metabolic & mechanic ultrastructural visible damage** at the level of **organ of Corti,** initially causing a **loss of outer hair cells,** leading to **neuronal degeneration**[Q].
  - **Outer hair cells** are **affected before the inner hair cells**[Q].

Clinical Features:
- Shouting to converse at workplace
- Aural fullness or muffled hearing after the work

Audiogram:
- **Audiogram in NIHL** shows a **typical notch, at 4 kHz,** both for **air & bone conduction**[Q].
- **As the duration of noise exposure increases,** the **notch deepens & widens to involve lower & higher frequencies**[Q].

Contd...

Noise-Induced Hearing Loss (NIHL)
Prophylaxis: • **Noise > 85 dB (A) at workplace: Pre-employment & annual audiograms** for early detection • **Ear protectors** should be used where **noise levels exceed 85 dB (A).** • **Rehabilitation:** If hearing impairment has already occurred

180. **Ans. b. Traumatic CSF rhinorrhea**   *(Ref: Dhingra 7/e p184; Scott-Brown 7/e p1636-1639)*
 Target sign is seen in traumatic CSF rhinorrhea.

> *"CSF rhinorrhoea: There is history of clear watery discharge from the nose on bending the head or straining. It may be seen on rising in the morning when patient bends his head (reservoir sign-fluid which had collected in the sinuses, particularly sphenoid, empties into the nose)."-Dhingra 7/e p184*

> *"CSF rhinorrhoea after head trauma is mixed with blood and shows double target sign when collected on a piece of filter paper. It shows central red spot (blood) and peripheral lighter halo."-Dhingra 7/e p184*

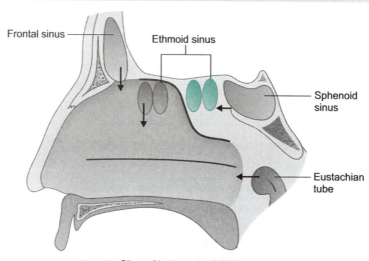

Fig. 45: Sites of leakage in CSF Rhinorrhea

CSF Rhinorrhea
• **Leakage of CSF into the nose** is called CSF rhinorrhoea. • It may be **clear fluid** or **mixed with blood** as in acute head injuries. • **Underlying defect responsible for CSF leaks, regardless of the etiology: disruption in the arachnoid & dura mater coupled with an osseous defect** and **a CSF pressure gradient** that is continuously or intermittently greater than the tensile strength of the disrupted tissue[Q].
Etiology: • Penetrating & closed-head trauma are **responsible for 90% of all cases of CSF leaks[Q].**
Clinical features: • CSF rhinorrhea following a traumatic injury is classified as **immediate** (within 48 hours) or **delayed[Q].** • Majority of patients with a CSF leak due to accidental trauma (e.g., motor vehicle accident) **present immediately[Q].** • Most of the patients (95%) with a delayed CSF leak present within 3 months after the injury[Q]. • Typical history of a CSF leak is that of **clear, watery discharge, usually unilateral[Q].** • Diagnosis is made more easily in patients with recent trauma or surgery than in others.
Diagnosis: • **Rhinoscopy:** Visualization of CSF leakage from paranasal sinuses • **Tissue test:** Unlike nasal mucus, **CSF does not cause a tissue to stiffen**. • **Reservoir sign: Fluid** which had collected **in the sinuses**, particularly **sphenoid, empties into the nose** (history of clear watery discharge from nose on bending the head or straining)

AIIMS November 2017

Contd...

CSF Rhinorrhea
• **Filter paper test:** Sample of nasal discharge on a filter paper exhibits a light CSF border and a dark central area of blood, double ring sign or halo sign or double target sign (in traumatic CSF leak, where blood & CSF are mixed)
• **Queckenstedt test:** Compression of jugular veins leads to increased CSF leakage due to increase in ICP[Q].
• **Beta-2 transferrin:** Preferred biochemical marker of CSF. It helps in distinguishing CSF from other nasal discharge[Q].
• **High-resolution fine-slice CT scan:** Investigation of choice for locating a defect in CSF rhinorrhea[Q].
Treatment
• **Early cases of post-traumatic CSF rhinorrhoea** are **managed conservatively by placing the patient in the semi-sitting position, avoiding blowing of nose, sneezing & straining**[Q].
• **Prophylactic antibiotics** are also administered to prevent meningitis.
• **Persistent cases of CSF rhinorrhoea** are **treated surgically by nasal endoscopic or intracranial approach**[Q].
• **Nasal endoscopic approach is useful for leaks from the frontal sinus, cribriform plate, ethmoid or sphenoid sinuses**[Q].

181. **Ans. a. Interstitial keratitis + Eighth nerve deafness + Hutchinson incisor** *(Ref: Fitzpatrick 6/e p2164-2212; Rooks 8/e p34.1-34.20; Dermatology by Jean L. Bolognia 3/e p1377; Neonatal and Infant Dermatology By Lawrence F. Eichenfield (2014)/p173)*

Hutchinson's triad is Interstitial keratitis + Eighth nerve deafness + Hutchinson incisor.

"Congenital syphilis: Late manifestations (i.e., appearing after 2 years of age) involve the central nervous system (neurosyphilis, which may be asymptomatic), bones (frontal bossing, saddle nose, concave central face, saber shins, Clutton's joints), teeth (Hutchinson peg-shaped notched central incisors, mulberry multicuspid first molars), skin (rhagades, nodular syphilids, gummata), eyes (interstitial keratitis, optic atrophy), and ears (eighth-nerve deafness). Hutchinson's triad of defects includes interstitial keratitis, defects of the incisors, and sensorineural hearing loss."- Neonatal and Infant Dermatology By Lawrence F. Eichenfield (2014)/p173

Clinical Presentation of Syphilis	
Early Congenital Syphilis	• Earliest feature: Snuffles (rhinitis)[Q] • Lesions are vesicobullous[Q] & snail track ulcers on mucosa
Late Congenital Syphilis	• Characterized by Hutchinson's triad (interstitial keratitis + 8th nerve deafness + Hutchinson's teeth i.e. pegged central upper incisors)[Q] • Saddle nose, sabre tibia, mulberry molars[Q] • Bull dog's jaw (protrusion of jaw) • Rhagades[Q] (linear fissure at mouth, nares) • Frontal bossing, hot cross bun deformity of skull • Clutton's joint[Q] (painless swelling of joints, most commonly both knee) • Palatal perforation[Q] • Higaumenakis sign (periosteitis leads to unilateral enlargement of sterna end of clavicle)
Primary Syphilis	• Painless, indurated, non-bleeding, usually single punched out ulcer (hard chancre)[Q] • Painless, rubbery shotty lymphadenopathy[Q]
Secondary Syphilis	• Bilateral symmetrical asymptomatic localized or diffuse mucocutaneous lesion[Q] (macule, papule, papulosquamous & rarely pustule) • Non-tender generalized lymphadenopathy[Q] • Highly infectious condylomata lata[Q], in warm moist intertriginous areas • Moth eaten alopecia, arthritis, proteinuria[Q]
Tertiary Syphilis	• Gumma, neurosyphilis / tabes dorsalis[Q] • Osteitis, periosteitis • Aortitis, aortic insufficiency, coronary stenosis & nocturnal angina[Q]

SKIN

182. **Ans. a. Scabies** *(Ref: Bolognia 3/e p1423-1424; Fitzpatrick 6/e p2540)*

History of pruritus over fingers and lesions present in the finger webs as given in the picture is highly suggestive of scabies.

AIIMS ESSENCE

"The hallmark of scabies is intractable pruritus, characteristically more severe at night. The itching, often disproportionately severe, is associated with lesions that initially appear on the web spaces, then the sides of the fingers, the flexor surfaces of the wrists, elbows and anterior axillary folds. Other common sites of lesions are the penis and scrotum, the areolae in women, the buttocks, and the sacral and periumbilical areas. Lesions may be eczematous and often are excoriated, but the pathognomonic lesion is the burrow, a short, wavy, dark line. The classical features are often obscured by excoriations, impetiginization or eczematization."- Fitzpatrick 6/e p2540

Scabies

- Infestation caused by **Acarus or Sarcoptes scabie[Q]**
- Usually a disease of **children**, with no gender predilection
- Mainly involving **lower socio economic strata** living in **poor hygiene & crowding**
- **Transmitted by close physical contact** from **human to human** or from **pets to human.**
- **Several cases in same household[Q]**

Epidemiology:
- **Incubation period: 2-4 weeks[Q]**
- **MC symptom: Itching (worse at night)**
- Family history of similar **itchy eruptions in close contact[Q]**

Morphology of Lesions & Variants

Primary lesions	Secondary lesions	Variants or Types
• **Burrow**: **Serpentine (S-shaped) path traversed** by parasite in **stratum corneum[Q]**. It is **pathognomic of lesion** • **Papules & papulovesicles**: Due to hypersensitivity to the mite • **Fine pin-head size follicular papules**	• **Pustules due to 2° infection** is one of commonest form of presentation • **Eczematized exudative crusted lesions**, in infants & children are predominant lesions • **Nodular lesions** are seen on **scrotum[Q]** (**MC**), groin & anterior axillary fold (**Nodular scabies**)	• **Crusted Norwegian scabies** is **most severe[Q]** form seen in **immunocompromised** or **mentally ill patients**, and showing hyperkeratotic crusted lesions on whole body. • **Scabies incognito** is **wrongly treated with steroids.**

Site of predilection:
- **In adults web of fingers[Q]**, flexure aspect of wrist, ulnar aspect of forearm, anterior axillary fold, umbilicus, periumbilical fold, **genitals[Q]** (penis & scrotum in males, nipple & areola in females), upper thigh, lower part of buttocks
- Back is rarely affected

> - **Scalp, face, palms** & **soles** are **characteristically spared** in **adults[Q]**.
> - In **infants, scalp, face, palms** & **soles** are **typically involved[Q].**

- An anatomical circle, encompassing the **axial, elbow flexures, wrists, hands & genital region** has been referred to as the **circle of Hebra.**
- **Site of predilection for scabies** is **circle of Hebra[Q]**.
- Scabies & scabies in circle of hebra (both) simulate sabra dermatitis seen in prickly pears (eg. cactus with spines & glochids) pickers.

Treatment
- **Drug of choice: Permethrin[Q]** (1st) > **BHC[Q]** (2nd)
- **Oral drug** (only): **Ivermectin[Q]**
- Other drugs: **Benzyl benzoate[Q]** 25%, **Crotamiton[Q]** 10%, Malathion, Monosulfiram
- In 2° infection: IV antibiotics

> - **Scabicides should be applied to the whole body** (below jaw line in adults) **to all members of family whether symptomatic or not[Q]**
> - Ordinary laundering of cloths & bed linen. Mites any way die in unworn clothes in ~ 7 days.

---

183. **Ans. a. Basal cell carcinoma** *(Ref: Harrison 19/e p500; Robbins 9/e p1157)*

Lesion near inner canthus with raised, pearly borders and central crust and with telangiectasia on surface of the lesion is highly suggestive of basal cell carcinoma.

"Basal cell carcinomas usually present as pearly papules containing prominent dilated subepidermal blood vessels (telangiectasias). Some tumors contain melanin and superficially resemble melanocytic nevi or melanomas. Advanced lesions may ulcerate, and extensive local invasion of bone or facial sinuses may occur after many years of neglect or in unusually aggressive tumors, explaining the archaic designation rodent ulcers."- Robbins 9/e p1157

"BCC arises from epidermal basal cells. BCC also can present as a small, slowly growing pearly nodule, often with tortuous telangiectatic vessels on its surface, rolled borders, and a central crust (nodular BCC). The occasional presence of melanin in this variant of nodular BCC (pigmented BCC) may lead to confusion with melanoma. Morpheaform (fibrosing), infiltrative, and micronodular BCC, the most invasive and potentially aggressive subtypes, manifest as solitary, flat or slightly depressed, indurated whitish, yellowish, or pink scar-like plaques."- Harrison 19/e p500

Basal Cell Carcinoma (Rodent Ulcer)

- **Locally invasive** carcinoma, **arises from** the **basal layer**[Q] of the epidermis
- **MC type of skin cancer**[Q]
- **90%** of **BCC** are seen **in the face**[Q], above a **line from** the **corner of mouth to lobule of ear**[Q].
- **MC site: Nose >Inner canthus**[Q] of the eye, also known as **Tear cancer**[Q].

Types of BCC

• **Nodular: MC type of BCC**[Q], characterized by small slow growing **pearly nodules**, with **telengiectatic vessels** on surface. **Central depression** with **umbilication**[Q] is a classic sign.	• **Pigmented** (Mimic malignant melanoma) • **Cystic** • **Superficial**

Characteristic Features of BCC

• **Low grade malignancy**[Q] • **More common in fair** & **dry skinned** people • **Nuclear palisading**[Q] on histology	• **Exposure to sunlight**[Q] is an important etiological factor • Has been seen following prolonged administration of **Arsenic**[Q]

Spread:
- BCC usually **spreads by local invasion**[Q], rarely metastasizes
- **Rodent ulcer**[Q]: It gradually **destroys the tissues** it comes **in contact with**.
- **Lymphatic spread** is **not seen**[Q] (Regional LNs are not enlarged)
- Blood spread is extremely rare.

Diagnosis:
- Diagnostic procedure for BCC is **wedge biopsy**[Q].

Treatment:
- **Non-aggressive tumor** on **trunk** or **extremities: Excision** or **Electro dissection & curettage**[Q]
- **Large, aggressive,** located at **vital areas** or **recurrent: Moh's micrographic surgery**[Q]

184a. Ans. c. Hyperthyroidism *(Ref: Harrison 19/e p1651; Schwartz 10/e p1531)*

The findings in the given picture is noninflamed, indurated plaque with a deep pink or purple color and an "orange skin" appearance, over the anterior and lateral aspects of the lower leg. This suggest the diagnosis of pretibial myxedma, which is seen in patients of Grave's disease (hyperthyroidism).

"Bilateral leg swelling occurs in patients with congestive heart failure, hypoalbuminemia secondary to nephrotic syndrome or severe hepatic disease, myxedema caused by hypothyroidism or pretibial myxedema associated with Graves' disease, and with drugs such as dihydropyridine calcium channel blockers and thiazolidinediones."-Harrison 19/e p1651

"Thyroid dermopathy occurs in <5% of patients with Graves' disease, almost always in the presence of moderate or severe ophthalmopathy. Although most frequent over the anterior and lateral aspects of the lower leg (hence the term pretibial myxedema), skin changes can occur at other sites, particularly after trauma. The typical lesion is a noninflamed, indurated plaque with a deep pink or purple color and an "orange skin" appearance. Nodular involvement can occur, and the condition can rarely extend over the whole lower leg and foot, mimicking elephantiasis. Thyroid acropachy refers to a form of clubbing found in <1% of patients with Graves' disease. It is so strongly associated with thyroid dermopathy that an alternative cause of clubbing should be sought in a Graves' patient without coincident skin and orbital involvement."- Harrison 19/e p2295

"Graves' disease is characterized by thyrotoxicosis, diffuse goiter, and extra- thyroidal conditions including ophthalmopathy, dermopathy (pretibial myxedema), thyroid acropachy, gynecomastia, and other manifestations."- Schwartz 10/e p1531

Grave's Disease (Diffuse Toxic Goiter)

- **MC cause** of **hyperthyroidism,** caused by **stimulatory autoantibodies** to **TSH-R**[Q].
- **Autoimmune disease** with strong **familial predisposition**[Q]
- More common in **females** with peak incidence between **40-60** years
- Characterized by **thyrotoxicosis, diffuse goiter** & **extrathyroidal conditions**[Q] (ophthalmopathy, dermopathy, thyroid acropachy & gynecomastia)

Contd...

Etiopathogenesis:

- **Autoimmune process** with possible **triggers** (post-partum state, iodine excess, lithium therapy & bacterial or viral infections)
- Associated with **HLA-B8, HLA-DR3, HLA-DQA1*0501 & CTLA-4**[Q]
- **HLA-DRB1*0701** is **protective** against it
- **Thyroid stimulating antibodies**[Q] stimulate thyrocytes to grow & synthesize excess thyroid hormone, which is **hallmark of Grave's disease**
- Associated with **type I diabetes mellitus, Addison's disease, pernicious anemia & myasthenia gravis**

Histopathology:

- **Hyperplastic gland** with columnar epithelium & minimal colloid
- Nuclei exhibit **mitosis**
- **Papillary projections** of **hyperplastic epithelium**[Q]

Clinical Features:

- **Hyperthyroid symptoms**[Q] (heat intolerance, increased sweating & thirst, weight loss despite adequate caloric intake)
- **Symptoms of adrenergic stimulation**[Q] (palpitations, nervousness, fatigue, emotional lability, hyperkinesis & tremors)
- **MC GI symptom** is **increased frequency** of **bowel movements & diarrhea**[Q]

  - **Female patients** often develop **amenorrhea, decreased fertility & increased** incidence of **miscarriage**[Q]
  - **Children** experience **rapid growth** with **early bone maturation**[Q]
  - **Older patients** present with **CVS complications (AF & CHF)**[Q]

- Weight loss, facial flushing, warm & moist skin, tachycardia, cutaneous vasodilatation, **collapsing pulse** is seen on examination
- A **fine tremor, muscle wasting & proximal muscle** group **weakness** with **hyperactive tendon reflexes** often are present[Q]

  - Overlying **bruit** or **thrill** at **upper pole**[Q] due to **increased vascularity**
  - **Loud venous hum**[Q] in supraclavicular space
  - **Ophthalmopathy** (orbital proptosis) occurs in **50%, dermopathy** in **1-2%.**[Q]
  - Dermopathy is characterized by deposition of **glycosaminoglycans** leading to **thickened skin** in **pretibial region & dorsum of foot**[Q] (pretibial myxedema).

- **Gynecomastia** is common in **young men**[Q]
- Rare bony involvement leads to **subperiosteal bone formation & swelling in metacarpals**[Q] (**thyroid acropachy**)

Diagnosis:

- **Suppressed TSH** with or without an elevated free T4 or T3 level. **If eye signs are present,** other tests are generally not needed[Q].
- **In absence** of **eye signs, elevated RAIU** with **diffusely enlarged gland**[Q] confirms the diagnosis
- **Elevated TSH-R** or **thyroid-stimulating antibodies (TSAb)** are **diagnostic**[Q] of Grave's disease & increased in about **90%** patients
- **Anti-Tg & Anti-TPO antibodies** are **non-specific** & elevated in upto **75%** cases.
- **MRI of orbits** are useful in evaluating **Grave's ophthalmopathy**

Treatment:

- Treatment modalities: **Antithyroid drugs**, thyroid ablation with radioactive ^{131}I & **thyroidectomy**[Q].

184b. Ans. a. Diabetes mellitus   *(Ref: Harrison 19/e p2430)*

The given lesions are indurated, annular, yellowish brown plaques with atrophic centre and ectatic blood vessels visible through the thinned skin, present over shin is highly suggestive of necrobiosis lipoidica diabeticorum (seen in diabetes mellitus).

> *"Necrobiosis lipoidica diabeticorum is an uncommon dis-order, accompanying diabetes in predominantly young women. This usually begins in the pretibial region as an erythematous plaque or papules that gradually enlarge, darken, and develop irregular margins, with atrophic centers and central ulceration. They are often painful."- Harrison 19/e p2430*

Dermatologic Manifestations of Diabetes Mellitus	
Xerosis & pruritus	• **MC skin manifestations of DM, usually relieved by skin moisturizers**. • Protracted wound healing & skin ulcerations are frequent complications.
Diabetic dermopathy	• Also termed as **pigmented pretibial papules**, or **"diabetic skin spots"** • Begins as an **erythematous macule or papule** that evolves into an **area of circular hyperpigmentation.** • Result from **minor mechanical trauma** in **pretibial region** • More common in **elderly men with DM**
Bullosa diabeticorum	• Bullous diseases (**shallow ulcerations or erosions** in the **pretibial region**)

Contd...

Necrobiosis lipoidica diabeticorum	• Uncommon disorder, accompanying **diabetes in predominantly young women.** • Usually **begins in the pretibial region** as an **erythematous plaque or papules** that **gradually enlarge, darken & develop irregular margins,** with **atrophic centers & central ulceration.** They are often **painful.**
Vitiligo	• Occurs at increased frequency in individuals with **type 1 DM.**
Acanthosis nigricans	• **Hyperpigmented velvety plaques** seen on **the neck, axilla, or extensor surfaces** • Feature of **severe insulin resistance & accompanying diabetes.**
Granuloma annulare	• **Erythematous plaques** on the extremities or trunk
Lipoatrophy & lipohypertrophy	• Occur **at insulin injection sites** but are now unusual with the use of human insulin.
Scleredema	• Areas of **skin thickening on the back or neck at** the **site of previous superficial infections**

185. Ans. c. Chikungunya *(Ref: IJDVL: Year 2010| Volume:76 |Issue:6 | Page:671-676-Cutaneous manifestations of chikungunya during a recent epidemic in Calicut, north Kerala, south India; Harrison 19/e p1313)*

Clinical history of fever, joint pain and rash and after one week of NSAIDs use, the patient developed brownish discoloration over nose as given in the image, the most probable diagnosis is pigmentation caused by Chikungunya. Nose pigmentation is striking in the cases of CKG, which has not been reported in any other viral exanthem. For fixed drug eruption, mucocutaneous junction (lip, glans) is most frequently involved, genital skin (glans) is the most commonly involved site.

"Chikungunya (CKG) is acute febrile illness with incapacitating polyarthralgia, headache, vomiting, sore throat, conjunctivitis and skin eruptions. It is usually self limiting and rarely fatal. The most common cutaneous lesion described in CKG is erythematous maculopapular rash affecting trunk, limbs and face. The abundance of Aedes albopictus and mutations in glycoprotein envelope (E1) gene of CHIKV may be the contributory factors for repeated outbreaks. Nose pigmentation was striking in several cases of CKG, which has not been reported in any other viral exanthem. Its presence and persistence for about three to six month after an attack of CKG helps to make a clinical and retrospective diagnosis of CKG. Hence, this may be considered as a marker of CKG, and we suggest 'chik sign' for this peculiar pigmentation."-*Ref: IJDVL: Year: 2010| Volume : 76 |Issue : 6 | Page : 671-676-Cutaneous manifestations of chikungunya during a recent epidemic in Calicut, north Kerala, south India*

186. Ans. a. Coxsackie *(Ref: Harrison 19/e p1292; Ananthanarayan 10/e p497; Jawetz 27/e p522)*

The given picture is of hand-foot-mouth disease caused by Coxsackie virus.

"Hand-Foot-Mouth Disease: After an incubation period of 4–6 days, patients with hand-foot-and-mouth disease present with fever, anorexia, and malaise; these manifestations are followed by the development of sore throat and vesicles on the buccal mucosa and often on the tongue and then by the appearance of tender vesicular lesions on the dorsum of the hands, sometimes with involvement of the palms. The vesicles may form bullae and quickly ulcerate. About one-third of patients also have lesions on the palate, uvula, or tonsillar pillars, and one-third have a rash on the feet (including the soles) or on the buttocks. The disease is highly infectious, with attack rates of close to 100% among young children. The lesions usually resolve in 1 week. Most cases are due to coxsackievirus A16 or enterovirus 71."-*Harrison 19/e p1292*

"Hand-foot-and-mouth disease is characterized by oral and pharyngeal ulcerations and a vesicular rash of the palms and soles that may spread to the arms and legs. Vesicles heal without crusting, which clinically differentiates them from the vesicles of herpes viruses and poxviruses. This disease has been associated particularly with coxsackievirus A16 but also with B1 (and enterovirus 71)."-*Jawetz 27/e p522*

Coxsackie virus
• Characteristic feature of this group: **Ability to infect suckling but not adult mice**[Q]. • Coxsackie viruses are **highly infective for newborn mice**, in contrast to most other human enteroviruses. • Certain strains (**B1–6, A7, 9, 16 & 24**) also **grow in monkey kidney cell culture**[Q].
Pathogenesis: • Virus has been recovered from the blood in the early stages of natural infection in humans. • Virus is also found in the throat for a few days early in the infection and in the stools for up to 5–6 weeks.
Clinical Findings • **Incubation period: 2-9 days**[Q] • Clinical manifestations of infection range from mild febrile illness to CNS, skin, cardiac & respiratory diseases. • **Fever, malaise, headache, nausea & abdominal pain** are common **early symptoms**[Q]. • Patients almost always recover completely from non-poliovirus paresis.

Contd...

Diseases caused by Coxsackie virus	
Aseptic meningitis	• **Aseptic meningitis:** Caused by **all types of group B** Coxsackie viruses & by many **group A** Coxsackie viruses, most commonly **A7 & A9**[Q].
Herpangina	• **Severe febrile pharyngitis** caused by certain **group A viruses**[Q]. • Characterized by **abrupt onset of fever & sore throat with discrete vesicles on posterior half of palate, pharynx, tonsils, or tongue**[Q]. • **Self-limited** & most frequent in **small children**[Q].
Hand-foot-and-mouth disease	• Characterized by **oral & pharyngeal ulcerations** and a **vesicular rash of palms & soles that may spread to arms & legs**[Q]. • **Vesicles heal without crusting**, which clinically **differentiates from vesicles of herpes viruses & poxviruses**[Q]. • Associated with **coxsackievirus A16 & B1** (and **enterovirus 71**)[Q]. • **Virus** may be **recovered from** the **stool, pharyngeal secretions & vesicular fluid**.
Pleurodynia	• Also known as **epidemic myalgia**, caused by **group B viruses**[Q]. • **Fever & stabbing chest pain** are usually abrupt in onset but are sometimes preceded by malaise, headache & anorexia[Q]. • **Abdominal pain** in approximately half of cases & chief complaint in children. • **Self-limited** with **complete recovery**[Q]
Myocarditis	• **Coxsackie virus B infections** are a cause of primary myocardial disease in **adults & children**[Q]. • **Infections may be fatal in neonates** or may cause **permanent heart damage** at any age[Q].
Generalized disease of infants	• **Extremely serious disease** in which the infant is overwhelmed by simultaneous **viral infections of** multiple organs, including **heart, liver & brain**[Q]. • Clinical course may be **rapidly fatal**, or the **patient may recover completely**. • Caused by **group B Coxsackie viruses**[Q].

Diagnosis:

Recovery of Virus
• Virus can be **isolated from throat washings** during the first few days of illness & **from stools during the first few weeks**[Q].   • In **coxsackievirus A21 infections**, the **largest amount of virus is found in nasal secretions**[Q].   • In cases of **aseptic meningitis**, **strains** have been **recovered from CSF & alimentary tract**[Q].   • In **hemorrhagic conjunctivitis** cases, **A24 virus is isolated from conjunctival swabs, throat swabs & feces**[Q].   • Specimens can be **inoculated into tissue cultures & suckling mice**[Q].   • In tissue culture, a **cytopathic effect appears within 5–14 days**[Q].

ANVESTHESIA

187. Ans. b. A-beta   *(Ref: Morgan 4/e p266; Miller 8/e p1037, 7/e p917, 921, 924)*

Type A-beta nerve fiber is least susceptible to local anesthetics.

Fiber type (Erlanger & Gassers)	Function	Fiber Diameter (mm)	Conduction velocity (ms)	Local Anesthetic Sensitivity
Aα	Proprioception, somatic motor[Q]	12-20[Q]	70-120[Q]	++
Aβ	Touch, pressure, motor	5-12	30-70	++
Aγ	Motor to muscle spindles[Q]	3-6	15-30	++
Aδ	**Pain, cold, touch**[Q]	2-5	12-30	+++
B	Preganglionic autonomic[Q]	<3	3-15	++++
C (Dorsal root)	**Pain, temperature**[Q], some mechano-reception, reflex responses	0.4-1.2[Q]	0.5-2[Q]	++++
C (Sympathetic)	Postganglionic sympathetic	0.3-1.3[Q]	0.7-2.3[Q]	++++

Differential Block
• **Differential block depends on concentration of local anesthetic.**   • A drug at **lower concentration** will produce **only sensory block** while at **higher concentration** can produce **motor block**.

Contd...
- **Nerve fiber type** also has a **significant effect on the action of LA**[Q].
- **Factors which determine the sensitivity of nerve fibres to LA** are fiber diameter & myelination, therefore **type B fibres (myelinated)** are more readily blocked than type C (non myelinated) in spite of being of thinner diameter than B[Q].

Sequence of Differential Block
• Sequence of block: Type B →type C → type A[Q]
• Sequence of block in functional terms: Autonomic (mediated by C & B fibers) → Sensory (mediated by C & Aδ fibers) → Motor[Q]
• Sequence of recovery: Motor → sensory → autonomic.
• Sequence of blockade among sensory fibres: Temperature (cold before hot) → pain → touch → deep pressure → proprioception[Q].

Intrinsic susceptibility of Nerve Fibers to Local Anesthetic Block
• **LAs** preferentially **block smaller diameter fibers first**[Q]
• **Myelinated nerves** tend to be **blocked before unmyelinated nerves** of the same diameter.
• **Blockade by LAs** is **more marked at higher frequencies of depolarization**.
• **Sensory (pain) fibers** have a **high firing rate** & relatively **long action potential duration**[Q].
• **Motor fibers fire at a slower rate** & have **shorter action potential duration**[Q].

188. **Ans. d. Face mask with a reservoir** *(Ref: Benumof and Hagberg's Airway Management By Carin A. Hagberg 3/e p304, 305, 307)*

Highest concentration of oxygen is delivered through face mask with a reservoir.

Oxygen Therapy Devices
• Oxygen therapy is aimed to increase the fraction of inspired oxygen concentration available to a patient.

Classification of Oxygen Therapy Devices	
Low Flow (Variable Performance)	**High Flow (Fixed Performance)**
• Low-flow systems **do not provide the patients entire ventilatory requirements** through the delivery devices[Q]. • Patients **rate & depth of breathing determines FiO_2 and not fixed**[Q]. • **Example:** • Nasal prongs or cannula • Simple face mask or Hudson mask • Non-rebreather face mask • Tracheostomy mask (without entrainment device)	• **Whole ventilatory requirement** of the patient **is provided** by the delivery devices[Q]. • **Deliver accurate oxygen concentration**[Q] • Performance is **not affected by changes in** patients **tidal volume & respiratory rate**[Q] • It works on **Venturi principle**[Q] (The pressure drop induced by the increase in velocity of a fluid passing through a narrow orifice can be used to entrain room air or a nebulizer solution in specific ratio). • **Example:** • Venturi mask, multivent mask, Aquapac • Tracheostomy mask & face mask used in with entrainment device • Ventilators • Continuous positive air pressure (CPAP)

Approximate FiO_2 Delivered by Nasal Cannula	
Flow Rate (L/min)	Approximate FiO_2
1	0.24
2	0.28
3	0.32
4	0.36
5	0.40
6	0.44

Approximate FiO_2 Delivered by Simple Face Mask	
Flow Rate (L/min)	Approximate FiO_2
5-6	0.4
6-7	0.5
7-8	0.6

Approximate FiO_2 Delivered by Mask with Reservoir Bag	
Flow Rate (L/min)	Approximate FiO_2
6	0.6
7	0.7
8	0.8
9	0.8+
10	0.8+

Facemask
• Facemask is **designed to fit the contour of face**
• Used to **ventilate patient without intubation**
• Consist of three part: Mount, body & edge
• **Transparent masks** are **better (Secretions** & **vomitus** are **easily detected & tackled)**
• **Facemask increases** the **dead space (Adult** sized face mask increases the dead space by **80-200 ml).**
• Anesthesia by using facemask is usually **associated with lower incidence of sore throat & respiratory infections.**

Complications of the Use of Facemask
• Contact Dermatitis
• Pressure to branches of trigeminal nerve & facial nerve
• Damage to eyes & face, conjunctival edema

• **Controlled ventilation with mask** leads to **significant air leak** into **esophagus & stomach,** increasing the risk of **vomiting & aspiration** especially in **hiatus hernia, pregnancy, full stomach & intestinal obstruction patients**[Q].
• **Bag & mask ventilation** is **contraindicated in congenital diaphragmatic hernia** & **trachea-esophageal fistula**[Q].

189. Ans. c. 3 minutes of deep breathing *(Ref: Miller 7/e p1577)*

The recommended duration of pre-oxygenation before intubation is 3 minutes of deep breathing.

"Hypoxemia can occur in the time between induction of anesthesia and attainment of airway security and is particularly likely if airway management proves difficult. It makes sense to maximize oxygen stores before induction to prolong the period before the onset of hypoxemia in the event of serious difficulty with airway management. The principal oxygen stores are in the lungs. These stores can be increased by using a maneuver called "preoxygenation" (also know as denitrogenation), which is achieved by having the patient breath 100% oxygen from a close-fitting facemask before induction of anesthesia. Several techniques of preoxygenation have been described, and the most effective technique should be used. Deep breathing with a high fresh gas flow for 1.5 minutes and tidal breathing for 3 minutes are equally effective." -Miller 7/e p1577

Oxygenation and Preoxygenation
• Hypoxemia can occur between induction of anesthesia & attainment of airway security.
• **Maximize oxygen stores before induction** to prolong the period before the onset of hypoxemia in the event of serious difficulty with airway management.
• **Oxygen stores in lungs** can be **increased by "preoxygenation",** achieved by having the **patient breath 100% oxygen from a close-fitting facemask before induction of anesthesia.**
• **Deep breathing** with a **high fresh gas flow for 1.5 minutes & tidal breathing for 3 minutes** are equally effective.
• **End-tidal oxygen concentration** should be used as a guide to the adequacy of preoxygenation, with a value of **90%** being well accepted.
• **Preoxygenation in semi-sitting position prolongs the time to development of hypoxemia** by increasing functional residual capacity in relation to supine position, particularly in an **obese patient**.
• Use of **positive end-expiratory pressure** (PEEP) **during induction** may further **improve oxygenation.**

190. Ans. a. 10–15 seconds *(Ref: Current Diagnosis and Treatment Critical Care 3/e p255)*

Tracheal secretions should be suctioned limiting the time to less than 10-15 seconds. The patient should be preoxygenated with 100% oxygen for at least a minute, and the total suction time should be limited to no more than 10–15 seconds on each attempt.

"Minimal negative pressure should be used, and the suction catheter should be introduced gently. During suctioning, PaO2 may fall rapidly, particularly if the patient is receiving high concentrations of inspired O2 and suctioning is performed for more than 10–15 seconds." -Current Diagnosis and Treatment Critical Care 3/e p255

Tracheostomy Suctioning Procedure
• Wash hands, put on an apron & gloves protective eyewear is also advisable.
• Explain the procedure to patient & position the patient upright.
• Ensure a non-fenestrated inner cannula is in place if the patient has a double cannula tube.
• Turn on suction–use minimum pressure required to clear secretions to reduce risk of mucosal damage: • **Adults**: 13.5–20 kPa [**100-150** mm Hg] • **Adolescents**: 10–16 kPa [**80-120** mm Hg] • **Children**: 10–13 kPa [**80-100** mm Hg] • **Neonates**: 8–10 kPa [**60-80** mm Hg]

Contd...

AIIMS November 2017

Contd...

Tracheostomy Suctioning Procedure
• Select a **suction catheter** for **no more than half the diameter of the tracheostomy tube**
• Consider preoxygenating the patient prior to suctioning if the patient is critically unwell with high oxygen requirements or the suction procedure has caused them respiratory compromise previously.
• Using an intertie technique, introduce the catheter into the tracheostomy. **In adults** it is recommended that the **catheter is inserted to the level of carina** and then **withdrawn 1–2 cm before suction is applied**. There is little evidence for the benefits and risks of deep versus shallow suctioning in neonates & young infants. Measuring the tube & **only introducing the catheter 1.5 cm or less beyond the top of tube may minimize trauma to carina.**
• Slowly & smoothly withdraw the catheter
• Dispose of the catheter safely and replace the patient's oxygen or HME.
• **Steps 7 & 8 should take no longer than 10–15 seconds in total**, and **suctions should ideally be performed no more than 3 litres during any 1 episode.** Allow the patient sufficient time to recover between suctioning.

191. Ans. b. Lorazepam   *(Ref: Miller 8/e p841; Katzung 12/e p443; Clinical Anesthesia by Paul G. Barash 6/e p457)*

Lorazepam can be used as intravenous induction agent.

"The slow onset and prolonged duration of action of lorazepam limit its usefulness for preoperative medication or induction of anesthesia, especially when rapid and sustained awakening at the end of surgery is desirable."-Katzung 12/e p443

Induction Characteristics & Dosage Requirements for Currently Available Sedative & Hypnotic Drugs			
Drug Name	**Induction Dose (mg/kg)**	**Onset (sec)**	**Duration (min)**
Thiopental	3-6	<30	5-10
Methohexital	1-3	<30	5-10
Propofol	1.5-2.5	15-45	5-10
Midazolam	0.2-0.4	30-90	10-30
Diazepam	0.3-0.6	45-90	15-30
Lorazepam	0.03-0.06	60-120	60-120
Etomidate	0.2-0.3	3-12	3-12
Ketamine	1-2	10-20	10-20

Benzodiazepines
• Benzodiazepines commonly used in the perioperative period include **midazolam, lorazepam & diazepam**.
• **Action** can **readily be terminated by** administration of their **selective antagonist, flumazenil[Q]**.
• **Most desired effects** are **anxiolysis & anterograde amnesia[Q]**

Pharmacokinetics:
- **Highly lipid-soluble benzodiazepines rapidly enter the CNS**, which accounts for **rapid onset of action, followed by redistribution to inactive tissue sites** & subsequent **termination of drug effect[Q]**.
- Despite its prompt passage into the brain, **midazolam** is considered to have a **slower effect-site equilibration time than propofol & thiopental**. In this regard, **IV doses of midazolam should be sufficiently spaced to permit the peak clinical effect** to be recognized before a repeat dose is considered.
- **Midazolam** has the **shortest context-sensitive half-time**, which makes it the **only one of the three benzodiazepine drugs suitable for continuous infusion[Q]**.

Organ System Effects of Benzodiazepines	
CNS Effects	• **Decrease CMRO$_2$ & cerebral blood flow[Q]** • **Potent anticonvulsants**, used in **status epilepticus, alcohol withdrawal & local anesthetic-induced seizures[Q]**. • **CNS effects** can be **promptly terminated by flumazenil[Q]**
Cardiovascular Effects	• Midazolam decreases systemic BP than comparable doses of diazepam, most likely **due to peripheral vasodilation** inasmuch as **cardiac output is not changed[Q]**.
Respiratory Effects	• **Produce minimal depression of ventilation**, although **transient apnea may follow rapid IV administration of midazolam** for induction of anesthesia, especially in the presence of opioid premedication. • **Decrease ventilatory response to CO$_2$** • **Airway obstruction** can **induced by hypnotic effects**
Other Effects	• **Pain during IV & IM injection** and **subsequent thrombophlebitis** are **most pronounced with diazepam[Q]**

Contd...

Contd...

Benzodiazepines

Clinical Uses & Dosage:
• **Benzodiazepines** are **most commonly used for preoperative medication, IV sedation & suppression of seizure activity**[Q].
• **Slow onset & prolonged duration of action** of **lorazepam** limit its usefulness for **preoperative medication** or **induction of anesthesia**, especially when rapid and sustained awakening at the end of surgery is desirable.
• **Amnestic, anxiolytic & sedative effects of benzodiazepines** make this class of drugs the **most popular choice for preoperative medication**[Q].
    • **Midazolam** (1–2 mg IV) is **effective for premedication, sedation** during regional anesthesia & **brief therapeutic procedures**[Q].
    • **Midazolam** has a **more rapid onset, with greater amnesia & less postoperative sedation, than diazepam**[Q].
    • **Midazolam** is **MC used oral premedication for children**; 0.5 mg/kg **administered orally 30 minutes before induction** of anesthesia **provides reliable sedation & anxiolysis in children** without producing delayed awakening[Q].
• **Synergistic effects** between **benzodiazepines, opioids & propofol**, can be **used to achieve better sedation & analgesia** but **enhance** their **combined respiratory depression** & may lead to **airway obstruction or apnea**[Q].
• Benzodiazepine effects are **more pronounced with increasing age, dose reduction & careful titration** may be necessary **in elderly patients**[Q].

Dexmedetomidine
• **Dexmedetomidine** is a **centrally active selective alpha-2 agonist** with **strong sedative properties**[Q] • **Introduced for sedating critically ill/ventilated patients in intensive care units. It is also being used as an adjunct to anaesthesia**[Q]. • **Analgesia & sedation** are produced with **little respiratory depression**[Q]. • Sympathetic response to stress and noxious stimulus is blunted.
Pharmacokinetics: • Administered by **IV infusion**; **Half-life: 2–3 hours**[Q] • Dexmedetomidine undergoes **rapid hepatic metabolism** involving **conjugation, N-methylation & hydroxylation, followed by conjugation**[Q]. • **Metabolized in the liver & excreted,** mainly as metabolites, **in the urine.**
Anesthetic Properties: • **Sedation, hypnosis;** at high doses **anxiolysis, sympatholysis & analgesia**[Q]

Dexmedetomidine: Organ System Effects	
CNS Effects	• **Hypnosis, analgesia, sedation & decrease in cerebral blood flow** • Potential to lead to the development of **tolerance & dependence**[Q].
CVS Effects	• **Decreases HR, systemic vascular resistance & hypotension**[Q]

Side-effects: • **Side effects** are similar to those with **clonidine** (**hypotension, bradycardia & dry mouth**[Q]).
Uses: • As premedication (**anxiolysis**[Q]) • Adjuvant to reduce the dose of analgesics (**Analgesic property**[Q]) • Adjuvant to reduce the dose of IV & inhalational anesthetics (**Sedative property**[Q]) • **To attenuate cardiovascular response to intubation** (it causes **hypotension & bradycardia**[Q])
Contraindications: • **Hypovolemia**[Q], hypotension, heart block & congestive heart failure[Q] (it causes **hypotension & bradycardia**[Q])

192. **Ans. a. Assess the patient, give bag and mask ventilation and look for spontaneous breathing** *(Ref: Benumof and Hagberg's Airway Management By Carin A. Hagberg 3/e p1068)*

In self-extubation, assess the patient, give bag and mask ventilation and look for spontaneous breathing.

Unplanned Extubation
• Unplanned extubation of mechanically ventilated patients is relatively common • **Self-extubation** refers to the patient's action, who **deliberately removes the endotracheal tube** (**MC type of unplanned extubation, typically occur at night**) • **Accidental extubation** is attributed either to **personnel's inappropriate manipulation** of the tube during patient care or to a **non-purposeful patient's action**, e.g. **coughing (mostly occur in the morning)**

Contd...

Contd...

Risk Factors for Unplanned Extubation	
Patient factors	**Staff factors**
• **Male** • **Delirium** • **Light sedation** • **Difficulty in securing tube** (e.g. facial swelling, facial burns) • **Previous unplanned extubation**	• Junior staff • Nurse-to-patient ratio • Inadequately secured endotracheal tube and/or checks

Management:
- Attend to potential life-threats using an ABC approach
- **Many patients (>50%) do not require reintubation if oxygenation & ventilation remains adequate (consider oxygen via NP or mask, high flow nasal prongs or NIV)**
- Check previous airway grade, obtain difficult airway trolley & call for assistance if likely difficult grade of intubation
- **If stridor present, may need a smaller ETT than previously used due to laryngeal trauma/ oedema**
- Ensure the incident is documented & entered into a risk monitoring system; need to address cause of self-extubation

Complications of Unplanned Extubation	
• Effects of extubation with ETT cuff up • Hemodynamic effects: **hypotension, arrhythmias** • **Laryngeal injury, bleeding or edema** • **Airway obstruction** • **Acute pulmonary oedema** due to loss of CPAP/PEEP in a patient with left ventricular failure	• **Respiratory failure** • **Aspiration** • Reintubation & associated sequelae (e.g. prolonged stay, complications of mechanical ventilation, etc)

RADIOLOGY

193. Ans. a. Pneumothorax *(Ref: The Chest X-Ray By Gerald de Lacey (2012)/e p101)*

The given chest X-ray shows increased lucency on the right side with absent vascular markings, collapse of the right lung and mediastinal shift to the left suggestive of right sided pneumothorax.

Condition	Chest X-ray	Findings
Pneumothorax		• **Visible visceral pleural edge** is seen as a **very thin, sharp white line** • **No lung markings** are **seen peripheral to this line** • **Peripheral space** is **radiolucent compared to adjacent lung** • Lung may completely collapse • Mediastinum should not shift away from the pneumothorax unless a <u>tension pneumothorax</u> is present
Hydropneumothorax		• An **upright chest X-ray** will show **air fluid levels**. • **Horizontal fluid level** is usually **well-defined & extends across the whole length of hemithorax**. • **Supine radiograph: Sharp pleural line** is bordered by **increased opacity lateral to it within the pleural space**
Pleural effusion		• **Blunting of costophrenic angle & cardiophrenic angle** • Fluid within horizontal or oblique fissures • A **meniscus** will be seen, on frontal films **seen laterally & gently sloping medially** • With **large volume effusions, mediastinal shift** occurs away from the effusion may occur towards the effusion) • **Lateral films** are able to **identify a smaller amount of fluid, as the costophrenic angles are deepest posteriorly.**

Contd...

Contd...

Condition	Chest X-ray	Findings
Consolidation		• Right middle lobe consolidation (RML): • Opacification of RML abutting the horizontal fissure • Indistinct right heart border • Loss of medial aspect of right hemidiaphragm • Air bronchograms • When the **fissures are outwardly convex**, the appearance is referred to as the **bulging fissure sign**.

194. Ans. b. Typical carcinoid *(Ref: Clinical Radiation Oncology By Leonard L. Gunderson (2015)/p880)*

Positron emission tomography with 2-deoxy-2[fluorine-18] fluoro-D-glucose integrated with computed tomography (18F-FDG PET/CT) has emerged as a powerful imaging tool for the detection of various cancers and is based on the increased glucose uptake and glycolysis of cancer cells. The tumor 18F-FDG uptake is analyzed in terms of Standardized Uptake Value (SUV). Typical carcinoids and bronchoalveolar carcinoma are less FDG avid compared to other malignant tumors in lung. The mean SUV of typical carcinoid in many studies is between 2 to 4. Means SUV of large cell neuroendocrine tumor is 12, small cell cancer is 11.6 and atypical carcinoid is 8.1.

Tumor	Mean SUV
Typical carcinoid	2 to 4
Atypical carcinoid	8.1
Small cell cancer	11.6
Neuroendocrine tumor	12

"Patients with suspected lung mass require a thorough history and physical examination. Routine blood tests and chemistry tests may give clues to the presence of associated syndromes. The differential diagnosis, in addition to bronchopulmonary carcinoid, includes lung carcinoma and metastasis from an extra-pulmonary primary tumor. CT and bronchoscopy are two of the most valuable diagnostic procedures. Upto 80% of carcinoids manifest with type 2 somatostatin receptors, and the receptors can be targeted by radioactive octreotide or pentetreotide. Somatostatin receptor scintigraphy with indium-111-radiolabeled octreotide has demonstrated reliable uptake in primary tumors and been used to detect early recurrences. FDG-PET scans are often normal." - Clinical Radiation Oncology By Leonard L. Gunderson (2015)/p880

195. Ans. a. Aneurysm *(Ref: Schwartz 10/e p1730)*

The image shown is digital subtraction angiography of right internal carotid artery showing balloon-like outpouching suggestive of aneurysm.

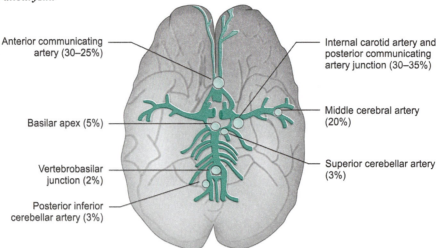

Cerebral Aneurysm
• An **aneurysm** is a **focal dilatation of vessel wall** and is **most often a balloon-like outpouching**, but may also be fusiform. • Aneurysms **usually occur at branch points of major vessels** (e.g., **internal carotid artery bifurcation**), or **at the origin of smaller vessels** (e.g., **posterior communicating artery or ophthalmic artery**).

Contd...

Contd...

- Approximately **85% of aneurysms** arise from **anterior circulation (carotid)** & **15% from posterior circulation (vertebrobasilar)**[Q].

Prevalence of Cerebral Aneurysm by Location	
Prevalence	**Aneurysm Location**
Anterior circulation 85%	• **30% Anterior communicating artery (MC)**[Q] • **25% Posterior communicating artery**[Q] • **20% Middle cerebral artery bifurcation**[Q] • 10% Other
Posterior circulation 15%	• **10% Basilar artery**, **most frequently** at the **basilar tip**[Q] • 5% Vertebral artery, usually at posterior inferior cerebellar artery

- **Aneurysms** are **thin walled** & **at risk for rupture**[Q].
- **Major cerebral vessels & aneurysms, lie in the subarachnoid space. Rupture results in SAH**[Q].
- Aneurysmal tear may be small & seal quickly, or it may not.
  - **SAH** may consist of a **thin layer of blood in CSF spaces**, or **thick layers of blood around the brain & extending into brain parenchyma**, resulting in a **clot with mass effect**[Q].
  - Because the **meningeal linings of brain are sensitive**, SAH usually results in a **sudden, severe "thunderclap" headache**[Q].
  - A patient will classically describe **"the worst headache of my life"**[Q]
- Presenting neurologic symptoms may range from **mild headache to coma to sudden death**.

PSYCHIATRY

196. Ans. a. Akathisia   *(Ref: Kaplan 11/e p862; Harrison 19/e p2624; Goodman Gilman 12/e p438)*

Inner restlessness and urge to move after intake of antipsychotics like haloperidol is highly suggestive of akathisia.

"Akathisia is subjective feelings of restlessness, objective signs of restlessness, or both. Examples include a sense of anxiety, inability to relax, jitteriness, pacing, rocking motions while sitting, and rapid alternation of sitting and standing. Akathisia has been associated with the use of a wide range of psychiatric drugs, including antipsychotics (Haloperidol), antidepressants, and sympathomimetics." -Kaplan 11/e p862

Extrapyramidal Disturbances of Anti-Psychotic drugs
• These are the **major dose limiting side effects**[Q] • **More prominent with high potency drugs like fluphenazine, haloperidol, pimozide etc**[Q]. • **Least with thioridazine, clozapine, olanzapine**, and **low doses of resperidone**[Q].

Types of Extrapyramidal Disturbances caused by Anti-Psychotic drugs	
Parkinsonism	• With typical manifestations-**rigidity, tremor, hypokinesia, mask like facies, shuffling gait**[Q] • Appears **between 1-4 weeks of therapy**[Q] • Treatment: Central anticholinergic drugs[Q]
	Rabbit syndrome • A rare form of extrapyramidal side effect is **perioral tremors "rabbit syndrome"** • Occurs years after of therapy • **Treatment: Central anticholinergic drugs**[Q]
Acute muscular dystonia	• **Bizarre muscle spasms, mostly involving linguo-facial muscles-grimacing, torticollis, locked jaw**[Q] • Occurs **within few hours of single dose** or at the **most in the first week of therapy**[Q] • **More common in children below 10 years and in girls, particularly after parenteral administration**[Q] • **Treatment: Central anticholinergic**[Q], **promethazine**[Q] or hydroxyzine
Akathisia	• Restlessness, feeling of discomfort, apparent agitation manifested as **compelling desire to move about but without anxiety**[Q] • **Between 1-8 weeks of therapy**[Q] • No specific antidote is available • **Treatment: First line drug is Propranolol**[Q]

Contd...

AIIMS ESSENCE

Contd...

Extrapyramidal Disturbances of Anti-Psychotic drugs	
Malignant neuroleptic syndrome	• **Occurs rarely with high doses of potent agents**[Q] • Marked rigidity, immobility, tremor, fever, semi-consciousness, fluctuating BP and heart rate, myoglobin may be present in blood-lasts 5-10 days after drug withdrawal and may be fatal[Q]. • **Treatment: Stop neuroleptic, Bromocriptine**[Q]
Tardive dyskinesia	• **Occurs late in therapy (Chronic therapy), sometimes even after withdrawal of neuroleptic**[Q] • Manifests as purposeless involuntary facial and limb movements like constant chewing, pouting, puffing of cheeks, lip licking, choreoathetoid movements[Q] • **More common in elderly women**[Q] • Probably a manifestation of progressive neuronal degeneration along with supersensitivity to DA • **Accentuated by anticholinergics & temporarily suppressed by high doses of neuroleptics**[Q]

197. Ans. d. Delusion of grandiosity, persecution and reference *(Ref: Kaplan 11/e p1268)*

The given description suggests that the patient is having delusion of grandiosity, persecution and reference.

Delusion of grandeur	• Exaggerated conception of one's importance, power, or identity.
Delusion of persecution	• **False belief of being harassed or persecuted**; often found in litigious patients who have a pathological tendency to take legal action because of imagined mistreatment. • **MC delusion.**
Delusion of reference	• **False belief** that **behavior of others refers to oneself or that events, objects, or other people** have a **particular & unusual significance,** usually of a **negative nature** • **Derived from idea of reference,** in which **persons falsely feel that others are talking about them** (e.g., belief that people on television or radio are talking to or about the person).

Delusion
• **False belief, based on incorrect inference about external reality,** that is **firmly held despite objective & obvious contradictory proof or evidence** & despite the fact that other members of culture do not share the belief.

Risk factors associated with Delusion	
• Advanced age • Sensory impairment or isolation • Family history • Social isolation	• Personality features (unusual interpersonal sensitivity) • **Recent immigration**

Types of Delusion	
Delusion of control	• False belief that a **person's will, thoughts, or feelings** are being **controlled by external forces**[Q]
Delusion of grandeur	• **Exaggerated conception of one's importance, power, or identity**[Q].
Delusion of infidelity	• False belief that **one's lover is unfaithful.** Sometimes called **pathological jealousy**[Q].
Delusion of persecution	• False belief of **being harassed or persecuted**; often found in litigious patients who have a pathological tendency to take legal action because of imagined mistreatment. • **MC delusion**[Q]
Delusion of poverty	• False belief that one is **bereft** or will be **deprived of all material possessions**[Q].
Delusion of reference	• **False belief that behavior of others refers to oneself or that events, objects, or other people** have a **particular & unusual significance,** usually of a **negative nature**[Q] • **Derived from idea of reference,** in which **persons falsely feel that others are talking about them**[Q] (e.g., belief that people on television or radio are talking to or about the person).

Contd...

Contd...

Delusion of self-accusation	• False feeling of **remorse & guilt**; Seen in **depression with psychotic features**[Q].
Erotic delusion	• Also known as **erotomania, de Clérambault syndrome** or **psychose passionelle**
	• **Delusional conviction** that **another person, usually of higher status, is in love with him or her**[Q].
	• Such patients also tend to be **solitary, withdrawn, dependent, and sexually inhibited** as well as to have **poor levels of social or occupational functioning**[Q].
	• Generally **unattractive women in low-level jobs** who **lead withdrawn, lonely lives**; they are **single & have few sexual contacts**[Q].
Somatic (Hypochondrial) delusion	• Delusions involving bodily functions/and or sensations
	• **False belief of carrying severe disease or other malfunctions**[Q]

DSM-5 Diagnostic Criteria for Delusional Disorder
• The individual has **one or more delusions** that **persist for at least a month or more**.
• Criterion A for schizophrenia is not and never has been met.
• **Aside from the delusion(s) direct effects, functioning is not obviously impaired & behavior is not noticeably strange.**
• Any manic or major depressive episodes have been brief, compared to the length of the delusional period.
• The disturbance cannot be attributed to the physiological effects of a substance, another medical condition, or another mental disorder.
• The severity of the delusions should be noted and it should also be specified if delusions involve bizarre content, or are clearly implausible. Additionally, there are a few subtypes with specific delusional themes that should be specified:
• **Erotomanic type:** This involves delusions about **another person being in love with the affected individual.**
• **Grandiose type:** Individuals with the grandiose type of delusional disorder believe they have a **great talent (which is unrecognized) or made a great, important discovery.**
• **Jealous type:** This involves delusions about **his or her lover being unfaithful**.
• **Persecutory type:** This subtype pertains to individuals with delusions involving their beliefs that they are **being conspired against, spied or cheated on, poisoned or drugged, harassed or followed, or generally obstructed in the pursuit of long-term goals.**
• **Somatic type:** Individuals with the somatic type of delusional disorder have **delusions involving bodily functions/ and or sensations.**
• **Mixed type:** There is not one delusional theme that persists over others.
• **Unspecified type:** The dominant delusional belief cannot be clearly determined or does not fall into the descriptions of the specific types.

198. **Ans. a. Capgras syndrome**   *(Ref: Kaplan 11/e p321, 319)*

As per the given description (wife is replaced by the nurse), patient is suffering from Capgras syndrome. The delusion in Capgras syndrome is the belief that a familiar person has been replaced by an impostor.

*"The category unspecified type is reserved for cases in which the predominant delusion cannot be subtyped within the previous categories. A possible example is certain delusions of misidentification, for example, **Capgras syndrome,** named for the French psychiatrist who described **the illusion des sosies, or the illusion of doubles**. The delusion in Capgras syndrome is the belief that a familiar person has been replaced by an impostor. Others have described variants of the Capgras syndrome, namely, the delusion that persecutors or familiar persons can assume the guise of strangers (Frégoli's phenomenon) and the very rare delusion that familiar persons can change themselves into other persons at will (intermetamorphosis). Each disorder is not only rare but may also be associated with schizophrenia, dementia, epilepsy, and other organic disorders. Reported cases have been predominantly in women, have had associated paranoid features, and have included feelings of depersonalization or derealization. The delusion may be short lived, recurrent, or persistent."-Kaplan 11/e p321*

*"**Delusional disorder with delusions of infidelity has been called conjugal paranoia when it is limited to the delusion that a spouse has been unfaithful. The eponym Othello syndrome has been used to describe morbid jealousy that can arise from multiple concerns. The delusion usually affects men, often those with no prior psychiatric illness. It may appear suddenly and serve to explain a host of present and past events involving the spouse's behavior. The condition is difficult to treat and may diminish only on separation, divorce, or death of the spouse."- Kaplan 11/e p319*

199. Ans. b. Digit span forward up to 7 digits with 2 skips allowed *(Ref: Kaplan 11/e p1213; DeJong's The Neurologic Examination 7/e p78)*

Test for immediate memory is digit span forward up to 7 digits with 2 skips allowed.

> *"Memory: Memory usually is evaluated in terms of immediate, recent, and remote memory. Immediate retention and recall are tested by giving the patient six digits to repeat forward and backward. The examiner should record the result of the patient's capacity to remember. Persons with unimpaired memory usually can recall six digits forward and five or six digits backward. The clinician should be aware that the ability to do well on digit-span tests is impaired in extremely anxious patients. Remote memory can be tested by asking for the patient's place and date of birth, the patient's mother's name before she was married, and names and birthdays of the patient's children."-Kaplan 11/e p1213*

> *"Digit span forward is a good test of attention, concentration, and immediate memory. The examiner gives the patient a series of numbers of increasing length, beginning with 3 or 4, at a rate of about one per second; the patient is asked to repeat them. The numbers should be random, nor following any identifiable pattern, for example, a phone number. Backward digit span, having the patient repeat a series of numbers in reverse order, is a more complex mental process that involves working memory; it requires the ability to retain and manipulate the string of numbers. Expected performance is 7 ± 2 forward and 5 ± 1 backward. Reverse digit span should not be more than two digits less than the forward span. Forward digit span is also a test of repetition and may be impaired in aphasic patients. Another test of attention and concentration is a three-step task. For instance, tear a piece of paper in half, then tear half of it in half, then tear one half in half again, so that there are three different sizes. Give the patient an instruction such as, "Give the large piece of paper to me, put the small piece on the bed, and keep the other piece." Another multistep task might be, "Stand up, face the door, and hold out your arms."-DeJong's The Neurologic Examination 7/e p78*

200. Ans. b. Dysthymia *(Ref: Kaplan 11/e p363)*

Presence of a depressed mood that lasts most of the day and is present almost continuously with associated feelings of inadequacy, guilt, irritability, and anger; withdrawal from society; loss of interest; and inactivity and lack of productivity is highly suggestive of dysthymia.

> *"The most typical features of dysthymia, also known as persistent depressive disorder, is the presence of a depressed mood that lasts most of the day and is present almost continuously. There are associated feelings of inadequacy, guilt, irritability, and anger; withdrawal from society; loss of interest; and inactivity and lack of productivity."-Kaplan 11/e p363*

> *"Cyclothymic disorder is symptomatically a mild form of bipolar II disorder, characterized by episodes of hypomania and mild depression. In DSM-5, cyclothymic disorder is defined as a "chronic, fluctuating mood disturbance" with many periods of hypomania and of depression. The disorder is differentiated from bipolar II disorder, which is characterized by the presence of major (not minor) depressive and hypomanic episodes."-Kaplan 11/e p365*

Dysthymia
• Also known as **persistent depressive disorder**[Q]
• **Most typical features**: **Presence of a depressed mood** that lasts most of the day & present almost continuously; **Feelings of inadequacy, guilt, irritability, and anger; withdrawal from society; loss of interest; inactivity & lack of productivity**[Q].
• **Early onset**, beginning in **childhood or adolescence** & in most cases by the **age of 20 years**[Q].
• More common among **unmarried & young persons with low incomes**[Q].

DSM-5 Diagnostic Criteria for Dysthymia
• **Depressed mood for most of the day**, for more days than not, as indicated by either subjective account or observation by others, **for at least 2 years** (In **children & adolescents**, mood can be irritable & duration must be **at least 1 year**)
• Presence, while depressed, of ≥2 of the following:
• Poor appetite or overeating; Insomnia or hypersomnia; Low energy or fatigue; Low self-esteem; Poor concentration or difficulty making decisions; Feelings of hopelessness.
• During the 2-year period (1 year for children or adolescents) of the disturbance, individual has never been without symptoms in Criteria A & B for >2 months at a time.
• **Criteria for a major depressive disorder** may be **continuously present for 2 years.**

Contd...

AIIMS November 2017

Contd...

Dysthymia
• There has **never been a manic episode or a hypomanic episode** & criteria have never been met for cyclothymic disorder. • Disturbance is **not better explained by a persistent schizoaffective disorder**, **schizophrenia, delusional disorder**, or other specified or unspecified schizophrenia spectrum and other psychotic disorder. • Symptoms are **not attributable to the physiological effects of a substance** (e.g., a drug of abuse, a medication) or **another medical condition** (e.g., hypothyroidism). • **Symptoms cause clinically significant distress or impairment in social, occupational, or other important areas of functioning.**
Treatment: • Options: **Cognitive therapy, behavior therapy & pharmacotherapy** (SSRIs, venlafaxine & bupropion). • **Combination of pharmacotherapy** & some form of **psychotherapy** may be the **most effective treatment**.   • **Individual insight-oriented psychotherapy** is **MC treatment method used for dysthymia**, considered as the **treatment of choice**.

201. Ans. a. Biological relationship *(Ref: The First Interview by James Morison 3/e p181: Kaplan 11/e p210-211)*

Biological relationship needs not be essential for good history, e.g., Informant of a patient who is staying in a rehabilitation home for long can be given by the caretaker rather than by a biological relation.

Reliability of Information
• Reliability of information includes: • **Corroborative:** Information **corroborative with findings of the clinician** • **Consistency: Repeatability of the information** by the informant • **Continuity:** Ability to convey the **gradual evolution of symptoms** of the patient over the years. • **Informants who are educated** will have **high health seeking behaviour & observational skills** and will be **able to verbalize the symptoms.** • **Duration of stay with patient** is an important aspect **in identifying the symptoms** and it is independent of the biological relationship

Note

Note

Note

AIIMS MAY 2017

Multiple Choice Questions

ANATOMY

1. The following coronal section of the abdomen is showing the relations of epiploic foramen. Which of the following structure forms its superior boundary as indicated in the figure below?

   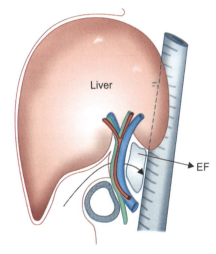

   a. Lesser omentum
   b. Duodenum
   c. Inferior vena cava
   d. Caudate lobe of liver

2. The following is the representation of a cervical vertebra. Which part lies in relation with the third part of vertebral artery?

   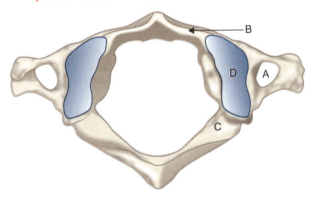

   a. A
   b. B
   c. C
   d. D

3. Nucleus pulposus of intervertebral disc is a derivative of which of the following germ layers?

   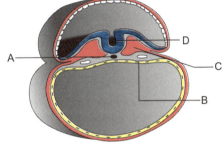

   a. A
   b. B
   c. C
   d. D

4. Which of the following part of scapula can be palpated in the infraclavicular fossa?

   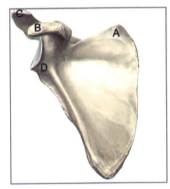

   a. A
   b. B
   c. C
   d. D

5. The following picture shows various foramina at the skull base. Mandibular nerve passes through which of the following foramen?

   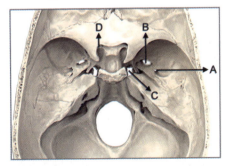

   a. A
   b. B
   c. C
   d. D

6. A patient came with inability to move his 4th and 5th digit, cannot hold a pen and he was not able to hold a piece of paper between his fingers. Which of the following site given below is the probable cause of injury to the nerve in the question?

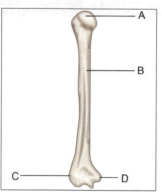

a. A　　　　　　　　b. B
c. C　　　　　　　　d. D

7. A 5 years old child presented with absence of thymus, hypoparathyroidism and tetany. Which of the following marked area is defective in this case?

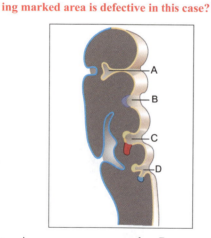

a. A　　　　　　　　b. B
c. C　　　　　　　　d. D

8. An area has been marked in the coronal section of the brain below. Defect in this area will lead to what pathology?

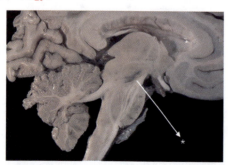

a. Alzheimer's disease　　b. Huntington's chorea
c. Paralysis agitans　　　d. Dementia

9. The muscle labeled in the following cross section is responsible for which movement of the jaw?

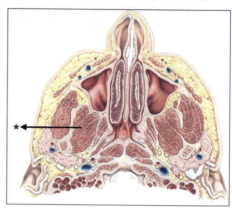

a. Protraction　　　　b. Elevation
c. Retraction　　　　 d. Depression

10. The arrow marked structure in the given picture connects, which of the following structure?

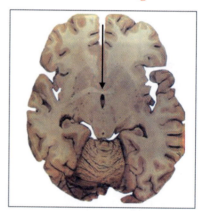

a. Hippocampus　　　b. Amygdala
c. Mammillary bodies　d. Insular cortex

11. The muscle marked in diagram is supplied by the nerve, whose nucleus is situated at the level of:

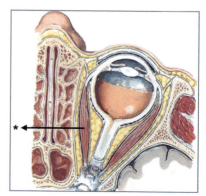

a. Superior colliculus
b. Facial colliculus
c. Inferior colliculus
d. Superior olivary nucleus

12. In this cut section through the ischioanal fossa, correctly identify the pelvic diaphragm:

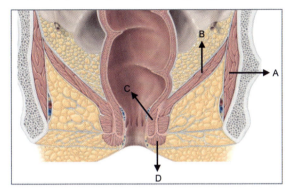

a. A
b. B
c. C
d. D

13. In this cross-sectional image, the axon of the neuron pointed with an arrow is inhibitory to which of the following?

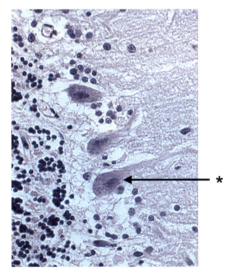

a. Vestibular nuclei
b. Cerebellar nuclei
c. Red nucleus
d. Basal ganglia

14. Direct hernia arises from the Hesselbach triangle, boundary of which is formed by the conjoint tendon. The following diagram shows attachments of transversus abdominis muscle. Identify the correct label showing the conjoint tendon:

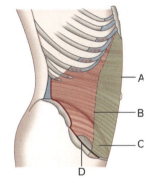

a. A
b. B
c. C
d. D

PHYSIOLOGY

15. A spirometry curve of a patient has been provided below. Calculate the FEV_1/FVC ratio from the curve:

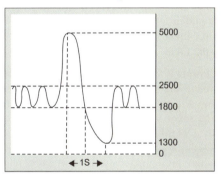

a. 60–69%
b. 70–79%
c. 80–89%
d. 90–99%

16. Bezold-Jarisch reflex is mediated by:
a. Serotonin
b. Angiotensin
c. Prostaglandin
d. Histamine

17. Two vessels are compared as shown below. Assuming constant pressure along both the vessels and linear flow pattern, what will be the flow across the vessel 1 compared to vessel 2?

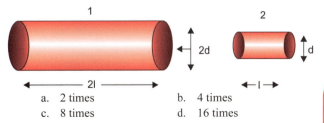

a. 2 times
b. 4 times
c. 8 times
d. 16 times

18. Identify the accessory protein marked in the diagram below:

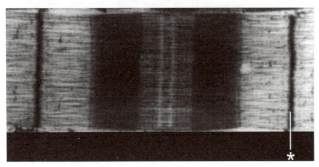

   a. Nebulin
   b. Alpha actinin
   c. Titin
   d. Tropomyosin

19. A patient inhales a tidal volume of 500 mL. The intrapleural pressure was measured as – 4 cm of water before inspiration and – 9 cm of water after inspiration. Calculate the pulmonary compliance in this patient:
   a. 0.1 L/cm   b. 0.3 L/cm
   c. 0.2 L/cm   d. 0.4 L cm

20. Following is the graph showing renal tubular transport maxima for glucose excretion in a diabetic patient. What will be the urinary glucose in a patient with a blood sugar of 200 mg/dL and a glomerular filtration rate of 90 mL/min?

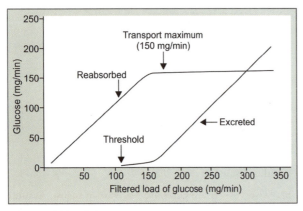

   a. 20 mg/min
   b. 30 mg/min
   c. 60 mg/min
   d. 100 mg/min

21. What will be the oxygen carrying capacity of an 18-year-old patient with a hemoglobin of 14 g/dL?
   a. 7
   b. 14
   c. 18
   d. 28

22. Calculate the tetanizing frequency of the frog's gastrocnemius muscle from the graph shown below:

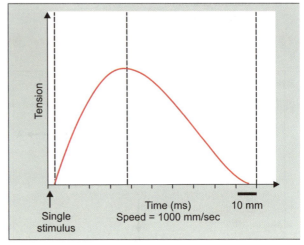

   a. 25–30 Hz
   b. 30–35 Hz
   c. 35–40 Hz
   d. 40–50 Hz

23. The 'a' wave in jugular venous pulse represents:
   a. Passive atrial filling
   b. Ventricular filling
   c. Right atrial contraction
   d. Ventricular relaxation

BIOCHEMISTRY

24. A lady presented with fatigue and tingling sensation in both hands and legs. On examination, she is found to have a fissured red tongue, lesions at angle of mouth and peripheral neuropathy with a decreased RBC glutathione reductase activity. What is the likely deficient vitamin?
   a. Riboflavin
   b. Vitamin B12
   c. Thiamine
   d. Vitamin B6

25. Maximum thermic effect of food is seen with:
   a. Carbohydrates   b. Protein
   c. Fat
   d. Not dependent on macronutrients

26. Thiamine deficiency results in decreased energy production because TPP interferes with:
   (AIIMS May 2017, All India 2010)
   a. Its coenzyme for pyruvate and alpha ketoglutarate dehydrogenase
   b. Transketolase activity
   c. Energy production from amino acid
   d. Alcohol metabolism

27. Which of these is an example of anaplerotic reaction?
    a. Pyruvate to oxaloacetate
    b. Pyruvate to Acetyl CoA
    c. Pyruvate to lactic acid
    d. Pyruvate to acetaldehyde

28. A girl complaints of acute abdominal pain on and off with tingling sensation of limbs. She had a history of eating paint from the wall of newly built house. Which of the following enzyme deficiency will be the cause of her condition?
    a. ALA dehydratase
    b. ALA synthase
    c. Coproporphyrinogen synthase
    d. Heme synthase

29. In uncontrolled diabetes mellitus, elevated triglyceride and VLDL levels are seen due to:
    a. Increased activity of lipoprotein lipase and decreased activity of hormone sensitive lipase
    b. Increased activity of hormone sensitive lipase and decreased activity of lipoprotein lipase
    c. Increase in peripheral LDL receptors
    d. Increased activity of hepatic lipase

30. Which of the following is true about mitochondrial DNA?
    a. It codes for more than 20% of respiratory chain enzymes are coded
    b. It has 3×10^9 base pairs
    c. One set is inherited from both maternal and paternal chromosomes each
    d. It is less prone to mutations than human DNA

31. Anaerobic glycolysis of which of these produces 3 ATPs per unit glucose consumed?
    a. Amino acid
    b. Fructose
    c. Galactose
    d. Glycogen

32. Restriction Fragment Length Polymorphism (RFLP) was used in order to identify the five different species of Staphylococci in a surgical ICU. Which of the following site does the restriction enzymes act?
    a. TAGATA/ATCTAT
    b. ATGGAC/TACGTG
    c. AATATA/TATAAT
    d. GATTAC/CATTAG

33. Low insulin to glucagon ratio is seen in all of these **except**:
    a. Glycogen synthesis
    b. Glycogen breakdown
    c. Gluconeogenesis
    d. Ketogenesis

34. Phenylbutyrate is used in management of urea cycle disorders. What is its role?
    a. Activates enzymes of urea cycle
    b. Excretion of products of urea cycle
    c. Maintains energy production
    d. Scavenges nitrogen

PATHOLOGY

35. An elderly male patient presented with blurring of vision. Fundus examination revealed cotton wool spots on retina and systemic examination showed decreased peripheral sensations and decreased urine output. What finding is the following renal biopsy showing?

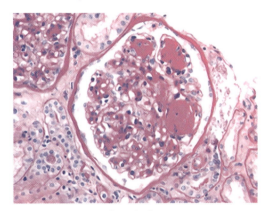

    a. Kimmelstiel-Wilson lesion
    b. Crescents
    c. Amyloid deposits
    d. Hyaline atherosclerosis

36. A 43 years old male presented with facial puffiness and a history of frothy urine for 4 days. Acute kidney injury is suspected. A renal biopsy was done and direct immunofluorescence and electron microscopic image is as shown below. What is the likely diagnosis?

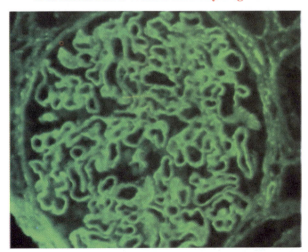

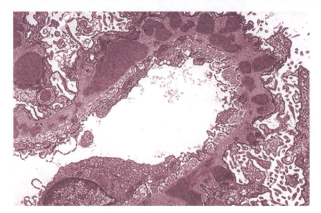

a. Membranous glomerulopathy
b. Membranoproliferative nephritis
c. Minimal change disease
d. Focal segmental glomerulosclerosis

37. A 70 years old male presented with severe intractable diarrhea. His bone marrow and renal biopsy was done which is as shown below. What is the most appropriate diagnosis?

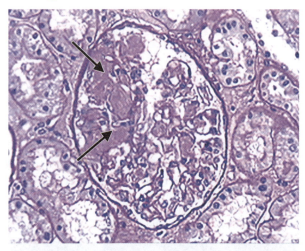

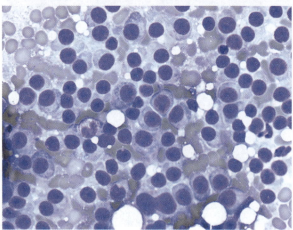

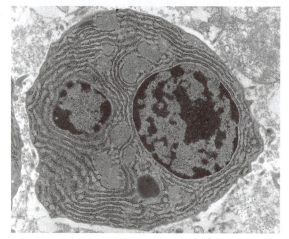

a. Multiple myeloma b. Amyloidosis
c. Urate nephropathy d. Lymphoma

38. A 35 years old patient with history of high-grade fever and tonsillitis 2 months back now presents with cervical lymphadenopathy. Peripheral smear shows lymphocytosis with WBC count 22 × 10⁹/L. Monospot test was negative. Tonsillectomy was done and it showed large cells mixed with lymphocytes. The cells were positive for CD20, EBV-LMP1, MUM1, CD79a. Background cells were positive for CD3. The cells are negative for CD15. The most probable diagnosis is:

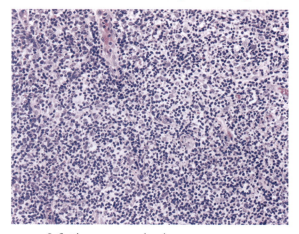

a. Infectious mononucleosis
b. Hodgkin lymphoma
c. EBV positive diffuse large B-cell lymphoma
d. EBV positive mucocutaneous ulcer

39. A new marker for mantle cell lymphoma especially useful in Cyclin D1 negative cases is:
 a. SOX11 b. Annexin V
 c. MYD88 d. ITRA 1

40. On histopathological examination of lymph node as shown below, which of the following zone is represented by the marked area?

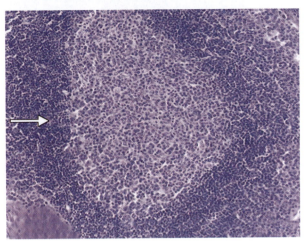

a. Germinal center b. Marginal zone
c. Mantle zone d. Paracortical area

41. Which of the following is true about intracellular iron homeostasis in iron deficiency anemia?
    a. Transferrin receptor-1 iron responsive elements increase transferrin receptor mRNA concentration and synthesis
    b. Transferrin receptor-1 iron responsive elements decrease transferrin receptor mRNA concentration and synthesis
    c. Apoferritin mRNA iron response element decreases and ferritin synthesis decreases
    d. Apoferritin mRNA iron response element decreases and ferritin synthesis increases

42. In the following liver biopsy, which special stain has been used?

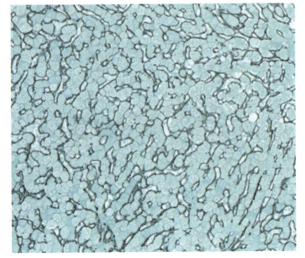

a. Masson's trichrome stain
b. Grimelius silver stain
c. Steiner silver stain
d. Sweet's reticulin stain

43. In a 30 years old female patient with polyarthritis, testing reveals nucleolar pattern of ANA staining. What is the likely course of this patient?
    a. Malar rash, alopecia and renal failure
    b. Sclerodactyly, esophageal dysmotility and Raynaud's phenomenon
    c. Sjogren's syndrome
    d. Painful genital and oral blisters and ulcers

44. Which of the following is anaplastic lymphoma kinase (ALK) positive neoplasm?
    a. Synovial sarcoma
    b. Fibromatosis
    c. Ewing sarcoma
    d. Inflammatory myofibroblastic tumor

45. Which of the following is a tool used in gene editing?
    a. CRISPR b. Gene Xpert
    c. Big Data d. HealthCare App

46. All the following markers are expressed on the surface of T-cells at some stage of development *except*:
    a. CD1a b. PAX5
    c. CD 34 d. Tdt

47. What will be the corrected reticulocyte count in a patient with a hemoglobin of 5 and absolute reticulocyte count of 9%?
    a. 1 b. 3
    c. 4.5 d. 6

48. Which of the following is a negative acute phase reactant?
    a. Ferritin b. Haptoglobin
    c. Albumin d. C-reactive protein

49. A 68 years old man had severe chest pain. The patient died on the way to the hospital. In the hospital, at autopsy tetrazolium chloride staining of the heart was done. What will be the color of viable myocardium?
    (AIIMS May 2017, November 2016)
    a. Red b. Blue
    c. Dark brown d. Pink

50. If the Rb gene phosphorylation is defective, which of the following will happen?
    a. Cell cycle will stop at G1 phase
    b. Cell cycle will stop at G2 phase
    c. The cell cycle will progress and the cell will divide
    d. There will be no effect on cell cycle as for Rb gene phosphorylation is not needed

51. A 20 years old boy presented with persistent cervical lymphadenopathy for the past 1 year. Histopathology of lymph node shows Reed-Sternberg cells with focal nodularity and background of T reactive lymphocytes. The cells were positive for CD20, LCA, EMA and negative for CD15 and CD30 and EBV negative. Diagnosis is:

a. Nodular lymphocyte predominant Hodgkin's lymphoma
b. Lymphocyte rich Hodgkin's lymphoma
c. Diffuse large B-cell lymphoma
d. Small cell lymphoma

52. **What does the red cell distribution width represents?**
a. Anisocytosis
b. Poikilocytosis
c. Level of hypochromia
d. Anisochromia

53. **In thymus, which gene is responsible for recognition of self-antigens?**
a. AIRE
b. Rb
c. Notch1
d. CPK

54. **Which of the following can change the gene expression by methylation and acetylation without affecting the content of the gene?**
a. Epigenetics
b. Translocation
c. Inversion
d. Transduction

55. **Acetone free methyl alcohol is present in Leishman's stain for:**
a. It fixes cells to the slide
b. It colors the red cells
c. It prevents the cells from sticking to the slide surface
d. It stops metabolic and enzymatic activity of the cell

56. **In order to avoid liver biopsy, which of the following can be used as biochemical marker to diagnose liver fibrosis?**
a. SGOT and SGPT
b. Serum hyaluronic acid and laminin
c. Serum ALP and GGT
d. Unconjugated and conjugated bilirubin

PHARMACOLOGY

57. **Which of these drugs is an antidote for fibrinolytic therapy?** *(AIIMS May 2017, November 2015)*
a. Epsilon aminocaproic acid
b. Protamine
c. Heparin
d. Streptokinase

58. **A drug X was given continuous intravenous infusion at 1.6 mg/min. The clearance of the drug is 640 mL/min. With a half-life of 1.8 hours, what would be the steady state plasma concentration of drug?**
a. 0.002 mg/mL
b. 0.004 mg/mL
c. 2.88 mg/mL
d. 3.55 mg/mL

59. **Lente insulin is composed of:**
a. 30% Amorphous + 70% Crystalline insulin
b. 30% Crystalline + 70% Amorphous insulin
c. Same as NPH insulin
d. Only 70% amorphous insulin

60. **Storage of drug in the tissues is suggested by:**
a. Large volume of distribution
b. Small volume of distribution
c. Excretion in urine
d. Excretion in saliva

61. **Which of the following disease modifying anti-rheumatoid drugs acts by increasing extracellular adenosine?**
a. Leflunomide
b. Hydroxychloroquine
c. Azathioprine
d. Methotrexate

62. **A 70 years old hypertensive patient with stage 5 chronic kidney disease was diagnosed recently with Type 2 diabetes mellitus. He doesn't want to take injectable insulin. Which of the following oral hypoglycemic agents will be preferred in this patient, which won't require any renal dose modification?**
a. Linagliptin
b. Repaglinide
c. Vildagliptin
d. Glimepiride

63. **A patient is administered 200 mg of a drug. 75 mg of the drug is eliminated from the body in 90 minutes. If the drug follows first order kinetics, how much drug will remain after 6 hours?**
a. 12.5 mg
b. 25 mg
c. 30 mg
d. 50 mg

64. **Mechanism of action of Oseltamivir (Tamiflu) as an antiviral agent is:**
a. Inhibition of M2 receptor
b. Neuraminidase inhibition
c. Inhibition of RNA dependent DNA polymerase
d. Apoptosis of infected cells

65. **Which of the following is a bactericidal drug against Mycobacterium leprae?**
a. Erythromycin
b. Ofloxacin
c. Cotrimoxazole
d. Amoxicillin

66. **Mechanism of action of protease inhibitors is:**
a. Inhibition of translation
b. Inhibition of assembly of viral proteins
c. Inhibition of proviral RNA synthesis
d. Inhibition of conversion of RNA to DNA

67. **Idiosyncratic side-effects of carbamazepine are all *except:***
a. Steven-Johnson syndrome
b. Agranulocytosis
c. Rash
d. Blurred vision

68. **Which of the following drugs is a P-glycoprotein inducer?**
a. Azithromycin
b. Ketoconazole
c. Itraconazole
d. Rifampicin

69. What drug is used for prophylaxis against Pneumocystis jirovecii in patients on chemotherapy?
    a. Cotrimoxazole
    b. Amoxicillin
    c. Dexamethasone
    d. Cephalosporin

70. Patient is a known case of epilepsy, taking levetiracetam 1 gm BD. He is now seizure free from 2 years but he developed agitation and anger issues interfering with day to day activities as a result of the drug intake. What should be the next best step?
    a. Stop levetiracetam and start on a different antiepileptic
    b. Discontinue the drug as he is seizure free
    c. Slowly taper the drug over next 6 months
    d. Continue levetiracetam since a 5-year seizure free interval is needed

71. In an animal model, the phenomenon of vasomotor reversal of dale can be demonstrated by:
    a. Stimulation of alpha-1 followed by stimulation of beta-2
    b. Block of alpha-1 followed by stimulation of beta-2
    c. Stimulation of alpha-1 followed by block of beta-2
    d. Stimulation of beta-1 receptor followed by block of beta-2 receptor

MICROBIOLOGY

72. Identify the bacteria seen in following stained slide:

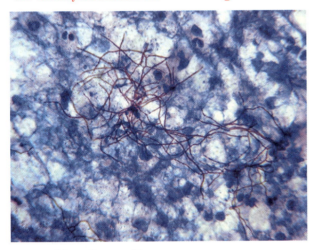

   a. Nocardia asteroides
   b. Actinomyces israelii
   c. Mycobacterium tuberculosis
   d. Mycobacterium leprae

73. Disease caused by Staphylococcus aureus which is not mediated through a toxin is:
    a. Food poisoning
    b. Septicemic shock
    c. Toxic shock syndrome
    d. Staphylococcal scalded skin syndrome

74. A 2 weeks old infant has conjunctivitis, which later developed into respiratory distress and pneumonia. Chest X-ray showed bilateral lung infiltrates. WBC count was 14,300/dL. Which of the following is most likely organism?
    a. Chlamydia trachomatis
    b. Streptococcus agalactiae
    c. Gonococcus
    d. Haemophilus influenzae

75. The egg seen in the following fecal examination belongs to which helminth?

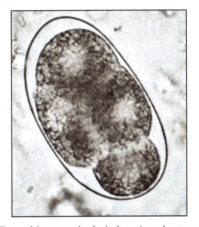

   a. Enterobius vermicularis   b. Ancylostoma duodenale
   c. Ascaris lumbricoides   d. Trichuris trichiura

76. Identify the protozoa whose life cycle and cell division has been depicted here:

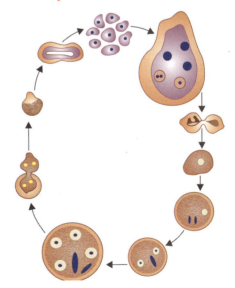

   a. Balantidium coli
   b. Escherichia coli
   c. Entamoeba histolytica
   d. Trypanosoma cruzi

77. Identify the life cycle of helminth as shown below:

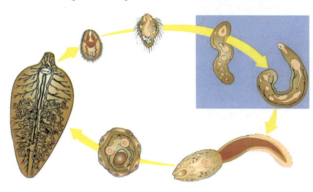

a. Fasciola hepatica b. Schistosoma
c. Clonorchis sinensis d. Fasciolopsis buski

78. Wet mount of the scraping from a genital ulcer in a young sexually active female has been shown below. Identify the diagnosis.

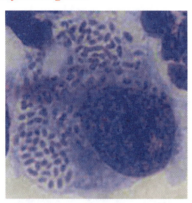

a. Klebsiella granulomatis b. Neisseria gonorrhoeae
c. Haemophilus ducreyi d. Gardnerella vaginalis

79. A patient comes after a dog bite with hydrophobia, tearing and altered sensorium. You suspect rabies in this patient. Corneal impression has been taken. What test will you do on it for most accurate diagnosis?
(AIIMS May 2017, November 2016)
a. Indirect immunofluorescence
b. RT-PCR for virus
c. Histopathological examination for Negri bodies
d. Antibodies against Rabies virus

80. A 22 years old male presented with history of fever, sore throat and enlarged neck lymph nodes. He was ordered a Paul-Bunnell test with a suspicion of Infectious mononucleosis. What is the immunological basis behind the use of this test?
a. Heterophile antibody test
b. Complement mediated agglutination reaction
c. Homophile antibody test
d. Latex agglutination test

81. 1,3-beta D-glucan assay can identify all the following organisms *except*:
a. Invasive aspergillosis
b. Pneumocystis jiroveci pneumonia
c. Invasive candidiasis
d. Invasive cryptococcosis

82. Rhinosporidium seeberi belongs to:
a. Fungus
b. Bacteria
c. Aquatic protistan protozoa
d. Virus

83. Hydrolysis of IgG with papain will lead to formation of following fragments:
a. 1 Fc and 2 Fab fragments
b. 2 Fc and 1 Fab fragment
c. 1 variable chain and 1 constant chain
d. 1 Fab and 1 hypervariable region

84. MHC Class II proteins are expressed by:
a. B-cells, dendritic cells and macrophages
b. Platelets
c. T-cells
d. All nucleated cells

85. A patient was brought to emergency with complaints of high-grade fever and altered sensorium. He was diagnosed to be suffering from meningococcal meningitis. Which of the following is the most appropriate empirical treatment option?
a. Ceftriaxone b. Piperacillin–Tazobactam
c. Penicillin G d. Cotrimoxazole

FORENSIC MEDICINE

86. An adult came to casualty with complaints of rapid heart rate. On examination everything else was normal except for episodic tachycardia and occasional extra-systole and amblyopia. Which of the following is the cause of it?
a. Nicotine b. Cannabis
c. Atropine d. Cocaine

87. A 70 years old male patient presents with amblyopia, exertional chest pain, episodic tachycardia and extra systoles on ECG. What is the probable cause?
a. Cocaine poisoning
b. Chronic nicotine poisoning
c. Arsenophagia
d. Cannabis ingestion

88. Keeping in Jack-knife position for long leads to death by:
a. Wedging b. Burking
c. Positional asphyxia d. Traumatic asphyxia

89. Which of the following is not true regarding teeth features and ethnicity?

a. Upper third molar is most commonly absent in Mongolians
b. Carabelli cusps are seen in Caucasians
c. Negros have wide molar cusps and deep, shovel shaped cusps in incisors
d. Prominent lingual ridge and labial ridge is seen in Mongolians

90. A young patient presented to casualty with history of some substance abuse. His pulse was 130 beats per minute and respiratory rate was 30 per minute. Blood gas analysis revealed metabolic acidosis and his urea was 100 mg/dL and creatinine was 4 mg/dL. Urinalysis revealed calcium oxalate crystals. He improved symptomatically after management with intravenous fluids, gastric lavage, sodium bicarbonate, calcium gluconate and 4-methylpyrazole administration. What is the most likely substance that he consumed?
   a. Formaldehyde b. Methyl alcohol
   c. Ethylene glycol d. Paraldehyde

91. Which of the following is correct regarding corporobasal index of sacrum?
   a. Breadth of 1st sacral vertebra × 100/breadth of 5th lumbar vertebra
   b. Breadth of 5th lumbar vertebra × 100/breadth of all sacral vertebra
   c. Breadth of 5th lumbar vertebra × 100/breadth of base of sacrum
   d. Breadth of 1st sacral vertebra × 100/breadth of base of sacrum

92. Autopsy of a female brought dead to the casualty was performed. No specific signs were seen. On external examination, only a mark on the chin was seen as shown below and on internal examination, following appearance was seen. What is the likely cause of death?

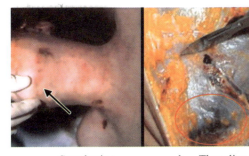

   a. Smothering b. Throttling
   c. Hanging d. Ligature strangulation

PSM

93. A new test in red line has been designed to diagnose a disease condition. The test is being applied to both normal and diseased population. The graph of which is given below. Which of the following is correct regarding the test?

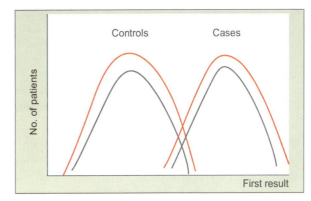

   a. High sensitivity and high specificity
   b. High sensitivity and low specificity
   c. Low sensitivity and low specificity
   d. Low sensitivity and high specificity

94. The following figures represent the frequencies of a disease in 3 different areas. Identify the correctly matched outbreak pattern in each area:
   Area A - 48–50 cases per week, last week 43 cases
   Area B - 1–3 cases per week, last week 13 cases
   Area C - 10–13 cases per year, last week 1 case
   a. Endemic-Epidemic-Pandemic
   b. Epidemic-Endemic-Sporadic
   c. Endemic-Epidemic-Sporadic
   d. Pandemic-Endemic- Sporadic

95. The following diagram represents the natural history of a communicable disease. Which of the following point marks the onset of symptoms?

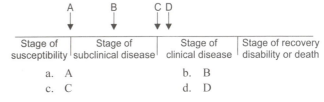

   a. A b. B
   c. C d. D

96. A patient with cough was sputum AFB negative but chest X-ray was suggestive of TB. What should be the next step according to RNTCP?
   a. Line probe assay
   b. Culture
   c. Nucleic acid amplification test
   d. Tuberculin test

97. A researcher said he has discovers a new drug which is effective in chronic hypertensives with a p value of < 0.10. Which of the following is true regarding the same?
   a. The test is 90% reproducible
   b. 90% of test results could have occurred by chance
   c. Not more than 10% of the people benefitted by the drug could be due to chance
   d. 90% of patients will be benefitted by giving the drug

98. A radiotherapist prescribes a new drug combination of chemotherapy and immunotherapy for metastatic melanoma. It prolongs the survival. Which of the following is true in this situation?
    a. Incidence reduces and prevalence increases
    b. Incidence remains the same and prevalence increases
    c. Incidence reduces and prevalence remains the same
    d. Incidence increases and prevalence reduces

99. What will be the mean CD4 count in a sample of 100 patients with distribution of CD4 counts as shown below?

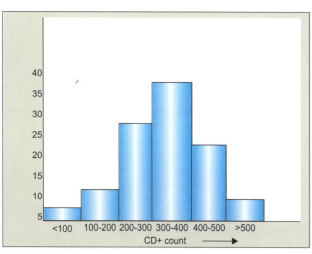

    a. <250
    b. 200–300
    c. >350
    d. 300–400

100. According to the new biomedical waste disposal guidelines, What type of wastes are disposed in the dustbin shown below?

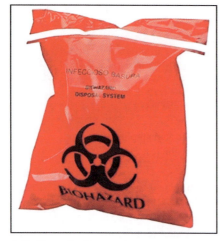

    a. Infectious plastic wastes
    b. Sharps
    c. Animal waste
    d. Human anatomical waste

101. A research was undertaken by a group of psychiatrists and obstetricians to assess postpartum depression in mothers giving birth to male versus female children according to the Edinburgh depression scale (EPDS). What test should be used to compare the outcomes?
    a. Student's t-test
    b. Paired t-test
    c. Chi-square test
    d. Pearson's correlation coefficient

MEDICINE

102. A 50 years old smoker and hypertensive was diagnosed to have non-small cell lung carcinoma with brain metastases. He is on enalapril and hydrochlorothiazide for hypertension. On investigation, he had a serum Sodium 120 mg/dL, Urinary Sodium 110 mg/dL, Serum creatinine 0.8 mg/dL, Serum osmolarity 285 mOsm/L, Urinary osmolarity 350 mOsm/L, Urinary K^+ 9 mg/dL, Blood sugar 112 mg/dL and BP of 150/90 mm Hg. Which of the following is the most probable cause for his hyponatremia?
    a. Cerebral salt wasting
    b. Diuretic induced
    c. SIADH
    d. Pseudohyponatremia

103. A young girl with the diagnosis of acute promyelocytic leukemia (APML) was treated medically. On day 3 of treatment, she developed tachypnea and fever. Chest X-ray shows bilateral pulmonary infiltrates. Which of the following drug should be given next?
    a. Dexamethasone
    b. Cytarabine
    c. Dacarbazine
    d. Doxorubicin

104. ECG is recorded with phonocardiogram to identify the different heart sounds. Second heart sound will appear at which point in the following diagram?

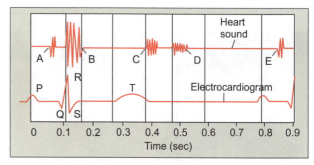

    a. Point A
    b. Point B
    c. Point C
    d. Point D

105. A 60 years old patient who had myocardial infarction 2 weeks back, the lipid profile is done for a patient and reveals HDL 32 mg/dL, LDL 126 mg/dL, TG 276 mg/dL. Which of the following is preferred for this patient?
    a. Rosuvastatin + Fenofibrate
    b. Fenofibrate alone
    c. Rosuvastatin 10 mg
    d. Atorvastatin 80 mg

AIIMS May 2017

106. All the following are seen in myasthenia gravis *except*:
   a. Ptosis
   b. Muscle fatigability
   c. Absent DTRs
   d. Normal pupillary reflex

107. Which of the following complications of stroke need not to be treated?
   a. Fever
   b. Spasticity
   c. Dysphagia
   d. Neglect

108. A 40 years old female currently on a drug for psychiatric illness and hypertension presents with NYHA class III heart failure with dyspnea, pedal edema and K⁺ levels of 5.5 mEq/L and creatinine 2.5 mg%. Which of the following drug is best avoided?
   a. Carvedilol
   b. Enalapril
   c. Spironolactone
   d. Digoxin

109. A patient presents to emergency and ECG was recorded as shown below. What will be the immediate management?

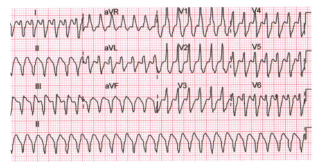

   a. Adenosine
   b. DC cardioversion
   c. Diltiazem
   d. Lignocaine

110. A 20 years old female came with complaints of headache, vomiting and decrease in movement of right leg. In the past, she had episodes of violent and aggressive behaviour and abdominal pain. Which of the following is the most probable diagnosis?
   a. Conversion disorder
   b. Mitochondrial disorder
   c. Acute inflammatory demyelinating paralysis
   d. Acute intermittent porphyria

111. A 40 years old male with history of fall and one episode of vomiting near an alcohol shop. He was brought to casualty and he was awake with open eyes and had retrograde amnesia. Which of the following is most likely cause?
   a. Diffuse axonal injury
   b. Concussion
   c. Drunkenness
   d. Cerebral venous thrombosis

112. The definition of pyrexia of unknown origin includes all *except*:
   a. Diagnosis requires fever persisting for 3 weeks
   b. Fever undiagnosed after 1 week of in-patient workup
   c. Absence of immunological compromise
   d. Temperature of 38.3°C or more

113. A female patient has TSH elevated above normal and subnormal free T4. What is the likely diagnosis?
   a. Primary hypothyroidism
   b. Secondary hypothyroidism
   c. Hyperthyroidism
   d. Subclinical hypothyroidism

114. A 23 years old boy, a badminton player, sustained injury of left ankle. He was immobilized for 3 months, the cast was removed and patient was able to walk normally. Later he complained of pain and swelling in the left calf, left ankle and foot. His mother massaged him for 30 minutes. After a while he developed acute onset of breathlessness and was brought to emergency and died. Most likely cause of death is:
   a. Pulmonary thromboembolism
   b. Congestive cardiac failure
   c. Massive stroke
   d. Hypovolemic shock

115. CURB-65 score includes all *except*:
   a. Age > 65 years
   b. Confusion and elevated blood urea nitrogen > 7 mmol/L
   c. Respiratory rate > 30/min
   d. Systolic BP < 100 mm Hg and Diastolic BP < 60 mm Hg

116. A 40 years old patient came with complaints of spikes of fever and difficulty in breathing. Transesophageal ECHO found out the vegetations in the heart. The culture was positive for Burkholderia cepacia. Drug of choice for Burkholderia cepacia pneumonia is:
   a. Aminoglycoside and colistin
   b. Carbapenems with 3rd generation cephalosporins
   c. Tigecycline and cefipime
   d. Cotrimoxazole with 3rd generation cephalosporins

117. All of the following clinical features are seen in Zika fever *except*:
   a. Guillain-Barré syndrome
   b. Petechial rash
   c. Fever with arthralgia
   d. Petechial rash

118. Hand to knee gait in polio is due to involvement of which muscle?
   a. Gastrocnemius
   b. Gluteus medius
   c. Quadriceps
   d. Hamstring

119. A 50 years old male presented with frontal bossing, enlarged nasal bone, enlarged jaw and spade like fingers. Which of the following test will you do for diagnosis?
   a. IGF1
   b. ACTH
   c. TSH
   d. Serum cortisol

120. A patient presents with ascending muscle weakness for 2 days. On examination, the limb is flaccid. What investigation should be done first?
   a. Serum potassium
   b. Serum creatinine
   c. Serum magnesium
   d. Serum calcium

121. Window period for thrombolysis in a stroke patient is:
    a. 1.5 hours
    b. 2.5 hours
    c. 3.5 hours
    d. 4.5 hours

122. A patient had a femur fracture for which internal fixation was done. Two days later, the patient developed sudden onset shortness of breath with low-grade fever. What is the likely cause?
    a. Pneumothorax
    b. Fat embolism
    c. Pleural effusion
    d. Congestive heart failure

SURGERY

123. A 27 years old lady with 20 weeks pregnancy presented with a thyroid nodule on right side. FNAC from the nodule was suggestive of papillary carcinoma. Which of the following is contraindicated in her management?
    a. Total thyroidectomy plus neck node dissection
    b. Right lobectomy
    c. Radioactive iodine ablation
    d. Total thyroidectomy

124. The following is a thyroid scan. The most probable diagnosis can be:

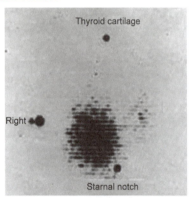

    a. Papillary carcinoma thyroid
    b. Lateral aberrant thyroid
    c. Hypersecreting adenoma
    d. Graves disease

125. A young lady presented with a midline neck swelling as seen below which moves with deglutition and swallowing. It is stable in size for last one year. What is the most likely diagnosis?

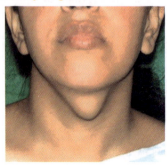

    a. Branchial cyst
    b. Cervical lymphadenopathy
    c. Thyroglossal cyst
    d. Thyroid adenoma

126. What is the sensitivity of axillary ultrasound in identifying axillary metastases in clinically node negative carcinoma breast?
    a. 10–20%
    b. 20–30%
    c. 30–40%
    d. 55–60%

127. A 36 years old patient underwent breast conservation therapy and chemotherapy for a 1.5 × 1.2 cm ER positive breast cancer with one positive axillary lymph node. She is now on tamoxifen. How will you follow-up the patient?
    a. Annual bone scan
    b. Assessment of tumor markers 6 monthly
    c. Routine clinical examination 3 monthly in 1st year with annual mammogram
    d. Routine clinical examination 3 monthly and 6 monthly liver function tests

128. A 45 years old female presented with a history of painless breast lump of size 6 × 5 cm in left upper quadrant with no axillary lymph nodes. A true-cut biopsy was suggestive of ductal carcinoma in situ. She undergoes surgery with resection of all tumor tissue with adequate margins and postoperative HPE showing DCIS with high grade necrosis with 4 mm clearance on margins. Which of the following is needed?
    a. Adjuvant chemotherapy
    b. Adjuvant chemoradiotherapy
    c. Adjuvant radiotherapy
    d. No additional treatment

129. A 56 years old patient came to casualty with history of massive hemoptysis. His routine investigations and chest X-ray was normal. Which of the following is not done to prevent hemoptysis?
    a. Bronchial artery embolization
    b. Pulmonary artery embolization
    c. Bronchoscopic laser cauterization
    d. Lobectomy of the affected segment

130. A woman was brought to the casualty 8 hours after sustaining burns on the abdomen, both the limbs and back. What will be the best formula to calculate amount of fluid to be replenished?
    a. 2 mL/kg × %TBSA
    b. 4 mL/kg × %TBSA
    c. 8 mL/kg × %TBSA
    d. 4 mL/kg × %TBSA in first 8 hours followed by 2 mL/kg/hour × %TBSA

131. In the patient as shown below, chest wall closure has been achieved by using which flap?

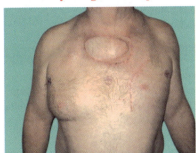

   a. Transversely oriented rectus abdominis muscle flap
   b. Vertically oriented rectus abdominis muscle flap
   c. Pectoralis major myocutaneous flap
   d. Serratus anterior muscle flap

132. A 1.5 years old child was brought to emergency with history of burn by hot water on both hands and palms. The lesion was pink, oozing and painful to air and touch. Which of the following is the best management for this patient?
   a. Paraffin gauze and dressing
   b. Collagen dressing
   c. Excision and grafting
   d. Apply 1% silver sulfasalazine ointment and keep the wound open

133. All the following are true about imaging in primary survey of a trauma patient *except*:
   a. Cervical X-ray is not mandatory
   b. Chest X-ray and pelvic X-ray are taken as a part of primary survey
   c. Hemodynamically unstable patients should not be sent for CT scan
   d. All patients should have chest X-ray-PA view only

134. A patient met with a RTA with paralysis of both upper and lower limb. Patient has not passed urine and tenderness elicited in the cervical region. What will you advise?
   a. The doctor should order a cervical X-ray and shift the patient from the trolley by himself
   b. The patient should not be shifted and portable X-ray machine should be used after neck stabilization
   c. The doctor will instruct the radiographer to take cervical and chest X-ray
   d. The doctor will instruct the radiographer to take cervical X-ray AP and lateral view without any cervical support

135. A patient of motor vehicle accident was admitted to the casualty. He does not speak but moans every now and then, eyes are closed but opens to pain, the right limb is not moving but the left limb shows movement to pain. Both the legs are in extended posture. What will be the GCS score?
   a. 5
   b. 7
   c. 9
   d. 11

136. A young boy presented to the casualty with history of fever, pain abdomen and vomiting. On examination, he was febrile with a pulse rate of 104/min. The resident was eliciting the sign shown below. Identify the sign:

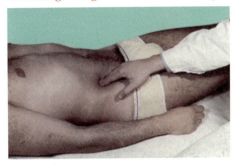

   a. Rovsing's sign
   b. Ballance's sign
   c. McBurney's point tenderness
   d. Psoas sign

137. A patient underwent laparoscopic cholecystectomy and was discharged on the same day. On postoperative day 3, he presented to the hospital with fever. Ultrasonography showed a 5 × 5 cm collection in the right sub diaphragmatic region. What will be the management?
   a. Observe with antibiotic cover
   b. Re-explore the wound with T-tube insertion
   c. Pigtail insertion and drainage
   d. ERCP and proceed

138. Kraissl's lines are:
   a. Collagen and elastin lines in stab wounds
   b. Point of maximum tension in a fracture
   c. Point of tension in hanging
   d. Relaxed tension lines in skin

139. A middle-aged female presented with recurrent bloody diarrhea. Colonoscopy reveals multiple geographic ulcers and histopathological examination is shown below. What is the likely diagnosis?

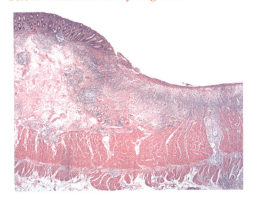

a. Crohn's disease   b. Adenocarcinoma colon
   c. Pseudomembranous colitis
   d. Ulcerative colitis

140. **Maximum risk of carcinoma pancreas is seen in which of these?**
   a. Hereditary atypical multiple mole melanoma syndrome
   b. Hereditary pancreatitis
   c. Peutz-Jegher's syndrome
   d. Familial adenomatous polyposis

141. **A 55 years old patient presented with dysphagia. Identify the diagnosis from upper GI biopsy of esophagus showed in the following picture:**

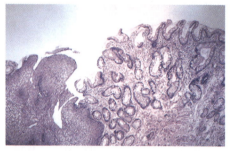

   a. Squamous cell carcinoma   b. Eosinophilic esophagitis
   c. Barrett's esophagus   d. Adenocarcinoma

142. **A person met with road traffic accident and came to casualty with contusion on anterior chest wall with Pulse rate-90/minute, BP-120/80 mm Hg, respiratory rate-16/minute. Normal heart sounds are heard but breath sounds were decreased on the left side and trachea was deviated towards right. Which of the following is the first line management?**
   a. Needle thoracostomy
   b. Pericardiocentesis
   c. Chest tube insertion and drainage
   d. Immediate exploratory thoracotomy

143. **A middle aged male patient presents with fever and diarrhea for 1 week and acute onset pain abdomen for 6 hours. An erect abdominal X-ray was taken as shown. What is the likely diagnosis?**

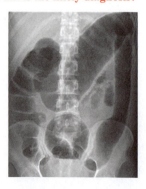

   a. Pseudomembranous colitis
   b. Adenocarcinoma colon
   c. Pneumatosis intestinalis
   d. Toxic megacolon

OBSTETRICS AND AND GYNECOLOGY

144. **According to WHO guidelines, which of the following is true about management of second stage of labor?**
   a. Manual support of perineum to maintain continuous deflexion of head
   b. Episiotomy should be performed as a routine
   c. A warm cloth should be applied to the perineum to prevent trauma
   d. Delivery should be ideally performed in a lithotomy position

145. **A lady delivered a normal vaginal delivery and was discharged. On third day she came back with fever, tachycardia and seizures. Fundus showed papilledema with no focal deficits. What is the most likely diagnosis?**
   a. Cortical vein thrombosis
   b. Meningitis
   c. Subarachnoid hemorrhage
   d. Acute migraine

146. **Which of the following is the most useful parameter according to WHO in assessing adequacy of sperms for fertilization?**
   a. Spermatocyte count
   b. Spermatocyte motility
   c. Semen volume
   d. Spermatocyte morphology

147. **In endometriotic lesions, histology represents its:**
   a. High estrogen
   b. Low insulin
   c. High levels of prolactin
   d. High cholesterol

148. **A Rh-negative mother, who has Indirect Coombs Test (ICT), negative was given Anti-D during 28 weeks of pregnancy. Which of the following is the ideal one?**
   a. Give another dose of Anti-D 72 hours postpartum depending on the baby blood group
   b. Give another dose of Anti-D 72 hours postpartum irrespective of baby blood group
   c. No need of additional dose since she is ICT negative
   d. All of the above

149. **A 32 years old female came for routine PAP smear testing. The report came as carcinoma in situ. What is the next step?**
   a. HPV-DNA testing
   b. Hysterectomy
   c. Conization
   d. Colposcopy and biopsy

AIIMS May 2017

150. A midwife at a PHC did per vaginal examination of a women in labor with 8 cm cervical dilation and 70% cervical effacement with the fetal head at +1 station. This +1 station implies the position of fetal head is:
    a. 1 cm above the ischial spine
    b. 1 cm below the ischial spine
    c. At the level of ischial spine
    d. 1 cm below the cervical os

151. A 61 years old post-menopausal woman with a family history of ovarian cancer presents with pain abdomen. She is on hormone replacement therapy. An abdominal ultrasound revealed a smooth cyst in the right ovary. What should be done next?
    a. Observe and reassure the patient
    b. Laparoscopic surgery to visualize the nature of the cyst
    c. Drilling of cysts
    d. Check CA-125 levels and advise regular follow-up if normal

152. Maximum risk of ureter injury is seen after:
    a. Vaginal hysterectomy
    b. Wertheim's hysterectomy
    c. Laparoscopic abdominal hysterectomy
    d. Anterior colporrhaphy

153. A 24 years old female presented with amenorrhea for 3 months. LH and FSH levels are elevated three times the normal value. What is the next best step?
    a. Urinary HCG level
    b. Check serum estradiol levels
    c. Progesterone challenge test and look for withdrawal bleeding
    d. Ultrasound of abdomen and pelvis

154. True about significant variable decelerations is:
    a. Drop in fetal heart rate to less than 90 bpm for 60 sec
    b. Drop in fetal heart rate to less than 100 bpm for 60 sec
    c. Drop in fetal heart rate to less than 80 bpm for 60 sec
    d. Drop in fetal heart rate to less than 70 bpm for 60 sec

155. Which of the following abnormalities can be diagnosed in the 1st trimester of pregnancy?
    a. Anencephaly
    b. Encephalocele
    c. Meningocele
    d. Microcephaly

156. A middle-aged woman came to OPD with a twin pregnancy. She already had 2 first trimester abortion and she has a 3 years old female child who was born at the end of ninth month of gestation. Which of the following is her accurate representation? G = gravid, P = para?
    a. G4P1 1+2+1
    b. G4P1 0+1+2
    c. G5P1 2+0+1
    d. G5P0 1+0+2

157. What is the next step in management of a 32 years old woman with a 5 years history of primary infertility with bilateral tubal block seen at cornu on hysterosalpingogram? *(AIIMS May 2017, November 2011)*
    a. In vitro fertilization
    b. Laparoscopy and hysteroscopy
    c. Intracytoplasmic sperm injection
    d. Tuboplasty

158. A pregnant woman at 36-week of gestation is admitted in your ward. During the morning rounds, she is lying supine as shown in the figure. What syndrome has been depicted below?

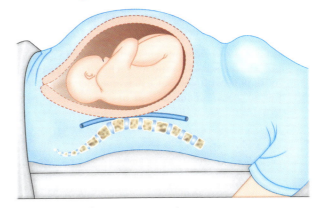

    a. Superior vena cava syndrome
    b. Supine vena cava syndrome
    c. Abdominal aorta syndrome
    d. Inferior vena cava syndrome

159. A midwife at a PHC is monitoring pregnancy and maintaining the partograph of pregnancy progression. At how much cervical dilation should the partograph plotting be started?
    a. 4 cm
    b. 5 cm
    c. 6 cm
    d. 8 cm

PEDIATRICS

160. All of the following are sequelae of fetal alcohol syndrome *except*:
    a. Macrocephaly
    b. Holoprosencephaly
    c. Microcephaly
    d. Thinning of corpus callosum

161. Which of the following is true regarding congenital CMV infection?
    a. Diagnosed only by persistent presence of IgM antibody after 6 months
    b. It is the most common cause on nonsyndromic sensory neural hearing loss
    c. All babies born are symptomatic
    d. Mothers of developing countries who transmit the virus are usually symptomatic

162. A 5 years old child brought to the hospital with history of loose stools but no history of fever or blood in stools. Mother says he is irritable and drinks water hastily when given. On examination eyes are sunken and in skin pinch test, the skin retracted within two seconds but not immediately. What is the treatment for this child?
   a. Administer the first dose of IV antibiotic and immediately refer to higher center
   b. Give oral fluids and ask the mother to continue the same and visit again next day
   c. Consider severe dehydration, start IV fluids, IV antibiotics and refer to higher center
   d. Give Zinc supplementation and oral rehydration solution only and ask mother to come back if some danger signs develop

163. A 6 years old child presents with fever, pancytopenia, generalized weakness and weight loss. On examination, he is pale with generalized lymphadenopathy. Peripheral smear of the patient has been shown below. What is the likely diagnosis?

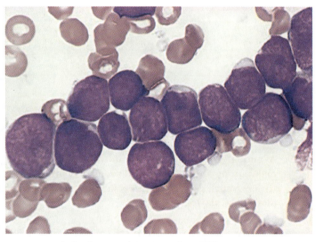

   a. Aplastic anemia   b. ALL
   c. AML   d. JMML

164. An 18 months child weighing 11.5 kg comes to the PHC with fever and respiratory difficulty. On examination, the child is lethargic, with a respiratory rate of 46 bpm and no chest retractions. What is the most appropriate management of this child?
   a. Prescribe oral antibiotics, warn of danger signs and send home
   b. Intravenous fluids alone
   c. Intravenous antibiotics and observation
   d. Give intravenous antibiotics and refer to a higher center

165. A patient presented with fever and cough with expectoration. Raised total leukocyte count was seen on hemogram. The chest X-ray has been shown below. What is the likely causative organism?

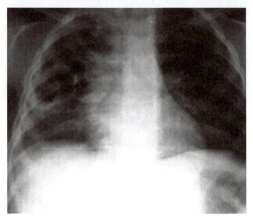

   a. Haemophilus influenzae
   b. Streptococcus pneumoniae
   c. Staphylococcus aureus
   d. Mycoplasma

ORTHOPEDICS

166. In a surgery, the orthopedic surgeon asks you for bone holding forceps. Correctly identify bone holding forceps among the instruments in the tray as shown below:

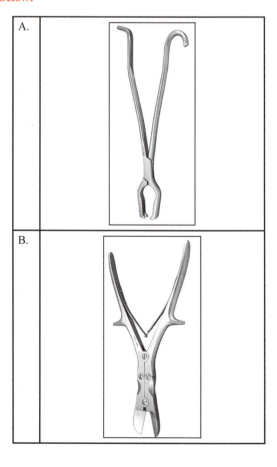

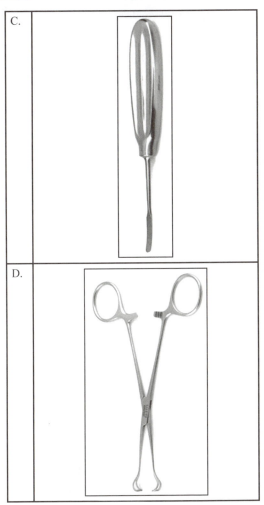

a. Brachial artery
b. Radial artery
c. Ulnar artery
d. Cubital vein

169. Haglund's deformity is seen in which joint?
    a. Elbow
    b. Wrist
    c. Knee
    d. Ankle

170. Which of the following is true regarding Galeazzi's fracture dislocation?
    a. Interosseous membrane tear with ulnar shaft fracture
    b. Radial collateral ligament tear with interosseous membrane tear with radial shaft fracture
    c. Interosseous membrane tear with triangular fibro-cartilage complex (TFCC) tear and ulnar shaft fracture
    d. Interosseous membrane tear with triangular fibro-cartilage complex (TFCC) tear and radial shaft fracture

171. A 75 years old male after a fall in bathroom had hip dislocation as seen in the pelvic X-ray below. What will be the position of the left lower limb?

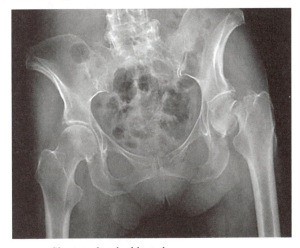

    a. Shortened and adducted
    b. Shortened, abducted and externally rotated
    c. Abducted and internally rotated
    d. Extended, abducted and externally rotated

167. Which part of 2nd metatarsal is involved in the March fracture?
    a. Head   b. Neck
    c. Shaft   d. Base

168. In the fracture seen in the X-ray below, what is the most commonly expected vascular injury?

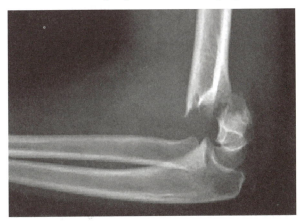

172. What is the most common sequelae of traumatic shoulder dislocation in young adults?
    a. Rotator cuff tear
    b. Recurrent shoulder dislocation
    c. Adhesive capsulitis
    d. Subscapular tendinitis

173. What is the management of the fracture shown below?
(AIIMS May 2017, November 2016)

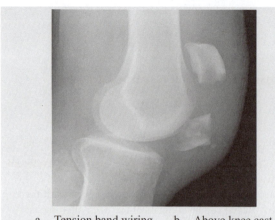

a. Tension band wiring b. Above knee cast
c. Intramedullary nailing d. Patellectomy

174. Which movement of the hip is being demonstrated by the examiner in the following diagram?

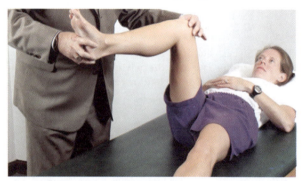

a. Internal rotation b. Adduction
c. External rotation d. Abduction

175. A patient presented with chronic low back pain and hyperpigmented nose and ears. Schober's test is positive. On spinal X-ray, the following appearance is seen. What is the most likely diagnosis?

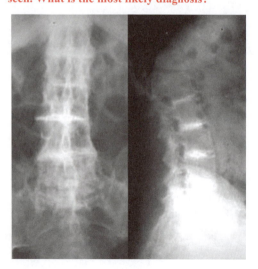

a. Hypoparathyroidism b. Ankylosing spondylitis
c. Ochronosis d. Fluorosis

OPHTHALMOLOGY

176. Identify the phenomenon seen in the eye below:

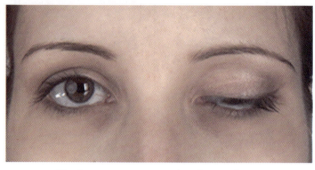

a. Ptosis b. Proptosis
c. Lagophthalmos d. Entropion

177. A 63 years old patient comes to you 1 year after cataract surgery with complaints of decreased vision. The following clinical picture was obtained. What is the likely diagnosis?

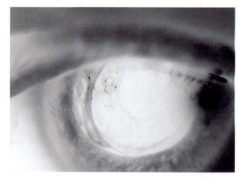

a. After cataract b. UGH syndrome
c. Irvine-Gass syndrome d. Endophthalmitis

178. The following picture of the eye was taken. It shows corneal abrasion, foreign body, corneal ulcer and perforation. Hypotonic maculopathy can result from all *except*:

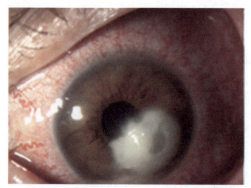

a. Suprachoroidal hemorrhage
b. Uveal bleb leak
c. Cyclodialysis
d. Filtration site leak

179. Which ophthalmological investigation is being done here?

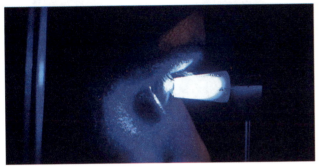

a. Tonometry
b. Pachymetry
c. Laser interferometry
d. B-mode ultrasound

180. Interruption of the optic chiasm will lead to:
a. Bitemporal hemianopia
b. Binasal hemianopia
c. Homonymous hemianopia
d. Normal vision

ENT

181. A 5 years old child present with gradually progressive hoarseness in voice for the last 2 weeks with worsening hoarseness for 3 months and stridor for 2 weeks. What is the most likely diagnosis?
a. Vocal cord nodule
b. Croup
c. Acute epiglottis
d. Respiratory papillomatosis

182. Which of the following vessel is not ligated in case of epistaxis control?
a. Maxillary artery
b. Anterior ethmoidal artery
c. Internal carotid artery
d. External carotid artery

183. Identify the line marked on face in the picture below?

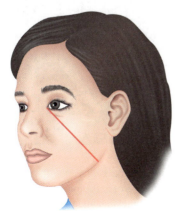

a. Sebileau's line
b. Frankfurt's line
c. Ohngren's line
d. Donaldson line

184. Audiogram of a 30 years old female is given below. Most likely diagnosis is:

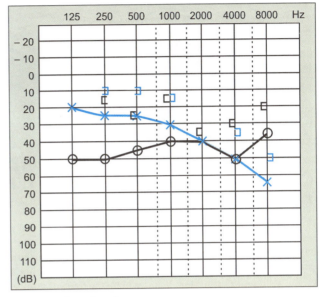

a. Otosclerosis
b. Meniere's disease
c. Ototoxicity
d. Noise induced hearing loss

SKIN

185. A middle-aged lady presented to the OPD with painful blisters on the skin and oral mucosa. Direct immuno fluorescence was done as shown below. All the following are true about the disease pathogenesis *except*?

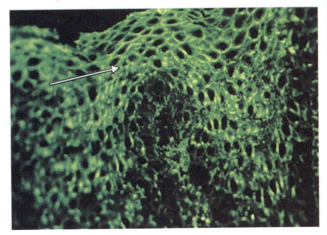

a. Due to IgG against Desmoglein-1
b. Intercellular deposits of IgG and C3
c. Due to IgG against hemidesmosomes
d. Due to IgG against Desmoglein-3

186. A histopathological image of the skin biopsy of a patient given below is suggestive of:

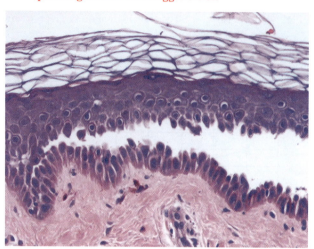

   a. Leprosy   b. Lichen planus
   c. Pemphigus vulgaris   d. Psoriasis

187. A young female presented with vaginal itching and green frothy genital discharge. Strawberry vagina is seen on examination. What will be the drug of choice?
   a. Doxycycline   b. Oral fluconazole
   c. Metronidazole   d. Amoxicillin

188. A child presented with scaly plaques on head with itching, mild discharge and hair loss. What investigation should be done next?

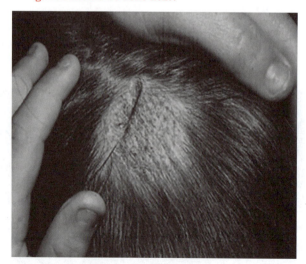

   a. KOH mount
   b. Gram stain
   c. Tzanck smear
   d. Slit skin preparation

189. A young girl presented to the OPD with patchy hair loss for 2 weeks as shown below. There was no scarring or erythema. What is the likely cause?

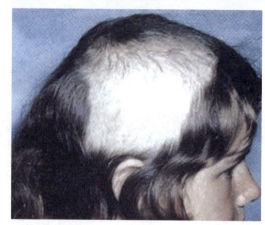

   a. Telogen effluvium
   b. Alopecia areata
   c. Trichotillomania
   d. Tinea capitis

190. A 12 years old boy came with complaints of 4 hypopigmented patches on back and on left arm. The patches had loss of sensation. Which of the following is the treatment for this case?
   a. Rifampicin (450 mg) + Dapsone (50 mg) + Clofazimine (150 mg) monthly and 50 mg daily
   b. Rifampicin (600 mg) + Dapsone (150 mg) only
   c. Rifampicin (450 mg) + Dapsone (50 mg) + Clofazimine (150 mg) monthly and 50 mg alternate days
   d. Rifampicin (600 mg) + Dapsone (150 mg) + Clofazimine (300 mg) monthly and 50 mg daily

191. Identify the following congenital lesion on face:

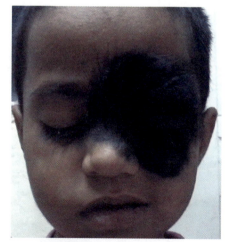

   a. Hematoma
   b. Melanoacanthoma
   c. Epidermal verrucous nevi
   d. Congenital melanocytic nevus

192. A 11 years old child presented with itchy and hyper-pigmented plaques in cubital and popliteal fossa as shown below. Most probable diagnosis is:

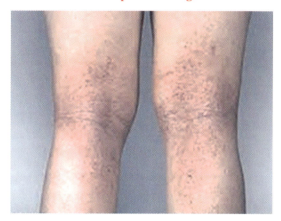

a. Atopic dermatitis
b. Psoriasis
c. Solar keratosis
d. Pemphigus vulgaris

ANESTHESIA

193. All are true about the procedure done with the following needle *except*:

a. Breath holding is not required for the procedure
b. The bevel of the needle face upwards while inserting the needle
c. Done in lateral recumbent position
d. Coagulopathy is not an absolute contraindication

RADIOLOGY

194a. A complex renal cyst was incidentally detected on ultrasound in a patient following which he underwent a CT for an insurance workup. What is the likely diagnosis?

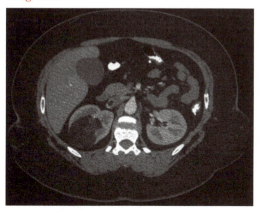

a. Oncocytoma
b. Angiomyolipoma
c. Perinephric cyst
d. Renal cell carcinoma

194b. A 65 years old male banker came for an ultrasound to renew his medical insurance. In right kidney, a complex cyst was found and the picture of CT scan is given below. Most likely diagnosis is:

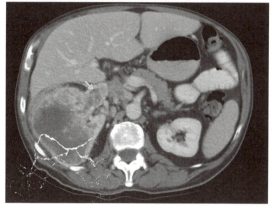

a. Oncocytoma
b. Angiomyolipoma
c. Perinephric cyst
d. Renal cell carcinoma

195. A young female with history of renal calculi complains of bone pain and abdominal cramps. On investigation, multiple fractures were discovered and serum calcium and PTH was raised. Which of the following will be the best investigation to arrive at a definitive diagnosis?

a. CECT neck
b. Sestamibi scan
c. Radioiodine scan
d. Ultrasound neck

196. A patient with pain abdomen for 2 hours presents to the casualty and the following X-ray was obtained. What is the most likely diagnosis?

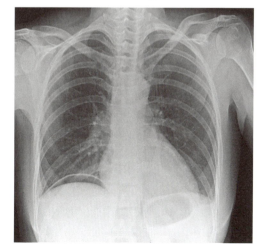

a. Pneumoperitoneum
b. Subphrenic abscess
c. Pneumomediastinum
d. Amebic liver abscess

197. Chest X-ray shown below is showing all the features *except*:

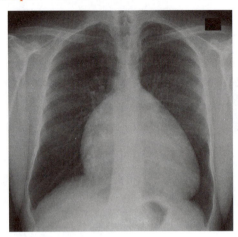

a. Right atrial enlargement
b. Narrow vascular pedicle
c. Decreased pulmonary blood flow
d. Pulmonary venous hypertension

PSYCHIATRY

198. Which of the following is a mood stabilizer with an anti-suicidal effect?
   a. Lithium
   b. Valproate
   c. Carbamazepine
   d. Lamotrigine

199. A state of mutism and akinesis where patient is aware of his surroundings and somewhat alert is best described as: *(AIIMS May 2017, All India 2006)*
   a. Delirium
   b. Stupor
   c. Oneiroid state
   d. Twilight state

200. A 20 years old female has thoughts of cutting her fingers, she plans and imagines doing it but never actually does it. She says that she is not having any guilt of having such thought. And also says the thoughts are distressing her and she is unable to control them. The thoughts vanish either by ending with a seizure or automatically subsides on its own. Which of the following is the cause?
   a. Thought insertion
   b. Obsession
   c. Forced thinking
   d. Thought crowding

Explanations

ANATOMY

1. **Ans. d. Caudate lobe of liver** *(Ref: Gray's 41/e p1107)*

    Caudate lobe of liver forms the superior boundary of epiploic foramen.

    > "The epiploic foramen (foramen of Winslow, aditus to the lesser sac), is a short, vertical slit, usually 3 cm in height in adults, in the upper part of the right border of the lesser sac. It leads into the greater sac. The hepatoduodenal ligament, which is formed by the thickened right edge of the lesser omentum extending from the flexure between the first and second parts of the duodenum, forms the anterior margin of the foramen. The anterior border contains the common bile duct (on the right), portal vein (posteriorly) and hepatic artery (on the left) between its two layers. Superiorly the peritoneum of the posterior layer of the hepatoduodenal ligament runs over the caudate lobe of the liver which forms the roof of the epiploic foramen."-Gray' 41/e p1107

    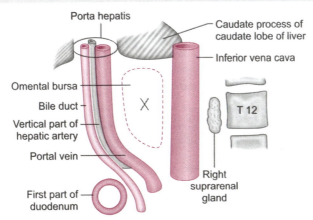

    ### Epiploic Foramen (Foramen of Winslow, aditus to the lesser sac)

    - Epiploic foramen is the **space connecting the greater sac & lesser sac, lying between portal vein & IVC.**

Boundaries of Epiploic Foramen	
Anterior	Hepatoduodenal ligament & portal triad (portal vein, hepatic artery, CBD; cystic duct also present in free edge of lesser omentum[Q]
Posterior	IVC & right suprarenal gland[Q]
Superior	Caudate process of caudate lobe[Q] of liver & inferior layer of coronary ligament
Inferior	1st part of duodenum & transverse part of hepatic artery[Q]
Left lateral	Splenorenal & gastrosplenic ligament[Q]

    ### Pringle Maneuver (Total Inflow Occlusion)

    - **Total clamping** of **hepatic pedicle**, by placing an **atraumatic clamp** across the **foramen of Winslow**[Q].
        - **Appropriate-sized vascular clamp** or **loop snare** easily **controls hemorrhage** from **portal vein** (effectively) & **hepatic arteries**[Q].
        - It **doesn't control bleeding** from **IVC & hepatic veins**[Q].
    - Inflow occlusion durations of up to **30 minutes** can be **tolerated safely** in **cirrhotic livers** and possibly up to **60 minutes** in **early disease**.
    - If prolonged occlusion is required, intermittent clamping can be used with **repeated clampings** of **10-20 minutes** duration, each followed by **5 minutes declamping**.

2. **Ans. c. C** *(Ref: Gray's 41/e p283)*
Third part of vertebral artery, which passes over the posterior aspect of atlas vertebra is represented by 'C'.

A	Transverse foramen
B	Anterior arch and articular facet for dens
C	Groove for vertebral artery
D	Articular surface for occipital condyle

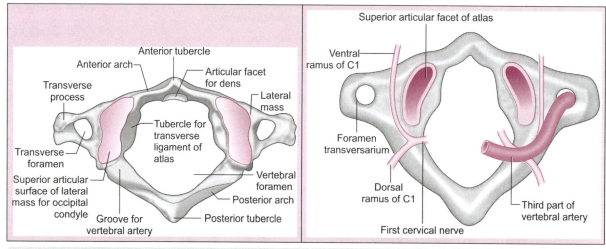

"The vertebral artery arises from the superoposterior aspect of the first part of the subclavian artery. It passes through the foramina in the transverse processes of all of the cervical vertebrae except the seventh, curves medially behind the lateral mass of the atlas and enters the cranium via the foramen magnum. At the lower pontine border it joins its fellow to form the basilar artery. Occasionally it may enter the cervical vertebral column via the fourth, fifth or seventh cervical vertebra." —Gray's 41/e p283

"The third part issues medial to rectus capitis lateralis, and curves backwards and medially behind the lateral mass of the atlas, with the first cervical ventral spinal ramus lying on its medial side. In this position it lies in a groove on the upper surface of the posterior arch of the atlas, and it enters the vertebral canal below the inferior border of the posterior atlanto-occipital membrane. This part of the artery, covered by semispinalis capitis, lies in the suboccipital triangle." —Gray's 41/e p283

"The vertebral artery ascends in the neck through the foramina in the transverse processes of the upper six cervical vertebrae. It passes medially above the posterior arch of the atlas and then ascends through the foramen magnum into the skull. On reaching the anterior surface of the medulla oblongata of the brain at the level of the lower border of the pons, it joins the vessel of the opposite side to form the basilar artery." —Snells 9/e p599

Vertebral Artery

- Vertebral artery ascends in the neck through foramina in the transverse processes of upper six cervical vertebrae[Q].
- It passes medially above the posterior arch of atlas & then ascends through foramen magnum into skull[Q].
- On reaching the anterior surface of medulla oblongata of brain at the level of lower border of pons, it joins the vessel of the opposite side to form the basilar artery[Q].

Parts of Vertebral Artery		
Cervical part	First part	Extends from origin to foramen transversarium of C6 vertebra[Q]. This part lies in the scalenovertebral triangle.
Vertebral part	Second part	Lies within foramen transversaria of upper six cervical vertebrae
Suboccipital part	Third part	Extends from foramen transversarium of C1 vertebra to the foramen magnum of skull[Q].
		This part lies within the suboccipital triangle[Q].
Intracranial part	Fourth part	Extends from foramen magnum to the lower border of pons[Q].

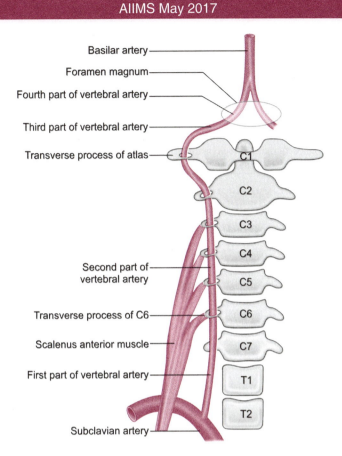

Fig. 1: Course of vertebral artery

3. **Ans. a. A** *(Ref: Gray's 41/e p756; Langman 13/e p153; Snells 9/e p707)*

Nucleus pulposus of intervertebral disc is a derivative of notochord depicted by A. Nucleus pulposus is central gelatinous portion of an intervertebral disc derived from proliferation of notochord cells.

\multicolumn{2}{c}{The image shown is the description of the embryo during Gastrulation (Week 2–3).}
A	**Notochord**, which forms the nucleus pulposus (remnant) in adults.
B	Endoderm
C	Mesoderm
D	Ectoderm

"Vertebral centra are derived from caudal and cranial sclerotomal halves. An intervertebral disc is formed from the free somitocele cells within the epithelial somite which migrate with the caudal sclerotomal cells. The sclerotomal mesenchyme which forms the centra of the vertebrae replaces the notochordal tissue which it surrounds. In contrast, the notochord expands between the developing vertebrae as localized aggregates of cells and matrix which form the nucleus pulposus of the intervertebral disc."-*Gray's 41/e p756*

"The mesenchymal cells of the sclerotome rapidly divide and migrate medially during the fourth week of development and surround the notochord. The caudal half of each sclerotome now fuses with the cephalic half of the immediately succeeding sclerotome to form the mesenchymal vertebral body. Each vertebral body is thus an intersegmental structure. The notochord degenerates completely in the region of the vertebral body, but in the intervertebral region, it enlarges to form the nucleus pulposus of the intervertebral discs. The surrounding fibrocartilage, the annulus fibrosus, of the intervertebral disc is derived from sclerotomic mesenchyme situated between adjacent vertebral bodies."–*Snells 9/e p707*

Notochord Formation	

- **Midline structure** located **between** the **primitive streak & prochordal plate**^Q
- Gives rise to **nucleus pulposus in the region of each intervertebral disc**^Q.
- **Passes through several stages** that are as follows:
  - **Primitive node, primitive knot or Henson's node**^Q (thickened cranial end of primitive streak).
  - **Blastopore**^Q (central depression in the primitive knot)
  - **Notochordal process**^Q (head process): Cells in the primitive streak multiply and pass cranially reaching up to the caudal margin of prochordal plate. The cells undergo several stages of arrangement ending in the formation of a **solid cord** called the **notochord**^Q.

4. **Ans. b. B**   *(Ref: Gray's 41/e p787, 803)*
   Coracoid process of scapula, as depicted by 'B' can be palpated in the infraclavicular fossa.

A	Spine of scapula
B	Coracoid process
C	Acromion process
D	Infraglenoid tubercle

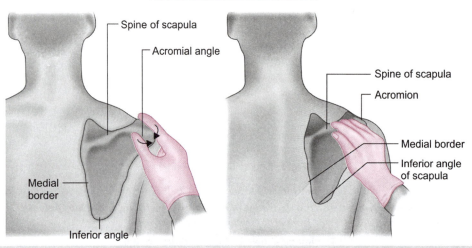

"The coracoid process lies about 2.5 cm below the clavicle at the junction of the lateral fourth with the rest of the bone and is connected to its under surface by the coracoclavicular ligament. It is covered by the anterior fibres of deltoid and can be identified only on deep pressure through the lateral border of the infraclavicular fossa." — *Gray's 41/e p787*

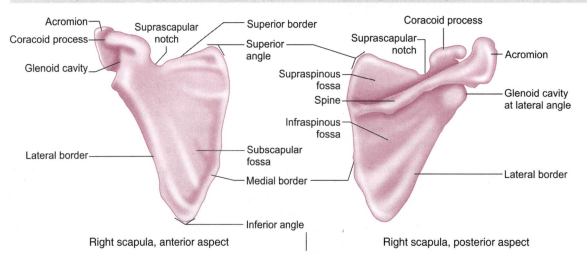

Parts and Surface marking of Scapula	
Spine	• From acromioclavicular joint palpate across the **upper part of posterior surface of scapula**. It is a **long thin projection**, which runs medial to lateral, at **T3 level**[Q].
Acromion process	• Located on the **lateral part of the shoulder**, right above the shoulder joint[Q].
Coracoid process	• Palpate under the **lateral part of clavicle**[Q] (about **2.5 cm below the anterior edge of clavicle**).
Medial (vertebral) border	• Palpable below the spine of scapula
Lateral (axillary) border	• Lateral (or outer) edge of scapula **located between inferior angle & shoulder joint**[Q].

5. **Ans. b. B**   *(Ref: Gray's 41/e p422, 1442)*
   Behind the foramen rotundum is the foramen ovale (labeled as 'B'), which transmits the mandibular nerve.

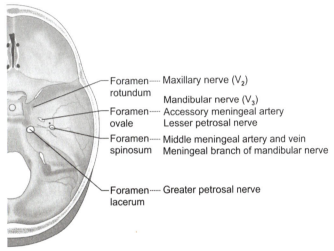

A	Foramen spinosum
B	Foramen ovale
C	Foramen lacerum
D	Optic foramen

*"The greater wing of the sphenoid bone contains three consistent foramina and other small variable foramina. **The foramen rotundum, situated just below and behind the medial end of the superior orbital fissure, leads forwards into the pterygopalatine fossa, and contains the maxillary nerve. Behind the foramen rotundum is the foramen ovale, which transmits the mandibular nerve:** it is occasionally divided into two or three components. Accessory named foramina, the foramen of Vesalius and the cavernous foramen, may occur close to the foramen ovale. The small foramen of Vesalius occurs in some 20% of skulls: it is consistently symmetrical and lies anteromedial to the foramen ovale and lateral to the foramen rotundum and vidian canal. It transmits an emissary vein through which the cavernous sinus and pterygoid plexus communicate. **The foramen spinosum lies posterolateral to the foramen ovale and transmits the middle meningeal artery and veins.** The vessels groove the floor and lateral wall of the middle cranial fossa. The foramen ovale and foramen spinosum open into the underlying infratemporal fossa."-Gray's 41/e p422*

Foramen	Structures passing through
Foramen spinosum (MEN)	• **Middle meningeal artery & vein**[Q] • Emissary vein • **Nerves spinosus (Meningeal branch of mandibular nerve**[Q]**)**
Foramen ovale (MALE)	• **Mandibular nerve**[Q] • **Accessory meningeal artery**[Q] • **Lesser petrosal nerve**[Q] • **Emissary vein**[Q] from cavernous sinus to pterygoid plexus
Carotid canal	• **Internal carotid artery & vein & sympathetic plexus**[Q] around it

Contd...

Contd...

Foramen	Structures passing through
Foramen rotundum	• Maxillary nerve[Q]
Stylomastoid foramen	• Facial nerve[Q] • Posterior auricular artery[Q]
Internal acoustic meatus	• Facial nerve[Q] • Vestibulocochlear nerve[Q] • Nerves intermedius or pars intermedia of Wrisberg[Q] • Labyrinthine vessels[Q]
Foramen lacerum	• Internal carotid artery & artery to pterygoid canal[Q] • Nerve to pterygoid canal[Q] • Greater & deep petrosal nerve[Q]
Optic canal	• Optic nerve[Q] • Ophthalmic artery & central retinal vein[Q]
Foramen magnum	**Through Anterior Part** • Apical ligament of dens[Q] • Membrana tectoria[Q] **Through Posterior Part** • Medulla oblongata[Q] • Spinal roots of accessory nerve[Q] • Vertebral arteries[Q] • Anterior spinal artery[Q] • Posterior spinal artery[Q]
Jugular foramen	• Glossopharyngeal (IX), Vagus (X), Cranial accessory (XI) nerve[Q] • Internal jugular vein[Q]

6. Ans. d. D *(Ref: Gray's 41/e p172, 40/e p798, 837; Apley 9/e p283; Snell's 9/e p433)*

The clinical picture in which patient is not able to move 4th & 5th digit, cannot hold the pen and not able to hold paper between fingers is typically seen in ulnar nerve injury at elbow, which passes posterior to the medial epicondyle (labeled as 'D') of humerus. Fracture dislocation of the medial epicondyle can lead to ulnar nerve injury.

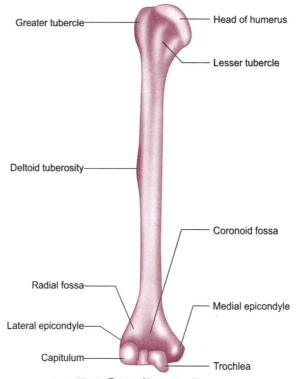

Fig. 2: Parts of humerus bone

A	**Head of humerus:** In relation to axillary nerve and vessels	
B	**Shaft:** In relation to Radial nerve posteriorly, and brachial artery	
C	**Lateral epicondyle:** In relation to radial nerve	
D	**Medial epicondyle:** In relation to ulnar nerve	

"The ulnar nerve is in a vulnerable position as it lies between the medial epicondyle and the olecranon: it lies on bone covered only by a thin layer of skin. It is easily damaged if the ulnar groove is shallow and the nerve may become more prominent than the medial epicondyle or the olecranon when the elbow is fully flexed."- Gray's 40/e p837

"Fractures of the humerus are comparatively common and may occur at almost any level. The humerus is fractured by muscular action probably more frequently than any other long bone: usually the shaft is broken below the attachment of deltoid. The radial nerve may be injured in its groove or may very rarely become involved later in the growth of callus. Fractures at the proximal end of the humerus may rarely damage the axillary nerve, and similarly fractures of the medial epicondyle may be complicated by damage to the ulnar nerve. Supracondylar fractures are relatively common in children: the end of the proximal fragment can sometimes injure the brachial artery or median nerve."-Gray's 40/e p798

"The ulnar nerve is most commonly injured at the elbow, where it lies behind the medial epicondyle, and at the wrist, where it lies with the ulnar artery in front of the flexor retinaculum. The injuries at the elbow are usually associated with fractures of the medial epicondyle. The superficial position of the nerve at the wrist makes it vulnerable to damage from cuts and stab wounds."-Snell's 9/e p433

Injury	Common nerve involved
Surgical neck of humerus	• **Axillary nerve[Q]**
Shaft of humerus	• **Radial nerve[Q]**
Medial condyle of humerus	• **Ulnar nerve[Q]**
Monteggia fracture dislocation	• **Posterior interosseus nerve[Q]**
Volkmann's ischemic contracture	• **Anterior interosseus nerve[Q]**
Lunate dislocation	• **Median nerve[Q]**
Hip dislocation	• **Sciatic nerve[Q]**

Complications of Epicondyle Fracture	
Lateral Epicondyle Fracture	**Medial Epicondyle Fracture**
• **Nonunion & malunion**: If the condyle is left capsized, nonunion is inevitable; **with growth, elbow becomes increasingly valgus & tardy ulnar nerve palsy** is then likely to develop[Q]. • The fracture is a **Salter-Harris Type IV injury** and so **imperfect reduction can result in growth arrest[Q]**. • **Recurrent dislocation**: Occasionally condylar displacement results in **posterolateral dislocation of elbow[Q]**.	**Early**: • **Lateral dislocation of elbow** occasionally occurs with a severe valgus strain & **avulsion of medial condyle[Q]**. • **Ulnar nerve damage** is not uncommon, but recovery is usual unless nerve is left kinked in joint[Q]. **Late**: • **Stiffness of elbow** is common & extension often limited for months[Q].

Nerve	Test	Muscle
Ulnar nerve	**Book test[Q]**	**Adductor pollicis[Q]**
	Card test[Q]	**Palmar interossei[Q]**
	Froment's sign[Q]	**Flexor pollicis substitutes for adductor pollicis[Q]**
	Igawa test[Q]	**Dorsal interossei[Q]**
Median Nerve	**Ape thumb[Q]**	**Thenar muscles[Q]**
	Pen test[Q]	**Adductor pollicis brevis[Q]**
	Pincer grasp (Kiloh Nevin sign)[Q]	**Flexor digitorum profundus + Flexor pollicis longus[Q]** (Anterior interosseus nerve)
	Pointing index (Ochsner clasp/ Benediction test)[Q]	**Flexor digitorum superficialis + Lateral half of Flexor digitorum profundus[Q]**
Radial Nerve	**Thumb & finger drop[Q]**	**Extensors[Q]** (Posterior interosseus nerve)
	Wrist drop[Q]	**Extensors of wrist[Q]**

Ulnar Nerve	

- **Ulnar nerve** arises from **medial cord of brachial plexus** (C8 & T1), gives off **no cutaneous or motor branches in the axilla or in the arm**[Q].
- As it **enters the forearm from behind the medial epicondyle**, it **supplies flexor carpi ulnaris & medial half of flexor digitorum profundus (FDP)**[Q].
- In the **distal third of forearm**, it gives off its **palmar & posterior cutaneous branches**[Q].
- **Palmar cutaneous branch** supplies the **skin over hypothenar eminence**; **posterior branch** supplies the skin over the **medial third of dorsum of hand & medial one and a half fingers**[Q].
- Having entered the palm by passing in **front of flexor retinaculum, superficial branch** of ulnar nerve **supplies the skin of palmar surface of medial one & a half fingers**[Q].
  - **Deep branch** supplies **all the small muscles of hand except muscles of thenar eminence & first two lumbricals**, which are **supplied by median nerve**[Q].
  - **Ulnar nerve** is **most commonly injured at elbow**, where it **lies behind the medial epicondyle & at the wrist**, where it **lies with ulnar artery in front of flexor retinaculum. Injuries at the elbow** are usually **associated with fractures of medial epicondyle**[Q].
  - With ulnar nerve injuries, the **higher the lesion**, the **less obvious the clawing deformity of hand**[Q].
- **Superficial position** of the nerve at the wrist makes it **vulnerable to damage from cuts & stab wounds**[Q].

Injuries to Ulnar Nerve at the Elbow	**Motor:** • **Flexor carpi ulnaris & medial half of FDP** muscles are **paralyzed**[Q]. • **Paralysis of flexor carpi ulnaris** can be observed by asking the patient to make a tightly clenched fist. Normally, the synergistic action of flexor carpi ulnaris tendon can be observed as it passes to the pisiform bone; **tightening of tendon will be absent if the muscle is paralyzed**[Q]. Profundus tendons to ring & little fingers will be functionless & terminal phalanges of these fingers are not capable of being markedly flexed. • **Flexion of wrist joint** will result in **abduction**, owing to **paralysis of flexor carpi ulnaris**[Q]. • **Medial border of front of forearm** will show **flattening** owing to **wasting of** underlying **ulnaris & profundus muscles**[Q]. • **Small muscles of hand** will be **paralyzed, except the muscles of thenar eminence & first two lumbricals** (supplied by **median nerve**). Patient is **unable to adduct & abduct the fingers & is unable to grip a piece of paper placed between the fingers**[Q]. • It is **impossible to adduct the thumb** because the **adductor pollicis muscle is paralyzed**. If the **patient is asked to grip a piece of paper between thumb & index finger,** he or she does so by strongly contracting the flexor pollicis longus & flexing the terminal phalanx **(Froment's sign**[Q]**)**. • **Metacarpophalangeal joints** become **hyperextended** because of **paralysis of lumbrical & interosseous muscles,** which normally flex these joints. Because **1st & 2nd lumbricals** are **not paralyzed (supplied by median nerve), hyperextension of MCP** joints is **most prominent in 4th & 5th fingers**[Q]. **Interphalangeal joints** are **flexed,** owing again to **paralysis of lumbrical & interosseous muscles,** which normally extend these joints through the extensor expansion. **Flexion deformity at interphalangeal joints of 4th & 5th fingers**[Q] is obvious because 1st & 2nd lumbrical muscles of index & middle fingers are not paralyzed. • In **long-standing cases,** the **hand assumes the characteristic "claw" deformity (main en griffe)**[Q]. • **Wasting of paralyzed muscles** results in **flattening of hypothenar eminence & loss of convex curve** to medial border of hand. • Examination of dorsum of hand: **Hollowing between metacarpal bones** caused **by wasting of dorsal interosseous muscles**[Q]. **Sensory:** • **Loss of skin sensation** over **anterior & posterior surfaces** of **medial third of hand & medial one & a half fingers**[Q]. **Vasomotor & trophic changes:** • **Skin areas** involved in sensory loss are **warmer & drier** than normal because of **arteriolar dilatation & absence of sweating** resulting from loss of sympathetic control.
Injuries to Ulnar Nerve at the Wrist	**Motor:** • **Small muscles of hand** will be **paralyzed & show wasting, except** for the **muscles of thenar eminence & first two lumbricals**[Q]. • **Claw hand** is much **more obvious in wrist lesions** because **FDP muscle is not paralyzed** & marked flexion of terminal phalanges occurs[Q].

Contd...

	Sensory:
	• **Sensory loss** confined to **palmar surface** of medial third of hand & medial one and a half fingers & to **dorsal aspects** of **middle & distal phalanges** of same fingers[Q].
	Vasomotor & trophic changes:
	• Same as described for injuries at the elbow.

7. **Ans. c. C** *(Ref: Langman 13/e p88; Gray's 41/e p618; Nelson 19/e p728)*

Absence of thymus, hypoparathyroidism and tetany (suggestive of developmental anomaly of parathyroid) is suggestive of DiGeorge syndrome, which results from dysmorphogenesis of the 3rd and 4th pharyngeal pouches during early embryogenesis, leading to hypoplasia or aplasia of the thymus and parathyroid glands and signs and symptoms of hypocalcemia. Thymus develops from 3rd branchial pouch and there is absence of thymus in the patient, out of 3rd and 4th branchial pouch, the better answer is 3rd pouch.

*"**Thymic hypoplasia (DiGeorge syndrome)** results from dysmorphogenesis of the 3rd and 4th pharyngeal pouches during early embryogenesis, leading to hypoplasia or aplasia of the thymus and parathyroid glands. Other structures forming at the same age are also frequently affected, resulting in anomalies of the great vessels (right-sided aortic arch), esophageal atresia, bifid uvula, congenital heart disease (conotruncal, atrial, and ventricular septal defects), a short philtrum of the upper lip, hypertelorism, an antimongoloid slant to the eyes, mandibular hypoplasia, and low-set, often notched ears. The diagnosis is often first suggested by hypocalcemic seizures during the neonatal period."- Nelson 19/e p728*

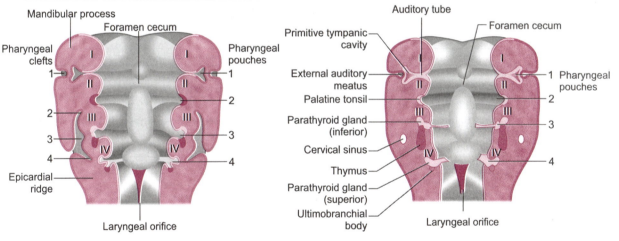

Ectodermal Cleft	
Cleft	**Fate**
1st	• Ventral part is obliterated
	• **Dorsal part** form: **Epithelium** of **external auditory meatus**[Q]; **Ear drum**[Q] & **Pinna**[Q]
2nd, 3rd, 4th	• 2nd arch over grows & cover 2nd, 3rd, 4th cleft to form **cervical sinus**[Q]
	• **Normally cervical sinus disappear** but may **persist as brachial cyst**[Q]

Endodermal Pouch	
Pouch	**Fate**
1st	• **Ventral: Tongue**[Q]
	• **Dorsal: Tubotympanic recess**[Q] (together with 2nd pouch dorsal part). **Proximal part** form **auditory (Eustachian) tube**[Q] & distal part form **middle ear cavity & tympanic antrum**[Q]
2nd	• **Ventral: Tonsil**[Q]; **Dorsal: Tubotympanic recess**[Q]
3rd	• **Thymus**[Q] & **inferior parathyroid gland**[Q]
4th	• **Superior parathyroid gland**[Q]
	• **Thyroid gland** from thyroid gland from thyroglossal duct at foramen caecum
5th	• **Ultimobranchial body** forming **parafollicular cells** (C-Cells) of thyroid[Q]
	• **Disappears**

Arch	Nerve of Arch	Muscles of Arch	Skeletal Element
1st	Trigeminal (V): mandibular[Q] & maxillary division	• Mylohyoid[Q] • Mastication muscles[Q]: Temporalis[Q], Masseter[Q], Lateral & Medial pterygoids[Q] • Anterior belly of digastric[Q] • Tensor palatine & tensor tympani	• Malleus[Q] • Incus[Q] • Anterior ligament of malleus • Spheno-mandibular ligament[Q]
2nd	Facial nerve[Q] (VII)	• Stapedius[Q], Stylohyoid[Q], Posterior belly of digastric[Q] • Facial expression muscles[Q]: Auricularis, Buccinator[Q], Frontalis[Q], Platysma, Orbicularis oris & oculi[Q]	• Stapes[Q] • Styloid process[Q] • Stylohyoid ligament[Q] • Smaller (lesser) cornu of hyoid[Q] • Superior part of body of hyoid[Q]
3rd	Glossopharyngeal Nerve[Q] (IX)	• Stylopharyngeus[Q]	• Greater cornu of hyoid • Lower part of body of hyoid
4th	Vagus (X): Superior laryngeal Nerve[Q]	• Constrictors of pharynx[Q] • Cricothyroid & levator palatine	• Cartilage of larynx[Q] • Thyroid cartilage • Epiglottic cartilage[Q]
6th	Vagus (X): Recurrent laryngeal Nerve	• Intrinsic muscles of larynx except cricothyroid[Q]	–

Aortic Arch Derivatives	
Aortic Arch	Derivatives
1st	• Maxillary artery[Q] • May also contribute to form external carotid artery[Q]
2nd	• Hyoid & stapedial artery
3rd	• Proximal part: CCA[Q] • Distal part: Joins dorsal aorta to form internal carotid artery[Q] (first part)
4th	• Left 4th: Arch of aorta[Q] • Right 4th: Proximal part of right subclavian artery, distal part of right subclavian artery is formed by right dorsal aorta & right 7th intersegmental artery[Q] • Left subclavian artery is formed by left 7th intersegmental artery[Q]
5th	• In 50% it never forms, in another 50% it forms incompletely & soon degenerates
6th	• Left- Proximal: Left pulmonary artery; Distal: Ductus arteriosus • Right- Proximal: Right pulmonary artery; Distal: Degenerates

8. **Ans. c. Paralysis agitans** *(Ref: Gray's 41/e p370; Vishram Singh 2/e p84)*

The area marked with the star is dark, blackish area in the region of mid-brain, which represents substantia nigra. Lesions of substantia nigra produce Parkinson's disease, also called paralysis agitans. Paralysis agitans, which literally means "shaking palsy," is another term used for Parkinson's disease. In Parkinson's disease, the levels of dopamine in the substantia nigra and striatum decrease dramatically as a result of the degeneration of pars compacta neurones.

"Parkinson's disease is the most common pathological condition affecting the basal ganglia. It is characterized by akinesia, muscular rigidity and tremor due to degeneration of the dopaminergic neurones of the substantia nigra pars compacta (which project to the striatum in the nigrostriatal pathway). As a consequence, dopamine terminals are lost in the striatum and dopamine levels are severely depleted. Dopamine receptors, which are located upon medium spiny neurones, and are the target of the nigrostriatal pathway, are spared." -*Gray's 41/e p370*

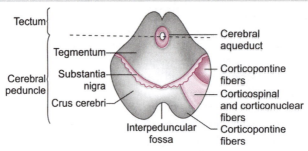

AIIMS May 2017

Substantia Nigra
• It is a **basal ganglia structure located in the midbrain** that plays an **important role in reward & movement**[Q].
• Substantia nigra is Latin for **"black substance"**, reflecting the fact that **parts of the substantia nigra appear darker than neighboring areas** due to **high levels of neuro-melanin in dopaminergic neurons**[Q].

Parts of Substantia Nigra	
Pars compacta	**Pars Reticulata**
• **Pars compacta** serves mainly as an **input to the basal ganglia circuit, supplying the striatum with dopamine**[Q].	• **Pars reticulata**, though, **serves mainly as an output**, conveying signals from the basal ganglia to numerous other brain structures[Q].

9. Ans. a. Protraction *(Ref: Gray's 41/e p569)*

Protraction of jaw is carried out by the bilateral action of lateral pterygoid muscle, which is represented by star in the diagram, originating by two heads from sphenoid bone and getting inserted at anterior surface of mandibular condyle.

"Lateral pterygoid is a short, thick muscle consisting of two parts. The upper head arises from the infratemporal surface and infratemporal crest of the greater wing of the sphenoid bone. The lower head arises from the lateral surface of the lateral pterygoid plate. From the two origins, the fibres converge, and pass backwards and laterally, to be inserted into a depression on the front of the neck of the mandible (the pterygoid fovea)."– Gray's 40/e p539

"Actions of Lateral Pterygoid: When left and right muscles contract together the condyle is pulled forward and slightly downward. If only one lateral pterygoid contracts, the jaw rotates about a vertical axis passing roughly through the opposite condyle and is pulled medially toward the opposite side. This contraction together with that of the adjacent medial pterygoid (both attached to the lateral pterygoid plate) provides most of the strong medially directed component of the force used when grinding food between teeth of the same side. It is arguably the most important function of the inferior head of lateral pterygoid."– Gray's 40/e p539

10. Ans. b. Amygdala *(Ref: Gray's 41/e p262; DeJong's The Neurological Examination by William W. Campbell 7/e p58)*

The white fibers marked in the given figure are anterior commissure. The fibers of the anterior commissure can be traced laterally and posteriorly on either side beneath the corpus striatum into the substance of the temporal lobe. It serves in this way to connect the two temporal lobes, but it also contains decussating fibers from the olfactory tracts, and is a part of the neospinothalamic tract for pain. The anterior commissure also serves to connect the amygdala.

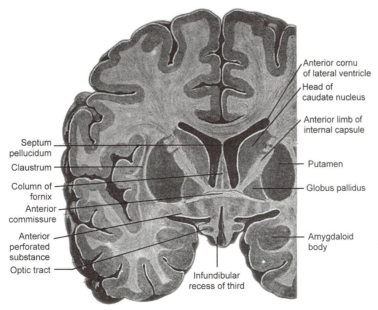

"The anterior commissure arose phylogenetically as part of the rhinencephalon; it connects the olfactory bulbs (of the temporal lobes), amygdala, and basal forebrain region of the two sides. It lies in the lamina terminalis forming part of anterior part of third ventricle, above the optic chiasm, behind and below the rostrum of the corpus callosum."- DeJong's The Neurological Examination by William W. Campbell 7/e p58

"Fibres of the olfactory tracts cross in the ventral or lower part of the lamina terminalis and, together with fibres from the piriform and prepiriform areas and the amygdaloid bodies, form the rostral part of the anterior commissure."

- Gray's 41/e p262

11. **Ans. a. Superior colliculus**   *(Ref: Gray's 41/e p312*

Medial rectus has been labeled in the image above, which is supplied by oculomotor nerve. Nucleus of oculomotor nerve is situated at the level of superior colliculus.

"The third nerve nucleus is located in the midbrain near the cerebral aqueduct at the level of the superior colliculus".
- Ophthalmology By Myron Yanoff, Jay S. Duker 3/e p1010

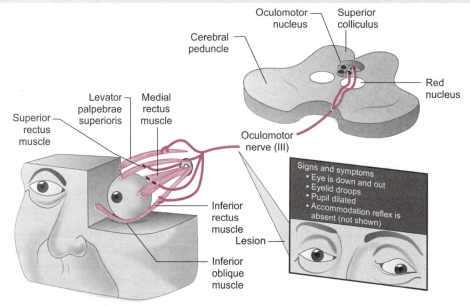

"The oculomotor nerve is the third cranial nerve. It innervates four of the extraocular muscles (superior, inferior and medial rectus and inferior oblique), and also conveys parasympathetic fibres, which relay in the ciliary ganglion. The nerve emerges at the midbrain, on the medial side of the crus of the cerebral peduncle and passes along the lateral dural wall of the cavernous sinus, dividing into superior and inferior divisions, which run beneath the trochlear and ophthalmic nerves. The two divisions enter the orbit through the superior orbital fissure, within the common tendinous ring of the recti, separated by the nasociliary branch of the ophthalmic nerve."

"The main oculomotor nucleus is situated in the anterior part of the grey matter that surrounds the cerebral aqueduct of the midbrain. It lies at the level of superior colliculus." –Snell's 7/e p340

12. **Ans. b. B**   *(Ref: Gray's 41/e p1223)*
Pelvic diaphragm is depicted by label B.

A	Obturator internus & obturator fascia (lateral wall)
B	Pelvic diaphragm (medial wall)
C	Internal anal sphincter
D	Subcutaneous part of external anal sphincter

The pelvic diaphragm is formed by the important levatores ani muscles and the small coccygeus muscles and their covering fasciae. It is incomplete anteriorly to allow passage of the urethra in males and the urethra and the vagina in females. –Snells 9/e p207

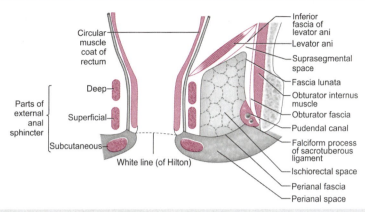

"*Levator ani is a broad muscular sheet of variable thickness which is attached to the internal surface of the true pelvis and forms a large portion of the pelvic floor. The muscle is subdivided into named portions according to their attachments and the pelvic viscera to which they are related (ischiococcygeus, iliococcygeus and pubococcygeus). These parts are often referred to as separate muscles, but the boundaries between each part cannot be easily distinguished and they perform many similar physiological functions.*"-Gray's 41/e p1223

Boundaries of Ischiorectal Fossa	
Lateral	• Fascia covering the **obturator internus muscle & ischial tuberosity**[Q]
Medial	• Fascia covering the **levator ani muscle & external anal sphincter**[Q]
Posterior	• **Sacrotuberous ligament**[Q], on the posterior surface of which is gluteus maximus
Anterior	• **Posterior border of perineal membrane**[Q]
Floor	• Perineal skin
Roof	• Meeting point of fascia covering **obturator internus & inferior fascia of pelvic diaphragm**[Q].

Levator Ani Muscle	
Origin	• **Linear origin** from back of the **body of pubis**, a **tendinous arch** formed by **thickening of fascia covering obturator internus & spine of ischium**[Q].
Insertion	• Groups of fibers sweep downward & medially to their insertion as follows: – **Anterior fibers:** Levator prostatae or **sphincter vaginae** form a sling around the prostate or vagina and are **inserted into perineal body**[Q]. – **Intermediate fibers: Puborectalis** forms a sling around the junction of rectum & anal canal. **Pubococcygeus** passes posteriorly to be inserted into **anococcygeal body**[Q]. – **Posterior fibers: Iliococcygeus** is inserted into the **anococcygeal body & coccyx**[Q].
Action	• Levatores ani of two sides forms an **efficient muscular sling** that **supports & maintains the pelvic viscera** in position[Q]. • **Resist the rise in intrapelvic pressure** during straining & expulsive efforts of abdominal muscles[Q] • **Important sphincter action on anorectal junction** & serves as a **sphincter of vagina**[Q].
Nerve supply	• **Perineal branch of 4th sacral nerve** & from perineal branch of **pudendal nerve**[Q]

13. **Ans. b. Cerebellar nuclei**   *(Ref: Gray's 41/e p336; Ganong 25/e p248)*

The arrow-marked cell bodies are Purkinje cells, a class of GABAergic neurons located in the cerebellum. Purkinje cells send inhibitory projections to the deep cerebellar nuclei, and constitute the sole output of all motor coordination in the cerebellar cortex.

"*The cerebellar cortex has three layers: an external molecular layer, a Purkinje cell layer that is only one cell thick, and an internal granular layer. There are five types of neurons in the cortex: Purkinje, granule, basket, stellate, and Golgi cells. The Purkinje cells are among the biggest neurons in the CNS. They have very extensive dendritic arbors that extend throughout the molecular layer. Their axons, which are the only output from the cerebellar cortex, project to the deep cerebellar nuclei, especially the dentate nucleus, where they form inhibitory synapses. They also make inhibitory connections with neurons in the vestibular nuclei.*"- Ganong 25/e p248

> "**Cerebellum: The molecular layer is approximately 300–400 μm thick.** It contains a sparse population of neurones, dendritic arborizations, non-myelinated axons and radial fibres of neuroglial cells. **Purkinje cell dendritic trees extend towards the surface and spread out in a plane perpendicular to the long axis of the cerebellar folia. Purkinje cell dendrites are flattened. The lateral extent of the Purkinje cell dendrites is some 30 times greater in the transverse plane than it is in a plane parallel to the cerebellar folia.**" - Gray's 41/e p336

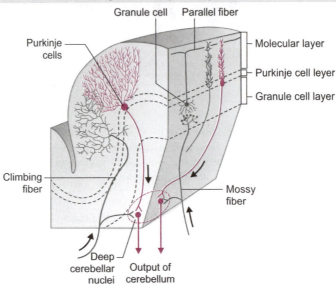

Fig. 3: Arrangement of neurons in cerebellar cortex

Cerebellum	
• **Cerebellum** consists of a **cortex of gray matter** & a **central core of white matter**. • Contains **three well-defined layers**: Granular layer, Purkinje cell layer & molecular layer (from inside to outside)	
Granular layer	• **Densely packed with granule cells**, small neurons whose axons extend into the molecular layer[Q].
Purkinje cell layer	• **One of the largest neurons** in the human brain (**Betz cells being the largest**[Q]) • Consists of a **single row of Purkinje cells**, large neurons with a single axon extending deep into cerebellum & multiple dendrites branching extensively in the molecular layer[Q].
Molecular layer	• Contains mostly **axons of granule cells & dendrites of Purkinje cells**. • Cells in molecular layer are **primarily glial cells**[Q].

Cerebellar Lesions	
Deficit	**Manifestation**
Ataxia[Q]	• Reeling, wide-based gait
Decomposition of movement[Q]	• **Inability to correctly sequence fine, coordinated acts**[Q]
Dysarthria[Q]	• **Inability to articulate words correctly**, with slurring & inappropriate phrasing
Dysdiadochokinesia	• **Inability to perform rapid alternating movements**
Dysmetria[Q]	• **Inability to control range of movement**
Hypotonia[Q]	• Decreased muscle tone
Nystagmus[Q]	• **Fast component** maximal **toward the side of cerebellar lesion**[Q]
Scanning speech[Q]	• **Slow enunciation** with a tendency to hesitate at beginning of a word or syllable
Tremor[Q]	• **Coarse, 2–4 Hz, classically intentional tremors**[Q]

AIIMS May 2017

14. **Ans. c. C** *(Ref: Gray's 41/e p1080)*
    Label 'C' represents conjoint tendon.

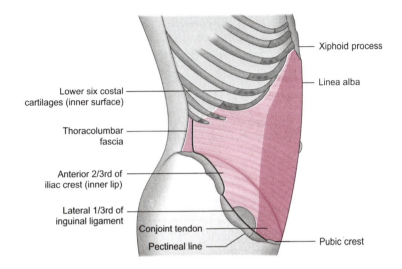

"The conjoint tendon is formed from the lower fibres of internal oblique and the lower part of the aponeurosis of transversus abdominis. It is attached to the pubic crest and pectineal line. It descends behind the superficial inguinal ring and acts to strengthen the medial portion of the posterior wall of the inguinal canal. The attachment to the pectineal line is frequently absent. Medially, the upper fibres of the tendon fuse with the anterior wall of the rectus sheath, and laterally some fibres may blend with the interfoveolar ligament." -Gray's 41/e p1080

PHYSIOLOGY

15. **Ans. c. 80–89%** *(Ref: Ganong 25/e p630)*
    FEV_1/FVC ratio calculated from the given curve is between 80–89%.

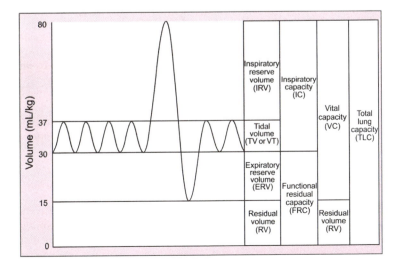

FEV1/FVC Ratio

- The **FEV1/FVC ratio** is **used in the diagnosis of obstructive & restrictive lung disease**[Q].
- It **represents the proportion of a person's vital capacity** that they are **able to expire in the first second of forced expiration to the full vital capacity**[Q].
- **Normal values** are approximately **80%**[Q].
- It is usually **decreased in obstructive lung disease**[Q] & **normal or increased in restrictive lung disease**[Q] (as **FEV1 & FVC** are equally reduced)

  - Here, **Forced Vital Capacity, FVC** = 5000–1300 = **3700 mL**
  - Forced expiratory volume in 1st second, FeV1 = 5000 – 1800 = **3200 mL**
  - **FeV1%** = FeV1/FVC × 100 = 3200/3700 × 100 = **86.5%**

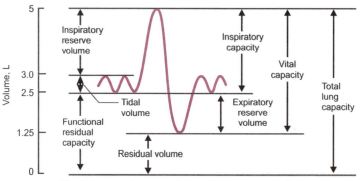

Fig. 4: Lung volumes and capacity measurements

Lung Volume		Lung Capacities	
Tidal volume (TV): • Air that moves into the lung with each normal inspiration or volume of air that moves out of lung with each expiration	500 ml[Q]	**Inspiratory capacity: IC = TV+IRV** • Total amount of air that can be breathed in.	3800 ml[Q]
Inspiratory reserve volume (IRV): • Air inspired with a maximal Inspiratory effort in excess of tidal volume.	3300 ml[Q]	**Vital capacity: VC = TV + IRV + ERV** • Maximal amount of air that can be expelled out forcefully after a maximal (deep) inspiration.	4800 ml[Q]
Expiratory reserve volume (ERV): • Air expelled with a maximal expiratory effort in excess of tidal volume.	1000 ml[Q]	**Functional residual capacity: FRC = ERV+RV** • Volume of air remaining in the lung after normal expiration.	2200 ml[Q]
Residual volume (RV): • Amount of air remaining in the lungs even after forced expiration.	1200 ml[Q]	**Total lung capacity: TLC = TV + IRV + ERV + RV** • Amount of air present in the lung after a maximal inspiration. • This is maximum volume to which the lungs can be expanded.	6000 ml[Q]

16. **Ans. a. Serotonin** *(Ref: Ganong 25/e p592; Miller 7/e p409)*

The Bezold-Jarisch reflex involves a variety of cardiovascular and neurological processes which cause hypopnea (excessively shallow breathing or an abnormally low respiratory rate) and bradycardia (abnormally low resting heart rate). Serotonin can elicit Bezold-Jarisch reflex.

> *"Endogenous substances such as prostaglandins, bradykinin and serotonin could also elicit a Bezold-Jarisch like reflex."-Myocardial Ischemia: Mechanisms, Reperfusion, Protection by Morris Karmazyn (2013)/p5*

> *"Bezold-Jarisch reflex may occasionally be elicited by severe hemorrhage. Reduced circulatory volume may cause increased parasympathetic activity with decreased blood pressure and heart rate. Serotonin released from activated platelets may exacerbate this response."-Post-Anesthesia Care: Symptoms, Diagnosis, and Management by James W. Heitz (2016)/p31*

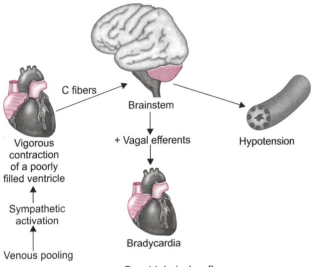

Fig. 5: Bezold-Jarisch reflex

Bezold-Jarisch reflex

- **Bezold-Jarisch reflex** responds to **noxious ventricular stimuli** sensed by **chemoreceptors & mechanoreceptors within the LV wall** by inducing the **triad of hypotension, bradycardia & coronary artery dilatation**[Q].

  - The **activated receptors communicate** along **unmyelinated vagal afferent type C fibers**. These fibers **reflexively increase parasympathetic tone**. Because it invokes **bradycardia**, the Bezold-Jarisch reflex is thought of as a **cardioprotective reflex**[Q].

- This reflex has been **implicated in** the physiologic response to a range of cardiovascular conditions such as **myocardial ischemia or infarction, thrombolysis, or revascularization & syncope**[Q].
- **Natriuretic peptide receptors** stimulated by **endogenous ANP or BNP** may **modulate the Bezold-Jarisch reflex**[Q].
- Bezold-Jarisch reflex may be **less pronounced in** patients with **cardiac hypertrophy or atrial fibrillation**[Q].

  - Stimulation of arterial baroreceptors or ventricular baroreceptors by any of a host of chemicals—**veratrum alkaloids, nicotine, capsaicin, anti-histamine, serotonin**[Q], **snake and insect venoms**—can also **trigger the Bezold-Jarisch reflex**[Q].
  - It usually occurs in **nitrate therapy & use of serotonin agonists**[Q].

17. **Ans. c. 8 times** *(Ref: Ganong 25/e p573, 24/e p575)*

The flow across the vessel 1 is eight times of the flow across vessel 2.

Poiseuille Hagen Formula

- Mathematic expression of the relationship between the flow in a long narrow tube, the viscosity of the fluid, and the radius of the tube:

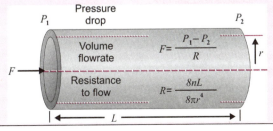

<table>
<tr><td colspan="2" align="center">**Poiseuille Hagen Formula**</td></tr>
<tr><td colspan="2" align="center">$F = (P_A - P_B) \times (\pi/8) \times (1/\eta) \times (r^4/L)$</td></tr>
<tr><td colspan="2">
Where
F = flow
$P_A - P_B$ = pressure difference between two ends of the tube
η = viscosity
r = radius of tube
L = length of tube
Because flow is equal to pressure difference divided by resistance (R),
$R = 8\eta L/\pi r^4$
</td></tr>
</table>

- Because **flow varies directly** and **resistance inversely with the fourth power of the radius, blood flow, and resistance in vivo are markedly affected by small changes in the caliber of the vessels**. Thus, for example, flow through a vessel is doubled by an increase of only 19% in its radius; and when the radius is doubled, resistance is reduced to 6% of its previous value.
- This is why **organ blood flow is so effectively regulated by small changes in the caliber of the arterioles** and why variations in arteriolar diameter have such a pronounced effect on systemic arterial pressure.

$$F = (P_A - P_B) \times (\pi/8) \times (1/\eta) \times (r^4/L)$$

Hence, Blood flow is:
- Directly proportional to pressure difference $(P_A - P_B)$
- Directly proportional to 4th power of radius of vessel
- Inversely proportional to viscosity (mu) of fluid
- Inversely proportional to length of vessel

Here, In this question,
Radius of tube 1 = 2R
Length of tube 1 = 2L
Flow rate = $2^4/2$ R/L = 8 R/L, i.e. 8 times tube 2.

18. **Ans. b. Alpha actinin** *(Ref: Ganong 25/e p101, 24/e p99; Guyton 13/e p75)*

The protein marked in the diagram is linking Z-line and actin, is called as actinin. Titin anchors thick filament (myosin) to actin, while nebulin and tropomyosin (or tropomodulin) are parts of thin filament (actin).

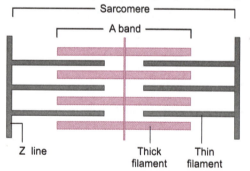

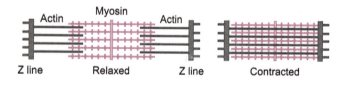

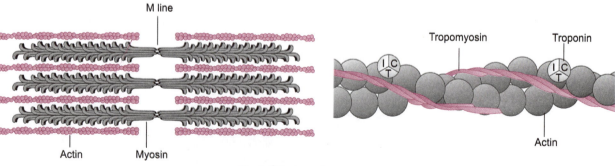

Fig. 6: Structure of sarcomere

"Some additional structural proteins that are important in skeletal muscle function include actinin, titin, and desmin. Actinin binds actin to the Z lines. Titin, the largest known protein (with a molecular mass near 3,000,000 Da), connects the Z lines to the M lines and provides scaffolding for the sarcomere. It contains two kinds of folded domains that provide muscle with its elasticity. At first when the muscle is stretched there is relatively little resistance as the domains unfold, but with further stretch there is a rapid increase in resistance that protects the structure of the sarcomere. Desmin adds structure to the Z lines in part by binding the Z lines to the plasma membrane."-Ganong 25/e p101

Actinin
• It is a **microfilament protein of spectrin gene superfamily**[Q]
• **α-Actinin is necessary for the attachment of actin filaments to the Z-lines in skeletal muscle cells, and to the dense bodies in smooth muscle cells**[Q].
• The **functional protein** is an **anti-parallel dimer**, which **cross-links the thin filaments in adjacent sarcomeres, & coordinates contractions between sarcomeres in the horizontal axis**[Q].
• In non-muscle cells, the **cytoskeletal isoform** is **found along microfilament bundles & adherens-type junctions**, where it is **involved in binding actin to the membrane**[Q].

Types of Proteins in Myofibrils		
Contractile	**Regulatory** (All localized to the **thin filament**)	**Structural**
• **Actin (thin filament)**: Contains a **myosin-binding site** where the myosin heads can attach, is **anchored to the Z discs**[Q]. • **Myosin (thick filament)**: Motor protein, have **cross-bridges for movement** and has an **attachment site for actin & ATP**[Q].	• **Troponin**: Holds the tropomyosin proteins in place & binds to calcium on activation[Q]. • **Tropomyosin**: Blocks the myosin-binding sites on the actin proteins so the myosin heads cannot attach[Q]. • **Nebulin** is an **actin-binding protein, regulates thin filament length** during sarcomere assembly[Q].	• **Titin: Anchors the thick filament to the Z disc** & M line[Q]; Responsible for elasticity. • **Desmin: Connects Z-line to plasma membrane**[Q]. • **Actinin: Binds actin to Z-lines**[Q] • **Dystrophin**: Provides **scaffolding for fibrils**[Q].

Physiologic Anatomy of Muscle Fiber
• Each **muscle fiber** is a **single cell** that is **long multinucleated, cylindric** & surrounded by a cell membrane, sarcolemma.
• Muscle fibers are **made up of myofibrils** in turn are made up of individual filaments made up of contractile proteins.

Muscle contractile Proteins	
Actin	• **Thin filaments** are **polymers made up of two chains of actin** that form a long double helix[Q].
Myosin	• **Thick filaments** are **made up of myosin**[Q] • **Heads of myosin** molecules **form cross-bridges with actin**[Q]
Troponin (I, T, C)	• Troponin molecules are **small globular units located at intervals along** the **tropomyosin molecules.**

Troponin T	• **Binds the troponin** components to tropomyosin[Q]
Troponin I	• **Inhibits the interaction of myosin with actin**[Q]
Troponin C	• **Contains the binding sites for Ca²⁺** that helps to initiate contraction[Q]

Tropomyosin	• Tropomyosin molecules are long filaments **located in groove between two chains in actin**[Q]
Additional structural proteins (actinin, titin & desmin)	• **Actinin binds actin to Z lines**[Q] • **Titin (largest known protein) connects Z lines to M lines** & **provides scaffolding for sarcomere**[Q] • **Desmin binds Z lines to plasma membrane**[Q]

Contd...

Contd...

Physiologic Anatomy of Muscle Fiber
• **LIght I band** is **divided by dark Z line**; **d<u>A</u>rk <u>A</u> band** has **lighter H band in its center**[Q].
• A transverse **M line** is seen **in the middle of H band & this line plus narrow light areas on either side** of it are called **pseudo-H zone**[Q].
• **Area between two adjacent Z lines** is called a **sarcomere**[Q].

• **Thick filaments** are **made up of myosin; thin filaments** are made up of **actin, tropomyosin & troponin**[Q].
      • **Thick filaments** are **lined up to form A bands**[Q]
      • **Array of thin filaments** extends out of A band & into less dense staining **I bands**[Q].

• **Lighter H bands** in center of A bands are the regions where, when the muscle is relaxed, thin filaments do not overlap thick filaments[Q].
• **Z lines** allow for **anchoring of thin filaments**[Q].

19. Ans. a. 0.1 L/cm *(Ref: Ganong 25/e p629)*

The pulmonary compliance in this patient is 0.1 L/cm H_2O.

Pulmonary Compliance
• **Measure of the lung's ability to stretch & expand** (distensibility of elastic tissue).
• **Static lung compliance** is the change in volume for any given applied pressure.
• **Dynamic lung compliance** is the compliance of the lung at any given time during actual movement of air.
• **Low compliance** indicates a **stiff lung** (one with **high elastic recoil**) and can be thought of as a thick balloon – this is the case often seen in fibrosis.
• **High compliance** indicates a **pliable lung** (one with **low elastic recoil**) and can be thought of as a grocery bag – this is the case often seen in emphysema or COPD.
• **Compliance is highest at moderate lung volumes**, and much lower at volumes, which are very low or very high.
• Compliance of the lungs demonstrate **lung hysteresis** (compliance is different on inspiration & expiration for identical volumes)
• **Pulmonary surfactant increases compliance** by **decreasing the surface tension of water.**

Pulmonary compliance $= \Delta V / \Delta P$,
    • ΔV is the **change in volume** or amount of air inhaled in mL or L
    • ΔP is the **change in intrapleural pressure in cm H_2O**
    • Here, $\Delta P = (-4) - (-9) = 5$ cm H_2O
    • $\Delta V = 500$ mL
    • **Compliance = 500/5 = 100 mL/cm = 0.1 L/cm H_2O**

20. Ans. b. 30 mg/min *(Ref: Ganong 25/e p681)*

The urinary glucose in a patient with a blood sugar of 200 mg/dL and a glomerular filtration rate of 90 mL/min will be 30 mg/min.

Renal Transport Maximum (T_m or T_{max})
• Refers to the **point at which increase in tubular concentration of a substance does not result in an increase in tubular reabsorption due to saturation of ion channels**[Q].
• **Quantity of a substance excreted = (filtration + secretion)–reabsorption**[Q]
• **Proximal convoluted tubule** of nephron has protein channels that **reabsorb glucose**, and others that **secrete para-aminohippuric acid (PAH)**. However, its ability to do so is **proportionate to the channel proteins available** for the transport[Q].

Contd...

AIIMS May 2017

Contd...

Renal Transport Maximum (T_m or T_{max})

Glucose is not secreted, so excretion = filtration - reabsorption[Q].
• Both **filtration & reabsorption** are **directly proportional to concentration of glucose in plasma[Q].** • However, while the **maximum reabsorption** is about **260 mg/min** in healthy nephrons, **filtration has effectively no limit** (within reasonable physiological ranges). • Therefore, if the **concentration** rises **above 260 mg/min,** the **body cannot retain all the glucose, leading to glucosuria[Q].** (In this question, **above 150 mg/min- decreased due to diabetes**)

PAH is not reabsorbed and is secreted, so excretion = filtration + secretion.
• As with glucose, the **transfer is at the proximal tubule**, but **in the opposite direction**: from the peritubular capillaries to the lumen. • **At low levels, all the PAH is transferred,** but **at high levels, the transport maximum is reached & PAH takes longer to clear[Q].**

• In practice, the transport maximum is not all-or-nothing. As the concentration approaches the transport maximum, some of the channels are overwhelmed before others are. For example, with glucose, some sugar appears in the urine at levels much lower than 300 mg/dL.

• The **point at which the effects start to appear** is called **"threshold",** and the **difference between threshold & transport maximum** is called **"splay".**

> • Hence, renal threshold and renal transport maxima are slightly different entities.
> • **Total amount of glucose filtered per minute = Plasma sugar x GFR** = 200 mg/dL × 90 mL/min = 2 mg/ml × 90 mL/min = 180 mg/min
> • **Total amount of glucose reabsorbed = Transport maximum = 150 mg/min**
> • **Amount of glucose excreted = Amount filtered – Amount reabsorbed** = 180-150 = **30 mg/min**

21. **Ans. c. 18** *(Ref: Ganong 25/e p640)*

Oxygen carrying capacity of hemoglobin of 14 g/dL is 18 mL.

> *"When blood is equilibrated with 100% O_2, the normal hemoglobin becomes 100% saturated. When fully saturated, each gram of normal hemoglobin contains 1.39 mL of O_2. However, blood normally contains small quantities of inactive hemoglobin derivatives, and the measured value in vivo is thus slightly lower. Using the traditional estimate of saturated hemoglobin in vivo, 1.34 mL of O_2, the hemoglobin concentration in normal blood is about 15 g/dL (14 g/dL in women and 16 g/dL in men). Therefore, 1 dL of blood contains 20.1 mL (1.34 mL × 15) of O_2 bound to hemoglobin when the hemoglobin is 100% saturated. The amount of dissolved O_2 is a linear function of the PO_2 (0.003 mL/dL blood/ mm Hg PO_2)."-Ganong 25/e p640*

Maximum amount of oxygen that can combine with the hemoglobin of the blood
• **Each gram of hemoglobin can bind with a maximum of 1.34 milliliters of oxygen[Q]** (1.39 milliliters when the hemoglobin is chemically pure, but impurities such as methemoglobin reduce this[Q]). • Here, **Hb = 14**, • Hence, **oxygen carrying capacity** = 1.34 × 14 = **18 mL O_2/dL**

22. **Ans. a. 25–30 Hz** *(Ref: Ganong 25/e p107; Guyton 12/e p80)*

Tetanizing frequency of the frog's gastrocnemius muscle from the given graph is 25-30 Hz.

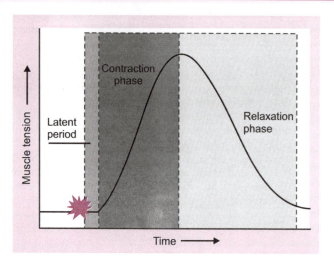

Tetany
• **Tetany** is the **continuous contraction of muscle fibers, without latent period & relaxation period**^{Q}.   • Tetanizing frequency depends on contraction time^Q.   • Twitch duration = Contraction period = 40 millisecond = 0.04 sec (1 millisecond = 0.001 second)   • Tetanizing frequency = 1/Contraction period = 1/0.04 = 25 Hz

23. **Ans. c. Right atrial contraction**   *(Ref: Harrison 19/e p1444; Ganong 25/e p542)*
The 'a' wave in jugular venous pulse represents right atrial contraction.

> *"The venous waveform is divided into several distinct peaks. The a wave reflects right atrial presystolic contraction and occurs just after the electrocardiographic P wave, preceding the first heart sound (S1). A prominent a wave is seen in patients with reduced right ventricular compliance; a cannon a wave occurs with atrioventricular (AV) dissociation and right atrial contraction against a closed tricuspid valve. In a patient with a wide complex tachycardia, the appreciation of cannon a waves in the jugular venous waveform identifies the rhythm as ventricular in origin. The a wave is not present with atrial fibrillation."- Harrison 19/e p1444*

BIOCHEMISTRY

24. **Ans. a. Riboflavin**   *(Ref: Harrison 19/e p96e-4; Harper 30/e p556; Ghai 8/e p118)*
Cheilosis, glossitis, angular stomatitis with decreased RBC glutathione reductase activity is typically seen in riboflavin deficiency.

> *"Laboratory diagnosis of riboflavin deficiency can be made by determination of red blood cell or urinary riboflavin concentrations or by measurement of erythrocyte glutathione reductase activity, with and without added FAD."- Harrison 19/e p96e-4*

> *"Riboflavin deficiency: Activity of glutathione reductase in erythrocytes gives a functional index of flavin coenzyme activity; cofactor-induced increase of 20% above the basal level indicates deficiency."- Ghai 8/e p118*

> *"Riboflavin nutritional status is assessed by measurement of the activation of erythrocyte glutathione reductase by FAD added in vitro."-Harper 30/e p556*

25. **Ans. b. Protein**   *(Ref: Harper 30/e p542; Guyton 11/e p886; Biochemistry by Pankaja Naik 4/e p347)*
The production of heat by the body increases as much as 30% above the resting level during the digestion and absorption of food. This effect is called the thermic effect of food or diet-induced thermogenesis. Maximum thermic effect of food is seen with proteins (20-30%) >carbohydrates (5-6%) > fat (2.5-4%).

Thermic Effect of Food

- **Production of heat by body increases** as much as 30% above the resting level **during the digestion & absorption of food.** This effect is called the **thermic effect of food** or **diet-induced thermogenesis.**

Food	Average Absorption	Respiratory Quotient	Calories	Thermic effect
Carbohydrates	98%^{Q}	1^Q	4^Q	5-6%
Fat	95%	0.7%^{Q}	9^Q	2.5-4%^{Q}
Protein	92%^{Q}	0.8%	4^Q	20-30%^{Q}

26. **Ans. a. Its coenzyme for pyruvate and alpha ketoglutarate dehydrogenase** *(Ref: Harper 30/e p173, 555, 556)*

Thiamine deficiency results in decreased energy production because TPP interferes with its coenzyme for pyruvate and alpha ketoglutarate dehydrogenase.

*"Pyruvate, formed in the cytosol, is transported into the mitochondrion by a proton symporter. Inside the mitochondrion, it is **oxidatively decarboxylated to acetyl-CoA by a multienzyme complex** that is associated with the inner mitochondrial membrane. This **pyruvate dehydrogenase complex** is analogous to the **alpha-ketoglutarate dehydrogenase complex of the citric acid cycle.** Pyruvate is decarboxylated by the pyruvate dehydrogenase component of the enzyme complex to a hydroxyethyl derivative of the thiazole ring of enzyme-bound thiamin diphosphate, which in turn reacts with oxidized lipoamide, the prosthetic group of dihydrolipoyl transacetylase, to form acetyl lipoamide. Thiamin is vitamin B1 and in deficiency, glucose metabolism is impaired, and there is **significant (and potentially life-threatening) lactic and pyruvic acidosis.**"-Harper 30/e p173*

"Thiamin has a central role in energy-yielding metabolism, and especially the metabolism of carbohydrate. Thiamin diphosphate is the coenzyme for three multi-enzyme complexes that catalyze oxidative decarboxylation reactions: pyruvate dehydrogenase in carbohydrate metabolism; α-ketoglutarate dehydrogenase in the citric acid cycle; and the branched-chain keto-acid dehydrogenase involved in the metabolism of leucine, isoleucine, and valine. It is also the coenzyme for transketolase, in the pentose phosphate pathway."- Harper 30/e p555

"The activation of apo-transketolase (the enzyme protein) in erythrocyte lysate by thiamin diphosphate added in vitro has become the accepted index of thiamin nutritional status."- Harper 30/e p556

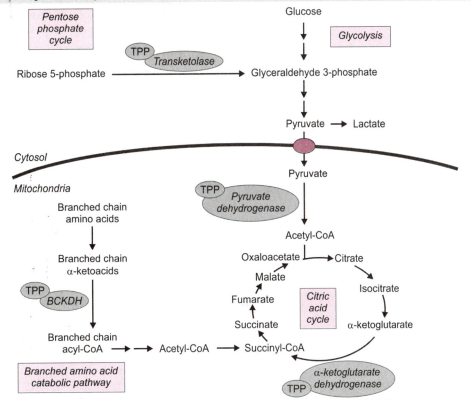

Fig. 7: Metabolic pathways requiring thiamin pyrophosphate (BCKDH: Branched α-ketoacid dehydrogenase, complex; CoA: Coenzyme A; TPP: thiamin Pyrophosphate)

AIIMS ESSENCE

Thiamin (Vitamin B1)
• **Thiamin diphosphate (TDP)**[Q] also known as **Thiamin pyrophosphate (TPP)**[Q] is **biologically active & storage form of vitamin B1,** formed by **transfer of pyrophosphate group from ATP.**

Physiological Role:

- **Thiamin** has a **central role in energy yielding metabolism** and especially of **carbohydrates.**
- **Thiamin requirements increase in excess intake of carbohydrates** and its **deficiency leads to decreased energy production.**

Thiamin diphosphate	• Thiamin diphosphate is the coenzyme for:
	1. **3 multi-enzyme complexes that catalyze oxidative decarboxylation reactions:**
	  – **Branched-chain ketoacid dehydrogenase**[Q] involved in the metabolism of **leucine, isoleucine & valine**
	  – **Alpha-ketoglutarate dehydrogenase**[Q] in the **citric acid cycle**
	  – **Pyruvate dehydrogenase**[Q] in carbohydrate metabolism
	2. **Transketolase**[Q] reaction in the **pentose phosphate pathway**

Thiamin triphosphate	• **Thiamin triphosphate** has a **role in nerve conduction**; it phosphorylates, and so **activates a chloride channel**[Q] in the nerve membrane

Thiamine Deficiency Diseases:

- Chronic peripheral Neuritis, Beriberi & Wernicke Encephalopathy with Korsakoff's Psychosis

Beriberi	Wernicke Encephalopathy with Korsakoff's Psychosis
• **Wet beriberi:** Patients present with an **enlarged heart, tachycardia, high-output congestive heart failure**, peripheral edema & peripheral neuritis[Q]. • **Dry beriberi:** Symmetric peripheral neuropathy of the motor and sensory systems, with diminished reflexes. **Neuropathy affects the legs most markedly**[Q] • **Infantile beriberi:** Occurs in infants born to thiamin deficiency mothers and show tachycardia, vomiting, convulsions & death.	• Alcoholic patients with **chronic thiamin deficiency** also may have **CNS manifestations** known as *Wernicke's encephalopathy*[Q]. • *Wernicke's encephalopathy*: Consists of **horizontal nystagmus, ophthalmoplegia** (due to weakness of one or more extraocular muscles), **cerebellar ataxia, & mental impairment**[Q]. • When there is an **additional loss of memory** and a **confabulatory psychosis**, the syndrome is known as *Wernicke-Korsakoff syndrome*[Q].

27. **Ans. a. Pyruvate to oxaloacetate** *(Ref: Harper 30/e p164)*

Carboxylation of pyruvate to oxaloacetate is an example of anaplerotic reactions.

"Anaplerotic reactions are chemical reactions that form intermediates of a metabolic pathway. Examples of such are found in the citric acid cycle (TCA cycle). In normal function of this cycle for respiration, concentrations of TCA intermediates remain constant; however, many biosynthetic reactions also use these molecules as a substrate."

"Anaplerosis is the act of replenishing TCA cycle intermediates that have been extracted for biosynthesis (in what are called cataplerotic reactions). *The term amphibolic is used to describe a biochemical pathway that involves both catabolism and anabolism. The citric acid cycle (the Krebs cycle) is a good example of amphibolic pathway."*

"The TCA cycle is a hub of metabolism, with central importance in both energy production and biosynthesis. Therefore, it is crucial for the cell to regulate concentrations of TCA cycle metabolites in the mitochondria. Anaplerotic flux must balance cataplerotic flux in order to retain homeostasis of cellular metabolism."

"Net transfer into the citric acid cycle occurs as a result of several reactions. Among the most important of such anaplerotic reactions is the formation of oxaloacetate by the carboxylation of pyruvate, catalyzed by pyruvate carboxylase. This reaction is important in maintaining an adequate concentration of oxaloacetate for the condensation reaction with acetyl-CoA. If acetyl-CoA accumulates, it acts as both an allosteric activator of pyruvate carboxylase and an inhibitor of pyruvate dehydrogenase, thereby ensuring a supply of oxaloacetate."- Harper 30/e p164

Examples of Anaplerotic Reactions

- Carboxylation of pyruvate to oxaloacetate[Q]
- Transamination of aspartate to oxaloacetate by aspartate amino transferase[Q]
- Hydration of glutamate to alpha-ketoglutarate by glutamate-dehydrogenase[Q]
- Beta-oxidation of fatty acids to succinyl-CoA[Q]
- In purine synthesis & purine nucleotide cycle: **Adenylosuccinate to fumarate** catalyzed **by adenylosuccinate lyase**.

28. **Ans. a. ALA dehydratase** *(Ref: Harper 30/e p325, 329; Harrison 19/e p2689, 427e-2)*

ALA dehydratase is a zinc-containing enzyme and is sensitive to inhibition by lead (present in the paints). High levels of lead can affect heme metabolism by combining with SH groups in enzymes such as ferrochelatase and ALA dehydratase.

"A zinc metalloprotein, ALA dehydratase is sensitive to inhibition by lead, as can occur in lead poisoning." -Harper 30/e p325

"High levels of lead can affect heme metabolism by combining with SH groups in enzymes such as ferrochelatase and ALA (delta-amino levulinic acid) dehydratase. This affects porphyrin metabolism. Elevated levels of protoporphyrin are found in red blood cells, and elevated levels of ALA and of coproporphyrin are found in urine." - Harper 30/e p329

"The most common presentation of lead poisoning is an encephalopathy; however, symptoms and signs of a primarily motor neuropathy can also occur. The neuropathy is characterized by an insidious and progressive onset of weakness usually beginning in the arms, in particular involving the wrist and finger extensors, resembling a radial neuropathy. Sensation is generally preserved; however, the autonomic nervous system can be affected. Laboratory investigation can reveal a microcytic hypochromic anemia with basophilic stippling of erythrocytes, an elevated serum lead level, and an elevated serum coproporphyrin level. A 24-h urine collection demonstrates elevated levels of lead excretion." - Harrison 19/e p2689, 427e-2

"Lead Poisoning: Abdominal pain, irritability, lethargy, anorexia, anemia, Fanconi's syndrome, pyuria, azotemia in children with blood lead level (BPb) >80 µg/dL; may also see epiphyseal plate "lead lines" on long bone X-rays." - Harrison 19/e p 427e-2

Lead poisoning

- **Metallic lead & all its salts are poisonous.**
- **Principal toxic salts of Lead: Lead acetate**[Q] **(Saturn salt or sugar of lead), lead carbonate**[Q] **(safeda), lead chromate**[Q], **lead tetra oxide (red lead, vermillion, sindur), lead mono oxide** (litharge), **bold lead sulphide (Least toxic)**
  - **Fatal dose: Lead acetate: 20 gm; Lead carbonate: 40 gm**
  - **Fatal period: 1-2 days**

Metabolism:
- **Absorbed through ingestion or inhalation;** organic lead (e.g., **tetraethyl lead) absorbed dermally**[Q].
- In blood, **95–99% sequestered in RBCs**—thus, must **measure lead in whole blood**[Q] (not serum).
- **Distributed widely in soft tissue,** with **half-life ~30 days**
- **15%** of dose **sequestered in bone** with half-life of >20 years.
- **Excreted mostly in urine**[Q]
  - **Interferes with mitochondrial oxidative phosphorylation, ATPases, calcium-dependent messengers; enhances oxidation & cell apoptosis**[Q].
  - At cellular level **lead interacts with sulfhydryl groups** and **interferes in action of enzymes essential for heme synthesis,** for **hemoglobin & cytochrome production. It causes hemolysis**[Q].

Main source:
- Manufacturing of **auto batteries, lead crystal;** demolition or sanding of lead-painted houses, bridges; stained glass–making, plumbing, soldering; exposure to the combustion of leaded fuels[Q].

Signs and symptoms of Lead Poisoning	
Acute Poisoning	**Chronic Lead Poisoning (Plumbism, saturnism)**
<ul><li>Astringent or metallic taste</li><li>Dry throat and thirst</li><li>**Abdominal pain**^{Q}, nausea & vomiting, sometimes diarrhea.</li><li>**Peripheral circulatory collapse**^{Q}</li><li>**Headache, lethargy & weakness, insomnia, paresthesia, depression, coma** & **death**^{Q}.</li><li>**Cerebellar ataxia is common in children in acute lead poisoning**^{Q}</li></ul>	<ul><li>**Facial pallor: Earliest & most consistent sign**^{Q}</li><li>Weakness</li><li>**Punctate basophilic or basophilic stippling**^{Q}</li><li>**Lead line (Burtonian lines in gums)**^{Q}</li><li>**Colic (Dry belly ache)**^{Q} **& constipation is late symptom**^{Q}</li><li>**Sterility** in males and females.</li><li>**Wrist drop & foot drop**^{Q}</li><li>**Vasoconstriction** leads to **hypertension & arteriolar degeneration**^{Q}.</li><li>**Lead encephalopathy**^{Q}</li></ul>

Diagnosis:

- **Porphyrinuria** (mainly **due to coproporphyrin III inhibition**^{Q})

Blood tests	**Urine tests**
<ul><li>**>200 punctate basophilia stippling cells/mm³ is diagnostic**^{Q}</li><li>**Zinc protoporphyrin & free erythrocyte protoporphyrin > 50 mg/100 ml**^{Q}</li><li>**Increased lead & aminolaevulinic acid (>25 mg/100 ml)**^{Q}</li></ul>	<ul><li>**Increased coproporphyrin (CPU) levels. In nonexposed person it is <150 µg /liter**^{Q}</li><li>**Aminolaevulinic acid > 5 µg**</li><li>Presence of **0.25 mg lead /liter is diagnostic**^{Q}</li></ul>

X-ray Findings in Lead Poisoning	
	<ul><li>**Radio-opaque bands /lines at metaphysis of long bones in children**^{Q}</li><li>**Radiopaque matter** in GI tract (ingested < 48 hours)</li></ul> • **X-ray in lead poisoning showing dense metaphyseal bands at distal femurs & proximal tibias.**

Treatment:

- **Gastric lavage with 1% solution of sodium or magnesium sulphate**^{Q}
- **Chelating agent: BAL, DMSA**^{Q}
    - **Most effective antidote: Calcium Disodium Versenate**^{Q}
    - **Intravenous calcium chloride causes deposition of lead in skeleton from blood**^{Q}.
- Peritoneal or hemodialysis.
- Symptomatic treatment

Chronic Lead Poisoning presents with "New-A B C D E F"	
New	***Neuropathy (leading to weakness, wrist drop) & Nephropathy**^{Q} **(Late** feature)*
A	***Anemia with punctate basophilia (i.e. basophilic stippling)**^{Q} **(Early** feature)*
B	**Burtonian or blue stippled lead line on gums**^{Q}
C	**Colic (abdominal pain) & Constipation**^{Q}
D	***Dry belly ache i.e. diarrhea is very rare**^{Q}* *Dyspepsia, Drop of wrist etc due to **neuropathy**^{Q}*
E	***Encephalopathy**^{Q}, Eosinophilia*
F	***Facial pallor**^{Q} **(earliest sign)***

29. Ans. b. Increased activity of hormone sensitive lipase and decreased activity of lipoprotein lipase *(Ref: Clinical Biochemistry By William J. Marshall, S. K. Bangert 6/e p223; Harper 30/e p262-263)*

In uncontrolled diabetes mellitus, elevated triglyceride and VLDL levels are seen due to increased activity of hormone sensitive lipase (which insulin inhibits) and decreased activity of lipoprotein lipase (which insulin stimulates).

"Insulin has a major role in the control of fat metabolism, and both type 1 and type 2 DM are associated with abnormalities of plasma lipids. **In type 1 DM, at presentation, or if glycemic control deteriorates, marked hypertriglyceridemia (manifest as an increase in VLDL, and often by chylomicronemia as well) is often present as a result of decreased activity of lipoprotein lipase (which insulin stimulates) and increased activity of hormone-sensitive lipase (which insulin inhibits), leading to increased flux of free fatty acids from adipose tissue that act as a substrate for hepatic triglyceride synthesis. Both these effects are reversed by insulin treatment.** Indeed, the degree of hypertriglyceridemia correlates with glycemic control. LDL concentration can also be increased, and that of HDL decreased."- *Clinical Biochemistry By William J. Marshall, S. K. Bangert 6/e p223*

"*Hormone-sensitive lipase is activated by ACTH, TSH, glucagon, epinephrine, norepinephrine, and vasopressin and inhibited by insulin, prostaglandin E_1, and nicotinic acid.*"- *Harper 30/e p262*

	Lipoprotein Lipase (LPL)	Hormone Sensitive Lipase (HSL)
Location	• **Extracellular**[Q]: Attached to **luminal surface capillary endothelium** of adipose tissue, heart skeletal muscle & lactating mammary gland[Q]	• Intracellular: Present inside adipocyte[Q]
Acts on	• **Triacylglycerol** present in chylomicron & VLDL[Q]	• **Diacylglycerol** derived from ATGL[Q]
Activators	• Insulin[Q]	• Glucagon, Epinephrine, ACTH[Q]

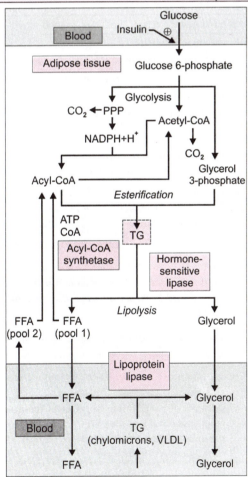

Fig. 8: Triacylglycerol metabolism in adipose tissue

Hormone-Sensitive Lipase (Cholesteryl Ester Hydrolase)

- **HSL** is an **intracellular neutral lipase** that is capable of hydrolyzing a variety of esters.
- The enzyme has a long & a short form.

Long form	• **Expressed in steroidogenic tissues**[Q] (testis) • **Converts cholesteryl esters to free cholesterol**[Q] for steroid hormone production.
Short form	• **Expressed in adipose tissue**[Q] • **Hydrolyzes stored triglycerides to free fatty acids**[Q]

- During fasting-state, increased FFA secretion by adipocyte cells was attributed to adrenaline hormone. Hence the name "**hormone-sensitive lipase**".
- **Main function** of hormone-sensitive lipase is **to mobilize the stored fats**[Q].

> • **Hormone-sensitive lipase** is **activated by ACTH, TSH, glucagon, epinephrine, norepinephrine, & vasopressin** and **inhibited by insulin, prostaglandin E₁ & nicotinic acid**[Q].

Lipase	Description
Lingual lipase	• Secreted from **lingual serous glands; activated in stomach by HCl**[Q] • Its action starts mainly in stomach.
Gastric lipase	• Secreted by **chief cells** in stomach[Q]
Pancreatic lipase	• **Requires co-lipase** for action; Produces 2-mono acyl glycerol[Q]
Adipose triglyceride lipase (ATGL)	• **Present in adipose tissues**[Q] • **Breaks TAG in adipose tissue to DAG** which is further acted upon by HSL[Q]
Endothelial lipase	• Synthesized & located in **vascular endothelial cells**[Q]. • Has **phospholipase A₁ activity**[Q]
Hepatic lipase	• **Hydrolyses triglycerides & phospholipids** in chylomicron remnants, VLDL & HDL[Q]

30. **Ans. a. It codes for more than 20% of respiratory chain enzymes are coded** *(Ref: Harper 30/e p378)*
Mitochondrial DNA is more prone to mutations than nuclear DNA. It codes for 13/67 (about 20%) of respiratory chain enzymes. It has only 16,569 bp (compared to 3.3 billion in nuclear genome) and is inherited exclusively from the ovum.

> *"The majority of the peptides in mitochondria (about 54 out of 67) are coded by nuclear genes. The rest are coded by genes found in mitochondrial (mt) DNA. Human mitochondria contain two to ten copies of a small circular double-stranded DNA molecule that makes up approximately 1% of total cellular DNA. This mtDNA codes for mt-specific ribosomal and transfer RNAs and for 13 proteins that play key roles in the respiratory chain."* - Harper 30/e p378

> *"An important feature of human mitochondrial mtDNA is that—because all mitochondria are contributed by the ovum during zygote formation—it is transmitted by maternal non-mendelian inheritance. Thus, in diseases resulting from mutations of mtDNA, an affected mother would in theory pass the disease to all of her children but only her daughters would transmit the trait."* - Harper 30/e p378

Major Features of Human Mitochondrial DNA

- **Circular, double-stranded** & composed of heavy (H) & light (L) chains; Contains **16,569 bp**

> **Encodes 13 protein subunits of respiratory chain** (of a total of about 67)
> - **7 subunits of NADH dehydrogenase**[Q] (complex I)
> - **Cytochrome b of complex III**[Q]
> - **3 subunits of cytochrome oxidase**[Q] (complex IV)
> - **2 subunits of ATP synthase**[Q]

- Encodes **large (16S) & small (12S) mt ribosomal RNAs**; Encodes **22 mt tRNA molecules**[Q]

Major Features of Human Mitochondrial DNA

- Genetic code differs slightly from the standard code:
  - UGA (standard stop codon) is read as **Trp**[Q]
  - AGA & AGG (standard codons for Arg) are read as **stop codons**[Q]
- Contains **very few untranslated sequences**[Q] (3% noncoding vs 93% in nuclear DNA)
- **High mutation rate**[Q] (5–10 times that of nuclear DNA)
- Comparisons of mtDNA sequences provide **evidence about evolutionary origins of primates** and other species
- **Inheritance is strictly maternal**[Q]

Human Nuclear and Mitochondrial Genomes

Characteristic	Nuclear genome	Mitochondrial genome
Size	~3.3×10^9 bp[Q]	16,569 bp[Q]
Number of DNA molecules per cell	23 in haploid cells; 46 in diploid cells	Several thousand copies per cell (polyploidy)
Number of genes encoded	~20,000–30,000[Q]	37 (13 polypeptides, 22 t-RNAs & 2 r-RNAs)[Q]
Gene density	~1 per 40,000 bp[Q]	1 per 450 bp[Q]
Introns	Frequently found in most genes[Q]	Absent[Q]
Percentage of coding DNA	~3%[Q]	~93%[Q]
Codon usage	The universal genetic code[Q]	AUA codes for methionine; TGA codes for tryptophan; AGA & AGG specify stop codons[Q]
Associated proteins	Nucleosome-associated histone proteins & non-histone proteins[Q]	No histones[Q]; but associated with several proteins (for example, TFAM) that form nucleoids
Mode of inheritance	Mendelian inheritance for autosomes & X chromosome; paternal inheritance for Y chromosome[Q]	Exclusively maternal[Q]
Replication	Strand-coupled mechanism that uses DNA polymerases α & δ[Q]	Strand-coupled & strand-displacement models; only uses DNA polymerase γ[Q]
Transcription	Most genes are transcribed individually[Q]	All genes on both strands are transcribed as large polycistrons[Q]
Recombination	Each pair of homologous recombines during the prophase of meiosis	Occurs at a cellular level

31. Ans. d. Glycogen   *(Ref: Harper 30/e p186)*

Anaerobic glycolysis of glycogen produces 3 ATPs per unit glucose consumed.

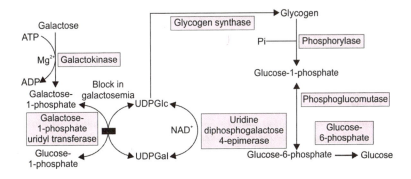

Energetics of Anaerobic Glycolysis

Enzyme	Reducing Equivalent/ATP from the step	ATP per molecule of Glucose
1, 3-Bisphosphaoglycerate kinase	1 ATP by substrate level phosphorylation	2 ATPs
Pyruvate kinase	1 ATP by substrate level phosphorylation	2 ATPs
The number of ATPs generated		4 ATPs
Consumption of ATPs in the hexokinase & phosphofructokinase		–2 ATPs
Number of ATPs from anaerobic glycolysis		4 –2 = 2 ATPs
Consumption of ATP at the level of hexokinase is not required when we start from glycogen as a substrate. As there is no glucose-6-phosphatase in muscle, glucose-6-phosphate directly enters into glycolysis. Hence, net ATPs are 4-1 = 3 ATPs.		

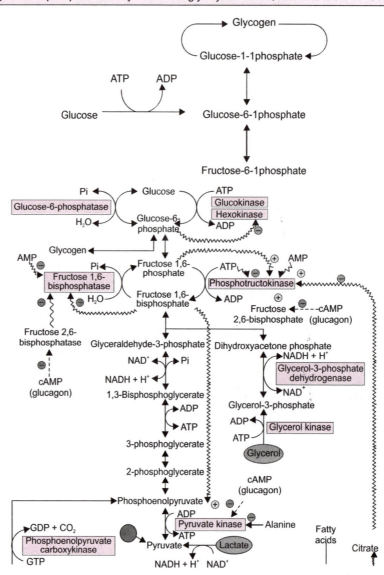

32. Ans. d. GATTAC/CATTAG   *(Ref: Harper 30/e p451, 463; Lippincott 6/e p840; Jawetz 27/e p119)*
Restriction endonucleases are enzymes that cut DNA at specific DNA sequences within the molecule — called the palindromic regions. A palindromic sequence is a sequence made up of nucleic acids within the double helix of DNA/ RNA that is same when read from 5' to 3' end on either, i.e. complimentary strands. In the given options, only GATTAC/ CATTAG (option d) is a palindrome.

"An inherited difference in the pattern of restriction enzyme digestion enzyme digestion (eg, a DNA variation occurring in more than 1% of the general population) is known as a restriction fragment length polymorphism, or RFLP."- Harper 30/e p463

"The genetic diversity of bacteria is reflected in their extensive range of restriction enzymes, which possess remarkable selectivity that allows them to recognize specific regions of DNA for cleavage. DNA sequences recognized by restriction enzymes are predominantly palindromes (inverted sequence repetitions). A typical sequence palindrome, recognized by the frequently used restriction enzyme EcoR1, is GAATTC; the inverted repetition, inherent in the complementarity of the G-C and A-T base pairs, results in the 5' sequence TTC being reflected as AAG in the 3' strand." -Jawetz 27/e p119

Restriction Endonucleases

- **Werner Arber** discovered **restriction modification system** in **bacteria.**[Q]
- It consists of **restriction endonucleases** & a **site-specific methylase**[Q].
- Restriction endonucleases **hydrolytically cleave polynucleotides internally at specific palindromic sites**[Q].
- **Palindrome** is a **sequence of duplex DNA** that is **same when the two strands are read in opposite directions.** Example: **GATCC & CCTAG**[Q]
- Restriction endonucleases belong to **class III hydrolases**[Q].
- **Restriction modification system protects bacteria against** invasion by **foreign viral (bacteriophage) DNA**[Q].

Types of Restriction Endonucleases

Type I	Type II
• Restriction endonucleases **cleave at random site**	• Restriction endonucleases **cleave at palindromic site**

Restriction Endonucleases as Molecular Biology Tools

- **Type II** restriction endonuclease discovered by **Hamilton Smith & Daniel Nathans**, are used as **biochemical tool of DNA manipulation**[Q].
- They are otherwise known as **molecular scissors**[Q].
- Restriction endonucleases are **named after the bacterium from which they are isolated**[Q].
- They **cut the DNA at specific palindromic site** to obtain **sticky/ staggered /cohesive end** (having **overhanging sequence**) & **blunt ends (not having overhanging sequence)**[Q].

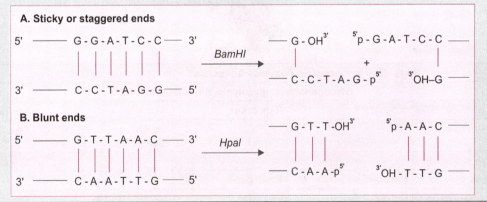

33. **Ans. a. Glycogen synthesis**   *(Ref: Harper 30/e p188)*

Low insulin to glucagon ratio implies a catabolic state, i.e. usage of body stores to form energy, typically seen in fasting state and diabetes mellitus. Hence, this state will promote glycogen breakdown, gluconeogenesis as well as ketone body formation, while at the same time inhibiting glycogen synthesis and storage.

"Insulin, secreted in response to increased blood glucose, enhances the synthesis of the key enzymes in glycolysis. It also antagonizes the effect of the glucocorticoids and glucagon-stimulated cAMP, which induce synthesis of the key enzymes of gluconeogenesis."-Harper 30/e p188

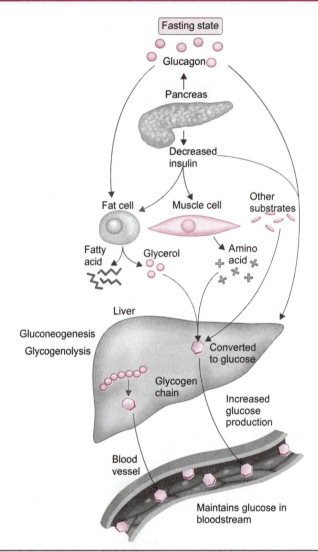

Regulatory and Adaptive Enzymes Associated with Carbohydrate Metabolism.				
Glycogenolysis, glycolysis, and pyruvate oxidation				
	Inducer	**Repressor**	**Activator**	**Inhibitor**
Glycogen synthase			Insulin, glucose 6-phosphate	Glucagon
Hexokinase				Glucose 6-phosphate
Glucokinase	Insulin^Q	Glucagon^Q		
Phosphofructo- kinase-1	Insulin	Glucagon	5'AMP, fructose 6-phosphate, fructose 2,6-bisphosphate, P$_i$	Citrate, ATP, glucagon
Pyruvate kinase	Insulin, fructose^Q	Glucagon^Q	Fructose 1,6-bisphosphate, insulin	ATP, alanine, glucagon, norepinephrine
Pyruvate dehydrogenase			CoA, NAD$^+$, insulin, ADP, pyruvate	Acetyl CoA, NADH, ATP (fatty acids, ketone bodies)

Contd...

Contd...

Gluconeogenesis				
Pyruvate carboxylase	Glucocorticoids, glucagon, epinephrine	**Insulin**^{Q}	Acetyl CoA	ADP
Phosphoenol pyruvate carboxykinase	Glucocorticoids, glucagon, epinephrine	**Insulin**^{Q}	Glucagon?	–
Glucose 6-phosphatase	Glucocorticoids, **glucagon**, epinephrine	**Insulin**^{Q}	–	–

34. Ans. d. Scavenges nitrogen *(Ref: Nelson 19/e p449; Inborn Metabolic Diseases: Diagnosis and Treatment by John Fernandes, Jean-Marie Saudubray 2/e p172; Lippincott 6/e p471)*

Phenylbutyrate is used to treat urea cycle disorders, because its metabolites offer an alternative pathway to the urea cycle to allow excretion of excess nitrogen. Urea cycle disorders result in the accumulation of precursors of urea, principally ammonia and glutamine. Phenylbutyrate provides an alternate means of detoxification of glutamine via acetylation, which bypasses the urea cycle.

"Phenylbutyrate is oxidised in the liver to phenylacetate, which is then conjugated with glutamine. The resulting phenylacetylglutamine is rapidly excreted by the urine and hence 2 mol nitrogenare lost for each mole of phenylbutyrate given."-*Inborn Metabolic Diseases: Diagnosis and Treatment by John Fernandes, Jean-Marie Saudubray 2/e p172*

"Phenylacetate conjugates with glutamine to form phenylacetylglutamine, which is readily excreted in the urine. One mole of phenylacetate removes 2 moles of ammonia as glutamine from the body."- Nelson 19/e p449

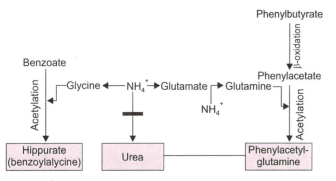

"Phenylbutyrate and sodium benzoate are orphan drugs approved for the treatment of hyperammonemia in patients with urea cycle disorders. Phenylbutyrate is a prodrug that is metabolized to phenylacetate, which is the active molecule that combines with glutamine to form phenylacetylglutamine, which is rapidly excreted by the kidneys and does not require metabolism via the urea cycle. Phenylbutyrate thus provides an ammonia sink, an alternative pathway for excretion of excess nitrogen and ammonia. The active metabolite phenylacetate is also effective therapeutically, but has a disagreeable odor and taste that affect compliance and acceptability." –*Lippincott 6/e p471*

Phenylbutyrate
• **Phenylbutyrate** is a **prodrug**. In the human body it is **first converted to phenylbutyryl-CoA & metabolized by mitochondrial beta-oxidation**, mainly **in the liver & kidneys**, to the active form, **phenylacetate**^{Q}.
• Phenylacetate conjugates with glutamine to form phenylacetylglutamine, which is readily excreted in the urine. One mole of phenylacetate removes 2 moles of ammonia as glutamine from the body^Q.
• **Sodium phenylbutyrate** is also a **histone deacetylase inhibitor & chemical chaperone**, leading respectively to research into its use as an **anti-cancer agent** and in **protein misfolding diseases** such as **cystic fibrosis**^{Q}.
• Administration during pregnancy is **not recommended** because **sodium phenylbutyrate treatment could mimic maternal phenylketonuria** due to the **production of phenylalanine**, potentially **causing fetal brain damage**^{Q}.

AIIMS ESSENCE

PATHOLOGY

35. **Ans. a. Kimmelstiel-Wilson lesion** *(Ref: Robbins 9/e p1118)*

The clinical findings are suggestive of diabetic retinopathy, neuropathy and nephropathy. The histopathology specimen above is showing pink, hyaline like nodules in the glomerulus, suggestive of Kimmelstiel-Wilson nodules, as well as mesangial sclerosis.

"Nodular Glomerulosclerosis. This is also known as inter-capillary glomerulosclerosis or Kimmelstiel-Wilson disease. The glomerular lesions take the form of ovoid or spherical, often laminated, nodules of matrix situated in the periphery of the glomerulus. The nodules are PAS-positive. They lie within the mesangial core of the glomerular lobules and can be surrounded by patent peripheral capillary loops or loops that are markedly dilated."- Robbins 9/e p1118

Diabetic Nephropathy

- **Kidneys** are **prime targets of diabetes**.
- Renal failure is second only to myocardial infarction as a cause of death from this disease.

Lesions encountered in Diabetic Nephropathy	

Glomerular lesions	• **Most important glomerular lesions**: **Capillary basement membrane thickening, diffuse mesangial sclerosis & nodular glomerulosclerosis**[Q].
	 • **Capillary Basement Membrane Thickening:**
	   – **Widespread thickening of glomerular capillary basement membrane**[Q] **(GBM)** occurs in virtually all cases of diabetic nephropathy
	   – Thickening continues progressively & concurrently with mesangial widening.
	   – Simultaneously thickening of tubular basement membranes occur
	 • **Diffuse Mesangial Sclerosis:**
	   – **Diffuse increase in mesangial matrix**[Q]
	   – Mesangial increase is associated with **overall thickening of GBM**[Q]
	   – Matrix depositions are **PAS-positive**[Q]
	   – **Progressive expansion of mesangium** correlate well with measures of **deteriorating renal function** such as increasing proteinuria[Q].
	 • **Nodular Glomerulosclerosis:**
	   – Also known as **inter-capillary glomerulosclerosis or Kimmelstiel-Wilson disease.**
	   – **Glomerular lesions** take the form of **ovoid or spherical**, often laminated, **nodules of matrix** situated in the **periphery of the glomerulus**[Q].
	   – Nodules are **PAS-positive**; **lie within mesangial core** of glomerular lobules & **surrounded by patent peripheral capillary loops** or loops that are markedly dilated[Q].
	   – Nodules show **features of mesangiolysis** with **fraying of mesangial/ capillary lumen interface** & disruption of sites at which the capillaries are anchored into the mesangial stalks leading to **capillary microaneurysms**[Q]
	   – **All lobules** in individual glomeruli **are not involved by nodular lesions**; **uninvolved lobules & glomeruli** show striking **diffuse mesangial sclerosis**[Q].

	– Accumulations of hyaline material in capillary loops ("fibrin caps") or **adherent to Bowman capsules** ("capsular drops")[Q]. – Both **afferent & efferent glomerular hilar arterioles** show **hyalinosis** leading to **renal ischemia, tubular atrophy, interstitial fibrosis & contraction of renal size**[Q]
Renal vascular lesions (Arteriolosclerosis)	• **Renal atherosclerosis & arteriolosclerosis** constitute part of the macrovascular disease in diabetics[Q]. • **Hyaline arteriolosclerosis** affects both **afferent & efferent arteriole**[Q].
Pyelonephritis & necrotizing papillitis	• **Pyelonephritis** usually **begins in interstitial tissue & spreads to affect the tubules**[Q]. • **Necrotizing papillitis** (**papillary necrosis** Special pattern of acute pyelonephritis, **more prevalent in diabetics**[Q]

AIIMS May 2017

36. Ans. a. Membranous glomerulopathy *(Ref: Robbins 9/e p915, 920; Harrison 19/e p1843)*

In the given clinical picture of Nephrotic syndrome, electron micrograph is showing subepithelial electron-dense deposits along the basement membrane and granular immunofluorescent deposits of IgG along glomerular basement membrane is highly suggestive of membranous glomerulopathy/ nephropathy/ glomerulonephritis.

*"**Membranous Glomerulonephritis:** By light microscopy the glomeruli either appear normal in the early stages of the disease or exhibit **uniform, diffuse thickening of the glomerular capillary wall.** By electron microscopy the thickening is seen to be caused by irregular electron dense also deposits containing immune complexes between the basement membrane and the overlying epithelial cells, with effacement of podocyte foot processes. Basement membrane material is laid down between these deposits, appearing as **irregular spikes protruding from the GBM. Immunofluorescence** microscopy demonstrates that the granular deposits contain both immunoglobulins and complement."- Robbins 9/e p915*

Membranous Glomerulopathy/ Nephropathy/ Glomerulonephritis	
Immunofluorescence Microscopy	**Electron Microscopy**
Characteristic granular immunofluorescent **deposits of IgG along glomerular basement membrane**	Electron micrograph showing **subepithelial electron-dense deposits** along the basement membrane

Deposits seen in various Types of Glomerulonephritis			
Subepithelial Deposits	**Subendothelial Deposits**	**Membranous Deposits**	**Mesangial Deposits**
• **Post-streptococcal** glomerulonephritis[Q] • **Membranous** glomerulonephritis[Q] • **Rapidly progressive** glomerulonephritis[Q] • **Heymann nephritis**[Q]	• **Lupus nephritis**[Q] • **Membranoproliferative** glomerulonephritis[Q] (Type I)	• **Membranoproliferative** glomerulonephritis[Q] (Type II)	• **IgA nephropathy**[Q] • **Henoch-Schonlein purpura**[Q]

Membranous Glomerulonephritis (MGN)
• **MGN or membranous nephropathy** accounts for approximately 30% of cases of nephrotic syndrome in adults   • **Peak incidence: 30-50 years;** Rare in childhood   • **MC cause of nephrotic syndrome in the elderly**[Q].
• Characterized by **diffuse thickening of the glomerular capillary wall** due to the **accumulation of electron-dense, Ig-containing deposits along the subepithelial side** of the **basement membrane**[Q]

Secondary membranous glomerulonephritis	
Infection	• **Hepatitis B & C, syphilis, malaria, schistosomiasis, leprosy, filariasis**
Cancer	• **Breast, colon, lung, stomach**, kidney, esophagus, neuroblastoma
Drugs	• **Gold**[Q], **mercury**[Q], **penicillamine**[Q], **NSAIDs**[Q], **probenecid**[Q]
Autoimmune diseases	• **SLE, rheumatoid arthritis, primary biliary cirrhosis, dermatitis herpetiformis, bullous pemphigoid, myasthenia gravis, Sjogren's syndrome, Hashimoto's thyroiditis**[Q]
Other systemic diseases	• **Fanconi's syndrome, sickle cell anemia, diabetes, Crohn's disease, sarcoidosis, Guillain-Barre syndrome**, Weber-Christian disease, angiofollicular lymph node hyperplasia

Pathogenesis:
- Form of **chronic immune complex–mediated disease**[Q]
- **Secondary MGN**: **Inciting antigens** can sometimes be identified in the **immune complexes**[Q].

Morphology:

Light microscopy	Electron microscopy	Immunofluorescence microscopy
• Uniform, diffuse thickening of the glomerular capillary wall[Q]	• Granular deposits[Q] (Ig + Complement) • Effacement of podocyte foot processes[Q]	• Granular/Lumpy bumpy electron dense immune complex deposits[Q]

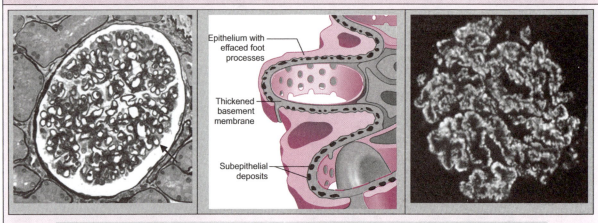

- On silver Methenamine stain: Prominent "spikes & domes" of silver staining matrix[Q]

Clinical Features:
- 80% of patients present with **nephrotic syndrome** & **nonselective proteinuria**[Q].
- **Spontaneous remissions** occur in **20-33% of patients**. Persistent proteinuria in 60% patients
- **10% die or progress to renal failure** within 10 years
- **40%** eventually **develop severe CKD or ESRD.**
- **Recurs in 40% patients who undergo transplantation**[Q]

Complications:
- MGN has the **highest reported incidences of renal vein thrombosis, pulmonary embolism** & DVT among the causes of nephrotic syndrome[Q].

Prognosis:
- **Male gender, older age, hypertension** & **persistence of proteinuria** are associated with **worse prognosis**[Q]
- **Concurrent sclerosis of glomeruli in renal biopsy** at the time of diagnosis is a **predictor of poor prognosis**[Q].

Summary of Salient Features of Major Glomerulonephritides

Disease	Clinical Presentation	Light Microscopy	Fluorescence Microscopy	Electron Microscopy
Post-infectious glomerulonephritis	**Nephritic syndrome**[Q]	Diffuse endocapillary proliferation; leukocytic infiltration	**Granular IgG & C3 in GBM** and mesangium; Granular IgA in some cases[Q]	Primarily **subepithelial humps**; subendothelial deposits in early disease stages.
Goodpasture syndrome	Rapidly progressive glomerulonephritis	Extracapillary proliferation with **crescents; necrosis**[Q]	**Linear IgG & C3; fibrin in crescents**[Q]	**No deposits**; GBM disruptions; fibrin[Q]
Membranous glomerulopathy	**Nephrotic syndrome**[Q]	**Diffuse capillary wall thickening**[Q]	**Granular IgG & C3; diffuse**[Q]	**Subepithelial deposits**[Q]
Minimal change disease	**Nephrotic syndrome**[Q]	Normal; lipid in tubules[Q]	Negative[Q]	Loss of foot processes; no deposits[Q]

Contd...

AIIMS May 2017

Contd...

Disease	Clinical Presentation	Light Microscopy	Fluorescence Microscopy	Electron Microscopy
Focal segmental glomerulosclerosis	**Nephrotic syndrome; non-nephrotic proteinuria**[Q]	**Focal & segmental sclerosis** and **hyalinosis**[Q]	Focal; IgM & C3[Q]	Loss of foot processes; epithelial denudation[Q]
Membranoproliferative glomerulonephritis (MPGN) Type I	**Nephrotic syndrome**[Q]	**Mesangial proliferation; basement membrane thickening; splitting**[Q]	IgG + C3; C1q + C4[Q]	Subendothelial deposits[Q]
Dense-deposit disease (MPGN type II)	**Hematuria Chronic renal failure**[Q]	Mesangial proliferative or membranoproliferative patterns of proliferation; **GBM thickening; splitting**[Q]	C3; no C1q or C4[Q]	Dense deposits[Q]
IgA nephropathy	**Recurrent hematuria or proteinuria**[Q]	Focal mesangial proliferative glomerulonephritis; **mesangial widening**[Q]	IgA ± IgG, IgM, & C3 in mesangium[Q]	Mesangial & paramesangial dense deposits[Q]

37. Ans. a. Multiple myeloma *(Ref: Robbins 9/e p599; Harrison 19/e p720)*

The light microscopy (first picture) is showing hyaline deposits in mesangium, likely amyloid deposits. The peripheral smear (second picture) is showing excess plasma cells in the bone marrow and the EM image (third picture) is showing plasma cells with multiple inclusions clinches the diagnosis of multiple myeloma. Secondary AL type amyloidosis is often seen in multiple myeloma.

"AL amyloidosis is most frequently caused by a clonal expansion of bone-marrow plasma cells that secrete a monoclonal immunoglobulin LC depositing as amyloid fibrils in tissues. Whether the clonal plasma ells produce an LC that misfolds and leads to AL amyloidosis or an LC that folds properly, allowing the cells to inexorably expand over time and develop into multiple myeloma, may depend upon primary sequence or other genetic or epigenetic factors. AL amyloidosis can occur with multiple myeloma or other B lymphoproliferative diseases, including non-Hodgkin's lymphoma and Waldenström's macroglobulinemia."- Harrison 19/e p720

"Multiple myeloma: Certain light chains (particularly those of the λ6 and λ3 families) are prone to cause amyloidosis of the AL type, which can exacerbate renal dysfunction and deposit in other tissues as well."- Robbins 9/e p599

Amyloidosis
• Amyloidosis is a pathological proteinaceous substance **deposited between cells**[Q] in various tissues and organs of the body in a variety of clinical settings.

Types of Amyloid Protein
1. AL (Amyloid Light chain): • This is **derived from plasma cells**[Q] and contains immunoglobulin light chains • Associated with **primary amyloidosis** & immunocyte dyscrasias with amyloidosis like **multiple myeloma**[Q]

2. AA (Amyloid Associate protein):
• It is unique non-immunoglobulin protein synthesized by **reticuloendothelial cells of liver**[Q].
• Associated with **secondary amyloidosis** & **reactive systemic amyloidosis**[Q].
    • **Chronic inflammatory conditions: Tuberculosis**[Q], **Bronchiectasis**[Q], **Osteomyelitis**[Q]
    • **Connective tissue disorders: Rheumatoid Arthritis (MC)**[Q], Ankylosing spondylitis[Q] & Primary biliary cirrhosis[Q]
    • **Non immune derived tumors: Renal cell carcinoma**[Q] **& Hodgkin's lymphoma**[Q]

Contd...

Types of Amyloid Protein
3. β_2 microalbumin (Aβ_2m): **Hemodialysis associated amyloidosis**[Q]
4. β_2 **Amyloid protein**: **Senile cerebral**[Q], **Alzheimer's disease**[Q]
5. **Transthyretin (ATTR)**: **Familial amyloidotic neuropathies**[Q] & **Systemic senile amyloidosis**[Q]
6. **Calcitonin associated amyloid (A cal)**: **Medullary CA thyroid**[Q]
7. **Islet amyloid peptide (AIAPP)**: **Type II DM**[Q]
8. **Atrial natriuretic factor associated amyloid**: Isolated atrial Amyloidosis & Misfolded prion protein (PrPsc) disease

Multiple Myeloma

- **Malignant proliferation of plasma cells in the bone marrow** results in the production of **large number of complete and incomplete immunoglobulins**[Q].
- **Classic triad of multiple myeloma**: Marrow plasmacytosis + Lytic bone lesions + Serum and/or urine M component[Q]

Pathology & Clinical Features:

Bone:

- **Proliferation of plasma cells in bone** and **activation of osteoclast activating factor**[Q] leading to **bone pain (MC)**[Q], pathological fractures & cord compression and hypercalcemia.

  - **Hypercalcemia** can lead to **metastatic calcification & osteoporosis**[Q].
  - **MC bones involved** are **vertebral column**[Q] > ribs > skull > pelvis.
  - Lesions are **punched out defects**[Q].

- Microscopic examination shows increased number of **plasma cells (>30% of marrow cellularity)**[Q].

  - Other cytologic variant include **flame cell**[Q] (with fiery red cytoplasm), **mott cell**[Q] and cells containing inclusion bodies which are **Russel bodies**[Q] **(cytoplasmic) & Dutcher bodies (nuclear)**[Q].

- Remember, multiple myeloma cause **osteolytic lesion**[Q] so, isotopic **bone scan is less useful** than plain radiograph for diagnosis.

Infections:

- Increased susceptibility to bacterial infections due to abnormal immunoglobulins[Q]

  - **MC infections** are **pneumonia & pyelonephritis**[Q]
  - **MC pathogen** is **S. pneumonia & S. aureus**[Q]

Renal Abnormalities:

- **Hypercalcemia** is **MC cause of renal failure** in multiple myeloma
- Renal damage is also contributed by **Bence Jones proteinuria (directly toxic to tubular cells), cast nephropathy & amyloidosis**[Q].
- **Earliest manifestation** of this tubular damage is adult **Fanconi anemia**[Q]

  - **Decreased anion gap**[Q] ($Na^+ - Cl^- + HCO_3^-$) as **M component** is **cationic resulting in retention of Cl$^-$**.

Hematologic abnormality:

- Suppression of normal hematopoietic cells in marrow results in **anemia (normocytic, normochromic)**[Q]
- **Hyperviscosity** leading to **neurological manifestation**[Q] like vertigo, tinnitus, headache, visual disturbances
- Interference with clotting factors & amyloid damage of endothelium leading to bleeding tendency[Q].

Electrophoresis

- **Protein electrophoresis** & **measurement of serum immunoglobulins** and **free light chains** are **useful for detecting & characterizing M spike, supplemented by immunoelectrophoresis**, which is **especially sensitive for identifying low concentrations of M component**, not detectable by protein electrophoresis[Q].

Multiple Myeloma	
Major Criteria	**Minor Criteria**
1. **Plasmacytoma** on tissue biopsy[Q] 2. **Bone marrow plasmacytosis** with **>30% plasma cells**[Q] 3. **Monoclonal globulin spike on serum electrophoresis** exceeding 3.5 gm/dl for IgG or 2 gm/dL for IgA, ≥ 1 gm/24 of k or l light-chain excretion on urine electrophoresis in the presence of amyloidosis[Q].	1. Bone marrow plasmacytosis 10% to 30%[Q] 2. Monoclonal globulin spike present but less than the level defined above[Q] 3. Lytic bone lesions[Q] 4. Suppressed uninvolved immunoglobulins; IgM <50 mg/dL, IgA <100 mg/dL, or IgG <600 mg/dL[Q]

Criteria for Diagnosis of Multiple Myeloma
• 1 Major & 1 minor criteria[Q] • 3 minor criteria that must include 1 & 2 of minor criteria[Q]

Prognostic Factors for Multiple Myeloma	
Tumor **Burden** – Related Factors	Tumor **Biology** – Related factors
• **Beta-2 microglobulin level**[Q] (single most important factor) • **Serum immunoglobulin level**[Q] (increased) • **Number of lytic bone lesions**[Q] • Hemoglobin level • Serum calcium level (**hypercalcemia**)[Q] • Percentage of bone marrow plasmacytosis • Albumin level	• Monosomy 13 or 13q • Plasma cell labeling index • **Renal failure (Azotemia)**[Q] • Mitotic activity • Immunoglobulin A myeloma • C reactive protein level • LDH level • Soluble IL-6 receptor level

38. **Ans. c. EBV positive diffuse large B-cell lymphoma** *(Ref: Robbins 9/e p596, 607; Harrison 19/e p705, 1189)*

History of high-grade fever, tonsillitis and cervical lymphadenopathy with peripheral smear showing lymphocytosis and cells positive for CD20, EBV-LMP1, MUM1, CD79a, negative for CD15 is highly suggestive of EBV positive diffuse large B-cell lymphoma. EBV-LMP1 positive DLBCL is a special variant of DLBCL. Mum-1 DLBCLs are usually advanced B-cell type and can have EBV positivity.

Hodgkins Lymphoma	• **CD15+ve & CD30+ve**
Infectious Mononucleosis	• **Non-malignant lesion, Monospot test positive (in majority) & Mum-1 Negative** • **Splenomegaly** in almost all the cases

"EBV⁺ tumor cells express latent membrane protein-1 (LMP-1), a protein encoded by the EBV genome that transmits signals that up-regulate NF-κB."-Robbins 9/e p607

"Infectious Mononucleosis: The commercially available monospot test for heterophile antibodies is somewhat more sensitive than the classic heterophile test. The monospot test is ~75% sensitive and ~90% specific compared with EBV-specific serologies."- Harrison 19/e p1189

"Pathologic characteristics of EBV-positive DLBCL: Monomorphic pattern displaying large cells with immunoblastic features, characterized by central prominent nucleoli. Positivity for CD20 is consistent with a B-cell lineage. Immunohistochemistry: MUM-1 (nuclear pattern). Most EBV-positive DLBCL of the elderly are positive for MUM-1, consistent with a nongerminal center cell phenotype."– http://theoncologist.alphamedpress.org/content/ 16/1/87.full

"EBV-positive DLBCL Immunophenotypic Features: The neoplastic cells are usually positive for the leukocyte common antigen CD45 as well as for B-cell markers CD20, CD19, CD79a, and PAX-5. The GC markers CD10 and BCL6 are usually negative, whereas IRF4/MUM1 is commonly positive, consistent with a post-GC phenotype. EBV-associated latent antigens such as LMP1 and EBNA-2 are positive in 94% and 28% of the cases, respectively. Up to 50% of the cases express CD30 but CD15 is negative. Ki-67 (or MIB-1), a marker of cellular proliferation, usually is expressed in higher than 70% of the malignant cells."– http://theoncologist.alphamedpress.org/content/16/1/87.full

Epstein-Barr virus–positive Diffuse Large B-cell lymphomas

- Defined as an **EBV-positive monoclonal large B-cell proliferation** that **occurs in patients >50 years of age** and in whom there is **no known immunodeficiency** or **history of lymphoma**[Q].
- Most EBV-positive DLBCL of the elderly patients have an **activated B-cell immunophenotype**[Q]
- It is now being identified in young patients without immuno deficiency.

Immunophenotype of EBV+ DLBL

- **Tumor cells** have **intact B-cell phenotype** with co-expression of CD20, CD79a, PAX5, MUM1[Q]
- Few shows **positivity for Bcl-6 & none express CD10**, indicative of a non-GCB immunophenotype.

EBV Positive DLBL	EBV Positive Mucocutaneous ulcer
• Seen in **immunocompetent** patients[Q] • Age **>50 years** • **70%** of patients present with **extranodal disease**[Q] (most commonly **skin, lung, tonsil & stomach**) with or without simultaneous lymph node[Q] • Cells are **positive for CD20, CD79a, IRF4/MUM1, EBV LMP1 and EBNA negative, CD15 negative**. Background are **predominantly T lymphocytes**[Q]	• Seen in **immunocompromised** patients[Q] • Age **30-50 years** • **Circumscribed ulcer** involving **oropharyngeal mucosa, skin, or GIT**[Q] (not mass forming) • **B-cell immunophenotype** with uniform expression of **CD30, MUM1, PAX5 & OCT-2** with **variable CD20, CD45, CD15, CD79a & BCL-6 expression**[Q].

Diffuse Large B-Cell Lymphoma

- DLBCL: MC type of non-Hodgkin's lymphoma[Q]
- More common in **males;** median age is **60 years**, also occurs in young adults & children.

Special Subtypes of DLBCL

Immunodeficiency-associated Large B-cell Lymphoma	Primary Effusion Lymphoma
• Occurs in the setting of **severe T-cell immunodeficiency** (advanced **HIV infection** & **allogeneic bone marrow transplantation**) • **Neoplastic B cells** are usually **infected with EBV**[Q] • **Restoration of T-cell immunity** may lead to **regression of these proliferations**[Q].	• Presents as a **malignant pleural** or **ascitic effusion**, mostly in patients with **advanced HIV infection** or **older adults**[Q]. • Tumor cells are **anaplastic in appearance** & fail to express surface B- or T-cell markers, but have **clonal IgH gene rearrangements**[Q]. • Tumor cells are **infected with KSHV/HHV-8**[Q]

Pathology:

- **Pathogenesis: Dysregulation of BCL6**; t(14;18) in 10-20% of tumors; **translocations** involving **MYC** in **5%**[Q]

Morphology

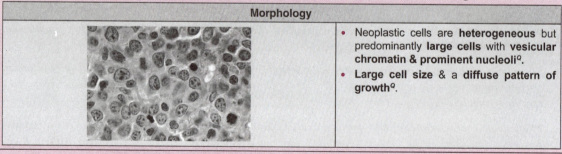

- Neoplastic cells are **heterogeneous** but predominantly **large cells** with **vesicular chromatin & prominent nucleoli**[Q].
- **Large cell size** & a **diffuse pattern of growth**[Q].

Diffuse Large B-Cell Lymphoma

Clinical Features:

- DLBCL typically presents as a **rapidly enlarging mass** at a nodal or extranodal site.
- **Waldeyer's ring** (oropharyngeal lymphoid tissue that includes tonsils & adenoids) is **involved commonly**[Q].
- Primary or secondary involvement of **liver & spleen** may take the form of **large destructive masses**[Q].
- **Extranodal sites:** GIT, skin, bone, brain & bone marrow

Immunophenotype:

- **CD19+ve, CD20+ve, CD10+ve, BCL6+, surface Ig+ve**[Q]

Contd...

Contd...

Diffuse Large B-Cell Lymphoma
Treatment:
• Initial treatment: Combination chemotherapy regimen; **most popular regimen** is **CHOP plus rituximab**[Q]
Prognosis:
• **Poor prognosis** with aggressive course **rapidly fatal without treatment**[Q]

39. Ans. a. SOX11 *(Ref: Robbins 9/e p592; Hematopathology By Elaine Sarkin Jaffe 2/e p414; Diagnostic Histopathology of Tumors By Christopher D. M. Fletcher 4/e p1393*

A new marker for mantle cell lymphoma especially useful in Cyclin D1 negative cases is SOX11.

"SOX11 expression is a highly specific for mantle cell lymphoma and identifies the cyclin D1-negative subtype."-Hematologica, 2009;94(11):1555-62

"The transcription factor SOX11 is a useful marker for the diagnosis of mantle cell lymphoma, including the cyclin D1-negative variant."-Hematopathology By Elaine Sarkin Jaffe 2/e p414

"SOX11, a transcription factor not normally expressed in B cells, is a sensitive and specific marker for mantle cell lymphoma; the staining shows nuclear localization. Cyclin D1-negative mantle cell lymphomas are often positive for SOX11-a feature that facilitates the diagnosis."-Diagnostic Histopathology of Tumors By Christopher D. M. Fletcher 4/e p1393

Mantle Cell Lymphoma (MCL)
• Tumor arising from **mantle zone** which surrounds germinal centres
• More common in **males**; seen in **5th to 6th decade**
Pathology:
• **MCL** has **pathognomonic chromosomal translocation t(11;14)**, leading to **constitutive cyclin D1 overexpression**[Q], which **promotes G1-to-S phase progression** during the cell cycle.
• **Cyclin D1 overexpression** has been detected in **90% of MCL patients**[Q].
• **Morphology of LN**: A homogenous population of **small lymphocytes** with **deeply cleaved nuclear contours**[Q]

Low-power view	High-power view
(Neoplastic lymphoid cells surround a **small, atrophic germinal center**, producing a **mantle zone pattern of growth**[Q])	(Homogeneous population of **small lymphoid cells with irregular nuclear outlines, condensed chromatin & scant cytoplasm**[Q])

Clinical Features:
• **MC presentation: Painless lymphadenopathy**[Q]
• Majority of patients have **generalized lymphadenopathy** at the time of diagnosis with **20-40%** have **peripheral blood involvement**[Q].
• **Sites of extranodal involvement**: Bone marrow, spleen, liver & gut.
• **Mucosal involvement** of **small bowel or colon** produces **polyp-like lesions**[Q] (lymphomatoid polyposis)
Immunophenotype:
• **CD20, CD79a & PAX-5** positive establish B lineage[Q]
• **CD5, CD43, FMC-7, cyclin D1 & SOX11 positive**[Q]
• **Surface IgM & IgD positive**[Q]

Contd...

Mantle Cell Lymphoma (MCL)
• CD5+ve & CD23–ve which help to **distinguish it from CLL/SLL**[Q]   • **SOX11** may be especially **useful in cyclin D1-negative cases of mantle cell lymphoma**[Q]
Treatment: • **Not curable with conventional chemotherapy**; most patients eventually succumb to **organ dysfunction caused by tumor infiltration**[Q].
Prognosis: • Associated with **poor prognosis**; median **survival is 3-4 years**

40. **Ans. c. Mantle zone**   *(Ref: Robbins 9/e p589; Gray's 40/e p74)*
    The marked structure in histopathological examination of lymph node is mantle zone.

    "The mantle zone is produced as surrounding cells are marginalized by the rapidly growing germinal centre. It is populated by cells similar to those found in primary follicles, mainly quiescent B cells with condensed heterochromatic nuclei and little cytoplasm (hence the deeply basophilic staining of this region in routine preparations), a few helper T cells, FDCs and macrophages."-Gray's 40/e p74

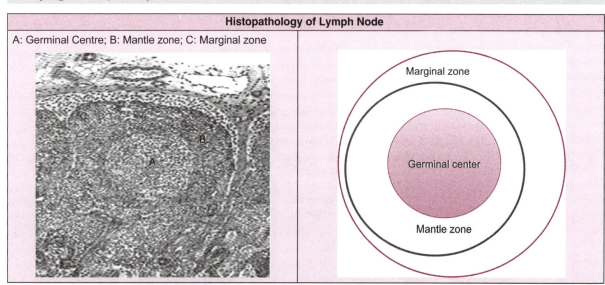

Histopathology of Lymph Node
A: Germinal Centre; B: Mantle zone; C: Marginal zone

Lymph Node
• The structures within a lymph node include: • Capsule & subcapsular sinus • **Cortex (B-cell zone with follicles & germinal centers)**: B-cell zone is further **divided into germinal centre, mantle zone & marginal zone.** • Paracortex (T cell zone) • Medullary sinuses, medullary cords & hilus

B-cell Zone Structures		
Germinal center	**Mantle zone**	**Marginal zone**
• **Round or oval zone containing pale staining cells**, surrounded by darker cells[Q] • CD19+ve, CD20+ve, CD10+ve, CD5–ve[Q]	• **Small unchallenged B-cells surrounding pale staining germinal centers**[Q] • CD19+ve, CD20+ve, CD10–ve, CD5+ve[Q]	• **Light zone surrounding follicles**; contains **post follicular memory B-cells** derived after stimulation of recirculating cells from T cell dependent antigen. • Named "marginal cells" due to **location at interface of lymphoid white pulp & non-lymphoid red pulp** in the spleen[Q] • Marginal zone is **rarely seen except in mesenteric LNs**[Q] • CD19+ve, CD20+ve, CD10–ve, CD5–ve[Q]

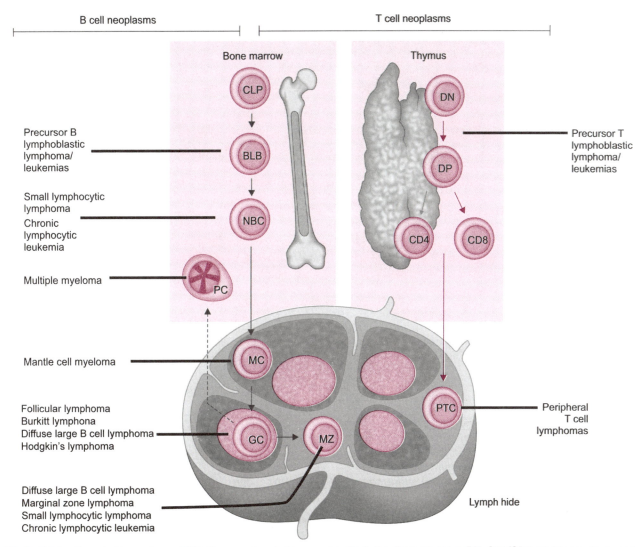

Fig. 9: Origin of lymphoid neoplasms CLP: Common lymphoid precursor; BLB: Pre-B lymphoblast; DN: CD4/CD8 double-negative pro-T cell; DP: CD4/CD8 double-positive pre-T cell; GC: Germinal-center B cell; MC: Mantle B cell; MZ: Marginal zone B cell; NBC: Naive B cell; PTC: Peripheral T cell

41. **Ans. a. Transferrin receptor-1 iron responsive elements increase transferrin receptor mRNA concentration and synthesis** *(Ref: Williams Hematology 9/e p624; Wintrobes 13/e p624)*

In iron deficiency anemia, transferrin receptor-1 iron responsive elements increase transferrin receptor mRNA concentration and synthesis.

> "The regulation of iron metabolism at the cytoplasmic mRNA level by interaction of iron regulatory protein (IRP-1) and the iron-responsive elements (IREs) to apoferritin mRNA and transferrin receptor mRNA. When the cytoplasmic iron concentration is low, IRP-1 binds to the IREs of both mRNAs. This represents the translation of Apoferritin mRNA, where the IRE is at the 5' end of the mRNA, thereby reducing the amount of apoferritin formed. It stabilizes and increases the translation of TfR mRNA where the IRE is at the 3' end of the mRNA, thereby increasing the amount of TfR formed. Conversely, when there is an abundance of iron in the cytoplasm, IRP-1 is displaced from both species of mRNA. This results in depression of apoferritin synthesis and destabilization and degradation of TfR mRNA."
> - *Williams Hematology 9/e p624*

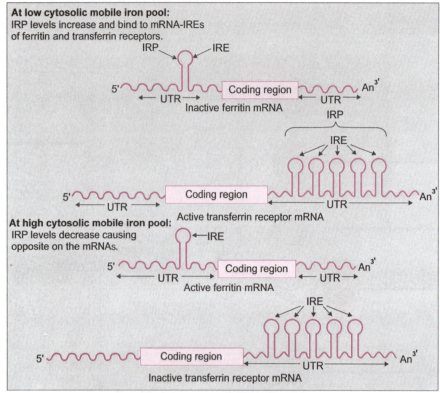

	Iron deficiency	Iron excess
Iron Uptake	↑	↓
Transferrin receptor synthesis	↑	↓
Transferrin mRNA concentration	↑	↓
Iron storage	↓	↑
Ferritin synthesis	↓	↑
Ferritin mRNA concentration	No change	No change

42. **Ans. d. Sweet's reticulin stain** *(Ref: Robbins 10/e p163)*

   Gordon and Sweet's silver staining method is used to stain reticulin fibers. In a properly stained slide, appearance is as follows- Red: nuclei, light red: cytoplasm, black: reticulin.

   > "Gordon and Sweet's Reticulin Stain: Identification of type III collagen; Evaluation of lobular architecture and hepatocyte plate thickness in dysplastic nodules, hepatocellular carcinoma, and nodular regenerative hyperplasia." - *Liver Pathology By Arief A Suriawinata /p8*

Gordon and Sweet's Stain for Reticulin
• **Connective tissue stain; Mechanism of staining: Argyrophil metallic impregnation**[Q]
• **Stains reticulin fibres** in **liver, spleen & lymph nodes**[Q]
• Properly stained slide: Red: nuclei, Light Red: cytoplasm, **Black: reticulin**[Q]
• Used to diagnose **hemangiopericytoma, endothelial cells tumors, myelofibrosis & liver fibrosis**[Q].

Special Stains for Liver	
Masson's trichrome stain	• Stain imparts a **blue color to collagen** against a **red background of hepatocytes** & other structures[Q].
	• It **stains type 1 collagen** that is normally present in portal tracts & vessel walls, but also highlights the presence and distribution of reactive fibrosis as a result of liver injury.
	• Used for **staging of chronic liver diseases**, helps to **delineate patterns of injury**, such as perisinusoidal fibrosis associated with steatohepatitis & periductal fibrosis in **primary sclerosing cholangitis**[Q].

Contd...

Contd...

Reticulin stain	• Reticulin stain uses silver impregnation to detect reticulin fibers, which are **made of type III collagen**[Q]. • **Reticulin fibers appear black** against a gray to light pink background[Q]. • In liver, such fibers are present as part of the extracellular matrix in the space of Disse. By highlighting these fibers, **stain helps in the assessment of architecture of hepatic plates**, such as **expansion in regenerative & neoplastic conditions, compression of plates in nodular regenerative hyperplasia & collapse of reticulin framework in necrosis**[Q].
Pearl's iron stain (Prussian blue reaction)	• Iron is stored in the hepatocytes as a soluble form (ferritin) & an insoluble form (hemosiderin). With the H&E stain, the latter is seen as coarsely granular brown refractile granules in the cytoplasm, whereas ferritin is not seen. • **Pearl's stain highlights hemosiderin** as **coarse blue granules**, while **ferritin** is seen as a **faint blue cytoplasmic blush**[Q].
Periodic acid— Schiff stain	• Useful for **identifying glycogen**, but **removing glycogen with diastase digestion enhances detection of non-digested material**, including the **alpha-1-antitrypsin globules, basement membrane, debris within macrophages & fungal organisms**, e.g. various glycogen storage diseases[Q]. • In patients with **alpha-1-antitrypsin deficiency**, accumulation is seen as **bright magenta globules**, typically in periportal hepatocytes[Q].
Congo-red stain	• Used to **assess amyloid deposition** and is **combined with polarization microscopy** to demonstrate the characteristic **apple-green birefringence**[Q].
Oil-red 'O' stain	• Used to highlight the **presence of fat globules**, with its most common application being **evaluation of pre-transplantation donor liver biopsies**[Q]. • Stain is **used on frozen sections** of liver tissue[Q].
Rhodamine stain	• Used to **detect copper-binding protein**, used to **evaluate Wilson disease**[Q]. • Stain can be used in the differential diagnosis of biliary (versus non-biliary) disease.

For Minerals, Pigments and Miscellaneous	
Name of stain	**Elements stained**
Von Kossa's stain (MC used) **Alizarin red S** at pH 4.2 (specific for Calcium)	**Calcium**[Q]
Prussian blue	**Iron**[Q]
Fontana Masson Silver stain	**Melanin**[Q]
Modified Fouchet's	**Bile pigments**[Q]
Orcein Modified rhodamine (method of choice)	**Copper**[Q]

For Connective Tissue and Lipids	
Name of stain	**Elements stained**
Trichrome Stain	**Collagen**[Q]
Verhoeff-Van Gieson stain (Best for Elastin)	**Elastic fibers**[Q]
Luna stain	Elastin & Mast cells
Silver Methenamine stain	**Reticulin**[Q]
Oil red 'O' stain (on Fresh specimen) **Sudan black** (on fixed specimen)	**Fat**[Q]
Mallory's PTAH stain	**Muscle striations**
Martius scarlet blue (MSB)	**Fibrin**[Q]
PAS, Silver Methenamine stain	**Basement membrane**[Q]
Bielschowsky (silver stain)	**Neurofibrillary tangles senile plaques**[Q]
Luxol fast blue	**Myelin**[Q]

43. **Ans. b. Sclerodactyly, esophageal dysmotility and Raynaud's phenomenon** *(Ref: Robbins 9/e p219, 226; Harrison 19/e p2163)*

Nucleolar ANA positivity is most likely suggestive of systemic sclerosis or scleroderma, which comprises of diffuse or limited disease—CREST syndrome (Calcinosis, Raynaud syndrome, Esophageal dysmotility, Sclerodactyly, Telangiectasia)

"Antinuclear antibodies (ANAs): Nucleolar pattern refers to the presence of a few discrete spots of fluorescence within the nucleus and represents antibodies to RNA. This pattern is reported most often in patients with systemic sclerosis."- *Robbins 9/e p219*

"Antinuclear autoantibodies are present in almost all patients with SSc and can be detected at disease onset. Autoantibodies against topoisomerase-I (Scl-70) and centromere are specific for SSc and are mutually exclusive. Topoisomerase-I antibodies are detected in 31% of patients with dcSSc, but in only 13% of patients with lcSSc; conversely, anticentromere antibodies are detected in 38% of patients with lcSSc, but in only 2% of patients with dcSSc. Nucleolar immunofluorescence pattern on serologic testing reflects antibodies to U3-RNP (fibrillarin), Th/To, or PM/Scl, whereas a speckled immunofluorescence pattern indicates antibodies to RNA polymerase III."– *Harrison 19/e p2163*

44. **Ans. d. Inflammatory myofibroblastic tumor** *Ref: Robbins 9/e p721; Diagnostic Histopathology of Tumors by Christopher D.M. Fletcher 4/e p810)*

Inflammatory myofibroblastic tumor is anaplastic lymphoma kinase (ALK) positive neoplasm.

"Inflammatory myofibroblastic tumor, though rare, is more common in children, with an equal male-to-female ratio. Presenting symptoms include fever, cough, chest pain, and hemoptysis. It may also be asymptomatic. Imaging studies show a single (rarely multiple) round, well-defined, usually peripheral mass with calcium deposits in about a quarter of cases. Grossly, the lesion is firm, 3 to 10 cm in diameter, and grayish white. Microscopically, there is proliferation of spindle-shaped fibroblasts and myofibroblasts, lymphocytes, plasma cells, and peripheral fibrosis. Some of these tumors have activating rearrangements of the anaplastic lymphoma kinase (ALK) gene, located on 2p23, and treatment with ALK kinase inhibitors have produced sustained responses in such cases."– *Robbins 9/e p721*

Anaplastic Lymphoma Kinase (ALK)

- **Anaplastic lymphoma kinase** also known as **ALK tyrosine kinase receptor** or **CD246** (cluster of differentiation 246) is an enzyme that in humans is **encoded by ALK gene.**
- The **2;5 chromosomal translocation** is associated with **60% anaplastic large-cell lymphomas** (ALCLs). **Translocation creates a fusion gene** consisting of **ALK gene & nucleophosmin (NPM) gene:** the 3' half of ALK, derived from chromosome 2 & coding for the catalytic domain, is fused to the 5' portion of NPM from chromosome 5[Q].

  - **EML4-ALK fusion gene** is responsible for approximately 3-5% of **non-small-cell lung cancer** (NSCLC). Also related to **Neuroblastomas[Q].**
  - **Germline mutations in anaplastic lymphoma kinase (ALK) gene** have recently been identified as a **major cause of familial predisposition to neuroblastoma[Q].**

Anaplastic Lymphoma Kinase (ALK) Positive Neoplasms

• **Anaplastic large-cell lymphomas[Q]**	• Esophageal SCC
• **Adenocarcinoma of lung[Q]**	• Breast cancer (inflammatory subtype)
• **Familial neuroblastoma[Q]**	• Colonic adenocarcinoma
• **Inflammatory myofibroblastic tumor[Q]**	• Glioblastoma multiforme
• Adult & pediatric RCC	• Anaplastic thyroid cancer

45. **Ans. a. CRISPR** *(Ref: Robbins 10/e p5-6)*

Clustered Regularly Interspaced Short Palindromic Repeats (CRISPRs) is a tool used in gene editing.

"Gene Editing: Exciting new developments that permit exquisitely specific genome editing stand to usher in an era of molecular revolution. These advances come from a wholly unexpected source: the discovery of clustered regularly interspaced short palindromic repeats (CRISPRs) and Cas (or CRISPR-associated genes). These are linked genetic elements that endow prokaryotes with a form of acquired immunity to phages and plasmids. Bacteria use this system to sample the DNA of infecting agents, incorporating it into the host genome as CRISPRs. CRISPRs are transcribed and processed into an RNA sequence that binds and directs the nuclease Cas9 to a sequences (e.g., a phage), leading to its cleavage and the destruction of the phage. Gene editing repurposes this process by using artificial guide RNAs (gRNAs) that bind Cas9 and complimentary to a DNA sequence of interest. Once directed to the target sequence by the gRNA, Cas9 induces double-strand DNA breaks."– *Robbins 10/e p5*

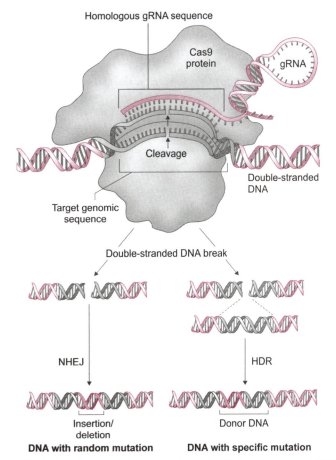

Fig. 10: Gene editing with clustered regularly interspaced short palindromic repeats (CRISPRs)/Cas9

In bacteria, DNA sequences consisting of CRISPRs are transcribed into guide RNA (gRNAs) with a constant region and a variable sequence of about 20 bases. The constant region of gRNAs bind to Cas9, permitting the variable region to form heteroduplexes with homologous host cell DNA sequences. The Cas9 nuclease then cleaves the bound DNA, producing a double-stranded DNA break. To perform gene editing, gRNAs are designed with variable regions that are homologous to a target DNA sequence of interest. Co-expression of the gRNA and Cas9 in cells leads to efficient cleavage of the target sequence. In the absence of homologous DNA, the broken DNA is repaired by non-homologous end joining (NHEJ), an error-prone method that often introduces disruptive insertions or deletions (indels). By contrast, in the presence of a homologous "donor" DNA spanning the region targeted by CRISPR/Cas9, cells instead may use homologous DNA recombination (HDR) to repair the DNA break. HDR is less efficient that NHEJ, but has the capacity to introduce precise changes in DNA sequence> potential applications of CRISPR/Cas9 couples with the repair of inherited genetic defects and the creation of pathogenic mutations."

Genome Editing

- A type of genetic engineering in which **DNA is inserted, deleted or replaced in the genome** of a **living organism** using **engineered nucleases**, or **"molecular scissors"**[Q]
- These **nucleases create site-specific double-strand breaks (DSBs)** at **desired locations** in the genome[Q].
- The **induced double-strand breaks** are **repaired through non- homologous end-joining (NHEJ)** or **homologous recombination (HR)**, resulting in **targeted mutations ('edits')**.

Four Families of Engineered Nucleases being used	
• Meganucleases	• Zinc finger nucleases (ZFNs)[Q]
• Transcription Activator-Like Effector-based Nucleases (TALEN)[Q]	• Clustered Regularly Interspaced Short Palindromic Repeats (CRISPR)-Cas system[Q]

Clustered Regularly Interspaced Short Palindromic Repeats (CRISPR)

- Segments of **prokaryotic DNA** containing **short, repetitive base sequences**^{Q}.
- **Form the basis of a genome editing technology** known as **CRISPR/Cas9** that **allows permanent modification of genes within organisms**^{Q}.
- In a **palindromic repeat**, the **sequence of nucleotides is the same in both directions**. Each repetition is followed by short segments of spacer DNA from previous exposures to foreign DNA (e.g., a virus or plasmid).
- **Small clusters of Cas** (CRISPR-associated system) **genes** are **located next to CRISPR sequences**^{Q}.

  - **CRISPR/Cas system** is a prokaryotic immune system that **confers resistance to foreign genetic elements** such as **those present within plasmids & phages** that **provide a form of acquired immunity**.

- RNA harboring the spacer sequence helps Cas proteins recognize and cut exogenous DNA. Other RNA-guided Cas proteins cut foreign RNA .
- A simple version of the CRISPR/Cas system, CRISPR/Cas9, has been modified to edit genomes.

  - By delivering the Cas9 nuclease complexed with a synthetic guide RNA (gRNA) into a cell, the cell's genome can be cut at a desired location, allowing existing genes to be removed and/or new ones added^Q.
  - **CRISPR/Cas genome editing techniques** have many potential applications, including **medicine & crop seed enhancement**^{Q}.

46. **Ans. b. PAX5**   *(Ref: Robbins 9/e p590)*

PAX5 is a B-cell transcription factor, essential in normal B-cell lymphopoiesis. T-cell never express PAX5 throughout its development. CD-1a, CD34 and Tdt are expressed on T-cells.

Lineage Antigen	
B cell	• **CD19, CD20, CD22, CD79a, cCD22, cCD79a**^{Q}
T cell	• **CD1, CD2, CD3, CD4, CD5, CD7, CD8, cCD3, lymphoid TdT**^{Q}
Myeloid	• **CD4, CD11b, CD13, CD15, CD33, CD117, cMPO**^{Q}
Monocytic	• **CD14, CD11b**^{Q}
Erythroid	• **Glycophorin A**^{Q}
Megakaryocyte	• **CD41, CD61, CDK41, CCD61**^{Q}

Lineage Independent Antigen	
Leucocyte common antigen	• **CD45**^{Q}
Stem cell antigen	• **CD34**^{Q}
Common acute lymphoblastic leukemia antigen	• **CD10**^{Q}

Immune Cell Antigens Detected by Monoclonal Antibodies	
Antigen Designation	**Normal Cellular Distribution**
PRIMARILY T-CELL ASSOCIATED	
CD1	**Thymocytes & Langerhans cells**^{Q}
CD3	**Thymocytes, mature T cells**^{Q}
CD4	**Helper T cells**^{Q}, subset of thymocytes
CD5	T cells & a small subset of B cells
CD8	**Cytotoxic T cells**^{Q}, subset of thymocytes & some NK cells
PRIMARILY B-CELL ASSOCIATED	
CD10	**Pre-B cells & germinal-center B cells**^{Q}; also called **CALLA**^{Q} (common acute lymphoblastic leukemia antigen)
CD19	**Pre-B cells & mature B cells**^{Q} but not plasma cells
CD20	**Pre-B cells after CD19 & mature B cells**^{Q} but not plasma cells
CD21	**EBV receptor**^{Q}; mature B cells & **follicular dendritic cells**^{Q}
CD23	**Activated mature B cells**^{Q}
CD79a	**Marrow pre-B cells & mature B cells**^{Q}

PRIMARILY MONOCYTE- OR MACROPHAGE-ASSOCIATED	
CD11c	Granulocytes, monocytes & macrophages; also expressed by hairy cell leukemias[Q]
CD13	Immature & mature monocytes & granulocytes[Q]
CD14	Monocytes[Q]
CD15	Granulocytes; Reed-Sternberg cells[Q] & variants
CD33	Myeloid progenitors & monocytes[Q]
CD64	Mature myeloid cells[Q]
PRIMARILY NK-CELL ASSOCIATED	
CD16	NK cells & granulocytes[Q]
CD56	NK cells[Q] & a subset of T cells
PRIMARILY STEM CELL–AND PROGENITOR CELL–ASSOCIATED	
CD34	Pluripotent hematopoietic stem cells[Q] & progenitor cells of many lineages
ACTIVATION MARKERS	
CD30	Activated B cells, T cells & monocytes[Q]; Reed-Sternberg cells[Q] & variants
PRESENT ON ALL LEUKOCYTES	
CD45	All leukocytes[Q]; also known as leukocyte common antigen (LCA)

47. **Ans. b. 3** *(Ref: Harrison 19/e p396; Clinical Hematology by Turgeon 4/e p77)*

Corrected reticulocyte count will be 3.

Corrected Reticulocyte Count

- **Reticulocyte count** needs to be **corrected for anemia** as it is a **percentage of the total RBC count** and **spuriously elevated when the number of RBCs fall in anemia.**
- Reticulocyte percentage may be increased due to **more reticulocytes in circulation** & fewer mature cells.

> **Corrected reticulocyte count = Reticulocyte % × Hematocrit/ Expected hematocrit or**
> **= Reticulocyte % × Hemoglobin/Expected hemoglobin**
> **= 9 × 5/15 = 3**

48. **Ans. c. Albumin** *(Ref: Robbins 10/e p86; Bailey 26/e p9)*

Albumin is a negative acute phase reactant whereas ferritin, CRP and haptoglobin are positive phase reactants.

> *"The serum levels of most proteins either increase or decrease during the acute phase response. Serum proteins that decrease levels during inflammation are called negative acute phase reactants (e.g., albumin and prealbumin) and are expected to return to normal as the inflammatory process resolves. Positive acute phase reactants are proteins that increase levels during times of stress because they are essential for the immune response. C-reactive protein, fibrinogen, protein S, and fibronectin are examples of positive acute phase reactants."* – *Acute & Chronic Wounds: Current Management Concepts By Ruth A. Bryant, Denise P. Nix 5/e p412*

Acute Phase Proteins (Acute Phase Reactants)

- **Acute phase proteins** are defined as those proteins whose **plasma concentrations increase (positive acute phase proteins)** or **decrease (negative acute phase proteins)** by at least 25% during inflammatory states.
- **Negative phase proteins** are **consumed for the production of positive phase proteins** during inflammatory reaction.

Positive Acute Phase Reactants	Negative Acute Phase Reactants
- **C-reactive protein[Q] (CRP)** - **Serum amyloid A[Q]** - **Haptoglobin[Q]** - **Ceruloplasmin[Q]** - α2-Macroglobulin[Q] - α1-Acid glycoprotein[Q] - **Fibrinogen[Q]** - **Complement (C3, C4)[Q]**	- **Albumin & prealbumin[Q]** - **Transferrin[Q]** - **Transthyretin[Q]** - Retinol-binding protein[Q]

49. **Ans. a. Red**   *(Ref: Robbins 9/e p544)*

Triphenyltetrazolium chloride (TTC) stain imparts a brick-red color to intact, non-infarcted myocardium where the dehydrogenase enzymes are preserved.

> "Early morphologic recognition of acute MI can be difficult, particularly when death occurs within a few hours of the onset of symptoms. **MIs less than 12 hours old are usually not apparent on gross examination.** However, **if the infarct preceded death by 2 to 3 hours, it is possible to highlight the area of necrosis by immersion of tissue slices in a solution of triphenyltetrazolium chloride.** This gross histochemical stain imparts a brick-red color to intact, non-infarcted myocardium where lactate dehydrogenase activity is preserved. Because dehydrogenases leak out through the damaged membranes of dead cells, **an infarct appears as an unstained pale zone. By 12 to 24 hours after infarction, an MI can usually be identified grossly as a reddish-blue area of discoloration caused by stagnated, trapped blood.** *Thereafter, the infarct becomes progressively more sharply defined, yellow-tan, and soft.* **By 10 days to 2 weeks, it is rimmed by a hyperemic zone of highly vascularized granulation tissue.** Over the succeeding weeks, the injured region evolves to a fibrous scar." – *Robbins 9/e p544*

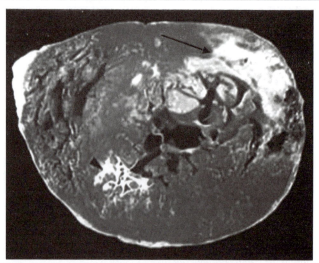

Myocardial Infarction (MI)
• MI is result of **acute plaque changes** that induces an **abrupt thrombotic occlusion**, resulting in **myocardial necrosis**.

Types of Myocardial infarction		
Subendocardial MI	**Transmural MI**	**Multifactorial Microinfarction**
• Ischemic necrosis limited to **1/3rd of ventricular wall**[Q] • Caused by **incomplete coronary artery occlusion**[Q]	• Ischemic necrosis **involves full thickness of ventricular wall**[Q] • Caused by **severe coronary atherosclerosis, with acute plaque rupture & superimposed occlusive thrombus**[Q]	• Occurs in setting of **microembolization, vasculitis or vascular spasm**[Q] • Can lead to **sudden cardiac death** (by fatal arrhythmia) or **ischemic dilated cardiomyopathy**[Q]

Pathogenesis of MI
Changes in atheromatous plaque[Q] (hemorrhage/ulceration/rupture) ↓ Exposure of underlying collagen and platelet aggregation[Q] ↓ Platelets release mediators which cause vasospasm[Q] ↓ Activation of extrinsic clotting pathway and increased thrombus formation[Q] ↓ Complete occlusion of coronary vessel by thrombus[Q]

Myocardial Response	
Feature	Time
Cessation of aerobic respiration or onset of ATP depletion	Seconds
Loss of contractility	<2 min^Q
ATP reduced to 50% of normal	10 min^Q
ATP reduced to 10% of normal	40 min^Q
Irreversible cell injury	20-40 min^Q
Microvascular injury	>1 hour^Q

Evolution of Morphological Changes in MI		
Time	Gross	Light Microscopy
Reversible injury		
0-30 min	None	None
Irreversible injury		
30 min to 4 hour	None	Waviness of fibers at border (earliest change)^Q
4-12 hour	None	Beginning of coagulative necrosis, edema and hemorrhage
12-24 hour	Dark mottling	On going coagulative necrosis, marginal contraction band necrosis, beginning of neutrophilic infiltration^Q
1-3 days	Mottling with yellow tan infarct centre	Coagulation necrosis, interstitial neutrophilic infiltrate^Q
3-7 days	Hyperemic borders, central yellow tan softening	Beginning of disintegration with dying neutrophils, early phagocytosis by macrophages^Q
7-10 days	Maximum yellow tan and soft depressed red-tan margin	Early formation of fibrovascular granulation tissue at margins^Q
10-14 days	Red grey depressed infarct borders	Well established granulation tissue & collagen deposition^Q
2-8 weeks	Grey-white scar progressive from border towards infarct core	Collagen deposition, ↓ Cellularity^Q
> 2 months	Scarring complete	Dense collagenous scar^Q

Diagnosis of MI:

- MI should be suspected in any patient developing **severe chest pain, rapid weak pulse, sweating, dyspnea & edema**. **Rapid pulse is first sign** and **dyspnea is first symptom of acute MI**. ECG shows **ST segment elevation** in **acute MI** whereas 'Q' wave indicates old MI^Q.
- Laboratory investigations show **nonspecific markers** like **increased ESR, leucocytosis & elevated C-reactive protein**^{Q}.

Specific Markers of MI			
Enzyme	Initiation of rise	Peak	Return to baseline
CK-MB	2-4 hours^Q	24 hours^Q	48-72 hours^Q
Troponin T and I (TnT, TnI)	2-4 hours^Q	48 hours^Q	7-10 days^Q
AST/SGOT	In 12 hours^Q	48 hours^Q	4-5 days^Q
LDH	24 hours^Q	3-6 days^Q	2 weeks^Q

AIIMS ESSENCE

Complications of MI	
Contractile dysfunction	• Leads to cardiogenic shock[Q] • Right ventricular infarcts can cause right-sided heart failure
Arrhythmias	• MC arrhythmia within one hour: Ventricular fibrillation[Q] • MC arrhythmia after one hour: Supraventricular tachycardia[Q]
Myocardial rupture	• MC occurs after 3-7 days of MI[Q] • MC site: Rupture of ventricular free wall[Q] • MC site of free wall rupture: Anterolateral wall at the **midventricular level**[Q] • Least common site: Rupture of papillary muscle[Q]
Ventricular aneurysm	• Late complication, can lead to **mural thrombus, arrhythmias** & **heart failure**[Q]
Pericarditis	• Develop on 2nd or 3rd day following transmural infarct as a result of underlying myocardial infarction (Dressler syndrome[Q])
Infarct expansion	• Occurs as a result of weakening of necrotic muscle[Q] (especially with anteroseptal infarcts)
Mural thrombus	• Can lead to **thromboembolism**
Papillary muscle dysfunction	• Most **post-infarct regurgitation** results from **ischemic dysfunction**[Q] of a papillary muscle

50. **Ans. a. Cell cycle will stop at G1 phase** *(Ref: Robbins 9/e p292)*

Rb is a tumor suppressor gene. It normally arrests cell division at G1-S phase. Phosphorylation of Rb gene allows the cell to divide, hence inhibition of phosphorylation (which is the constitutive scenario for Rb gene) arrests the cell in G1 phase.

"RB: Governor of Proliferation. RB, a key negative regulator of the G1/S cell cycle transition, is directly or indirectly inactivated in most human cancers. RB also controls cellular differentiation. It exists in an active hypophosphorylated state in quiescent cells and an inactive hyperphosphorylated state in cells passing through the G_1/S cell cycle transition. "- Robbins 9/e p292

Tumor Suppressor Genes	
RB (Retinoblastoma) gene	**p53 gene**
• Located on **chromosome no 13q14**[Q] • **Tumor suppressive pocket protein** that binds E2F transcription factors in hypophophorylated state[Q] • Key negative regulator of G_1/S cell cycle transition[Q] • **Tumors associated:** Retinoblastoma, osteosarcoma, Glioblastoma, small cell carcinoma of lung, CA breast & CA bladder[Q]	• Located on **chromosome no 17q13.1**[Q] • **p53 is universally expressed in all cells** & encodes a 53 kDa protein[Q] • **Regulates cell cycle progression, DNA repair, cellular senescence & apoptosis**[Q] • p53 activates CDK inhibitor (p21)→ Inhibits cyclin-CDK complexes →Inhibits phosphorylation of RB →arrests cell cycle at G_1S phase[Q] • **p53 gene** is the **tumor suppressor gene altered in >50% of human cancers**[Q] • p53 mutation causes: Brain tumors, CA breast, Leukemia, adrenal carcinoma & sarcoma[Q]

*Hypophosphorylated RB in complex with the E2F transcription factors binds to DNA, recruits chromatin-remodeling factors (histone deacetylases and histone methyltransferases), and inhibits transcription of genes whose products are required for the S phase of the cell cycle. When RB is phosphorylated by the cyclin D-CDK4, cyclin D-CDK6, and cyclin E-CDK2 complexes, it releases E2F. The latter then activates transcription of S-phase genes. **The phosphorylation of RB is inhibited by cyclin-dependent kinase inhibitors, because they inactivate cyclin-CDK complexes. Virtually all cancer cells show dysregulation of the G1-S checkpoint as a result of mutation in one of four genes that regulate the phosphorylation of RB; these genes are RB, CDK4, the genes encoding cyclin D proteins, and CDKN2A (p16). TGF-β, transforming growth factor-β.***

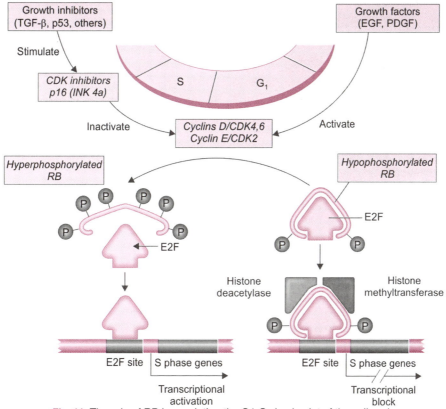

Fig. 11: The role of RB in regulating the G1-S checkpoint of the cell cycle

Cell Cycle
• Cell cycle is the sequence of events that results in cell division. • It consists of five phases. Sequence: $G_0 \to G_1 \to S \to G_2 \to M^Q$

G_0	G_1	S	G_2	M
• Quiescent state^Q • Cells that are not actively cycling are said to be in G0 state^Q	• Presynthetic phase^Q • Radiation exposure leads to chromo-somal aberration^Q	• Synthetic phase^Q • DNA synthesis occurs with doubling of nuclear content^Q • Called as "Point of no return"^{Q} • Most radioresistant phase^Q	• Pre-mitotic growth^Q • Radiation exposure leads to chromatid aberration	• Mitotic phase • Cell numbers are doubled^Q • Most radiosensitive phase^Q

• Radiation energy is absorbed by tissue causing ionization or excitation^Q, which are responsible for various biological effects.
• Susceptibility of various phases of cell cycle to radiation: $G_2M^Q > G_2 > M > G_1 >$ Early S > Late S Phase^Q.

Cell-cycle Checkpoints	
G_1/S Checkpoint	G_2/M Checkpoint
• Checks for DNA damage before replication in 'S' phase^Q • Arrest the cell cycle if damage is present^Q • Activates DNA repair mechanism^Q • DNA can be repaired only as long as the chromatids have not separated • Defects at G_1/S checkpoint are more important in cancer^Q	• Used for repair of DNA damage after replication^Q • Monitors the completion of DNA replication^Q • Checks weather cell can safely initiate mitosis & separate sister chromatids^Q • Defects in this checkpoint give rise to chromosomal abnormalities^Q • Important checkpoint in cells exposed to ionizing radiation • Cell exposed to ionizing radiation → Cell cycle arrested in G_2 →Repair mechanism activated^Q

Requirement of cell cycle Checkpoints		
Sensors of DNA Damage	**Signal Transducers**	**Effector Molecules**
• In G_1S & G_2M: RAD family & ATM (Ataxia telangiectasia mutates)	• In G_1S & G_2M: CHK kinase families	• In G_1S checkpoint: p53, which **induces the cell cycle inhibitor p21** • In G_2M checkpoint: Both p53 dependent & independent mechanisms

Cyclins & Cyclin-Dependent Kinases (CDK)		
Cyclins	**Cyclin-Dependent Kinases (CDK)**	**CDK Inhibitors (CDKI)**
• Proteins with **cyclic production & degradation** that derive cell cycle progression[Q]	• **Cyclin associated enzymes** that require the **ability to phosphorylate protein substrates by forming complexes with relevant cyclins**[Q]	• Proteins that **block the cell cycle by binding to cyclin-CDK complexes**[Q]

Cyclin-Dependent Kinases (CDK)	
Type	**Function**
CDK4	• Forms a **complex with cyclin D** that **phosphorylates** RB, allowing the **cell to progress through the G_1 restriction point**[Q].
CDK2	• Forms a **complex with cyclin E in late G_1**, which is **involved in G_1/S transition**[Q]. • Forms a **complex with cyclin A at the S phase that facilitates G_2/M transition**[Q].
CDK1	• Forms a **complex with cyclin B that facilitates G_2/M transition**[Q].

Checkpoints	Cyclin	CDK
G1-S	Cyclin D[Q]	CDK4/ CDK6[Q]
	Cyclin E[Q]	CDK2[Q]
G2-M	Cyclin A[Q]	CDK2/ CDK1[Q]
	Cyclin B[Q]	CDK1[Q]

Cell-cycle Inhibitors			
Family	**Checkpoints**	**Proteins**	**Functions**
CIP/KIP	G_1-S & G_2-M	p21, p27, p57	• **Block the cell cycle** by binding to **cyclin-CDK complexes**[Q] • **p21 is induced by p53**[Q] • **p27 responds to TGF-beta**[Q]
INK4/ARF (CDKN2A-D)	G_1-S	p15, p16, p18, p19	• **p16/INK41 binds to cyclin D-CDK4** & promotes inhibitory effects of RB[Q] • **p14/ARF increases p53 levels by inhibiting MDM2 activity**[Q]

Checkpoints Components	
Ataxia-telangiectasia mutated	**p53 gene**
• Activated by mechanisms that **sense double-stranded DNA breaks.** • **Transmits signals to arrest the cell cycle after DNA damage.** • **Acts through p53 in the G_1/S checkpoint**[Q]. • At the G_2/M checkpoint, it acts **both through p53-dependent mechanisms** and through the **inactivation of CDC25 phosphatase**, which **disrupts the cyclin B–CDK1 complex**[Q]. • Component of a network of genes that include *BRCA1* and *BRCA2*, which **link DNA damage with cell cycle arrest & apoptosis**[Q].	• Tumor suppressor gene **altered in the majority of cancers** • Causes **cell cycle arrest & apoptosis.** • Acts **mainly through p21 to cause cell cycle arrest.** • Causes **apoptosis by inducing the transcription of pro-apoptotic genes such as** *BAX*[Q]. • Levels of p53 are **negatively regulated by MDM2** through a feedback loop. • p53 is **required for the G_1/S checkpoint** and is a **main component of the G_2/M checkpoint**[Q].

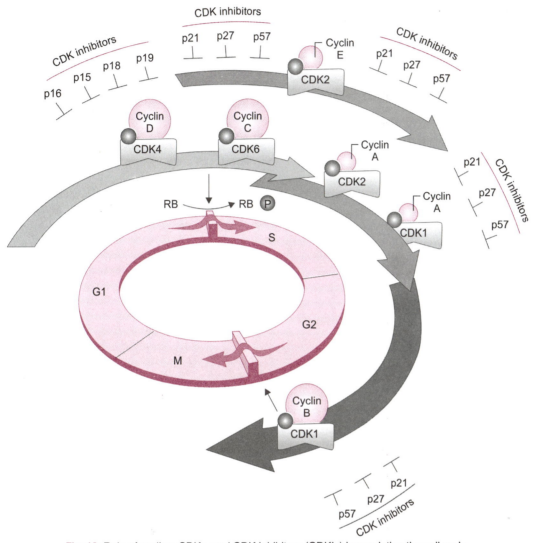

Fig. 12: Role of cyclins, CDKs, and CDK inhibitors (CDKIs) in regulating the cell cycle

51. **Ans. a. Nodular lymphocyte predominant Hodgkin's lymphoma** *(Ref: Robbins 9/e p609)*

Presence of Reed Sternberg cells is suggestive of Hodgkin's lymphoma, but classical Hodgkins lymphoma are CD15 and CD30 positive. Absence of these markers, along-with CD20 positivity points towards non- classical HL or Nodular lymphocyte predominant Hodgkin's lymphoma (NLPHL).

> *"**Lymphocyte Predominance Type:** This uncommon "nonclassical" variant of HL accounts for about 5% of cases. Involved nodes are effaced by a nodular infiltrate of small lymphocytes admixed with variable numbers of macrophages. "Classical" Reed-Sternberg cells are usually difficult to find. Instead, **this tumor contains so-called L&H (lymphocytic and histiocytic) variants, which have a multilobed nucleus resembling a popcorn kernel ("popcorn cell"). Eosinophils and plasma cells are usually scant or absent. In contrast to the Reed-Sternberg cells found in classical forms of HL, L&H variants express B-cell markers typical of germinal-center B cells, such as CD20 and BCL6, and are usually negative for CD15 and CD30.** The typical nodular pattern of growth is due to the presence of expanded B-cell follicles, which are populated with L&H variants, numerous reactive B cells, and follicular dendritic cells. **The IgH genes of the L&H variants show evidence of ongoing somatic hypermutation, a modification that occurs only in germinal center B cells.** In 3% to 5% of cases, this type transforms into a tumor resembling diffuse large B-cell lymphoma. **EBV is not associated with this subtype.**"-Robbins 9/e p609*

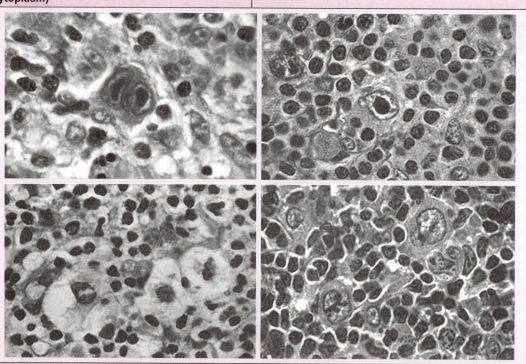

A. Diagnostic Reed-Sternberg cell (Two nuclear lobes, large inclusion-like nucleoli, abundant cytoplasm)	B. Reed-Sternberg cell, mononuclear variant
C. Reed-Sternberg cell, lacunar variant (folded or multilobated nucleus, lies within open space)	D. Reed-Sternberg cell, lymphohistiocytic variant.

Hodgkin's Lymphoma (HL)

- Arises in a single LN or chain (MC-cervical region[Q]), follow orderly spread to anatomically contiguous lymphoid tissues.
- Presence of distinctive neoplastic giant cells called Reed-Sternberg Cells, derived from germinal centre or post germinal centre of B-cells[Q].

Pathology:
- Activation of NF-κB is a common event in classical Hodgkin's Lymphoma[Q]
- Latent membrane protein-1 (LMP-1) of EBV up regulate NF-κB[Q].
- Reed-Sternberg cells secrete cytokines (IL-5, IL-10, M-CSF), chemokines (eotaxin) & other factors (Immunomodulatory factor galactin-1).

Reed-Sternberg Cells

- **Reed-Sternberg cells alone are not diagnostic**, since they are also seen in infectious mononucleosis, immunoblastic NHL, carcinoma & sarcoma[Q].
- **Histological diagnosis** is established by presence of Reed-Sternberg cells along with background of mixed inflammation consisting of neutrophils, plasma cells, eosinophils & histiocytes[Q].

> - *Reed–Sternberg cells are large and are either multinucleated or have a bilobed nucleus (thus resembling an "owl's eye" appearance[Q]) with prominent eosinophilic inclusion-like nucleoli[Q].*
> - *Reed–Sternberg cells are CD30 & CD15 positive, usually negative for CD20 & CD45[Q].*
> - *The presence of these cells is necessary in the diagnosis of Hodgkin's lymphoma – the absence of Reed–Sternberg cells has very high negative predictive value.*

Hodgkin's Lymphoma (HL)

Clinical Features:

- **MC presentation: Painless cervical lymphadenopathy**[Q]
- **Pel-Ebstein fever (Intermittent fever every alternate week**[Q]**)**
- **Paraneoplastic syndromes: Affected LN become painful with alcohol ingestion & secondary amyloidosis (AA type**[Q]**)**

WHO Classification of Hodgkin's Lymphoma	
Classical Variety (CD15+, CD30+)	**Non-Classical Variety (CD20+, CD15–, C30–)**
• Nodular sclerosis • Mixed cellularity • Lymphocyte rich • Lymphocyte depletion	• Lymphocyte Predominance

- **Prognosis: Lymphocytic predominant**[Q] **> Nodular sclerosis > Mixed cellularity > Lymphocyte depletion**
- **Nodular sclerosis is MC type all over the world**[Q] **whereas mixed cellularity is MC in India**[Q]
- **Nodular sclerosis is MC in females and mediastinal involvement**[Q] is particularly common

Hodgkin's Lymphoma	
Subtype	**Characteristic Features**
Nodular sclerosis	• **MC subtype**; usually **stage I or II** disease; frequent **mediastinal involvement**[Q] • **More common in females, most patients young adults**[Q]
Mixed cellularity	• **MC subtype in India**[Q]; >50% present as stage **III or IV** disease; **M > F;** • **Biphasic incidence**, peaking in young adults & again in >55 years • **Good prognosis**
Lymphocyte rich	• **Uncommon; M > F;** seen in **older adults; Good prognosis**[Q]
Lymphocyte depletion	• Uncommon; more common in **older males, HIV-infected individuals** & in **developing countries**; often presents with advanced disease • **Worst prognosis**[Q]
Lymphocyte predominance	• Uncommon; **young males** with **cervical or axillary lymph-adenopathy** • **Best prognosis**[Q]

Hodgkin's Lymphoma	Immuno-phenotype	Association with EBV	Morphology
Nodular sclerosis	CD15+, CD30+	Usually EBV–	• **Frequent lacunar cells (clear space around nucleus)** & occasional diagnostic **RS cells** • Background infiltrate composed of **T lympho-cytes, eosinophils, macrophages & plasma cells & fibrous bands**
Mixed cellularity	CD15+, CD30+	70% EBV+	• **Frequent mononuclear & diagnostic RS cells**
Lymphocyte rich	CD15+, CD30+	40% EBV+	• **Frequent mononuclear & diagnostic RS cell**
Lymphocyte depletion	CD15+, CD30+	Most EBV+	• **Reticular variant: Frequent diagnostic RS cells**
Lymphocyte Predominance	CD20+, CD15–, C30–	EBV–	• **Lymphocytic & Histiocytic (popcorn cell)**

AIIMS ESSENCE

Hodgkin's Lymphoma (HL)

Adverse Prognostic Factors of Hodgkin's Lymphoma	
• Age >45 years[Q] • Male gender[Q] • Hb <10.5 gm/dL[Q] • Leucocyte count >15,000/mm³[Q]	• Lymphocytopenia (Absolute lymphocyte count <600/μL; Lymphocytes <8% of leucocyte)[Q] • S. albumin <4 gm/dl[Q] • Stage IV[Q]

Hodgkin's Lymphoma	Non-Hodgkin's Lymphoma
• Localized to single axial group of LNs[Q] (MC-cervical) • Orderly spread to anatomically contiguous lymphoid tissues[Q]. • Mesenteric & Waldeyer's rings are rarely involved[Q] • Extranodal presentation is rare	• Involve multiple peripheral LNs[Q] • Non-contiguous spread • Mesenteric & Waldeyer's rings are commonly involved[Q] • Extranodal presentation is common[Q]

52. Ans. a. Anisocytosis *(Ref: Wintrobes 12/e p4; Robbins 8/e p164)*

Red cell distribution width (RDW) is a parameter that measures variation in red blood cell size or red blood cell volume. RDW is elevated in accordance with variation in red cell size (anisocytosis), i.e. when elevated RDW is reported on complete blood count, marked anisocytosis (increased variation in red cell size) is expected on peripheral blood smear review. Poikilocytosis is the variation in cell shape.

Red Cell Distribution Width

- **Measure the range of variation of RBC volume** that is reported as part of a standard complete blood count.
- **Higher RDW** values indicate **greater variation in size**.
- **Normal reference range** of RDW-CV in human red blood cells is **11.5–14.5%**.
- It is mainly **used to differentiate an anemia of mixed causes** from anemia of a single cause.
- The "width" in RDW refers to the **width of the volume curve (distribution width**, here presented as the Coefficient of Variation, or CV**), not the width of the cells.**

Normal RDW	High RDW
• Anemia in presence of a normal RDW may suggest **thalassemia**[Q]. • Anemia of chronic disease, hereditary spherocytosis, acute blood loss, aplastic anemia, and certain **hereditary hemoglobinopathies** may all present with a normal RDW[Q].	• Iron deficiency anemia: High RDW with low MCV[Q] • Folate & vitamin B12 deficiency anemia: High RDW & high MCV[Q] • Mixed deficiency (Iron + B12 or folate) anemia: High RDW & variable MCV[Q] • Recent hemorrhage: High RDW & normal MCV[Q]

53. Ans. a. AIRE *(Ref: Robbins 10/e p145, 9/e p121, 213; Harrison 19/e p2345)*

Recognition of self-antigens in thymus is called as central tolerance, which is regulated by AIRE (Autoimmune regulator) protein. Notch-1 signaling is used in maturation of T-cells and cell surface receptor expression.

"A protein called AIRE (autoimmune regulator) stimulates expression of some "peripheral tissue-restricted" self antigens in the thymus and is thus critical for deletion of immature T cells specific for these antigens. Mutations in the AIRE gene are the cause of an autoimmune polyendocrinopathy. In the CD4+ T-cell lineage, some of the cells that see self antigens in the thymus do not die but develop into regulatory T cells."–Robbins 9/e p213

Autoimmune Regulator (AIRE)

- A protein called **AIRE (autoimmune regulator) stimulates expression of** some "peripheral tissue-restricted" self-antigens in thymus[Q]
- Critical for **deletion of immature T cells specific for these antigens**[Q].
- **AIRE gene** is located on **chromosome 21q22**[Q]
- AIRE is **expressed primarily in the thymus**, where it **functions as a transcription factor** that **promotes the expression of many peripheral tissue antigens**[Q].
- **Self-reactive T cells** that recognize these antigens **are eliminated**[Q].

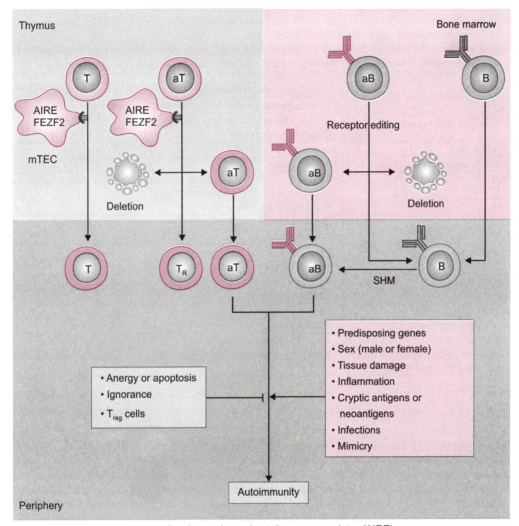

Fig. 13: Autoimmunity and autoimmune regulator (AIRE)

54. **Ans. a. Epigenetics** *(Ref: Harper 30/e p735, 438, 439; Harrison 19/e p102e-7)*
    Epigenetics can change the gene expression by methylation and acetylation without affecting the content of the gene.
    > "Epigenetics is defined as **changes that alter the pattern of gene expression that persist across at least one cell division** but are **not caused by changes in the DNA code**. Epigenetic changes include alterations of chromatin structure mediated by methylation of cytosine residues in CpG dinucleotides, modification of histones by acetylation or methylation, or changes in higher-order chromosome structure." – *Harrison 19/e p102e-7*

55. **Ans. d. It stops metabolic and enzymatic activity of the cell** *(Ref: Wintrobe's 13/e p43)*
    Acetone free methanol is used as a fixative in Leishman's stain. Fixation of the slide means preventing cell death by stopping metabolic and enzymatic activity, so that the cell is fixed in the state; it was sampled. It does not mean fixation of cells to the slide or smear.

Leishman's Stain	

- It is a **type of Romanowsky stain**, which contains an **acidic & a basic dye**[Q].
- **Acidic dye stains** the **basic components of cell & basic dye stains the acidic components** of cell[Q].

> - **Leishman's stain contains eosin & methylene blue in acetone free methyl alcohol**[Q].
> - **Methyl alcohol acts as a fixative**[Q].

- **Acetone** if present, will **destroy the cell membrane**[Q]
- **Methylene blue** ("polychromed"), **the basic dye** and **eosin, the acidic dye** exists as thiazine eosinate, which dissociates into the component dyes, when diluted with distilled water.
- **Methyl blue stains the nucleus** & basophilic granules of WBC, whereas **eosin stains** the **eosinophilic granules**.
- It is generally **used to differentiate & identify leucocytes, malaria parasites & trypanosomas**[Q].

Important Fixatives	
Routine Fixative	• **10% buffered normal formalin**[Q] (Most commonly used)
Electron microscopy	• **Glutaraldehyde**[Q] (Most commonly used)
	• **Osmium tetraoxide**[Q]
Adrenal medulla	• **Orth's fluid**[Q]
Bone marrow aspirate	• **Helly's fluid**[Q]
Bone marrow biopsy	• **Zenker's fluid**[Q] **& B-5** (Give **excellent nuclear detail, best for fixation of hematopoietic & reticuloendothelial tissues**)
Brain tissue	• **Formalin ammonium bromide**[Q]
Cell blocks	• **Bouin's fluid**[Q]
Cytoplasmic fixatives	• **Champy's fluid**[Q]
Nuclear fixatives	• **Carnoy's fluid**[Q]
	• **Clarke's fluid**[Q]
Karyotyping fixatives	• **Carnoy's fixative**[Q] (3:1 methanol to glacial acetic acid)
PAP's smear	• **95% ethanol**[Q]
Gastrointestinal biopsies	• **Bouin's fluid**[Q]
Testis & ovary	• **Susa's fixative**[Q]
HOPE Fixative (Hepes-glutamic acid buffer-mediated **O**rganic solvent **P**rotection **E**ffect)	• Gives formalin-like morphology
	• **Best for immunohistochemistry, enzyme histochemistry & nucleic acid**[Q]

56. **Ans. b. Serum hyaluronic acid and laminin** *(Ref: Harrison 19/e p1999; Zakim and Boyer's Hepatology 5/e p119)*

In order to avoid liver biopsy, serum hyaluronic acid and laminin can be used as biochemical marker to diagnose liver fibrosis.

> *"Biochemical markers of liver fibrosis (pro-collagen peptides type III and IV, the P1 fragment of laminin, hyaluronic acid, fibrosin, TNF-alphaR-II, sICAM-a, tissue inhibitor of matrix-metalloprotease-1 (TIMP-1), cytokeratin 18 and aspartate aminotransferase to platelet ration index (APRI) measured in serum have potential to provide a highly sensitive and cost-effective method for the assessment of schistosome-induced fibrosis."- Challenges in Infectious Diseases by I.W. Fong (2012)/p273*

Noninvasive Tests to Detect Hepatic Fibrosis

- These measures include multi-parameter tests aimed at detecting & staging the degree of hepatic fibrosis & imaging techniques.
- **FibroTest** is the best evaluated of the multi-parameter blood tests. The test **incorporates haptoglobin, bilirubin, GGT, apolipoprotein A-I, and α2-macroglobulin** and has been found to have **high positive & negative predictive values for diagnosing advanced fibrosis** in patients with **chronic hepatitis C, chronic hepatitis B & alcoholic liver disease** and patients taking **methotrexate for psoriasis**.
- **Transient elastography (TE)**, marketed as **Fibroscan**, and **magnetic resonance elastography (MRE)** both have gained U.S. FDA approval for use in the management of patients with liver disease.

- TE uses ultrasound waves to measure hepatic stiffness noninvasively. **TE has been shown to be accurate for identifying advanced fibrosis** in patients with **chronic hepatitis C, primary biliary cirrhosis, hemochromatosis, NAFLD & recurrent chronic hepatitis after liver transplantation.**
- **MRE has been found to be superior to TE for staging liver fibrosis** in patients with a variety of chronic liver diseases, but requires access to a magnetic resonance imaging scanner.

- **Serum hyaluronic acid & laminin concentrations** have showed **positive correlation with the stages of liver fibrosis**, and can be used as **non-invasive markers,** especially when **liver biopsy is contraindicated**[Q].
- The **combination of fibrosis markers** is **more valuable** than single marker.

PHARMACOLOGY

57. Ans. a. Epsilon aminocaproic acid *(Ref: Goodman Gilman 12/e p867; Katzung 13/e p599, 12/e p616; KDT 7/e p628, 6/e p608)*

Epsilon aminocaproic acid is an antidote for fibrinolytic therapy. Epsilon-aminocaproic acid is a synthetic inhibitor of the plasmin-plasminogen system. It is the only potent antifibrinolytic agent, which is commercially available.

"Aminocaproic acid is a lysine analog that competes for lysine binding sites on plasminogen and plasmin, blocking the interaction of plasmin with fibrin. Aminocaproic acid is thereby a potent inhibitor of fibrinolysis and can reverse states that are associated with excessive fibrinolysis."— *Goodman Gilman 12/e p867*

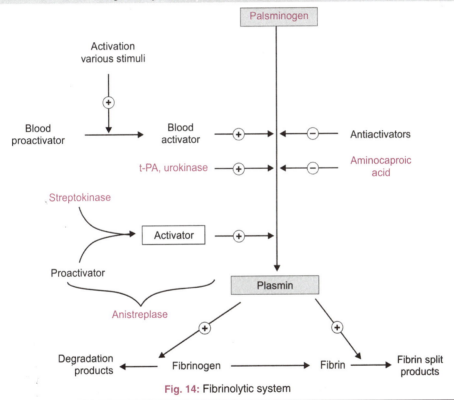

Fig. 14: Fibrinolytic system

Aminocaproic Acid
- EACA is a **synthetic inhibitor of plasmin-plasminogen system**[Q].
- It is the **only potent antifibrinolytic agent,** which is **commercially available**[Q].
Mechanism of Action:
- **Aminocaproic acid** is a **lysine analog that competes for lysine binding sites on plasminogen & plasmin, blocking the interaction of plasmin with fibrin**[Q].
- **Aminocaproic acid** is a **potent inhibitor of fibrinolysis & can reverse states** that are **associated with excessive fibrinolysis**[Q].
Therapeutic Uses:
- Used to reduce bleeding after prostatic surgery or after tooth extractions in hemophiliacs[Q].
- Used to treat the overdose and/ or toxic effects of the thrombolytics like tissue plasminogen activator & streptokinase[Q].
Side-effects:
- **Hypotension, cardiac arrhythmias, rhabdomyolysis & generation of thrombi**[Q].

Drug of Choice in Hematological Disorders	
• Heparin-induced thrombocytopenia	• Agartroban[Q]
• ITP (Idiopathic thrombocytopenic purpura)	• Steroids[Q]
• Chemotherapy induced leukopenia	• Sargramostim[Q]
• Chemotherapy induced thrombocytopenia	• Oprelvekin[Q]
• Chemotherapy induced anemia • Anemia due to chronic kidney disease	• Erythropoietin[Q]
• DVT prophylaxis • Chronic atrial fibrillation in mitral stenosis, advanced kidney disease & mechanical prosthetic heart valves	• Warfarin[Q]
• Initiation of therapy in DVT	• Heparin + Warfarin[Q]
• Heparin overdose	• Protamine[Q]
• Warfarin overdose	• Vitamin K[Q]
• Fibrinolytic overdose	• Epsilon Amino Caproic Acid[Q] (EACA)

58. Ans. a. 0.002 mg/mL   *(Ref: Goodman Gilman 12/e p28; Katzung 13/e p50, 12/e p46; KDT 7/e p32)*

Plasma Steady State Concentration (Cpss)

• **Plasma Steady State Concentration (Cpss)** is achieved after **repeated administration of drug** leading to a **balance between drug input & circulation.**
 • **Cpss** is **directly proportional to the dose rate & inversely proportional to the clearance of drug.**
     ◦ **Cpss = Dose rate/clearance**
     ◦ **Dose rate= 1.6 mg/ml; Clearance = 640 ml/min**
     ◦ **Cpss = 1.6/640 = 0.0025 mg/mL = 0.002 mg/mL**

59. Ans. a. 30% Amorphous + 70% Crystalline insulin   *(Ref: KDT 7/e p263)*

Lente insulin is a 7:3 mixture of long acting ultralente (crystalline) and short-acting semilente (amorphous) insulin zinc suspension.

"Lente insulin is a 7:3 mixture of ultralente (crystalline) and semilente (amorphous) insulin zinc suspension."– KDT 7/e p263

Insulin-Zinc Suspensions
• **Two types** of insulin-zinc suspensions have been produced.   • **Ultralente** or 'extended insulin zinc suspension: **With large particles, crystalline,** practically **insoluble in water & long acting.**   • **Semilente** or 'prompt insulin zinc suspension: With **smaller particles, amorphous & short-acting.**   ◦ The **7:3 mixture** of long acting **ultralente (crystalline)** and short-acting **semilente (amorphous) insulin zinc suspension is** called '**Lente insulin**' and is **intermediate- acting.**

Rapid Acting	Short Acting	Intermediate Acting	Long Acting
• **Lispro**[Q] • **Aspart**[Q] • **Glulisine**[Q]	• **Regular (soluble) insulin**[Q] • Velosulin[Q] (for use in insulin pump)	• **NPH** (Neutral protamine Hagedorn) or **isophane insulin**[Q] • Insulin zinc suspension or **Lente**[Q]	• Insulin glargine[Q] • Insulin detemir[Q] • Insulin degludec[Q] • **Protamine zinc insulin**

60. Ans. a. Large volume of distribution   *(Ref: Goodman Gilman 12/e p30; Katzung 13/e p42, 12/e p38, 48; KDT 7/e p17-18, 21)*

Storage of drug in the tissues is suggested by large volume of distribution (V_D). V_D is directly correlated with the amount of drug distributed into tissue; a higher V_D indicates a greater amount of tissue distribution. V_D may be increased by renal failure (due to fluid retention) and liver failure (due to altered body fluid and plasma protein binding). Conversely it may be decreased in dehydration.

"The apparent volume of distribution reflects a balance between binding to tissues, which decreases plasma concentration and makes the apparent volume larger, and binding to plasma proteins, which increases plasma concentration and makes the apparent volume smaller. Changes in either tissue or plasma binding can change the apparent volume of distribution determined from plasma concentration measurements."- Katzung 12/e p48

"A drug's volume of distribution therefore reflects the extent to which it is present in extravascular tissues and not in the plasma."- Goodman Gilman 12/e p30

*"**Volume of distribution** can vastly exceed any physical volume in the body because it is the volume apparently necessary to contain the amount of drug homogeneously at the concentration found in the blood, plasma, or water. Drugs with very high volumes of distribution, have much higher concentrations in extravascular tissue than in the vascular compartment, i.e., they are **not homogeneously distributed**. Drugs that are completely retained within the vascular compartment, on the other hand, have a minimum possible volume of distribution equal to the blood component in which they are distributed, for a drug that is restricted to the plasma compartment."*-Katzung 12/e p38

61. **Ans. d. Methotrexate** *(Ref: Harrison 19/e p2145; Katzung 13/e p627, 12/e p645)*
    Methotrexate has been shown to stimulate adenosine release from cells, producing an anti-inflammatory effect.

    *"**Methotrexate is the DMARD of choice for the treatment of RA** and is the anchor drug for most combination therapies. It was approved for the treatment of RA in 1986 and remains the benchmark for the efficacy and safety of new disease-modifying therapies. At the dosages used for the treatment of RA, methotrexate has been shown to stimulate adenosine release from cells, producing an anti-inflammatory effect."*-Harrison 19/e p2145

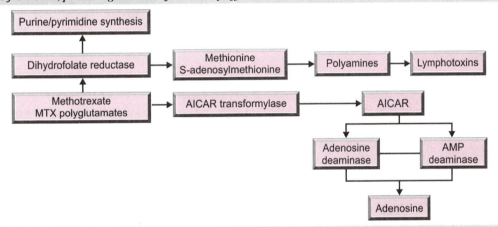

"Methotrexate's principal mechanism of action at the low doses used in the rheumatic diseases probably relates to inhibition of amino-imidazole carboxamide ribonucleotide (AICAR) transformylase and thymidylate synthetase. AICAR, which accumulates intracellularly, competitively inhibits AMP deaminase, leading to an accumulation of AMP. The AMP is released and converted extracellularly to adenosine, which is a potent inhibitor of inflammation."-Katzung 13/e p627

Leflunomide	• **Inhibitor of pyrimidine synthesis** • Effective as methotrexate in rheumatoid arthritis, including **inhibition of bony damage**.
Sulfasalazine	• Sulfasalazine is metabolized to sulfapyridine & 5-aminosalicylic acid. • **Sulfapyridine** is probably the **active moiety** when treating rheumatoid arthritis • Sulfasalazine or its metabolites **inhibit the release of inflammatory cytokines** (IL-1, -6, & -12, and TNF-α) • **Effective in rheumatoid arthritis** & reduces radiologic disease progression.
Chloroquine & Hydroxychloroquine	• Mechanism of the anti-inflammatory action in rheumatic diseases is unclear. • **Proposed mechanisms: suppression of T-lymphocyte responses** to mitogens, **decreased leukocyte chemotaxis, stabilization of lysosomal enzymes, inhibition of DNA & RNA synthesis & trapping of free radicals.** • **Improve symptoms** of rheumatoid arthritis

Methotrexate
• Methotrexate (MTX) is a **folic acid analog** that **binds with high affinity to the active catalytic site of dihydrofolate reductase (DHFR)**[Q].   • Mechanism of Action: • **MTX binds with high affinity to active catalytic site of dihydrofolate reductase (DHFR)**[Q].

Contd...

Contd...

- This **results in inhibition of synthesis of tetrahydrofolate (THF)**, the **key one-carbon carrier for enzymatic processes involved in de novo synthesis of thymidylate, purine nucleotides & amino acids serine & methionine**[Q].
- **Inhibition** of these **various metabolic processes interferes with the formation of DNA, RNA & key cellular proteins**[Q].
- **Intracellular formation of polyglutamate metabolites**, with the addition of up to 5–7 glutamate residues, is **critically important for the therapeutic action of MTX** & this process is **catalyzed by the enzyme folylpolyglutamate synthase (FPGS)**[Q].
- **Stimulate adenosine release from cells**, producing an **anti-inflammatory effect**[Q].
  - **MTX polyglutamates are selectively retained within cancer cells** & **display increased inhibitory effects on enzymes involved in de novo purine nucleotide & thymidylate biosynthesis**, making them important determinants of **MTX's cytotoxic action**[Q].

Mechanisms of Resistance to Methotrexate	
• **Impaired transport** of methotrexate into cells[Q] • **Production of altered forms of DHFR** that have **decreased affinity for the inhibitor**[Q] • **Increased concentrations of intracellular DHFR** through **gene amplification or altered gene regulation**[Q]	• **Decreased ability to synthesize methotrexate polyglutamates**[Q] • **Increased expression of a drug efflux transporter of the MRP class**[Q]

Clinical Uses:
- MTX is administered by the **intravenous, intrathecal, or oral route**[Q].
- Used for **acute lymphocytic leukemia; choriocarcinoma; breast, head, neck and lung cancers; osteogenic sarcoma; bladder cancer**[Q]
  - **Intraocular methotrexate** is used to **treat uveitis & uveitic cystoid macular edema**[Q].
  - **DMARD of choice** for the treatment of **rheumatoid arthritis**[Q]

Side-Effects:
- **Mucositis, diarrhea, myelosuppression with neutropenia & thrombocytopenia**[Q]

62. Ans. a. Linagliptin *(Ref: Goodman Gilman 12/e p1264; Katzung 13/e p1091, 12/e p761; FDA website: http://www.fda.gov/Safety/ MedWatch/SafetyInformation/ucm319215.htm)*

Linagliptin can be given safely in renal failure.

*"This suggests that **linagliptin has the ability to be safely dosed in chronic kidney disease patients. Chronic kidney disease is a major complication in type 2 diabetes** and presents one of the circumstances where using metformin can be challenging. The more severe the renal disease, the less likely one is to use metformin because of safety concerns. Linagliptin is an option for these patients."- http://www.medpagetoday.com/meetingcoverage/ada/27343*

Repaglinide	• Member of **meglitinide group of insulin secretagogues** • **Used cautiously in** individuals with **renal & hepatic impairment.**
Glimepiride (*sulfonylureas*)	• Sulfonylureas may cause **hypoglycemic reactions, including coma**, particular concern in elderly patients with **impaired hepatic or renal function.**

Dose Adjustment of Dipeptidyl Peptidase-4 (DPP-4) Inhibitors in Renal Impairment	
Sitagliptin	• **Mild impairment: No dose adjustment needed** • **Moderate impairment:** Creatinine clearance ≥30 to <50 mL/min, **reduce dose,** use sitagliptin 50 mg once daily. • **CrCl <30 mL/min or end-stage renal disease** requiring hemodialysis or peritoneal dialysis, use sitagliptin 25 mg once daily.
Saxagliptin	• **Reduce dose** to 2.5 mg in moderate to severe renal impairment
Linagliptin	• **No dose reduction required linagliptin for patients with renal impairment**[Q]
Vildagliptin	• **Reduce dose** to 50 mg once daily when CrCl <50 mL/min
Alogliptin	• **Reduce dose** to 12.5 mg once daily when CrCl <50 mL/min, 6.25 mg once daily when CrCl < 30 mL/min

Dipeptidyl Peptidase-4 (DPP-4) Inhibitors
• **Sitagliptin, saxagliptin, vildaglitin, alogliptin & linagliptin** are **inhibitors of DPP-4,** the enzyme that degrades incretin hormones[Q].
Mechanism of Action: • **Degrades incretin hormones**[Q]. • **Increase circulating levels of native GLP-1** & **glucose-dependent insulinotropic polypeptide (GIP)**[Q] • **Decreases postprandial glucose excursions** by **increasing glucose-mediated insulin secretion** & **decreasing glucagon levels**[Q].
Side Effects: • Nasopharyngitis, upper respiratory infections, headaches & hypoglycemia   • **Dosage should be reduced in patients with renal impairment** and may need to be **adjusted to prevent hypoglycemia if there is concurrent insulin secretagogue or insulin therapy**[Q].

Sitagliptin	• **Primarily (87%) excreted in urine** in part by **active tubular secretion** of drug. • **Limited hepatic metabolism**, mainly mediated by **cytochrome CYP3A4** isoform.
Saxagliptin	• **Minimally protein bound** • **Undergoes hepatic metabolism** by **CYP3A4/5** • **Major metabolite is active**, and **excretion** is by both **renal & hepatic pathways**. • **Dosage adjustment is recommended** for individuals with **renal impairment** & **concurrent use of strong CYP3A4/5 inhibitors**.

Linagliptin	• Most recently introduced drug in this class
	    • **Predominantly excreted via enterohepatic system** (**84.7%** of drug is eliminated in feces & 5% eliminated via urine)
	    • **Appears to be safe in patients with renal failure.**[Q]
	• **Approved for use as monotherapy** & in **combination with metformin, glimepiride & pioglitazone.**

Vildagliptin	• Vildagliptin elicits **dose-related decreases in fasting plasma glucose, postprandial glucose & HBA1C** when **added to metformin** monotherapy. • Associated with an **improvement in measures of β-cell function**, with **no weight gain** & **no increase in incidence of hypoglycemia.**

63. **Ans. c. 30 mg**   *(Ref: KDT 7/e p30)*

First Order Kinetics
• **In first order kinetics, constant fraction of drug is eliminated per unit time** • 75 mg out of 200 mg is eliminated in 90 minutes; 75/200 x 100 = 37.5% • 37.5% (fraction) of drug eliminated every 90 minutes • **Drug remains in the body at the end of 1st 90 minutes: 200–75 = 125** • 2nd 90 minutes: 37.5% of 125 will be eliminated = 125 x 37.5/100 = 47 • **Drug remains in the body at the end of 2nd 90 minutes (3 hours) = 125–47 = 78** • 3rd 90 minutes: 37.5% of 78 =29.25 • **Drug remains in the body at the end of 3rd 90 minutes (4.5 hours) = 78–29.25 = 48.75** • 4th 90 minutes: 37.5% of 48.75 = 18.3 • **Drug remains in the body at the end of 4th 90 minutes (6 hours) = 48.7 –18.3 = 30.4 (Approx. 30 mg)**

64. **Ans. b. Neuraminidase inhibition**   *(Ref: Goodman Gilman 12/e p1608; Katzung 13/e p861, 12/e p886; Harrison 19/e p215e-1)*

Mechanism of action of Oseltamivir (Tamiflu) as an antiviral agent is Neuraminidase inhibition.

"Zanamivir and oseltamivir are inhibitors of the influenza viral neuraminidase enzyme, which is essential for release of virus from infected cells and for its subsequent spread throughout the respiratory tract of the infected host." - Harrison 19/e p215e-1

"Oseltamivir carboxylate is a transition-state analog of sialic acid that is a potent selective inhibitor of influenza A and B virus neuraminidases." - Goodman Gilman 12/e p1608

666 AIIMS ESSENCE

"The neuraminidase inhibitors oseltamivir and zanamivir, analogs of sialic acid, interfere with release of progeny influenza virus from infected host cells, thus halting the spread of infection within the respiratory tract. These agents competitively and reversibly interact with the active enzyme site to inhibit viral neuraminidase activity at low nanomolar concentrations. Inhibition of viral neuraminidase results in clumping of newly released influenza virions to each other and to the membrane of the infected cell. Unlike amantadine and rimantadine, oseltamivir and zanamivir have activity against both influenza A and influenza B viruses."-Katzung 13/e p861

Specific Antiviral Therapy for influenza

- Neuraminidase inhibitors zanamivir, oseltamivir & peramivir are used for both **influenza A & B**[Q]
- Amantadine & rimantadine are used for **influenza A**[Q]

Oseltamivir	• **DOC for bird flu (H5N1)**[Q]
	• Treatment of **uncomplicated influenza A or B** in healthy adults.
Zanamivir	• **Administered by inhalational route**[Q]
	• Treatment of **uncomplicated influenza A or B** in healthy adults[Q].
Peramivir	• **Administered IV**[Q]
	• Activity against both **influenza A & B viruses**[Q]
Laninamivir	• **Long acting neuraminidase inhibitor**[Q]
	• Effective against **oseltamivir resistant virus**[Q]
Amantadine	• Active against **influenza A** only[Q]
Rimantadine	• **Longer acting than Amantadine**, active against **influenza A** only[Q]

Drug of Choice in Viral Diseases	
Disease	**Drug of Choice**
• **Viral hemorrhagic fever (Lass virus, Rift valley fever, Congo Crimean hemorrhagic fever, Hanta virus)** • **Respiratory syncytial virus** (in high risk patients) • **Measles**	Ribavirin[Q]
• **Seasonal influenza** • **Avian influenza (bird flu)**	Oseltamivir[Q]
• **Oseltamivir resistant influenza**	Zanamivir[Q]
• **Prion disease**	Flupirtine[Q]
• **Herpes simplex** • **Varicella**	Acyclovir[Q]
• **Acute herpes zoster**	Valacyclovir[Q]
• **Cytomegalovirus retinitis**	Gancicyclovir[Q]

65. **Ans. b. Ofloxacin** *(Ref: Harrison 19/e p1126; KDT 7/e p782, 783)*

Ofloxacin is a bactericidal drug against Mycobacterium leprae.

"Established agents used to treat leprosy include dapsone (50–100 mg/d), clofazimine (50–100 mg/d, 100 mg three times weekly, or 300 mg monthly), and rifampin (600 mg daily or monthly). Of these drugs, only rifampin is bactericidal. The sulfones (folate antagonists), the foremost of which is dapsone, were the first antimicrobial agents found to be effective for the treatment of leprosy and are still the mainstays of therapy."-Harrison 19/e p1126

"Other antimicrobial agents active against M. leprae in animal models and at the usual daily doses used in clinical trials include ethionamide/prothionamide; the aminoglycosides streptomycin, kanamycin, and amikacin (but not gentamicin or tobramycin); minocycline; clarithromycin; and several fluoroquinolones, particularly ofloxacin. Next to rifampin, minocycline, clarithromycin, and ofloxacin appear to be most bactericidal for M. leprae, but these drugs have not been used extensively in leprosy control programs."- Harrison 19/e p1126

Classification of Anti-leprosy Drugs	
Sulfones	• Dapsone (DDS)
Phenazine derivative	• Clofazimine
Antitubercular drugs	• Rifampin, Ethionamide
Other antibiotics	• Ofloxacin, Minocycline, Clarithromycin

AIIMS May 2017

Bactericidal Activity of Anti-leprosy Drugs	
Rifampin	• Upto **99.99%** M. leprae are **killed in 3-7 days** by 600 mg/day dose.
Ofloxacin	• Over **99.9% bacilli** were found to be **killed by 22 daily doses of ofloxacin monotherapy.**
Clarithromycin	• **Monotherapy with 500 mg daily** caused **99.9% bacterial killing in 8 weeks.**

66. Ans. b. Inhibition of assembly of viral proteins *(Ref: Goodman Gilman 12/e p1645; Katzung 13/e p851, 12/e p878; Harrison 19/e p1274; KDT 7/e p805)*

Mechanism of action of protease inhibitors is inhibition of assembly of viral proteins.

"Protease Inhibitors: These drugs prevent proteolytic cleavage of HIV gag and pol precursor polypeptides that include essential structural (p17, p24, p9, and p7) and enzymatic (reverse transcriptase, protease, and integrase) components of the virus. This prevents the metamorphosis of HIV virus particles into their mature infectious form."-Goodman Gilman 12/e p1645

"During the later stages of the HIV growth cycle, the gag and gag-pol gene products are translated into polyproteins, and these become immature budding particles. The HIV protease is responsible for cleaving these precursor molecules to produce the final structural proteins of the mature virion core. By preventing post-translational cleavage of the Gag-Pol polyprotein, protease inhibitors (PIs) prevent the processing of viral proteins into functional conformations, resulting in the production of immature, noninfectious viral particles. Unlike the NRTIs, PIs do not need intracellular activation."-Katzung 13/e p851

67. Ans. d. Blurred vision *(Ref: Goodman Gilman 12/e p595; Katzung 13/e p410, 12/e p410)*

Diplopia (not the blurring of vision) is a dose related side effect of carbamazepine, while others are idiosyncratic, reactions.

"The most common dose-related adverse effects of carbamazepine are diplopia and ataxia. The diplopia often occurs first and may last less than an hour during a particular time of day."- Katzung 13/e p410

"Considerable concern exists regarding the occurrence of idiosyncratic blood dyscrasias with carbamazepine, including fatal cases of aplastic anemia and agranulocytosis. Most of these have been in elderly patients with trigeminal neuralgia, and most have occurred within the first 4 months of treatment. The mild and persistent leukopenia seen in some patients is not necessarily an indication to stop treatment but requires careful monitoring. The most common idiosyncratic reaction is an erythematous skin rash; other responses such as hepatic dysfunction are unusual."- Katzung 13/e p410

Carbamazepine
• It is chemically related to imipramine & **teratogenic**[Q].   • Acts by **prolongation of inactive Na+ channels**[Q].   • **Water retention and hyponatremia can occur in the elderly as it enhances ADH action**[Q].   • On chronic administration, it **induces its own metabolism**[Q] like phenobarbitone.

Side effects:
 • MC dose-related adverse effects: Diplopia & ataxia[Q].
 • Other dose-related complaints: mild gastrointestinal upsets, unsteadiness, and, at much higher doses, drowsiness.
 • Hyponatremia & water intoxication[Q] have occasionally occurred and may be dose-related.
 	
      • **Considerable concern** exists regarding the occurrence of **idiosyncratic blood dyscrasias**[Q] with carbamazepine, including **fatal cases of aplastic anemia** and **agranulocytosis**[Q].
      • **MC idiosyncratic reaction** is an **erythematous skin rash**[Q]

Uses: • **Most effective drug for complex partial seizures**[Q].   • **Generalized tonic clonic & simple partial seizures**[Q]   • **DOC in Trigeminal neuralgia**[Q].   • As an alternative to lithium in **manic depressive illness** and **acute mania**[Q]

68. Ans. d. Rifampicin *(Ref: Clinical Pharmacology by Markus Müller 2/e p286; KDT 7/e p13-15)*

Rifampicin is a P-glycoprotein inducer. Ketoconazole & itraconazole are P-glycoprotein inhibitors

"Rifampicin induces the isoenzymes CYP3A4, 2C8, 2C9, 2C19, 2B6, and the transporter P-glycoprotein. When co-administered with drugs that are substrates of the same enzymes, their metabolism may be accelerated resulting in lower concentration and less efficacy."- Clinical Pharmacology by Markus Müller 2/e p286

P-glycoprotein					

- P-gp is associated with the phenomenon of **multiple drug resistance** (MDR)
- **Locations of P-glycoprotein:**
- **Apical domain of enterocytes** of **lower GIT** (jejunum, duodenum, ileum & colon) **limiting the absorption of drug substrates** from GIT[Q].
- **Liver:** Expression on **apical cell membrane of hepatocytes** leading to enhanced excretion of drug substrates into bile[Q]
- **Kidney:** Expression on **proximal tubular cells** leading to enhanced excretion of drug substrates into urine[Q]
- Expressed on **luminal side of capillary endothelial cells** that make up the **blood–brain barrier**, limiting the CNS entry of a variety of drug substrates[Q].
- **Placenta & testes** for **tissue–blood barriers**[Q]

P-glycoprotein					
Substrates			**Inducer**	**Inhibitor**	
Aldosterone	Domperidone	Nelfinavir	Amprenavir	Atorvastatin	**Saquinavir**[Q]
Amprenavir	Doxorubicin	Paclitaxel	Clotrimazole	Bromocriptine	**Tamoxifen**[Q]
Bilirubin	**Erythromycin**	**Quinidine**[Q]	Dexamethasone	Carvedilol	**Verapamil**[Q]
Cimetidine[Q]	**Etoposide**[Q]	**Ranitidine**[Q]	**Indinavir**[Q]	Cyclosporine	
Colchicine	Fexofenadine	Rhodamine	**Morphine**[Q]	**Clarithromycin**	
Cortisol	**Indinavir**[Q]	**Saquinavir**[Q]	**Nelfinavir**[Q]	**Erythromycin**[Q]	
CPT-11	**Itraconazole**[Q]	Sparfloxocin	Phenothiazine	**Itraconazole**[Q]	
Cyclosporine[Q]	Ivermectin	**Terfenadine**	Retinoic acid	**Ketoconazole**[Q]	
Dexamethasone	Loperamide	**Tetracycline**	**Rifampin**[Q]	Meperidine	
Digoxin[Q]	Methyl	**Vecuronium**	**Ritonavir**[Q]	Methadone	
Diltiazem[Q]	prednisolone	**Verapamil**[Q]	**Saquinavir**[Q]	**Nelfinavir**[Q]	
	Morphine	Vinblastine	St John's wort	Pentazocine	
				Progesterone	
				Quinidine[Q]	
				Ritonavir[Q]	

69. **Ans. a. Cotrimoxazole** *(Ref: Harrison 19/e p1362, 921, 943; Goodman Gilman 12/e p1470; Katzung 12/e p926)*

Drug of choice for prophylaxis and treatment of pneumocystis infection in both immunocompetent as well as immunocompromised is cotrimoxazole.

"Pneumocystis jirovecii Pneumonia Prophylaxis: TMP-SMX is the most effective prophylactic drug: few patients experience a Pneumocystis jirovecii pneumonia (PCP) breakthrough when they are reliably taking a recommended TMP-SMX chemoprophylactic regimen. Several TMP-SMX regimens have been used successfully."- Harrison 19/e p1362

"For patients who cannot tolerate TMP-SMX (usually because of hypersensitivity or bone marrow suppression), alternative drugs include daily dapsone, weekly dapsone-pyrimethamine, and monthly aerosol pentamidine."-Harrison 19/e p1362

"Because of the high and prolonged risk of Pneumocystis jirovecii pneumonia (especially among patients being treated for hematologic malignancies), most patients receive maintenance prophylaxis with trimethoprim-sulfamethoxazole (TMP-SMX) starting 1 month after engraftment and continuing for at least 1 year."-Harrison 19/e p921

"Several studies have demonstrated the effectiveness of low-dose therapy (150 mg/m² of body surface area of trimethoprim and 750 mg/m² of body surface area of sulfamethoxazole) for the prophylaxis of infection by P. jiroveci."- Goodman Gilman 12/e p1470

"Trimethoprim- sulfamethoxazole is also the standard chemoprophylactic drug for the prevention of P jiroveci infection in immunocompromised individuals."- Katzung 12/e p926

Drug of Choice in Protozoal Infections	
- Cyclospora, Isospora & Pneumocystis jiroveci	- **Cotrimoxazole**[Q]
- **Giardia lamblia**	- **Metronidazole**[Q]
- **Trichomonas vaginalis**	
- **Balantidium coli**	- **Tetracycline**[Q]

Contd...

AIIMS May 2017

Contd...

• Babesia	• Clindamycin + Quinine[Q]
• Cryptosporidium	• Nitazoxanide or Paromomycin[Q]
• Leishmania donovani	• Liposomal amphotericin B[Q]
• Toxoplasma gondii	• Pyrimethamine + Sulfadiazine + Folinic acid[Q]
• Toxoplasma gondii in pregnancy	• Spiramycin[Q]
• Trypanosoma cruzi (Chagas disease)	• Benznidazole[Q]
• Early African trypanosomiasis	• Suramin[Q]
• Late (CNS) African trypanosomiasis	• Melarsoprol[Q]

Pneumocystis jirovecii

- **Pneumocystis jiroveci** causes **pneumonia in immunocompromised patients**
- **P. jirovecii pneumonia (PCP)** develops in **HIV-positive** & immunocompromised patients secondary to **hematologic or malignant neoplasms, stem cell or solid organ transplantation & immunosuppressive medications**[Q].
- Incidence of PCP depends on **degree of immunosuppression**[Q] (inversely related to **CD4+ count**[Q])

Pathology:
- Pneumocystis organisms are **species specific;** Humans are **infected only by other humans who transmit P. jirovecii;** humans **cannot be infected with animal species** of Pneumocystis[Q]
- **Defects in cellular and/or humoral immunity** predispose to development of PCP[Q].
- **CD4+ T cells** are **critical in host defense against Pneumocystis**[Q].

Clinical Features:
- Initially a **vague sense of dyspnea alone** followed by **fever & nonproductive cough** with **progressive shortness of breath** ultimately resulting in **respiratory failure & death**[Q].
- **Extrapulmonary manifestations** are **rare** but can involve almost any organ, most notably **LNs, spleen & liver**.
- Untreated, **PCP is invariably fatal**[Q].

  - **Factors increasing the mortality risk: Age, degree of immunosuppression, preexisting lung disease, low serum albumin level**, need for **mechanical ventilation & pneumothorax**[Q].

Diagnosis:
- **H&E staining** of pulmonary tissue: **Foamy alveolar infiltrate** & a **mononuclear interstitial infiltrate**[Q].
- **Diagnosis** is **typically established in lung tissue** or **pulmonary secretions** by highly specific staining of the cyst—e.g., with **methenamine silver, toluidine blue O, or Giemsa** or by staining with a specific **immunofluorescent antibody**[Q].
- Differential staining of cell wall of cysts giving **"Cup in saucer" appearance** on **Grocotts stain**[Q]
- **Demonstration of organisms** in **bronchoalveolar lavage fluid** is almost **100% sensitive & specific for PCP**[Q].

  ### Radiographic Findings of P. jirovecii pneumonia (PCP)

  - **Radiographic Findings: Classic radiographic appearance** of PCP consists of **diffuse bilateral interstitial infiltrates** that are **perihilar & symmetric**[Q].
  - **HRCT: Diffuse ground-glass opacities** in virtually all patients with PCP.
  - A **normal chest CT** essentially **rules out the diagnosis of PCP**[Q].

Treatment:
- **Treatment of choice for PCP: TMP-SMX**[Q] (given either IV or PO for 14–21 days)
- **IV pentamidine** or combination of **clindamycin plus primaquine** for patients who cannot tolerate TMP-SMX[Q]

Prophylaxis:
- **TMP-SMX is the most effective prophylactic drug**[Q].
- **Alternative drugs: Daily dapsone, weekly dapsone-pyrimethamine & monthly aerosol pentamidine**[Q].

70. **Ans. c. Slowly taper the drug over next 6 months** *(Ref: Harrison 19/e p2556; Katzung 13/e p414)*

Stopping or switching an antiepileptic is based on seizure free period & compliance or adverse effects of the drug. Withdrawal of therapy should be gradual over 2-3 months, in the question 6 months. Anti-epileptic drug therapy should never be stopped abruptly. Even if new drug is to be added/replaced, the previous drug should be gradually stopped otherwise it can lead to breakthrough seizures.

"When to Discontinue Therapy: Overall, about 70% of children and 60% of adults who have their seizures completely controlled with antiepileptic drugs can eventually discontinue therapy. The following patient profile yields the greatest chance of remaining seizure free after drug withdrawal: (1) complete medical control of seizures for 1–5 years; (2) single seizure type, either focal or generalized; (3) normal neurologic examination, including intelligence; and (4) normal EEG. The appropriate seizure- free interval is unknown and undoubtedly varies for different forms of epilepsy. However, it seems reasonable to attempt withdrawal of therapy after 2 years in a patient who meets all of the above criteria, is motivated to discontinue the medication, and clearly understands the potential risks and benefits. In most cases, it is preferable to reduce the dose of the drug gradually over 2–3 months. Most recurrences occur in the first 3 months after discontinuing therapy, and patients should be advised to avoid potentially dangerous situations such as driving or swimming during this period."-Harrison 19/e p2556

71. **Ans. b. Block of alpha-1 followed by stimulation of beta-2**   *(Ref: KDT 7/e p131, 140)*

In an animal model, the phenomenon of vasomotor reversal of dale can be demonstrated by block of alpha-1 followed by stimulation of beta-2.

"Blockade of vasoconstrictor alpha-1 (also alpha-2) receptors reduces peripheral resistance and causes pooling of blood in capacitance vessels →venous return and cardiac output are reduced →fall in BP. Postural reflex is interfered with →marked hypotension occurs on standing →dizziness and syncope. Hypovolemia accentuates the hypotension. The alpha-blocker abolishes the pressor action of adrenaline (injected IV in animals), which then produces only fall in BP due to beta-2 mediated vasodilatation. This was first demonstrated by Sir HH Dale (1913) and is called vasomotor reversal of Dale. Pressor and other actions of selective alpha agonists (phenylephrine) are suppressed."- KDT 7/e p140

Vasomotor Reversal of Dale
• **Vasomotor reversal of Dale** is a **phenomenon is exaggerated fall in BP after alpha-receptor blockade**[Q].
• Phenomenon is **based on the biphasic action of adrenaline on BP**[Q].
• **Adrenaline acts on alpha-1 receptors at low dose & beta-2 at high dose**. When its given at a dose of say 5 mg IV, it will **stimulate alpha-1 receptors** first leading to **increase in BP**, then when its **dose gets reduced by metabolism beta-2 receptors get stimulated** which leads to **fall in BP**[Q].
• Now when **alpha-blockers** like **phentolamine is given** this will **block all alpha-receptors** thereby **preventing the initial action of adrenaline**. Therefor **all the available adrenaline** is **bound to act on beta-2 receptors**, thereby leading to **exaggerated fall in BP**[Q].

MICROBIOLOGY

72. **Ans. a. Nocardia asteroides**   *(Ref: Ananthanarayan 10/e p400; Jawetz 27/e p749; Harrison 19/e p1085, 1086)*

The given image is showing AFB stained filamentous bacteria, most likely Nocardia asteroides. Actinomyces is another filamentous bacteria, but does not stain positive with acid fast stain.

Nocardia: Members of this genus are filamentous, rod shaped bacteria that do not produce spores, do not exhibit motility and are catalase positive; they are Gram-positive and are also positive in Kinyoun's acid fast staining technique (weekly acid fast)."-Ananthanarayan 10/e p400

"Nocardiae are bacteria that clinically behave like fungi; weakly acid- fast, branching, filamentous gram-positive rods."- Jawetz 27/e p749

Actinomyces	Nocardia
• **Facultative anaerobes**[Q]	• **Obligate aerobes**
• Growth at **35–37°C**[Q]	• Variable temperatures
• **Endogenous infection**: Commensals in mouth, colon, vagina[Q]	• **Exogenous: Saprophytes**[Q]
• **Nonacid fast**[Q]	• **Acid fast**[Q]
• **DOC: Penicillin**[Q]	• **DOC: Sulfonamides**[Q]

Nocardia
• **Gram-positive, branching pleomorphic rods** with **intermittent or beaded staining patterns**[Q], especially when invading tissues.
• **Nocardiae** are **gram-positive weakly acid-fast branching rod- shaped bacteria** and can be **visualized by a modified Ziehl- Nielsen stain** like **Fite-Faraco method**[Q].

Nocardia
• **Nocardia asteroides** is **most frequently found species infecting humans**[Q]
• Most cases occur as an **opportunistic infection in immunocompromised patients.**

Staining & Culture Characteristics:
- Because it is **acid-fast to some degree**, it **stains only weakly Gram-positive**[Q].
- Visualized by a **modified Ziehl- Nielsen stain** like **Fite-Faraco method**[Q].
- **Stain black** with the **methenamine-silver stain.**
- In culture, **Nocardia are not fastidious** but do tend to **grow slowly.**
- Colonies will **grow on most bacterial, fungal, or mycobacterial media that lack antibiotics.**

  - **Blood & Sabouraud's agars** are good substrates for pathogenic organisms that usually **grow satisfactorily at temperatures between 35-37°C**[Q].
  - **Growth of N. asteroides** is facilitated by **10% carbon dioxide.**

Clinical Features:
- **MC form of human nocardial disease** is a **slowly progressive pneumonia**[Q], the common symptoms of which include **cough, dyspnea & fever**.
- Nocardia species are deeply involved in the process of **endocarditis** as one of its main pathogenic effects.
- Nocardia infection takes the form of **encephalitis** and/or **brain abscess formation** (In 25–33%)

  - **Cutaneous infections: Actinomycetoma** (especially **N. brasiliensis**), **lymphocutaneous disease, cellulitis, & subcutaneous abscesses**[Q].

Diagnosis:
- **First step in diagnosis: Examination of sputum or pus for crooked, branching, beaded, gram-positive filaments** 1 mm wide and up to 50 mm long[Q].
- **Most Nocardiae are acid-fast in direct smears if a weak acid is used for decolorization** (e.g., in the **modified Kinyoun, Ziehl-Neelsen & Fite-Faraco methods**)[Q].
- **Recovery from specimens** containing a mixed flora **can be improved with selective media (colistin-nalidixic acid agar, modified Thayer-Martin agar, or buffered charcoal-yeast extract agar)**[Q].

  - **Nocardiae grow relatively slowly**; colonies may take up to 2 weeks to appear and may not develop their **characteristic appearance, white, yellow, or orange, with aerial mycelia and delicate, dichotomously branched substrate mycelia**, for up to 4 weeks[Q].

- **Nocardia isolation from biological specimens** can be performed using **buffered charcoal-yeast extract agar (BCYE)**, the same **used for Legionella species**[Q].

73. **Ans. b. Septicemic shock**   *(Ref: Ananthanarayan 10/e p205; Jawetz 27/e p207; Harrison 19/e p956)*
Clinically, Staphylococcus aureus sepsis presents in a manner similar to that documented for sepsis due to other bacteria. Septicemic shock is not directly caused due to toxins and other virulence factors play a role like protein A, fibrinolysin and coagulase, which are anti-phagocytic, suppress host immunity and helps in spread of infection. Septicemia is mainly due to endotoxin like activity as seen in Gram-negative bacilli and not due to exotoxin.

"The common toxin-mediated staphylococcal diseases are as follows: Food poisoning, toxic shock syndrome, scalded skin syndrome."- Ananthanarayan 10/e p205

"S. aureus produces three types of toxin: cytotoxins, pyrogenic toxin superantigens, and exfoliative toxins. Both epidemiologic data and studies in animals suggest that antitoxin antibodies are protective against illness in TSS, staphylococcal food poisoning, and staphylococcal scalded-skin syndrome (SSSS). Illness develops after toxin synthesis and absorption and the subsequent toxin-initiated host response."-Harrison 19/e p956

Virulence Factors of Staphylococcus Aureus	
Cell associated polymers	• **Capsular polysaccharide: Decreases opsonisation**
	• **Teichoic acid:** Helps in **adhesion**[Q]
	• **Cell wall peptidoglycan**: Activates complement, **endotoxin like activity**[Q]

AIIMS ESSENCE

Virulence Factors of Staphylococcus Aureus	
Cell Surface proteins	• **Protein A:** Co-agglutination, chemotactic, anti-phagocytic • **Clumping Factor:** Adherence, responsible for **slide coagulase reaction**[Q]
Extracellular enzymes	• **Coagulase: Tube/ free coagulase test**[Q] • **Nuclease:** Characteristic thermostable DNA • **Fibrinolysin** (Staphylokinase): Helps in spread of infection, plasminogen activation; inactivate antimicrobial peptides • **Aureolysin:** Inactivate neutrophil proteolytic activity; inactivate antimicrobial peptides • **Others:** Protease, Hyaluronidase, Lipases etc.
Toxins	

	Cytolytic Toxins	• **Alpha-hemolysin:** Leukocidal & neurotoxic. • **Beta-hemolysin: Sphingomyelinase; Exhibits hot-cold phenomenon**[Q] • **Gamma-hemolysin:** Bicomponent protein • **Delta-hemolysin:** Diarrheal diseases, **detergent like effect**[Q] • **Leukocidin (Panton valentine toxin**[Q]**): Induce apoptosis** (at low concentration) & **lysis of various cell types**, including erythrocytes, lymphocytes, monocytes, epithelial cells. Bi-component, responsible for MRSA.
	Enterotoxins (A, B, C1-3, D, E, H)	• **Preformed, heat stable, responsible for food poisoning (<6 hours onset)**[Q] • **MC: Type A**[Q]
	Toxic shock syndrome toxin (Superantigen)	• **Activate T cells** & **macrophages** by binding to class II MHC, causes toxic shock syndrome • **MC TSST: Enterotoxin F (pyrogenic exotoxin C) > Enterotoxin B**
	Exfoliative/ Epidermolytic toxin	• Act as serine proteases; activate T cells, • **Causes epidermolysis & scalded skin syndrome**[Q]

Exotoxin	Mechanism of Action
Enterotoxin & TSST of S. aureus **Streptococcal pyrogenic exotoxin**	• Act as **super-antigen;** stimulate T-cell non-specifically, to release large amounts of cytokines[Q]
Diphtheria toxin **Exotoxin A of Pseudomonas**	• **Inhibits protein synthesis**[Q] (by inhibiting **EF-2**)
Anthrax toxin	• **Increases cAMP** in target cells, edema[Q]
Alpha toxin of Clostridium perfringens	• **Lecithinase & phospholipase** activity-causes **myonecrosis**[Q]
Tetanus toxin (tetanospasmin)	• Decrease in neurotransmitter (**GABA & glycine**) release from inhibitory **neurons-spasticity**[Q]
Botulinum toxin	• **Decrease in neurotransmitter** (acetylcholine) release from neurons **(flaccid paralysis)**[Q]
Heat labile toxin of ETEC and Cholera toxin (V. cholerae)	• Activation of **adenylate cyclase- Increases cAMP** in target cells-secretory diarrhea[Q]
Heat stable toxin	**Increases cGMP** in target cells leading to **secretory diarrhea**[Q]
Verocytotoxin (EHEC) **Shiga** toxin (Shigella dysenteriae type 1)	**Inhibit protein synthesis** by **inhibiting ribosome**[Q]

74. **Ans. a. Chlamydia trachomatis** *(Ref: Ananthanarayan 10/e p427; Jawetz 27/e p356; Nelson 20/e p1495; Harrison 19/e p1169)*

Among the given options, Chlamydia trachomatis is the only bacteria which causes both pneumonia and conjunctivitis.

"Infections during pregnancy can be transmitted to infants during delivery. Approximately 20–30% of infants exposed to C. trachomatis in the birth canal develop conjunctivitis, and 10–15% subsequently develop pneumonia."-Harrison 19/e p1169

AIIMS May 2017

"Chlamydia trachomatis: Of newborns infected by the mother, 10–20% may develop respiratory tract involvement 2–12 weeks after birth, culminating in pneumonia. Affected newborns have nasal obstruction or discharge, striking tachypnea, a characteristic paroxysmal staccato cough, an absence of fever, and eosinophilia. Interstitial infiltrates and hyperinflation can be seen on radiographs. The diagnosis should be suspected if pneumonitis develops in a newborn who has inclusion conjunctivitis and can be established by isolation of C trachomatis from respiratory secretions. In such neonatal pneumonia, an immunoglobulin M (IgM) antibody titer to C trachomatis of 1:32 or more is considered diagnostic. Oral erythromycin for 14 days is recommended; systemic erythromycin is effective treatment in severe cases."
-Jawetz 27/e p356

"Pneumonia due to C. trachomatis can develop in 10-20% of infants born to women with active, untreated chlamydial infection. Only about 25% of infants with nasopharyngeal chlamydial infection develop pneumonia. C. trachomatis pneumonia of infancy has a very characteristic presentation. Onset usually occurs between 1 and 3 mo of age and is often insidious, with persistent cough, tachypnea, and absence of fever. Auscultation reveals rales; wheezing is uncommon. The absence of fever and wheezing helps to distinguish C. trachomatis pneumonia from respiratory syncytial virus pneumonia. A distinctive laboratory finding is the presence of peripheral eosinophilia (>400 cells/ mm³). The most consistent finding on chest radiograph is hyperinflation accompanied by minimal interstitial or alveolar infiltrates."-
Nelson 20/e p1495

Infant Pneumonia caused by Chlamydia trachomatis
• **Pneumonia due to C. trachomatis** can develop in **10-20%** of infants born to women with active, untreated chlamydial infection[Q]. • Only about **25% of infants with nasopharyngeal chlamydial infection develop pneumonia**[Q].
Clinical Features: • **Conjunctivitis often precedes pneumonia**[Q] • Occurs between **2-12 weeks after birth**[Q] • Affected newborns have **nasal obstruction or discharge, striking tachypnea, a characteristic paroxysmal staccato cough, an absence of fever & eosinophilia. Auscultation reveals rales**; wheezing is uncommon[Q].   • **Absence of fever & wheezing** helps to **distinguish C. trachomatis pneumonia from respiratory syncytial virus pneumonia**[Q].

Diagnosis:
• Diagnosis should be suspected if **pneumonitis develops in a newborn having inclusion conjunctivitis** and can be established by isolation of **C. trachomatis from respiratory secretions**[Q].
• **IgM antibody titer to C. trachomatis of 1:32 or more is considered diagnostic**[Q].
    • **Distinctive laboratory finding: Peripheral eosinophilia (>400 cells/ mm³)**[Q].
    • **Most consistent finding on chest X-ray: Interstitial infiltrates & hyperinflation**[Q]

Treatment: • **Oral erythromycin**[Q] for 14 days is recommended; **systemic erythromycin** is effective treatment in **severe cases**.

75. Ans. b. Ancylostoma duodenale *(Ref: Paniker 7/e p183)*

The given egg in the image belongs to Ancylostoma duodenale (Hookworm). Eggs of Ancylostoma are oval, colorless, non-bile stained, and surrounded by a thin transparent hyaline shell. It has a segmented ovum with four blastomeres. Eggs of both the hookworms, Necator and Ancylostoma are similar in appearance.

"Egg of hookworm (Ancylostoma duodenale) is oval or elliptical, measuring 60 micron by 40 micron; colorless, not bile stained; Surrounded by thin transparent hyaline shell membrane; Floats in saturated salt saline; When released by the worm in the intestine, the egg contains an unsegmented ovum; During its passage down the intestine, the ovum develops. When passed in the feces, the egg contains a segmented ovum, usually with 4 or 8 blastomeres. There is a clear space between the segmented ovum and the egg shell."-Paniker 7/e p183

76. Ans. c. Entamoeba histolytica *(Ref: Paniker's 7/e p17; Jawetz 27/e p711; Harrison 19/e p1364)*

Entamoeba histolytica exists in three morphological forms, trophozoite, precyst and cyst. Tetranucleate cyst is the infective stage, which can divide to octanucleate cyst as in the given life cycle.

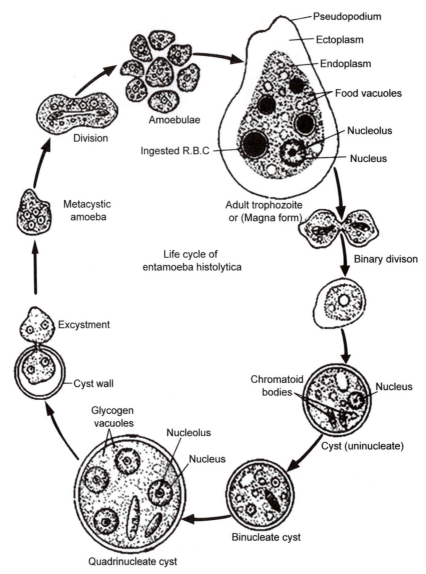

Fig. 15: Life cycle of entamoeba histolytica

Entamoeba Histolytica
• Entamoeba histolytica causes **intestinal amoebiasis & amebic liver abscess**. • **Host**: Humans are the only host[Q] • **Route of infection**: Feco-oral route[Q]; **Infective stage**: Quadrinucleate cyst[Q] • **Site of infection**: Large intestine[Q]
Life Cycle of Entamoeba Histolytica
• **Excystation occurs in small intestine** →8 metacystic trophozoites are released →carried to **large intestine**→Trophozoites colonizes large intestine mucosa →**Asymptomatic cyst passers /Amebic dysentery/ Amebic liver abscess** • **Encystation occurs in large intestine** →First precyst →Immature cyst →**Mature quadrinucleate cyst** released in feces (**diagnostic form**)

AIIMS May 2017

Pathogenesis:
- **Virulence factors: amebic lectin antigen[Q]**, cysteine proteinase, amebapore, neuraminidase & metalloproteinase
- Both **trophozoites & cysts** are found **in intestinal lumen**, but **only trophozoites invade tissue**.
- Trophozoites attach to colonic mucus & epithelial cells by **Gal/ GalNAc lectin[Q]**.
- **Earliest intestinal lesions: Microulcerations[Q] of mucosa** of large intestine

  - **MC form of invasive disease: Colitis[Q]**
  - **MC site of amebic colitis: Cecum & ascending colon[Q]**
  - **In colon: Flask-shaped ulcers[Q] (MC site: Cecum & ascending colon)[Q]**
  - **Synchronous hepatic abscess** is found in **one third** of patients with **active amebic colitis.**

Intestinal amoebiasis:
- **MC type of amebic infection**: **Asymptomatic cyst passage[Q]**
- Symptomatic amebic colitis develops 2–6 weeks after ingestion of cysts.
- A gradual onset of **lower abdominal pain & mild diarrhea** is followed by **malaise, weight loss & diffuse lower abdominal or back pain[Q]**.
- Cecal involvement may mimic **acute appendicitis[Q]**.
- **Complications:** Toxic megacolon, fulminant amebic colitis

Laboratory diagnosis:
- **Minimum 3 stool samples on consecutive days[Q]** (ameba are **shed intermittently[Q]**)
- **Stool microscopy: Trophozoite** (indicates **active infection[Q]**); **Quadrinucleate cyst** (indicates **carrier state**)
- Stool culture & stool antigen detection by ELISA

Appearance (Gross & Microscopic):
- **Proctoscopy: Small ulcers with heaped-up margins** & normal intervening mucosa[Q]

  - **Submucosal extension of ulcerations** under viable-appearing surface mucosa causes **classic "flask-shaped" ulcer** containing **trophozoites at margins of dead & viable tissues[Q]**.
  - **Human intestinal infection** is marked by a **paucity of inflammatory cells**, probably in part because of **killing of neutrophils by trophozoites[Q]**.

Treatment:
- **Metronidazole** is **mainstay of treatment[Q]**.
- **Luminal agents** include **iodoquinol, paromomycin & diloxanide furoate[Q]**.

77. **Ans. a. Fasciola hepatica**   *(Ref: Paniker 7/e p151; Jawetz 27/e p735; Harrison 19/e p1428)*

The given life cycle is of Fasciola hepatica in which adult worm is large, leaf-shaped fleshy with conical projection anteriorly containing oral sucker and rounded posteriorly. Eggs are large, ovoid, operculated, bile-stained.

Fasciola hepatica (Sheep liver fluke)

- **Largest & most common liver fluke** found **in humans**
- Found mainly in **sheep-rearing areas**, causes **'liver-rot' in sheep[Q]**

Morphology of Fasciola hepatica	
Adult Worm	**Egg**
- **Large, leaf-shaped fleshy** fluke[Q] - Length: 30 mm; Breadth: 15 mm - **Conical projection anteriorly** containing oral sucker[Q]	- Eggs are large, ovoid, **operculated, bile-stained[Q]** - Eggs contain **immature larva[Q] (miracidium)** - **Do not float** in saturated solution of common salt[Q] - **Freshly passed** eggs are **embryonated[Q]**

Life-Cycle:
- **Definitive host**: **Sheep**, goat, cattle & **man[Q]**
- **Intermediate host: Snail (Lymnaea & Succinea[Q])**; encystment occurs on **aquatic plant** which acts as **2nd intermediate host[Q]**
- **Mode of Infection: Eating metacercariae on watercress, aquatic vegetation[Q]**
- **Site of Infection:** Adult worms resides in **liver & bile duct of definitive host[Q]**

Contd...

Fasciola hepatica (Sheep liver fluke)
• **Adult worm** in biliary tree of definitive host →**Eggs** are laid in **biliary tree** & shed in feces →**Embryo matures in water** in 10 days →**Miracidium** escapes →Attaches & penetrate the **tissue of snail** →Converted into **cercariae in snail** → cercariae encyst on aquatic vegetation →**Metacercariae**→ Eating metacercariae on aquatic vegetation by definitive host → Metacercariae excyst in duodenum →Pierce gut wall to enter peritoneal cavity →**Penetrate Glisson's capsule** & traverse liver parenchyma →**Reach biliary passage** & mature into **adult worm**[Q].

Clinical Features:
- **Acute infection:** Abdominal pain, intermittent fever, eosinophilia, malaise & weight loss due to liver damage.
- **Chronic infection** may be **asymptomatic** or lead to **intermittent biliary tract obstruction**[Q].
- **Halzoun:** Allergic pharyngitis following the **consumption of raw liver of infected sheep**[Q].

Diagnosis:
- **Stool microscopy:** Demonstration of **operculated eggs in feces** or aspirated bile from duodenum is the **best method of diagnosis**[Q].

Treatment:
- **DOC: Oral triclabendazole**[Q]; Alternative drug: Bithionol

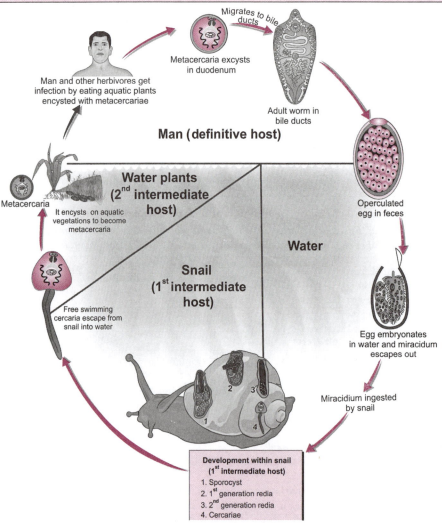

Fig. 16: Life cycle of fasciola hepatica

AIIMS May 2017

78. Ans. a. Klebsiella granulomatis *(Ref: Ananthanarayan 10/e p404; Jawetz 27/e p761; Harrison 19/e p198e-1; Robbins 9/e p371)*

Coccobacilli seen in the Giemsa-stained specimen suggest a diagnosis of granuloma inguinale or donovanosis. Donovan bodies are seen intracellularly in mononuclear cells. Granuloma inguinale, or donovanosis, is a chronic inflammatory disease caused by Calymmatobacterium granulomatis (Klebsiella granulomatis or Donovania granulomatis), a minute, encapsulated, coccobacilli that is closely related to the Klebsiella genus. The organism is sexually transmitted.

"Klebsiella granulomatis Laboratory Diagnosis: This can be made by demonstration of Donovan bodies in Wright-Giemsa stained impression smears from the lesions. They appear as rounded coccobacilli, 1-2 micron in size, within cystic spaces in large mononuclear cells. They show bipolar condensation of chromatin, giving a closed safety-pin appearance in stained smears. Capsules are usually seen as dense acidophilic areas around the bacilli. They are non-motile and Gram-negative."- Ananthanarayan 10/e p404

"Calymmatobacterium donovani: The organisms are demonstrable in Giemsa-stained smears of the exudate as minute, encapsulated coccobacilli (Donovan bodies) in macrophages. Silver stains (e.g., the Warthin-Starry stain) may also demonstrate the organism."- Robbins 9/e p371

Granuloma Inguinale
• **Granuloma inguinale or donovanosis**, is a chronic inflammatory disease **caused by *Calymmatobacterium granulomatis (Klebsiella granulomatis or Donovania granulomatis)*,** a minute, encapsulated, coccobacillus that is **closely related to *Klebsiella* genus[Q].** • **Calymmatobacterium granulomatis[Q]**, a pleomorphic, **gram-negative[Q]** rod. • Donovanosis is a **chronic, progressive bacterial infection**, involves **genital region**. • **Sexually transmitted infection** of **low infectivity**.
Etiology: • Characteristic **Donovan bodies** in **macrophages & stratum malpighii[Q]**. • Donovanosis is **associated with poor hygiene, more common in lower socioeconomic groups**
Clinical Features: • **Incubation period: 8 days to 12 weeks;** • A lesion starts as a **papule or subcutaneous nodule** that later **ulcerates after trauma[Q]**. • **Genitals** are affected in **90%** & **inguinal region** in **10%**. • Subcutaneous granulomas may develop in the inguinal region called **'pseudo-buboes[Q]'**

Four types of lesions have been described:	
1. **Classic ulcerogranulomatous lesion,** a **beefy red ulcer** that **bleeds readily when touched[Q]** 2. A **hypertrophic or verrucous ulcer** with a raised irregular edge[Q]	3. A **necrotic, offensive-smelling ulcer** causing **tissue destruction[Q]** 4. A **sclerotic or cicatricial lesion** with fibrous & scar tissue[Q].

• **Most common sites of infection: Prepuce, coronal sulcus, frenulum & glans** in men; labia minora & fourchette in women.
• **Cervical lesions** may **mimic cervical carcinoma**.

Diagnosis:
• **Diagnosis** is confirmed by **microscopic identification of Donovan bodies** in tissue smears[Q].
• **Donovan bodies** can be seen in large, **mononuclear (Pund) cells** as **gram-negative intracytoplasmic cysts filled with deeply staining bodies** that may have a **safety-pin appearance[Q]**.
• **PCR analysis with a colorimetric detection system** can now be used in routine diagnostic laboratories.

> • **Microscopic examination of active lesions** reveals marked epithelial hyperplasia at the borders of the ulcer, sometimes mimicking carcinoma (**pseudoepitheliomatous hyperplasia[Q]**).
> • **A mixture of neutrophils & mononuclear inflammatory cells is present at the base of the ulcer and beneath the surrounding epithelium[Q]**.
> • **Organisms** are demonstrable in **Giemsa-stained** smears of the **exudate** as **minute, encapsulated coccobacilli (Donovan bodies) in macrophages.[Q]**

Granuloma Inguinale
Treatment: • Drug of choice: Azithromycin[Q] • Alternatives; Cotrimoxazole, erythromycin & tetracycline

PAP Smear Findings in Sexually Transmitted Infections		
Granuloma inguinale	**Trichomonas vaginalis**	**Haemophilus ducreyi**
• Caused by **Calymmatobacterium granulomatis**[Q] • **Coccobacilli** seen in Giemsa-stained specimen[Q] • **Donovan bodies** are seen **intracellularly in mononuclear cells**[Q].	• In cervical smear, **transparent 'halo' around their superficial cell nucleus**[Q] • Three-dimensional clusters of neutrophils (**polyballs**[Q]) may be seen.	• **Moderate small gram-negative rods**[Q] • **School of fish appearance**[Q] is seen with 40–50 WBCs/hpf. • No clue cells observed.

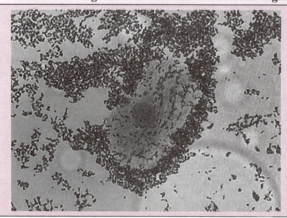
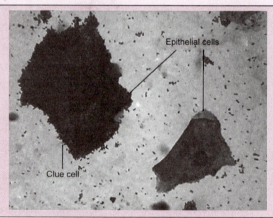

PAP Smear in Bacterial Vaginosis
• Finding of a **watery discharge & typical smell**[Q] • **'Clue cells'** (sloughed epithelial cells coated with Gram-variable pleomorphic coccobacilli): This is **sufficient evidence to diagnose infection with Gardnerella vaginalis**[Q].

79. Ans. b. RT-PCR for virus *(Ref: Ananthanarayan 10/e p538; Harrison 19/e p1302; Jawetz 27/e p610)*
RT-PCR techniques can accurately identify rabies genome in CSF, saliva, corneal scrapings or urine.

"Detection of rabies virus RNA by RT-PCR is highly sensitive and specific. This technique can detect virus in fresh saliva samples, skin, CSF, and brain tissues. In addition, RT-PCR with genetic sequencing can distinguish among rabies virus variants, permitting identification of the probable source of an infection."-Harrison 19/e p1302

"Reverse transcription-polymerase chain reaction testing can be used to amplify parts of a rabies virus genome from fixed or unfixed brain tissue or saliva. Sequencing of amplified products can allow identification of the infecting virus strain."- Jawetz 27/e p610

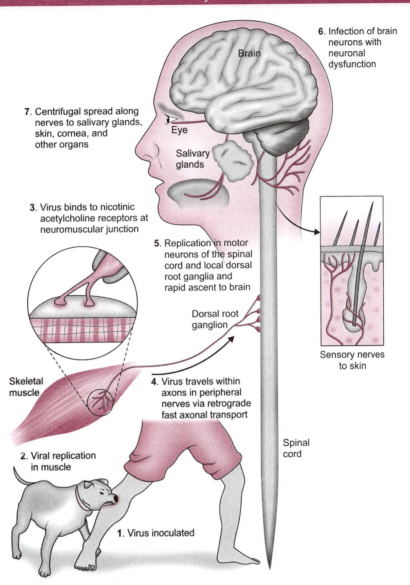

Fig. 17: Pathogenetic events following peripheral inoculation of Rabies virus

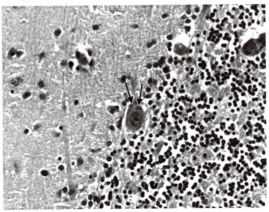

Fig. 18: Negri body seen in a Purkinje cell (arrows)

Rabies

- Rabies is a **rapidly progressive, acute infectious disease of CNS**[Q]
- **Zoonotic infection** occurs throughout the world **except in Antarctica** & on some islands[Q].
- Caused by infection with rabies virus, **transmitted from animal vectors** by the **bite of an infected animal (mainly dogs & sometimes from bats)**[Q]
  - **Aerosols generated** in laboratory or in **caves containing millions of Brazilian free-tail bats** have rarely **caused human rabies**[Q].
  - **Transmission** has resulted from **corneal transplantation, solid organ transplantation** & **vascular conduit** from undiagnosed donors[Q].

Etiologic Agent:
- Rabies virus is **single-strand RNA virus**[Q]
- **Family: Rhabdoviridae; Genera: Lyssavirus**[Q]

Pathogenesis:
- **Incubation period (IP): 20-90 days**[Q]
- During **IP, rabies virus** is **present** at or **close to site of inoculation**[Q].
  - Rabies virus **spreads centripetally along peripheral nerves toward CNS** at a rate of up to **~250 mm/day via retrograde fast axonal transport to spinal cord or brainstem**[Q].
  - In CNS, it **rapidly disseminates to other regions of CNS via fast axonal transport** along neuroanatomical connections[Q].
  - **Neurons are prominently infected in rabies; infection of astrocytes is unusual**[Q].
- **After established CNS infection, centrifugal spread along sensory & autonomic nerves** to other tissues, including salivary glands, heart, adrenal & skin occurs[Q].
  - **Rabies virus replicates** in acinar cells of salivary glands & is **secreted in saliva of rabid animals** that **serve as vectors of disease**[Q].

Pathology:
- **Pathologic changes** are mild in light of clinical severity & fatal outcome of disease.
- **Babes nodules: Microglial nodules** with **collection of lymphocytes in rabies**[Q]
- **Most characteristic pathologic finding: Negri body**[Q]

Negri bodies
- **Eosinophilic cytoplasmic inclusions in brain neurons** composed of **rabies virus proteins & viral RNA**[Q]
- Occur in a **minority of infected neurons**[Q]
- Commonly observed in **Purkinje cells of cerebellum** & in **pyramidal neurons of hippocampus; less frequently seen in **cortical & brainstem neurons**[Q].
- Negri bodies are **not observed in all cases** of rabies[Q].

- **Neuronal dysfunction** (rather than neuronal death) **is responsible for clinical disease in rabies**[Q].

Clinical Features:
- Rabies usually presents as **atypical encephalitis** with **relative preservation of consciousness**.
- Some patients present with **acute flaccid paralysis**.
- There are **prodromal, acute neurologic & comatose phases** that usually **progress to death** despite aggressive therapy.

Clinical Stages of Rabies

Phase	Typical Duration	Symptoms and Signs
Incubation period	20-90 days	• None
Prodrome	2-10 days	• Fever, malaise, anorexia, nausea, vomiting; paresthesias, pain, or pruritus at the wound site
Acute neurologic disease		
Encephalitic (80%)	2-7 days	• Anxiety, **agitation, hyperactivity, bizarre behavior, hallucinations, autonomic dysfunction, hydrophobia**[Q]
Paralytic (20%)	2-10 days	• **Flaccid paralysis** in limbs **progressing to quadriparesis** with **facial paralysis**[Q]
Coma, death	0-14 days	

Rabies
Diagnosis:
• Once rabies is suspected, **rabies-specific laboratory tests** should be performed **to confirm the diagnosis.**
• Diagnostically useful specimens: Serum, CSF, fresh saliva, skin biopsy samples from **neck & brain tissue**[Q] (rarely obtained before death).
• **Corneal impression smears** are of **low diagnostic yield** & are generally **not performed**[Q].
• **Negative ante-mortem rabies-specific laboratory tests never exclude a diagnosis of rabies**, and tests may need to be repeated after an interval for diagnostic confirmation[Q].
• **Rabies virus-specific antibodies in a previously unimmunized patient, serum neutralizing antibodies to rabies virus are diagnostic**[Q].
• **Presence of rabies virus–specific antibodies in CSF suggests rabies encephalitis**, regardless of immunization status[Q].
• **RT-PCR Amplification** Detection of rabies virus RNA by RT-PCR is **highly sensitive & specific**[Q].
• This technique can **detect virus in fresh saliva samples, skin, CSF, and brain tissues**[Q].
• **Direct fluorescent antibody testing** with rabies virus antibodies conjugated to fluorescent dyes is **highly sensitive & specific** and can be **performed quickly** and **applied to skin biopsies & brain tissue**[Q].
• In **skin biopsies, rabies virus antigen** may be **detected in cutaneous nerves at base of hair follicles**[Q].
Treatment:
• **No established treatment for rabies**[Q] (A palliative approach may be appropriate for some patients)
Prognosis:
• **Fatal disease** but **preventable with appropriate post-exposure therapy** during the **early incubation period**[Q].

80. **Ans. a. Heterophile antibody test** *(Ref: Ananthanarayan 10/e p111, 482; Harrison 19/e p1189)*

Epstein-Barr virus (EBV) infection induces specific antibodies to EBV and various unrelated non-EBV heterophile antibodies. These heterophile antibodies react to antigens from animal RBCs. Sheep RBCs agglutinate in the presence of heterophile antibodies and are the basis for the Paul-Bunnell test.

> *"Paul-Bunnell Test in Infectious Mononucleosis: The standard diagnostic procedure is Paul-Bunnell test. In infectious mononucleosis, heterophile antibodies agglutinate sheep erythrocytes. However, such antibodies may also occur after injection of sera and sometimes even in normal individuals. Infectious mononucleosis antibodies may be differentiated by adsorption tests. Inactivated serum (56°C for 30 minutes) in doubling dilutions is mixed with equal volumes of 1% suspension of sheep erythrocytes. After incubation at 37°C for four hours the tubes are examined for agglutination. An agglutination titre of 100 or above is suggestive of infectious mononucleosis."- Ananthanarayan 10/e p482*

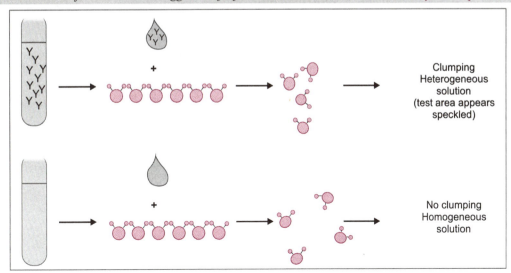

Fig. 19: Description of Paul-Bunnell test on positive and negative samples.

81. Ans. d. Invasive cryptococcosis *(Ref: Jawetz 27/e p665; Harrison 19/e p489, 1360; J. Clin. Microbiol, July 2014, vol. 52 no. 7 2328)*

(1-3)-β-D-glucan BG is a component of the cell walls of most fungi. The main exceptions are Mucorales and cryptococci, which release no or little BG to be detected in human serum. 1,3-beta D-glucan assay cannot identify invasive cryptococcosis.

"Another serum marker for the presence of invasive fungal infections is (1-3)-β-D-glucan (BG), which has been included in the relevant European Organization for Research and Treatment of Cancer (EORTC)/Mycoses Study Group diagnostic criteria. BG is a component of the cell walls of most fungi. The main exceptions are Mucorales and cryptococci, which release no or little BG to be detected in human serum."-J. Clin. Microbiol, July 2014, vol. 52 no. 7 2328

"β-(1,3)-d-glucan levels of ≥80 pg/mL are positive and associated with invasive candidiasis, aspergillosis, dimorphic pathogens, and other mycoses."-Jawetz 27/e p665

"There has been considerable interest in serologic tests such as assays for (1→3)-β-D-glucan, levels of which are frequently elevated in patients with PCP."-Harrison 19/e p1360

Cryptococcus neoformans
• **Cryptococcus neoformans** is **heavily encapsulated yeast**, not dimorphic & **found in soil, pigeon droppings**[Q]. • **C. neoformans** grows as **yeast (unicellular)** & **replicates by budding**[Q]. • **Cultured on sabouraud agar**[Q] • **Stains with India ink & mucicarmine**[Q]

Morphology:
• It makes **hyphae during mating** & eventually **creates basidiospores at the end of hyphae** before producing spores[Q].
   • **Under host-relevant conditions**, including **low glucose, serum, 5% carbon dioxide & low iron**, cells **produce a characteristic polysaccharide capsules**[Q].
   • When grown as yeast, **C. neoformans** has a **prominent capsule composed mostly of polysaccharides**[Q].
• **(1-3)-β-D-glucan BG is a component of the cell walls of most fungi. The main exceptions are Mucorales & cryptococci**, which **release no or little BG to be detected in human serum.**

Pathogenesis: • Acquired through **inhalation of aerosolized infectious particles** with **hematogenous dissemination to meninges**[Q].
Clinical Features: • **Meningoencephalitis, pneumonia, skin & soft tissue infections**[Q] • Characterized by **'Soap bubble' lesions in brain**[Q].

Diagnosis:
• A **diagnosis of cryptococcosis** requires the **demonstration of yeast cells in normally sterile tissues**[Q].
• **Visualization of the capsule of fungal cells in CSF mixed with India ink** is a **useful rapid diagnostic technique**[Q].
   • **Cryptococcal cells in India ink** have a **distinctive appearance because their capsules exclude ink particles (zone of clearance or 'halo' around the cells)**[Q]
   • For **identification in tissue, mucicarmine stain provides specific staining of polysaccharide cell wall in C. neoformans**[Q].
• **Cultures of CSF & blood** that are **positive for cryptococcal cells are diagnostic for cryptococcosis**[Q].
• A particularly useful test is **cryptococcal antigen (CRAg) detection in CSF & blood.** The assay is **based on serologic detection of cryptococcal polysaccharide** & is both **sensitive & specific**[Q].
• **Cryptococcal** capsules exhibit bright birefringence & **Maltese-cross** formation on polarizing microscopy[Q]

Drug of Choice in Fungal Infections	
• **Meningeal histoplasmosis** • **Endocarditis by Candida** • **Coccidioidomycosis** • **Severe or CNS Blastomycosis** • **Induction in Cryptococcal meningitis (for 2 weeks)** • **Mucormycosis** • **Exserohilum**	• **Amphotericin B**[Q]

• Non-meningeal histoplasmosis • Para-Coccidioidomycosis • Sporotrichosis • Mild or non-CNS Blastomycosis • Penicillium marneffei • Chromoblastomycosis • Eumycetoma & Actinomycetoma	• Itraconazole[Q]
• Maintenance in Cryptococcal meningitis (for 8 weeks) • Candida albicans	• Fluconazole[Q]
• Invasive aspergillosis • Fusarium • Pseudoallescheria boydii	• Voriconazole[Q]
• Allergic bronchopulmonary aspergillosis	• Prednisolone + Itraconazole/ Voriconazole[Q]
• Candida glabarata & Candida krusei	• Capsofungin[Q]

82. **Ans. c. Aquatic protistan protozoa**   *(Ref: Medical Microbiology by Patrick Murray 8/e p676)*
Rhinosporidium seeberi, most recently has been placed in the novel clade of aquatic protistan parasites, the Mesomycetozoa.

> "*Rhinosporidium seeberi:* This organism has been considered to be a protozoan, a fungus, and **most recently has been placed in the novel clade of aquatic protistan parasites, the Mesomycetozoa**. Because R. seeberi will not grow in synthetic media, this classification was **based on sequence analysis of the 18S small-subunit ribosomal DNA (rDNA) of this organism**. This analysis placed R. seeberi among the Mesomycetozoa (formerly DRIP: *Dermatocystidium*, Rosette agent, *Ichthyophonus*, and *Psorospermium*), a clade of fish parasite that form a branch of evolutionary tree near the animal-fungal divergence." - *Medical Microbiology by Patrick Murray 8/e p676*

83. **Ans. a. 1 Fc and 2 Fab fragments**   *(Ref: Harper 30/e p682; Jawetz 27/e p136)*
Hydrolysis of IgG with papain will lead to formation of 1 Fc and 2 Fab fragments. Papain hydrolyses IgG at the hinge region, which lyses IgG into one constant Fc region and two Fab fragments.

> "When studying the Ig molecule structure, it was identified experimentally that an antibody molecule, such as IgG, can be split into two fragments by the proteolytic enzyme, papain. When this happens, the peptide bonds in the hinge region are broken. The antigen-binding activity is associated with one of these fragments, the Fab portion. The second fragment is the Fc portion that is involved in placental transfer, complement fixation, attachment to various cells, and other biologic activities." - *Jawetz 27/e p136*

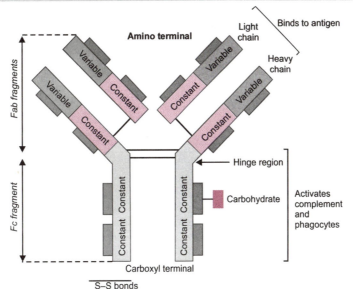

Fig. 20: Schematic representation of an IgG molecule, indicating the location of the constant and the variable regions on the light and heavy chains. Fab fragment is fragment antigen binding, Fc fragment is fragment crystallizable.

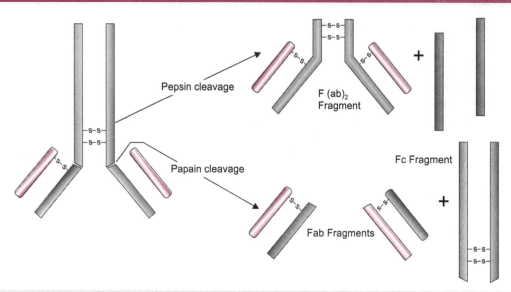

> "Fragmentation of IgG molecule, when digested by papain, produces three fragments, 2 Fab & 1 Fc. Digestion by pepsin leads to destruction of Fc, leaving a divalent fragment designated (Fab)₂."- *Fundamentals of Immunology By Otto G. Bier, Wilmar Dias Da Silva, Dietrich Götze, Ivan Mota 2/e p88*

> "Papain hydrolysis: The reaction by means of which IgG molecules are split into three fragments (2 Fab fragments, 1 Fc fragment) by treatment with papain in the presence of cysteine. The papain attacks a histidyl-threonine peptide bond on the heavy chain at the site."-*Illustrated Dictionary of Immunology by M.P. Arora/p410*

84. **Ans. a. B-cells, dendritic cells and macrophages**   *(Ref: Robbins 9/e p102, 191; Ananthanarayan 10/e p141)*

MHC Class II proteins are expressed by all antigen presenting cells, which includes B-cells, follicular dendritic cells and macrophages. MHC Class I proteins are expressed by all nucleated cells, which excludes platelets and RBCs.

> "HLA class I antigens (A, B and C) are found on the surface of virtually all nucleated cells. They are the principal antigens involved in graft rejection and cell-mediated cytolysis. Class I molecules may function as components of hormone receptors. HLA class II antigens are more restricted in distribution, being found only on cells of the immune system- macrophages, dendritic cells, activated T cells, and particularly on B cells."- *Ananthanarayan 8/e p 132*

Antigen Presenting Cells (APC)	
Professional APCs	**Nonprofessional APCs**

• Express MHC class II molecules[Q]
 • It includes:
   – Dendritic cells[Q]
   – Immature dendritic cells[Q]
   – Macrophages[Q]
   – B-cells[Q]
	• Do not express MHC class II for interaction with naïve T cells[Q].
	 • Stimulation by cytokines like IFN-γ[Q].
	
	 Nonprofessional APCs include
	 • Fibroblasts[Q] (skin) • Glial cells[Q] (brain)
	 • Thymic epithelial cells[Q] • Pancreatic beta cells[Q]
	 • Thyroid epithelial cells[Q] • Endothelial cells[Q]

Major Histocompatibility Complex

- In humans, **gene encoding MHC or HLA complex** are clustered on **a small segment (4 megabase region) of chromosome 6 short arm**[Q] **(6p 21.3)**[Q].
- HLA class I & class II genes whose products are critical for **immunological specificity & transplantation histocompatibility**[Q] & they play a major role in **susceptibility to a number of autoimmune diseases**.
- **Function: Binds peptide fragments of foreign protein for presentation to appropriate antigen specific T-Cells**[Q].

MHC is involved in	
• Transplantation reaction[Q] • Disease susceptibility (autoimmune[Q], infectious & inflammatory disease)	• Immune response & tolerance[Q] • Complement component[Q]

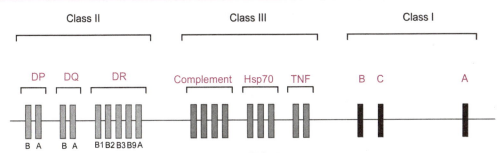

Fig. 21: MHC cluster

Feature	MHC-I	MHC-II	MHC-III
Expressed on (presented by)	All nucleated cells & platelets[Q]	Antigen presenting cells including Dendritic cells[Q] in lymph node & spleen, Langerhans cells[Q], Macrophages, B cells[Q] & activated T cells[Q]	Class III is **present in between I & II**
Encoded by (component loci)	3 closely linked loci designated HLA-**A**, HLA-**B** and HLA-**C**	HLA-D (HLA **DP, DQ, DR**)	C4B, BF, C2 TNF α & β
Encoding molecule	Cell surface glycoprotein involved in antigen presentation[Q]	Cell surface glycoprotein involved in antigen presentation[Q]	**Components of complement system**[Q]
Recognized by	**CD8+ T-cells**[Q], NK cell recognition	**CD4+ helper T-cells**[Q]	
Function	• Immune response against intracellular infection, tumors, allografts[Q] • Graft rejection[Q] • Cell mediated cytolysis[Q] • Component of hormone receptor[Q]	• Graft versus host response[Q] • Mixed leucocyte reaction (MLR) • Influence functional capacity of mature peripheral T cells[Q].	• MHC III include complement components linked to **formation of C3 convertases**, **heat shock proteins & tumor necrosis factors**.

85. **Ans. a. Ceftriaxone** *(Ref: Harrison 19/e p1000)*

Though penicillin is the drug of choice for susceptible strains in meningococcal meningitis, a 3rd generation cephalosporin like Ceftriaxone or cefotaxime is preferred as empirical therapy in patients with meningococcal septicemia. Once culture reports are available, antibiotic therapy should be based on the susceptibility.

"Empirical antibiotic therapy for suspected meningococcal disease consists of a third-generation cephalosporin such as ceftriaxone (75–100 mg/kg per day [maximum, 4 g/d] in one or two divided IV doses) or cefotaxime (200 mg/kg per day [maximum, 8 g/d] in four divided IV doses) to cover the various other (potentially penicillin-resistant) bacteria that may produce an indistinguishable clinical syndrome."-Harrison 19/e p1000

Neisseria meningitides (Meningococci)
• **Gram (-)ve, aerobic, non-motile, lens shaped diplococci**[Q] • **Oxidase positive**[Q] (key test for identifying Neisseria), catalase positive • **Ferments glucose & maltose** but not sucrose[Q] • Can grow both **intracellularly & extracellularly**[Q] • Categorized as **β-proteobacterium**[Q] on basis of genome sequencing
Classification: • On the basis of capsular polysaccharide, classified into 13 serogroups • 5 serogroups are responsible for most meningococcal diseases (**A,B,C,W,Y**)[Q] • **Group A- epidemic, Group B- both epidemic & outbreak, Group C- Localized outbreak**[Q]

AIIMS ESSENCE

Neisseria meningitides (Meningococci)
Virulence Factors: • Capsular polysaccharide   • Outer membrane protein (pilli)   • **Lipooligosaccharide, LOS (endotoxin)**[Q] not the lipopolysaccharide: **Morbidity & mortality** of meningococcal **bacteremia & meningitis** is **directly proportional to** amount of **circulating meningococcal endotoxin**   • IgA proteases & Transferrin binding protein
Pathogenesis: • **MC source of infection: Human nasopharyngeal carriers**[Q]   • **Mode of transmission: Droplet inhalation**[Q]   • **Spread of infection: MC route of spread to meninges** from nasopharynx is **hematogenous**[Q] > **direct olfactory nerve spread via cribriform plate**[Q]

Clinical Features:
 • **Incubation period: 3-4 days**[Q] (may vary from 2-10 days)
 • **Deficiency of** terminal or alternate complement pathway C_5-C_9[Q] **increases the risk of meningococcal infection**
        • **Meningitis** is the result of **blood borne dissemination**[Q] & not the direct invasion
        • **Early symptoms** are **non-specific** & suggest an influenza like illness with **fever, headache & myalgia** accompanied by **vomiting & abdominal pain**[Q].
 • **Rash**, if present may appear to be viral early in the course, until petechiae or purpuric lesions develop.
 • **Fulminant meningococcemia**, most rapid lethal form of septic shock, with **prominent hemorrhagic skin lesions & characteristic rash**[Q]
 • **Fatality** of typically **untreated cases: 80%**[Q]
 • With **early diagnosis and treatment, case fatality rates** have declined to **<10%.**
        • **Waterhouse-Friedrichsen syndrome:** Severe form of **fulminant meningococcemia with large purpuric rash (purpura fulminans), shock, DIC, bilateral adrenal hemorrhage & multi-organ failure**[Q].

Lab Diagnosis: • Diagnosis is established by **recovering meningococci from sterile body fluids** such as **blood, CSF** etc.   • **Specimen for cases: Blood & CSF; Specimen for carriers: Nasopharyngeal swab**[Q]   • Grow best on **Muller-Hinton**[Q] or chocolate agar at 35°C in 5-10% CO_2.   • **Thayer-martin media** is **selective media**[Q] used **for culturing throat or nasopharyngeal specimen**
Treatment: • **3rd generation cephalosporin** such as **cefotaxime or ceftriaxone**[Q] is **DOC** for **initial therapy**   • **Prophylaxis: Rifampicin is DOC for meningococcal prophylaxis**[Q]
Prevention: • **Vaccine: Quadrivalent vaccine Meningococcal polysaccharide vaccine** (serogroup **A, C, W, Y**)[Q]   • There is **no vaccine against serogroup B**[Q] as its capsule is non-immunogenic   • Vaccine is **ineffective in Age < 2 years**[Q], so given after 2 years

FORENSIC MEDICINE

86. Ans. a. Nicotine *(Ref: Reddy 34/e p572; 33/e p615)*

Nicotine chronic poisoning can lead to cough, wheezing, dyspnoea, anorexia, vomiting, diarrhea, anaemia, faintness, tremors, impaired memory, amblyopia, blindness, irregularity of the heart with extra-systoles and occasionally attacks pain suggesting angina pectoris.

"Nicotiana Tabacum Chronic Poisoning: Symptoms are cough, wheezing, dyspnoea, anorexia, vomiting, diarrhea, anaemia, faintness, tremors, impaired memory, amblyopia, blindness, irregularity of the heart with extra-systoles and occasionally attacks pain suggesting angina pectoris."-Reddy 24/e p572; 33/e p615

Nicotiana Tabacum

- **All parts are poisonous except the ripe seeds**.
- **Dried leaves (tobacco)** contain **1-8% of nicotine** and are used in the form of smoke or snuff or chewed.
- **Leaves contain active principles (toxic alkaloids) nicotine, anabasine & nornicotine[Q]**.
- **Nicotine:** Colorless, volatile, bitter, hygroscopic liquid alkaloid; used extensively in agricultural & horticultural work, for fumigating & spraying, as insecticides, worm powders, etc.
- **Fatal Dose: 50-100 mg** of nicotine; **Fatal Period: 5-15 minutes[Q]**.

Absorption & Excretion:
- **Nicotine** is **rapidly absorbed from all mucous membranes**, lungs & skin; **80-90% is metabolized by the liver[Q]**
- **Excreted by the kidneys[Q]**

Action:
- It **acts on autonomic ganglia**, which are **stimulated initially; depressed & blocked at later stage[Q]**.
- It also acts on the **somatic neuromuscular junction & afferent fibres from sensory receptors[Q]**.

Signs & Symptoms	
Acute Poisoning	**Chronic Poisoning**
• **GIT:** Burning acid sensation, nausea, vomiting abdominal pain, hypersalivation[Q] • **Cardiopulmonary: Tachycardia, hypertension, tachypnoea (early); bradycardia, hypotension, respiratory depression (late).** Cardiac arrhythmias may occur[Q]. • **CNS: Miosis, confusion, headache, sweating, ataxia, agitation, restlessness, hyperthermia (early); mydriasis, lethargy, convulsions, coma (late)[Q]**. • **Death** may occur from **respiratory failure[Q]**.	• Symptoms are **cough, wheezing, dyspnoea, anorexia, vomiting, diarrhea, anaemia, faintness, tremors, impaired memory, amblyopia, blindness**, irregularity of the heart with **extra-systoles** and occasionally attacks **pain suggesting angina pectoris[Q]**.

Withdrawal Symptoms

- **Intense urge to smoke, anxiety, impaired concentration & memory[Q]**, depression or hostility, headache, muscle cramps, sleep disturbances, increased appetite & weight gain, diaphoresis & rapid respirations.
- A short period (6 to 12 weeks) of maintenance often followed by a gradual reduction in 6 to 12 weeks is adopted.
- **Nicotine replacement therapy** (NRT) includes use of nicotine products including **gum, transdermal patch, nasal spray, lozenge & inhaler[Q]**.
- **Bupropion** can be used in those who are motivated to quit.
- **Clonidine & nortriptyline** can be used as **2nd line of treatment**.

Treatment:
- **Gastric lavage** with warm water containing **charcoal, tannin or potassium permanganate[Q]**
- A purge & colonic wash-out.
- **Mecamylamine (Inversine)** is a **specific antidote give orally[Q]**.
- **Protect airway: Atropine sulphate & hexamethonium chloride[Q]** to counteract peripheral autonomic disturbances and as respiratory stimulant
- Vasodilators, oxygen & sympotomatic treatment

87. Ans. b. Chronic nicotine poisoning   *(Ref: Harrison 19/e p2730; Reddy 34/e p572; 33/e p615)*

Symptoms of chronic nicotine poisoning are cough, wheezing, dyspnoea, anorexia, vomiting, diarrhea, anaemia, faintness, tremors, impaired memory, amblyopia, blindness, irregularity of the heart with extra-systoles and occasionally attacks pain suggesting angina pectoris.

	CVS effects	Ophthalmic effects
Atropine	Tachycardia, arrhythmias[Q]	Mydriasis, diplopia[Q]
Cannabis	**Tachycardia, palpitations, hypotension[Q]**	—
Cocaine	**Sinus tachycardia, hypertension, myocardial ischemia, tachyarrhythmias[Q]**	**Mydriasis, central retinal arterial occlusion, bilateral blindness[Q]**
Nicotine	**Tachycardia, extra-systoles[Q]**	**Tobacco amblyopia[Q]**
Arsenic	**MI, stroke[Q]**	**Vitamin A deficiency & night blindness[Q]**

See Q. No 86 AIIMS May 2017.

88. **Ans. c. Positional asphyxia** *(Ref: Reddy 34/e p131, 33/e p364; Knight's Forensic Pathology 4/e p365)*
Keeping in Jack-knife position for long leads to death by positional asphyxia.

> *"Postural or Positional Asphyxia: Occasionally, it results from indirect compression, when the body is subjected to force in such a manner that his thighs and the knees are driven against his chest, the so-called "Jack-Knife" position. There is usually marked congestion, cyanosis and petechiae in the face and neck."* - Reddy 33/e p364

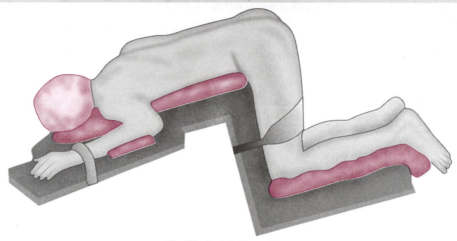

Fig. 22: Jack-knife position

Postural or Positional Asphyxia

- Occurs when the individual acquires a **certain body position** in which **breathing is impaired**, often because of **neck twisting with kinking** or **compression of trachea** and/or **elevation of the tongue into posterior hypopharynx. Normal venous return to heart** may be impaired[Q].
- **Body** is typically **inverted (upside-down)** & weight of abdominal contents press against the diaphragm pushing it upwards, thus **compressing the thoracic organs**, which combined with decreased respiratory movements, leads to **cardiorespiratory failure & death**[Q].
- It is **always accidental**[Q].

Causes:
- Most common in situations where a **violent or physically aggressive person** is physically or mechanically restrained **on their stomach, face down** or **in a prone position**.
- When a person **falls in a well & wedged between the walls**.
- An **intoxicated person may slide out of bed** so that his head & adjoining region hang down from the edge & remaining body rests at an upper level.
- From **forcible flexion of neck on the chest** or when he **collapses in a narrow space** & neck is bent or twisted.

> - **Indirect compression**, when the body is subjected to force in such a manner that thighs & knees are driven against his chest, the so-called **"Jack-Knife" position**[Q]. There is usually marked congestion, cyanosis & petechiae in the face & neck.

Diagnosis:
- Diagnosis is based on: **Body position must obstruct normal gas exchange**; It must **not be possible to move to another position**; Other causes of natural or violent death must be exclude.

89. **Ans. c. Negros have wide molar cusps and deep, shovel shaped cusps in incisors** *(Ref: Knight's Forensic Pathology 4/e p559)*

The presence of shovel shaped incisor is feature of mongoloids, and it is uncommon in Negroes. A congenital lack of the third upper molar is most common in Mongoloids, but can occur in any race. Small nodules on the lingual surface of maxillary molars, called 'Carabelli's cusp', are most common in Caucasian races and rare in the other major racial groups. Negroid races tend to have large teeth and often have more cusps on their molars, even up to eight, with two lingual cusps on the mandibular first premolars as an additional common finding.

AIIMS May 2017

*"Race is also a difficult criterion to determine from teeth. **The best-known feature is the 'shovel-shaped' upper central incisors of Mongoloid races**, first described in Leipzig by Muhlreiter in 1870. **The posterior surfaces of these teeth have a depression centrally, with two marginal bars, causing the back of the tooth to appear like a coal shovel with turned-up edges. The feature is found mainly amongst Chinese, Mongols, Eskimos and Japanese**, but is also found amongst non-Mongoloid races in lesser numbers. Some 91 per cent of Chinese, Japanese and Tibetans have such teeth, 95 per cent of Native Americans, 84 per cent of Eskimos, 46 per cent of Palestinian Arabs – and 90 per cent of Finns. **It is rare amongst Negroids and Australian Aboriginals."*- Knight's Forensic Pathology 4/e p559*

*"**In Caucasian races, the lateral incisors in the upper jaw are usually smaller than the central, especially in women, a feature absent or less marked in Negroid or Mongoloid races. Caucasians also have long pointed canine roots, a feature not seen in Mongoloids.** Enamel pearls, small nodules of enamel on the tooth surface, are much more frequent in Mongoloid teeth."*- Knight's Forensic Pathology 4/e p559*

*"**Small nodules on the lingual surface of maxillary molars, called 'Carabelli's cusp', are most common in Caucasian races and rare in the other major racial groups. The condition of bull-tooth or 'taurodontism' is most common in Mongoloid peoples: here the pulp cavity of molars is wide and deep, and the roots are fused and bent. A congenital lack of the third upper molar is most common in Mongoloids, but can occur in any race."*- Knight's Forensic Pathology 4/e p559*

*"**Negroid races tend to have large teeth and often have more cusps on their molars, even up to eight, with two lingual cusps on the mandibular first premolars as an additional common finding."*- Knight's Forensic Pathology 4/e p559*

90. **Ans. c. Ethylene glycol**   *(Ref: Reddy 34/e p542, 33/e p583)*

Most likely substance consumed by the patient was ethylene glycol as it can cause vomiting lethargy, ataxia, inebriation, convulsions and coma. In 12 to 24 hours tachycardia, tachypnoea and circulatory collapse, electrolyte imbalance and metabolic acidosis occur. In one to three days, hypocalcaemia, oliguria, tubular necrosis and renal failure occur. Urine contains crystals of calcium oxalate. For treatment gastric lavage, activated charcoal, ethanol in same dose as for methyl alcohol, 4-Methyl pyrazole, hemodialysis, IV sodium bicarbonate & 10% calcium gluconate IV is used.

*"**Ethylene Glycol Poisoning:** Initial symptoms are vomiting lethargy, ataxia, inebriation, convulsions and coma. In 12 to 24 hours tachycardia, tachypnoea and circulatory collapse, electrolyte imbalance and metabolic acidosis occur. In one to three days, hypocalcaemia, oliguria, tubular necrosis and renal failure occur. Urine contains crystals of calcium oxalate."*- Reddy 34/e p542, 33/e p583*

Ethylene Glycol
• **Ethylene glycol**: **Clear, colorless, odorless, non-volatile** liquid with a **bitter-sweet taste**[Q].
• Mainly used as an **antifreeze agent**; **Not absorbed through skin**[Q].
• **Metabolized to glycoaldehyde, glycolic acid & oxalic acid** and **inhibits oxidative phosphorylation**[Q].
• **Fatal dose: 100-200 ml; Fatal period: 3 days**[Q]

Signs & Symptoms of Ethylene Glycol Poisoning		
Initial symptoms	**In 12-24 hours**	**In 1-3 days**
Vomiting, **lethargy, ataxia,** inebriation, **convulsions & coma**[Q]	**Tachycardia, tachypnoe-a**[Q]**, circulatory collapse,** electrolyte imbalance & **metabolic acidosis**	**Hypocalcaemia, oliguria, tubular necrosis & renal failure**[Q]

• **Urine contains calcium oxalate crystals**[Q].

Postmortem Appearances:
• **Cerebral edema, chemical meningoencephalitis, liver & kidney damage** may be seen[Q].
• **Oxalate crystals** are seen in **brain, spinal cord & kidneys**[Q].

Treatment:
• **Gastric lavage, activated charcoal; Ethanol**[Q] in same dose as for methyl alcohol
• **Antidote is fomepizole**[Q] (**4-Methyl pyrazole**[Q])
• **Hemodialysis; IV sodium bicarbonate & IV 10% calcium gluconate**[Q]

91. Ans. d. Breadth of 1st sacral vertebra × 100/breadth of base of sacrum *(Ref: Reddy 34/e p62, 33/e p64)*

Corporobasal index is a sex-differentiating index used for sacrum.

$$Corporobasal\ index = \frac{Breadth\ of\ 1st\ sacral\ vertebra}{Breadth\ of\ base\ of\ sacrum} \times 100$$

Differences between Male & Female Vertebral Column		
Features	**Male**	**Female**
Atlas breadth	7.4-9.9 cm (mean 8.3 cm)	6.5-7.6 cm (mean 7.2 cm)
Length of vertebral column	70-73 cm	60 cm
Corporobasal index = Breadth of 1st sacral vertebra × 100/Breadth of base of sacrum	45 cm[Q]	40.5 cm[Q]

Differences between Male & Female pelvis		
Features	**Male pelvis**	**Female pelvis**
General framework	**Deep, funnel shaped** **Massive & rough**[Q]	**Shallow, bowl shaped** **Less massive & smooth**[Q]
True pelvis	**Narrow deep & funnel shaped**[Q]	**Wide & shallow**[Q]
Pelvic brim	**Heart shaped**[Q]	**Circular**[Q]
Ilium	**Smaller**[Q]	**Larger**[Q]
Iliac crest	Curve is more prominent, more sloped with less rounded margins	Curve is less prominent, less sloped with more rounded margins
Anterior superior iliac spine	**More prominent**[Q]	**Less prominent**[Q]
Pre auricular sulcus	**Not widely separated**[Q]	**Widely separated**[Q]
Acetabulum	**Wide & deep**, diameter about 52 mm	Prominent, **broad & deep**[Q]
Symphysis pubis	Higher & bigger in depth & narrow in width. **Margins of pubic arch** are **everted** & no parturition pits on the dorsal border	Small & narrow, diameter 46 mm **Lower, wider & rounded** Margins of pubic arch are **not everted** & **parturition pits** are present on dorsal border
Subpubic angle	**70°-75° (acute)** subpubic arch is **V shaped**[Q]	**90°** subpubic arch is **U shaped**[Q]
Greater sciatic notch	Smaller, deeper & narrower & less then right angle	Wider, larger & shallower & forming a right angle
Sciatic notch index = Width of sciatic notch x 100 Depth of sciatic notch	**4-5**[Q]	**5-6**[Q]
Obturator foramen	Large, oval shaped with base upwards	Small, triangular with the apex directed forwards
Ischial tuberosity	**More or less inverted**[Q]	**Everted**[Q]
Pubis (body)	**Narrow & triangular**[Q]	**Broad & square**[Q]
Pubis (ramus)	Is continuation of body	Narrow appearance
Pelvic index = AP diameter of pelvis/Transverse diameter x 100	**More**[Q]	**Less**[Q]
Kell index = Surface area of acetabulum/Surface area of illium x 100	**More**[Q]	**Less**[Q]

Differences between Male & Female sternum		
Features	**Male sternum**	**Female sternum**
Body	**Bigger, longer & more than twice** the length of manubrium[Q]	**Shorter & less than twice** the length of manubrium[Q]
Ashley's rule	Total length **>149 mm**[Q]	Total length **<149 mm**[Q]
Level of upper border	At the level of **lower part of body of 2nd** thoracic vertebrae[Q]	At the level of **lower part of 3rd** thoracic vertebrae[Q]
Manubrium	**Smaller**[Q]	**Bigger**[Q]
Sternal index	46.2[Q]	54.3[Q]
Sternal index = Length of manubrium x 100/length of body of sternum[Q]		

92. **Ans. b. Throttling**   *(Ref: Reddy 34/e p329, 33/e p352; Knight's Forensic Pathology 4/e p374)*

On external examination, a single abrasion is seen, likely due to assailant's fingers grasping the neck. Bruising of the neck is seen as well. On internal examination, we can see contused tissues of the neck with bleeding from strap muscles. All these features are suggestive of throttling. Hanging can be ruled out in absence of ligature mark. Absence of ligature mark rules out ligature strangulation.

"Throttling or Manual Strangulation: Asphyxia produced by compression of the neck by human hands is called throttling. Death occurs due to occlusion of carotid arteries. Occlusion of airway plays minor role."- Reddy 34/e p329, 33/e p352

"Postmortem Appearances: External-Bruises on the neck: The situation and extent of the bruised area on the neck will depend upon the relative positions of assailant and victim, the manner of grasping neck, and the degree of pressure exerted upon the throat. The bruises are produced by the tips or the pads of the fingers."- Reddy 34/e p0329, 33/e p352

Smothering: If the orifices are closed by the hand, there may be scratches, distinct nail marks, or laceration of the soft parts of the victim face. The lips, gum and tongue may show bruising or laceration. Slight bruising may be found in the mouth and nose, which should be confirmed by microscopy. The asphyxial signs and symptoms are severe, because death usually results due to slow asphyxia and often the fatal period is three to five minutes."- Reddy 334/e p337, 33/e p352

Throttling or Manual Strangulation
• **Asphyxia produced by compression of the neck by human hands** is called **throttling**[Q].
• **Death** occurs due to **occlusion of carotid arteries. Occlusion of airway** plays **minor role.**
• **Vagal inhibition** is much **more common in manual strangulation** than with a ligature[Q].

Usual Diagnostic Signs of Death due to Manual Strangulation	
• **Cutaneous bruising & abrasions**[Q]	• Fracture of **larynx, thyroid cartilage & hyoid bone**[Q]
• **Extensive bruising** with or without **rupture of neck muscles**[Q]	• **Cricoid cartilage** is almost **exclusively fractured in throttling**[Q]
• **Engorgement of the tissues at & above the level of compression**[Q]	• General signs of **asphyxia**[Q]

PSM

93. **Ans. b. High sensitivity and low specificity**   *(Ref: Park 24/e p149, 23/e p141)*

The line in red shows the new test. The new test curve distribution is shorter than old thus, the 95% CI range of new test will be more precise than the old test. For a particular cut off point, sensitivity of new test will be high, since the 95% CI is precise for new test than old test. So, high sensitivity is achieved at the expense of decrease in specificity.

Sensitivity	Proportion of persons with the condition who test positive: True positive /(True positive + False negative)[Q]
Specificity	Proportion of persons without the condition who test negative: True negative /(False positive + True negative)[Q]

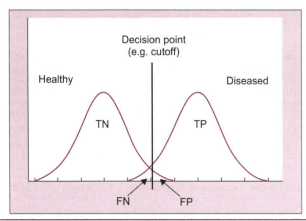

Assessment & Value of A Diagnostic Test		
	Condition Present	**Condition Absent**
Positive Test	a (True positive)	b (False positive)
Negative Test	c (False negative)	d (True negative)

Sensitivity	Proportion of persons with the condition who test positive: $a/(a+c)^Q$
Specificity	Proportion of persons without the condition who test negative: $d/(b+d)^Q$
Positive predictive value (PPV)	Proportion of persons with a positive test who have the condition: $a/(a+b)^Q$
Negative predictive value (NPV)	Proportion of persons with a negative test who do not have the condition: $d/(c+d)^Q$

Predictive Value
• Prevalence, sensitivity, and specificity determine predictive value^Q • PPV = Prevalence × Sensitivity /(Prevalence × Sensitivity) + (1 − Prevalence)(1 − Specificity)^Q • NPV = (1 − Prevalence)(Specificity) /(1 − Prevalence)(Specificity) + (1 − Sensitivity)(Prevalence)^Q

94. **Ans. c. Endemic-Epidemic-Sporadic** *(Ref: Park 24/e p98)*

Area A: Persistent prevalence of cases in high numbers in the area	Endemic
Area B: Usually less number of cases, sudden surge in cases last week	Epidemic
Area C: Very less number of cases annually, no increase in recent numbers	Sporadic

Term	Description	Example
Epidemic	Refers to an **increase, often sudden**, in the **number of cases of a disease above** what is **normally expected** in that population in that area^Q.	Cholera, Chickenpox
Endemic	Refers to the **constant presence and/or usual prevalence of a disease or infectious agent** in a population **within a geographic area**^{Q}.	Common cold

Term	Description	Example
Hyper-Endemic	Constant presence of a disease or infectious agent at **high incidence/prevalence** & **affects all age groups equally**[Q]	–
Holo-Endemic	**A high level of infection beginning early in life** & **affecting most of the children population**[Q]	Malaria
Sporadic	Refers to a disease that **occurs infrequently and irregularly**[Q]	Polio, Tetanus, Herpes Zoster, Meningococcal meningitis
Pandemic	An **epidemic usually affecting a large proportion of the population**, occurring over a **large geographical area** such as part of a **nation, continent or world**[Q]	Influenza pandemics of 1918 & 1957 Cholera El Tor in 1962 (still continuing) Acute hemorrhagic conjunctivitis in 1971 & 1981

95. Ans. d. D *(Ref: Park 24/e p40)*

Point C represents the onset of symptoms.

A	Exposure
B	Onset of pathologic changes
C	Onset of symptoms
D	Usual time of disease diagnosis

Natural history of disease timeline

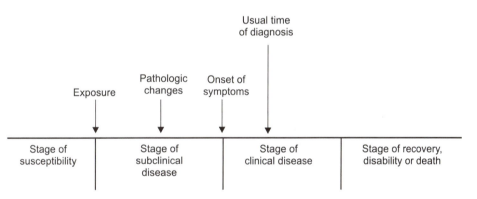

Natural History of Disease
• Progression of a disease process in an individual over time, in the absence of treatment. • **Process begins with appropriate exposure to re-accumulation of factors sufficient for disease process** to **begin in a susceptible host**. For an infectious disease, exposure is a microorganism. • For cancer, exposure may be a factor that initiates the process, such as asbestos fibers or components in tobacco smoke (for lung cancer). • **After the disease process has been triggered**, pathological changes then occur without the individual being aware of them. This stage of **subclinical disease**, extending from the time of exposure to onset of disease symptoms, is usually called the **incubation period** for infectious diseases, and the latency period for chronic diseases. During this stage, disease is said to be **asymptomatic**. • Although **disease is not apparent during the incubation period**, some **pathologic changes may be detectable with laboratory, radiographic, or other screening methods**. • **Most screening programs attempt to identify the disease process during this phase of its natural history**, since intervention at this early stage is likely to be more effective than treatment given after the disease has progressed and become symptomatic.

Contd...

Natural History of Disease

- **Onset of symptoms marks the transition from subclinical to clinical disease**. Most **diagnoses are made during the stage of clinical disease**. In some people, however, the disease process may never progress to clinically apparent illness.
- Ultimately, the disease process ends either in recovery, disability or death.
  - For an **infectious agent**, **infectivity** refers to the **proportion of exposed persons who become infected**.
  - **Pathogenicity** refers to **proportion of infected individuals who develop clinically apparent disease**.
  - **Virulence** refers to **proportion of clinically apparent cases** that are **severe or fatal**.

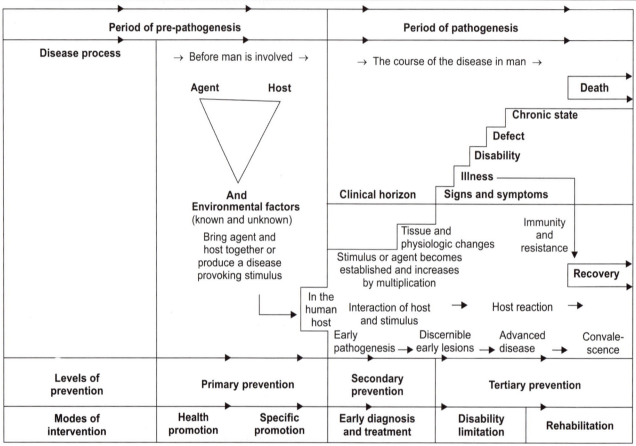

Fig. 23: Natural history of disease

96. Ans. c. Nucleic acid amplification test *(Ref: Park 24/e p447; RNTCP guidelines- 'Technical and Operational Guidelines for TB Control in India-2016'; Harrison 19/e p1113)*

A patient with cough was sputum AFB negative but chest X-ray was suggestive of TB. The next step according to RNTCP is Nucleic Acid Amplification Test (NAAT).

> "Cartridge Based Nucleic Acid Amplification Test (CB-NAAT): The CB-NAAT is known as the GeneXpert in most countries other than India. This is preferred first diagnostic test in children and people with TB and HIC co-infection." - *Human Diseases by Sasmita Panda, Surendra nath Padhi (2017)/p65*

> "With the availability of molecular diagnostic tools, rapid diagnosis of TB and detection of drug resistance have a made significant improvement in recent years. The Centre for Disease Control and Prevention (CDC) guidelines published in 2009 recommended the use of nucleic acid amplification testing (NAAT) as standard practice for aiding in established diagnosis in persons with suspected TB." - *Respiratory Infections, An Issue of Clinics in Laboratory Medicine By Michael J. Loeffelholz (2014)/p 298*

"*Nucleic Acid Amplification Technology:* Several test systems based on amplification of mycobacterial nucleic acid have become available in the past few years. **These tests are most useful for the rapid confirmation of TB in persons with AFB- positive specimens, but some also have utility for the diagnosis of AFB-negative pulmonary and extrapulmonary TB.** One system that permits rapid diagnosis of TB with high specificity and sensitivity (approaching that of culture) is the fully automated, real-time nucleic acid amplification technology known as the Xpert MTB/RIF assay. Xpert MTB/RIF can simultaneously detect TB and rifampin resistance in <2 h and has minimal biosafety and training requirements. Therefore, it can be housed in nonconventional laboratory settings. The WHO recommends its use worldwide as the initial diagnostic test in adults and children presumed to have MDR-TB or HIV-associated TB. Taking into account the availability of resources, the test may also be used in any adult or child presumed to have TB or as a follow-up test after microscopy in adults presumed to have TB but not at risk of MDR-TB or HIV-associated TB. Xpert MTB/RIF should be the initial test applied to CSF from patients in whom TB meningitis is suspected as well as a replacement test (over conventional microscopy, culture, and histopathology) for selected non-respiratory specimens—obtained by gastric lavage, fine-needle aspiration, or pleural or other biopsies—from patients in whom extrapulmonary TB is suspected. **This test has a sensitivity of 98% among AFB-positive cases and ~70% among AFB-negative specimens.**"
-Harrison 19/e p1113

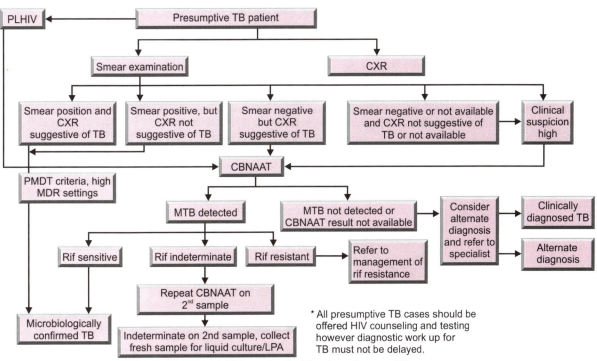

Fig. 24: Diagnostic algorithm for pulmonary TB

New Diagnostic Algorithm for Diagnosis of Pulmonary TB (2016)
• All presumptive TB patients to undergo two-sputum smear examinations[Q].
• **If first sputum is positive**, it will be categorized as **confirmed TB**[Q]
• If first smear is negative & chest X-ray is suggestive of TB, 2nd smear should be subjected to ZN staining and CB-NAAT simultaneously[Q].

CB-NAAT (Cartridge Based Nucleic Acid Amplification Test)
• Also called as **Gene-Xpert**[Q]
• **Detects DNA sequences specific for M. tuberculosis** as well as **rifampicin resistance by PCR**[Q].
• **Unprocessed sputum samples** can be **used** & **results** are readily **available** real time **within 90 minutes**.

97. Ans. c. Not more than 10% of the people benefitted by the drug could be due to chance *(Ref: Park 24/e p887, 23/e p849; High Yield Statistics/p123; Oxford handbook of Medical Statistics/p 248)*

- *The p (probability) value is used when we wish to see how likely is that a hypothesis is true. The hypothesis is usually that there is no difference between two treatments, known as "null hypothesis'.*
- *The p value gives the probability of any observed difference having happened by chance.*
- *p =0.5 means that the probability of any observed difference having happened by chance is 0.5 in 1 or 50:50.*
- *Similarly, a p value of <0.10 means that the probability of it happening by chance is 10%.*
- *In the question, the probability that the drug affected the chronic hypertensives by chance is less than 10%.* Hence, **90% of the subjects were benefitted by the drug.**

*"Type I error, also known as an **error of the first kind**, occurs **when the null hypothesis (H_0) is true, but is rejected**. It is **asserting something that is absent**, a false hit. A type I error may be compared with a so-called false positive (a result that indicates that a given condition is present when it actually is not present) in tests where a single condition is tested for. **The type I error rate or significance level is the probability of rejecting the null hypothesis, given that it is true. It is denoted by the Greek letter α (alpha) and is also called the alpha level**. Often, the significance level is set to 0.05 (5%), implying that it is acceptable to have a 5% probability of incorrectly rejecting the null hypothesis.*

Type I errors are philosophically a focus of skepticism and Occam's razor. A type I error occurs when we believe in falsehood ("believing in a lie"). In terms of folk tales, an investigator may be "crying wolf" without a wolf in sight (raising a false alarm) (H_0: no wolf)."

*"A **type II error**, also known as an **error of the second kind**, occurs when the null hypothesis is false, but erroneously fails to be rejected. It is failing to assert what is present, a miss. A type II error may be compared with a so-called false negative (where an actual 'hit' was disregarded by the test and seen as a 'miss') in a test checking for a single condition with a definitive result of true or false. A type II error is committed when we fail to believe a truth. In terms of folk tales, an investigator may fail to see the wolf ("failing to raise an alarm"). Again, H_0: no wolf. **The rate of the type II error is denoted by the Greek letter β (beta) and related to the power of a test (which equals 1−β).**"*

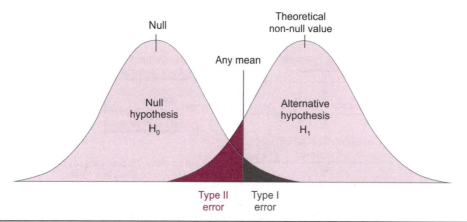

Type I Error	Type II Error
- The **null hypothesis is true but rejected (False positive)**[Q] - **Probability of type I error is given by p value**[Q] - **Significance (alpha) level is the maximum tolerable probability of type I errors**[Q] - **Keep type I error to be minimum; then results are declared to be statistically significant**[Q] - **Type I error is more serious than type II error**[Q]	- Null hypothesis is not false but is not rejected/accepted (false negative)[Q] - Probability of type II error is given by beta[Q]

98. Ans. b. Incidence remains the same and prevalence increases *(Ref: Park 24/e p66)*

A radiotherapist prescribes a new drug combination of chemotherapy and immunotherapy for metastatic melanoma. It prolongs the survival. In this case incidence remains the same and prevalence increases as survival is prolonged leading to increased number of people living with the disease in the community.

AIIMS May 2017

"Prevalence is the proportion of a population that has a condition at a specific time, but the prevalence will be influenced by both the rate at which new cases are occurring and the average duration of the disease. Incidence reflects the rate at which new cases of disease are being added to the population (and becoming prevalent cases). Average duration of disease is also important, because the only way you can stop being a prevalent case is to be cured or to move out of the population or die."

"Improvements in treatment may decrease the duration of illness and thereby decrease prevalence of disease. But if the treatment is such that by preventing death, and at the same time not producing recovery, may give rise to the apparently paradoxical effect of an increase in prevalence. Further, if duration is decreased sufficiently, a decrease in prevalence could take place despite an increase in incidence."- Park 24/e p67

Incidence
• **Incidence: Number of new case[Q]** occurring in a defined population during a specified period of time.
• It is **expressed as per 1000 per year[Q]**.
• **Incidence is a rate[Q]**
• Incidence is **not affected by duration of disease[Q]**
• **Use of in incidence** is generally **restricted to acute conditions[Q]**.
• This is a **much more accurate measure of risk than prevalence[Q]**.

Prevalence
• Prevalence is the **total current (Old+ new) cases in a given population over a point or period of time[Q]**.
• **Types:** Point prevalence (at a point of time) & Period prevalence (over a period of time)[Q]
• Prevalence = No. of total (old + new) cases of a disease in a year/ Total population × 100[Q]
• Prevalence = Incidence x Mean duration of disease[Q]
• **Prevalence is a proportion, not a ratio[Q]**: Numerator is a part of denominator, and is always expressed in percentage.
• **Prevalence can be determined from cross-sectional study[Q]**.

Relation between Incidence & Prevalence
• Given the assumption that **population is stable & incidence** and **duration are not changing**.
• **Prevalence = Incidence x Mean duration of disease[Q]**
• **Prevalence describes balance between incidence, mortality & recovery[Q]**.
• **Incidence reflects causal factors[Q]**.
• **Duration reflects prognostic factors[Q]**

99. **Ans. d. 300–400** *(Ref: Park 24/e p882, 884; High Yield Statistic/p67; Oxford Handbook of Medical Statistics/p182)*

In a normal distribution bell-shaped curve without any skew (if the given histogram is converted to a curve), the mean will lie at the midpoint, i.e., between 300–400.

CD4 Count	Interval midpoint (X)	No. of people (n)	Xn
0-100	50	5	250
100–200	150	10	1500
200–300	250	25	6250
300–400	350	35	12250
400–500	450	20	9000
>500	1050	5	5250
Total		100	34500

Arithmetic Mean = $X_1 n_1 + X_2 n_2 + X_3 n_3$....... = $\sum Xn/n$ = 34500/100 = **345 (Between 300-400)**

100. **Ans. a. Infectious plastic wastes** *(Ref: Park 24/e p830; Biomedical Waste Disposal Guidelines 2016)*

Infectious or contaminated waste is a recyclable waste and should be disposed in red colored dustbin according to new guidelines.

Biomedical Wastes, Categories and their Segregation, Collection, Treatment, Processing and Disposal Options

Category	Type of Waste	Type of bag/ container used	Treatment & Disposal Options
Yellow	• **Human anatomical waste**[Q] • **Animal anatomical waste**[Q] • **Soiled waste**[Q] • **Expired or discarded medicines**[Q] • **Chemical waste**[Q] • **Chemical liquid waste**[Q] • **Discarded linen, mattresses, beddings contaminated with blood or body fluid** • **Microbiology, biotechnology & other clinical laboratory waste**[Q]	• **Non-chlorinated plastic bags**[Q] • Separate collection system leading to effluent treatment system for chemical liquid waste	• **Incineration or plasma pyrolysis or deep burial**[Q]
Red	• **Contaminated waste (Recyclable):** tubing, bottles, IV tubes & sets, catheters, urine bags, syringes (without needles), **vaccutainers** with their needles cut & **gloves**[Q]	• **Red colored non-chlorinated plastic bags or containers**[Q]	• **Autoclaving or microwaving**[Q] or **hydroclaving** followed by **shredding or mutilation**[Q] or combination of **sterilization & shredding** • Plastic wastes should not be sent to landfill sites
White	• **Waste sharps including metals**[Q]	• **Puncture proof, leak proof, tamper proof containers**[Q]	• **Autoclaving or dry heat sterilizations** followed by **shredding or mutilation or encapsulation in metal containers or cement concrete**[Q]
Blue	• **Glassware**[Q] • **Metallic body implants**[Q]	• **Cardboard boxes with blue colored marking**[Q]	• **Disinfection or thorough autoclaving or microwaving or hydroclaving** and then sent for **recycling**[Q]

101. Ans. c. Chi-square test *(Ref: Park 24/e p889, 23/e p852; High Yield Statistics p143; Biostatistics by Mahajan 7/e p134)*

Chi-square test is used for comparison of two independent qualitative variables. Incidence of depression will be in nominal form (depression present or absent), whatever may be the value of the scale used for each patient. The other variable is number of male and female babies (two independent qualitative variables). Thus the comparison is best made through Chi-square test.

Student's t-test	Comparison of **two different groups** when **data is quantitative**
Paired t-test	Comparison of **pre-intervention & post-intervention quantitative data between same group**
Chi-square test	Comparison of **two independent qualitative variables**
Pearson's test	For correlation **between two parametric variables**

Number of Groups or Condition	Parametric Tests	Nonparametric Tests
Independent measures, **2 groups**	• **Unpaired t-test** or **Student t-test**[Q]	• **Chi-square test**[Q] (large or small sample with Yate's correction) • **Fischer's test**[Q] (small or large sample) • **Mann-Whitney U-test** (Wilcoxon Rank sum test)
Independent measures, **>2 groups**	• **ANOVA**[Q]	• **Kruskal-Wallis test**[Q] • **Chi-square test**[Q]
Repeated measures, **2 conditions or paired data**	• **Paired t-test**[Q]	• **Wilcoxon signed rank test**[Q] • **Mc-Nemar's test**[Q] • **Chi-square test**[Q]
Repeated measures, **>2 conditions**	• **ANOVA**[Q]	• **Friedman's test**[Q] • **Chi-square test**[Q]
Correlation test	• **Pearson**[Q]	• **Spearman**[Q] **(Rho)**
Regression	• Simple linear or nonlinear regression	• Nonparametric regression

Chi-square Test (c² Test)

- A 'non-parametric test' of significance[Q]
- Used to 'test significance of association between 2 or more qualitative characteristics'[Q]
- Used to compare proportions in 2 or more groups[Q]
- Used for non-Normal (non-Gaussian) distributions

Applications of Chi-square test		
Test of proportions	Test of association	Test of goodness of fit

Essential requirements for calculation of Chi-square test		
Random sample	Qualitative data	Lowest expected frequency not < 5

Student t-test

- Student t-test is used when the **outcome variable is normally distributed in the population (for quantitative data)** e.g., blood pressure, blood glucose

Paired t-test	Unpaired t-test (Independent t-test)
Comparing means (+ SD) in paired data (in same group of individuals before and after an intervention)	**Comparing means (+ SD) in two different groups of individuals**
Example: Blood sugar level in a sample of 10 patients is measured before giving and after giving the oral hypoglycemic. In this condition, **paired t-test is used (before & after)**	**Example:** Blood sugar concentration is measured in two different groups (A group of 10 patients and other group of 8 patients). To test the significance of difference between the means of the two groups, unpaired t-test is used.

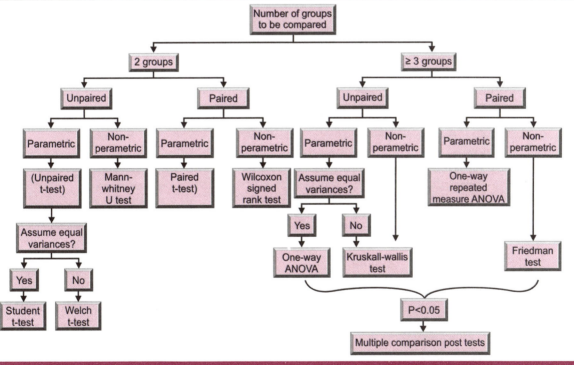

MEDICINE

102. **Ans. c. SIADH** *(Ref: Harrison 19/e p299, 610, 1794)*

   This patient is having increased urinary sodium, urine osmolality and near normal serum osmolality with euvolemia (normal blood pressure). In the setting of non-small cell lung cancer, this is likely to be due to SIADH. SIADH should be suspected in any patient with hyponatremia, hypo-osmolality and urine hyper-osmolality. Cerebral salt wasting syndrome patients are hypovolemic due to volume depletion hence these patients have hypotension. Diuretic induced hyponatremia will have urinary Na > 20 mmol/L and ECF volume will be decreased, leading to low blood pressure.

"Hyponatremia is a common electrolyte abnormality in cancer patients, and SIADH is the most common cause among patients with cancer." -Harrison 19/e p1794

"Ectopic vasopressin production by tumors is a common cause of the syndrome of inappropriate antidiuretic hormone (SIADH), occurring in at least half of patients with SCLC." -Harrison 19/e p610

"The diagnostic features of ectopic vasopressin production are the same as those of other causes of SIADH. Hyponatremia and reduced serum osmolality occur in the setting of an inappropriately normal or increased urine osmolality." -Harrison 19/e p610

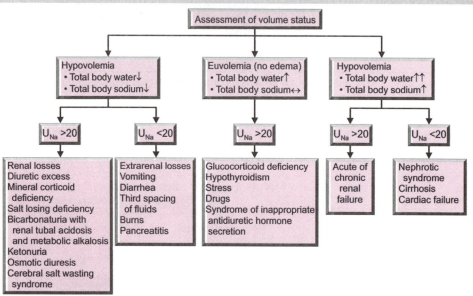

Fig. 25: Diagnostic approach to hyponatremia

Causes of Syndrome of Inappropriate Antidiuresis (SIADH)		
Neoplasms	**Infections**	**Neurologic**
• **Lung**[Q] • **Duodenum**[Q], **Pancreas**[Q] • **Ovary**[Q], **Bladder**[Q], **ureter**[Q] • **Thymoma**[Q], **Mesothelioma**[Q] • **Bronchial adenoma**[Q] • Carcinoid • Gangliocytoma, Ewing's sarcoma	• **Pneumonia**[Q], bacterial or viral • **Abscess**[Q], lung or brain • Cavitation (**aspergillosis**) • **Tuberculosis**, lung or brain • Meningitis, bacterial or viral • **Encephalitis**[Q], **AIDS**[Q]	• **Guillain-Barré syndrome**[Q] • **Multiple sclerosis**[Q] • **Delirium tremens**[Q] • **Amyotrophic lateral sclerosis**[Q] • Hydrocephalus, Psychosis • Peripheral neuropathy[Q]
Metabolic	**Vascular**	**Drugs**
• Acute intermittent porphyria	• Cerebrovascular occlusions, hemorrhage • Cavernous sinus thrombosis[Q]	• **Vasopressin**[Q] or desmopressin • **Chlorpropamide**[Q] • **Oxytocin, high dose**[Q] • **Vincristine, Carbamazepine**[Q] • **Nicotine, Phenothiazines**[Q] • **Cyclophosphamide**[Q] • **Tricyclic antidepressants**[Q] • Monoamine oxidase inhibitors[Q] • Serotonin reuptake inhibitors[Q]
Pulmonary		
• **Asthma, Pneumothorax**[Q] • Positive-pressure respiration		
Head trauma	**Congenital malformations**	
• **Closed** and **penetrating**[Q]	• **Agenesis corpus callosum** • **Cleft lip/palate**[Q] • Other midline defects	

Syndrome of Inappropriate ADH Secretion (SIADH)

- The term SIADH is applied to conditions with **vasopressin excess**.
- **Vasopressin excess** is termed **inappropriate** as this **increase occurs despite decreased plasma osmolality[Q]**.

> - **Increased vasopressin acts on renal tubules**, resulting in **increased absorption of water** (increased total body water), **concentrated urine[Q]** and **decreasing serum osmolality[Q]** and **hyponatremia[Q]**.
> - **Edema does not occur despite increased total body water[Q]** (due to unknown reasons)- **Clinical euvolemia[Q]**.

- **SIADH** is associated with **increased secretion of vasopressin** (ADH), which leads to increased absorption of water producing **dilutional hyponatremia (serum sodium typically < 135 mEq/l)** along with **concentrated or hyperosmolar urine[Q]**.
- **Excessive retention of water stimulates** compensatory mechanisms that enhance **'Natriuresis'[Q]**.
- **Natriuresis results in increased urinary sodium excretion rate (increased urinary sodium concentration)** and is believed to compensate for increased volume from inappropriate ADH secretion preventing a state of clinical hypervolemia, hypertension or edema.

> - **SIADH** should be suspected in patients who have **hyponatremia & concentrated urine** (osmolality > 300 mmol/kg) **in the absence of edema, orthostatic hypotension** and **features of dehydration[Q]**.

Cardinal features of SIADH

- **Hyponatremia[Q] (dilutional hyponatremia with Na⁺ <135 mmol/l)** - **Decreased plasma osmolality** (<280 mOsm/kg) with **inappropriately increased urine osmolality** >150 mOsm[Q]. - **High urine sodium (over 20 mEq/l)[Q]** - **Low blood urea nitrogen <10 mg/L[Q]** - **Hypouricemia (<4 mg/dL)[Q]**	- Clinical euvolemia - **Absence of signs of hypervolemia[Q]** (edema, ascites) - **Absence of signs of hypovolemia[Q]** (orthostatic hypotension, tachycardia, features of dehydration) - Absence of cardiac, liver or renal disease - Normal thyroid & adrenal function

Criteria for the diagnosis of SIADH

Essential	Supplemental
- **Decreased effective osmolality** of extracellular fluid (P_{osm} < 275 mOsmol/kg H_2O)[Q]. - **Inappropriate urinary concentration[Q]** (U_{osm} > 100 mOsmol/kg H_2O with normal renal function) at some level of hypo osmolality (Urinary concentration must be inappropriate for plasma hypo osmolality). - **Clinical euvolemia[Q]**, as defined by the absence of signs of hypovolemia (orthostasis, tachycardia, decreased skin turgor, dry mucous membranes) or hypervolemia (subcutaneous edema, ascites). - **Elevated urinary sodium** excretion while on normal salt and water intake[Q]. - **Absence of other potential causes of euvolemic hypo osmolality[Q]**: hypothyroidism, hypocortisolism (Addison's disease or pituitary ACTH insufficiency) and diuretic use.	- **Abnormal water load test[Q]** (inability to excrete at least 90% of a 20 mL/kg water load in 4 hours and/or failure to dilute U_{osm} to <100 mOsmol/kg H_2O). - **Plasma AVP level inappropriately elevated** relative to plasma osmolality[Q]. - **No significant correction of serum (Na⁺) with volume expansion** but **improvement after fluid restriction[Q]**

Treatment of SIADH:

- **Treatment of choice for SIADH: Water restriction[Q]**.
- In **acute SIADH**, the **keystone of treatment** is to **restrict total fluid intake to less than the sum total of insensible losses & urinary output[Q]**.
- If more **rapid correction of hyponatremia** is desired, the **fluid restriction** can be supplemented by **IV infusion of hypertonic saline[Q]**.
- **The drug of choice for SIADH** (when water restriction is unsuccessful) is **demeclocycline[Q]**.

Contd...

Syndrome of Inappropriate ADH Secretion (SIADH)
• **Demeclocycline** (a tetracycline) acts as an **ADH antagonist**[Q].
• **Desmopressin has no role in the management of SIADH**[Q].
• **Vaptans: New FDA approved agents for treatment of SIADH**[Q].

- **Vaptans** are a **new class of drugs** that have **emerged for treatment of hyponatremia**. These medications act as **Vasopressin receptors antagonists, blocking the action of AVP in renal tubule, pituitary** or **smooth muscles** depending upon receptor selectivity[Q].

Conivaptan[Q] (Intravenous use)	Tolivaptan[Q] (Oval use)
• Conivaptan is a **combined V1/V2 receptor antagonist** is FDA approved for **short-term IV use** for treatment of hospitalized patients with SIADH.	• Tolivaptan is a **V2 receptor antagonist** that has received FDA approval for oral use

103. Ans. a. Dexamethasone *(Ref: Harrison 19/e p686)*

In Acute Promyelocytic Leukemia, during treatment, Tretinoin decreases the frequency of DIC but produces another complication called the APL differentiation syndrome. Occurring within the first 3 weeks of treatment, it is characterized by fever, fluid retention, dyspnea, chest pain, pulmonary infiltrates, pleural and pericardial effusions, and hypoxemia. Glucocorticoids (dexamethasone), chemotherapy, and/ or supportive measures can be effective for management of the APL differentiation syndrome.

"Acute Promyelocytic Leukemia (APL) is a highly curable subtype of AML, and approximately 85% of these patients achieve long-term survival with current approaches. APL has long been shown to be responsive to cytarabine and daunorubicin, but previously patients treated with these drugs alone frequently died from DIC induced by the release of granule components by the chemotherapy-treated leukemia cells. However, the prognosis of APL patients has changed dramatically from adverse to favorable with the introduction of tretinoin, an oral drug that induces the differentiation of leukemic cells bearing the t(15;17), where disruption of the RARA gene encoding a retinoid acid receptor occurs. Tretinoin decreases the frequency of DIC but produces another complication called the APL differentiation syndrome. Occurring within the first 3 weeks of treatment, it is characterized by fever, fluid retention, dyspnea, chest pain, pulmonary infiltrates, pleural and pericardial effusions, and hypoxemia. The syndrome is related to adhesion of differentiated neoplastic cells to the pulmonary vasculature endothelium. Glucocorticoids, chemotherapy, and/ or supportive measures can be effective for management of the APL differentiation syndrome. Temporary discontinuation of tretinoin is necessary in cases of severe APL differentiation syndrome (i.e., patients developing renal failure or requiring admission to the intensive care unit due to respiratory distress). The mortality rate of this syndrome is about 10%."-Harrison 19/e p686

Treatment of Acute Promyelocytic Leukemia (APL)

- APL is a **highly curable subtype of AML** with 85% long-term survival.
- **Responsive to cytarabine & daunorubicin**, but **increased risk DIC**[Q] induced by release of granule components by the chemotherapy-treated leukemia cells.
- **Tretinoin** (an oral drug) **induces the differentiation of leukemic cells** bearing the t(15;17), where disruption of the *RARA* gene encoding a retinoid acid receptor occurs[Q].
- **Tretinoin decreases the frequency of DIC** but **produces another complication called the APL differentiation syndrome**[Q].

APL Differentiation Syndrome

- Occur within the **first 3 weeks of treatment**[Q]
- **Characterized by fever, fluid retention, dyspnea, chest pain, pulmonary infiltrates, pleural & pericardial effusions, and hypoxemia**[Q].
- **Cause:** Syndrome is **related to adhesion of differentiated neoplastic cells to pulmonary vasculature endothelium**[Q].
- **Treatment: Glucocorticoids, chemotherapy, and/ or supportive measures; Temporary discontinuation of tretinoin** in cases of **severe** APL differentiation syndrome[Q]
- **Mortality rate: 10%**

Treatment of Acute Promyelocytic Leukemia (APL)

- **Tretinoin** plus concurrent **anthracycline-based** (i.e., **idarubicin** or **daunorubicin**) **chemotherapy** appears to be among the **most effective treatment for APL**, leading to **CR rates of 90–95%**[Q].
  - **Arsenic trioxide** has **significant antileukemic activity** and is being explored as part of initial treatment in clinical trials of APL. Arsenic trioxide increases the **risk of APL differentiation syndrome** & may **prolong the QT interval**[Q].

104. Ans. b. Point B   *(Ref: Harrison 19/e p1448; Ganong 25/e p542)*

Second heart sound (S2) precedes or appears 0.09 sec after summit of "T" wave. In the given figure, A=E = S1; B= S2; C=S3; D=S4.

Two sounds are normally heard through a stethoscope during each cardiac cycle. The first is a low, slightly prolonged "lub" (first sound), caused by vibrations set up by the sudden closure of the AV valves at the start of ventricular systole. The second is a shorter, high-pitched "dup" (second sound), caused by vibrations associated with closure of the aortic and pulmonary valves just after the end of ventricular systole. A soft, low-pitched third sound is heard about one-third of the way through diastole in many normal young individuals. It coincides with the period of rapid ventricular filling and is probably due to vibrations set up by the inrush of blood. A fourth sound can sometimes be heard immediately before the first sound when atrial pressure is high or the ventricle is stiff in conditions such as ventricular hypertrophy. It is due to ventricular filling and is rarely heard in normal adults." -Ganong 25/e p542

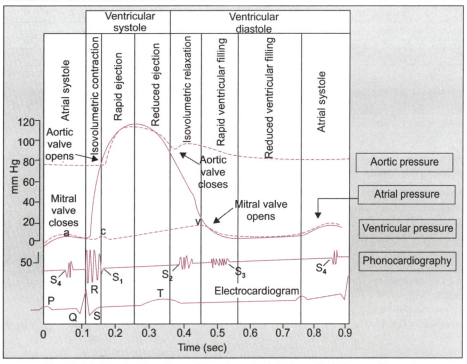

Fig. 26: Timing of various hemodynamic and related events during cardiac cycle

	Heart Sounds			
	S1	**S2**	**S3**	**S4**
Occurs during	Isometric contraction & ejection period, start of ventricular systole[Q]	Protodiastole & part of isometric relaxation, just after the end of ventricular systole[Q]	Rapid filling, beginning of middle third of diastole[Q]	Atrial systole, just before S1[Q]
Cause	Sudden closure of mitral & tricuspid (AV) valves[Q]	Closure of aortic or pulmonary (semilunar) valves[Q]	Rushing of blood into ventricles[Q]	Contraction of atrial musculature[Q]

Contd...

Contd...

	S1	S2	S3	S4
Characteris-tics	Long, soft & low pitched Resemble the word 'LUB'[Q]	Short, sharp & high pitched Resemble the word 'DUP'[Q]	Low pitched[Q]	Inaudible sound[Q]
Frequency	25-45 Hz[Q]	50 Hz[Q]	Low[Q]	<20 Hz[Q]
Duration	0.15 seconds[Q]	0.12 seconds[Q]	0.1 seconds[Q]	0.1 seconds[Q]
Relation to ECG	Later half of 'R' wave[Q]	Later half of 'T' wave[Q]	Between 'T' & 'P' wave[Q]	Following 'P' wave[Q]

105. Ans. d. Atorvastatin 80 mg *(Ref: Harrison 19/e p2447; CMDT (2017)/p1263-1264)*

When lipid-lowering agents are indicated, the treatment is started with HMG Co-A reductase inhibitors (statins). High intensity statin therapy should be started in the patients with presence of clinical atherosclerotic cardiovascular events (MI in this patient). In high intensity statin therapy, either atorvastatin (40-80 mg/day) or rosuvastatin (20-40 mg/day) should be given.

Rosuvastatin + Fenofibrate	• **Combination therapy is rarely indicated.** Only ezetimibe plus simvastatin has shown benefit in trials. • **Gemfibrozil (fibrates) & HMG Co-A reductase inhibitors increases the risk of muscle and liver disease** more than either drug alone.
Fenofibrate	• **Fibrates** are used to **reduce triglycerides and increase HDL levels.**

Indications of Lipid Lowering Agents	
Indications	**Treatment Recommendations**
Presence of clinical atherosclerotic cardiovascular disease	**High intensity statin or moderate intensity statin if age >75 years**[Q]
Primary elevation of **LDL cholesterol ≥190 mg/dL** (4.91 mmmol/L)	**High intensity statin**[Q]
Age 40-75 **Presence of diabetes** **LDL ≥70 mg/dL** (1.81 mmol/L)	**Moderate intensity statin** or high intensity statin if 10 year CVD risk 7.5% or higher[Q]
Age 40-75 years **No clinical atherosclerotic cardiovascular disease or diabetes** **LDL 70-189 mg/dL** (1.81-4.91 mmol/L) Estimated 10-year CVD risk 7.5% or higher	Treat with **moderate-to-high intensity statin**[Q]

High Intensity Statin Therapy	Moderate Intensity Statin Therapy

• **Lowers LDL cholesterol** by approximately **50%**
• Drugs used:
  – **Atorvastatin (40-80 mg**[Q])
  – **Rosuvastatin (20-40 mg**[Q])
	• **Lowers LDL cholesterol by 30-50%**
	• Drugs used:
	  – **Atorvastatin (10-20 mg**[Q])
	  – **Rosuvastatin (5-10 mg**[Q])
	  – **Simvastatin (20-40 mg**[Q])
	  – **Lovastatin (40 mg**[Q])

106. Ans. c. Absent DTRs *(Ref: Harrison 19/e p2701-2702)*

Deep tendon reflexes (DTRs) are present in patients of Myasthenia gravis.

"The limb weakness in myasthenia gravis (MG) is often proximal and may be asymmetric. Despite the muscle weakness, deep tendon reflexes are preserved."-Harrison 19/e p2702

Myasthenia Gravis (MG)
• **MG** is a **neuromuscular disorder** characterized by **weakness & fatigability of skeletal muscles**[Q]. • Associated with **thymomas**[Q] & certain **autoimmune diseases**[Q] • **More common in women**[Q] • **Peaks of incidence**: Women in **twenties & thirties**; men in **fifties & sixties**[Q].

Myasthenia Gravis (MG)

Pathophysiology:
- Decrease in number of available acetylcholine receptors (AChRs) at NM junctions due to an **antibody-mediated autoimmune attack** resulting in **decreased efficiency of NM transmission**[Q].

Clinical features:
- **Cardinal features**: Weakness & fatigability of muscles[Q].
- Weakness increases during repeated use (fatigue) or late in the day and may **improve following rest or sleep**.
- Distribution of muscle weakness has a **characteristic pattern**[Q].

> - **Cranial muscles (lids & extraocular muscles)** are typically **involved early** in the course of MG
> - **Diplopia & ptosis** are **common initial complaints**[Q].

- **Facial weakness** produces a **"snarling" expression** when the **patient attempts to smile**[Q].
- Weakness in chewing is most noticeable after prolonged effort, as in chewing meat.
- **Speech: Nasal timbre** (due to weakness of palate) & **dysarthric "mushy" quality**[Q] (due to tongue weakness)
- **Difficulty in swallowing** as a result of **weakness of palate, tongue, or pharynx**, giving rise to **nasal regurgitation or aspiration**[Q].
- **Bulbar weakness** is especially prominent in **MuSK antibody–positive MG**[Q].

> - In **~85%** of patients, **weakness becomes generalized**, affecting the limb muscles as well.
> - **Limb weakness** in MG is often **proximal** and may be **asymmetric**[Q].
> - Despite the muscle weakness, **deep tendon reflexes are preserved**[Q].

- If **weakness of respiration** becomes so severe as to **require respiratory assistance,** the patient is said to be in **crisis.**
- **Ocular MG:** Weakness restricted to extraocular muscles[Q]

Diagnosis:
- **Anti-AChR radioimmunoassay:** ~85% positive in generalized MG; 50% in ocular MG; **definite diagnosis if positive**; negative result does not exclude MG[Q]
- **~40% of AChR antibody–negative patients** with generalized MG have **anti-MuSK antibodies**[Q]

> - **Repetitive nerve stimulation: Decrement of >15% at 3 Hz**: highly probable[Q]
> - **Single-fiber electromyography: Blocking & jitter, with normal fiber density; confirmatory**, but not specific[Q]

- **Edrophonium chloride** 2 mg + 8 mg IV; **highly probable diagnosis** if unequivocally positive[Q]
- **For ocular or cranial MG:** exclude **intracranial lesions** by CT or MRI

Single most sensitive test for diagnosis of MG	**Single muscle electromyography**[Q]
Single most specific test for diagnosis of MG	**AChR antibodies**[Q]

Treatment:
- **Most useful treatments** for MG: **Anticholinesterase medications, immunosuppressive agents, thymectomy & plasmapheresis** or intravenous immunoglobulin **(IVIg)**[Q]

Test	Generalized MG (sensitivity)	Ocular MG (sensitivity)
AChR antibodies	80%	60%
Repetitive nerve stimulation	75%	48%
Single fiber EMG	99%	97%
Edrophonium (Tensilon) test	95%	85%

107. Ans. b. Spasticity *(Ref: Bradley's Neurology 7/e p797)*

Spasticity is seen in 20% of hemiplegic patients. Spasticity per se does not produce weakness and other aspects of motor control. Overzealous treatment affects the normal ambulation of patients. Hence, treating spasticity, as a rule is not always preferred, treating it is a double-edged sword. Spasticity as a consequence of a stroke may have a certain beneficiary compensatory aspect.

Fever	• **Fever** dramatically worsens brain injury during ischemia, as does hyperglycemia, so it is reasonable to suppress fever with antipyretics and surface cooling.
Spasticity	• **Overzealous treatment affects** the **normal ambulation** of patients. • **Treating spasticity as a rule is not always preferred**. • **Spasticity as a consequence of a stroke** might in many cases also have a certain **beneficiary compensatory aspect.**
Dysphagia	• **Dysphagia in stroke is predominantly oropharyngeal type**. • **Dysphagia is serious** and it **poses a significant risk for aspiration** and hence it has to be treated.
Neglect	• **Neglect** is an **inability to attend to, orient or explore** the hemisphere contralateral to a brain lesion. • Since right is dominant, for selective attention, this syndrome is **usually seen in right hemi stroke** (36-80% patients) and **affects awareness of left side.** • It has **negative impact on daily activities** & **on functional recovery. It should be treated.**

108. Ans. c. Spironolactone *(Ref: Harrison 19/e p1511; Katzung 13/e p262, 12/e p711, 263)*

In this case patient is having heart failure with hyperkalemia and renal dysfunction with psychiatric illness. Spironolactone and enalapril, both causes hyperkalemia but spironolactone causes CNS depression also. Digoxin causes hypokalemia. In this patient, spironolactone should be avoided.

"Potassium-sparing agents (spironolactone) can cause severe, even fatal, hyperkalemia in susceptible patients. Patients with chronic renal insufficiency are especially vulnerable and should rarely be treated with these diuretics." - Katzung 13/e p262

"Aldosterone antagonism is associated with a reduction in mortality in all stages of symptomatic NYHA class II to IV HFrEF. Elevated aldosterone levels in HFrEF promote sodium retention, electrolyte imbalance, and endothelial dysfunction and may directly contribute to myocardial fibrosis. The selective agent eplerenone (tested in NYHA class II and post–myocardial infarction heart failure) and the nonselective antagonist spironolactone (tested in NYHA class III and IV heart failure) reduce mortality and hospitalizations, with significant reductions in sudden cardiac death (SCD). Hyperkalemia and worsening renal function are concerns, especially in patients with underlying chronic kidney disease, and renal function and serum potassium levels must be closely monitored." - Harrison 19/e p1511

Spironolactone
• **Spironolactone** is **nonselective aldosterone antagonist** & **potassium sparing diuretic**[Q]

Spironolactone: Mechanism of Action
• **Pharmacologic antagonist of aldosterone in collecting tubules**[Q] • **Weak antagonism of androgen receptors**[Q] • **Weak inhibitor of testosterone synthesis**[Q]

Effects:
• Reduces Na^+ retention & K^+ wasting in kidney[Q]
• Poorly understood **antagonism of aldosterone in heart & vessels**[Q]

Spironolactone: Clinical applications	
• Treatment of **edema & hypertension**[Q] (Coadministered with thiazide or loop diuretics) • Treatment of **resistant hypertension due to primary hyperaldosteronism**[Q] (adrenal adenomas or bilateral adrenal hyperplasia) • **Refractory edema** associated with **secondary aldosteronism**[Q] (cardiac failure, hepatic cirrhosis, nephrotic syndrome & severe ascites).	• Spironolactone is **diuretic of choice** in patients with **hepatic cirrhosis**[Q]. • **Ventricular arrhythmias** in patients with heart failure[Q] • **Hypokalemia due to other diuretics**[Q] • **Post-myocardial infarction**[Q] • **Hirsutism in women**[Q]

Spironolactone	
Spironolactone: Adverse effects	
• Hyperkalemia[Q] • Cardiac arrhythmia[Q] • Menstrual abnormalities[Q] • Gynecomastia, impotence & BPH[Q] • Skin rashes[Q]	• Diarrhea, gastritis, gastric bleeding & peptic ulcers[Q] (contraindicated in peptic ulcers[Q]). • CNS: Drowsiness, lethargy, ataxia, confusion & headache[Q]

109. Ans. b. DC cardioversion *(Ref: Harrison 19/e p1494)*

ECG shown is suggestive of tachycardia with broad complexes and regular rhythm, i.e. likely monomorphic ventricular tachycardia. Management is DC cardioversion if patient is unstable and Amiodarone for stable patients. Adenosine is used in narrow complex or paroxysmal supraventricular tachycardia. Lignocaine is not indicated unless it is a post MI or ischemic VT.

"Sustained Monomorphic Ventricular Tachycardia: Initial management follows Advanced Cardiac Life Support (ACLS) guidelines. If hypotension, impaired consciousness, or pulmonary edema is present, QRS synchronous electrical cardioversion should be performed, ideally after sedation if the patient is conscious. For stable tachycardia, a trial of adenosine is reasonable, as this may clarify a supraventricular tachycardia with aberrancy. Intravenous amiodarone is the drug of choice if heart disease is present. Following restoration of sinus rhythm, hospitalization and evaluation to define underlying heart disease are required." - *Harrison 19/e p1494*

Sustained Monomorphic Ventricular Tachycardia

- **Sustained monomorphic VT** presents as a **wide QRS tachycardia** that has the same QRS configuration from beat to beat, indicating an identical sequence of ventricular depolarization for each beat.

  - **VT originates from a stable focus or reentry circuit[Q].**
  - In **structural heart disease**, the substrate is often an area of **patchy replacement fibrosis due to infarction, inflammation, or prior cardiac surgery** that creates anatomical or functional reentry pathways[Q].

- VT is related to **reentry or automaticity in a diseased Purkinje system[Q]**.
- **Idiopathic VT** can present as **sustained monomorphic VTs** due to **focal automaticity or reentry** involving a **portion of the Purkinje system[Q]**.

Diagnosis:
- In the presence of **known heart disease**, VT is the **most likely diagnosis of a wide QRS tachycardia[Q]**.
- **Presence of AV dissociation** is usually a **reliable marker for VT** but P waves can be difficult to define.
- A **monophasic R wave** or **Rs complex in AVR** or **concordance from V_1 to V_6** of monophasic R or S waves is **relatively specific for VT[Q]**.

Treatment:
- If **hypotension, impaired consciousness, or pulmonary edema** is present, **QRS synchronous electrical cardioversion should be performed**, ideally after sedation if the patient is conscious[Q].

  - **For stable tachycardia**, a **trial of adenosine** is reasonable[Q].
  - **Intravenous amiodarone** is **drug of choice if heart disease is present[Q]**.

- Following restoration of sinus rhythm, hospitalization and evaluation to define underlying heart disease are required.

  - If **VT recurs frequently or is incessant**, administration of **antiarrhythmic medications or catheter ablation** may be required to restore stability[Q].
  - **ICDs** are usually considered for **VT associated with structural heart disease[Q]**.

110. Ans. d. Acute intermittent porphyria *(Ref: Harrison 19/e p2526)*

Periodic abdominal pain (GI symptoms), peripheral neuropathy, headache (neurological symptoms) and psychiatric disorders (aggressive behavior) is highly suggestive of acute intermittent porphyria.

Acute Intermittent Porphyria (AD)
• **Autosomal dominant** condition **resulting from half-normal level of HMB synthase activity**[Q].
• **Precipitating factors**: Endogenous & exogenous **steroids, porphyrinogenic drugs, alcohol ingestion, low-calorie diets**[Q]
• More common in **women**

Clinical Features:
- **Asymptomatic** in majority of patients **prior to puberty**[Q]
- **MC symptom: Abdominal pain**[Q]
- Ileus, abdominal distention & decreased bowel sounds are common.

> - Nausea; vomiting; constipation; tachycardia; hypertension; mental symptoms; pain in limbs, head, neck, or chest; muscle weakness; sensory loss; dysuria; and urinary retention are characteristic[Q].
> - Tachycardia, hypertension, restlessness, tremors & excess sweating are due to **sympathetic overactivity**.

- **Peripheral neuropathy** is due to axonal degeneration and primarily **affects motor neurons**[Q].
- **Motor neuropathy** affects the **proximal muscles initially**, more often in the **shoulders & arms**[Q].
- **Mental symptoms**: Anxiety, insomnia, depression, disorientation, hallucinations, paranoia & **seizures**[Q]

Diagnosis:
- **ALA & PBG levels** are substantially **increased in plasma & urine**, especially **during acute attacks**[Q].

Treatment:
- **Acute attack**: **Narcotic analgesics** for abdominal pain & **phenothiazines** for nausea, vomiting, anxiety, and restlessness. **Chloral hydrate** for insomnia; **Carbohydrate loading (IV glucose)** effective in **milder acute attacks of porphyria** if hemin is not available[Q].
- **IV hemin is more effective** and should be used as **first-line therapy for all acute attacks**[Q].

Porphyrias					
Enzyme	**Location of enzyme**	**Associated porphyria**	**Type of porphyria**	**Inheritance**	**Symptoms**
d-aminolevulinate (ALA) synthase	Mitochondrion	X-linked sideroblastic anemia (**XLSA**)	Erythropoetic	X-linked	-
d-aminolevulinate (ALA) dehydratase	Cytosol	Doss porphyria/ ALA dehydratase deficiency/ plumbo porphyria	Hepatic	Autosomal recessive	Abdominal pain, neuropathy[Q]
Hydroxymeth-ylbilane (HMB) synthase (or PBG deaminase)	Cytosol	**Acute intermittent porphyria (AIP)**	Hepatic	Autosomal dominant	**Periodic abdominal pain, peripheral neuropathy,** psychiatric disorders, tachycardia[Q]
Uroporphyrinogen (URO) synthase	Cytosol	Congenital erythropoetic porphyria (CEP)	Erythropoetic	Autosomal recessive	**Severe photosensitivity** with erythema, swelling and blistering. Hemolytic anemia, splenomegaly[Q]
Uroporphyrinogen (URO) decarboxylase	Cytosol	Porphyria cutanea tarda (PCT)	Hepatic	Autosomal dominant	**Photosensitivity** with vesicles and bullae[Q]

Contd...

Contd...

Porphyrias					
Coproporphy-rinogen (COPRO) oxidase	Mitochondrion	Hereditary coproporhyria (HCP)	Hepatic	Autosomal dominant	**Photosensitivity, neurologic symptoms**, colic[Q]
Protoporphy-rinogen (PROTO) oxidase	Mitochondrion	Variegate porphyria (VP)	Mixed	Autosomal dominant	**Photosensitivity, neurologic symptoms**, developmental delay[Q]
Ferrochelatase	Mitochondrion	Erythropoetic protoporphyria (EPP)	Erythropoetic	Autosomal dominant	**Photosensitivity** with skin lesions; Gallstones, mild liver dysfunction Purpuric skin lesions[Q]

111. Ans. b. Concussion *(Ref: Harrison 19/e p2724, 457e-1, 2194)*

With history of fall, concussion and diffuse axonal injury are the probable outcomes. Diffuse axonal injury is associated with severe trauma. A brief period of both retrograde and anterograde amnesia is characteristic of concussion.

"Concussion: This form of minor head injury had in the past referred to an immediate and transient loss of consciousness that was associated with a short period of amnesia. Many patients, however, do not lose consciousness after a minor head injury but instead are dazed or confused, or feel stunned or "star struck," and the term concussion is now applied to all such cognitive and perceptual changes experienced after a blow to the head." - Harrison 19/e p457e-1

"A brief period of both retrograde and anterograde amnesia is characteristic of concussion, and it recedes rapidly in alert patients. Memory loss spans the moments before impact but may encompass the previous days or weeks (rarely months). With severe injuries, the extent of retrograde amnesia roughly correlates with the severity of injury." - Harrison 19/e p457e-1

"Diffuse axonal injury is associated with severe head trauma and may be seen on MRI as multiple areas of punctate hemorrhage in deep white matter and corpus callosum. Diffuse axonal injury is associated with poor prognosis." - Blueprints neurology 3/e p120

"Fortunately, very few alcoholics (perhaps as few as 1 in 500 for the full syndrome) develop Wernicke's (ophthalmoparesis, ataxia, and encephalopathy) and Korsakoff's (retrograde and anterograde amnesia) syndromes, although a higher proportion have one or more neuropathologic findings related to these conditions." - Harrison 19/e p2724

"Cerebral venous thrombosis is most frequently observed in the superior sagittal and transverse sinuses and is associated with headache and increased intracranial pressure." - Harrison 19/e p2194

112. Ans. b. Fever undiagnosed after 1 week of in-patient workup *(Ref: Harrison 19/e p135)*

According to new definition of fever of unknown origin, fever undiagnosed after 1 week of in-patient work up is not included.

Fever of Unknown Origin (FUO)
FUO is now defined as:
• Fever >38.3°C (101°F) on at least two occasions[Q]
• Illness duration of ≥3weeks [Q]
• No known immunocompromised state[Q]
• Diagnosis that remains uncertain after a thorough history-taking, physical examination, and the following obligatory investigations[Q]:
– Determination of **ESR & CRP** level; **Platelet count; leukocyte count** & differential[Q]
– Measurement of **Hb, electrolytes, creatinine, total protein, ALP, ALT, AST, LDH, creatine kinase, ferritin, antinuclear antibodies, rheumatoid factor; protein electrophoresis; urinalysis**[Q]
– **Blood cultures** (n = 3); **urine culture**[Q]
– **Chest X-ray;** abdominal USG; **Tuberculin skin test**[Q]

113. Ans. a. Primary hypothyroidism *(Ref: Harrison 19/e p2292)*

Elevated TSH with decreased T3/T4 in the patient is suggestive of primary hypothyroidism.

Elevated TSH with normal free T3/T4	• Subclinical hypothyroidism
Elevated TSH with decreased T3/T4	• Primary hypothyroidism
Decreased TSH and decreased T3/T4	• Secondary hypothyroidism
Decreased TSH and elevated T3/T4	• Primary hyperthyroidism
Elevated TSH and elevated T3/T4	• Secondary hyperthyroidism

Evaluation of Hypothyroidism

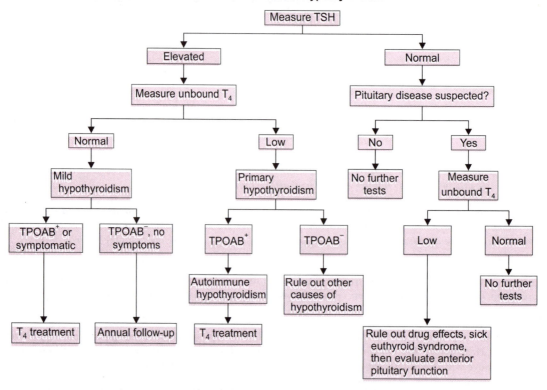

114. Ans. a. Pulmonary thromboembolism *(Ref: Harrisons 19/e p1632)*

History of immobilization for long duration suggests a probably subclinical deep venous thrombosis that had developed in the patient. On massaging, the thrombus of DVT got dislodged in the pulmonary circulation, causing pulmonary thromboembolism and death.

> *"Massive pulmonary embolism accounts for 5–10% of cases, and is characterized by extensive thrombosis affecting at least half of the pulmonary vasculature. Dyspnea, syncope, hypotension, and cyanosis are hallmarks of massive PE. Patients with massive PE may present in cardiogenic shock and can die from multisystem organ failure." - Harrisons 19/e p1632*

Pulmonary Embolism

- Risk factors for pulmonary embolism are the **risk factors for thrombi formation** within **venous circulation**.
- **Calf venous thrombosis**: Low risk for **embolism**[Q]
- **Thrombosis of larger veins**: High risk for **embolism**[Q] (due to **loosely attached thrombus** to **venous wall**)
    - MC site for DVT: Calf veins[Q]
    - MC source for pulmonary emboli: Proximal vein of lower extremity[Q] (femoro-popliteal & iliac vein)

Contd...

Contd...

Risk Factors for Pulmonary Thromboembolism		
• Age (Increasing age)[Q] • Obesity[Q] • Immobility (bed rest >4 days)[Q] • Pregnancy[Q] & Puerperium[Q] • High dose estrogen therapy[Q] • Nephrotic syndrome[Q]	• Surgery/trauma (especially of pelvis, hip or lower limb)[Q] • Malignancy (especially pelvis, abdominal, metastatic) • Heart failure / Recent MI[Q] • Inflammatory bowel disease[Q] • Polycythemia[Q]	• PNH[Q] or Lupus anticoagulant • Behcet's syndrome[Q] • Homocystinuria[Q] • Paralysis of lower limb • Varicose veins, Infection

Clinical features:
- Symptoms: Dyspnea (MC)[Q], chest pain, hemoptysis & cough
- Signs: Tachypnea (MC)[Q], fever, unilateral leg swelling, wheeze, pleural friction rub

  - Any patient with **high likelihood** of pulmonary embolism on clinical evaluation **straightaway undergoes imaging tests**, while a patient with **low clinical likelihood** should **first undergo D-dimer test[Q].**

Factors for Clinical Assessment of Pulmonary Embolism	
• Clinical **signs** & **symptoms of DVT[Q]** • An alternative diagnosis is less likely than pulmonary embolism • **Heart rate >100/min[Q]** • **Hemoptysis[Q]**	• **Immobilization** or **previous surgery in 4 weeks[Q]** • **Previous DVT/PE[Q]** • **Malignancy[Q]** (on treatment, treatment in past 6 months)

ECG Changes in Pulmonary Embolism (Sinus tachycardia: MC & non-specific finding on ECG[Q])	
Features of Acute Right Heart Strain	**Highly predictive of PE**
• Acute **right axis deviation[Q]** • **P pulmonale[Q]** • **Right bundle branch block[Q]** • **Inverted T waves[Q]** • ST segment change	• $S_1Q_3T_3$[Q]: Seen in **<12%** patients • S wave in lead I • Q wave in lead III • Inverted T wave in lead III • S wave in lead I, II, and III ($S_1S_2S_3$)

Diagnosis:
- **D-dimer: Excellent screening test for** the **diagnosis of PE[Q].**
- **Best investigation** in clinical suspicion of PE: **Multidetector CT[Q]**
- **Lung scanning** is now a **2nd line** diagnostic test for PE.

  - **Pulmonary angiography: Gold standard** for **diagnosis of PE[Q]** (but expensive & cumbersome)

Treatment:
- **Anticoagulation is foundation for successful treatment of DVT & PE[Q].**
- **Immediately effective anticoagulation is initiated with a parenteral drug**, **unfractionated heparin (UFH)[Q].**
- **Only FDA-approved indication for PE fibrinolysis is massive PE[Q].**
- **Pulmonary embolectomy:** Risk of intracranial hemorrhage with fibrinolysis has prompted a renaissance of surgical embolectomy.

115. **Ans. d. Systolic BP <100 mm Hg and Diastolic BP <60 mm Hg**   *(Ref: Harrison's 19/e p806)*
Pneumonia Severity Index (PSI) and CURB-65 criteria are used in patients of community-acquired pneumonia to decide severity of illness and which patients merit in-patient/ICU care. Systolic BP of <90 mm Hg (not < 100 mm Hg) is a part of the CURB65 criteria.

"The CURB-65 criteria include five variables: confusion (C); urea >7 mmol/L (U); respiratory rate ≥30/min (R); blood pressure, systolic ≤90 mmHg or diastolic ≤60 mmHg (B); and age ≥65 years. Patients with a score of 0, among whom the 30-day mortality rate is 1.5%, can be treated outside the hospital. With a score of 2, the 30-day mortality rate is 9.2%, and patients should be admitted to the hospital. Among patients with scores of ≥3, mortality rates are 22% overall; these patients may require ICU admission." -Harrison's 19/e p806

Community Acquired Pneumonia	
Pneumonia Severity Index (PSI)	**CURB-65**

• A prognostic model used to **identify patients at low risk of dying.**
• The PSI is less practical in a busy emergency room setting because of the need to assess 20 variables.
• **Only decision aid for risk stratification of patients with CAP**[Q]
	• A **severity-of-illness score**
	• The **CURB-65** criteria include **five variables**:
	  – **Confusion**[Q]
	  – **Urea > 7 mmol/L**[Q]
	  – **Respiratory rate ≥30/min**[Q]
	  – **Blood pressure, systolic <90** mm Hg or **diastolic <60** mm Hg[Q]
	  – **Age >65 years**[Q]

Calculator: Community-acquired Pneumonia Severity Index (PSI) for Adults		
Sex	**Demographic Factors**	**Comorbid Illness**
• Male: 0 points • Female: -10 points	• Age: 1 point for each year • Nursing home resident: 10 points	• Neoplastic disease: 30 points • Congestive heart failure: 10 points • Cerebrovascular disease: 10 points • Renal disease: 10 points
Physical examination findings	**Laboratory and Radiographic Findings**	
• Altered mental status: 20 points • Respiratory rate ≥ 30/min: 20 points • Systolic blood pressure <90 mm Hg: 20 points • Temperature <35° C or ≥ 40° C: 15 points • Pulse ≥ 125/min: 10 points	• Arterial pH <7.35: 30 points • BUN ≥ 30 mg/dL: 20 points • Sodium <130 mEq/L: 20 points • Glucose ≥ 250 mg/dL: 10 points • Hematocrit <30 percent: 10 points • Partial pressure of arterial oxygen <60 mm Hg or oxygen saturation <90%: 10 points • Pleural effusion: 10 points	

Pneumonia Score Interpretation		
Class I	0-50 points	0.1% mortality
Class II	51-70 points	0.6% mortality
Class III	71-90 points	0.9% mortality
Class IV	91-130 points	9.3% mortality
Class V	131-395 points	27.0% mortality

116. **Ans. d. Cotrimoxazole with 3rd generation cephalosporins** *(Ref: Harrison 19/e p1048; Katzung 13/e p802, 904, 12/e p904)*

Drug of choice for B. cepacia is TMP-SMX and alternative agents are ceftazidime, chloramphenicol.

"Burkholderia cepacia is intrinsically resistant to many antibiotics. Therefore, treatment must be tailored according to sensitivities. TMP-SMX, meropenem, and doxycycline are the most effective agents in vitro and may be started as first-line agents. Some strains are susceptible to third-generation cephalosporins and fluoroquinolones, and these agents may be used against isolates known to be susceptible. Combination therapy for serious pulmonary infection (e.g., in CF) is suggested when multidrug-resistant strains are implicated; the combination of meropenem and TMP-SMX may be antagonistic, however. Resistance to all agents used has been reported during therapy." -Harrison 19/e p1048

Burkholderia cepacia
• **B. cepacia** is the **cause of a rapidly fatal syndrome of respiratory distress & septicemia ("cepacia syndrome")** in **cystic fibrosis** patients[Q]. • **Predisposing factors: Cystic fibrosis & chronic granulomatous disease**[Q] • B. cepacia **inhabits moist environments** and is **found in rhizosphere**[Q]. • Possesses **multiple virulence factors & colonizing factors** capable of **binding to lung mucus**[Q] (**predilection of B. cepacia for the lungs in cystic fibrosis**).
Treatment: • **DOC for B. cepacia: TMP-SMX**[Q] • **Alternative agents: Meropenem & doxycycline**[Q]

Organism	Drug of Choice
• Streptococcus pneumoniae, S. viridans, Hemolytic streptococci group A, B, C, G • Staphylococcus (non-penicillinase producing) • Actinomyces, Bacillus cereus, Clostridium (ABC) • Peptococcus, Peptostreptococcus • Neisseria meningitidis • Treponema pallidum, T. pertenue • Leptospira	• Penicillin G[Q]
• MRSA, Coagulase negative Staphylococcus • Enterococcus faecium	• Vancomycin[Q]
• Enterococcus faecalis, Listeria	• Ampicillin[Q]
• Vibrio species	• Tetracycline[Q]
• **B**acillus anthracis • **B**orrelia burgdorferi, **B**. recurrentis • **C**hlamydia & **R**ickettsiae (**BCR**)	• Doxycycline[Q]
• Corynebacterium	• Erythromycin[Q]
• **H**emophilus ducreyi, **C**ampylobacter jejuni & **L**egionella (**HCL**) • Mycoplasma	• Azithromycin[Q]
• **B**urkholderia cepacia • **S**tenotrophomons maltophila • **N**ocardia (**BSNL**)	• Cotrimoxazole[Q]
• **P**roteus, **E**. coli, **K**lebsiella, **S**almonella (**PEKS**)	• Ceftriaxone[Q]
• **S**erratia, **E**nterobacter, **A**cinetobacter (**SEA**)	• Carbapenems[Q]
• **B**acteroides & **C**lostridium **d**ifficile (**BCD**)	• Metronidazole[Q]
• Burkholderia pseudomallei (meliodosis)	• Ceftazidime[Q]
• Helicobacter pylori	• PPI + Amoxicillin + Clarithromycin[Q]

117. **Ans. b. Petechial rash**   *(Ref: Harrisons 19/e p1307, 1314)*
 Maculopapular rash and not petechial rash is commonly seen in Zika virus disease.

> "Zika virus is an emerging pathogen that is transmitted among nonhuman primates and humans by Aedes mosquitoes. Human infections are usually benign and are most likely misdiagnosed as dengue or influenza. Zika virus infection is characterized by influenza-like clinical signs, including fever, headaches, and malaise. A maculopapular rash, conjunctivitis, myalgia, and arthralgia usually accompany or follow those manifestations." - *Harrisons 19/e p1314*

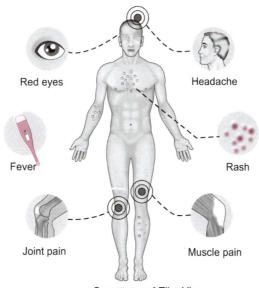

Fig. 27: Symptoms of Zika Virus

Zika Virus Outbreak

Microbiology:
- Zika virus belongs to **family Flaviviridae & genus Flavivirus**; **Single stranded RNA virus**[Q]

History:
- It is named after the **Zika Forest, Uganda** in 1947.
- **Reservoir: Monkeys**[Q]

Transmission:
- **Mosquito borne: Mainly spread by the Aedes aegypti**[Q]
- **Mother-to-child transmission through placenta** (common in first trimester),
- **Sexual transmission** is also possible

Current Outbreak:
- **Zika virus current outbreak began in April 2015 in Brazil.**
- Subsequently it spread to other countries in South America, Central America, and the Caribbean.
- Imported cases have also been reported from Europe and the United States and Australia.
- In February 2016, WHO declared Zika virus outbreak a public health emergency of international concern.

Situation in India:
- **No cases have been reported so far**, but there is evidence of sero-prevalence (i.e. Indian patients have in the past tested positive for Zika virus antibodies).
- As the vector is prevalent, so India may be affected in near future.

Clinical Manifestations:
- **Majority** patients are **asymptomatic**[Q]
- **Zika fever: Minor illness such as fever and a maculopapular rash**[Q].

> - **Symptoms of Zika virus: Maculopapular rash**[Q] **(90%), Fever**[Q] **(65%), Arthritis or arthralgia**[Q] **(65%), Non-purulent conjunctivitis (55%), Myalgia**[Q] **(48%), Headache (45%), Retroorbital pain (39%), Edema (19%) & Vomiting (10%)**

- Symptoms normally last for **2–7 days.**
- **Congenital transmission** leads to **newborn microcephaly**[Q]
- In very few cases, **Guillain-Barre syndrome**[Q] has been reported.

Laboratory Diagnosis:
- **IgM ELISA** is available. But it cross reacts with Dengue antibodies
- **Plaque-reduction neutralization test** may be more specific.
- **RT-PCR** is done in acutely ill patients

Treatment and Vaccine:
- **No effective treatment & vaccine is available so far**[Q].
- Usually **mild** and **requires no specific treatment.**
- **Only symptomatic treatment available** such as fluid replacement & analgesic (acetaminophen).

118. **Ans. c. Quadriceps** *(Ref: Textbook of Orthopedics by John Ebenzar 4/e p74)*
Hand to knee gait is typically seen in polio in which the person places on hand on the knee to walk to prevent it from buckling due to quadriceps paralysis.

Muscles involved in Poliomyelitis	
In Early stages	**Post Polio Residual Paralysis**
- **Rigidity & tenderness of neck muscles**[Q] - **Asymmetric paralysis**[Q] - **Most commonly affected muscle is quadriceps and it is partially affected**[Q] - Muscle **most commonly affected in hand** is **opponens pollicis**[Q] - **Bulbar polio** results in paralysis of respiratory & cardiovascular centres	- Wasting, paralysis & deformity of lower limb muscles - **Deformity at hip:** Flexion, abduction & external rotation - **Deformity at knee:** Triple deformity of flexion, posterior subluxation & external rotation - **Foot: Equinovarus is most deformity followed by equinovalgus, Calcaneovalgus, calcaneovarus** - **Upper limb:** Shoulder and elbow muscles

AIIMS May 2017

119. Ans. a. IGF1 *(Ref: Harrisons 19/e p2262, 2269)*

Clinical findings of frontal bossing, enlarged nasal bone, enlarged jaw and spade like fingers is suggestive of acromegaly. Screening Investigation of choice for diagnosis of acromegaly is IGF-1 (Insulin like growth factor).

"Age-matched serum IGF-I levels are elevated in acromegaly. Consequently, an IGF-I level provides a useful laboratory screening measure when clinical features raise the possibility of acromegaly. Due to the pulsatility of GH secretion, measurement of a single random GH level is not useful for the diagnosis or exclusion of acromegaly and does not correlate with disease severity. The diagnosis of acromegaly is confirmed by demonstrating the failure of GH suppression to <0.4 µg/L within 1–2 h of an oral glucose load (75 g)."- Harrisons 19/e p2269

Acromegaly

- **Acromegaly** is the clinical syndrome resulting from **hypersecretion of GH or somatomedins like IGF-1[Q]**.

  - **MC cause** of acromegaly: **GH secreting pituitary adenoma[Q]**
  - **MC cause** of GHRH-mediated acromegaly: Chest or abdominal **carcinoid tumor[Q]**.

Causes of Acromegaly

Excess GH secretion	Excess GH-Releasing Hormone secretion
- **Pituitary:** Densely or sparsely granulated **GH cell adenoma (MC)[Q]** > **Mixed GH cell & prolactin cell adenoma** > Mammosomatotrope cell adenoma - **Extra-pituitary tumor:** Pancreatic islet cell tumor[Q], lymphoma	- **Central:** Hypothalamic hamartoma[Q], choristoma, ganglioneuroma - **Peripheral:** Bronchial carcinoid[Q], Pancreatic islet cell tumor[Q], Small cell lung cancer[Q], Adrenal adenoma, Medullary thyroid carcinoma, Pheochromocytoma

Clinical Features:

- Protean manifestations are indolent and often are **not clinically diagnosed for 10 years or more**.

  - **Acral bony overgrowth** results in **frontal bossing, increased hand and foot size, mandibular enlargement with prognathism & widened space between the lower incisor teeth[Q]**.

- In **children & adolescents**, initiation of GH hypersecretion before epiphyseal long bone closure is associated with development of **pituitary gigantism[Q]**.

  - **Soft tissue swelling** results in **increased heel pad thickness, increased shoe or glove size, ring tightening**, characteristic **coarse facial features**, and a **large fleshy nose[Q]**.
  - **Generalized visceromegaly:** Cardiomegaly, macroglossia & thyroid gland enlargement[Q].

- **CVS: Coronary heart disease, cardiomyopathy** with arrhythmias, **left ventricular hypertrophy**, decreased diastolic function & **hypertension[Q]**
- **Respiratory: Upper airway obstruction with sleep apnea**, soft tissue laryngeal airway obstruction & central sleep dysfunction[Q].
- **Diabetes mellitus**, insulin resistance, **hypertriglyceridemia[Q]**.

  - **Colonic:** Increased risk of **colon polyps & colonic malignancy[Q]**
  - **Local tumor effects: Visual field defects, diplopia, headache[Q]**

- **Others:** Hyperhidrosis, a deep & hollow-sounding voice, oily skin, arthropathy, kyphosis, **carpal tunnel syndrome, proximal muscle weakness & fatigue**, acanthosis nigricans & **skin tags[Q]**.

Diagnosis:

- **Screening investigation of choice in acromegaly: IGF-1[Q]**
- **Confirmatory & Gold standard: Oral Glucose Tolerance tests[Q]**

  - Diagnosis of acromegaly is confirmed by demonstrating the failure of GH suppression to < 0.4 µg/L within 1–2 hour of an oral glucose load[Q] (75 gm).

Acromegaly
Treatment:
• **Goal of treatment**: **Control GH & IGF-I hypersecretion**, **ablate or arrest tumor growth**, ameliorate comorbidities, restore mortality rates to normal & preserve pituitary function[Q].
• **Initial treatment**: **Surgical resection of GH-secreting adenomas** (**Transsphenoidal surgical resection**[Q]) • **Unresectable cases or relapse**: **Octreotide or lanreotide**[Q] (Somatostatin analogue) or **Pegvisomant**[Q] (GH receptor antagonist)

120. Ans. a. Serum potassium *(Ref: Harrisons 19/e p2697, 462e-16)*

Hypokalemia can cause flaccid ascending paralysis, which is a differential diagnosis for GBS. It can also cause periodic paralysis. Hypocalcemia and hypomagnesemia usually cause tetany and hypercalcemia won't cause ascending paralysis. A low serum potassium level during an attack, excluding secondary causes, establishes the diagnosis of Hypokalemic Periodic Paralysis.

Hypokalemic Periodic Paralysis (HypoKPP)
• Rare inherited neuromuscular disorder, related to **defect in muscle ion channels**
• More common in **males; Begins in late adulthood or teenage years**

Gene Mutations in Hypokalemic Periodic Paralysis	
HypoKPP type 1	**HypoKPP type 2**
• **MC form**[Q] • **Autosomal-dominant** with incomplete penetrance. • These patients have mutations in **voltage-sensitive, skeletal muscle calcium channel gene, CALCL1A3**	• Responsible for 10% of cases • These patients have mutations in **voltage-sensitive sodium channel gene (SCN4A).**

Clinical Features:
• Manifest by episodes of **painless muscle weakness, provoked by** meals high in **carbohydrates or sodium** and may accompany **rest following prolonged exercise**[Q].
• **Weakness** usually **affects proximal limb muscles more than distal**[Q]. • **Ocular & bulbar muscles** are **less likely to be affected**[Q].
• **Respiratory muscles** are usually **spared,** but when they are involved, the **condition may prove fatal**[Q].
• **Weakness** may take as long as **24 hours to resolve**[Q].
• **Life-threatening cardiac arrhythmias** related to **hypokalemia** may occur during attacks.
• As a **late complication**, patients commonly develop severe, **disabling proximal lower extremity weakness**[Q].

Diagnosis:
• **A low serum potassium level during an attack, excluding secondary causes, establishes the diagnosis**[Q].
• **Inter-attack muscle biopsies** show the presence of **single or multiple centrally placed vacuoles or tubular aggregates**[Q].
• **Provocative tests with glucose & insulin** to establish a diagnosis are usually not necessary and are **potentially hazardous**[Q].

Treatment:
• **Acute paralysis** improves after the **administration of potassium**[Q] (**Oral KCl** every 30 min; IV therapy is rarely necessary)
• Administration of **potassium in a glucose solution** should be **avoided** because it may further **reduce serum potassium levels**[Q].

121. Ans. d. 4.5 hours *(Ref: Harrison 19/e p2562)*

Window period for thrombolysis in a stroke patient is 4.5 hours.

"Based on these data, rtPA is approved in the 3- to 4.5-h window in Europe and Canada, but is still only approved for 0–3 h in the United States and Canada. Use of IV tPA is now considered a central component of primary stroke centers. It represents the first treatment proven to improve clinical outcomes in ischemic stroke and is cost-effective and cost-saving."

Harrison 19/e p2562

AIIMS May 2017

"Intravenous thrombolysis is usually practiced within the window period of 4.5 hours (Hacke W, 2008; ECASS III)."-
Neurological Practice: An Indian Perspective by Noshir H. Wadia, Satish V Khadilkar 2/e p175

"Stroke is a major cause of mortality and morbidity, and thrombolysis has served as a catalyst for major changes in the management of acute ischaemic stroke. Intravenous alteplase (recombinant tissue plasminogen activator) is the only approved thrombolytic agent at present indicated for acute ischaemic stoke. While the licensed time window extends to 3h from symptom onset, recent data suggest that the trial window can be extended up to 4.5 h with overall benefit."-
https://www.ncbi.nlm.nih.gov/pmc/articles/PMC3513874/

"In Early 2009, the AHA/ASA guidelines for the administration of rtPA following acute stroke were revised to expand the window of the treatment from 3 to 4.5 hours to provide more patients with an opportunity to receive benefit form this effective therapy."- Evidence-Based Neurology: Management of Neurological Disorders by Bart Demaerschalk, Dean Wingerchuk 2/e p55

Administration of IV Recombinant Tissue Plasminogen Activator (rtPA) for Acute Ischemic Stroke	
Indication	**Contraindication**
• Clinical diagnosis of stroke[Q] • Onset of symptoms to time of drug administration ≤ 4.5 hours[Q] • CT scan showing no hemorrhage or edema of >1/3 of the MCA territory[Q] • Age ≥ 18 years[Q] • Consent by patient or surrogate	• Sustained BP >185/110 mm Hg despite treatment[Q] • Platelets <100,000; HCT <25%; glucose <50 or >400 mg/dL[Q] • Use of heparin within 48 hours & prolonged PTT, or elevated INR[Q] • Rapidly improving symptoms[Q] • Prior stroke or head injury within 3 months[Q] • Prior intracranial hemorrhage[Q] • Major surgery in preceding 14 days[Q] • Minor stroke symptoms[Q] • Gastrointestinal bleeding in preceding 21 days[Q] • Recent myocardial infarction[Q] • Coma or stupor[Q]

Administration of IV Recombinant Tissue Plasminogen Activator (rtPA)
• **IV access with two peripheral IV lines[Q]** (avoid arterial or central line placement) • Review eligibility for rtPA • **Administer 0.9 mg/kg IV** (maximum 90 mg) IV as 10% of total dose by bolus, followed by remainder of total dose over 1 h • **Frequent cuff blood pressure monitoring[Q]** • **No other antithrombotic treatment for 24 hours[Q]** • **For decline in neurologic status or uncontrolled blood pressure, stop infusion, give cryoprecipitate, and reimage brain emergently[Q]** • **Avoid urethral catheterization for ≥2 hours [Q]**

122. **Ans. b. Fat embolism** *(Ref: Harrisons 19/e p1632; Robbins 9/e p128; Apley's 9/e p681; Rockwood 6/e p553)*
Fat embolism is a common cause of pulmonary embolism after pelvic or long bone fractures. PE can lead to sudden onset breathlessness and fever.

"Fat embolism is a common phenomenon following limb fractures. Circulating fat globules larger than 10 μm in diameter occur in most adults after closed fractures of long bones and histological traces of fat can be found in the lungs and other internal organs."-Apley's 9/e p681

"Early warning signs of fat embolism (usually within 72 hours of injury) are a slight rise of temperature and pulse rate. In more pronounced cases, there is breathlessness and mild mental confusion or restlessness. Pathognomonic signs are petechiae on the trunk, axillae and in the conjunctival folds and retinae. In more severe cases there may be respiratory distress and coma, due both to brain emboli and hypoxia from involvement of the lungs. The features at this stage are essentially those of ARDS."- Apley's 9/e p681

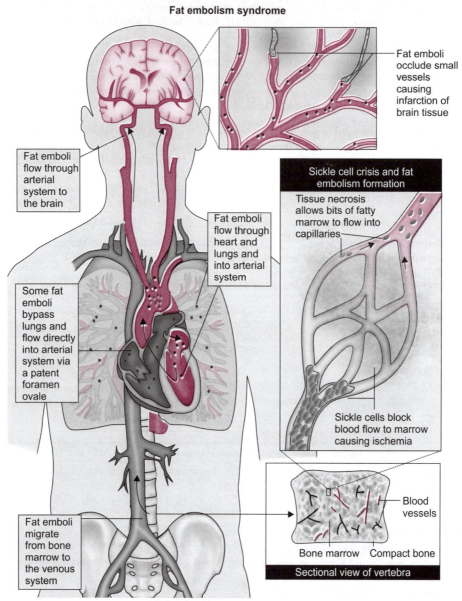

Fig. 28: Fat embolism syndrome

Fat Embolism Syndrome
Pathophysiology: • Fat embolism is seen in **multiple fracture & in fractures involving lower limbs especially femur**[Q]. • Circulating **fat globules >10 micron**[Q] in diameter occur in most adults after **close fracture of long bones**[Q] & histological traces of fat can be found in the lungs & other internal organs.
Clinical presentation: • **Classic triad: Hypoxemia + Neurologic abnormalities + Petechial Rash** • Usually manifests itself **within 24-48 hours**[Q]. • Early **warning signs** (within 72 hours of injury): Slight rise in temperature (**pyrexia**) & pulse rate (**tachycardia**)[Q]   • In more pronounced cases there is **breathlessness**, mild mental confusion or restlessness, **petechiae on chest, axillae, retina & conjunctival folds**[Q]; progressive to **marked respiratory distress** & coma in severe cases.

Fat Embolism Syndrome

Diagnosis:

- In addition to the classic clinical features, signs of **retinal artery emboli (Striate hemorrhage & exudates^Q)** may be present.
- **Sputum & urine: Presence of fat globules^Q.**
- Chest X-ray: **Patchy pulmonary infiltration (Snow storm appearance)** ^{Q}

Laboratory Tests
No characteristic laboratory test, **suggestive findings are:**

• **Thrombocytopenia^Q**	• **Tachycardia^Q**
• **(platelets <1.5 lacks)**	• **Pyrexia^Q**
• **PO$_2$ <60 mm Hg^Q**	• **Fall in hemoglobin value^Q**

Management:

- **Supportive pulmonary care, definitive fracture management & effective treatment of shock** are the **corner stones** of current fat embolism management^Q.

Respiratory support	Treatment of shock	Fracture stabilization
• Ranges from **oxygen administration** to **full respiratory support** with mechanical ventilation • **Oxygen** is the **only therapeutic tool** of **proven use^Q**	• Maintain adequate intravascular volume • **Aggressive fluid resuscitation^Q** • **Appropriate CVP monitoring** to avoid fluid overload^Q. • **Albumin** for **fluid resuscitation** along with a **balanced electrolyte solution^Q** because it not only restores blood volume but also binds free fatty acids.	• **Maintain adequate intravascular volume** • Since **movement at** the **fracture site** has been shown to **increase** the **fat emboli** in circulation, **early immobilization of lower extremity fractures^Q** is advocated

Additional Therapies	
• **Steroids**: Prophylactic corticosteroids **benefit high risk patients** • **Heparin: Increase** serum **lipase activity** & decrease number of circulating fat globules • **Hypertonic glucose**: Metabolically **decrease production** of **free fatty acids**	• **Dextran^Q**: To **reduce red cell aggregation, expand plasma volume, decrease blood viscosity** & **reduce platelet adherence** • **Aprotinin**: Decrease platelet aggregation & serotonin release • **Alcohol**: Reduces serum lipase activity

SURGERY

123. Ans. c. Radioactive iodine ablation *(Ref: Sabiston 20/e p2063; Schwartz 10/e p1543, 1546; Bailey 27/e p819-820, 26/e p767-768; William's Endocrinology 10/e p479)*

Radioactive iodine ablation is contraindicated in pregnancy because of severe teratogenic effects.

"Radioactive iodine therapy is contraindicated during pregnancy."-Sabiston 20/e p2063

"Radioactive iodine is contraindicated in pregnancy, which should be avoided for a year, and in lactating mothers." Textbook of Endocrine Surgery 3/p99

"Radioactive iodine treatment is contraindicated during pregnancy, as is oral iodide therapy, because it can cause fetal goiter and hypothyroidism."-Stoelting's Anesthesia and Co-Existing Disease 6/e p388

Radioactive Iodine (I^{131}) Therapy

- I^{131} is an **effective agent** for **delivering high radiation doses** to the **thyroid tissue^Q**
- It **emits mainly beta radiation (90%)**, which **penetrates** only **0.5 mm^Q** of the **tissue** and thus allow therapeutic effects on the thyroid **without any damage** to the surrounding structures, particularly the **parathyroids.**

Mechanism of Action:

- I^{131} emits **beta particles^Q** & **gamma rays**.
- **Beta rays** are utilized for their **destructive effects** on **thyroid^Q** cells.
- **X-rays** are useful for **tracer studies.**

Radioactive Iodine (I[131]) Therapy	
Indications in Carcinoma Thyroid	**Contraindications of I[131] Therapy**
1. **Distant metastasis**[Q] at diagnosis 2. **Incomplete tumor resection**[Q] 3. Patients at **high risk** for **mortality** or **recurrence**[Q]	• **Childhood**[Q] • **Pregnancy**[Q] • **Lactation**[Q]

Papillary Carcinoma of Thyroid

- Accounts for **80%** of all thyroid malignancies in **iodine-sufficient areas**[Q]
- **MC thyroid cancer** in **children** and **individuals** exposed to **external radiation**[Q].
- More often in **women, 30-40** years.

Pathology:
- **Grossly: Hard** and **whitish** and **remain flat** on sectioning with a blade with macroscopic **calcification, necrosis**, or **cystic changes**

> - **Multifocality**[Q] is **common** (up to **85%** of cases) on **microscopic examination**.
> - **Multifocality** is associated with an **increased risk** of **cervical nodal metastases**[Q], **rarely invade adjacent structures** such as the trachea, esophagus, and RLNs.

- **Rarely encapsulated**[Q] (PCT are **seldom encapsulated**)
- **Other variants: Tall cell**[Q], **insular**[Q], columnar, diffuse sclerosing, clear cell, **trabecular**, and poorly differentiated types; account for about **1%**; associated with a **worse prognosis**.

Histological characteristics of Papillary Carcinoma Thyroid

- **Papillary projections**[Q]: PTC contains branching papillae of cuboidal epithelial cells
- **Orphan Annie eye nuclei**:
  - The nuclei contain finely dispersed chromatin, which imparts an **optically clear** or **empty appearance**, giving rise to term **ground glass** or **Orphan Annie eye nuclei**[Q].
  - **Invaginations** of **cytoplasm** in cross-sections: **Intranuclear inclusions**[Q] (pseudo-inclusion) or **intranuclear grooves**[Q].
  - **Diagnosis** of PTC is **based on** these **nuclear characteristics**[Q] even in the absence of papillary structures.
- Psammoma bodies[Q]: Microscopic, calcified deposits representing clumps of sloughed cells

Clinical Features:
- Most patients are **euthyroid** and present with a **slow-growing painless mass**[Q] in the neck.
- Dysphagia, dyspnea & dysphonia are associated with locally advanced invasive disease.
- **Lymph node metastases** are **common**[Q], especially in **children** and **young adults**, and may be the presenting complaint.

> - "**Lateral aberrant thyroid**" almost always denotes a **cervical lymph node** that has been **invaded by metastatic cancer**[Q].

- **Distant metastases** are **uncommon** at initial presentation, but may ultimately develop in up to **20%** of patients.
- The **MC sites of metastasis: Lungs**[Q] >bone >liver >brain.

Diagnosis:
- **Diagnosis is** established by **FNAC** of the **thyroid mass** or **lymph node**[Q].
- Once thyroid cancer is diagnosed on FNAC, a **complete neck ultrasound** to evaluate the **contralateral lobe** and for **LN metastases** in the central & lateral neck compartments.

Treatment:
- **Total** or **near-total thyroidectomy**[Q]
- During thyroidectomy, **enlarged central neck nodes** should be **removed**[Q].
- **Biopsy-proven lymph node metastases** detected clinically or by imaging in the lateral neck in patients with papillary carcinoma are managed with **modified radical neck dissection**.

Prognosis:
- PTC have an **excellent prognosis** with a **>95% 10-year survival rate**[Q].

124. **Ans. c. Hypersecreting adenoma** *(Ref: Grainger & Allison Diagnostic Radiology 5/e p860; Bailey 27/e p811, 26/e p746; Essentials of Nuclear Medicine Imaging by Fred A Milter/p605; Manual of Endocrinology and Metabolism by Norman Lavin 4/e p495*

The given thyroid scan is showing increased focal uptake in the right upper lobe of thyroid and decreased uptake in rest of the thyroid gland. This is suggestive of hypersecreting thyroid adenoma. There is no ectopic thyroid tissue, so lateral aberrant thyroid and lateral extension is ruled out. Malignancy is ruled-out as there is no cold nodule.

> "Scintigraphy: A single toxic nodule shows high uptake of tracer with the remaining normal thyroid tissue showing poor or virtually no activity." - *Grainger & Allison Diagnostic Radiology 5/e p860*

> "Toxic adenoma (hyperfunctioning solitary nodule): Thyroid hormone from an adenoma is secreted independent of TSH stimulation. The excessive release of thyroid hormone suppresses the pituitary release of TSH, resulting in diminished activity in the remainder of the gland. On thyroid scan, the toxic adenoma appears as a hot nodule surrounded by little or no thyroid tissue." - *Manual of Endocrinology and Metabolism by Norman Lavin 4/e p495*

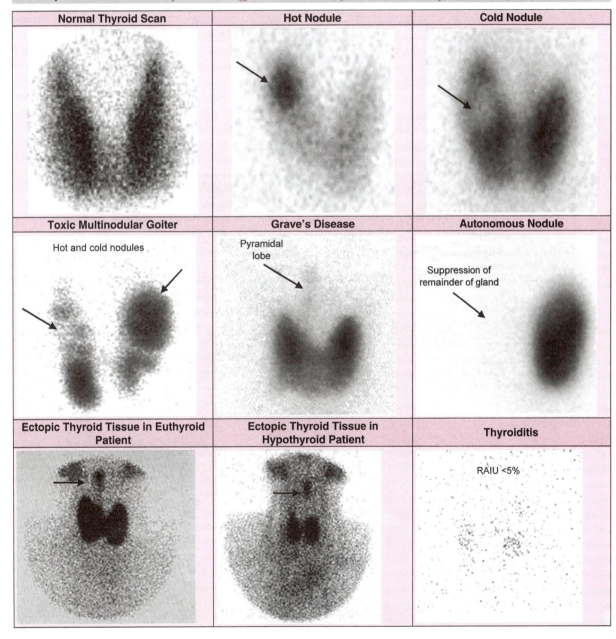

125. Ans. c. Thyroglossal cyst *(Ref: Sabiston 20/e p1861; Schwartz 10/e p1522; Bailey 27/e p755, 26/e p701)*
Thyroglossal cyst is the only midline neck swelling which moves with both deglutition and swallowing.

> *"Thyroglossal Cyst: The diagnosis usually is established by observing a 1- to 2-cm, smooth, well-defined midline neck mass that moves upward with protrusion of the tongue."- Schwartz 10/e p1522*

> *"Thyroglossal Cyst: The cysts almost always arise in the midline but, when they are adjacent to the thyroid cartilage, they may lie slightly to one side of the midline. Classically, the cyst moves upwards on swallowing and with tongue protrusion, but this can also occur with other midline cysts such as dermoid cysts, as it merely indicates attachment to the hyoid bone."-Bailey 27/e p755, 26/e p701*

Thyroglossal Cyst
• It is **cystic swelling** developed in the remnant of the **thyroglossal duct** or **tract**
• It may be **present** in **any part** of the **thyroglossal tract**[Q] (thyroglossal tract extends from foramen caecum to the isthmus of thyroid)

Common Sites of Thyroglossal Cyst	
• **Subhyoid (MC)**[Q]	• In the floor of mouth
• In the region of the thyroid cartilages	• Beneath the foramen caecum
• Suprahyoid	

Clinical Features:
- It is a **midline swelling**[Q], except in the region of the thyroid cartilage, where the thyroglossal tract is pushed to one side, usually to the left.
- Though it's a **congenital swelling**[Q] most common **age of presentation** is between **15-30 years**[Q].
- Cyst can be **moved sideways** but not vertically.

Peculiar characteristic which helps in distinguishing thyroglossal cyst from other neck swelling
• **Moves up with protrusion of tongue**[Q] as the thyroglossal tract is attached to the tongue.
• **Moves with deglutition**[Q] so do all thyroid swellings, subhyoid bursitis.

- Cyst is lined by pseudostratified columnar epithelium and squamous epithelium with **heterotopic thyroid tissue** present in **20%** of cases.

Complications of Thyroglossal Cyst	
Recurrent infections[Q]	Carcinomatous change, usually **papillary carcinoma**[Q]
Formation of **thyroglossal fistula**[Q]	

Treatment of Thyroglossal Cyst	
Sistrunk operation: En-bloc cystectomy & excision of the **central hyoid bone**[Q] to minimize recurrence.	

AIIMS May 2017

126. Ans. d. 55–60% *(Ref: Schwartz 10/e p527; De Vita 10/e p1122)*

Sensitivity of axillary ultrasound in identifying axillary metastases in clinically node negative carcinoma breast is 55–60%.

"Ultrasonography can also be utilized to image the regional lymph nodes in patients with breast cancer. The sensitivity of examination for the status of axillary nodes ranges from 35% to 82% and specificity ranges from 73% to 97%. The features of a lymph node involved with cancer include cortical thickening, change in shape of the node to more circular appearance, size larger than 10 mm, absence of a fatty hilum and hypoechoic internal echoes."- Schwartz 10/e p527

"The status of the regional lymph nodes is one of the most important prognostic factors in early stage breast cancer. Ultrasound may add to clinical examination and improve the sensitivity of node detection (combined sensitivity ranges from 60–80% in various trials, as it is based on subjective findings and operator dependence), but surgical staging using US guided FNA or SLNB/ALND is required for all patients."-De Vita 10/e p1122

"PET can detect axillary lymph node involvement with higher sensitivity in patients with higher node stages: 41% in pN1, 67% in pN2, and 100% in pN3. USG is 41.2% sensitivity and 93% specificity for detecting metastatic axilla."- Breast Imaging by Debra Ikeda 3/e p446

127. Ans. c. Routine clinical examination 3 monthly in 1st year with annual mammogram *(Ref: De Vita 10/e p1145 (ASCO 2006 Updated guidelines); Bailey 27/e p879, 26/e p816; MD Anderson Handbook of Surgical Oncology 5/e p71-72)*

Breast cancer follow-up should be done with history & physical examination Every 3 to 6 months for the first 3 years, every 6 to 12 months, 4 and 5 years, annually thereafter; Mammography annually, beginning no earlier than 6 months after radiation therapy. There is currently no routine role for repeated measurements of tumour markers or imaging other than mammography.

"Follow up of breast cancer: Patients with breast cancer used to be followed for life to detect recurrence and dissemination. This led to large clinics with little value for either patient or doctor. It is current practice to arrange yearly or two-yearly mammography of the treated and contralateral breast. There is a move to return the patient early to the care of the general practitioner with fast-track access back to the breast clinic if suspicious symptoms appear. There is currently no routine role for repeated measurements of tumour markers or imaging other than mammography."- Bailey 27/e p879, 26/e p816

Breast Cancer Follow-Up	
Recommended for Routine Surveillance	
History/physical examination	• Every 3 to 6 months for the first 3 years, every 6 to 12 months, 4 and 5 years, annually thereafter[Q]
Mammography	• Annually, beginning no earlier than 6 months after radiation therapy[Q]
Breast self-examination	• All women should be counseled to perform monthly[Q]
Pelvic examination	• Annually[Q]
Coordination of care	• Continuity of care with breast cancer specialist and appropriate other health care providers
Not Recommended for Routine Surveillance	
Routine blood test	• Complete blood count & LFT are not recommended[Q]
Imaging studies	• CXR, bone scans, liver USG, CT scans, FDG-PET scans & breast MRI are not recommended for routine breast cancer surveillance[Q]
Tumor markers	• Cancer antigen 15.3, 27.29 & CEA are not recommended[Q]

128. Ans. c. Adjuvant radiotherapy *(Ref: Sabiston 20/e p851-855; Schwartz 10/e p537; Bailey 26/e p810)*

In this case, patient is 45 years old (Score 2) with size 5 cm (Score 3), margin of 4 mm (Score 2), necrotic features without high grade (Score 2), the total score is 9. Usually for score 7-9, if local excision is done radiotherapy should be given. If simple mastectomy is done, there is no need of adjuvant treatment. In this patient next best step would be adjuvant radiotherapy.

Silverstein-Van Nuy's Prognostic Index for DCIS			
Parameters	**Score 1**	**Score 2**	**Score 3**
Size	≤1.5 cm	1.6 to 4 cm	> 4 cm
Margin	≥10 mm	1 to 9 mm	<1 mm
Class	Grade 1 or 2 without necrosis	Grade 1 or 2 with necrosis	Grade 3
Age	>60	40–60	<40

- Scores 4, 5, 6, 7 with >3 mm margin: **Excision alone**[Q]
- Scores 7 with < 3 mm margin, 8 with > 3 mm margin, 9 with >5 mm margin: **Excision + RT**[Q]
- Score 9 with < 5mm margin & score 10, 11, 12: **Mastectomy**[Q]

"Women with DCIS and evidence of extensive disease (>4 cm of disease or disease in more than one quadrant) usually require mastectomy. For women with limited disease, lumpectomy and radiation therapy are generally recommended. For non-palpable DCIS, needle localization or other image-guided techniques are used to guide the surgical resection. Specimen mammography is performed to ensure that all visible evidence of cancer is excised. Adjuvant tamoxifen therapy is considered for DCIS patients with ER-positive disease."- Schwartz 10/e p537

Ductal Carcinoma In Situ

- **DCIS** is **predominantly** seen in the **female breast** (accounts for **5% of male breast** cancers)
- DCIS carries a **high risk for progression** to an **invasive cancer**[Q].
- DCIS is **classified** on the basis of **nuclear grade & presence of necrosis**[Q]

Histological Types of DCIS	
Low Grade: Cribriform, Papillary & Micropapillary[Q]	**High Grade: Solid & Comedocarcinoma**[Q]

Pathology:
- **Proliferation of epithelium** that lines the minor ducts, resulting in **papillary growths within** the **duct lumina**.
  - Papillary growths (**papillary growth pattern**) eventually coalesce & fill the duct lumina so that only scattered, rounded spaces remain between the clumps of atypical cancer cells, which show **hyperchromasia & loss of polarity (cribriform growth pattern)**.
  - Eventually pleomorphic cancer cells with **frequent mitotic figures obliterate** the **lumina & distend** the **ducts (solid growth pattern)**.
  - With continued growth, these cells outstrip their blood supply & become **necrotic (comedo growth pattern)**.

Diagnosis:
- **Calcium deposition** occurs in the areas of necrosis and is a **common feature** seen on **mammography**[Q].
- DCIS most frequently **presents** as **mammographic calcifications**[Q].

- **Most sensitive investigation** for diagnosis of DCIS: **MRI**[Q] **> Mammography**[Q]

Treatment of DCIS	
Non-palpable DCIS	Section by **needle localization** technique with **specimen mammography** to ensure that all visible evidence of cancer is excised
Low grade DCIS (cribriform or papillary subtype <0.5 cm in diameter)	**Lumpectomy** alone if margins are widely free of disease
DCIS with limited disease	Lumpectomy + Radiotherapy[Q]
DCIS with extensive disease (>4 cm in diameter or disease in >1 quadrant)	Mastectomy[Q]

129. Ans. d. Lobectomy of the affected segment *(Ref: Harrison's 19/e p247; Sabiston 20/e p1598; Schwartz 10/e p662, 663)*

All of the given options are used for control of hemoptysis in the following order: Bronchoscopic laser cauterization → Bronchial artery embolization → Pulmonary artery embolization → Lobectomy of the affected segment.

> "Large-volume hemoptysis, referred to as massive hemoptysis, is variably defined as hemoptysis of >200–600 mL in 24 h. Massive hemoptysis should be considered a medical emergency."- *Harrison's 19/e p246*

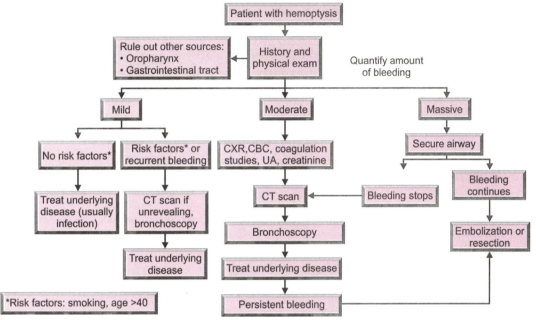

Fig. 29: Decision tree for evaluation of hemoptysis
(CBC, complete blood count; CT, computed tomography; CXR, chest X-ray; UA, urinalysis)

> "For the most part, the treatment of hemoptysis varies with its etiology. However, large-volume, life-threatening hemoptysis generally requires immediate intervention regardless of the cause. The first step is to establish a patent airway, usually by endotracheal intubation and subsequent mechanical ventilation. As large-volume hemoptysis usually arises from an airway lesion, it is ideal to **identify the site of bleeding by either chest imaging or bronchoscopy (more commonly rigid rather than flexible). The goals are then to isolate the bleeding to one lung and not to allow the preserved airspaces in the other lung to be filled with blood so that gas exchange is further impaired. Patients should be placed with the bleeding lung in a dependent position (i.e., bleeding-side down), and, if possible, dual lumen endotracheal tubes or an airway blocker should be placed in the proximal airway of the bleeding lung.** These interventions generally require the assistance of anesthesiologists, interventional pulmonologists, or thoracic surgeons." -*Harrison's 19/e p247*

> "If the bleeding does not stop with treatment of the underlying cause and the passage of time, severe hemoptysis from bronchial arteries can be treated with angiographic embolization of the responsible bronchial artery. This intervention should be entertained only in the most severe and life-threatening cases of hemoptysis because of the risk of unintentional spinal-artery embolization and consequent paraplegia. Endobronchial lesions can be treated with a variety of bronchoscopically directed interventions, including cauterization and laser therapy. In extreme circumstances, surgical resection of the affected region of the lung is considered. Most cases of hemoptysis resolve with treatment of the infection or inflammatory process or with removal of the offending stimulus."-*Harrison's 19/e p247*

130. Ans. b. 4 mL/kg × %TBSA *(Ref: Sabiston 20/e p514; Schwartz 10/e p230; Bailey 27/e p624, 26/e p392)*

According to Parkland's formula, total amount of fluid replenished in 24 hours will be 4 mL/kg × % TBSA.

> "Perhaps the simplest and most widely used formula is the Parkland formula. This calculates the fluid to be replaced in the first 24 hours by the following formula: total percentage body surface area × weight (kg) × 4 = volume (mL). Half this volume is given in the first 8 hours and the second half is given in the subsequent 16 hours."-*Bailey 27/e p624, 26/e p392*

AIIMS ESSENCE

Resuscitation Formulas			
Formula	Crystalloid Volume	Colloid Volume	Free water
Parkland[Q]	4 mL/kg per % TBSA burn	None	None
Brooke[Q]	1.5 mL/kg per % TBSA burn	0.5 mL/kg per % TBSA burn	2.0 L
Galveston[Q] (pediatric)	5000 mL/m² burned area + 1500 mL/m² total area	None	None

> **Half of fluid** is given in **first 8 hours** & other half in **next 16 hours**[Q]

Fluid Resuscitation

- **IV fluid resuscitation:** In **children** with burn **>10%**[Q] TBSA & **adult** with burn **>15%**[Q] TBSA
- **Regimen** of **fluid resuscitation follows** the **fluid loss**, which is at its **maximum in first 8 hours** & slows such that by 2-36 hours the patient can be maintained on her/his normal daily requirement.

> **Fluids used in Resuscitation**
> - **Ringer Lactate** is **most commonly used**[Q].
> - Some centers use **human albumin, FFP** or **hypertonic saline**[Q]

- If **oral resuscitation** is to be commenced, it is important that the **water given is not salt free. Hyponatremia** & **water intoxication can be fatal**[Q].
- In **children, maintenance fluid** must be given, usually **dextrose-saline.**[Q]
- **Simplest** & **most widely used formula: Parkland formula**[Q]

> - **Hypertonic saline** has been **effective in treating burn shock**[Q].
> - It produces **hyperosmolarity** & **hypernatremia.**
> - This reduces the shift of intracellular water to the extracellular space.
> - Advantage includes **less tissue edema** & a resultant **decrease in escharotomies** & **intubation**[Q].

- **Protein** should be given **after the first 12 hours** of burn.
- The commonest **colloid based formula** is **Muir & Barclay formula**[Q].

Monitoring of resuscitation:
- The key to monitoring is **urine output**[Q].

> - **Urine output** should be **0.5-1.0 ml/kg/hour**[Q] (i.e. 30-60 ml per hour[Q]).

Other measures for monitoring:
- Acid base balance & Hematocrit
- In **cardiac dysfunction:** Transesophageal USG & Central line[Q]

Venous Access for Infusion:
- **In adults:** Ideal sites are **veins in hand, antecubital fossa** or **neck.**
- **Saphenous vein cut down** is useful **in patient with difficult access** & is **used in preference to central venous cannulation.**
- **CVP line** is used for **CVP monitoring,** helps in **estimating fluid overload**[Q].

131. Ans. c. Pectoralis major myocutaneous flap *(Ref: Sabiston 20/e p1953; Schwartz 10/e p1873; Grabb and Smith Plastic Surgery 7/e p921)*

In the patient as shown in the question, chest wall closure has been achieved by using pectoralis major myocutaneous flap. Pectoralis major myocutaneous flap is one of the most commonly used flaps in chest wall reconstruction. Flaps frequently used for chest wall reconstruction include one or both the pectoralis major muscles, latissimus dorsi muscles, and rectus abdominis muscles, as well as the greater omentum.

"Reconstruction of the Chest Wall: The choice of muscle depends on the location of the defect; options include the latissimus dorsi, serratus anterior, and pectoralis major muscle flaps. Other muscle flaps with limited but specific uses are the trapezius and superiorly based rectus abdominis. The greater omentum can be transposed on the right gastroepiploic artery as a pedicle flap to provide well-vascularized tissue with the bulk and pliability to obliterate dead space, but it is a secondary choice because of the risks of intra-abdominal complications."-Sabiston 20/e p1953

"The pectoralis major muscle is the workhorse pedicled flap for coverage of the sternum, upper chest, and neck."-Schwartz 10/e p1873

Type of Flap	Uses
Pectoralis Major Myocutaneous (**PMMC**) flap	**Head & neck reconstruction**[Q]
	Sternal & chest wall reconstruction, especially **anterior & superior central chest**[Q]
Transverse Rectus Abdominis Muscle flap	**Breast reconstruction**[Q]
Vertical Rectus Abdominis Muscle (**VRAM**) flap	Used to cover **defects of sternum, chest wall, pelvis & perineal areas**[Q]
Latissimus dorsi flap	**Breast reconstruction**[Q]
	Chest wall reconstruction especially **lateral or anterolateral defects of upper 1/3rd of chest wall**[Q]
Serratus anterior flap	**Head & neck reconstruction**[Q]
	Non-sternal & lower chest wall defects[Q]

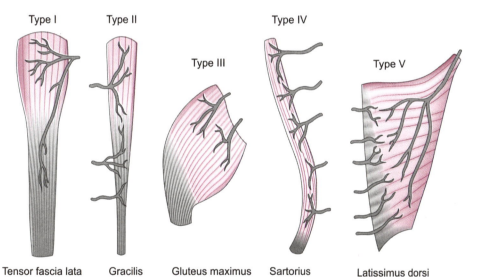

Fig. 30: Mathes & nahai classification of muscles flap

Mathes & Nahai Classification of Muscles Flap (According to vascular supply)		
Type	Description	Example
I	**Single dominant pedicle**[Q]	• Tensor fascia lata
II	**Single dominant** pedicle with **minor pedicles**[Q]	• Gracilis • Trapezius
III	**Two dominant** pedicles[Q]	• Gluteus maximum • Rectus abdominis • Serratus anterior
IV	**Multiple segmental pedicles** without a single dominant pedicle[Q]	• Sartorius • External Oblique
V	**Single dominant pedicle** with **secondary segmental pedicles**[Q]	• Pectoralis major • Latissimus dorsi • Internal oblique

132. Ans. a. Paraffin gauze and dressing *(Ref: Kirk General Surgical Operations 6/e p548; Bailey 27/e p624-626, 26/e p392-394)*
Paraffin gauze and dressing is the best management for this patient having superficial burns caused by hot water.

Paraffin gauze and dressing	• Collagenase is the **most commonly employed enzymatic debriding agent** currently commercially available in the United States. • It is **slow acting, requiring several days to one week to adequately debride** or heal intermediate-depth partial thickness wounds.
Collagen dressing	• **Sterile liquid paraffin reduces crusting.** • **Superficial burns** are **covered by paraffin dressing gauze** followed by **bulky absorptive dressing to leave it unchanged for 1 week or it get soaked.** Subsequently twice per week until the wound is healed.
Excision and grafting	• **Excision & skin grafting** is the **last resort of burns management for large area burns** and in **late stages in cases of contractures.** • **Tangential shaving (excision) of the dead tissue** is done **until we observe punctuate bleeding in deep burns before grafting,** not superficial burns.
1% silver sulfasalazine ointment	• **Silver sulfadiazine (1%)** is **most commonly used burn wound dressing** applied once or twice daily and can be soothing. SSD • **Silver sulfadiazine** and related agents should **not be used in women who are pregnant** or **breastfeeding** or **in infants <2 months old.**

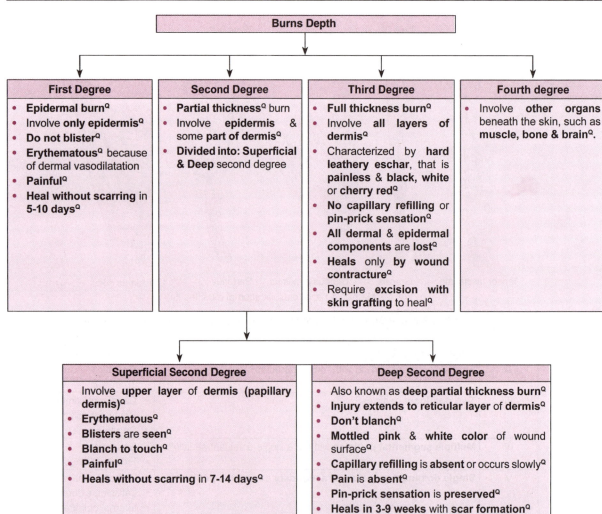

Management of Burns	
Superficial Burns	• **Clean** the burn wound & **remove the roof** of all blisters[Q] • **Expose superficial burns of face** but apply sterile liquid paraffin to reduce crusting. • For **burns of perineum**, **clean & expose** but apply **silver sulfadiazine cream**. Nurse the patient **without dressings** on a sterile sheet on air or water-bed. • **Cover superficial burns** of other areas with **two layers of paraffin gauze** & a **bulky absorptive dressing**[Q]. Leave this dressing for 1 week unless it becomes soaked, whereupon you should change it. Change the dressing at 1 week and subsequently twice per week until the wound is healed.
Deep Dermal Burns	• **Tangentially shave** with a graft knife **between 2nd & 5th day**[Q]. • Continue to shave until you observe punctuate bleeding from the surface. • Achieve hemostasis and apply a split skin graft. Re-dress at 4 days. • When fully healed, apply a pressure garment for 6 months or longer if necessary to minimize hypertrophy & contracture of the resulting scars. • **Treat areas that are not healed at 3 weeks as full thickness burns**
Full Thickness Burns	**Escharotomy**: • Note the **areas of full thickness burns** that are **circumferential around digit limb** or **trunk**. If the **viability** of the distal pan is **jeopardized**, or if **respiration is hindered**, as with partial circumferential burns of the chest wall, **carry out an escharotomy**[Q]. • Give IV dose of diazepam. **Incise along the full length of full thickness burn**[Q]. • Repeat the longitudinal escharotomy at different sites of the circumference until satisfactory perfusion of the distal part. • Dress the wounds with paraffin gauze or silver sulfadiazine **Grafting**: • **Identify site of grafting not >20% BSA. Identify donor site of skin graft**[Q] • **Excise the chosen area of full-thickness burn till bed consists of viable tissue**[Q]. • Harvest a split skin graft and mesh it to expand. • Apply the mesh graft to the burn wound site and dress with several layers of paraffin gauze and an absorbent dressing. Re-dress after 4 days. • Do not excise further burn until the donor site has healed and is ready for re-harvesting, or another donor site is available

133. **Ans. d. All patients should have chest X-ray-PA view only** *(Ref: ATLS Guidelines 9/e p6-9, 13; Sabiston 20/e p413-417; Schwartz 10/e p161, 173)*

In primary survey, cervical X-ray is not mandatory as imaging of the cervical spine can be done later after complete evaluation of spinal cord injuries. Patients with blunt trauma are always sent for plain radiographs of chest and pelvis with anteroposterior (AP) views, as the patient will be in supine position and not the PA views. CT scan is avoided in hemodynamically unstable patients.

"Transport of a hypotensive patient out of the emergency department for computed tomographic (CT) scanning is hazardous; monitoring is compromised, and the environment is suboptimal for dealing with acute problems. The surgeon must accompany the patient and be prepared to abort the CT scan with diversion to the operating room." - Schwartz 10/e p173

Advanced Trauma Life Support (ATLS) Guidelines
• All trauma patients are managed based on **Advanced Trauma Life Support** guidelines. • **Steps: Triage → Primary survey → Emergency resuscitation → Adjuncts to primary survey → Secondary survey → Adjuncts to secondary survey**[Q] • **Primary Survey includes: Airway & cervical spine stabilization → Breathing & ventilation → Circulation & blood loss control → Disability & neurologic evaluation → Exposure/Environment**[Q] • **Massive transfusion protocol:** Resuscitation of the patients with **packed red blood cells, fresh-frozen plasma (FFP) & platelets in 1:1:1 ratio** has **favorable outcomes**[Q].

Contd...

Contd...

Advanced Trauma Life Support (ATLS) Guidelines

- **Imaging of cervical spine can be done later after complete evaluation of spinal cord injuries.**
- Patients with blunt trauma are always sent for **plain radiographs of chest & pelvis with anteroposterior (AP) views,** as the patient will be in supine position and **not the PA views.**

- **CT scan is avoided in hemodynamically unstable patients.** Further contrast induced organ damages also potentiates owing to low circulatory volume.

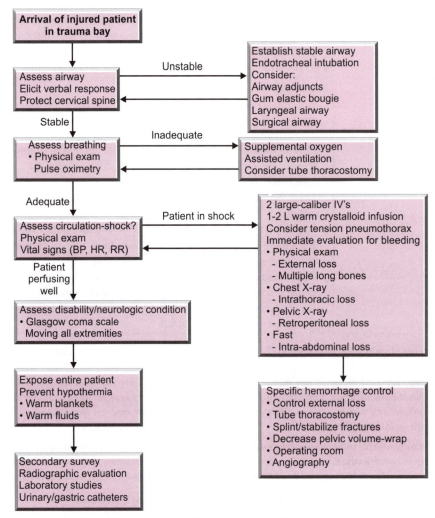

Fig. 31: Algorithm for the initial assessment of the injured patient

134. Ans. b. The patient should not be shifted and portable X-ray machine should be used after neck stabilization

(Ref: Sabiston 20/e p421; Schwartz 10/e p161; ATLS Manual 9/e p6, 182)

In a trauma patient, cervical stabilization is the first step in management along with airway. Hence any imaging should be done after hard neck collar support and long spine board. In fact, a cross table lateral cervical spine X-ray is considered, in the same trolley itself without shifting the patient. A surgeon should accompany the patient if needed, so that patient can be transferred immediately to OT if any hemodynamic instability occurs.

"Simultaneously, all patients with blunt trauma require cervical spine immobilization until injury is excluded. This is typically accomplished by applying a hard collar or placing sandbags on both sides of the head with the patient's forehead taped across the bags to the backboard. Soft collars do not effectively immobilize the cervical spine. For penetrating neck wounds, however, cervical collars are not believed useful because they provide no benefit, but may interfere with assessment and treatment."-Schwartz 10/e p161

Management of Cervical Spine Injury in a Trauma Patient

- The **spine should always be immobilized** assuming a spine injury until proven otherwise
- Blunt & penetrating trauma result in different forms of spinal cord injury.
- **Blunt trauma** causes **cord injury through direct impingement** or **indirect compression due to vertebral fracture or dislocation.**
- **Penetrating trauma** causes **direct cord laceration** or indirectly through **ischemia or fracture**.

> - **Spine immobilization should be done** and after immobilization X-ray attempted with a portable machine[Q]
> - X-rays in the acute trauma are **usually taken with the help of portable X-ray machine**, which includes **AP views of cervical, chest & pelvis**, as unnecessary mobilization & shifting of the patient might aggravate injury even with immobilization by cervical collar[Q].

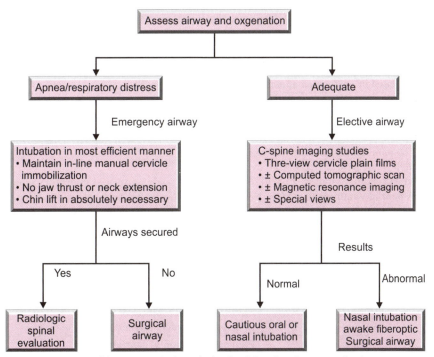

Fig. 32: Management of cervical spine injury in a trauma patient

135. **Ans. c. 9** *(Ref: Harrison 19/e p1730; Sabiston 20/e p411; Schwartz 10/e p1712; Bailey 27/e p331, 26/e p312)*
Here, E = 2 (eyes opening to pain); V = 2 (moans or Incomprehensible sounds) ; M = 5 (Movement of one limb toward pain, Extended posture doesn't imply M2 in presence of pain localization). Hence, GCS = E2V2M5 = 9.

136. **Ans. c. McBurney's point tenderness** *(Ref: Sabiston 20/e p1299; Schwartz 10/e p1244; Bailey 27/e p1303, 26/e p1202-1203)*
The given clinical picture is suggestive of acute appendicitis. In the image, resident is eliciting McBurney's point tenderness in the patient of acute appendicitis.

"Gentle superficial palpation of the abdomen, beginning in the left iliac fossa moving anticlockwise to the right iliac fossa will detect muscle guarding over the point of maximum tenderness, classically McBurney's point."- Bailey 27/e p1303, 26/e p1203

"Patients with appendicitis usually move slowly and prefer to lie supine due to the peritoneal irritation. On abdominal palpation, there is tenderness with a maximum at or near McBurney's point."- Schwartz 10/e p1244

"Abdominal examination typically reveals a quiet abdomen with tenderness and guarding on palpation of the right lower quadrant. The location of the tenderness is classically over McBurney point, which is located one-third the distance between the anterior superior iliac spine and the umbilicus."-Sabiston 20/e p1299

"Ballance's sign: A fixed area of percussible dullness in the left upper quadrant due to coagulation of blood from the injured spleen[Q]."

Acute Appendicitis
• **Acute appendicitis** is the **MC general surgical emergency[Q]**   • Worldwide, **perforated appendicitis** is the **leading general surgical cause** of **death[Q].**
Pathophysiology: • **Obstruction of the lumen[Q]** is believed to be the **major cause** of **acute appendicitis[Q].**   • **Obstruction of the lumen** may be **caused by inspissated stool** (fecalith[Q] or appendicolith[Q]), **lymphoid hyperplasia[Q], vegetable matter** or **seeds[Q], parasites**, or a **neoplasm[Q].**   • Obstruction of the appendiceal lumen contributes to **bacterial overgrowth** and **continued secretion of mucus** leads **to intraluminal distention** and **increased wall pressure.** Luminal distention produces the **visceral pain** sensation experienced by the patient as **periumbilical pain[Q].**   • **Subsequent impairment of lymphatic** and **venous drainage** leads to **mucosal ischemia.**
Bacteriology: • **MC bacteria isolated** in **perforated appendicitis: Bacteroides fragilis[Q]** (80%) >**E. coli[Q]** (77%).

Clinical Features:
 • **Diagnosis** can be **made primarily** on the basis of the **history & physical examination** in **most cases[Q].**
 • **Typical presentation**: Periumbilical pain followed by **anorexia** and **nausea.**
 	
    • The **pain** then **localizes to** the **right lower quadrant** as the inflammatory process progresses to involve the parietal peritoneum overlying the appendix.
    • **Most reliable symptom** of **acute appendicitis: Classic pattern of migratory pain**
    • A **bout of vomiting** may occur. **Fever ensues, followed by** the development of **leukocytosis.**
    • **Occasional patients** have **urinary symptoms** or **microscopic hematuria**
 	
 • **Tenderness** is **directly over** the **appendix**, at **McBurney's point[Q].**
 • **Rectal** and **pelvic examinations** are **most likely** to be **negative** (Tenderness on P/R examination in **pelvic appendix**)[Q]

Dunphy's sign[Q]	Pain on coughing[Q]
Rovsing's sign[Q]	**Pain** in the **right lower quadrant** during **palpation of** the **left lower quadrant[Q]**
Obturator sign[Q]	**Pain** on **internal rotation of** the **hip[Q]** Suggestive of **pelvic appendix[Q]**
Iliopsoas sign[Q]	**Pain on extension** of the **right hip[Q]** Suggestive of **retrocecal appendix[Q]**

Diagnosis:

Laboratory Studies
• **WBC count** is **elevated**, with **more than 75% neutrophils** in **most patients[Q].**   • **Normal WBC count** and **differential** is found in **10%** of **patients** with acute appendicitis[Q].   • **High WBC count (>20,000/mL)** suggests **complicated appendicitis with gangrene** or **perforation[Q].**   • **Microscopic hematuria** is **common in appendicitis** (**gross hematuria** may **indicate** the presence of a **kidney stone**)[Q]

Acute Appendicitis

Ultrasound:
- USG has a **sensitivity of 85%** and a **specificity > 90%** for the diagnosis of acute appendicitis in patients of abdominal pain.
- **Characteristic findings**: Appendix ≥ 7 mm diameter, a **thick-walled**, **non-compressible luminal structure** seen in cross section (**target lesion**), or the **presence of an appendicolith[Q]**.
- Commonly used in **children & pregnant patients[Q]** with equivocal clinical findings suggestive of acute appendicitis.

Plain X-ray:
- A **calcified appendicolith** is **visible** in only **10-15%** of patients with acute appendicitis.
- **Failure of the appendix to fill during** a **barium enema** has been **associated with appendicitis[Q]** (this finding lacks sensitivity and specificity because up to 20% of normal appendices do not fill).

CT Scan

- **CT scan**: **Sensitivity** of **90%** and a **specificity** of **80-90%** for the diagnosis of **acute appendicitis** in patients with abdominal pain[Q].
- **Classic findings** on CT: **Distended appendix >7 mm** in diameter and **circumferential wall thickening** and **enhancement** (appearance of a **halo** or **target**)[Q]
- **CT detects appendicoliths** in **50%** of patients with appendicitis.
- **Most valuable for older patients** and in patients with atypical symptoms

Treatment:
- Most patients are managed by prompt **appendectomy[Q]**.

137. **Ans. c. Pigtail insertion and drainage** *(Ref: Sabiston 20/e p1503; Schwartz 10/e p; Bailey 27/e p1204, 26/e p1112; Blumgart 5/e p615-644; Shackelford 7/ e p1380-1388)*

This patient is most likely having a biliary leak from the cystic duct stump, which has formed a large 5 × 5 cm collection. Such a patient needs to be managed with intravenous antibiotics as well as drainage of the collections (as it acts as source of infection). Ultrasound guided pigtail insertion is the easiest method to obtain adequate drainage of the bile leak.

"In the delayed presentation of a bile duct injury, three major goals guide therapy. First, control of infection with drainage of any fluid collections will minimize the inflammatory process. Inflammation in the porta hepatis leads to fibrosis, which acts only to increase stricture formation. Broad-spectrum antibiotics, decompression of the biliary tree, and drainage, whether per- cutaneous or operative, of any fluid collections will achieve this goal. With control of sepsis, there is no urgency for biliary reconstruction." -Sabiston 20/e p1503

Goals of Therapy in Iatrogenic Bile Duct Injury

1. **Control of infection limiting inflammation:**
   - Parenteral antibiotics[Q]
   - **Percutaneous drainage** of periportal fluid collection[Q]
2. **Clear and thorough delineation of entire biliary anatomy:**
   - MRCP/PTC[Q]
   - ERCP (especially if cystic duct stump leak suspected)[Q]
3. **Re-establishment of biliary enteric continuity:**
   - Tension-free, mucosa-to-mucosa anastomosis[Q]
   - Roux-en-Y hepaticojejunostomy[Q]
   - Long-term transanstomotic stents if involving bifurcation or higher[Q]

Bile Duct Injury and Ligation

- **Most benign strictures** follow **iatrogenic bile duct injury[Q]**
- **Most commonly** during **laparoscopic cholecystectomy[Q]**
- **Incidence** of bile duct injury during **open** cholecystectomy is **0.1-0.2%[Q]**
- **Incidence** of bile duct injury during **laparoscopic** cholecystectomy is **0.3-0.85%[Q]**

Bile Duct Injury and Ligation

Pathogenesis:

Risk Factors for Bile Duct Injury	
• **Acute** or **chronic inflammation**[Q]	• **Anatomic variation**[Q]
• **Obesity**[Q]	• **Bleeding**[Q]

- **Bile duct injury** rate increased in **acute cholecystitis, pancreatitis, cholangitis,** and **obstructive jaundice**[Q].

  - As **surgeon experience** increases **beyond 20 cases**, the bile duct **injury rate decreases**[Q].
  - **Errors** leading to laparoscopic bile duct injuries stem from '**misperception**'[Q], not errors of skill, knowledge or judgment.
  - The **primary cause of error** in **97% cases** was a '**visual perceptual illusion**'[Q], whereas only **3% injuries** were due to **faults of technical skills**[Q].

- Surgical technique with **inadequate exposure** and **failure to identify** structures **before ligating** or **dividing** them are the most common cause of **significant biliary injury**[Q].
- The **routine** use of **intra-operative cholangiography** may **limit the extent** of **bile duct injury**, but does **not** seem to **prevent it**[Q].
- If a **bile duct injury** is **suspected** during cholecystectomy, a **cholangiogram must be obtained** to identify the anatomy[Q].
- **Classic Laparoscopic Injury:** A long length of **common duct** is excised up to the **proximal common hepatic duct**, which is either occluded or left to drain bile into the peritoneal cavity.

Clinical Features:

- About **25%** of **major ductal injuries** are **recognized intraoperatively**[Q] because of bile leakage, an abnormal cholangiogram, or late recognition of the anatomy.
- **MC presentation** of a **complete occlusion** of the common hepatic or bile duct is **jaundice** with or without **abdominal pain**[Q].
- Patients may also present **months or years after** prior surgery with **cholangitis** or **cirrhosis** secondary to a biliary tract injury.

Diagnosis:

- **USG** or **CT** should be performed in patients with signs of **abdominal pain** or **peritonitis, sepsis,** or any other clinical suspicion of **biloma**[Q].
- Patients must be stabilized with **immediate parenteral antibiotics** and **image-guided percutaneous drainage** of any fluid collections[Q].
- **Cholangiography** should be performed to establish the **presence of ductal stricture**, identify the **level** of the stricture, and identify the **nature of the injury** when necessary[Q].
- **PTC** is the **imaging method of choice** for **most postoperative biliary strictures**[Q]

  - **ERCP** may be easier to obtain in a patient with a biliary stricture and cholangitis who **requires urgent cholangiography** and **biliary decompression**.
  - However, this is **only useful** in patients **with bile duct continuity**.
  - **Cystic duct leaks** or **small tangential injuries** can be treated with **endoscopic stenting**.
  - In situations in which the **biliary stricture** is **too tight** to pass with ERCP, **PTC** may be performed for proximal biliary decompression.

- **CT arteriography** should be considered in the **preoperative evaluation** of patients with benign biliary strictures.
- **Unrecognized injury** to the **hepatic artery** or a **portal vein branch** occurs with a frequency of **12-47%** concomitant with a bile duct injury.
- In patients presenting with **late strictures** with evidence of **liver dysfunction**, a **CT arteriogram** should be performed to evaluate for **evidence of portal hypertensio**n.

---

138. **Ans. d. Relaxed tension lines in skin**   *(Ref: Grabb and Smith's Plastic Surgery 7/e p1-3; Gray's 41/e p157)*

Kraissl's lines are relaxed tension lines in skin)

*"**Kraissl's lines** are essentially **exaggerated wrinkle lines** obtained by studying the loose skin of elderly faces whilst contracting the muscles of facial expression. These lines for the most part correspond to **Relaxed skin tension lines (RSTLs)**, but slight variation exists on the face, especially on the lateral side of the nose, the lateral aspect of the orbit, and the chin." - Gray's 41/e p157*

"Blaschko's lines refer to the way in which patterns of naevi and related dermatological pathologies are distributed or develop along certain preferred cutaneous pathways. They do not appear to correspond to vascular or neural elements of the skin, and may be related to earlier developmental boundaries of a 'mosaic' nature." - Gray's 41/e p157

Line Systems in Plastic Surgery

Line	Description
Langer's Line	• **Langer's lines (cleavage lines)** are **topological lines drawn**[Q] on a map of the human body. • Orientation of these lines corresponds to natural orientation of **collagen fibers** in the dermis & generally **parallel to the orientation of underlying muscle fibers**[Q]. • **Wounds against Langer lines** generally have **poor cosmetic outcome**[Q]. • **Represent skin tension in rigor mortis**[Q] • Do not relate to the lines of choice in making elective incisions; **often run at right angles to the relaxed skin tension lines** in the face[Q].
Kraissl's Lines	• **Kraissl's lines** are **essentially exaggerated wrinkle lines**[Q] obtained by studying the loose skin of elderly faces whilst contracting the muscles of facial expression. • **Correspond to relaxed skin tension lines** with **slight variation on face**, especially on the lateral side of the nose, lateral aspect of orbit & chin[Q]. • Kraissl's lines **coincide with wrinkle lines** (not always) & tend to be **perpendicular to the muscle action**[Q].
Borge's Relaxed Skin Tension Lines	• Tension is present in all directions in the skin but mainly in one direction, which follows the relaxed skin tension lines first described by Borges. • **Relaxed skin tension lines** (RSTLs) **correspond to the directional pull** (which forms furrows) when the skin is relaxed: they **do not always correspond to wrinkle lines**[Q]. The • **Tension across the RSTL is constant** even during sleep but **can be altered** (increased, decreased or abolished) **by underlying muscle contraction**[Q]. • Direction of the RSTLs can be determined by pinching the skin in different directions.

139. Ans. a. Crohn's disease   *(Ref: Robbins 9/e p798-799; Sabiston 20/e p1258; Bailey 27/e p1242, 26/e p1153)*
History of recurrent bloody diarrhea with multiple geographic ulcers and histopathological findings showing transmural inflammation is highly suggestive of Crohn's disease.

"The microscopic features of active Crohn disease include abundant neutrophils that infiltrate and damage crypt epithelium. Clusters of neutrophils within a crypt are referred to as crypt abscesses and are often associated with crypt destruction. Ulceration is common in Crohn disease, and there may be an abrupt transition between ulcerated and adjacent normal mucosa. Even in areas where gross examination suggests diffuse disease, microscopic pathology can appear patchy. Repeated cycles of crypt destruction and regeneration lead to distortion of mucosal architecture; the normally straight and parallel crypts take on bizarre branching shapes and unusual orientations to one another. Epithelial metaplasia, another consequence of chronic relapsing injury, often takes the form of gastric antral-appearing glands, and is called pseudopyloric metaplasia. Noncaseating granulomas, a hallmark of Crohn disease, are found in approximately 35% of cases and may occur in areas of active disease or uninvolved regions in any layer of the intestinal wall."

-Robbins 9/e p799

Feature	Crohn's Disease	Ulcerative Colitis
A. Macroscopic features		
1. Distribution	Segmental with **skip areas**[Q]	**Continuous** without skip areas[Q]
2. Location	Commonly **terminal ileum** and/or **ascending colon**	Commonly **rectum,** sigmoid colon and extending upwards
3. Extent	Usually involves the **entire thickness** of the affected segment of bowel wall	Usually **superficial,** confined to mucosal layers
4. Ulcers	**Serpiginous ulcers**, that may develop into deep **Fissures**[Q]	**Superficial mucosal ulcers** without fissures
5. **Pseudopolyps**	Rarely seen	**Commonly present**[Q]
6. **Fibrosis**	**Common**	Rare
7. Shortening	Due to fibrosis	Due to contraction of muscularis

Contd...

Contd...

B. Microscopic features

1. Depth of inflammation	Typically **transmural**[Q]	**Mucosal**[Q] **& Submucosal**
2. Type of inflammation	**Non-caseating granulomas**[Q] and infiltrate of mononuclear cells (lymphocytes, plasma cells and macrophage)	**Crypt abscess** and non-specific acute & chronic inflammatory cells (lymphocytes, plasma cells neutrophils, eosinophils, mast cells)
3. Mucosa	Patchy ulceration	Hemorrhagic mucosa with ulceration
4. Submucosa	Widened due to edema and lymphoid aggregates	Normal or reduced in width
5. Muscularis	Infiltrated by inflammatory cells	Usually spared, except in cases of **Toxic Megacolon**[Q]
6. Fibrosis	Present	Usually absent

C. Complications

1. Fistula formation	**Internal** & external fistulae in 10% case	Extremely **rare**[Q]
2. Malignant changes	Less common but present	May occur in disease of more than 10 years duration (**more common**[Q])
3. Fibrous strictures	**Common**[Q]	Never[Q]
4. Toxic megacolon	-	**Risk present**[Q]
5. Named Features	• **Hose pipe** appearance[Q] • **Cobble-stone** appearance[Q] • **Halo sign** on CT[Q] • **String sign of Kantor**[Q] • **Raspberry/rosethorn appearance**[Q]	• **Garden hose** appearance[Q] • **Pseudopolyps**[Q] • **Pipestem colon (Ahaustral)**[Q]

Remember:
- **Earliest change** in **Crohn's disease**: **Apthoid ulceration**[Q].
- **Earliest Change** in **Ulcerative colitis**: **Blurring of mucosal stripe & granular appearance**[Q].
- **Surgery** is **palliative** in **Crohn's disease**[Q] whereas **curative in ulcerative colitis**[Q].

Crohn's Disease

- **Chronic, transmural inflammatory disease** of the GIT for which the **cause is unknown**[Q].
- Can **involve any part of the alimentary tract** from the **mouth to the anus** but most commonly affects the **small intestine & colon**[Q].

  - Involvement of **both large & small intestine: 55%**[Q]
  - Involvement of **only small intestine: 30%**[Q]
  - Involvement of **only large intestine: 15%**[Q]

- Crohn's disease primarily **attacks young adults**[Q] in the **2nd & 3rd decades** of life.
- **More common** in smokers & urban dwellers[Q]
- **Two genders** are **affected equally** with **strong familial association**[Q]

  - **Upper GI Crohn's disease** is most frequently found in the **gastric antrum & duodenum**[Q].
  - In patients with **colonic disease, rectal sparing** is **characteristic**[Q].

Etiology: Unknown
- **Infectious agents** proposed as **potential causes: Mycobacterium paratuberculosis** & **measles virus**[Q].
- The identification in 2001 of the **CARD-15/NOD2 mutation**[Q] (on chromosome **16q,** also known as **IBD-1 locus**) provided the first definitive genetic link to the condition & is **relatively specific** for Crohn's disease.

IBD-1 (chromosome 16q)	Relatively specific for **Crohn's disease**[Q]
IBD-2 (chromosome 12q)	More common in **Ulcerative colitis**[Q]

Contd...

Contd...

Crohn's Disease

Pathology:
- **Diseased bowel** separated by areas of **grossly appearing normal bowel (skip areas)**[Q]
- **Extensive fat wrapping** caused by the **circumferential growth** of the **mesenteric fat**[Q] around the bowel wall.
- **Thickened, firm, rubbery**, and almost **incompressible bowel wall**[Q].
- **Involved segments** are **adherent to adjacent intestinal loops** or other viscera, with **internal fistulas**[Q].
- **Mesentery** of the involved segment is **thickened,** with **enlarged lymph nodes**[Q].

> - **Earliest gross pathologic lesion** is a **superficial aphthous ulcer**[Q] noted in the mucosa.

- **Linear ulcers** may coalesce to produce **transverse sinuses** with **islands of normal mucosa** in between (**cobblestone appearance**[Q])
- **Inflammatory reaction** is **characterized by extensive edema, hyperemia**[Q] **lymphangiectasia**, an intense infiltration of mononuclear cells, and **lymphoid hyperplasia**[Q].

> - **Characteristic histologic lesions** of Crohn's disease are **noncaseating granulomas** with **Langerhans' giant cells**[Q].
> - **Granulomas** appear later in the course and are found in the **wall of the bowel** or in **regional lymph nodes**[Q] in 60-70% of patients

Clinical Features:
- **MC symptom** is **intermittent & colicky abdominal pain**, most commonly noted in the **lower abdomen**[Q].
- **Diarrhea** is the next most frequent symptom and is present, at **least intermittently**, in about 85% of patients.
- In contrast to ulcerative colitis, patients with Crohn's disease **typically have fewer bowel movements,** and the **stools rarely contain mucus, pus, or blood**[Q].

> - **Main intestinal complications** of Crohn's disease include **obstruction** and **perforation**[Q].
> - **Fistulas occur between** the **sites of perforation** and **adjacent organs**, usually **at the site of a previous laparotomy**[Q].

- **Long-standing Crohn's disease** predisposes to **cancer of the small intestine** and **colon**[Q].
- **Perianal disease (fissure, fistula, stricture, or abscess**[Q]) is common

> - In **Crohn's disease**, **ileum** is the **MC site** of **fistula (enterocutaneous & enterovesical)**, MC site of **perforation** & MC site of **carcinoma**[Q].

Diagnosis:
- **Enteroclysis: IOC** for **diagnosis** of **Crohn's** disease[Q]

> - **Earliest radiographic findings** in **enteroclysis** are **aphthous ulceration**, a coarse villous pattern of the mucosa, and thickened folds
> - **Ulcerations** on the **mesenteric aspect** with **sacculation** on the **antimesenteric surface**)

- **Serology:** Anti-Saccharomyces cerevisiae (**ASCA**[Q]) autoantibodies have **specificity of 92%** for **Crohn's disease**.

140. **Ans. c. Peutz-Jegher's syndrome** *(Ref: Robbins 9/e p894; Sabiston 20/e p1542)*
Maximum risk of carcinoma pancreas is seen in Peutz-Jegher's syndrome.

> *"The risk of pancreatic cancer in the setting of Peutz-Jeghers syndrome is more than 100 times greater than that in unaffected individuals."-Sabiston 20/e p1542*

Inherited Predisposition to Pancreatic Cancer		
Disorder	**Gene**	**Increased Risk of Pancreatic Cancer (Fold)**
Peutz-Jeghers syndrome	*STK11/LKB1* (19p13)[Q]	130[Q]
Hereditary pancreatitis	*PRSS1*[Q] (7q35) (Cationic trypsinogen gene)	50–80
Familial atypical multiple mole melanoma syndrome (FAMMM)	*p16(CDKN2A)* (9p21)[Q]	20–35
HNPCC (Lynch II variant)	*hMSH2* (2p22), *hMLH1* (3p21)[Q]	8-10
Hereditary breast and ovarian cancer	*BRCA2* (13q12-q13)[Q]	4–10
Familial adenomatous polyposis	APC[Q]	4[Q]

Peutz-Jegher's Syndrome (AD)

- **Hamartomatous** polyps (usually <100) throughout the GIT, **most common** in **jejunum**[Q]
- Associated with **hypermelanotic macule** in the **perioral region**, **buccal mucosa**[Q].
- **Mucocutaneous pigmentation** occurs **during infancy** & most commonly noted in **perioral** & **buccal** region.

  - Pigment spots usually appear in **first few years** of life, reach a **maximum level** in **early adolescence** and **can fade** in **adulthood**[Q].
  - Pigmentation on **buccal mucosa remains throughout** the **life**[Q].
  - Pigmented macules of PJS have **no malignant potential**[Q].

- **Polyposis** develops by **age 20**, occur most commonly in the jejunum (**jejunum**[Q] >colon >stomach).

Histology:
- Smooth muscle extends into superficial epithelial layer in a tree like manner known as **arborization**[Q].
- **Pseudoinvasion (epithelial cell trapping)**[Q] is noted in up to 10% of polyps >3 cm.

Genetics:
- **Autosomal dominant**; Chromosome **19p13.3** encodes the serine threonine kinase **LKB1/STK11**[Q].

Extra-intestinal Features:
- **Increased risk** for **extra-intestinal cancer** of **pancreas (maximum risk**[Q] among rest of inherited factors**), thyroid, breast** (may be bilateral), lung, gall bladder, biliary tract (**cholangiocarcinoma**)[Q].
- Increased risk of **gynecologic malignancies** of **ovary** (bilateral **sex cord tumors** with annular features) & **uterus (well-differentiated adenocarcinoma** of cervix, known as **adenoma malignum**)[Q]
- In men there is increased risk of **feminizing Sertoli cell tumors** of **testis**.

Treatment:
- **As malignant change rarely occurs, resection is only necessary for serious bleeding or intussusception.**
- Large single polyps can be removed by enterotomy, or short lengths of heavily involved intestine can be resected.

141. **Ans. c. Barrett's esophagus** *(Ref: Robbins 9/e p757, 758)*

The histopathological image of esophagus is showing intestinal type epithelium with goblet cells, typical of Barrett's esophagus.

"Esophageal adenocarcinoma usually occurs in the distal third of the esophagus and may invade the adjacent gastric cardia. Initially appearing as flat or raised patches in otherwise intact mucosa, large masses of 5 cm or more in diameter may develop. Alternatively, tumors may infiltrate diffusely or ulcerate and invade deeply. Microscopically, Barrett esophagus is frequently present adjacent to the tumor. Tumors most commonly produce mucin and form glands, often with intestinal-type morphology; less frequently tumors are composed of diffusely infiltrative signet-ring cells (similar to those seen in diffuse gastric cancers) or, in rare cases, small poorly differentiated cells (similar to small-cell carcinoma of the lung)."- Robbins 9/e p758

Barrett's Esophagus

- **Distal squamous mucosa** is **replaced by metaplastic specialized (intestinalized columnar) epithelium**, e.g. **goblet cells**, as a response to **chronic injury**; may regress after treatment[Q]
- Also called **columnar lined esophagus**[Q]
- **Metaplasia** of esophageal **squamous epithelium into columnar** in **distal**[Q] esophagus
- **MC type** of columnar epithelium is **intestinal epithelium (Intestinal metaplasia**[Q])

Etiology:
- Usually due to **chronic GERD**[Q]
- **Columnar epithelium of Barrett's** may be **more resistant to acid, pepsin & bile**[Q]
- Often associated with **sliding hiatal hernia**[Q]

Clinical Features:
- Higher incidence in **whites, males & obese**
- **Symptoms: long history of heartburn** & other reflux symptoms; more massive reflux with more numerous and longer episodes than most reflux patients
- Major risk factor for **esophageal adenocarcinoma**[Q]

Barrett's Esophagus

Diagnosis:
- Characteristic **endoscopic appearance plus characteristic histologic findings**[Q]
- **8 random biopsies recommended**
- Report should include type of epithelium present and **presence/absence of dysplasia, grade of dysplasia,** & **extent of dysplasia**[Q]
    - **Barrett's esophagus** requires **both endoscopically visible segment of columnar lining** of distal esophagus and **intestinal metaplasia** showing **goblet cells on biopsy**[Q]

Endoscopy:
- **Red velvety GI type mucosa** between **pale squamous mucosa** of lower esophagus & **lush pink gastric mucosa**[Q]
- May have **tongues extending up from GE junction or a broad band displacing GE junction proximally**

Positive Stains:
- **Goblet cells contain acid mucin, usually sialomucin**[Q] (Alcian blue+ at pH 2.5, although stain generally not needed or recommended), **columnar cells contain neutral mucins (PAS+); intestinal metaplastic cells are often CK7+/CK20-;** also **CDX2+.**
- **Guanylyl cyclase C+, Hep+**
- In routine practice, **only H&E is used for diagnosis**

Treatment:
- **Anti-reflux therapy**[Q]
- **Endoscopy every 1-2 years to detect dysplasia or early adenocarcinoma** with **4 quadrant biopsies using jumbo forceps at intervals of 2 cm** or less throughout the length of the Barrett's segment **plus any suspicious lesions**[Q]

142. Ans. c. Chest tube insertion and drainage *(Ref: Bailey 26/e p304, 25/e p341; Sabiston 20/e p230-231; Schwartz 10/e p164; Harrison 19/e p1719)*

This case is a classical description of post RTA traumatic pneumothorax of left hemithorax, with decreased breath sounds and trachea shifted to the right. Presence of heart sounds indicates absence of cardiac tamponade. Tension pneumothorax is ruled out, as the patient is not having hypotension (BP-120/80 mm Hg). So the first line management is chest tube insertion and drainage

"Traumatic pneumothoraxes can result from both penetrating and non-penetrating chest trauma. Traumatic pneumothoraxes should be treated with tube thoracostomy unless they are very small."- Harrison 19/e p1719

Features	Cardiac Tamponade	Tension Pneumothorax
Presenting	Shock[Q] (Shortness of breath[Q] may be seen)	Respiratory distress[Q] (Shock may be the presenting feature but less common)
Neck veins	Distended[Q]	Distended[Q]
Trachea	Midline[Q]	Deviated[Q]
Breath sounds	Normal[Q]	Decreased or absent on side of injury[Q]
Percussion Note	Normal[Q]	Hyper-resonant[Q]
Heart sound	Muffled[Q]	Normal[Q]

Traumatic Pneumothorax

- Traumatic pneumothoraxes can result **from penetrating & non-penetrating chest trauma.**
- It should be **treated with tube thoracostomy** unless it's very small.
    - **Iatrogenic pneumothorax** is a **type of traumatic pneumothorax** that is becoming more common.
    - **Leading causes** are **transthoracic needle aspiration, thoracentesis,** and the **insertion of central intravenous catheters**[Q].
    - **Most** can be **managed with supplemental oxygen** or **aspiration**[Q], but if these measures are unsuccessful, a tube thoracostomy should be performed.

143. Ans. d. Toxic megacolon *(Ref: Sabiston 20/e p313, 1289; Essentials of Radiology By Fred A. Mettler 3/e p149)*

History of diarrhea for long duration (suggestive of ulcerative colitis) with acute history of abdominal pain and dilated transverse and descending colon is suggestive of toxic megacolon. Ulcerative colitis is a predisposing factor for toxic megacolon.

AIIMS ESSENCE

"Pneumatosis intestinalis: The diagnosis is usually made radiographically by plain abdominal or barium studies. On plain films, pneumatosis intestinalis appears as radiolucent areas within the bowel wall, which must be differentiated from luminal intestinal gas. The radiolucency may be linear or curvilinear or appear as grape-like clusters or tiny bubbles. Alternatively, barium contrast or CT studies can be used to confirm the diagnosis. Visualization of intestinal cysts has also been described by ultrasound."-Sabiston 20/e p1289

"Pseudomembranous colitis: CT scanning is diagnostic and typically shows a boggy, edematous, and thickened colon wall (>3 mm) in 88%, pancolitis in 50%, serous ascites in 35%, pericolic inflammation in 35%, a clover leaf or accordion sign in 20%, and megacolon (transverse colon >8 cm) in 25% of cases. Sigmoidoscopy shows pseudomembranes in 90% of cases versus 23% in mild cases."-Sabiston 20/e p313

Toxic Megacolon

- Toxic megacolon is a **serious life-threatening condition** that can occur in patients with **ulcerative colitis, Crohn's colitis**, and **infectious colitides** such as **pseudomembranous colitis**[Q]
- This **decompensation** results in a **necrotic thin-walled bowel** in which **pneumatosis**[Q] can often be seen radiographically.

Diagnosis:
- **Plain abdominal radiographs** are critical for diagnosing toxic megacolon and for following its course.
- **Transverse colon is usually the most dilated >6 cm on supine films**.
- **Multiple air-fluid levels** in the colon are common; **normal colonic haustral pattern** is either **absent or severely disturbed.**
- Deep mucosal ulcerations may appear as air-filled crevices between large pseudopolypoid projections extending into the colonic lumen.

Organ	Diameter in Megacolon
Cecum	**>12 cm**[Q]
Ascending colon	>8 cm
Transverse colon	**>6 cm**[Q]
Rectosigmoid or descending colon	>6.5 cm

Management:
- **Medical treatment** is associated with a **high rate of recurrence** with subsequent **urgent operation**[Q] has been reported.
- **Aggressive preoperative stabilization** is required, using **volume resuscitation** with **crystalloid solutions** to prevent dehydration secondary to third-space fluid losses, stress-dose steroids for patients previously on steroid therapy, and **broad-spectrum antibiotics**[Q].

  - **Total abdominal colectomy** with **ileostomy** and preservation of the rectum is **treatment of choice** for **toxic megacolon**[Q].
  - It serves the **main purpose of removing the diseased colon** and **avoiding a difficult** and **morbid pelvic dissection**[Q].

OBSTETRICS AND GYNECOOLOGY

144. Ans. a. Manual support of perineum to maintain continuous deflexion of head *(Ref: Williams 24/e p447, 537, 538; FIGO GUIDELINES 'Management of the second stage of labor' 2012)*

In second stage of labor, either the 'hands on' (guarding the perineum & deflexing the baby's head) or the 'hands poised' (with hands off the perineum and baby's head but in readiness) technique can be used to facilitate spontaneous birth. Encourage active pushing once the urge to bear down is present, with encouragement to adopt any position for pushing preferred by the woman, except lying supine which risks aortocaval compression and reduced uteroplacental perfusion. Lithotomy position reduces uteroplacental blood flow, can contribute to fetal distress, and provides no mechanical advantage to enhance descent. Conduct the delivery with support for the perineum to avoid tears, and use of episiotomy only where a tear is very likely.

"Second stage of labor: This stage begins with complete cervical dilatation and ends with fetal delivery. The median duration is approximately 50 minutes for nulliparas and about 20 minutes for multiparas, but it is highly variable. In a woman of higher parity with a previously dilated vagina and perineum, two or three expulsive efforts after full cervical dilatation may suffice to complete delivery. Conversely, in a woman with a contracted pelvis, with a large fetus, or with impaired expulsive efforts from conduction analgesia or sedation, the second stage may become abnormally long."-Williams 24/e p447

AIIMS May 2017

"When the head distends the vulva and perineum enough to open the vaginal introitus to a diameter of 5 cm or more, a gloved hand may be used to support the perineum. The other hand is used to guide and control the fetal head to avoid expulsive delivery."- Williams 24/e p537

"Alternatively, if expulsive efforts are inadequate or expeditious delivery is needed, the modified Ritgen maneuver may be employed. With this, gloved fingers beneath a draped towel exert forward pressure on the fetal chin through the perineum just in front of the coccyx. Concurrently, the other hand presses superiorly against the occiput. Originally described in 1855, the Ritgen maneuver allows controlled fetal head delivery. It also favors neck extension so that the head passes through the introitus and over the perineum with its smallest diameters."- Williams 24/e p538

Second Stage of Labor (NICE/WHO guidelines)
• **Do not perform perineal massage** in **2nd stage of labor**[Q].
• Either the **'hands on' (guarding the perineum & deflexing the baby's head)** or the **'hands poised'** (with hands off the perineum and baby's head but in readiness) technique can be **used to facilitate spontaneous birth**[Q].
• **Do not offer lidocaine spray to reduce pain** in 2nd stage of labor[Q].
• **Do not carry out a routine episiotomy** during spontaneous vaginal birth[Q].
• **Do not offer episiotomy routinely at vaginal birth after previous third- or fourth-degree trauma**[Q].

145. Ans. a. Cortical vein thrombosis *(Ref: Chestnut's Obstetric Anesthesia 5/e p716; Harrison 19/e p910; Williams 24/e p1193)*

The patient is having clinical features of raised intracranial tension, which is commonly seen in cortical vein thrombosis. It is one of the common neurological complications seen in puerperium. Meningitis (neck rigidity is seen), subarachnoid hemorrhage and migraine (no seizures) will usually not present with these complaints and are not more frequent after pregnancy.

"The incidence of cerebral cortical vein thrombosis is increased during pregnancy and in the puerperium, and is estimated to be 10 to 20 per 100, 000 deliveries in developed countries. The incidence appears higher in developing countries. Often it is difficult to distinguish cortical vein thrombosis from post-dural puncture headache (PDPH), because the headache of cortical vein thrombosis may have a postural component. Preceding dural punctures have been reported, and it has been hypothesized that the reductions in CSF pressure and cerebral vasodilatations that accompany dural puncture predispose to thrombosis development. Associated features may include focal neurological sings, seizures and coma."-Chestnut's Obstetric Anesthesia 5/e p716.

Cortical Vein Thrombosis (CVT)
• **Incidence** of CVT is **increased** during **pregnancy** & in **puerperium**[Q]
• **Incidence** appears **higher in developing countries**[Q].
Predisposing Factors:
• **Prothrombotic conditions, OCPs, pregnancy, puerperium**[Q]
• **Malignancy, infection & head injury**[Q]
Clinical Features:
• **MC presenting symptom: Headache**[Q] (of gradual, acute, or thunderclap onset)
• Associated features may include **focal neurological sings, seizures and coma**[Q].
Diagnosis:
• Diagnosis is done with **MR venography**[Q].
Treatment:
• **Anticonvulsants for seizures**; **heparinization** is recommended by most, its efficacy is controversial.
• **Antimicrobials** for septic thrombophlebitis
• **Fibrinolytic therapy** is **reserved for those women failing systemic anticoagulation**.

146. Ans. d. Spermatocyte morphology *(Ref: WHO 'Normal Semen analysis' 5/e (2010); Speroff 8/e p1270-1271; Novaks 15/e p1142)*

Evaluation and assessment of semen is very important for both diagnosis of male infertility and selection of patients for treatment with IVF or ICSI. It has been shown that sperm morphology assessed strictly is most strongly related to fertilization rate than other parameters. In the WHO guidelines for Normal semen analysis, Sperm morphology, i.e. > 4% normal forms is the only strict criteria for sperm adequacy.

AIIMS ESSENCE

"Sperm morphology reflects the quality of spermatogenesis. Strict sperm morphology remains the best available predictor of sperm function (the capacity to fertilize a mature oocyte)."- Speroff 8/e p1270

"The percentage of sperm with normal morphology correlated strongly with the probability of achieving pregnancy."- Essential Reproductive Medicine (2005)/p373

Semen Characteristics	WHO 1999	WHO 2010
Volume (ml)	≥ 2 ml	≥ 1.5 ml[Q]
Sperm count	≥ 20 million/ml	≥ 15 million/ml[Q]
Total sperm count	≥ 40 million per ejaculate	≥ 39 million per ejaculate[Q]
Total motility	≥ 50 %	≥ 40%[Q]
Progressive motility	≥ 25%	≥ 32%[Q]
Vitality	≥ 75%	≥ 58%[Q]
Morphology (Normal form)	14%	≥ 4%[Q] normal forms (Strict criteria)
Leukocyte count (10⁴/ml)	<1	<1[Q]

Semen Analysis (WHO-2010)
• Semen analysis is the **cornerstone of male factor infertility evaluation**.
• Semen sample should be **collected after at least 3 days of abstinence** and is **best evaluated within 1 hour of ejaculation**
• Two specimens should be collected within 2-3 weeks intervals, if markedly different, additional specimens should be collected.
• Assisted reproductive technologies such as in vitro fertilization (IVF) require that **motile sperm be isolated from seminal plasma within 1 hour if ejaculation** to protect sperm from the inhibitory effects of seminal plasma on fertilization.

Common Indications for Semen Analysis
• As a part of **couple's infertility investigation**
• **After vasectomy to verify that the procedure was successful**
• **Testing human donors** for sperm donation

Semen Characteristics	
Volume	• **Lower reference limit: 1.5 ml** • **Low volume:** Due to **partial or complete blockage of seminal vesicles**
Count	• Over **15 million sperm per ml** is considered normal
Liquefaction	• Process when the gel formed by proteins from the seminal vesicle is broken up and the semen becomes more liquid • In the nice guidelines, a liquefaction time <60 minutes is within normal range • Semen analysis should be done after liquefaction with thorough mixing
Morphology	• ≥ 4% (or 5th centile) of the observed sperm should have normal morphology.
pH	• 7.2-7.8 • **Acidic ejaculate: When one or both of the seminal vesicles are blocked** • **Basic ejaculate:** Seen in infection

147. **Ans. a. High estrogen** *(Ref: Robbins 10/e p 721, 9/e p1012; Shaw's 15/e p466)*

In endometriotic lesions, histology represents its high estrogen activity. Whatever the initial genesis of endometriosis, its further development depends on the presence of hormones, mainly estrogen.

"Recent studies suggest that the endometriotic tissue is not just misplaced but it is also abnormal. As compared to normal endometrium, endometriotic tissue exhibits increased levels of inflammatory mediators, particularly prostaglandin E2, and increased estrogen production due to high aromatase activity of stromal cells. These changes enhance the survival and persistence of the endometriotic tissue with a foreign location (a key feature in the pathogenesis of endometriosis) and help to explain the beneficial effects of COX-2 inhibitors and aromatase inhibitors in the treatment of endometriosis."- Robbins 10/e p 721

"Molecular analyses have provided additional insights into the pathogenesis of endometriosis. The endometriotic implants show certain differences when compared to the endometria of women without endometriosis. These include the following: Release of proinflammatory and other factors, including PGE2, IL-1β, TNFα, IL-6 and -8, NGF, VEGF, MCP-1, MMPs, and TIMPs; Increased estrogen production by endometriotic stromal cells, due in large part to high levels of the key steroidogenic enzyme aromatase, which is absent in normal endometrial stroma. Estrogen enhances the survival and persistence of endometriotic tissue, and inhibitors of aromatase are beneficial in the treatment of endometriosis. A link between inflammation and estrogen production is made plausible by the ability of prostaglandin E2 to stimulate local synthesis of estrogen."- Robbins 9/e p1012

Endometriosis

- Presence of **ectopic functional endometrial tissue** is known as endometriosis. They contain **both gland** & **stroma** and respond to hormonal stimulation.

> - **Prevalence** in general population: **10%**[Q]
> - Prevalence among **infertile couple**: **30-40%**[Q]

Theories:
1. **Implantation theory** by Sampson
2. **Coelomic metaplasia** (Meyer & Ivanoff)
3. Direct implantation
4. **Metastatic theory**: **Halban's theory** of metastasis through vascular or lymphatic channel
5. **Histogenesis** by induction

Sites:
- **Ovary, Pouch of Douglas, uterosacral ligament, broad ligament**, peritoneum of bladder, sigmoid colon, intestinal coil.

Pathology:

> - **Endometriotic implants** → **Estrogen influence**[Q] → Proliferation → No secretory change, **shedding of blood** → **Cystic structure** due to **pent up secretions** → **Fibrosis** due to blood[Q].

- **Powder Burn Appearance**[Q]: **Appearance of endometriotic implant** is **dark red, bluish or black cystic puckering due to fibrosis, small black dot**[Q]

> - The **ovary** have **endometriotic cyst** of varying size, **bluish thickening of tunica albuginea**[Q]. The epithelial lining of cyst is columnar, adjacent to epithelium is a layer of large, polyhedral, Phagocytic cell laden with blood pigment hemosiderin, also known as **Pseudoxanthoma cells**[Q].

Clinical Features:

> - **Dysmenorrhea, Pain, Infertility, Menstrual irregularity**[Q]
> - **Dyspareunia** (specially when present in **pouch of Douglas**)[Q]

- **Pelvic Examination: Tenderness, nodule** in POD, **cobble stone feel**[Q] of uterosacral ligament, fixed retroverted uterus, bluish or blackish puckered spot in posterior fornix.

- **Diagnosis:**

> - **Laparoscopy** is **gold standard** for diagnosis of **endometriosis**[Q].
> - **Powder burn** or **matchstick spots** are seen on laparoscopy[Q].

Laparoscopic Findings
- **Unless disease** is **visible in** the **vagina** or **elsewhere, laparoscopy** is the **standard technique for visual inspection of pelvis** and **establishment of a definitive diagnosis**[Q]
- **Characteristic findings** include typical **"Powder burn or gun shot"** lesions on the **serosal surface** of peritoneum[Q].
- In the presence of **ovarian endometrioma >3cm in** diameter and **deeply infiltrative disease, histology** should be **obtained to identify endometriosis** and **to exclude rare instance of malignancy**[Q].

- **CA-125 >35 U/mL** may be used as **evidence of recurrence**[Q].

Complications:
- **Malignancy: MC type** is **endometroid adenocarcinoma**[Q]
- **Infertility**[Q]
- **Ureteric obstruction** & hydronephrosis

Contd...

Treatment of Endometriosis	
Medical	**Surgical**
• **NSAIDs** in patients with **pelvic pain**, if the diagnosis of endometriosis has not been definitively (excision & biopsy) established.	• **Laparoscopic surgical approaches** include **excision of ovarian adhesions** & of endometriomas[Q].
• **Achieve an anovulatory state by hormonal contraception:** Progestins (**Medroxyprogesterone acetate**), **danazol, gestrinone, or GnRH**	• **Endometriomas: Excision** is considered to be far superior in terms of permanent removal of the disease & pain relief.
• **GnRH** can be combined **with estrogen & progestogen** without loss of efficacy but with fewer hypoestrogenic symptoms.	• **Operative laparoscopic surgery** can provide **pain relief & improved fertility.**
	• **Radical surgical options** could include **singular or bilateral oophorectomy.**

148. Ans. a. Give another dose of Anti-D 72 hours postpartum depending on the baby blood group *(Ref: Williams 24/e p 311–312, 643; RCOG Guidelines)*

ACOG (2010) recommends anti-D immune globulin to be given prophylactically to all Rh D-negative, unsensitized women at approximately 28 weeks, and a second dose given after delivery if the infant is Rh D-positive. Before the 28-week dose of anti-D immune globulin, repeat antibody screening is recommended to identify individuals who have become alloimmunized. Following delivery, anti-D immune globulin should be given within 72 hours.

*"In the United States, **anti-D immune globulin is given prophylactically to all Rh D-negative, unsensitized women at approximately 28 weeks, and a second dose is given after delivery if the infant is Rh D-positive (American College of Obstetricians and Gynecologists, 2010)**. Before the 28-week dose of anti-D immune globulin, repeat antibody screening is recommended to identify individuals who have become alloimmunized (**American Academy of Pediatrics and American College of Obstetricians and Gynecologists 2012**). Following delivery, anti-D immune globulin should be given within 72 hours. Importantly, if immune globulin is inadvertently not administered following delivery, it should be given as soon as the omission is recognized, because there may be some protection up to 28 days postpartum (Bowman, 2006). **Anti-D immune globulin is also administered after pregnancy-related events that could result in fetomaternal hemorrhage.**"-Williams 24/e p312*

Prevention of Rh-D Alloimmunization
• **Rh-D immunoglobulin** is given by **IM injection, used to prevent the immunological condition known as Rh disease (or hemolytic disease of newborn)**[Q].
• It contains **IgG anti-D (anti-RhD) antibodies that take out any fetal RhD-positive erythrocytes,** which have **entered the maternal blood stream from fetal circulation, before the maternal immune system can react to them,** thus **preventing maternal sensitization**[Q].
Indication:
• **Rh –ve mother with Rh +ve father to prevent hemolytic disease of the fetus**[Q]
Dose:
• **IM dose of anti-D immune globulin: 1500 IU protects haemorrhage of 30 mL blood/15 mL of fetal red cells**[Q].
Prophylaxis:
• **Given prophylactically to all Rh D-negative unsensitized women at approximately 28 weeks**, and a **second dose is given after delivery if the infant is Rh D-positive**[Q].
• Before the 28-week dose of anti-D immune globulin, repeat antibody screening is recommended to identify individuals who have become alloimmunized.
• **Following delivery, anti-D immune globulin should be given within 72 hours**[Q].
Special cases:
• In 1% of pregnancies, **volume of fetomaternal hemorrhage exceeds 30 mL, higher dose of Anti D Immunoglobulin is required.** Example: Abdominal trauma, placental abruption, placenta previa, intrauterine manipulation, multifetal gestation, or manual placenta removal.

AIIMS May 2017

Prevention of Rh-D Alloimmunization

- **Rh-D immunoglobulin** is **given by IM injection, used to prevent the immunological condition known as Rh disease (or hemolytic disease of newborn)**[Q].
  - It contains **IgG anti-D (anti-RhD) antibodies** that take out any fetal RhD-positive erythrocytes, which have **entered the maternal blood stream from fetal circulation, before the maternal immune system can react to them,** thus **preventing maternal sensitization**[Q].

Indication:
- **Rh –ve mother with Rh +ve father to prevent hemolytic disease of the fetus**[Q]

Dose:
- IM dose of anti-D immune globulin: **1500 IU protects haemorrhage of 30 mL blood/15 mL of fetal red cells**[Q].

Prophylaxis:
- **Given prophylactically to all Rh D-negative unsensitized women at approximately 28 weeks**, and a **second dose is given after delivery if the infant is Rh D-positive**[Q].
- Before the 28-week dose of anti-D immune globulin, repeat antibody screening is recommended to identify individuals who have become alloimmunized.
  - **Following delivery, anti-D immune globulin should be given within 72 hours**[Q].

Special cases:
- In 1% of pregnancies, **volume of fetomaternal hemorrhage exceeds 30 mL, higher dose of Anti D Immunoglobulin is required.** Example: Abdominal trauma, placental abruption, placenta previa, intrauterine manipulation, multifetal gestation, or manual placenta removal.

149. **Ans. d. Colposcopy and biopsy** *(Ref: ASCCP Consensus Guidelines for Managing Abnormal Cervical Cancer Screening Tests and Cancer Precursors, 2014; Shaw 15/e p 405; Novak's 15/e p576, 589)*

HSIL (High grade squamous intraepithelial lesion) category includes CIN 2 & CIN 3 (moderate dysplasia, severe dysplasia and carcinoma in situ). Any women with cytologic specimen suggesting the presence of HSIL should undergo colposcopy and directed biopsy.

"HSIL (High grade squamous intraepithelial lesion): Any women with cytologic specimen suggesting the presence of HSIL should undergo colposcopy and directed biopsy. This is because two thirds of patients with this cytologic finding will have CIN 2 or greater. After colposcopically directed biopsy and determination of the distribution of the lesion, excisional or ablative therapy, that address the entire transformation zone should be performed."- Novak's 15/e p576

Cervical Intraepithelial Neoplasia (CIN)

- Invasive squamous cell cervical cancers are preceded by a long phase of pre-invasive disease, collectively referred to as CIN.
- Histopathologically a **part or the full thickness of cervical squamous epithelium is replaced by cells showing varying degree of dysplasia,** with intact basement membrane.
- **CIN may be suspected through cytological examination using Pap smear test** or through **colposcopic examination. Cervical cytology is the most efficacious & cost-effective method for cancer screening**[Q].
- **Final diagnosis of CIN** is established by the histopathological examination of a **cervical punch biopsy** or **excision specimen.**
- Additionally, **HPV testing** can be performed in order to better triage women with early cytologic changes.

Comparison of Cytology Classification System

Bathesda	CIN	Dysplasia	Limit of histologic Changes
LSIL (Low grade squamous intraepithelial lesion)	CIN 1	Mild	Basal 1/3rd of squamous epithelium
HSIL (High grade squamous intraepithelial lesion)	CIN 2	Moderate	Basal ½ to 2/3rd
	CIN 3	Severe	Whole thickness except one or two superficial layers
		Carcinoma-in-situ	Whole thickness

Contd...

Contd...

Cervical Intraepithelial Neoplasia (CIN)		
Treatment of CIN		
CIN 1	• **Spontaneous regression rate in CIN 1: 60-85%** • Regressions typically occur **within a 2-year follow-up with cytology & colposcopy.**	
	Observation	• Biopsy diagnoses of CIN 1 with satisfactory colposcopy and who agree to the evaluation every 6 months
	Ablative treatment	• If the **lesions progress** during follow-up **or persist** at 2 years
	• Treatment options: LEEP & Cryosurgery[Q]	
CIN 2 & 3	• **All CIN 2 & 3 lesions require treatment**[Q] • **Preferred treatment for CIN 2 & 3: LEEP**[Q]	

Techniques of Treatment for Squamous Intraepithelial Lesions		
Ablative	**Excisional**	
• Cryotherapy • Laser ablation (vaporization)	• Laser excisional conization • Cold knife conization	• LEEP

Cryotherapy	• Cryotherapy destroys the surface epithelium of the cervix by crystallizing the intracellular water • **Cryotherapy should be considered acceptable therapy when the following criteria are met: CIN, grade 1 to 2; Small lesion ; Ectocervical location only; Negative ECC findings; No endocervical gland involvement on biopsy**
Laser vaporization	**Laser vaporization is particularly applicable in the following situations:** 1. **Large lesions** that the cryoprobe cannot adequately cover[Q] 2. **Irregular cervix** with a **"fish mouth" appearance** & deep clefts[Q] 3. **Extension of disease to vagina** or **satellite lesions on vagina**[Q] 4. Lesions with **extensive glandular involvement** in which the treatment must reach beyond the deepest gland cleft [Q]
Loop Electrosurgical Excision Procedure (LEEP)	• **LEEP is a valuable tool for diagnosis & treatment of CIN**[Q] • **Preferred treatment for CIN 2 & 3**[Q] • **Advantage:** Perform **diagnostic & therapeutic operation simultaneously** during one outpatient visit[Q].
Conization	**Conization is indicated for diagnosis in women with HSIL based on a Pap test under the following conditions:** 1. **Limits of the lesion cannot be visualized with colposcopy.** 2. **SCJ is not seen at colposcopy.** 3. ECC histologic findings are positive for **CIN 2 or CIN 3.** 4. **Lack of correlation** between cytology, biopsy & colposcopy results. 5. **Microinvasion** is suspected based on biopsy, colposcopy, or cytology results. 6. Colposcopist is **unable to rule out invasive cancer.**

Hysterectomy	• **Hysterectomy is currently considered too radical for treatment of CIN.**
	• **Indications of hysterectomy in CIN:**
	   1. **Microinvasion**[Q]
	   2. **CIN 3 at limits of conization specimen**[Q]
	   3. Poor compliance with follow-up
	   4. **Other gynecologic problems** requiring hysterectomy, such as fibroids, prolapse, endometriosis, & PID[Q]

150. **Ans. b. 1 cm below the ischial spine** *(Ref: Williams 24/e p 449)*

Station describes descent of the fetal biparietal diameter in relation to a line drawn between maternal ischial spines. Thus +1 station implies fetal head is 1 cm below the ischial spine.

"The level—or station—of the presenting fetal part in the birth canal is described in relationship to the ischial spines, which are halfway between the pelvic inlet and the pelvic outlet. When the lowermost portion of the presenting fetal part is at the level of the spines, it is designated as being at zero (0) station. In the past, the long axis of the birth canal above and

Contd...

Contd...

below the ischial spines was arbitrarily divided into thirds by some and into fifths (approximately 1 cm) by other groups. In 1989, the American College of Obstetricians and Gynecologists adopted the classification of station that divides the pelvis above and below the spines into fifths. Each fifth represents 1 cm above or below the spines. Thus, as the presenting fetal part descends from the inlet toward the ischial spines, the designation is –5, –4, –3, –2, –1, then 0 station. Below the spines, as the presenting fetal part descends, it passes +1, +2, +3, +4, and +5 stations to delivery. Station +5 cm corresponds to the fetal head being visible at the introitus. If the leading part of the fetal head is at 0 station or below, most often the fetal head has engaged—thus, the biparietal plane has passed through the pelvic inlet. If the head is unusually molded or if there is an extensive caput formation or both, engagement might not have taken place although the head appears to be at 0 station." -Williams 24/e p 449

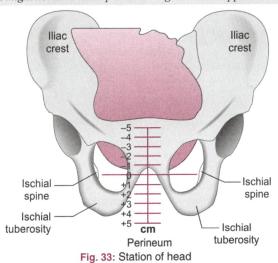

Fig. 33: Station of head

Station of Head in Relation to Ischial Spines
• Level of ischial spine is halfway between pelvic inlet & outlet. This level is known a **station zero**^{Q} **(0)**.
• Levels above & below the spines are **divided into fifth to represent centimeters**^{Q}.
• The station is said to be **'0'** if the **presenting part is at the level of ischial spines**. The station is stated in **minus figures**, if it is **above the spines** (–1 cm, –2 cm, –3 cm, –4 cm & –5 cm) and in **plus figures** if it is **below the spines** (+1 cm, +2 cm, +3 cm, +4 cm & +5 cm)^Q

151. Ans. d. Check CA-125 levels and advise regular follow-up if normal *(Ref: Shaw's 15/e p369)*

This is a post-menopausal patient with a simple (smooth) cyst in the ovary. Such a cyst doesn't need further investigations, but this patient has two risk factors for malignancy: Family history of ovarian tumor and history of Hormonal therapy. Hence, CA-125 levels should be evaluated and the RMI-I score (Risk of Malignancy index) calculated before proceeding for regular follow up. If RMI score exceeds 200, further imaging/ laparoscopic surgery will be needed in this patient.

Risk of Malignancy Index (RMI-I) NICE Guidelines
• **RMI-I combines three pre-surgical features**: Serum **CA125**, menopausal status **(M)** & ultrasound score **(U)**.
• RMI is product of ultrasound scan score, menopausal status & serum CA125 level (IU/mL).
• **RMI = U × M × CA125**
• **Ultrasound** result is scored **1 point for each of the following characteristics**: multilocular cysts, solid areas, **metastases, ascites and bilateral lesions.** U = 0 (for an ultrasound score of 0), U = 1 (for an ultrasound score of 1), U = 3 (for an ultrasound score of 2–5).
• The **menopausal status is scored as 1 = pre-menopausal and 3 = post- menopausal**; The classification of 'post-menopausal' is a woman who has had no period for more than 1 year or a woman over 50 who has had a hysterectomy.
• Serum CA125 is measured in IU/mL and can vary between 0 and hundreds or even thousands of units.

Management	
RMI score **>200**	**High risk**, with **referral** to specialist gynecological cancer service & **staging CT** advised
RMI score **25–200**	**Intermediate risk**, with **MRI recommended** to further evaluate the lesion
RMI score **<25**	**Low risk**, with **repeat clinical assessment advised**, with MRI if ultrasound features are borderline.

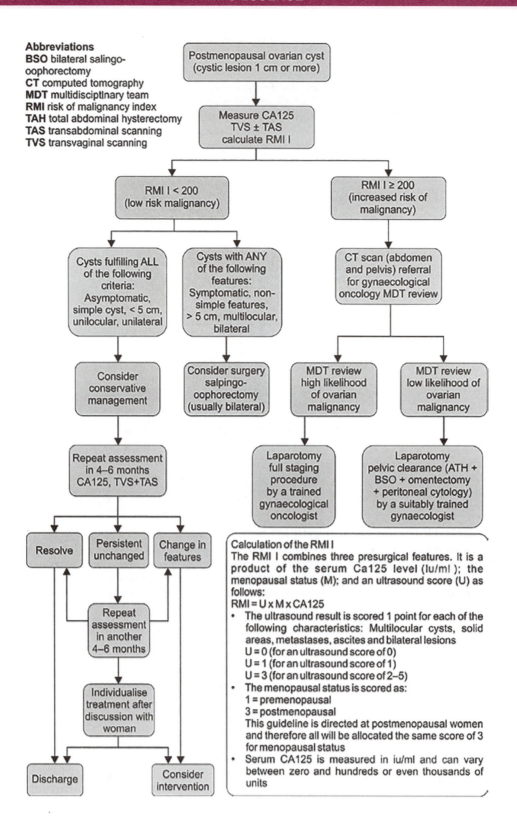

Management of Ovarian Cysts

Indications for Surgery in Ovarian Cysts
• **Persistent complex ovarian cysts** • Persistent cysts that are **causing symptoms** • **Complex ovarian cysts >5 cm** • Simple ovarian cysts **>10 cm** or **>5 cm in postmenopausal patients** • Women who are **menopausal or perimenopausal**

- **Follow-up imaging in women of reproductive age for incidentally discovered simple cysts on ultrasound is not needed until 5 cm, as these are usually normal ovarian follicles.**

  - For simple cysts **>5 cm but <7 cm** in premenopausal females, cysts should be **followed yearly**.
  - For simple cysts **>7 cm, further imaging with MRI or surgical assessment** is mandated as, because of their large size, these cysts cannot be reliably assessed by ultrasound alone.

- For the corpus luteum, a dominant ovulating follicle that typically appears as a cyst with circumferentially thickened walls and crenulated inner margins, follow up is not needed if the cyst is <3 cm in diameter.

  - **In postmenopausal patients, any simple cyst >1 cm but <7 cm needs yearly follow-up, while those >7 cm need MRI or surgical evaluation**, similar to reproductive age females.
  - **For multiloculate cysts with thin septation <3 mm, surgical evaluation is recommended.**

- **Presence of multiloculation suggests a neoplasm**, although **thin septation** implies that the **neoplasm is benign**.
- Ovarian cysts are considered large when they are >5 cm and giant when they are >15 cm.

152. **Ans. b. Wertheim's hysterectomy**   *(Ref: Shaw's 15/e p184, 414; Novaks 15/e p870)*

Radical or Wertheim's hysterectomy is associated with the highest risk of ureteric injury. The risk of ureteral injury at vaginal hysterectomy is higher (0.6%) than with an open abdominal approach (0.07%). The main reason is the inability to see and sometimes palpate the ureter during vaginal surgery as compared to an open procedure.

"Ureteral injuries are a potential complication of any open or endoscopic pelvic operation. Gynecologic surgery accounts for more than 50 percent of all ureteral injuries resulting from an operation, with the remaining occurring during colorectal, general, vascular and urologic surgery. The ureter is injured in roughly 0.5 to 2 percent of all hysterectomies and routine gynecologic pelvic operations and in 10 percent (range, 5 to 30 percent) of radical hysterectomies. Ureteral complications from radical hysterectomy have declined over the years because of improved patient selection, limiting of surgery to mostly low-stage disease, decreased use of preoperative radiation and modifications in surgical technique that limit extreme skeletonization of the ureter. Of ureteral injuries from gynecologic surgery, roughly 50 percent are from radical hysterectomy, 40 percent are from abdominal hysterectomy and less than 5 percent result from vaginal hysterectomy. All gynecologic ureteral injuries occur to the distal one third of the ureter (or in other words, the segment of ureter closest to bladder and in the pelvis)."-http://urology.wustl.edu/en/Patient-Care/ReconstructiveSurgery/Urologic-Complications-from-Surgery

Ureteric Injury	
Type of Surgical Operations	**Incidence**
Vaginal vault suspension surgery	2–4%[Q]
Radical or Wertheim's hysterectomy	1.3%[Q]
Obstetric hysterectomy	1.17%
Laparoscopic assisted vaginal hysterectomy (LAVH)	0.45–1%
Burch colposuspension	0.41%
Abdominal hysterectomy	0.2%
Vaginal hysterectomy	0.1%
Caesarean section	0.09%
Other laparoscopic surgery	0.03%

153. Ans. b. Check serum estradiol levels *(Ref: Shaw's 15/e p70; Novak's 15/e p1036*

LH and FSH levels by the third month of pregnancy are steady at a low level. HCG takes over the function of LH after fertilization and inhibits production on LH. Inhibin A produced by fetal trophoblasts suppresses maternal FSH secretion. Hence, 3 times elevation of LH and FSH points towards premature ovarian failure. Serum estradiol levels should be measured to confirm the diagnosis.

> *"Women with hypoestrogenic amenorrhea have either ovarian failure or hypothalamic-pituitary dysfunction. Serum concentrations of FSH and LH of more than 40-50 mIU/ml are diagnostic of ovarian failure. Serial assessment may be necessary because of the pulsatile nature of pituitary gonadotropin secretion. Most women under age of 40 years belonging to this category have premature ovarian failure. Overt primary ovarian insufficiency is defined as the presence of amenorrhea for 4 months or more accompanied by two serum FSH levels in the menopausal range for a woman who is less than 40 years of age. Serum estradiol values will be low in gonadal failure cases like premature ovarian failure."- Novak's 15/e p1036*

Premature Ovarian Failure

- Premature ovarian failure is a **primary ovarian defect** characterized by **absent menarche[Q] (primary amenorrhea)** or **premature depletion of ovarian follicles before the age of 40 years (secondary amenorrhea)**.
- **Triad for diagnosis**: Amenorrhea + Hypergonadotropism + Hypoestrogenism[Q].
- **Characterized by high FSH, LH & serum prolactin and low serum estradiol levels[Q]**

Causes of Premature Ovarian Failure

- **Genetic:**
  - **Turner's syndrome**
  - **Gonadal dysgenesis** 46XX, 46XY
  - **Trisomy 18 & 13**
  - X-chromosome deletion, translocation.
- **Autoimmune:**
  - Autoantibodies antinuclear antibodies
  - Lupus anticoagulant
  - **Polyglandular autoimmune syndrome** (antibodies against thyroid, parathyroid adrenal, islet cells of pancreas)
- **Infection: Mumps, tuberculosis**

- **Iatrogenic:** Radiation therapy, chemotherapy (cyclophosphamide), surgery
- **Metabolic:**
  - Galactosemia (In galactosemia, enzyme **galactose-l-phosphate uridyl transferase**, is **absent**. **Follicles are destroyed to the toxic effects or galactose**)
  - **17α-hydroxylase deficiency**
- **Environmental**: Smoking.
- **FSH receptor** absent or post-receptor defect **(Savage's syndrome)**.
- **Idiopathic**

Clinical Features:

- **History of amenorrhea** in **<35 years of age; primary (25%) or secondary (75%)**
- **Features of hypoestrogenic state: Hot flushes, vaginal dryness, dyspareunia** & psychological symptoms[Q]

Diagnosis:

- Serum **gonadotropin level (FSH>40 mIU/mL)** is **high & Serum E2 level is low (<20 pg/mL)[Q]**
- **Karyotype abnormality**: In patients **<30 years, rule out chromosomal abnormality[Q]**.
- Organ specific humoral antibody **(antithyroid commonest)[Q]**
- **Possibility of autoimmune disorders** should be considered **<35 years of age (antithyroid antibodies, rheumatoid factor & ANA should be measured)[Q]**

  - **Ovarian biopsy: Not essential for diagnosis**
  - In **autoimmune variety**: Perifollicular lymphocyte infiltration
  - In **resistant ovarian syndrome**: Follicles are present, **FSH receptor is either absent or defective**.

Management:

- **Hormone replacement therapy; corticosteroids** in proved case of autoimmune disorders
- **Induction of ovulation**: By administration of **sequential estrogen & progesterone** or by use of **GnRH agonist**, followed by **administration of gonadotropins for ovulation induction**
- **IVF with donor's oocyte** with total replacement of hormones can increase the chance of pregnancy.
- In the **presence of 'Y' chromosome** of **gonadectomy to avoid malignancy**

AIIMS May 2017

751

154. Ans. d. Drop in fetal heart rate to less than 70 bpm for 60 sec   *(Ref: Williams 24/e p341, 477)*
Significant variable decelerations is drop in fetal heart rate to less than 70 bpm for 60 sec.

"Significant variable decelerations have been defined as those decreasing to less than 70 bpm and lasting more than 60 seconds."-William's 24/e p477

Classification of Variable Decelerations	
Mild	• >80 bpm irrespective of duration or <30 seconds irrespective of depth or 70–80 bpm lasting for 60 seconds
Moderate	• >70 bpm lasting for 30–60 seconds or 70–80 bpm lasting for ≥ 60 seconds
Severe	• <70 bpm lasting at least 60 seconds

Electronic FHR monitoring: Decelerations		
Early Deceleration	**Late Deceleration**	**Variable Deceleration**
• Visually apparent usually symmetrical **gradual decrease & return of FHR associated with a uterine contraction**[Q]. • A **gradual FHR decrease** is defined as **from the onset to the FHR nadir of ≥ 30 sec**[Q]. • The **nadir of deceleration** occurs at the same time as the **peak of contraction**[Q].	• Visually apparent usually symmetrical **gradual decrease & return of FHR associated with a uterine contraction**[Q]. • A gradual FHR decrease is defined as from the onset to the FHR nadir of ≥ 30 sec. • **Deceleration is delayed in timing**, with the **nadir of deceleration** occurring **after** the **peak of contraction**[Q].	• **Visually apparent abrupt decrease in FHR**[Q]. • An **abrupt FHR decrease** is defined as **from the onset to FHR nadir of < 30 sec**[Q]. • **Decrease in FHR is ≥15 bpm, lasting ≥ 15 sec & <2 min in duration**[Q]. • When **variable decelerations** are associated with uterine contraction, their **onset, depth & duration** commonly **vary with successive uterine contractions**. • Likely **due to umbilical cord compression**. • **Can lead to fetal asphyxia** when severe or **may progress to late decelerations** or **severe fetal bradycardia**, both of which indicate the **need for urgent intervention**[Q]. • **Variable decelerations, if non-repetitive & brief (< 30 seconds) do not indicate fetal compromise or the need for obstetrical intervention**[Q]. • In contrast, **repetitive variable decelerations, at least three in 20 minutes**, even if mild, have been **associated with an increased risk of cesarean delivery for fetal distress**[Q].

155. Ans. a. Anencephaly   *(Ref: Williams 24/e p201; High Risk Pregnancy: Management Options By David K. James 4/e p112; Dutta 8/e p736)*
Anencephaly can be diagnosed in the 1st trimester of pregnancy. Anencephaly is earliest recognized congenital anomaly, usually detectable in a first trimester sonogram at 11–14 weeks.

"Anencephaly is diagnosed by the absence of cranial vault (calvarium) and telencephalon. Brain tissue is angiomatous. Early diagnosis is possible at about 13 weeks."- Dutta 8/e p736

"Anencephaly can be diagnosed reliably on routine 11-14 weeks ultrasound examination. Acrania is the main feature of anencephaly in the first trimester. Fetus with acrania may have normal brain or one that shows varying degree of disruption."- High Risk Pregnancy: Management Options By David K. James 4/e p112

"Anencephaly is characterized by absence of the cranium and telencephalic structures, with the skullbase and orbits covered only by angiomatous stroma. Acrania is absence of the cranium, with protrusion of disorganized brain tissue. Both are generally grouped together, and anencephaly is considered to be the final stage of acrania. These lethal anomalies can be diagnosed in the late first trimester, and with adequate visualization, virtually all cases may be diagnosed in the second trimester. An inability to view the biparietal diameter should raise suspicion. Hydramnios from impaired fetal swallowing is common in the third trimester."-Williams 24/e p201

"Ultrasound Diagnosis: Currently, anencephaly is diagnosed at the time of the nuchal translucency scan (12-14) weeks or even earlier in the majority of cases. At this gestational age, the stage is that of exencephaly, with the cerebral hemispheres visible above the orbits, on a frontal or midsagittal view of the fetal head."-Ultrasound of Congenital Fetal Anomalies By Dario Paladini 2/e p82

Acrania	Anencephaly
• **Absence of cranium**, with **protrusion of a disorganized mass of brain tissue** that resembles a "shower cap" (arrows)[Q] • Characteristic **triangular facial appearance**[Q].	• **Absence of forebrain & cranium** above skull base & orbit. • **Long white arrow** points to **fetal orbit** & **short white arrow indicates nose**[Q].

Anencephaly
• **Absence of a major portion of brain, skull & scalp** that occurs during embryonic development.   • It is **a cephalic disorder** that **results from a neural tube defect** that occurs when **rostral (head) end of neural tube fails to close**, usually between 23rd & 26th day following conception.   • **Largest part of brain consisting mainly of cerebral hemispheres**, including neocortex, which is responsible for cognition[Q].   • The **remaining structure is usually covered only by a thin layer of membrane-skin, bone, meninges, etc. are all lacking**[Q]

156. **Ans. b. G4P1 0 + 1 + 2** *(Ref: Williams 24/e p161; Dutta 8/e p107)*

The nomenclature for this question is based on a system called GTPAL system.

TPAL terminology= A system used to describe obstetrical history. (T = Term births, P = Preterm births (prior to 37 weeks gestation), A = Abortions, L = Living children). The GPA terminology is combined with TPAL terminology → GTPAL terminology. So, Patient describe in the question will be represented as (live is included as Para 1) G4 P1 (0+1+2).

"Gravida and parity: Gravida denotes a pregnant state both present and past, irrespective of the period of gestation. Parity denotes a state of previous pregnancy beyond the period of viability."- Dutta 8/e p107

"Gravida and para refers to pregnancies and not to babies. As such, a woman who delivers twins in first pregnancy is still a gravida one para one. A pregnant woman with previous history of two abortions and one term delivery can be expressed as fourth gravida but primipara. It is customary in clinical practice to summarize the past obstetric history by two digits (the first one relates with viable births and second one relates with abortions) connected with a plus sign affixing the letter 'P'. Thus, P_{2+1} denotes the patient had two viable births and one abortion. In some centres, it is expressed by four digits connected by dashes. $P_{A-B-C-D}$, where A denotes number of term (37-42 weeks) pregnancies; B: Number of preterm (28 to <37 weeks) pregnancies; C: Number of miscarriages (<28 weeks) and D: The number of children alive at present. A pregnant woman with previous history of four births or more is called grand multipara."-Dutta 8/e p107

157. **Ans. b. Laparoscopy and hysteroscopy** *(Ref: Shaw's 15/e p 214; Speroff 8/e p1108)*

Bilateral tubal block at cornu should be confirmed using Laparoscopy and hysteroscopy (Chromopertubation test), which is the gold standard. Treatment of choice will be tuboplasty, but other causes like spasm should be ruled out as hysterosalpingogram is not a very reliable test.

"Laparoscopy is considered as gold standard for diagnosing tubal and peritoneal diseases.it allows visualization of all pelvic organ and permits detection and potential concurrent treatment of intramural and subserosal uterine fibroids, peritubal and periovarian adhesion and endometriosis. Direct visualization on laparoscopy using chromopertubation involves the transcervical instillation of dye such as indigo carmine or methylene blue to directly visualize tubal patency and fimbrial architecture."- http://www.ijsrp.org/research-paper-0715/ijsrp-p4374.pdf

Bilateral Fallopian Tube Obstruction
• **Bilateral fallopian tube obstruction** is a **major cause of female infertility**[Q] (~20%).

Causes:
• **Pelvic inflammatory disease**[Q] (MC cause), **endometritis, intra-abdominal infections** & **formation of adhesions** etc.

Evaluation:
• A **HSG** will demonstrate that **tubes are open** when the **radiopaque dye spills into the abdominal cavity**[Q].
• **Sonography** can demonstrate tubal abnormalities such as a **hydrosalpinx indicative of tubal occlusion**[Q].
• **During surgery, typically laparoscopy, status of the tubes can be inspected and a dye such as methylene blue can be injected** in a process termed **chromotubation** into the uterus and shown to pass through the tubes when the cervix is occluded[Q].
• **Laparoscopic chromotubation** has been described as the **gold standard of tubal evaluation**[Q].
• Tubal insufflation is only of historical interest as an older office method to indicate patency; it was used prior to laparoscopic evaluation of pelvic organs.

Treatment:

Treatment of Fallopian Tube Obstruction	
Proximal Tubal Obstruction	**Distal Tubal Obstruction**
• **Reconstructive surgery** done for proximal tubal obstruction **tubocornual anastomosis**[Q]. • **Tubocornual anastomosis:** – **The cornual portion of the tube is resected followed by anastomosis.** – Since this procedure is performed by laparotomy rather than laparoscopically & intrauterine pregnancy rate is relatively low, IVF is often a better alternative. – Reconstructive surgery for proximal tubal occlusion not very effective & risk of subsequent ectopic pregnancy is high therefore IVF is preferable if available.	• In contrast to patients with proximal tubal obstruction where findings from HSG are often false positive the **HSG findings & laparoscopic tubal lavage are typically concordant**[Q]. • **Surgery for the treatment of tubal factor infertility is most successful in women with distal tubal obstruction**[Q]. • **Surgical procedures for distal tube obstruction:** – **Fimbrioplasty:** Lysis of fimbrial adhesions or dilatations fimbrial strictures. – **Neosalpingostomy:** Creation of new opening in a distally occluded tube.

In-vitro Fertilization
• **IVF** is a **proven method of treatment of tubal factor infertility** and has the following advantages & disadvantages with tubal reconstruction.

In-vitro Fertilization	
Advantage	**Disadvantages**
• **Good per cycle success rate** • **Less surgically invasive than tubal surgery** • **Can overcome other subfertility factors, if present** • Site and extent of tubal damage are not important to outcome	• **High per cycle cost and possible need for multiple cycle** • Need for IVF each time a pregnancy is desired • Requires **frequent injection & monitoring** • Increases risk of **multiple gestation** • Increases risk of **ovarian hyperstimulation syndrome**

158. **Ans. b. Supine vena cava syndrome**   *(Ref: Williams 24/e p61)*

Supine vena cava syndrome or aortocaval compression syndrome is compression of the abdominal aorta and inferior vena cava by the gravid uterus when a pregnant woman lies on her back, i.e. in the supine position.

"Supine Hypotension: In approximately 10 percent of women, supine compression of the great vessels by the uterus causes significant arterial hypotension, sometimes referred to as the supine hypotensive syndrome. Also when supine, uterine arterial pressure—and thus blood flow—is significantly lower than that in the brachial artery. This may directly affect fetal heart rate patterns. These changes are also seen with hemorrhage or with spinal analgesia." -Williams 24/e p61

Supine Hypotension or Supine Hypotensive Syndrome
• In approximately **10%** of women, **supine compression of great vessels by uterus causes significant arterial hypotension**, sometimes referred to as the **supine hypotensive syndrome**[Q]. • In supine position, **uterine arterial pressure & blood flow** is significantly lower than in brachial artery, this may **directly affect fetal heart rate patterns**[Q]. • It is a **frequent cause of low maternal BP (hypotension)** resulting in **loss of consciousness** and in extreme circumstances **fetal demise**[Q].
Cause: • **Aortocaval compression** is thought to be the cause of supine hypotensive syndrome.
Clinical Features: • It is characterized by **pallor, tachycardia, sweating, nausea, hypotension & dizziness** and **occurs** when a **pregnant woman lies on her back & resolves** when she is **turned on her side**[Q].
Management: • Patients should be placed in a **left lateral recumbent position**[Q].

159. Answer is None >a. 4 cm *(Ref: Williams 24/e p452)*

Partograph recording is usually started after a cervical dilation of 3 cm (not the 4 cm), i.e. the active stage of labor. As 3 cm is not given in the option, we have to choose 4 cm.

> "A partograph was designed by the World Health Organization (WHO) for use in developing countries. According to Orji (2008), the partograph is similar for nulliparas and multiparas. Labor is divided into a latent phase, which should last no longer than 8 hours, and an active phase. The active phase starts at 3 cm dilatation, and progress should be no slower than 1 cm/hr. A 4-hour wait is recommended before intervention when the active phase is slow. Labor is graphed, and analysis includes use of alert and action lines." - *Williams 24/e p452*

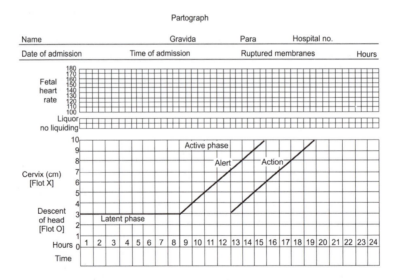

Partograph
• Partograph is a **composite graphical record of cervical dilatation in centimeters & descent of head against duration of labor in hours**[Q]. • **Introduce as an early warning system** to detect labour that was progressing normally, **for timely transfer to a referral center**[Q].
In a partograph the labor process is divided into
• **Latent phase** that **ends** when the **cervix is 3 cm dilated**[Q] • **Active phase starts with cervical dilation of 3 cm**. Cervix should **dilate at least 1cm/hour in this active phase**[Q]

- **Cervical dilation rate (cervicograph)** is **plotted in relation to alert line & action line**[Q].
- Concept of Alert line & Action line **given by Philpott**[Q]

Alert line	Action line
- Alert line **starts at the end of latent phase (3 cm cervical dilation)** & ends with full dilation of the cervix (10 cm) in 7 hours (1cm/hour dilation rate)[Q]	- Action line is **drawn four hours to the right of the alert line.** An interval of 4 hours is allowed to diagnose delay in active phase and then **appropriate intervention is done**[Q].

- **Labor** is considered **abnormal when cervicograph crosses the alert line & falls on zone 2**[Q].
- **Intervention is required** when it **crosses the action line & falls on zone 3**[Q].

PEDIATRICS

160. Ans. a. Macrocephaly   *(Ref: Nelson's 20/e p895)*

Fetal alcohol syndrome is associated with microcephaly rather than macrocephaly. Holoprosencephaly can occur in extreme forms of fetal alcohol syndrome along with midline hypoplasia.

"Fetal Alcohol Syndrome (FAS): No single malformation or characteristic malformation complex has been described in few cases of FAS in which neuropathology has been reported. The neuropathologic changes are varied and nonspecific and include microcephaly, hydrocephalus, leptomeningeal, white matter and periventricular neuroglial heterotopias, agenesis of corpus callosum and the cerebellar vermis, incomplete holoprosencephaly, and neural tube defects."
Neuropathology by Richard A. Prayson 2/e p460

Fetal Alcohol Syndrome (FAS)

- High levels of alcohol ingestion during pregnancy can be **damaging to embryonic & fetal development**
- **MC teratogen to** which **fetus** can be exposed: **Alcohol**

Features of Fetal Alcohol Syndrome	
- **Symmetric IUGR & postnatal growth deficiency (short stature**[Q]**)** - **Mental retardation**[Q] - **Microcephaly**[Q] - **Incomplete holoprosencephaly**[Q] - **Agenesis of corpus callosum and the cerebellar vermis**[Q] - Fine motor dysfunction - Behavioral abnormalities	- Irritability in infancy, **hyperactivity in childhood**[Q] - **Mid-face dysmorphism**[Q] (abnormal frontal lobe development), short palpebral fissures, maxillary hypoplasia, short nose, smooth philtrum, thin & smooth upper lip - **Joint abnormalities**: Abnormal position and/or function - **Cardiac anomalies: VSD >ASD**, tetralogy of Fallot[Q]

Teratogenic Drugs	
Drug/ Chemical Name	**Teratogenic Effect**
Alcohol	**Fetal alcohol syndrome**, congenital cardiac, CNS, limb anomalies, IUGR[Q]
ACE inhibitors (captopril, enalapril)	**Fetal toxicity** including **intrauterine renal insufficiency**[Q]
Amphetamines	Learning disability, motor incoordination, **hepatic calcification**[Q]
Androgens	**Cleft lip-palate, tracheoesophageal fistula**, CHD, masculinization[Q]
Barbiturates	**Abruption placentae**, **microcephaly**, limb defects, urinary tract malformations[Q]
Busulfan	**Corneal opacities, cleft palate, hypoplasia of ovaries, thyroid & parathyroid**[Q]
Carbamazepine	**Neural tube defects (Spina bifida)**[Q]
Carbimazole	**Scalp defects, choanal atresia, esophageal atresia**[Q]
Chloroquine	**Deafness** after prolonged use[Q]
Cocaine	**Microcephaly, IUGR**[Q]

Danazol	Virilization[Q]
Diazepam	**Cleft lip-palate**, apnea, hypothermia[Q]
Dicumarol	Bleeding, **depressed nasal bridge, stippling of phalanges, choanal atresia**; cardiac, renal & ophthalmic defects[Q]
Diphenylhydantoin	**Facial, cardiac & limb anomalies**[Q]
Folic acid antagonists (Aminopterin)	**CNS defects**, facial anomalies[Q]
Gentamicin	**Eighth nerve damage**[Q]
Heroin	**Intrauterine death, LBW, sudden infant death**
Indomethacin	**LBW, platelet dysfunction**
Iodides	**Hypothyroidism, goiter**[Q]
Lithium	**Ebstein's anomaly, macrosomia**[Q]
Misoprostol	**Moebius' syndrome**[Q]
Phenytoin	**Congenital anomalies, IUGR, neuroblastoma, bleeding**[Q] (Vitamin K deficiency)
Progestins	**Masculinization, advances bone age**
Quinine	**Deafness, thrombocytopenia**[Q]
Tetracyclines	**Yellow-brown discoloration of teeth, hypoplasia of enamel, retarded skeletal growth, congenital cataracts**[Q]
Thalidomide	**Phocomelia, deafness**[Q]
Tolbutamide	Fetal death, **thrombocytopenia**[Q]
Valproate	**CNS, cardiac & facial anomalies, limb defects**[Q]
Vitamin D (heavy dose)	**Supravalvular aortic stenosis, ventricular opacities, elfin facies**[Q]
Warfarin	**Fetal warfarin syndrome, fetal bleeding, hypoplastic nasal structures**[Q]

161. **Ans. b. It is the most common cause on nonsyndromic sensory neural hearing loss** *(Ref: Nelson 20/e p1592, 3074; Ghai 8/e p272)*

Asymptomatic congenital CMV infection is likely a leading cause of sensorineural hearing loss, which occurs in approximately 7-10% of all infants with congenital CMV infection, whether symptomatic at birth or not. The definitive method for diagnosis is virus isolation or PCR and not IgM antibody detection, which is non-specific and may be due to acquired CMV infection after birth.

"The most common infectious cause of congenital SNHL is cytomegalovirus (CMV), which infects 1/100 newborns in the USA."- Nelson 20/e p3074

"Asymptomatic congenital CMV infection is likely a leading cause of sensorineural hearing loss, which occurs in approximately 7-10% of all infants with congenital CMV infection, whether symptomatic at birth or not."- Nelson 20/e p1592

"Symptomatic congenital CMV infection was originally termed cytomegalic inclusion disease. Only 5% of all congenitally infected infants have severe cytomegalic inclusion disease, another 5% have mild involvement, and 90% are born with subclinical, but still chronic, CMV infection."-Nelson 20/e p1592

"The definitive method for diagnosis of congenital CMV infection is virus isolation or demonstration of CMV DNA by PCR, which must be performed during the 1st 2 weeks of life because viral excretion afterwards may represent infection acquired at birth or shortly thereafter. Urine and saliva are the best specimens for culture and saliva, and cord blood is best for PCR."-Nelson 20/e p1592

"Infections resulting from exposure to CMV in the maternal genital tract at delivery or in breast milk occur despite the presence of maternally derived, passively acquired antibody. Approximately 6-12% of seropositive mothers transmit CMV by contaminated cervical-vaginal secretions and 40% by breast milk to their infants, who usually remain asymptomatic and do not exhibit sequelae."-Nelson 20/e p1592

Congenital CMV Infection
• **Symptomatic congenital CMV infection** was originally termed **cytomegalic inclusion disease**[Q].
• **Severe** cytomegalic inclusion disease-**5%**; **Mild** involvement-**5%**; **Subclinical** chronic infection-**90%**

Cause:
- Congenital infections that are **symptomatic & most severe** & resulting in sequelae are **more likely to be caused by primary rather than reactivated infections in pregnant women**[Q].
- **Re-infection with a different strain** of CMV can lead to **symptomatic congenital infection**[Q].

Clinical Features:
- **Characteristic signs & symptoms** of clinically manifested infections: **IUGR, prematurity, hepatosplenomegaly & jaundice, blueberry muffin–like rash, thrombocytopenia & purpura, microcephaly & intracranial calcifications**[Q].
- **Other neurologic problems: Chorioretinitis, sensorineural hearing loss** & mild increases in CSF protein[Q].

> - **Asymptomatic congenital CMV infection** is likely a **leading cause of SNHL,** which occurs in **7-10% of** all infants with congenital CMV infection, **whether symptomatic at birth or not**[Q].

Diagnosis:
- **Definitive diagnosis**: By virus isolation or **demonstration of CMV DNA by PCR** (performed **during 1st 2 weeks of life**)[Q]
- **Urine & saliva** are **best specimens for culture**; saliva & cord blood is **best for PCR**[Q].

> - **IgG antibody test: Little diagnostic value** (positive result also reflects maternal antibodies); **Negative result excludes the diagnosis of congenital CMV infection**[Q].
> - **IgM tests lack sensitivity & specificity; unreliable for diagnosis of congenital CMV infection**[Q].

Treatment:
- **Ganciclovir prevents hearing deterioration & improves or maintains normal hearing function** at 6 months of age & may **prevent hearing deterioration** that occurs after 1 year of age[Q].

162. **Ans. d. Give Zinc supplementation and oral rehydration solution only and ask mother to come back if some danger signs develop** *(Ref: Ghai 8/e p293-294, 296, 755; IMNCI Guidelines; Nelson 20/e p1869-1874)*
The child in this given scenario is having some dehydration, as the child is restless and irritable, drink water readily and skin pinch goes back slowly (< 2 seconds) with sunken eyes. Treatment includes oral rehydration therapy, zinc supplementation and continued breastfeeding according to the WHO IMNCI protocol plan B.

Parameters	No Dehydration	Some Dehydration	Severe Dehydration
Appearance	Well, alert	Restless, irritable	Lethargic, or unconscious; floppy
Eyes	Normal	Sunken	Very sunken
Thirst	Drinks normally, not thirsty	Thirsty, drinks eagerly	Drinks poorly or not able to drink
Skin pinch	Goes back **quickly (<1 second)**	Goes back **slowly (1 second)**	Goes back **very slowly (≥ 2 seconds)**

WHO IMNCI Protocol Plan B for Some Dehydration
- Treat with **fluid & foods** along with **zinc supplementation**. Treat the child with **ORS solution**.
- **Breastfed children should continue breastfeeding**.
- Other children should receive their usual milk or some nutritious food after 4 hours of treatment with ORS.
- Advise mother when to **return immediately** if child develops **general danger signs**.
- Follow up in 5 days if not improving.

> - **Antibiotics, oral or intravenous is not required** in this patient. They are **indicated only if child is having bloody diarrhea, persistent diarrhea** or any other severe manifestation like **fever** or **pneumonia**.

AIIMS ESSENCE

Acute Diarrhea Management
• The **cornerstone of acute diarrhea management** is **rehydration by using oral rehydration solutions (ORS)**.

Principles of Acute Diarrhea Management
1. Correction of **dehydration, electrolytes & hypoglycemia**ℚ
2. **Evaluation for infections** using appropriate investigations and their management ℚ
3. **Nutritional therapy**ℚ

Physiological Basis for Oral Rehydration Therapy

- In most cases of acute diarrhea, **sodium & chloride are actively secreted from the gut mucosa** due to pathogen-induced dysfunction of several actively functioning absorption pumps.
- However, **glucose dependent sodium pump remains intact** and **functional transporting one molecule of glucose** and **dragging along a molecule of sodium** and **one of water across intestinal mucosa** resulting in repletion of sodium and water losses.

  - The **glucose dependent sodium & water absorption** is the **principle behind replacing glucose** and **sodium in 1:1 molar ratio in the WHO oral rehydration solution (ORS)**ℚ.
  - **Use of low osmolality ORS causes reduction of stool output, decrease in vomiting and decrease in the use of unscheduled IV fluids without increasing the risk of hyponatremia.**
  - For this reason, the **recommendation for use of standard WHO ORS** (having osmolarity of **311** mmol/l) **was changed to low osmolarity WHO ORS** (having osmolality of **245** mmol/l) ℚ

Home available fluids for Acute Diarrhea

• Fluids that contain salt (preferable)	• **Oral rehydration solution**
	• Salted drinks (e.g. Salted rice water or salted yoghurt drink)
	• Vegetable or chicken soup with salt
• Fluids that do not contain salt (acceptable)	• Plain water, water in which a cereal has been cooked (e.g. unsalted rice water), unsalted soup, yoghurt drinks without salt, green coconut water, weak unsweetened tea, unsweetened fresh fruit juice
• Unsuitable home available fluids	• Commercial carbonated beverages, commercial fruit juices, sweetened tea

Zinc Supplementation

- It is helpful in **decreasing severity & duration of diarrhea** and also **risk of persistent diarrhea**ℚ.
- Zinc is recommended to be supplemented as **sulphate, acetate or gluconate formulation**, at a dose of **20 mg** of elemental zinc per day for children >**6 months for a period of 14 days**ℚ.

---

163. Ans. b. ALL *(Ref: Wintrobes Clinical Hematology 12/e p1892-1908; Robbins 9/e p590-593)*

The given image is showing a classical image of a Lymphoblast, i.e. an abnormal immature cell with high nucleo-cytoplasmic ratio, prominent nucleoli and scant, agranular cytoplasm; typically seen in acute lymphoblastic leukemia (ALL).

"Compared with myeloblasts, lymphoblasts have more condensed chromatin, less conspicuous nucleoli, and smaller amounts of cytoplasm that usually lacks granules."- Robbins 9/e p592

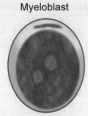

	Myeloblast	Lymphoblast
Size	Larger	Smaller
Cytoplasm	Moderate	Scanty
Auer rod	May be present	Absent
Nuclear chromatin	Fine	Coarse
Nucleoli	Prominent, 1-4	Indistinct

	Lymphoblasts	Myeloblasts
General characteristics	Blast population tends to be **homogenous**[Q]	Blast population tends to be **heterogenous**[Q], with the exception of the undifferentiated form
Size	Variable, **mainly small**[Q]	Variable **mainly large**[Q]
Nucleus	**Central, mainly round**[Q]; sometimes indented, particularly in the form in adults. **NC ratio very high** in the form occurring **in children**[Q]. **NC ratio lower** in the form occurring **in adults**[Q]	Tending to be **eccentric, round, oval or angulated**, sometimes convoluted, particularly in the form with a monocytic component. **NC ratio high** in **undifferentiated blast cells** and in some megakaryoblasts. **NC ratio mainly low** in the form with **differentiation**[Q]
Chromatin	Fine with dispersed condensation[Q]	Fine, granular, delicately dispersed[Q]
Nucleoli	Absent in small lymphoblasts[Q]	Almost always **present, large & prominent, double or triple**[Q]
Cytoplasm	Scanty, basophilic[Q]. Sometimes with a single long projection (hand-mirror cell)	Abundant in monoblasts. With **protrusions in erythroblasts & megakaryoblasts**[Q]
Granules	Rarely present, azurophilic. Always **negative for peroxidase, esterases & toluidine blue**[Q]	**Peroxidase in neutrophil & eosinophil lineages**. **Nonspecific esterase** in **monocyte lineage**[Q]. **Toluidine blue in the basophil lineage**[Q]
Auer rods	Always absent[Q]	Can be **present**. Typically present in **hypergranular promyelocytic form**[Q]
Vacuolation	Can be present[Q]	Can be present[Q]. Almost always present in forms **with a monocytic component**[Q]

Acute Lymphoblastic Leukemia (ALL)

- ALL is **neoplasms of immature B (pre-B)** or **T (pre-T) cells,** which are referred to as **lymphoblasts**
- B-ALLs (85%) typically manifest as **childhood acute "Leukemias"**[Q]
- T-ALLs tend to present in **adolescent males as thymic "lymphomas"**[Q]

Epidemiology:
- ALL: MC cancer of children[Q]; Peak Incidence: 3rd year[Q]; **Whites**> blacks; **Boys**>girls
- **Highest incidence in Hispanics**

> **Mature B-cell ALL** is an **uncommon type ALL**[Q] (1-2% of ALL cases) **in children.**

Pathology:
- **T-ALLs** have **gain of function mutations in NOTCH-1**[Q]
- **B-ALLs** have **loss of function mutations PAX5**[Q], **E2A**[Q] **& EBF**[Q], or **t(12;21)**[Q] involving genes **ETV6** & **RUNX1**, 2 genes that are needed in very early hematopoietic precursor.

Contd...

Acute Lymphoblastic Leukemia (ALL)

- **Mature B-cell ALL** is associated with **t(8;14)** & **over expression of the c-myc oncogene**
- **T-ALL are aggressive lymphomas**[Q]
- In **T-ALL**, cells are **positive for markers of blasts like-Tdt,**[Q] **CD34** & **T cell markers CD1, CD2, CD5, CD7**[Q]

Classification of ALL			
Immunologic Subtype	% of Cases	FAB Subtype	Cytogenetic Abnormalities
Pre-B ALL	75	L1, L2[Q]	t(9;22), t(4;11), t(1;19)
T-cell ALL	20	L1, L2[Q]	14q11 or 7q34
B-cell ALL	5	L3[Q]	t(8;14), t(8;22), t(2;8)

Clinical Features:

- **Abrupt stormy onset**; Symptoms related to **depression of marrow function**[Q]
- **Fatigue due to anemia; Fever due to neutropenia & Bleeding due to thrombocytopenia**[Q]

  - **Marrow expansion & infiltration of sub-periosteum: Sternal tenderness**[Q]
  - Generalized **lymphadenopathy, hepatosplenomegaly & testicular enlargement** due to **neoplastic infiltration**[Q]

- **CNS features:** headache, vomiting & nerve palsies due to meningeal spread

  - **T-ALL commonly presents with Mediastinal mass (Superior mediastinal syndrome)**[Q]

Diagnosis:

- **Hypercellular bone marrow** with **>20% lymphoblasts**[Q]
- Compared with myeloblasts, **lymphoblasts have more condensed chromatin, less conspicuous nucleoli & scanty agranular cytoplasm**[Q]
- Cytochemistry: **Myeloperoxidase (MPO)–ve, Sudan Black B (SBB)–ve**[Q]

FAB (French American British) Classification			
ALL-subtype	L1	L2	L3 (Mature B-cells)
• Morphology	• **Small homogenous blasts**[Q] • **Little cytoplasm**[Q] • **Regular nucleus** • **Small indistinct nucleoli**	• **Large heterogeneous blasts** • One or more nucleoli	• **Large homogenous blasts** • **Abundant basophilic cytoplasm** • **Prominent cytoplasmic vacuolation** • Resemble **Burkitt lymphoma**[Q]
• **Age group**	• **Children**	• **Adults**	• **Adults**
• **Prognosis**	• **Good**[Q]	• **Intermediate**[Q]	• **Poor**[Q]
• Cytochemistry	• **PAS+**	• **PAS+**	• **PAS-, SBB+**[Q]

- **Both B-cell ALL & Burkitt lymphoma** are characterized by **FAB L3**[Q] **morphology**

Prognostic Factors in ALL		
Determinants	Favorable	Unfavorable
WBC counts	<10 × 10^9/L (Low)[Q]	>200 × 10^9/L (High)[Q]
Age	3-7 years[Q]	<1 year, >10 years
Gender	Female[Q]	Male[Q]
Ethnicity	White[Q]	Black[Q]
Node, liver, spleen enlargement	Absent	Massive[Q]
Testicular enlargement	Absent	Present[Q]

Contd...

Acute Lymphoblastic Leukemia (ALL)		
Determinants	**Favorable**	**Unfavorable**
Central nervous system	Absent	**Overt (blasts + pleocytosis)**
FAB morphologic features L1	L1^Q	L2^Q
Ploidy	**Hyperdiploidy^Q**	**Hypodiploidy <45**
Cytogenetic markers	Trisomies 4, 10 and/or 17 t(12;21) (TEL-AML1)	t(9;22) (BCR-ABL) t(4;11) (MLL-AF4)
Time to remission	<14 days^Q	> 28 days^Q
DNA index	> 0.16^Q	< 0.16^Q
Immunophenotype	Early Pre-B cell	T cell

164. Ans. a. Prescribe oral antibiotics, warn of danger signs and send home *(Ref: IMNCI Guidelines, Ghai 8/e p755)*

This child is having fast breathing (respiratory rate >46/minute) without danger signs like lower chest wall indrawing or stridor. Hence, the child will be classified to have pneumonia (non-severe). So, the child should be prescribed appropriate antibiotic and advise mother about supportive measures and when to return for follow-up.

Fast breathing in children	
Age	**Respiratory rate**
<2 months	**> 60**/minute
2-12 months	**> 50**/minute
12 months-5 years	**> 40**/minute

Signs	**Classify as**	**Treatment**
Any general danger sign or Lower chest wall indrawing or Stridor in calm child	• **Severe pneumonia**	• **Refer urgently to hospital for injectable antibiotics & oxygen**, if needed • Give **first dose of appropriate antibiotic**
Fast breathing	• **Pneumonia**	• **Prescribe appropriate antibiotic** • **Advise mother about other supportive measures and when to return for a follow-up visit**
No fast breathing	• **Other respiratory illness**	• Advise mother about other **supportive measures** and when to return if symptoms persist or get worse

165. Ans. c. Staphylococcus aureus *(Ref: Nelson 20/e p2090; Harrison 19/e p958)*

The chest X-ray above is showing a pneumatocele in the right lung, which are most commonly seen in pneumonias caused by Staphylococcus aureus.

"Respiratory tract infections caused by S. aureus occur in selected clinical settings. S. aureus is a cause of serious respiratory tract infections in newborns and infants; these infections present with shortness of breath, fever, and respiratory failure. Chest x-ray may reveal pneumatoceles (shaggy, thin-walled cavities). Pneumothorax and empyema are recognized complications."-Harrison 19/e p958

"S. aureus pneumonia can be suspected on the basis of chest roentgenograms that reveal pneumatoceles, pyopneumothorax, or lung abscess."-Nelson 20/e p2090 .

Pneumatocele
• **Intrapulmonary air-filled cystic spaces** that can have a variety of sizes & appearances. • May contain air-fluid levels • Usually the result of **ventilator-induced lung injury in neonates** or **post-pneumonic^Q**.

Contd...

Contd...

Pneumatocele
Etiology: • **Majority as a result of pneumonia**[Q] (post-pneumatic pneumatocele). • **Causative agents: Staphylococcus aureus**[Q] **(MC)**, Streptococcus pneumoniae , Haemophilus influenzae , Escherichia coli, Group A streptococci, Klebsiella pneumoniae , Adenovirus , Primary pulmonary tuberculosis
Clinical Features: • Pneumatoceles are **typically asymptomatic** and, if secondary to pneumonia, remain **visible after septic symptoms have resolved**[Q]. • Occasionally, large pneumatoceles may **compress adjacent lung & mediastinum** enough to cause respiratory or cardiovascular symptoms.
Diagnosis: • **Diagnosed by chest X-ray**[Q] • When mature, pneumatoceles appear as **thin walled cystic spaces within the lung parenchyma, containing air.** • Tend to **appear within 1st week of infection** & usually **resolved by 6th week**[Q].   • **Features that make the diagnosis of a pneumatocele more likely than abscess: Smooth inner margins**; Contain little if any fluid; **Wall**, if visible, is **thin & regular**; **Persist despite of absence of symptoms**[Q].

ORTHOPEDICS

166. Ans. a. a *(Ref: Jaypee's Instrument and Operative Procedures (2013)/p117)*

Lane bone holding forceps (Option A)	Bone cutting forceps (Option B)	Periosteal elevator (Option C)	Babcock's forceps (Option D)
• Two-bladed instrument with a handle **for compressing or grasping tissues** in surgical operations	• **Strong & stout instrument** used for **cutting the bones**	• **Used to elevate the periosteum from the surface of bone** during removal of periosteum	• **Light & non-traumatic instrument** used to **hold delicate structures like bladder & bowel**

167. Ans. b. Neck *(Ref: Apley's 9/e p932; Campbell's Operative Orthopaedics 12/e p4201; Rockwood and Green's Fractures in Adults 7/e p525)*

Most common site of stress fracture or March fracture is second metatarsal neck.

"Metatarsal stress fractures are common in distance runners and ballet dancers. The second metatarsal neck is the most likely site for stress fractures, but all metatarsals are susceptible."-Rockwood and Green's Fractures in Adults 7/e p525

"Stress Injury (March Fracture): In a young adult (often a military recruit or a nurse) the foot may become painful and slightly swollen after overuse. A tender lump is palpable just distal to the midshaft of a metatarsal bone. Usually the second metatarsal is affected, especially if it is much longer than an 'atavistic' first metatarsal."- Apley's 9/e p932

"Military recruits in their first few weeks of training also are vulnerable to so called march fractures. Patients often note the gradual onset of pain directly over the second metatarsal neck region 2 to 4 weeks after beginning a running or aerobics program."- Campbell's Operative Orthopaedics 12/e p4201

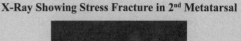

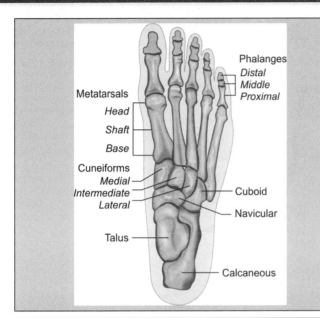

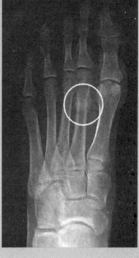

Stress Fracture
• A **stress or fatigue fracture** is one occurring **in the normal bone** of a healthy patient, due to **small repetitive stresses** of two main types: **bending & compression**. • Commonly occurs in **athletes** or **new military recruits**[Q] • **March fracture: Fatigue** or **stress fracture of metatarsals** often encountered in **military personnel**[Q].
Sites affected: • MC bones affected: Metatarsals >Fibula >Tibia[Q] • MC site: **2nd metatarsal neck**[Q]
Clinical features: • History of **unaccustomed & repetitive activity** or **one of a strenuous physical exercise** programme. • A **common sequence of events** is: *pain after exercise – pain during exercise – pain without exercise.* • Affected site may be swollen or red. It is sometimes **warm & usually tender**; the callus may be palpable. **'Springing' the bone** (attempting to bend it) is often **painful**.
Imaging: • **X-Ray:** Plain x-rays taken a **few weeks later** may show a **small transverse defect in the cortex** and/or **localized periosteal new-bone formation**.
MRI
• **The earliest changes, particularly in 'spontaneous' undisplaced osteoarticular fractures, are revealed by MRI**[Q]. • This investigation **should be requested in older patients (possibly with osteoporosis) complaining of sudden onset of pain over the anteromedial part of the knee**[Q].

Treatment:
• **Most stress fractures need no treatment** other than an **elastic bandage & avoidance of the painful activity** until the lesion heals
   • An **important exception** is **stress fracture of the femoral neck**. This should be **suspected in all elderly people** who **complain of pain in the hip** for which no obvious cause can be found.
   • If the **diagnosis is confirmed by bone scan**, the **femoral neck should be internally fixed with screws as a prophylactic measure.**

168. Ans. a. Brachial artery *(Ref: Apley 9/e p371, 760; Rutherford's Vascular Surgery 8/e p2497)*

The given X-ray is showing a supracondylar fracture. Most commonly injured vessel in supracondylar fracture is brachial artery.

*"The **brachial artery** is by far the most frequently injured upper extremity artery in children and damage to this vessel is frequently associated with a **supracondylar** humerus fracture, especially in younger children."- Rutherford's Vascular Surgery 8/e p2497*

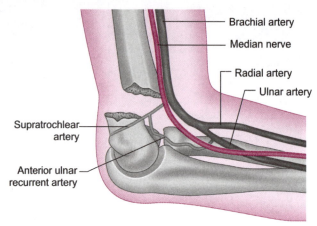

Fig. 34: Supracondylar fracture humerus

169. **Ans. d. Ankle**   *(Ref: Campbell's Operative Orthopaedics 12/e p3963; Apley's 9/e p617)*
     *Prominence of posterosuperior portion of calcaneus leading to heel pain is called **Haglund deformity**.*

"A Haglund deformity, or pump bump, is caused by chronic inflammation of the adventitious superficial pretendinous Achilles bursa that separates the Achilles tendon from the overlying skin."- Campbell's Operative Orthopaedics 12/e p3963

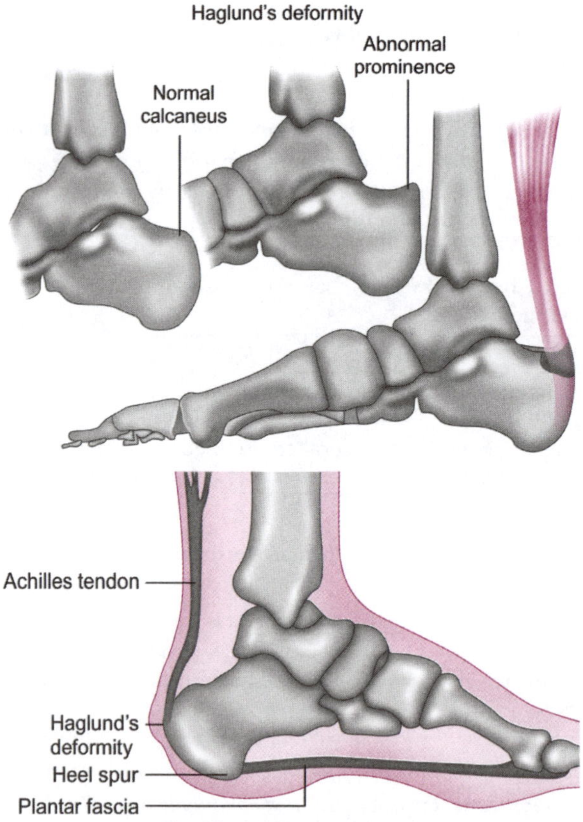

Fig. 35 : Haglund deformity

Haglund Deformity
• Caused by **chronic inflammation of adventitious superficial pretendinous Achilles bursa** that separates the Achilles tendon from the overlying skin.   • Known as **pump bump, achillodynia, retrocalcaneal bursitis, winter heel, cucumber heel**[Q]
Clinical Features: • Seen in young patients in **2nd & 3rd decade**   • Complain of **painful bumps** on the backs of their heels.   • **Posterolateral portion of calcaneum** is **prominent & shoe friction causes retrocalcaneal bursitis**[Q].   • Symptoms are **worse in cold weather** and when wearing high-heeled shoes
Diagnosis: • On Radiograph: **Bony prominence** on **posterosuperior aspect of calcaneal tuberosity**[Q]   • **MRI**: **Degenerative changes** within the **Achilles tendon**[Q].
Treatment: • Conservative: Attention to **footwear** (open-back shoes are best) & **padding of heel.**   • Operative: Removal of bump or dorsal wedge osteotomy of calcaneum

170. Ans. d. Interosseous membrane tear with triangular fibrocartilage complex (TFCC) tear and radial shaft fracture *(Ref: Apley's 9/e p790; Campbell's Operative Orthopaedics 12/e p1385)*

Galeazzi's fracture is a fracture of lower one-third of radius with dislocation of distal radioulnar joint. It is associated with tearing of interosseous membrane and triangular fibrocartilage complex (TFCC).

"Components of Distal Radioulnar Joint (DRUJ): The distal radius and ulna are linked to each other by the interosseus membrane, the capsule of DRUJ and the triangular fibrocartilage complex (TFCC). The triangular fibrocartilage plate is connected as its apex to the base of the ulnar styloid process and laterally to the inferomedial ridge of the radius. Its outer fibers blend with those of the ligaments around the ulnar aspect of the wrist. It has been proposed that major cause of dislocation and poor response to conservative management in Galeazzi fracture is because of injury to TFCC and interosseus membrane."

Galeazzi's Fracture
• It is a **fracture of lower one-third of radius with dislocation of distal radioulnar joint**[Q].
Mechanism of injury: • **Fall on the hand; Probably with a superimposed rotation force**[Q].   • **Radius fractures in its lower third & inferior radio-ulnar joint subluxates or dislocates**[Q].
Clinical features: • **More common** than Monteggia   • **Striking feature: Prominence or tenderness over the lower end of ulna**[Q]   • It may be possible to demonstrate the **instability of radio-ulnar joint** by 'ballotting' the distal end of the ulna ('piano-key sign') or by rotating the wrist[Q].
X-ray: • **A transverse or short oblique fracture** is seen in lower third of radius, **with angulation or overlap. Distal radio-ulnar joint is subluxated or dislocated**[Q].
Treatment: • **Perfect reduction is essential for complete restoration of all functions**; called **fracture of necessity** because **surgery is absolutely necessary**   • Restore the length of the fractured bone.   • **Children: Closed reduction is often successful**   • **Adults**: Reduction by open operation & compression plating of radius.

AIIMS ESSENCE

171. Ans. b. Shortened, abducted and externally rotated *(Ref: Apley's 9/e p848)*

The given X-ray is shows fracture neck of femur, which is common in older patients due to unsteadiness of gait and reduced bone mineral density. If the fracture is displaced, the attitude of limb is shortened, abducted and externally rotated.

"Femoral neck fractures are common in elderly patients with osteoporosis. The leg is shortened, abducted and held in external rotation."-Emergency Medicine by Jahn Ma 2/e p597

"Femoral Neck Fractures: Examination reveals a markedly shortened, abducted, significantly rotated lower limb."-Textbook of Adult Emergency Medicine By Peter Cameron 4/e p188

Femoral Neck Fractures: With partially or completely displaced fractures, the patient will present with severe pain and lie with the extremity in a slightly shortened, abducted and externally rotated fashion."- Musculoskeletal Imaging By Thomas Pope/p294

Fracture Neck of Femur (Intracapsular Fracture)

- **MC site of fractures in elderly: Fracture neck of femur**[Q]
- Femoral neck fractures are a **subset of proximal femoral fractures**. Femoral **neck** is the **weakest part**[Q] of femur.
- Femoral neck fractures are considered **intracapsular fractures** (also called **proximal femoral fractures**).

Mechanism of Injury:
- **MC mechanism in elderly** is due to **fall**[Q].
- In **young patients**, significant **high force trauma**[Q] (e.g. motor vehicle collisions) is required.

Risk Factors:
- **Osteoporosis, osteomalacia, diabetes, stroke** (disuse), **alcoholism & chronic debilitating disease**[Q].
- In addition, **old people** often have **weak muscles & poor balance** resulting in an **increased tendency to fall**[Q].

Pathology Anatomy & Classification:
- Femoral neck fractures are prone to **avascular necrosis & slow union**[Q]
- Classification according to **level of fracture line in the neck: Subcapital; Transcervical: Basicervical**[Q]
- **In children,** proximal femoral fractures are classified as per **Delbert's classification; transcervical fracture is most common**[Q].
- **Evans** and **Boyd & Griffin classification** are used for **intertrochanteric fracture**[Q].

Subcapital	Transcervical	Basicervical
• Femoral head & neck junction	• Mid-portion of femoral neck	• Base of femoral neck

Garden Classification[Q] (According to Degree of Displacement)	
Non-displaced	**Displaced**
• **Grade I: Incomplete** or **valgus impacted** fracture[Q] • **Grade II: Complete fracture without bone displacement**[Q].	• **Grade III: Complete fracture with partial displacement** of fracture fragments[Q]. • **Grade IV:** Complete fracture with **total displacement** of fracture fragments[Q].

Classification of Subcapital Fractures	
Pauwels Classification[Q]	**Linton Classification**[Q]
• **Type I:** Obliquity ranging from **0 to 30°** • **Type II:** Obliquity ranging from **30 to 50°** • **Type III:** Obliquity of **≥ 70°**	• **Stage I: Incomplete** • **Stage II: Complete** but **undisplaced** fracture • Stage III: Complete, **partially displaced** fracture • Stage IV: **Displaced & totally free** fracture

Fracture Neck of Femur (Intracapsular Fracture)

Clinical Features:

- **History of a fall in elderly person** (osteoporotic females) followed by **pain in the hip & inability to walk**[Q]
- **Pain in groin**[Q] (in **femoral triangle area**); **Tenderness**[Q] over anterior & lateral aspects of hip joint[Q].

> - In **displaced fracture, leg is shortened, abducted & held in external rotation**[Q].

- **Greater trochanter** is **elevated**[Q] on the injured side.
- **All movements** are **extremely painful**[Q] except in the rare case of an impacted type of fracture.
- With an **impacted fracture** the **patient may still be able to walk**
- Femoral neck fractures **in young adults** result from **road traffic accidents** or **falls from heights** and are often **associated with multiple injuries.**

Diagnosis:

- Diagnosis can be made by **pelvic X-ray & MRI**[Q]
- **Occult fracture neck of femur** is diagnosed by **MRI**.

Treatment:

- **Surgery within 24 hours**[Q] is the **treatment of choice**

Patients Age	Treatment Option
<60 years	• **Open reduction & internal fixation** under radiological control using **multiple cancellous screws**[Q] (MC method) or **dynamic hip screw**[Q].
>60 years	• **Hemiarthroplasty**[Q] (removing the head of femur & replacing it by metal prosthesis like Austin-Moore's[Q] prosthesis). • This enables the patient to be ambulant & start early weight bearing
> 60 years with pre-existing hip arthritis	• **Total hip replacement**[Q]

- After surgery, **early ambulation** to **prevent DVT** & **decubitus ulcers**[Q]

Complications:

- **Avascular necrosis:** in **30%** of **displaced** fractures & **10%** of **undisplaced** fractures
- **Non-union: 30%** of all fractures
- **Osteoarthritis**

---

172. Ans. b. Recurrent shoulder dislocation *(Ref: Apley's 9/e p354; Rehabilitation of the Hand and Upper Extremity By Terri M. Skirven 6/e p1189)*

Most common sequelae of traumatic shoulder dislocation in young adults are recurrent shoulder dislocation. Anterior dislocation Type 1 is the most common type of traumatic shoulder dislocation and its most common sequelae in young adults is recurrent dislocation in around 1/3rd patients. In fact, more than 90% patients < 20 years have some shoulder instability as sequelae.

> *"The mechanism of injury for traumatic anterior dislocations is usually falls, trauma, atheletic injuries, or domestic or work inuries, typically with the arm in an abducted and externally rotated position. Recurrent instability is the most common complication after traumatic anterior shoulder dislocation. The rate of recurrence has been reported to range from less than 25% to approaching 100%, and is related to the patients age at the time of dislocation, patient sex, the degree of trauma and capsulolabroligamentous injury, bony lesions including Hill-Sachs lesions, anteroinferior glenoid rim fractures, greater tuberosity fractures, rotator cuff tears and presence of neurological injury. In one study, 21 patients who were younger than 13 years all had recurrent anterior dislocations, suggesting that younger age at the time of initial dislocation correlated with a higher recurrence rate of persistent disability."- Rehabilitation of the Hand and Upper Extremity By Terri M. Skirven 6/e p1189*

Anterior Dislocation of Shoulder	
• **Shoulder** is the **MC joint to undergo recurrent & /or nonrecurrent (traumatic) dislocation**[Q].	
• **Anterior dislocation** is the **MC type of shoulder dislocation**[Q] accounting for ~ 97% of cases.	
• **Subcoracoid**[Q] is the **MC subtype.**	

Mechanism of Injury:
- Two type of injury may lead to it:
  - **External rotation or horizontal abduction force on humerus**[Q] this movement occurs in throwing ball or slapping.
  - **Direct posterior or posteriorlateral blow on shoulder** e.g. a fall on elbow directed backward & outward.
- In young patients **lesion of anterior capsule is most commonly an avulsion of labrum from front of glenoid & neck of scapula (Bankart's lesion)**[Q].

Pathology (in recurrent cases):
- **Bankart's lesion** is **stripping off fibrocartilage labrum from anterior glenoid & neck of scapula**[Q].
- **Hill Sachs lesion** is **compression fracture of posterolateral humeral head**[Q] due to impression (friction) of glenoid rim, which occurs during repeated dislocation.

Clinical Features:
- Reproduction of patient's symptom in a position of **abduction, external rotation and extension**[Q].
- Patient keeps his arm **slightly abducted hanging by the side of body**[Q].
- Normal round contour of shoulder is lost & it becomes flat.
- Fullness/bulge is seen below the clavicle

Dugas test	• It is **not possible for the patient to bring the elbow close to the body** & put the hand on his opposite shoulder[Q].
Callaway's Test	• In dislocation **vertical circumference of axilla is increase compared to the normal side**[Q].
Hamilton ruler test	• Because of **flattening of shoulder**, it is **possible to place a ruler on the lateral side of arm and it touches acromian & lateral condyle of humerus simultaneously** (in normal it would not due to shoulder contour)[Q].

- **AP X-ray** show **overlapping shadow of humeral head & glenoid fossa**; and later view show humeral head out of line with the socket.

Management:
- Commonly used reduction techniques are **stimson's gravity method, Hippocratic method and Kocher's method**[Q].

Kocher's method[Q]	• Reduction, in general (by **Kocher's method**) is done by increasing the deformity by traction and then doing opposite movements. • So the steps of reduction are **traction in slight abduction & external rotation to increase deformity followed by adduction and internal rotation**[Q].
Stimson's method	• Patient is **left prone with the arm hanging over the side of bed**. Thus weight of limb helps in reduction.
Hipprocatic method	• In Hipprocatic method, **gently increasing traction & counter traction is applied.**

173. **Ans. a. Tension band wiring** *(Ref: Apley 9/e p887-888)*

The given X-ray shows displaced transverse fracture of patella, which is treated by tension band wiring.

*"Displaced transverse fracture: The lateral expansions are torn and the entire extensor mechanism is disrupted. **Operation is essential.** Through a longitudinal incision the fracture is exposed and the **patella repaired by the tension-band principle. The fragments are reduced and transfixed with two stiff K-wires; flexible wire is then looped tightly around the protruding K-wires and over the front of the patella.** The tears in the extensor expansions are then repaired. A plaster back-slab or hinged brace is worn until active extension of the knee is regained; either may be removed every day to permit active knee-flexion exercises."- Apley 9/e p888*

174. Ans. a. Internal rotation *(Ref: Gray's 41/e p132; Apley 9/e p496)*

The examiner here is trying to move the leg of the patient at the hip joint along a longitudinal axis. There is internal rotation at the hip when the ankle is bent outwards and knee inwards.

Movement	
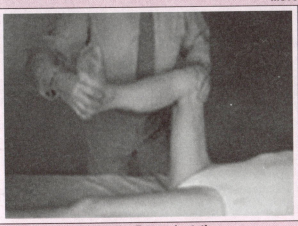	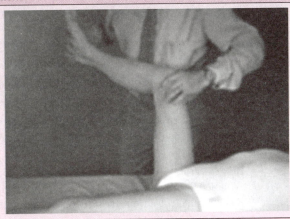
Testing for External rotation	Testing for internal rotation

- To test rotation, both the legs lifted by the ankles are rotated first internally (medially) and then externally (laterally). The patellae are watched to estimate amount of rotation
- **Rotation in flexion is tested with the hip & knee, each flexed 90°.**
- **If internal rotation is full with the hip extended, but restricted in flexion**, this suggests **pathology in the anterosuperior portion of the femoral head** probably **avascular necrosis** (the so called **'sectoral sign'**).
- In **young person, pain on internal rotation with the hip flexed** may indicate a **torn acetabular labrum**.
- Internal rotation is checked by rotating the foot laterally in flexion position of hip and knee joint. Range of motion is 40°.
- External rotation is checked by rotating the foot medially. Normal range of motion is 45°.

Movement		
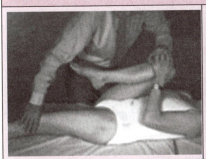	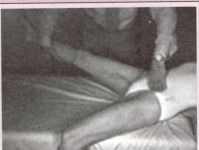	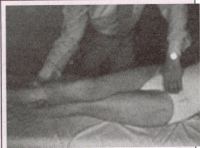
Forcing one hip into full flexion will straighten out the lumbar spine	Testing for abduction. The pelvis is kept level by placing the opposite leg over the edge of the examination couch with that hip also in abduction (the examiner's left hand checks the position of the anterior spines) before abducting the target hip.	Testing for adduction.

175. Ans. c. Ochronosis *(Ref: Harrison 19/e p2172, 434e-4; Apley 9/e p82)*

Positive Schober's test and Diffuse skeletal hyperostosis (DISH) and intervertebral disk calcification as seen in the set of X-rays here can be seen in various spondyloarthropathies like ankylosing spondylitis (AS) as well as other less-common metabolic, infectious, and malignant causes of back pain. It includes infectious spondylitis, spondylodiscitis, and sacroileitis, and primary or metastatic tumor. Ochronosis can produce a phenotype that is clinically and radiographically similar to AS. Along with low back pain, presence of hyperpigmented nose and ears point towards ochronosis.

AIIMS ESSENCE

"Alkaptonuria may go unrecognized until middle life, when degenerative joint disease develops. Prior to this time, about half of patients might be diagnosed for the presence of dark urine. Foci of gray-brown scleral pigment and generalized darkening of the concha, anthelix, and, finally, helix of the ear usually develop after age 30. Low back pain usually starts between 30 and 40 years of age. Ochronotic arthritis is heralded by pain, stiffness, and some limitation of motion of the hips, knees, and shoulders. Acute arthritis may resemble rheumatoid arthritis, but small joints are usually spared. Pigmentation of heart valves, larynx, tympanic membranes, and skin occurs, and occasional patients develop pigmented renal or prostatic calculi. Pigment deposition in the heart and blood vessels leads to aortic stenosis necessitating valve replacement, especially after 60 years of age."- Harrison 19/e p2172, 434e-4

Alkaptonuria (AR)

- **Autosomal recessive disease** due to **deficiency of homogentisic acid oxidase[Q]**.
- Alkaptonuria is characterized by **appearance of homogentisic acid in the urine, dark pigmentation of connective tissues (ochronosis) and calcification of hyaline & fibrocartilage**

Pathology:

- **Inborn error: Absence of homogentisic acid oxidase in liver & kidney.**
- With deficiency of this enzyme **homogentisic acid accumulate, polymerizes** and gets **deposited at various sites as black pigment- Ochronosis[Q]**.

Clinical features:

- Patients usually remain **asymptomatic until the 3rd or 4th decade**
- Patients present with **low back pain & stiffness of spine** and (later) **larger joints.**

Ochronotic Arthritis[Q]

- **Black pigment deposition** in **intervertebral discs of vertebra[Q]**
- Later knee, shoulder & hips are affected
- **Small joints of hand & feet are spared[Q]**

- **Black ochronotic pigmentation** in **sclera (between cornea & canthi), ear & nose cartilage[Q]**.

- **Pigmentation** of **heart valves, larynx, tympanic membranes & skin** occurs[Q]
- Occasional patients develop **pigmented renal** or **prostatic calculi[Q]**.

- **Pigment deposition** in **heart & blood vessels** leads to **aortic stenosis** necessitating **valve replacement**, after 60 years of age.
- **Clothes** may become **stained by homogentisic acid** in the sweat.

Diagnosis:

- **Urine turns black on standing[Q]** especially when **pH of urine is alkaline.**

- **X-rays: Narrowing & calcification of intervertebral discs** at multiple levels & **spinal osteoporosis**
- **Later stage: Large peripheral joints** may show **chondrocalcinosis & severe osteoarthritis.**

Treatment:

- Administration of **vitamin C or ascorbic acid[Q]** prevents oxidation of homogentesic acid
- Otherwise **no specific therapy**

OPHTHALMOLOGY

176. Ans. a. Ptosis *(Ref: Kanski's 8/e p40; Parson's 22/e p460)*

Ptosis is drooping of the upper lid to a level that covers more than 2 mm of the superior cornea. Ptosis is generally unilateral, in over 70% of individuals.

"Ptosis: This is drooping of the upper lid to a level that covers more than 2 mm of the superior cornea. Ptosis is generally unilateral, in over 70% of individuals. This may be due to hypoplasia or dystrophy of the levator palpebrae superioris and has been shown to be associated with anomalies of the genes PTOS1, PTOS2, and ZFH-4. Elevation of the upper lid is largely a function of the levator palpebrae superioris, assisted by the frontalis and Muller muscle. Ptosis is the term given to a drooping of the upper lid, usually due to paralysis or defective development of the levator palpebrae superioris."-Parson's 22/e p460

Proptosis	<ul><li>An **abnormal protrusion of the globe** is called **exophthalmos or proptosis**.</li><li>**Exophthalmos:** Reserved for describing the prominence of eyes secondary to thyroid disease</li><li>**Proptosis:** Used to signify a **protrusion of eyeball due to all other causes**.</li><li>**Causes: Space-occupying lesions** within the orbit, **herniation or extension** of cranial or sinus contents into the orbit.</li></ul>
Lagophthalmos	<ul><li>Characterized by **incomplete closure of palpebral aperture** when an attempt is made to shut the eyes.</li><li>Due to **contraction of lids from cicatrization** or a **congenital deformity, ectropion, paralysis of orbicularis, proptosis** due to exophthalmic goitre, orbital tumour</li></ul>
Entropion	<ul><li>**Rolling inwards of the lid margin** is called entropion</li><li>Produced by a **disparity in length & tone between anterior skin- muscle** and **posterior tarsoconjunctival laminae of eyelid**.</li></ul>

Ptosis

- Ptosis is drooping of upper lid to a level that covers **>2 mm of superior cornea**[Q].
- **Unilateral in over 70% of individuals.**
- Associated with anomalies of genes **PTOS1, PTOS2 & ZFH-4.**
- Ptosis is usually due to **paralysis or defective development** of **levator palpebrae superioris**[Q] (Elevation of upper lid is largely a **function of levator palpebrae superioris, assisted by frontalis & Muller muscle**)

Classification of Ptosis

Congenital	Acquired
<ul><li>**Simple**</li><li>**Complicated:** associated with ocular motor anomalies, blepharophimosis syndrome & Marcus Gunn ptosis</li></ul>	<ul><li>**Neurogenic**: Oculomotor nerve palsy, Horner's syndrome, Marcus Gunn jaw winking syndrome, 3rd cranial nerve palsy.</li><li>**Myogenic**: Oculopharyngeal muscular dystrophy, Myasthenia gravis, myotonic dystrophy, ocular myopathy, simple congenital ptosis & blepharophimosis syndrome.</li><li>**Aponeurotic**: Involutional (LPS weakness) or post-operative.</li><li>**Mechanical**: Edema or tumors of the upper lid.</li></ul>

Management:
- **Surgery is the treatment of choice** and is **carried out between 3 and 5 years of age** if the **ptosis is partial**[Q], but if the visual axis is covered at least a temporary procedure should be carried out as soon as possible to avoid sensory deprivation amblyopia.
- **Type of surgery performed** is determined by **amount of ptosis, levator action & associated anomalies** such as a **Marcus Gunn phenomenon**[Q].

Ptosis			
Surgical Treatment of Various Types of Ptosis			
Ptosis surgery	**Requisite levator action**	**Amount of ptosis that can be treated**	**Indications**
Fasanella-Servat[Q]	Good	<2 mm	**Horner syndrome**[Q]
Levator resection — anterior approach[Q]	Moderate	Any	**Larger resections** in congenital or acquired ptosis
Levator resection— conjunctival approach[Q]	Moderate	Any	**Moderate** congenital or acquired ptosis
Levator resection with aponeurotic reinsertion	Moderate	Any	**Acquired** ptosis[Q]
Frontalis suspension[Q]	Poor	>2 mm	**Congenital**-especially **Marcus Gunn ptosis** or for **temporary relief**[Q]

177. Ans. a. After cataract *(Ref: Yanoff and Duker 4/e p407; Kanski's 8/e p294; Parson's 22/e p285)*

Greyish white opacities seen in the given picture are called as Elschnig pearls and are suggestive of secondary cataract or after cataract.

*"**Posterior capsular opacification (PCO)**, also called **'after' or 'secondary' cataract**, is the **opacity which follows extracapsular extraction of the lens**. In this operation the posterior and part of the anterior capsule are left in situ. In many cases these remnants are fine, forming a thin membrane which is difficult to see, particularly following operation with modern suction and infusion devices. In other cases, especially **when the cataract was not mature, some soft, clear cortex sticks to the capsule. This becomes partially absorbed by the action of the aqueous but often becomes shut off by adhesion of the remains of the anterior to the posterior capsule.** In such cases the cubical cells which line the anterior capsule also persist; they continue to fulfill their function of forming new lens fibres, although those formed under these abnormal conditions are abortive and opaque. **Sometimes these fibres, enclosed between the two layers of capsule, form a dense ring behind the iris (the ring of Sommerring)**; it may cause subsequent trouble by becoming dislocated into the anterior chamber. **At other times, the subcapsular cells proliferate and instead of forming lens fibres, develop into large balloon-like cells which some-times fill the pupillary aperture (Elschnig pearls).** If these remnants lie in the pupillary area a dense membrane is formed so that vision is impaired. If the previous operation has been followed by iritis, exudates also adhere to the lens remnants and organize, thus contributing a fibrous membrane in addition." -Parson's 22/e p285*

*"**The basic pathogenic factor of the Sommerring's ring is the anterior capsular break, which may then allow exit of central nuclear and cortical material out of the lens, with subsequent Elschnig pearl formation.**" - Yanoff and Duker 4/e p407*

Types of 'After' Cataract			
Anterior Capsular Opacification	**Posterior capsular opacification**	**Sommerring ring**	**Elschnig pearls**
Irvine-Gass syndrome	<ul><li>Also known as **pseudophakic cystoid macular edema** or **post-cataract CME**</li><li>One of the most common **causes of visual loss after cataract surgery**</li><li>**Typical time of onset: 3–4 weeks post-operatively**</li><li>**Predisposing factors**: Intraoperative complications (e.g. **vitreous loss or severe iris trauma**), **vitreous traction** at the wound, **diabetic retinopathy** & pre-existing epiretinal membrane.</li></ul>			

Endophthalmitis	• **Most dreaded postoperative complication** • **Early onset within 7 days** and commonly caused by **Staphylococcus aureus** • Presents with **pain, redness, corneal edema, corneal exudates, hypopyon** & vitritis with low IOP.
Uveitis-Glaucoma-Hyphema (UGH) Syndrome	• Complication of **intraocular chafing from intraocular lens (IOL) implants** leading to a spectrum of **iris transillumination defects** & pigmentary dispersion to microhyphemas & hyphemas with elevated IOP. • Characterized by **chronic inflammation, CME, secondary iris neovascularization, recurrent hyphemas & glaucomatous optic neuropathy** leading to a loss of vision. • Result of **mechanical irritation of anterior segment structures** from an intraocular lens. • Patients often present with **intermittent decreased or blurred vision, intermittent white-out of vision, photophobia, redness** & ocular pain in the involved eye. • **Patient's ocular discomfort** may be **out of proportion to ocular findings.** • **Raised IOP**, microhyphema or hyphema, anterior chamber cell & flare or **hypopyon, iris neovascularization, iris-lens contact, iris transillumination defects**, dislocated or malpositioned IOL, misplaced haptic, vitreous hemorrhage if the posterior capsule is not intact, and or CME may be seen. • **Surgical intervention** is often required as definitive treatment.

Secondary Cataract or Posterior Capsule Opacification (PCO)

- **MC postoperative complication** of cataract surgery[Q]
- Occurs at a rate between **3–50% in the first 5 postoperative years**[Q].

  - **PCO** results from **migration & proliferation of residual lens epithelial cells (LECs) onto the central posterior capsule.** When the **cells invade the visual axis as pearls, fibrotic plaques, or wrinkles**, the patient experiences a **decrease in visual function**, and ultimately in **visual acuity**[Q].

- **Epithelium of crystalline lens** consists of a sheet of **anterior epithelial cells ('A' cells)** that are in continuity with the cells of **equatorial lens bow ('E' cells).** The latter cells comprise the germinal cells that undergo mitosis as they peel off from the equator. They constantly form new lens fibers during normal lens growth.
- The **'A' cells**, when disturbed, tend to **remain in place** & not migrate. They are **prone to a transformation into fibrous-like tissue.**

  - In contrast, **in pathologic states**, the **'E' cells of equatorial lens bow tend to migrate posteriorly along the posterior capsule**; e.g. **in posterior subcapsular cataracts** & pearl form of PCO. In general, instead of undergoing a fibrotic transformation, they tend to **form large, balloon-like bladder cells** (the **cells of Wedl**).
  - These are the cells that are **clinically visible as 'pearls' (Elschnig pearls)**. These **equatorial cells** are the **primary source of classic secondary cataract**, especially the **pearl form of PCO.**

- The **'E' cells** are also those **responsible for formation of** a **Sommerring's ring**, which is a **doughnut-shaped lesion composed of retained/ regenerated cortex**[Q] and cells that may form following any type of disruption of the anterior lens capsule. This lesion was initially described in connection with ocular trauma.

  - **Basic pathogenic factor of Sommerring's ring** is the **anterior capsular break**, which may then **allow exit of central nuclear & cortical material out of the lens, with subsequent Elschnig pearl formation**[Q].
  - A **Sommerring's ring**[Q] forms every time any form of extracapsular cataract extraction **(ECCE) is done,** whether manually, automated, or with phacoemulsification (phaco). For practical purposes it is useful to **consider this lesion as the basic precursor of classic PCO, especially the 'pearl' form**[Q].
  - The **LECs have higher proliferative capacity in the young** compared with the old, therefore, the **incidence of PCO formation is higher in younger patients**[Q].

178. Ans. a. Suprachoroidal hemorrhage *(Ref: Kanski 8/e p637; Yanoff and Duker 4/e p1157)*

Suprachoroidal hemorrhage is a bleed into the suprachoroidal space from ruptured posterior ciliary vessels. It doesn't cause hypotony maculopathy.

Hypotony Maculopathy
• Hypotony maculopathy is **low IOP associated with chorioretinal folds near macula, optic nerve head edema & vessel tortuosity[Q].**
• May occur after **ocular inflammation, trauma, or surgery[Q].**
• MC cause: Glaucoma filtering surgery; Mitomycin C increases the risk[Q].

Causes of Hypotonic Maculopathy			
Postoperative Hypotony	Traumatic Hypotony	Bilateral Hypotony	Miscellaneous forms of Hypotony
• **Mitomycin C** toxicity of the ciliary body[Q] • **Overfiltration[Q]** • **Bleb leak** [Q] • **Wound leak** [Q] • **Iridocyclitis[Q]** • **Cyclodialysis[Q]** • **Ciliochoroidal detachment[Q]** • Retinal detachment	• **Scleral perforation[Q]** • **Retinal detachment[Q]** • **Cyclodialysis[Q]** • **Iridocyclitis[Q]** • **Ciliochoroidal detachment[Q]**	• Osmotic dehydration • Diabetic coma • Uremia • Myotonic dystrophy	• **Ciliary body hypoperfusion[Q]** from vascular occlusive disease

Clinical Features:
- Patient typically presents with **loss of central vision & distortion** as well as **relative hyperopia** due to reduction of anteroposterior diameter of eye.
- **Clinical Examination: Optic nerve swelling** associated with **folding of retina & choroid** in posterior pole; Macular fold often radiates outward from fovea.

Diagnosis:
- **Low IOP[Q]**
- **Fluorescein angiography: Chorioretinal folds & differentiate choroidal folds** from retinal folds; Characteristic findings include an **irregular increase in background choroidal fluorescence** producing a **series of fluorescent streaks** corresponding to the crest of choroidal folds[Q]

Management:
- **Conservative:** Aqueous suppressants, topical antibiotics, corticosteroids
- **Surgical intervention** is undertaken immediately in cases of trauma, including scleral rupture or retinal detachment.

179. Ans. a. Tonometry *(Ref: Yanoff and Duker 4/e p56, 1021; Kanski's 8/e p307; Parson's 22/e p127)*

The process shown in the image is applanation tonometry, using Goldmann's tonometer. The applanation tonometer is used to measure intraocular pressure. It relies on the principle that for an ideal, dry, thin-walled sphere, the pressure inside a sphere is proportional to the force applied to its surface.

"An applanation tonometer is more accurate than an indentation tonometer and is based on the Imbert-Fick principle. Instead of measuring the amount of indentation, the applanation tonometer assesses the amount of force needed to flatten or applanate a known area of the cornea. In this process, the factor of ocular rigidity is offset by an induced capillary force acting in the opposite direction."- Parson's 22/e p127

Applanation Tonometer
• Applanation tonometer is **used to measure intraocular pressure.** It relies on the principle that **for an ideal, dry, thin-walled sphere, pressure inside a sphere is proportional to the force applied to its surface.**
• Based on Imbert–Fick principle (force necessary to applanate a perfectly elastic, infinitely thin, dry sphere divided by the area flattened ($P = F/A$) equals the pressure inside the sphere)

Applanation Tonometer

- Tonometer's head is applied to the surface of cornea and a variable force is applied using a sensitive spring system regulated by a dial. The dial is turned in either direction until the inner edges of the two semicircles, which are visualized using a **cobalt blue light**
- Examiner then reads the value on the dial (expressed in mmHg) to determine the IOP.
- **IOP measurements with Goldmann tonometer** are limited by presence of **corneal astigmatism >3 diopters**. This potential error can be **avoided by using average of two measurements taken 90° apart** (vertical & horizontal axes at right angles) or by aligning the tonometer biprisms so that the red line on the prism holder is opposite to the known corneal axis of least astigmatism.
- **Perkins & Draeger tonometer**: A modified version of Goldmann tonometer, portable and used when the patient is supine.

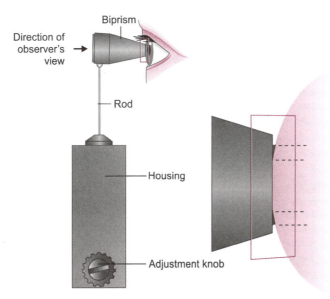

Fig. 36: Goldman applanation tonometry
(A-i: Basic features of tonometer; A-ii: Enlargement of A shows tear film meniscus created by contact of biprism and cornea)

Pachymetry	Ophthalmic B-Mode Ultrasound	Laser interferometry
• Used for **assessment of central corneal thickness** (CCT). • Ultrasound pachymetry is **easy, portable** & **most widely used method of measuring CCT**	• B-scan ultrasonography is an important adjuvant for clinical assessment of various ocular & orbital diseases. • B-scan is a **two dimensional imaging system** which utilizes high frequency sound waves ranging from **8-10 MHz**. • 'B' stands for **bright echoes**.	• **Used for high precision measurements** (distance, angles etc). • It uses very small, stable & accurately defined wavelength of laser as a unit of measure. • **Optical coherence tomography** (OCT) is a medical imaging technique **using low-coherence interferometry to provide tomographic visualization of internal tissue microstructures.**

AIIMS ESSENCE

Tonometers	
Tonometers	
Indentation	**Applanation**

• **Measures amount of deformation of globe**
• **Affected by scleral rigidity**
• Example: **Schiotz**
	• Measures flattening
	• Based on Imbert fick law
	• **Two types:**
	  – **Variable force (Goldman)**
	  – **Variable area (Maklakov)**

Types of Tonometers	

• **Goldmann: Gold standard**
• **Perkins: Hand held** tonometer
• **Draeger**: Portable and counter balanced
• **Pulsair: Non-contact type**, sterilization not required
• **Mackay-Marg: Useful for scarred/irregular cornea; Accurate over soft contact less as well**
• **Tono-pen:** Hand held form of Mackay Marg
• **Pneumatic tonometer:** Also useful for scarred or edematous cornea.
	• **Maklakov:** Variation in applanation surface, **constant force rather than constant area application used.**
	• **Dynamic contour tonometry (Pascal):**
	  – Based on a totally different principle that by surrounding & matching the contour of a sphere, pressure outside equals pressure inside.
	  – **Advantage: Not affected by corneal thickness**
	• **Diaton tonometer: Pen like handheld device, non-contact type.**

Rebound Tonometer/Impact-Rebound Tonometer
• A new **handheld tonometer**, the **Icare tonometer** is able to measure IOP without the use of topical anesthetic. • IOP is determined by measuring the force produced by a small plastic probe as it rebounds from the cornea. • The rebounded tonometer has been shown to have similar accuracy to the Tono-Pen, and it is comparable with Goldman for IOPs over a reasonable range in adults.

> • **Icare tonometer proven valuable as a screening tool in children[Q].**
> • **Ability to evaluate IOP without use of topical anaesthesia potentially provides the opportunity to monitor IOP at home[Q].**

180. **Ans. a. Bitemporal hemianopia** *(Ref: Gray's 41/e p1992; Parson's 22/e p506, 508; Kanski's 8/e p820; Yanoff and Duker 4/e p911)*

Interruption of the optic chiasma will lead to bitemporal homonymous hemianopia because optic chiasma contains crossed over medial fibers from both optic nerves, which are responsible for temporal field of vision.

> *"Hemianopia denotes loss of half of the field of vision. The commonest clinical form is homonymous hemianopia, in which the right or left half of the binocular field of vision is lost, owing to loss of the temporal half of one field and the nasal half of the other. This condition is due to a lesion situated in any part of the visual paths from the chiasma to the occipital lobe. A focus of disease in this area causes loss of vision of the corresponding halves of each retina (hence the designation homonymous) and therefore loss of the opposite halves of the visual fields."-Parson's 22/e p506*

> *"Lesions of the optic chiasma: Bitemporal hemianopia is usually caused by tumours in the region of the sella turcica, pressure by a suprasellar aneurysm or by chronic arachnoiditis; these press upon the chiasma, so that the fibres going to the nasal halves of each retina are destroyed. Tumours of the pituitary body are most common; but suprasellar tumours, particularly craniopharyngiomata derived from Rathke pharyngeal pouch and suprasellar meningiomata must be considered. Other lesions are gliomas of the third ventricle, ectopic pinealomas, dermoid tumours and third ventricular dilatation due to obstructive hydrocephalus."- Parson's 22/e p508*

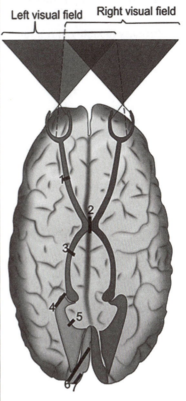

ENT

181. Ans. d. Respiratory papillomatosis *(Ref: Dhingra 7/e 345, 6/e p305; Scott-Brown 7/e p1176)*

Most likely diagnosis in a 5 years old child who present with gradually progressive hoarseness in voice for the last 2 weeks with worsening hoarseness for 3 months and stridor for 2 weeks is respiratory papillomatosis. Acute epiglottitis and croup usually present with fever and acute illness. Vocal nodule develops after voice abuse.

Juvenile Papilloma (Recurrent Laryngeal Papillomatosis or Recurrent Respiratory Papillomatosis)
• Disease of **viral origin**[Q] characterized by presence of **multiple recurrent papillomas in the larynx**[Q] • Common in **anterior part of glottis**[Q], especially **anterior commissure**[Q] (MC site: **Vocal fold**[Q]) • More common in children **<5 years of age**[Q], equally common in males & females • **First born vaginally delivered child** of a **teenage mother** is most prone (**Vertical transmission**[Q])
Etiology: • Associated with **HPV infection (HPV-6 & HPV-11)**[Q] • **HPV-11: More aggressive disease** & more prone to malignant change.
Pathology: • **Multiple sessile or pedunculated papilloma, friable & bleed on touch**[Q]
Transmission: • The exact mode is not known. • **Recognized association** between **maternal genital warts** (condylomata acuminata) & **recurrent laryngeal papillomatosis** both conditions being caused by HPV-6 & HPV-11.
Clinical Features: • **Presenting features: Hoarseness & abnormal cry**[Q] • **Dyspnea, stridor**[Q] & eventually complete airway obstruction may occur.

Juvenile Papilloma (Recurrent Laryngeal Papillomatosis or Recurrent Respiratory Papillomatosis)
Treatment: • **Surgery: Primary modality of treatment**[Q]   • **Endoscopic surgical removal** is the **preferred treatment**[Q]   • **CO$_2$ laser**: MC used modality[Q]   • **Recurrence is common** and multiple procedures are often required[Q]

Other Treatments Options	
• Systemic interferon • Photodynamic therapy • Intralesional injection of antiviral drug (cidofovir)[Q]	• Interferon alpha-2a • 13-cis-retinoic acid

Prognosis:
- **More severe in juvenile onset disease** as compared to adult onset
- **Remission** of recurrent papillomatosis may take place **at any time; more likely to undergo remission in larynx (48%)** than in tracheobronchial tree
- **Malignant transformation is rare** but may be seen (**squamous cell carcinoma**).

182. **Ans. c. Internal carotid artery**   *(Ref: Dhingra 7/e p201; 6/e p194; Scott-Brown 7/e p1602)*

Surgical ligation of vessels or embolization is the last resort to control epistaxis when all other methods fail. Internal carotid artery is not ligated in case of epistaxis control, as it is the main vessel supplying the central nervous system.

"Endoscopy identifies the source of posterior epistaxis in over 80 percent of the cases. Ligation should be performed as close as possible to the likely bleeding point. Thus the hierarchy of ligation is: Sphenopalatine artery; internal maxillary artery; external carotid artery; anterior/posterior ethmoidal artery."-Scott-Brown 7/e p1602

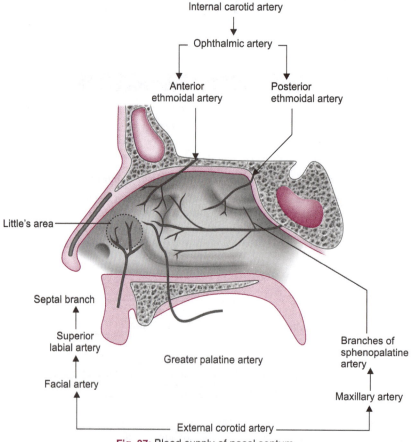

Fig. 37: Blood supply of nasal septum

Surgical Management of Epistaxis

- Surgical treatment is often **performed endoscopically** and can include **ligation of sphenopalatine** or **anterior ethmoid artery**[Q].
- **Angiographic embolization**[Q] is increasingly common, with results that approximate those of surgical treatment.
- The rate of severe complications (e.g. stroke, blindness) with embolization is approximately four percent.

Arterial Ligation

- **Choice of specific vessel** or vessels to be ligated **depends on the location of epistaxis**[Q].
- **External carotid artery**[Q]: Usually ligated just **distal to superior thyroid artery**[Q].
- **Internal maxillary artery**[Q]: It is closer to bleeding site, hence more chances of success (lesser collaterals). The internal maxillary artery and 3 of its terminal branches (i.e. sphenopalatine, descending palatine, pharyngeal) are elevated with nerve hooks, then clipped.
- **Sphenopalatine artery**[Q] at its exit from the sphenopalatine foramen.
- **Ethmoidal artery**[Q]: If bleeding occurs high in the nasal vault, consider ligation of anterior ethmoidal artery, posterior ethmoidal artery, or both.

183. Ans. c. Ohngren's line *(Ref: Hamilton Bailey Physical Signs 19/e p338; Dhingra 7/e p233, 6/e p207)*

Ohngren's line is a line that connects the medial canthus of eye to the angle of mandible.

Ohngren's line

- **Ohngren's line** is a *line that* **connects the medial canthus of** *eye to the* **angle of mandible**.
- The line **defines a** *plane orthogonal* **to a** *sagittal plane that* **divides the** *maxillary sinus into* **anterior-inferior part & superior-posterior part.**
- Tumours that arise **in anterior-inferior part, i.e. below Ohngren's line**, generally have a **better prognosis** than those in the other group.

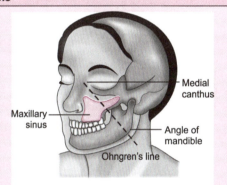

Sebileau's line	Frankfurt's line	Donaldson line
• **Sebileau's lines dividing the sino-nasal area in regions & sites.** • **Horizontal Sebileau's line** in the **Lederman's classification divides the structure into superior structure, mesostructure & inferior structure.**	• **Skull is oriented** so that the **inferior margins of orbits and superior margins of external acoustic meatus are horizontal**. This is known as **Frankfurt plane** and the **line joining them** is known as **Frankfurt line.**	• **Anatomical landmark used in endolymphatic sac surgery is Donaldson's line.** • This is an **imaginary line drawn posteriorly from the course of horizontal semicircular canal.** • The line should **course perpendicular to posterior semicircular canal.** • **Endolymphatic sac is located inferior to this line.**
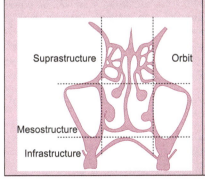	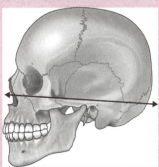	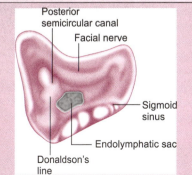

184. **Ans. a. Otosclerosis** *(Ref: Scott-Brown's 7/e p3185; Dhingra 7/e p96, 6/e p29)*

Most likely diagnosis is otosclerosis as the given audiogram shows conductive pattern of hearing loss (BC >AC) with Carhart's notch, a dip in bone conduction at 2,000 Hz is seen.

Audiometry in Otosclerosis	
<ul><li>**Conductive hearing loss** occurs in otosclerosis[Q] **(BC >AC)**</li><li>**Impedance audiometry**: Patients with **early disease** may show **type A tympanogram**[Q]</li><li>**Progressive stapes fixation** results in **As type curve**[Q]</li><li>**Acoustic reflex**: It is one of the **earliest sign of otosclerosis** & precedes the development of an air-bone gap[Q]</li><li>In **early stages of otosclerosis**, a **characteristic diphasic on-off pattern** is seen in which there is a **brief increase in compliance at the onset and the termination of stimulus** occurs. This is pathognomic for otosclerosis[Q].</li><li>In later stages, stapedial reflex is absent[Q].</li><li>**Carhart's notch: A dip in bone conduction at 2,000 Hz**[Q]</li></ul>	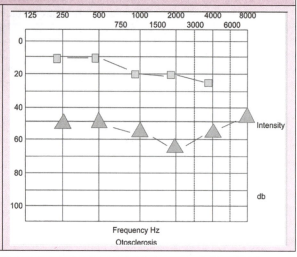

Symbols Used in Audiogram
<ul><li>**Blue line for left ear**[Q]</li><li>**Red line for right ear**[Q] (Remember **R-R**)</li><li>**Continuous line** for **air conduction**[Q]</li><li>**Broken line for bone conduction**[Q] (Remember **B-B**)</li></ul>

Audiogram Key

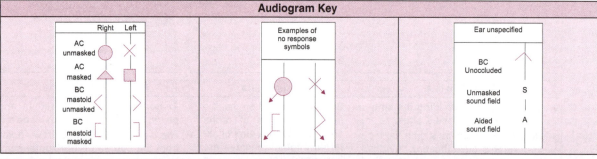

Audiogram		
Normal hearing	**Conductive hearing loss**	**Sensorineural hearing loss**
<ul><li>This is the **PTA graph seen in normal persons.**</li><li>In normal persons, **hearing threshold values with both air & bone remain between 0 and 10 dB**</li></ul>	<ul><li>Sound cannot properly conduct through outer and/or middle ear to reach the normal-hearing cochlea</li><li>**AC thresholds** will be **abnormal in presence of normal BC thresholds** in **disorders of outer and/or middle ear only**</li><li>Air-bone gap ≥15 dB difference between AC & BC</li><li>In the graph, **bone-air gap is seen** which means a **patient can hear by bone under 10-20 dB,** while with **air hearing is much below,** depending on severity, indicating **conductive hearing loss.**</li></ul>	<ul><li>**SNHL: Disorder of inner ear and/or auditory nerve**</li><li>**AC thresholds will be equal to BC thresholds (no air-bone gap)** & both will be abnormal</li><li>Both **bone & air conduction** value are **decreased** and may **even overlap each other.**</li><li>In this graph air-bone is not seen. Thus in SNHL, air bone gap is <15-20 dB.</li></ul>

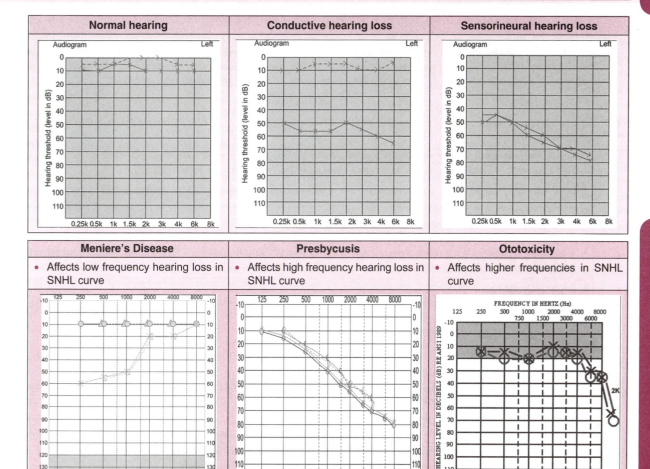

SKIN

185. **Ans. c. Due to IgG against hemidesmosomes** *(Ref: Harrison 19/e p370, 18/e p426-428; Fitzpatrick 7/e p432-441; Rooks 8/e p40.27, 13.19, 10.12-10.28)*

Skin as well as mucosal involvement in this patient, along with Fishnet pattern seen in DIF points towards a diagnosis of Pemphigus vulgaris. Pemphigus vulgaris is caused by IgG antibodies against Desmoglein 1 and 3, and there is intercellular IgG and complement deposition in fishnet pattern. IgG against hemidesmosomes and deposition in the basal layer is seen in Bullous pemphigoid.

Disorder	Immunofluorescence	Pattern	Target antigen
Pemphigus vulgaris	Intercellular, intraepidermal[Q]	IgG, fish net[Q]	Desmoglein 3[Q] (Mucosal type) Desmoglein 3 & 1[Q] (Mucocutaneous type)
Pemphigus foliaceus	Intercellular, intraepidermal[Q]	IgG, fish net[Q]	Desmoglein 1[Q]
Paraneoplastic pemphigus	Intercellular and subepidermal[Q]	IgG, fish net[Q]	Plakins (desmoplakin, envoplakin, periplakin, BP 230)
Bullous pemphigoid	Basement membrane zone[Q]	IgG, linear[Q]	BP230 > BP180
Herpes gestationalis	Basement membrane zone[Q]	IgG, linear[Q]	BP230 > BP180
Dermatitis herpetiformis	Dermal papillae[Q]	IgA, granular[Q]	(?) Epidermal tissue trnasglutaminase[Q]
Linear IgA disease	Basement membrane zone[Q]	IgA, linear[Q]	BP180

AIIMS ESSENCE

186. Ans. c. Pemphigus vulgaris *(Ref: Harrison 19/e p370, 18/e p426-428; Fitzpatrick 7/e p432-441; Rooks 8/e p40.27, 13.19, 10.12-10.28)*

Histopathological image shown above is showing a suprabasal split between the keratinocytes and basal layer. The attached basal keratinocytes give an appearance of 'Tomb stoning'. These findings are characteristically seen in Pemphigus vulgaris. Acantholytic cells can be seen at higher power in the blister cavity and the edge of blister.

See Q. No. 185 AIIMS May 2017

187. Ans. c. Metronidazole *(Ref: Harrison 19/e p1409; Goodman Gilman 12/e p1420; Paniker's Parasitology 6/e p41; Jawetz 27/e p713)*

History of vaginal itching and green frothy genital discharge in a young female with strawberry vagina on examination is highly suggestive of Trichomoniasis. The drug of choice for Trichomoniasis is metronidazole.

"Metronidazole remains the drug of choice for the treatment of trichomoniasis."- Goodman Gilman 12/e p1420

Trichomonas Vaginalis
• **Trichomonas vaginalis** is an **anaerobic, flagellated protozoa, exists only as a trophozoite (no cyst stage**[Q]**)**
• It has **four free flagella** that arise from a single stalk and a **fifth flagellum**, which forms an **undulating membrane**[Q].
• **MC pathogenic protozoan infection** of humans **in industrialized countries.**
Life Cycle and Epidemiology:
• **T. vaginalis** is a **pear-shaped, actively motile organism**, replicates by **binary fission**, and **inhabits the lower genital tract of females & urethra & prostate of males**.
• **Sexual transmission** accounts for virtually all cases of trichomoniasis.
• **Prevalence is greatest** among persons with **multiple sexual partners**
Clinical Manifestations:
• Many **men** infected with T. vaginalis are **asymptomatic**, although some **develop urethritis, epididymitis or prostatitis.**
• **Women: Usually symptomatic** & manifests with **malodorous vaginal discharge (often yellow), vulvar erythema** & itching, dysuria or urinary frequency & dyspareunia[Q].
• **'Frothy', greenish vaginal discharge** with **a 'musty' malodorous smell** is **characteristic**[Q].
• **Vaginal walls** are **tender** with **multiple small punctuate strawberry spots on the vaginal vault & portio vaginialis of cervix** known as **strawberry vagina**[Q].
Diagnosis:
• Detection of **motile** flagellated **trichomonads by microscopic examination of wet mounts of vaginal or prostatic secretions** has been the **conventional means of diagnosis.**
• Culture done on **Feinberg-Whittington media**[Q]
• **Classically, with a cervical smear**, infected women have a **transparent 'halo' around their superficial cell nucleus**[Q].
• **T. vaginalis** was traditionally diagnosed via a **wet mount, in which 'corkscrew' motility was observed**[Q].
• **Direct immunofluorescent antibody staining** is **more sensitive (70–90%)** than wet-mount examinations.
• A new **NAAT, APTIMA**, is **FDA approved and is highly sensitive & specific for urine** and for endocervical & vaginal swabs from women.
Treatment:
• **DOC: Metronidazole**[Q] **(tinidazole** is also effective)
• **All sexual partners must be treated concurrently to prevent reinfection**, especially from asymptomatic males.

188. Ans. a. KOH mount *(Ref: Fitzpatrick 8/e p2284-2285, 7/e p1811-1814; Roxburgh's 17/e p41)*

Kerion and Favus, which are types of Tinea infections often, cause scarring alopecia and present as scaly plaques with itching. Investigation of choice is KOH mount to look for fungal filaments.

Tinea Capitis
• **Dermatophytosis of scalp** & associated hair[Q]
• **Most commonly caused by Microsporum canis > Trichophyton tonsurans** (never caused by Epidermophyton)

Contd...

Contd...

Clinical features:
- Most commonly found in **pre-pubertal children** between **3 to 14 years** of age[Q]; Rare in adults
- Characterized by **patchy alopecia**[Q]

Classification:
- **Ectothrix pattern:** Fungus grows completely **within** the **hair shaft**, replacing the intrapilary keratin, leaving the **cortex (cuticle surface) intact**[Q].
- **Endothrix pattern:** Infection establish in perifollicular stratum corneum, spreading around and into the hair shaft. **Cortex (cuticle surface)** is **breached**[Q].

Non-inflammatory Types (Causing Non-scarring Alopecia)	
Black Dot (Endothrix pattern)	**Gray Patch (Ectothrix)**
• **Organism: Trichophyton violaceum & Trichophyton tonsurans**[Q] • **Multiple black dots** are seen with **non-scarring hair loss**[Q] • **Hair becomes weak & breaks right at the surface of scalp; Broken tips** are seen as **black dots**[Q]	• **Organism: Microsporum canis**, M. ferrugineum, M. audouinii[Q] • **Characterized by grey patch** (grey coloured areas of alopecia with scales) **& broken hair**[Q] (breaking 3-4 mm above scalp surface)

Inflammatory Types (Causing Scarring Alopecia)	
Kerion (either ectothrix or endothrix pattern)	**Favus (Endothrix with air spaces inside hair)**
Organism: Trichophyton mentagrophytes & T. verrucosum, Microsporum canis[Q] Characterized by **boggy inflammatory tender mass studded with broken hairs, follicular orifice oozing with pus & easily pluckable hairs**[Q] Pruritus, pain, fever, **occipital & posterior cervical lymphadenopathy & scarring alopecia** may occur[Q].	**Organism: Trichophyton schoenleini**[Q] Presence of **foul smelling yellowish cup shaped crusts (scutula) entangling many scalp hair**[Q]. Often results in **cicatricial alopecia**[Q].

Diagnosis:
- **Diagnosis** is made by first examining **scale & hair** on microscope slide in **potassium hydroxide (KOH) wet mount**. It is **single most important test for diagnosis**[Q].

Treatment:
- **Drug of choice: Oral griseofulvin**[Q] (if species is not mentioned)

Drug of choice in Tinea Capitis	
Microsporum species	• **Oral griseofulvin**[Q]
Trichophyton species	• **Oral terbinafine**[Q]

189. Ans. c. Trichotillomania *(Ref: Rook's 9/e p86.17-86.1; Fitzpatrick 6/e p735)*

Patchy hair loss in young female for 2 weeks without scarring or erythema as given in the picture is highly suggestive of trichotillomania.

*"Trichotillomania (Greek, "hair pulling madness") is a common, but difficult to manage, **cause of focal scalp hair loss**. It is classified as an **impulse control disorder in which patients pull, pluck, or cut their hair**. Clinical presentation is usually quite distinctive, with a **confluence of very short sparse hairs within an otherwise normal area of the scalp**. Microscopic examination of the ends of cut or plucked hairs generally reveals either the tapered tips of newly regrowing anagen hairs or bluntly cut hairs. (A hair pull here is usually negative because the telogen hairs have generally all been dislodged). The differential diagnosis includes alopecia areata and tinea capitis, and because patients generally deny any role in the hair loss, these usually need to be definitively ruled out. A scalp biopsy can be diagnostic, showing the characteristic increase in the number of catagen hairs (rarely seen in biopsies of normal scalp), trichomalacia, and melanin within the follicular canal secondary to traumatic hair removal and the absence or sparsity of a perifollicular inflammatory infiltrate."- Fitzpatrick 6/e p735*

Contd...

Trichotillomania (TTM)
• **TTM** is a common, but difficult to manage, **cause of focal scalp hair loss**[Q].   • It is classified as an **impulse control disorder**[Q] in which **patients pull, pluck, or cut their hair**[Q].   • Patients have an **irresistible urge to pluck hair**[Q] resulting in **localized or full alopecia** of scalp

Characteristic Features:
 • Clinical presentation is usually quite distinctive, with a **confluence of very short sparse hairs within an otherwise normal area of the scalp**[Q].
 • Plucking causes **hair shaft fractures.** Some **hair** are broken **short & some long** leading to **"varying lengths of hair inside area of hair loss"** [Q]
 • **Hair is never completely lost in patch**[Q]
 	
         • **Orentreich/Friar-tuck/Tonsure sign:** Loss of central area hair (easier to pull) with **sparing of margins of scalp**[Q]
         • **Microscopic examination** of ends of cut or plucked hairs generally reveals either **tapered tips of newly regrowing anagen hairs or bluntly cut hairs**[Q].

Diagnosis:
 • **Scalp biopsy can be diagnostic**[Q]
 	
         • Characteristic **increase in number of catagen hairs** (rarely seen in biopsies of normal scalp)
         • **Trichomalacia & melanin within** the **follicular canal secondary to traumatic hair removal**[Q]
         • **Absence** or **sparsity of a perifollicular inflammatory infiltrate**[Q]

Treatment: • **Behavior modification** in children   • Adolescents & adults (**primarily females**) are **reluctant to accept the diagnosis** & require **psychological intervention and/or medication** to help modify their behavior (**Clomipramine** may be particularly effective).

190. **Ans. c. Rifampicin (450 mg) + Dapsone (50 mg) + Clofazimine (150 mg) monthly and 50 mg alternate days** *(Ref: Neena Khanna 4/e p267, National leprosy eradication program (nlep.ni.in)*

The clinical history fits the patient into multibacillary leprosy and requires extensive multidrug therapy for 12 months. Since the patient is aged 12 years, doses are Rifampicin (450 mg) + Dapsone (50 mg) + Clofazimine (150 mg) monthly and 50 mg alternate days.

Feature	Paucibacillary (PB)	Multibacillary (MB)
Skin lesions	• **1–5** lesions	• **>5**
Peripheral nerve involvement	• **No nerve/only one nerve** with or without 1 to 5 lesions	• **>1 nerve** irrespective of number of skin lesions
Skin smear	• **Negative** at all sites	• **Positive** at any site

Leprosy Regimen			
Type	**Drugs Used**	**Duration**	**Follow-up**
Adult MB Leprosy	• **Rifampicin: 600 mg once a month** supervised • **Clofazimine: 300 mg once a month** supervised & **100 mg on alternate days** or **50 mg daily** self-administered • **Dapsone: 100 mg once a month** supervised with **100 mg daily** self-administered	**12 months** (12 blister packs)	Once a year for **5 years**

Contd...

Contd...

Type	Drugs Used	Duration	Follow-up
Child (ages 10-14) MB Leprosy	• **Rifampicin: 450 mg once a month** supervised • **Clofazimine: 150 mg once a month** supervised & **50 mg on alternate days** • **Dapsone: 50 mg once a month** supervised with **50 mg daily** self-administered	**12 months** 12 blister packs)	Once a year for **5 years**
Child (ages 6-9) MB Leprosy	• **Rifampicin: 300 mg once a month** supervised • **Clofazimine: 100 mg once a month** supervised & **50 mg twice weekly** • **Dapsone: 25 mg once a month** supervised & **50 mg daily** self-administered	**12 months** (12 blister packs)	Once a year for **5 years**
Adult PB Leprosy	• **Rifampicin: 600 mg once a month** supervised • **Dapsone: 100 mg daily** self-administered • (For adults with body weight <45 kg, dose of rifampicin should be 450 mg once monthly & dapsone 50 mg daily)	**6 months** (six blister packs)	Once a year for **2 years**
Child PB leprosy	• **Rifampicin: 300 mg (0-5 years)** or **450 mg (6-14 years) once a month** supervised • **Dapsone: 25 mg (0-5 years)** or **50 mg (6-14 years)** daily	**6 months** (six blister packs)	Once a year for **5 years**

Note
• The appropriate dose for **children <10 years** of age can be **decided on the basis of body weight**. [**Rifampicin: 10 mg/kg body weight, clofazimine: 1 mg/kg body weight daily and 6 mg/kg monthly, dapsone: 2 mg/kg body weight daily.**] The standard child blister pack may be broken up so that the appropriate dose is given to children under 10 years of age. Clofazimine can be spaced out as required. • Rarely, it may be considered advisable to **treat a patient with a high bacillary index (BI) for >12 months**. This decision may only be taken by specialists, at referral units, after careful consideration of the clinical & bacteriological evidence.

191. Ans. d. Congenital melanocytic nevus   *(Ref: Bolgonia Dermatology 3/e p1873)*

The lesion seen is clearly a hyperpigmented lesion, and is present since birth. The lesion looks hairy as well, hence most likely to be a congenital melanocytic nevus.

• **Hematoma**	• Not present at birth & not associated with hypertrichosis • Resolves with time
• **Melanoacanthoma**	• Present in patients **>40 years** as **hyperpigmented verrucous plaques on the face & trunk**
• **Epidermal verrucous nevi**	• **Not hyperpigmented;** Has a **warty surface** and **follows Blaschko's line**

Congenital Melanocytic Nevi
• **Derived from epidermal melanocytes & nevus cells** have a **predilection for deeper penetration**. • **Present at birth**; May be single, but is most often multiple.

Types of Congenital Melanocytic Nevi (CMN)		
Small	**Medium Sized**	**Large or Giant**
• Size: <1.5 cm	• Size: 1.5–19.9 cm	• Size: ≥20 cm

Contd...

Contd...

Congenital Melanocytic Nevi

Characteristic Features:
• **Usually solitary, color** varies from **brown to black**; lesions usually **darken & enlarge with age**[Q]
• **Located in** the area of **head & neck 15%** of the time (can occur anywhere on the body)
    • Bathing trunk nevus (Size >20 cm): Higher malignant potential[Q]
    • With age, the lesions also become **raised & develop rugosities** (cerebriform appearance[Q]).
• **Coarse hair develops on 90%** of the lesions and may have a **vortex distribution**[Q].
• **Larger lesions** may have **satellite lesions at the periphery**[Q].
    • As compared with a melanocytic nevus, congenital melanocytic nevi are **usually larger in diameter** and may have **excess terminal hair**, a condition called **hypertrichosis**[Q].

Complications: • **Malignant potential**, especially if large • **Meningeal involvement & spina bifida**, seen in lesions located over vertebral column.
Treatment: • **Surgical excision** is the standard of care. • Some individuals advocate the use of hair removal laser for the treatment of congenital nevi.

192. Ans. a. Atopic dermatitis *(Ref: Fitzpatrick 8/e p165, 7/e p147; Rooks 7/18.1-30; Harrison 19/e p344)*

Most probable diagnosis in this child, who presents with itchy and hyperpigmented plaques in cubital and popliteal fossa is atopic dermatitis.

> *"Atopic Dermatitis (AD): The clinical presentation often varies with age. Half of patients with AD present within the first year of life, and 80% present by 5 years of age. About 80% ultimately co-express allergic rhinitis or asthma. The infantile pattern is characterized by weeping inflammatory patches and crusted plaques on the face, neck, and extensor surfaces. **The childhood and adolescent pattern is typified by dermatitis of flexural skin, particularly in the antecubital and popliteal fossae.**"- Harrison 19/e p344*

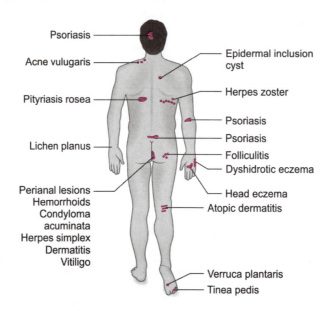

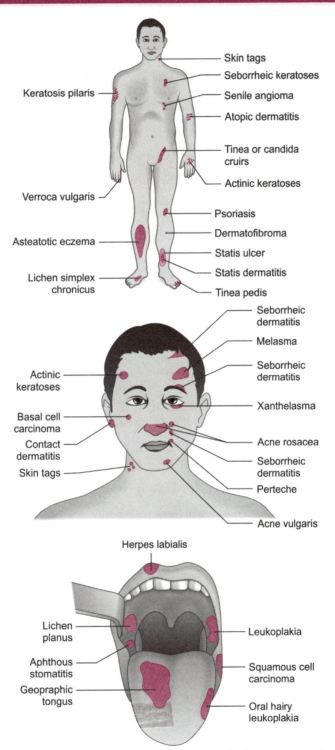

Fig. 38: Distribution of some common dermatologic diseases and lesions

Atopic dermatitis (AD)
• AD is a **cutaneous expression of the atopic state**, characterized by a **family history of asthma, hay fever or dermatitis**[Q] in ~ 70% of patients.

Contd...

Contd...

Atopic dermatitis (AD)

Etiopathogenesis:
- **Genetic predisposition**: When **both parents are affected, over 80%** and when only one parent is affected ~50% of their children manifest the disease
- **Increased IgE synthesis; increased serum IgE; increased specific IgE** to food, aeroallergens, bacteria & bacterial products.
- **Increased expression of CD23** (low affinity IgE receptor) on monocyte & B- cells
- **Impaired delayed type hypersensitivity reactions.**

Clinical Presentation:
- The clinical presentation varies with the age, **half of the patients present within the first year of life, & 80% presents by 6 years of age**[Q].

> - **Infantile pattern is characterized by** weeping inflammatory patches & crusted plaques that occur on face, neck & extensor surfaces (Infantile eczema)[Q]
> - **Childhood & adolescent pattern** is marked by **dermatitis of flexural skin** particularly in **antecubital & popliteal fossa**[Q].

- Clinical course lasting longer than **6 weeks**[Q].
- AD **may resolve spontaneously**, but over half of affected children will have dermatitis in adult life, i.e. **course is marked by exacerbation & remissions**.

Pruritus and Scratching made worse by	
- **Environmental alterations** - **Denny Morgan fold**[Q] (Extra-fold of skin beneath lower eyelid).	- Change in temperature, sundry (In rainy season) & rough (woolen) clothing and leading to **excoriation, lichenification, dryness.**

- **Increased tendency for vasoconstriction** like **perioral pallor & white dermatographism**[Q].

Atopic dermatitis Associated with	
- **Alopecia areata**[Q] - **Susceptibility to skin infections**[Q], - **Antenna sign** (Follicular openings are filled with horny plugs)	- **Head light sign** (Inflammation of skin on and around lips) - **Hertoghe's sign** (Thinning of lateral half of eyebrows)

Clinical Phase of Atopic Dermatitis		
Infantile phase	**Childhood phase**	**Adult phase**
- Rarely starts before 4-6 weeks of age & usually **begins between 2-3 months**[Q] of age - **First begin on face**[Q] & may quickly spread to other areas. Although, often then **napkin area is relatively spared**[Q], as a result of area being kept moist. - **Excoriation & lichenification** appear at about 6 months of age, when the ability to scratch develops - **Initially the disorder involves flexural distribution**. But when the child starts to crawl, **exposed extensor aspect of knees, are most involved**[Q].	- From **one & half to two years onwards**[Q] - Most characteristically involve **elbow & knee flexures**[Q], wrist & ankle. - Sides of neck show a reticulate pigmentation known as **atopic dirty neck.** - **Uncommon extensor distribution & inability to lichenify**[Q] (even after prolonged rubbing) are very difficult to treat and take longer time to remit.	- **Lichenification, especially of flexures & hands** (similar to that in later childhood) - Involvement of vermilion of lip (like dermatitis) - **Nipple** involvement in young / adolescent women - **Photosensitivity** with ultraviolet & infrared radiation.

Atopic dermatitis (AD)

Hanifin & Rajka Diagnostic Criteria for Atopic Dermatitis (Three major and three minor criteria should be present)	
Major criteria	**Minor criteria**
• **Pruritus[Q]** • **Involvement of face & convexities in infants[Q]** (<2 years) and **distribution over flexures** (popliteal and antecubital fossa) in **older children.** • Tendency to chronicity • **Personal or family history of atopy[Q]** such as **asthma, allergic rhinitis or atopic dermatitis[Q].**	• **Facial pallor[Q]/suborbital shadowing** • **Infra orbital fold (Dennie's line)[Q]** • Ichthyosis vulgaris with accentuation over palmar crease • **Recurrent skin infections[Q]** (**pyoderma[Q]**, warts, molluscum contagiosum) • Tendency to non specific dermatosis of hand • Immediate skin test • Delayed blanching to cholinergics • **Raised serum total IgE** • Anterior subcapsular cataract • Keratoconus

ANESTHESIA

193. **Ans. d. Coagulopathy is not an absolute contraindication** *(Ref: Harrison 19/e p443-e2; Morgan 5/e, p948; Millers 8/e p1699, 7/e p1621)*

The given needle is a spinal needle used for lumbar puncture, diagnostic as well as for spinal analgesia or anesthesia. Coagulopathy is an absolute contraindication for spinal anesthesia. Lumbar puncture can be performed in both lateral decubitus as well as sitting position. Breath holding is not necessary for lumbar puncture.

Spinal Anesthesia	
Absolute Contraindications	**Relative Contraindications**
• Patient refusal • **Sepsis at the site of injection[Q]** • **Hypovolemia[Q]** • **Coagulopathy[Q]** • **Indeterminate neurologic disease[Q]**	• Infection distinct from the site of injection • **Unknown duration of surgery[Q]** • **Increased intracranial pressure[Q]**

"The LP needle (typically 20- to 22-gauge) is inserted in the midline, midway between two spinous processes, and slowly advanced. The bevel of the needle should be maintained in a horizontal position, parallel to the direction of the dural fibers and with the flat portion of the bevel pointed upward; this minimizes injury to the fibers as the dura is penetrated."- Harrison 19/e p443-e2

"Breath holding is not required. Breath holding during lumbar puncture can only help in ensuring cooperation of the patient by helping him to cope with the sudden pain due to needle prick, since it acts as a distraction. It is certainly not an essential part of lumbar puncture."-Blueprints Neurology by Frank W. Drislane 4/e p8

"Lumbar puncture for SAB may be performed with the patient sitting or in the lateral decubitus position."- Smith and Aitkenhead's Textbook of Anaesthesia 6/e p525

Contd...

Contd...

Lumbar Puncture
• **Normal extent of spinal cord: From foramen magnum to lower border of L1 vertebra in adults**[Q] **& to upper border of L3 vertebra in infants**[Q]
• **LP** is therefore performed **at or below the L3–L4 interspace**[Q]
• Patients with an **altered level of consciousness**, a **focal neurologic deficit, new-onset seizure, papilledema**, or an **immunocompromised state** are at **increased risk for potentially fatal cerebellar or tentorial herniation** following LP. **Neuroimaging** should be **obtained in these patients prior to LP to exclude a focal mass lesion** or diffuse **swelling**[Q].
• **A low platelet count of <20,000/μL** is considered to be a **contraindication to LP**[Q].

<table>
<tr><td colspan="2">During lumbar puncture, the needle passes through the following anatomic structures before it enters the subarachnoid space:</td></tr>
<tr>
<td>
• **Skin**[Q]
• **Subcutaneous tissue**[Q]
• **Supraspinous ligament**[Q]
• **Interspinous ligament**[Q]
</td>
<td>
• **Ligamentum flavum**[Q]
• **Dura mater**[Q]
• **Arachnoid mater**[Q]
</td>
</tr>
</table>

Positioning:

- Performed on a **firm surface** in **left lateral decubitus (preferred)** or **sitting position**[Q]
- If performed **at bedside**, patient should be positioned **at the edge of bed**[Q] (not in middle).
- Patient is asked to **lie on his or her side, facing away from examiner** & to **"roll up into a ball."**[Q]
- **Neck** is **gently anteflexed** & **thighs pulled up toward abdomen**[Q]
- **Shoulders & pelvis** should be **vertically aligned without forward or backward tilt**[Q].
- **Breath holding** is **not necessary**[Q].

> - **Performed at or below the L3–L4 interspace**[Q]
> - **Useful anatomic guide: Line drawn between posterior superior iliac crest**, which **correspond closely to level of L3–L4 interspace**[Q].

- **Interspace** is chosen following **gentle palpation to identify spinous processes** at each lumbar level.
- An **alternative to lateral recumbent position** is the **seated position**.
- Patient **sits at the side of bed**, with **feet supported on a chair**.
- Patient is **instructed to curl forward**, trying to **touch the nose to umbilicus**.
- LP is sometimes **more easily performed in obese patients if they are sitting**.
- **Disadvantage of seated position: Measurement of opening pressure** is **not accurate**[Q].

Technique:

- **Proper local disinfection** reduces the risk of introducing skin bacteria into subarachnoid space (SAS).
- Local anesthetic (**1% lidocaine**), **3–5 mL total**, is injected into subcutaneous tissue.
- **LP** should be **delayed for 10–15 min** following the injection of anesthetic to decrease pain from the procedure.

> - **LP needle** (typically **20-22 gauge**[Q]) is **inserted in midline, midway between two spinous processes**[Q] & slowly advanced.
> - **Bevel of needle** should be **maintained in a horizontal position, parallel to direction of dural fibers** & with **flat portion of bevel pointed upward**[Q]; this **minimizes injury to fibers as dura is penetrated.**

Contd...

Contd...

Lumbar Puncture
• When **LP** is performed **in sitting position**, **bevel** should be **maintained in vertical position**.
• In most adults, **needle is advanced 4–5 cm** before the SAS is reached; examiner recognizes **entry as a sudden release of resistance, a "pop."[Q]**
• If no fluid appears despite apparently correct needle placement, then the **needle may be rotated 90°–180°**. If there is **still no fluid**, stylet is reinserted & needle is advanced slightly[Q]. If the **needle cannot be advanced** because it hits bone, if the patient **experiences sharp radiating pain down one leg**, or if **no fluid appears ("dry tap")**, needle is **partially withdrawn & reinserted at a different angle**.
• Once the **SAS is reached**, a **manometer is attached to needle** & opening pressure measured.
• **Upper limit of normal opening pressure** with the **patient supine** is **180 mm H$_2$O** in adults but may be **as high as 200–250 mm H$_2$O in obese adults[Q]**.
• CSF is **allowed to drip into collection tubes**; it **should not be withdrawn with a syringe[Q]**.

CSF Obtained for	
• **Cell count with differential[Q]** • **Protein & glucose concentrations[Q]** • **Culture[Q]** (bacterial, fungal, mycobacterial, viral) • **Smears** (e.g., Gram's & acid-fast stained smears) • **Antigen tests[Q]** (e.g., latex agglutination) • **Antibody levels** against microorganisms[Q]	• **PCR amplification** of DNA or RNA of microorganisms (e.g., herpes simplex virus, enteroviruses)[Q] • **Immunoelectrophoresis** for determination of γ-globulin level & **oligoclonal banding[Q]** • **Cytology[Q]**

• Although **15 mL of CSF** is **sufficient to obtain all of the listed studies[Q]**, yield of fungal & mycobacterial cultures & cytology increases when larger volumes are sampled (20–30 mL may be safely removed from adults).

> • A **bloody tap** due to penetration of a meningeal vessel (a **"traumatic tap"**) may result in confusion with subarachnoid hemorrhage (SAH).
> • **Specimen of CSF should be centrifuged immediately** after it is obtained[Q]
> • **Clear supernatant following CSF centrifugation supports the diagnosis of a bloody tap**, whereas **xanthochromic supernatant suggests SAH[Q]**.
> • **Bloody CSF due to penetration of a meningeal vessel clears in successive tubes**, whereas **blood due to SAH does not[Q]**.
> • **Xanthochromic CSF** may also be present **in patients with liver disease** & when **CSF protein concentration is markedly elevated (>1.5–2 g/L)[Q]**.

• **Prior to removing LP needle, stylet is reinserted to avoid the possibility of entrapment of a nerve root in the dura** as the needle is being withdrawn; **entrapment could result in a dural CSF leak, causing headache[Q]**.

RADIOLOGY

194a. Ans. b. Angiomyolipoma *(Ref: Campbell 10/e p1499; Bailey 27/e po1416, 26/e p1303)*

In the given CT image, the renal mass is containing fat content, which is suggestive of angiomyolipoma, which is a fat containing benign renal neoplasm.

"Angiomyolipoma is the only benign renal tumor that is confidently diagnosed on cross-sectional imaging. The presence of fat (confirmed on non-enhanced thin-cut CT by a value of −20 Hounsfield Units [HU] or less) within a renal lesion is considered the diagnostic hallmark. Findings of more than 20 pixels with attenuation less than −20 HU and of more than 5 pixels with attenuation less than −30 HU have been shown to have a positive predictive value of 100%. Ultrasonography shows a well-circumscribed, highly echogenic lesion with shadowing. On angiography (or CT-angiography) aneurysmal dilation is found in 50% of angiomyolipomas. The size of the aneurysms has been reported to correlate with the risk of rupture. MRI can be used in difficult cases or in lieu of CT, with findings on fat-suppressed images being highly suggestive of the diagnosis."-Campbell 10/e p1499

Angiomyolipoma

- **AML** is a **benign** clonal neoplasm consisting of varying amounts of **mature adipose tissue, smooth muscle & thick-walled vessels**[Q]

  - Approximately **20%-30%** are found in patients with **tuberous sclerosis (TS)**[Q]
  - **AML in TS** is more likely to be **bilateral** and **multicentric**, presents with **accelerated growth rates** and **symptomatic presentation**[Q]

- Who do not have TS **(70-80%)**, pronounced **female predominance**, present **later** during **5th** or **6th decade**[Q]
- **Pregnancy** appears to **increase the risk of hemorrhage**[Q] from AML

  - **Massive retroperitoneal hemorrhage** from AML **(Wunderlich's syndrome)**[Q] is seen in **10%** of patients. It's the most significant and feared complication.

Diagnosis:
- IOC for diagnosis of angiomyolipoma: CT scan

  - **CT scan: Presence of fat**[Q] within a renal lesion virtually **excludes the diagnosis of RCC** and is considered **diagnostic of AML**. Presence of fat (confirmed on non-enhanced thin-cut CT by a value of **−20 HU or less) within a renal lesion** is considered the **diagnostic hallmark**.
  - **Lack of calcification**[Q]

- **USG:** Well circumscribed, **highly echogenic lesion**, often associated with **shadowing.**
- **Angiography:** Aneurysmal dilation[Q] is found in **50% of AMLs**

DSA-angiography

- **Arterial phase**: a **sharply marginated hypervascular mass** with a dense early arterial network & tortuous vessels giving the **"sunburst" appearance**[Q]
- **Venous phase**: whorled **"onion peel" appearance** of peripheral vessels[Q]
- **Micro-** or **macro-aneurysms** & absent AV shunting[Q].

- **MRI:** Fat saturated techniques demonstrate **high signal intensity on non-fat-saturated sequences & loss of signal following fat saturation**[Q].

  - Positive immunoreactivity for **HMB-45**[Q], is **characteristic** for **AML** (used to differentiate AML from sarcoma)

Contd...

Angiomyolipoma
Treatment:
• **Asymptomatic** AML upto **4 cm: Follow up** with imaging at 6-12 months.
• **Symptomatic** or **>4 cm:** Intervention is required.
• **Nephron sparing approach** for small symptomatic AML by selective **embolization**[Q] (most preferred) or **partial nephrectomy**
• **Total nephrectomy** for larger lesions or **life threatening hemorrhage**[Q]

Oncocytoma
• Represents **3-7%** of all solid renal masses
• Most renal oncocytomas **cannot be differentiated** from eosinophilic **malignant RCC**[Q] by clinical or radiographic means
Pathology:
• In grossly, tumors are light brown or tan, **homogeneous**, and **well circumscribed**, not truly encapsulated
• A **central scar** without prominent necrosis or hypervascularity.
• Ultrastructurally, **packed** with **numerous large mitochondria,** which contributes to their **distinctive staining characteristics**[Q]
Diagnosis:
• **CT scan: Central stellate scar**[Q]
• **Angiography: Spoke-wheel pattern**[Q] of feeding arteries
• **MRI:** well-defined capsule, central stellate scar, and distinctive intensities on T1 & T2 images
Treatment:
• A **nephron-sparing approach**[Q] is preferred.

194b. Ans. d. Renal cell carcinoma *(Ref: Smith 17/e p334; Campbell 10/e p1419-1491; Bailey 27e p1417-1419, 27/e p1417-1419, 26/e p1304-1307)*

Most likely diagnosis for an asymptomatic complex cyst in a 65 years old male as given in CT image, which appears as exophytic mass is renal cell carcinoma.

"CT scanning is more sensitive than US or IVU for detection of renal masses. A typical finding of RCC on CT is a mass that becomes enhanced with the use of intravenous contrast media. In general, RCC exhibits an overall decreased density in Hounsfield units compared with nor- mal renal parenchyma but shows a heterogeneous pattern of enhancement or increased attenuation (slightly decreased from the surrounding parenchyma) when contrast is used. In addition to defining the primary lesion, CT scanning is also the method of choice in staging the patient by visualizing the renal hilum, perinephric space, renal vein and vena cava, adrenals, regional lymphatics, and adjacent organs." -Smith 17/e p334

Renal Cell Carcinoma
(Gravitz tumor, Hypernephroma, Internist's tumor, Radiologist's tumor)[Q]
• **MC malignant tumor** of adult kidney & **most lethal**[Q] of all malignancies
• More common in **males,** in **6th & 7th** decade
• Majority are sporadic
• Hereditary variants are **VHL syndrome, Hereditary clear cell carcinoma** & **Hereditary papillary carcinoma**[Q]
• Tumor usually involve **upper pole**[Q]
Risk Factors:
• **Most significant risk factors** are **smoking & tobacco chewing**[Q]
• Other risk factors are obesity, hypertension, exposure to **Asbestos,** petroleum products & **cadmium,** chronic renal failure (specially due to **analgesic nephropathy)**[Q]

Contd...

Contd...

Renal Cell Carcinoma
(Gravitz tumor, Hypernephroma, Internist's tumor, Radiologist's tumor)[Q]

Spread:
- Characteristic feature of RCC is tendency to **invade renal vein.** Further extension produces a **continuous cord of tumor** in IVC and even in **right side of heart[Q].**
- **MC route is hematogenous[Q]**

> - **MC sites of distant metastasis: Lungs (cannon ball deposits & pulsating secondaries)[Q]>** bone> liver> brain.

- **Lymphatic spread** occurs when tumor extends beyond renal capsule.

Notable features of RCC
1. Encapsulated in spite of being malignant (**pseudocapsule**)
2. **Spontaneous regression[Q]**
3. **Refractoriness** to **cytotoxic agents[Q]**
4. **Response** to biological response modifiers (**IL-2 & IFN-alpha)[Q]**
5. **Prolonged** period of **stable disease[Q]**

Clinical Features
- **Classical triad of gross hematuria, abdominal mass & pain** is seen in **10%** cases[Q] **(Too late triad)**
- **MC & consistent presentation: Hematuria[Q].**
- Other symptoms: Fever, weight loss, malaise, **acute & non-reducing varicocele, lower limb edema** due to IVC obstruction.

RCC: Paraneoplastic Syndromes (20%)
1. **Raised ESR: MC** paraneoplastic manifestation[Q]
2. **Hypercalcemia:** Due to production of **PTH-rp[Q];** Only **paraneoplastic syndrome** in which **medical therapies** are proven **useful.**
3. **Hypertension[Q] (Renin** production from tumor)
4. **Polycythemia[Q] (Erythropoietin** production from tumor)
5. **Stauffer's syndrome: Non-metastatic hepatic dysfunction[Q]** due to raised **IL-6[Q]** leading to **increased ALP, PT & bilirubin;** Hepatic function **normalizes after nephrectomy[Q]**
6. Others are: **Cushing syndrome,** hypoglycemia, anemia, gynecomastia, amenorrhea

Diagnosis:
- **IOC for diagnosis: CECT** (95% accurate)[Q]

> - **MRI is most accurate** non-invasive investigation for detecting **tumor thrombus** in **renal vein** or **IVC. Distinguishes tumor thrombus** from **bland thrombus[Q]**
> - **Inferior venocavogram[Q]** is **most sensitive & specific** but **invasive** means to detect involvement of IVC.

Contd...

Renal Cell Carcinoma
(Gravitz tumor, Hypernephroma, Internist's tumor, Radiologist's tumor)[Q]

- **Renal arteriography** is done before **renal sparing surgery** (partial nephrectomy), but 3-D helical CT is also sufficient.
- Specific **plain X-ray** finding is **central calcification[Q]**.

FNAC is not routinely done in RCC, indications are:
1. Suspected **secondaries[Q]**
2. Suspected **lymphoma[Q]**
3. Clinical suspicion of **renal abscess[Q]**
4. To prove pathological diagnosis in **disseminated** or **unresectable disease[Q]**

Prognostic factors:
- **Pathologic stage[Q]** is single **most important** prognostic factor
- **Lymph node involvement** is a **poor** prognostic factor

Staging & grading:
- **TNM** (preferred) & **Robson's[Q]** staging are used for RCC.
- **Fuhrman[Q]** histological system is used for **grading.**

Treatment:

Localized RCC
- **TOC** is **open radical nephrectomy[Q]**
- Chemotherapy & radiotherapy is not effective

- Patient with **Stauffer's syndrome** are also candidate for **radical nephrectomy[Q]**.
- **Radical nephrectomy** or **debulking** is done **for cytoreduction** in both **locally advanced & metastatic RCC[Q]**.

Indications of nephron sparing surgery
- **Bilateral RCC** or **VHL syndrome[Q]**
- RCC involving a **solitary functioning kidney[Q]**
- Unilateral carcinoma and a functioning opposite kidney affected by a condition that might threaten its future function (e.g. RAS)
- **Low stage** or **≤4 cm RCC[Q]** at any location

Locally Advanced & Metastatic RCC
- **Sunitinib** is the **first line treatment** for **metastatic RCC** (response rate-31%)[Q]
- Combined **IL-2** & **IFN-alpha** is the **2nd line** treatment for **metastatic RCC** (response rate:15%)[Q]
- Chemotherapy with **vinblastine[Q],** as it is single most effective agent
- **Removal of thrombus** should be considered in **renal or IVC extension[Q]**
- **Radiotherapy** for **symptomatic bone metastasis[Q]**

195. Ans. b. Sestamibi scan   *(Ref: Sabiston 20/e p930; Harrison 19/e p2474; Bailey 27/e p827, 26/e p773)*

History of renal stones, bone pains and abdominal cramps with history of fractures is highly suggestive of hyperparathyroidism. Most common cause of primary hyperparathyroidism is parathyroid adenoma. Sestamibi scan is the best investigation to delineate parathyroid abnormalities.

"Sestamibi single photon emission computed tomography, owing to its improved spatial resolution, has become the most commonly used preoperative imaging study in parathyroid disease."-Sabiston 20/e p930

"However, the major limitation of ultrasound is that its accuracy is highly operator dependent; ultrasound sensitivity for detecting abnormal parathyroid glands ranges from 70% to 96%. Additionally, mediastinal parathyroid lesions cannot be identified on neck ultrasound because the ultrasound cannot penetrate the sternum or clavicles. However, when used in combination with sestamibi, the sensitivity for identifying a single parathyroid adenoma increases to 80% to 95%."-Sabiston 20/e p930

"Preoperative ⁹⁹ᵐTc sestamibi scans with single- photon emission CT (SPECT) are used to predict the location of an abnormal gland and intraoperative sampling of PTH before and at 5-min intervals after removal of a suspected adenoma to confirm a rapid fall (>50%) to normal levels of PTH."- Harrison 19/e p2474

Accuracy of Imaging Techniques in Parathyroid Localization	
Ultrasound	• Modern USG using high-resolution (7.5-10 MHz) probe is only slightly less sensitive than nuclear medicine. • Highest reported **sensitivity** for identifying an adenoma **is 82%** and **specificity of 78-100%.**
Sestamibi scan	• **Overall sensitivity for identifying parathyroid adenoma** with technetium (Tc) 99m-Sestamibi ranges from **80-95%.**
CT	• **Sensitivity** for identifying parathyroid adenoma is **similar to USG** with **specificity ranging from 92-95%.**

Primary Hyperparathyroidism

- PHPT arises from **increased PTH production**[Q] from abnormal parathyroid glands and results from a disturbance of normal feedback control exerted by serum calcium.
- More common in **women**[Q]

> • **Solitary adenoma**[Q] is the **MC cause** (in **80%**)
> • **Parathyroid adenomas** are **most commonly located** in **inferior** parathyroid glands.

- **Increased PTH production** leads to **hypercalcemia via**: **Increased GI absorption** of calcium; **Increased** production of **vitamin D3; Reduced renal calcium clearance**

Etiology:
- Exposure to **low-dose therapeutic ionizing radiation & familial predisposition**[Q]
- Renal leak of calcium
- **Declining renal function** with age
- **Alteration** in the **sensitivity** of parathyroid glands to suppression by calcium
- **Lithium therapy**

Genetics:
- **Most cases** of PHPT are **sporadic**
- Also associated with **MEN1, MEN2A,** isolated familial HPT, and familial HPT with jaw-tumor syndrome.

Clinical Features:
- Patients with PHPT formerly presented with the "classic" pentad of symptoms:

> | | |
> |---|---|
> | • **Kidney stones**[Q] | • **Psychic moans**[Q] |
> | • **Painful bones**[Q] | • **Fatigue overtones**[Q] |
> | • **Abdominal groans**[Q] | |

- Alteration in the "typical" patient with PHPT due to widespread use of automated blood analyzers.
- Patients are more likely to be minimally symptomatic or asymptomatic.
- Currently, **most patients** present with **weakness,** fatigue, **polydipsia, polyuria, nocturia, bone & joint pain, constipation**[Q], decreased appetite, nausea, heartburn, pruritus, depression, and memory loss.

Contd...

Contd...

Primary Hyperparathyroidism
• Renal **calculi** are typically composed of **calcium phosphate** or **oxalate**[Q].

Osteitis fibrosa cystica in advanced PHPT
• **Pathognomonic radiologic findings** on **x-rays** of **hands**, characterized by: • **Subperiosteal resorption**[Q] (most apparent on the **radial aspect**[Q] of **middle phalanx**[Q] of 2nd & 3rd fingers) • **Bone cysts**[Q] • **Tufting of distal phalanges**[Q]

Diagnosis:
- **Elevated serum calcium** and **intact PTH** or two-site PTH levels, **without hypocalciuria** establishes the **diagnosis of PHPT** with virtual certainty[Q].
- **Decreased serum phosphate** (50%) & **elevated 24-hour urinary calcium** (60%) **in PHPT**[Q]

Localization:
- **99mTc-labeled sestamibi: Most widely used & accurate modality**[Q] (sensitivity >80% for detection of parathyroid adenomas)

Treatment:
- **Parathyroidectomy** for patients having **"classic" symptoms** of PHPT or **<50 years**[Q]
- **SERM** & **bisphosphonates** are used to **lower serum calcium** & **increase BMD in PHPT.**

Indications for Parathyroidectomy in Asymptomatic Primary HPT	
1. Serum **calcium >1 mg/dL above** the **upper limits** of normal 2. **Life-threatening hypercalcemic** episode 3. **Creatine clearance** reduced by **30%** 4. **Kidney stones** on abdominal x-rays 5. Markedly **elevated 24-h urinary calcium excretion (≥400 mg/d)**	6. Substantially **decreased bone mineral density** at the lumbar spine, hip, or distal radius 7. Age **<50 years** 8. Long-term medical surveillance not desired or possible

196. Ans. a. Pneumoperitoneum   *(Ref: Sabiston 20/e p1126)*

The given chest X-ray is clearly showing gas under the right dome of diaphragm, suggestive of pneumoperitoneum.

Pneumoperitoneum
• **Pneumoperitoneum** describes **gas within the peritoneal cavity** • **MC cause** of pneumoperitoneum: **Perforation of hollow viscus** (leading to release of air from bowel and collection just below the diaphragm)

- **Best projection** to demonstrate **pneumoperitoneum: Chest X-ray**[Q]
- If the **patient cannot get into** an **erect position** then **left lateral decubitus** projection is required[Q].

- Patient should be in that position for **10 min**[Q] at least for **air to rise up**.
- By careful technique even **1 ml of air can be detected**[Q]

Causes of Pneumoperitoneum	

1. **Perforation of GI Tract:**
  – **Peptic ulcer**[Q]
  – Inflammation (**Diverticulitis, appendicitis, toxic megacolon, necrotizing enterocolitis**)[Q]
  – **Infarction**
  – Malignant neoplasm
  – **Pneumatosis cystoides rupture**[Q]
  – Iatrogenic (**Endoscopy**)[Q]
1. **Penetrating abdominal injury**[Q]
	2. **Iatrogenic:**
	  – **Surgery, peritoneal dialysis,**
	  – **Drainage catheter, biopsy**
	4. **Through female genital tract:**
	  – Spontaneous
	  – Iatrogenic (perforation, culdocentasis, tubal patency test)[Q]
	5. **Gas forming peritonitis**[Q]
	6. **Pneumothorax** with **pleuroperitoneal fistula**

Contd...

Pneumoperitoneum

Supine Film Signs of Pneumoperitoneum

Football sign	• Collection of **air in the centre of abdomen over a fluid collection**[Q]
Rigler's sign	• Visualization of **both aspects of bowel** wall being **outlined by air** on either side[Q]
Cupola sign	• Large amount of gas under the **diaphragm**[Q]
Triangle sign	• Air between bowel loop[Q]

Bowel Related Signs	Peritoneal Ligament Related Signs	Right Upper Quadrant Signs
• Double wall sign[Q] (Rigler's sign) • Telltale triangle sign[Q] (triangle sign)	• Football sign[Q] • Silver sign[Q]: Visualization of falciform ligament • Lateral umbilical ligament sign (also known as inverted "V" sign) • Urachus sign	• Lucent liver sign[Q] • Hepatic edge sign[Q] • Fissure for ligamentum teres sign[Q] • Morison's pouch sign[Q] (Doge cap sign) • Cupola sign[Q]

Chilaiditi Syndrome

• **Interposition of colon between liver & diaphragm** can **mimic pneumoperitoneum**[Q]

197. Ans. d. Pulmonary venous hypertension *(Ref: Chest X-ray Made Easy (Elsevier) 3/e p110)*

The given chest X-ray is of Ebstein's anomaly (with box shaped heart) shows cardiomegaly, narrow vascular pedicles, hyperlucent lung fields (less prominent vascular markings suggestive of decreased pulmonary flow), not the pulmonary hypertension in this case. Pulmonary venous hypertension will show prominent hilar vessels, plethoric lung fields.

> "Ebstein's anomaly: On roentgenographic examination, heart size varies from slightly enlarged to massive box-shaped cardiomegaly caused by enlargement of the right atrium. In newborns with severe Ebstein anomaly, the heart may totally obscure the pulmonary fields." -Nelson 19/e p1584

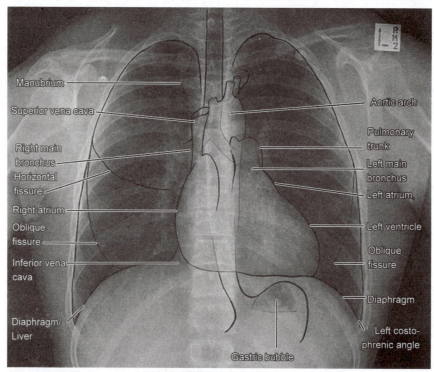

Fig. 39: Normal chest X-ray

Features of Increased Pulmonary Blood Flow

- **Blood vessels become visible in the outer third of lung field (At least 6 vessels can be traced to the outer third).** When hilar and intrapulmonary vessels are uniformly changed, it is very suggestive of shunt lesions.
- **Ratio of right descending pulmonary artery to trachea >1**
- **Right descending pulmonary artery diameter >14 mm suggests increased blood flow and >17 mm is very strongly suggestive**
- **Prominent end-on vessels seen at hilum**
- Enface vessels below 10th posterior rib
- Prominent vessels seen below crest of diaphragm
- **Ratio of vessels to adjacent bronchus >2:1**

Signs of Pulmonary Venous Hypertension
(In order of appearance with increasing pulmonary venous pressures)

• **Vascular Redistribution**	• **Alveolar edema**
– **Upper lobe venous distension**[Q]	– **Airspace opacities**[Q]
• **Intestitial edema**	– **Perihilar bat wing distribution**[Q]
– **Kerly B lines**[Q]	– **Clears rapidly with diuretics**[Q]
– **Perihilar haze**[Q]	• **Pleural effusions**[Q]
– **Bronchial cuffing**[Q]	

PSYCHIATRY

198. Ans. a. Lithium *(Ref: Kaplan's 11/e p236; Niraj Ahuja 7/e p78; Goodman Gilman 12/e p447)*

Lithium is a mood stabilizer with an anti-suicidal effect. Lithium is the drug of choice for bipolar disorders as it is a mood stabilizer as well as it has an anti-suicidal effect. Hence it is also used as a response-augmenting agent with antidepressants in resistant major depression. is a mood stabilizer with an anti-suicidal effect.

"Clinical studies have shown that lithium reduces the incidence of suicide in Bipolar 1 disorder patients six-fold to seven-fold."- Kaplan's 11/e p236

"Li⁺ is the only mood stabilizer with data on suicide reduction in bipolar patients, and Li⁺ also has abundant efficacy data for augmentation in unipolar depressive patients who are inadequate responders to antidepressant therapy."- Goodman Gilman 12/e p447

Lithium

- **Mood stabilizer with an anti-suicidal effect:** Reduces the incidence of suicide in Bipolar 1 disorder patients six-fold to seven-fold[Q].

FDA Approved (Well established) Indications of Lithium	
• **Treatment of acute mania**[Q]	• **Prophylaxis of bipolar mood disorders**[Q]

Pharmacokinetics:
- Very **rapidly absorbed from GIT,** peak serum levels occur between 30 minutes to 3 hours, absorption is complete in 8 hours
- It is **not protein bound**[Q]
- **Maximum levels occur in thyroid**[Q] (3-5 times serum level), **saliva** (2 times), **milk** (0.3-1.0 times) & **CSF** (0.4 times)
- The steady state levels are achieved in 7 days

> - There is **no metabolism of lithium in the body**[Q] and is **excreted almost entirely by kidneys**[Q].
> - As proximal reabsorption is influenced by sodium balance, **depletion of sodium results in retention, causing higher blood levels of lithium**[Q].

Contd...

Contd...

Lithium		
Serum Concentration of Lithium		
Therapeutic level	**Prophylactic level**	**Toxic level**
0.8-1.2 mEq/L[Q]	0.6-1.2 mEq/L[Q]	>2.0 mEq/L[Q]

Side effects of Lithium	
Neurological	• **Tremors (MC)**[Q] • Muscle weakness; **Increased deep tendon reflexes (DTRs)**[Q] • **Seizures, convulsions**[Q]**, drowsiness, delirium, coma**[Q]
Renal	• **Nephrogenic diabetes insipidus, polyuria, polydipsia**[Q] **(inhibits action of ADH on distal tubules)** • **Tubular changes, nephrotic syndrome**[Q]
Cardiovascular	• **T wave depression** (effects are **similar to hypokalemia**)[Q]
Endocrine	• **Goiter, hypothyroidism, abnormal thyroid function**[Q] **(interfering with iodination of thyroid)** • **Weight** gain (pedal edema is also common)
GIT	• Nausea, vomiting, **diarrhea**[Q] • Metallic taste, abdominal pain
Dermatological	• Acneiform eruptions, papular eruptions & exacerbation of psoriasis
During pregnancy & lactation	• Teratogenic, increased incidence of **Ebstein's anomaly**[Q] (when taken in first trimester) • **Secreted in milk**[Q] with 30-100% of the maternal blood lithium levels, can cause toxicity in infant

• **Leucocyte count is increased by lithium therapy.**

Contraindications of Lithium	
• Presence of clear evidence of **cardiac**, renal, **thyroid or neurological dysfunction**[Q] • During **first trimester** of pregnancy & **lactation**[Q]	• **Concomitant administration of thiazide diuretics, tetracycline or anaesthetics**[Q] • **Presence of blood dyscrasia**[Q]

• **Lithium should be stopped 2 days before surgery**[Q]**.**

199. Ans. b. Stupor   *(Ref: Kaplan's 11/e p341; Niraj Ahuja 7/e p239)*

A state of mutism and akinesis where patient is aware of his surroundings and somewhat alert is best described as stupor. Akinetic mutism, i.e. severe reduction of speech and action in an awake and alert person is referred to as Stupor.

"Stupor: (1) State of decreased reactivity to stimuli and less than full awareness of one's surroundings; as a disturbance of consciousness, it indicates a condition of partial coma or semicoma. (2) In psychiatry, used synonymously with mutism and does not necessarily imply a disturbance of consciousness; in catatonic stupor, patients are ordinarily aware of their surroundings."-Kaplan's Synopsis of Psychiatry

Oneiroid state	• Also called **dreamlike state or nightmare-like state**, often as part of schizophrenia • Defined by the **fantastic psychological suffering**. It is characterized by **ambivalent, contradictory speech, criminal action, senses global, changing, catastrophe & celebration simultaneously.** • Frequently met with **vivid hallucination & illusion** which are **perceived not as a real fact in the world** but as a presentation, like a movie **(pseudo-hallucination)**
Twilight state	• A dreamy state lacking touch with present reality, occurring in **epilepsy, hysteria, alcoholism, brain trauma & schizophrenia,** and sometimes induced with narcotics. • A condition of **disordered consciousness during which actions may be performed without conscious volition & without any remembrance afterward.** • The patient may show **abnormal violent behavior in this period.** • Described as **disturbed consciousness with hallucination** • Characterized by **sudden onset, very short duration & abrupt end with** total **amnesia for the total period of disorder of consciousness.**
Delirium	• **Acute reversible mental disorder** characterized by **confusion & some impairment of consciousness** • Associated with **emotional lability, hallucinations or illusions, and inappropriate, impulsive, irrational, or violent behavior.**

Stupor

- It is the **lack of critical mental function** and a **level of consciousness wherein a sufferer is almost entirely unresponsive** and **only responds to base stimuli such as pain[Q].**
- Those in a stuporous state are **rigid, mute and only appear to be conscious,** as the **eyes are open & follow surrounding objects[Q].**

Causes of Stupor	
• **Infectious diseases** • **Complicated toxic states** (e.g. heavy metals) • Severe hypothermia • Mental illnesses (e.g. **schizophrenia,** severe clinical depression) • **Epilepsy**	• Vascular illnesses (e.g. hypertensive encephalopathy) • **Shock** • **Neoplasms** (e.g. brain tumors) • **Vitamin D deficiency**

- **If not stimulated externally, a patient** with st**upor will be in a sleepy state most of the time.** In some extreme cases of severe depressive disorders the patient **can become motionless, lose their appetite and become mute[Q].**

200. Ans. c. Forced thinking *(Ref: Kaplan's 11/e p236; SIMS Psychopathology 5/e p298; Lishman's Organic Psychiatry 4/e p557)*

Forced thinking is a rare epileptic phenomenon, usually seen in patients with frontal lobe epilepsy. It is a rare type of aura that refers to recurrent intrusive thoughts, ideas, or crowding of thoughts. The above profile fits into the criteria for epileptic forced thinking, which is a rare phenomenon seen in patients with frontal lobe epilepsy.

Obsession	• It usually comes with a **compulsion or attempt to stop these thoughts** • Obsessions are thoughts that **recur & persist despite efforts to ignore or confront them.**

Thought insertion	• Usually **seen in** patients with **Schizophrenia,** in which patients describe that **thoughts have been inserted by some external agency.**
Thought crowding	• **Seen in** patients with **Schizophrenia,** with **multiple thoughts, too fast & excessive in amount** and **patient can localize the origin of thoughts, from the back of his head or by some external agency.**

Forced Thinking (FT)

- **Forced thinking** is a **rare epileptic phenomenon,** usually **seen in patients with frontal lobe epilepsy.**
- FT is a **rare type of aura** that **refers to recurrent intrusive thoughts, ideas, or crowding of thoughts.**
- FT is generally considered **as a type of psychic auras.**

  - Patients may experience **distortion of thoughts** such as **forced thinking,** which describes a **feeling of being compelled to think about a specific topic or word;** or **crowding of thoughts** which describes a **feeling of racing, disorganized thoughts.**
  - Subtle but disturbing changes in the quality of perception are reported, including **derealization & depersonalization, distortions in the perception of time & changes in the significance of objects.**

- FT, which originates in the **frontal lobe** may differ from FT of **temporal lobe origin.**

Forced Thinking	
Frontal Lobe Origin	**Temporal Lobe Origin**
• **Accompanied by an attempt to act on the thought** (forced acts such as real behavior of the same content, vocalization & gaze attraction), where it takes on **colder & more ideational aspect,** particularly **more intentional,** as **thoughts that impose them** and then **need to find a way to materialize.**	• **Requires the limbic system for expression.** • **Content of FT** is set in **a much more intense** and **vivid experiential, emotional & affective contexts** • Content of FT originating in the temporal lobe may be **vaguer expression.**

Note

Note

Note

Note

Note

Note

AIIMS NOVEMBER 2016

Multiple Choice Questions

ANATOMY

1. The following type of epithelium is found in which body part?

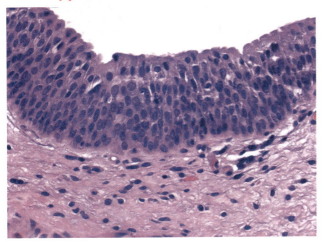

   a. Bile duct
   b. Common bile duct
   c. Skin
   d. Urinary bladder

2. Which of the following are the set of structures that pierce the given structure in the image?

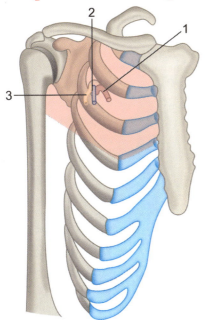

   a. Basilic vein, lateral pectoral nerve, medial pectoral nerve
   b. Thoracoacromial artery, cephalic vein, medial pectoral nerve
   c. Thoracoacromial artery, cephalic vein, lateral pectoral nerve
   d. Cephalic vein, lateral pectoral nerve, medial pectoral nerve

3. Parasympathetic nervous system comprises of:
   a. Cranial nerves III, V, VII, X and sacral nerves S1, S2, S3, S4, S5
   b. Cranial nerves III, VII, IX, X and sacral nerves S2, S3, S4
   c. Cranial nerves V, VII, IX, X and sacral nerves S2, S3, S4
   d. Cranial nerves III, V, VII, X and sacral nerves S2, S3, S4

4. The given image is the pictorial representation of spaces of neck enclosed by cervical fascia. The spaces are labeled as A, B, C and D. Which of these is the danger space of the neck?

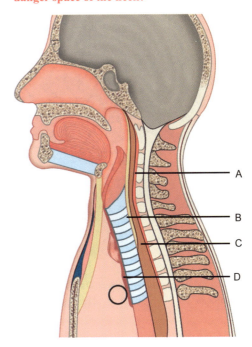

   a. A
   b. B
   c. C
   d. D

5. In the given cross-section of axilla, the structures marked are:

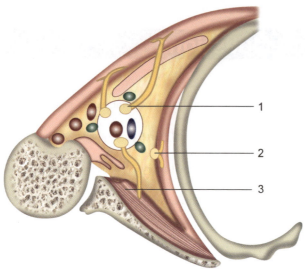

a. 1-Lateral cord of brachial plexus, 2-long thoracic nerve, 3-subscapularis
b. 1-Posterior cord of brachial plexus, 2-nerve to serratus anterior, 3-subscapularis
c. 1-Medial cord of brachial plexus, 2-long thoracic nerve, 3-subscapularis
d. 1-Lateral cord of brachial plexus, 2-long thoracic nerve, 3-serratus anterior

6. What will happen when the area marked in the sagittal section of brain below gets affected?

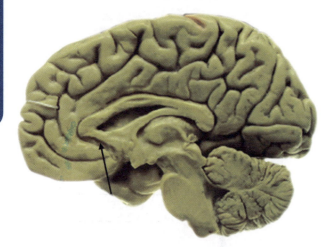

a. Lower limb paralysis
b. Visual agnosia
c. Aphasia
d. Diplopia

7. Which of the following muscle is supplied by the nucleus present beneath the area marked by the arrow below?

Mark the image

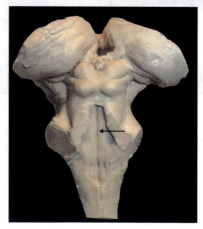

a. Risorius
b. Lateral rectus
c. Inferior oblique
d. Medial pterygoid

8. Extra-embryonic mesoderm is derived from:
a. Epiblast
b. Primary yolk sac
c. Secondary yolk sac
d. Hypoblast

9. Anterior two third of the tongue is demarcated from the posterior one third by:
a. Passavant's ridge
b. Circumvallate papillae
c. Sulcus terminalis
d. Filiform papilla

10. All of the following structures lie in the relation to the left ureter *except:*
a. Mesentery of sigmoid colon
b. Bifurcation of common iliac artery
c. Quadratus lumborum
d. Gonadal vessels

11. In the following image of anterior abdominal wall, the correct matching of marking is:

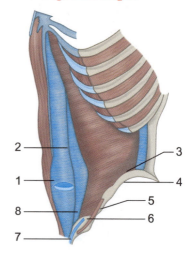

a. 1. Linea alba, 2- linea semilunaris, 3-outer lip of iliac crest, 4-inner lip of iliac crest, 5-inguinal ligament, 6-superficial inguinal ring
b. 1. Linea alba, 2- linea semilunaris, 3-inner lip of iliac crest, 4-outer lip of iliac crest, 5-inguinal ligament, 6-deep inguinal ring
c. 1. Linea semilunaris, 2- linea alba, 3-outer lip of iliac crest, 4-inner lip of iliac crest, 5-inguinal ligament, 6-superficial inguinal ring
d. 1. Linea semilunaris, 2- linea alba, 3- inner lip of iliac crest, 4- outer lip of iliac crest, 5-inguinal ligament, 6-deep inguinal ring

12. **All of the following muscles have parallel oriented fibers *except*:**
    a. Sartorius
    b. Rectus abdominis
    c. Sternohyoid
    d. Tibialis anterior

PHYSIOLOGY

13. **Area marked by the arrow in the given figure contain all the following, *except*:**

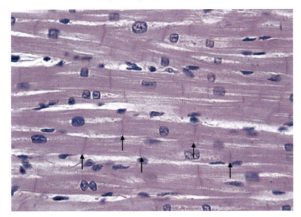

    a. Zona occludens
    b. Fascia adherens
    c. Macula adherens
    d. Gap junction

14. **The peripheral processes of spiral ganglion end at:**

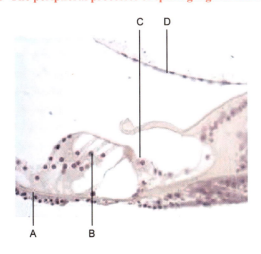

    a. A
    b. B
    c. C
    d. D

15. **Endo-cochlear potential is:**
    a. +45 mV
    b. –45mV
    c. –60mV
    d. +85 mV

16. **The following image shows cell counts in different squares of a Neubauer's chamber after charging with 20 times diluted blood. What is the total leukocyte count?**

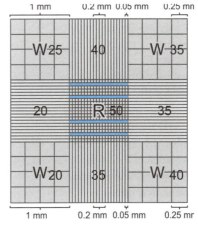

    a. 6000/mm³
    b. 2400/mm³
    c. 3000/mm³
    d. 14200/mm³

17. **In the following electron micrograph of the sarcomere, correctly identify the area labeled as "E":**

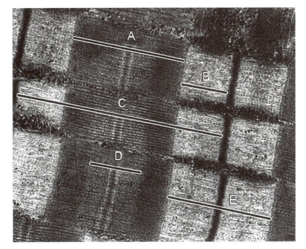

    a. A-band
    b. I-band
    c. M-band
    d. H-zone

18. Countercurrent mechanism is not seen in:
    a. Kidney
    b. Testes
    c. Eye
    d. Intestine

19. Which of the following nerve root is the control center for the stapedial reflex?
    a. Superior olivary complex
    b. Lateral lemniscus
    c. Inferior colliculus
    d. Medial geniculate body

20. All of the following increases calcium absorption from the gut *except:*
    a. Phytates
    b. Vitamin D
    c. Alkaline pH in gut
    d. Protein in diet

21. Which of the following is the function of Hyperpolarizing Cyclic Nucleotide (HCN) gated channels?
    a. Cardiac rhythm generation
    b. Generation of mitochondrial action potential
    c. Myocardial muscle contraction
    d. Memory formation

22. In the following sections of the adrenal gland, which of the following hormone is secreted by the region marked as "A"?

    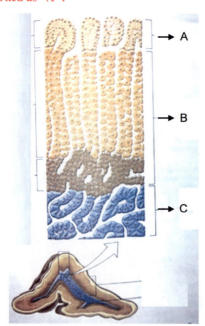

    a. Aldosterone
    b. Cortisol
    c. Testosterone
    d. Epinephrine

23. In the following graph, the curve A represents the normal relationship between alveolar ventilation and pCO_2, when pO_2 is 100 mm Hg. If pH is changed from 7.4 to 7.3, where will the original curve shift?

    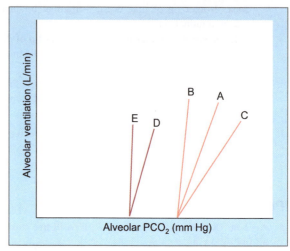

    a. A
    b. B
    c. C
    d. D

24. Which of the following is rapid source of energy by resynthesizing ATP for exercising muscles is?
    a. Glycolysis
    b. Glycogenolysis
    c. TCA cycle
    d. Phosphocreatine

25. Which of the following hormones will be affected most after the change in sex hormone binding globulin?
    a. Testosterone
    b. Estrogen
    c. Progesterone
    d. DHEA

26. Migratory motor complexes in the gut reappear after intervals of:
    a. 60 minutes
    b. 90 minutes
    c. 120 minutes
    d. 150 minutes

27. Diffusion capacity of carbon monoxide is decreased in all except:
    a. Polycythemia
    b. Interstitial lung disease
    c. Emphysema
    d. Pulmonary vascular disease

28. Potential generated due to movement of freely diffusible ions across a semi-permeable membrane is calculated using:

a. Nernst equation
b. Gibbs equation
c. Goldman-Hodgkin-Katz equation
d. Fick principle

29. During starvation, graph of three substances are plotted as below. The scale for A and B is on the left and the scale for C is on the right. Which of the substances are represented by the curve B?

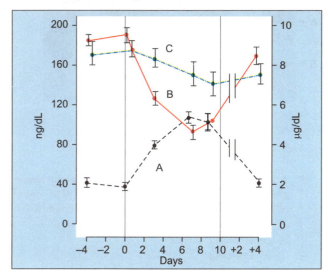

a. RT$_3$
b. T$_3$
c. T$_4$
d. DIT

BIOCHEMISTY

30. CG islands in our DNA are important for:
    a. Methylation
    b. Acetylation
    c. t-RNA synthesis
    d. DNA replication

31. The pH of a solution containing 5 millimole/liter of H$^+$ ions is closest to what value?
    a. 1.7   b. 2.3
    c. 3.5   d. 4.2

32. A patient has normal blood glucose level as estimated by glucose-oxidase peroxidase method, shows positive Benedicts test in urine. Which of the following is the most likely cause?
    a. Fructosemia
    b. Denaturation of glucose
    c. Galactosemia
    d. False positive

33. Ammonia from brain is removed as:
    a. Urea   b. Alanine
    c. Glutamate   d. Glutamine

34. Respiratory Quotient (RQ) of a person on pure carbohydrate diet will be:
    a. 0.7
    b. 1
    c. 1.2
    d. 1.5

35. Common intermediate in synthesis of steroid hormones is:
    a. Cortisone
    b. 7 Dihydrocholesterol
    c. 7 Hydroxycholesterol
    d. Pregnenolone

36. At physiological pH, which of these amino acids has a positive charge?
    a. Valine
    b. Aspartic acid
    c. Arginine
    d. Isoleucine

37. Which of the following is maximum in HDL as compared to other lipoproteins?
    a. Cholesterol
    b. Apoproteins
    c. Triglycerides
    d. Fatty acids

38. HCO$_3$/H$_2$CO$_3$ is the best buffer because it is:
    a. pKa near physiological pH
    b. Its components can be increased or decreased in the body as needed
    c. Good acceptor and donor of H$^+$ ions
    d. Combination of a weak acid and weak base

39. All of the following processes take place in mitochondria *except*:
    a. Beta-oxidation of fatty acids
    b. DNA synthesis
    c. Fatty acid synthesis
    d. Protein synthesis

40. Which of the following is most effective for gluconeogenesis in starvation? *(AIIMS November 2016, May 2012)*
    a. Acetyl Co-A stimulation of pyruvate carboxylase
    b. Fructose-1, 6-biphosphate stimulation of phosphofructokinase-1
    c. Citrate stimulation of acetyl carboxylase
    d. Fructose-2, 6-biphosphate stimulation of phosphofructokinase-2

41. Which of the following vitamin is synthesized in vivo, in the body by humans?
    a. Niacin
    b. Pantothenic acid
    c. Cyanocobalamin
    d. Folic acid

PATHOLOGY

42. A 58 years old man suffered road traffic accident and came to the hospital. He had multiple fractures in his lower limbs, ribs and lung contusion. Ultimately he succumbed to his injuries. At autopsy, a biopsy from the lung showed the following appearance. What is the most likely cause of his death?

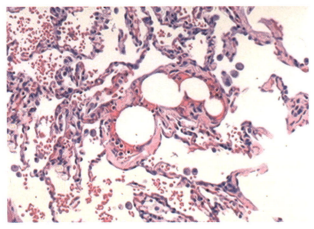

   a. Emphysema
   b. Congestive heart failure
   c. Fat embolism
   d. Pulmonary embolism

43. A 56 years old female presented in the month of December with chronic fatigue and cyanosis of nose with blue lips and arthralgia. A peripheral blood smear showed the following image. What is the most likely cause of the findings seen?

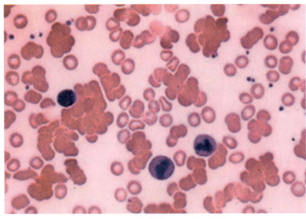

   a. Clumps of RBCs due to IgG mediated cold autoimmune hemolytic anemia
   b. Clumps of RBCs due to IgM mediated cold autoimmune hemolytic anemia
   c. RBC lysis due to hemoglobinopathy
   d. Clumps of RBCs due to IgG mediated warm autoimmune hemolytic anemia

44. In the given Leishman's stained blood smear, identify the cell, which is raised markedly in worm infestations:

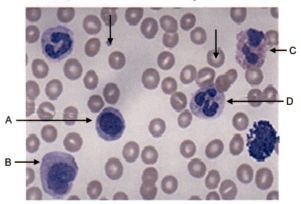

   a. A
   b. B
   c. C
   d. D

45. A 26 years old female presented with pallor and hemoglobin of 9.5 mg/dL, PCV 30 mm Hg and RBC count of 2 million/mm^3. What is the most likely diagnosis?
   a. Iron deficiency anemia
   b. Sideroblastic anemia
   c. Thalassemia
   d. Folic acid deficiency

46. A 32 years old slum dweller presented with complaints of diarrhea and constipation with a 2 kg weight loss for last 2 months. On examination, the patient had a dry tongue and poor skin turgor. An endoscopic biopsy from the gut revealed the following microscopic appearance. What is the most likely diagnosis?

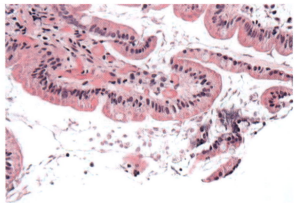

   a. Entamoeba histolytica
   b. Whipple's disease
   c. Giardiasis
   d. Helicobacter pylori

47. Given below is the histopathology of liver biopsy of a patient with hemochromatosis. Which of the following stain has been used?

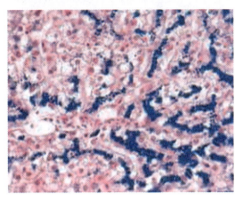

a. Alcian blue b. Prussian blue
c. Crystal violet d. Von kossa

48. Which of the following is the most consistent feature of rapidly progressing glomerulonephritis (RPGN)?
    a. Crescent formation
    b. Mesangial cell proliferation
    c. IgA deposition
    d. Loss of foot processes

49. A 40 years old HIV positive patient presented to the emergency with fever, neck pain and vomiting. He ultimately died and the appearance of the brain at autopsy and the micrograph is shown below. Identify the most likely pathogen involved:

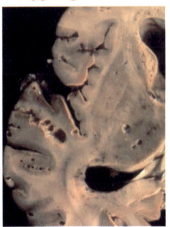

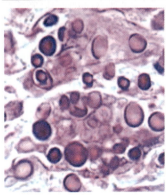

a. Toxoplasmosis
b. Echinococcus multilocularis
c. Herpes meningitis
d. Cryptococcus

50. A post-renal transplant patient presented with decreased urine output. A urinalysis was done and the microscopic image is shown below. Identify the structure marked with an arrow:

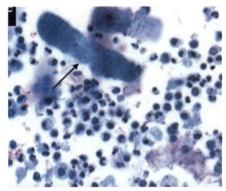

a. Hyaline casts
b. Renal tubular epithelial cells
c. Decoy cells
d. Clue cells

51. Damage to the part of brain represented in the micrograph below will lead to what speech abnormality?

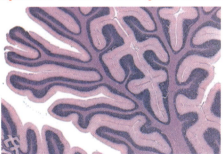

a. Sensory aphasia b. Speech apraxia
c. Aphonia d. Dysarthria

52. During autopsy of a patient died due to suspected myocardial infarction, the heart was stained with triphenyltetrazolium tetrachloride dye. What will be the color of the viable myocardium?
    a. White *(AIIMS May 2017, November 21016)*
    b. Red
    c. Blue
    d. Dark Brown

53. The resolving power of a microscope depends upon all of the following *except*:
    a. Size of the aperture
    b. Focal length of the eyepiece
    c. Thickness of the film
    d. Wavelength of light source used

54. MHC antigens are absent on:
    a. Platelet
    b. Erythrocyte
    c. Neutrophil
    d. Monocyte

55. Stain useful for identifying premalignant lesions of the lip is:
    a. Toluidine blue
    b. Alizarin red
    c. Hematoxylin and eosin
    d. Giemsa

PHARMACOLOGY

56. A pharmacological experiment was conducted to study effect of three drugs on heart rate and blood pressure. The following graphs were obtained before and after giving the drug. Which of the following statements is correct?

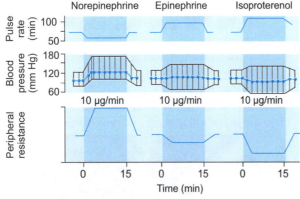

    a. A is isoprenaline
    b. B is epinephrine
    c. C is norepinephrine
    d. Action of C is antagonized by muscarinic blockers

57. Which of the following statements is true about the following dose response?

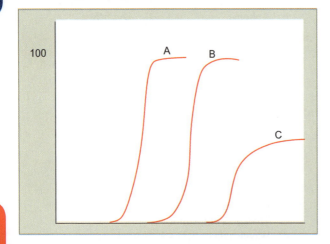

    a. Both A and B are full agonists
    b. B is more potent than A
    c. C is a noncompetitive antagonist
    d. A is more efficacious than B, but potency is same

58. A healthy volunteer was taken for a blood experiment. A history was taken from the volunteer before the experiment regarding exposure of NSAIDs, which he specifically denied. But on testing, the BT was found to be increased All of the following can be causative agent except:
    a. Theophylline
    b. Cephalosporin
    c. Anti-depressants
    d. Multivitamins containing Vitamin K

59. Which of the following drug can be used in benzodiazepine toxicity?
    a. Barbiturate   b. Ethyl alcohol
    c. Protamine sulphate   d. Flumazenil

60. Which of the following drugs can be given in renal failure safely?
    a. Saxagliptin   b. Linagliptin
    c. Vildagliptin   d. Sitagliptin

61. Metformin causes a severe, sometimes life-threatening side effect of lactic acidosis. All of the following factors increase the risk of lactic acidosis *except*:
    a. Advanced age
    b. Smoking
    c. Liver dysfunction
    d. Renal failure

62. Drug advertisement letter is a necessary component of each drug formulation and contains various information about the drug like drug dosing, frequency and half-life. Which of the following information need not be given in the drug advertisement letter?
    a. Research papers and other articles proving efficacy of the drug
    b. Date of expiry of the drug
    c. Rare, but serious life threatening adverse-effects
    d. Common, not so serious adverse-effects

63. All of the following are potentially serious side effects of thioamide group of antithyroid drugs *except*:
    a. Hepatic dysfunction
    b. Severe rash
    c. Agranulocytosis
    d. Anaphylaxis

63b. A patient is started on thioamide. Which of the following is not a life-threatening/serious side-effect of thioamide?
    a. Hepatic toxicity   b. Aplastic anemia
    c. Agranulocytosis   d. Lung fibrosis

64. Which of the following correctly represents the sequence of the rate of topical drug absorption?
    a. Postauricular skin > scalp > scrotum > dorsal aspect of hand > sole
    b. Postauricular skin > scrotum > scalp > dorsal aspect of hand > sole
    c. Scalp > scrotum > postauricular skin > dorsal aspect of hand > sole
    d. Scrotum > scalp > postauricular skin > dorsal aspect of hand > sole

65. Which of the following sites is least commonly preferred for insulin injection?
    a. Anterior thigh   b. Lateral thigh
    c. Dorsum of arm   d. Around umbilicus

66. Which of the following is not true for rifabutin as compared to rifampicin?
    a. Rifabutin has the longer half-life than rifampicin
    b. Rifabutin has lesser incidence of drug-interactions
    c. Rifabutin is more efficacious against MAC as compared to rifampicin
    d. Rifabutin is more efficacious for pulmonary TB as compared to rifampicin

67. Which of the following is not used in osteoporosis?
    a. Milnacipran   b. PTH
    c. Strontium ranelate d. Denosumab

68. Pigmentation of nail is caused by all of these drugs *except:*
    a. Cyclophosphamide   b. Chlorpromazine
    c. Chloroquine   d. Amiodarone

69. Digoxin is obtained from a plant product and has a half-life of 36 hours. How does this information help us in formulating treatment?
    a. To adjust maintenance dose of digoxin required to keep the blood levels within therapeutic range
    b. Intravenous administration in emergency and urgent dosing
    c. Long half-life permits alternate day dosing
    d. It requires a high loading dose to be administered

MICROBIOLOGY

70. In the following gram stained specimen, identify the bacteria seen:

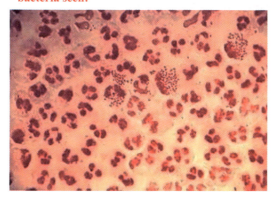

    a. Streptococcus pneumoniae
    b. Hemophilus influenzae
    c. Staphylococcus aureus
    d. Neisseria gonorrhoeae

71. Schizonts and late trophozoite stages of plasmodium falciparum not seen in peripheral blood smear because:
    a. They are sequestered in the spleen
    b. Due to adherence to the capillary endothelium, they are not seen in peripheral blood
    c. Due to antigen-antibody reaction and removal
    d. They are seen in mosquito blood

72. Which of the following is the most common systemic symptom during migration of larval phase of Helminths like Ancylostoma, Strongyloides and Ascaris?
    a. Asymptomatic
    b. Pneumonitis
    c. Liver failure
    d. Larva migrans

73. A 15 years old boy presented with fever and chills for 3 days. On examination he was found to have delayed skin pinch time and dry oral mucosa. A peripheral blood smear revealed the following picture. Identify the pathogen involved?

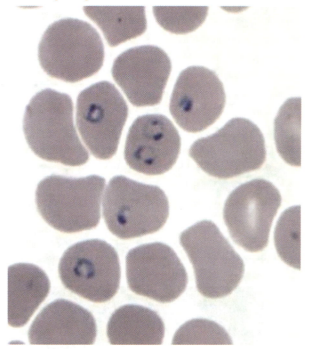

    a. Babesia
    b. Plasmodium vivax
    c. Plasmodium falciparum
    d. Salmonella typhi

74. The following are images of an intestinal nematode. Which of these are true about it?

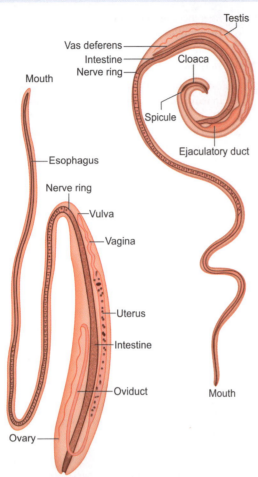

a. Transmitted through percutaneous and auto-inoculation
b. Embryonated egg is the infectious stage for this worm
c. The adult worm usually lives in the small intestine
d. Triclabendazole is the drug of choice

75. A patient with benign hypertrophy of prostate was admitted in the hospital for 3 weeks. He subsequently developed suspected catheter associated-urinary tract infection. The tip of the catheter was sent for culture and was grown on blood agar. After 24 hours, the blood agar shows the following appearance. What is the most likely causative agent for the UTI?

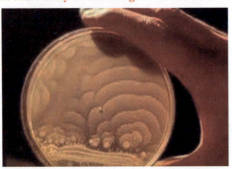

a. Escherichia coli
b. Klebsiella pneumoniae
c. Proteus mirabilis
d. Pseudomonas

76. Which of the following Treponema is seen in the silver impregnation micrograph below?

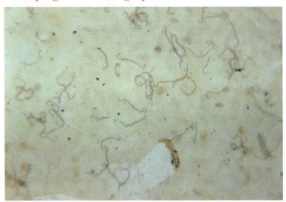

a. Leptospira interrogans
b. Treponema pallidum
c. Ehrlichia chaffeensis
d. Borrelia burgdorferi

77. In a suspected patient of dengue, all of these are acceptable investigations at day 3 of presentation *except*:
a. Viral culture and isolation in C6/36 cell line
b. ELISA for antibody against dengue virus
c. NS1 antigen detection
d. RT-PCR

78. A patient presented to the hospital with severe hydrophobia. You suspect rabies, obtained corneal scrapings from the patient. What test should be done on this specimen for a diagnosis of rabies?
a. Negri bodies   *(AIIMS May 2017, Nov 2016)*
b. Antibodies to rabies virus
c. RT-PCR for rabies virus
d. Indirect immunofluorescence

79. Which of the following is an obligate intracellular pathogen?
a. Coxiella burnetii
b. Listeria monocytogenes
c. Klebsiella
d. Legionella pneumophila

FORENSIC MEDICINE

80. St. Anthony's fire refers to poisoning by:
a. Ergot alkaloids
b. Spanish fly
c. Crotalaria juncea
d. Aflatoxin

81. A 19 years old patient presented to the emergency with altered sensorium. A noncontrast CT revealed hydrocephalus, requiring urgent neurosurgical intervention. The patient had nobody accompanying or any identity proof. Under which of these sections of Indian Penal Code (IPC) can the neurosurgeon perform the procedure without obtaining an informed consent from a guardian?

a. Section 87
b. Section 89
c. Section 90
d. Section 92

82. The following patient was brought for an autopsy. What is the cause of the discoloration of the region pointed by the arrow?

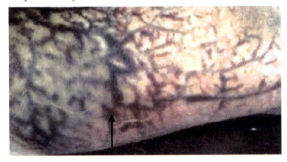

a. Hematoma formation
b. Methemoglobin
c. Sulfhemoglobin
d. Loss of blood

83. A doctor used the same needle used in a patient with HIV to inject in another patient. The latter patient on testing found to be infected with HIV. The doctor is punishable for this negligence according to which section of Indian penal code?
a. Section 166B
b. Section 202
c. Section 203
d. Section 269

84. A 38 years old female presented to the emergency with extensive burns. The patient had grade 3 burns on the face, back, upper arms and forearms along with singeing of hairs. Which of the following is not a proof of inhalation burns?
a. Yellow colored sputum
b. Blackish soot deposit on posterior part of tongue
c. Hoarseness & stridor of voice
d. Singeing of eyebrows and facial hair

85. All of the following are suggestive of domestic violence in a child *except*:
a. Wormian bones
b. Microfractures in the sub-epiphyseal region
c. Corner fractures
d. Bucket handle fractures of metaphyses

86. An abandoned dead male fetus was found and bought by police for autopsy. The following was the report "The head to feet length is 63 cm, eyes are open, pupillary membrane is absent, Crown Rump Length is 23 cm, testes are at the superficial inguinal ring and weight of the fetus is 1000 gm." What is the estimated age of the fetus?

a. 5 months
b. 6 months
c. 7 months
d. 8 months

87. Correctly match the following:

Declaration	Motive
1. Declaration of Geneva	i. Global health
2. Declaration of Helsinki	ii. Hippocratic oath
3. Declaration of Tokyo	iii. Medical Ethics
4. Declaration of Oslo	iv. Inhuman practices and torture

a. 1-iii, 2-ii, 3-iv, 4-i
b. 1-ii, 2-iii, 3-iv, 4-i
c. 1-iv, 2-i, 3- ii, 4-iii
d. 1-ii, 2-iv, 3-iii, 4-i

88. A farmer ingested some unknown poisonous seeds and had pain and vomiting. Soon he developed paralysis of his lower limbs, which ascends till it affected the respiratory muscles and he died within two days. Identify the likely cause:
a. Abrus precatorium
b. Solanum lycopersicum
c. Conium maculatum
d. Strychnine nux vomica

89. A lady was brought from village, unconscious, about 12 hours after ingesting some kind of unknown poison. Her heart rate was 103/min, blood pressure in 90/50 mm Hg and respiratory rate is 19/min. Her breath smelled like kerosene. All of the following should be done in her management, *except*:
a. Gastric lavage should be done
b. Atropine should be administered till signs of recovery
c. Vasopressors should be administered intravenously
d. Immediate airway management

90. All of these stains are used in tattooing *except*:
a. Osmium blue
b. Prussian blue
c. Vermillion
d. India ink

PREVENTIVE SOCIAL MEDICINE

91. CA-125 is a marker for screening of ovarian cancer. To characterize this test, histopathological confirmation of ovarian cancer was done in a cohort of patients. 60/100 women who tested positive for this test actually had ovarian cancer and 20/100 women who tested negative had ovarian cancer. What is the negative predictive value of this test?
a. 20/100
b. 40/100
c. 60/100
d. 80/100

92. A study was conducted to see the effect of pulse oximeter readings in neonates with and without micropore. A plot between the two values was drawn as shown in the figure. Which of the following conclusion of the figure is correct?

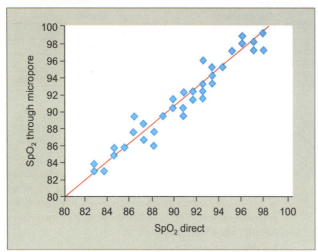

   a. There is positive correlation between two groups
   b. There is negative correlation between two groups
   c. There is no correlation between two groups
   d. The data is insufficient to comment

93. A study was conducted to find out number of positive lymph nodes in a population of breast cancer patients who underwent axillary dissection. A graph was plotted between the number and frequency of positive nodes as below. Which of the following is the correct statement?

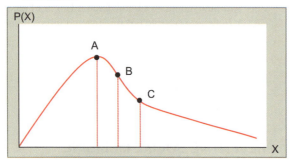

   a. A; Mode B: Median C: Mean
   b. A: Mode B: Mean C: Median
   c. A: Median B: Mode C: Mean
   d. A: Mean B: Median C: Mode

94. Which of the following is the best for determining the threshold for diagnosis of a positive test?
   a. Analysis of variance
   b. Pearson coefficient
   c. Receiver-operating characteristic curve
   d. Pre-test probability

95. A study was done in 3 states to see the mean blood pressure in each community. Health workers were assigned and they visited each house in the three communities. Mean blood pressure in each community was found and compared. What type of study design is represented here?
   a. Cohort study
   b. Cross-sectional study
   c. Field trial
   d. Case control study

96. A 42 years old woman from a dry state who ingested rye for long time presented with complaints of weakness in both the lower limbs, nausea and fatigue. Over due course of time, she is completely unable to walk. What is the most likely cause?
   a. Argemone mexicana
   b. Amanita
   c. Ergot alkaloids
   d. Lathyrus sativus

97. A scatter diagram was plotted as shown below to study the relationship between two quantitative variables. What is the correct interpretation?

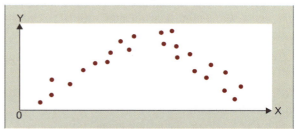

   a. There is correlation between the two variables and the Pearson's coefficient is 1
   b. There is correlation between the two variables and the Pearson's coefficient is 1
   c. There is no correlation between the two variables
   d. There is no relation between the two variables

98. According to the new RNTCP guidelines, the following is not a suspect of tuberculosis:
   a. Confirmed extra-pulmonary tuberculosis patient with cough of 2 weeks or more
   b. HIV-positive patient with cough of any duration
   c. Contacts of sputum positive tuberculosis patient with cough of any duration
   d. Any individual having cough of duration 2 weeks or more

99. A study was conducted to find average intra-ocular pressure. IOP was measured in 400 people and the mean was found to be 25 mm Hg with a standard deviation of 10 mm Hg. What is the range in which IOP of 95% of the population would be lying?

a. 22-28 mm Hg
b. 20-30 mm Hg
c. 24-26 mm Hg
d. 23-27 mm Hg

100. In a cohort study, to study association between factor and disease, the risk ratio was calculated to be equal to 1. What does this signifies?
    a. There is no association present between the factor and the disease
    b. There is positive association between the factor and the disease
    c. There is negative association between the factor and the disease
    d. Data insufficient to comment

MEDICINE

101. A 34-years old male patient presented with complaints of dyspnea and productive cough with postural variation. The patient gives a history of 20 pack years of smoking. The patient also has a history of recent binge drinking. A chest X-ray was taken and is shown below. What is the next step in management?

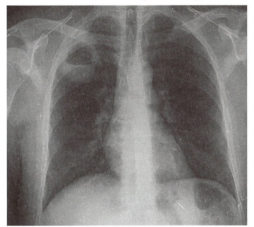

    a. Gemcitabine and carboplatin-based chemotherapy
    b. Lobectomy
    c. Intravenous clindamycin and fluids
    d. Antitubercular therapy

102. Identify the diagnosis from the following electrocardiogram:

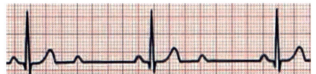

    a. 2:1 heart-block
    b. Trifascicular block
    c. First degree heart block
    d. Atrial fibrillation

103. A 59 years old male patient presented with complaints of right-sided facial weakness and loss of sensation on right side of the face with left sided hemiparesis. Examination reveals Horner's syndrome, nystagmus, vertigo, ataxia and dysphagia. The patient is not able to balance himself. What is the most common cause of this presentation?
    a. Due to occlusion of right posterior inferior cerebellar artery
    b. Due to occlusion of basilar artery
    c. Due to occlusion of left posterior inferior cerebellar artery
    d. Due to occlusion of anterior inferior cerebellar artery

104. Hypereosinophilic syndrome is a disease characterized by elevated eosinophil count in the blood for at least 6 months, without any recognizable cause, with involvement of either heart, nervous system or bone marrow. What should be the eosinophil count for diagnosis?
    a. $>500/mm^3$
    b. $>1000/mm^3$
    c. $>1500/mm^3$
    d. $>2000/mm^3$

105. A patient presented with history of vomiting for last three days. On examination, signs of dehydration were present. On further investigation, the patient was found to have raised creatinine, a pH = 7.22, pCO_2 = 21 mm Hg, HCO_3 = 9 mEq, Na^+ = 138 mEq/L and K^+ = 3.4 mEq/L. Identify the acid base abnormality observed in this patient:
    a. Metabolic acidosis
    b. Metabolic alkalosis
    c. Mixed metabolic acidosis and respiratory alkalosis
    d. Mixed respiratory acidosis and metabolic alkalosis

106. Calculate the base deficit in a patient of weight 75 kg with a pH = 6.96, pCO_2 = 30 mm Hg and HCO_3^- = 6 mEq/L:
    a. 300 mEq
    b. 400 mEq
    c. 500 mEq
    d. 800 mEq

107. About anti-epileptic drugs, which of the following is an incorrect match?

Focal seizures	Lamotrigine, Carbamazepine, Phenytoin	Valproate
Absence seizure	Carbamazepine	Ethosuximide, Valproate
Myoclonic seizures	Valproate, Lamotrigine	Clonazepam
Generalized tonic clonic seizures	Valproate, Lamotrigine, Topiramate	Phenytoin, Carbamazepine

    a. 1
    b. 2
    c. 3
    d. 4

108. An 80 kg male patient presented to the emergency with hypotension and you have been instructed to start him on an inotrope at a dose of 10 mcg/kg/min. Each 5 mL amp of the drug contains 200 mg drug. You choose 2 ampules of the drug and decide to mix it with saline to make a 250 mL solution. What should be the flow rate of the drug solution to maintain the BP of the patient (assuming 16 drops = 1 mL)?
   a. 4 drops/min
   b. 8 drops/min
   c. 10 drops/min
   d. 16 drops/min

109. An 86 years old lady presented with severe constipation. She was a known hypertensive on medications for 10 years. In clinic, her BP was 157/98 mm Hg with a heart rate of 58/min. On taking here BP in the supine position it was found to be 90/60 mm Hg. She had the recent history of depression. She is taking atenolol, thiazide, imipramine, haloperidol and docusate. What will be the next best step in the management?
   a. Change atenolol and thiazide to calcium channel blocker and ACE inhibitor and add bisacodyl for constipation
   b. Change imipramine and haloperidol to fluoxetine and risperidone and add bisacodyl for constipation
   c. Only add bisacodyl for constipation and continue rest of the medications
   d. Discontinue all her medications and start her on steroids

110. A 42 years old male patient presented with jaundice. His AST was 48 U, ALT was 51 U, ALP, GGTP were normal. Ultrasound of liver was suggestive of cirrhosis. Viral markers were done and the following results were obtained.

Test	Result
Anti-HAV	Negative
Anti-HBsAg	Negative
Anti-HBeAg	Negative
Anti-HBcAg IgG	Positive
Anti-HBcAg IgM	Negative
HBsAg	Negative
Anti-HCV	Positive
Anti-HEV	Negative

What is the next best step in management of this patient?
   a. Start interferon therapy
   b. Liver biopsy
   c. RT-PCR for hepatitis C virus
   d. PCR for HBV-DNA

111. A 25 years old unidentified male from roadside was brought by police to emergency room with disorientation, altered sensorium and vomiting. He had a BP of 90/70 mm Hg, heart rate of 110/min, temperature –36.4°C and respiratory rate of 11/min. On examination, he had bilateral pin-point pupils. What is the most probable diagnosis?
   a. Pontine hemorrhage
   b. Hypothermia
   c. Dhatura poisoning
   d. Opioid poisoning

112. Continuous murmur can be heard in all except:
   a. VSD with aortic regurgitation
   b. Coronary AV fistula
   c. Pulmonary AV fistula
   d. Patent ductus arteriosus

113. Metered Dose Inhalers are used in management of asthma. To use a MDI, it is recommended to shake well before use, breathe out, bring the inhaler to your mouth, start to breathe in slowly, press the top of you inhaler once and keep breathing in slowly until you have taken a full breath and then hold your breath for 10 seconds. Some patients might need a second puff of MDI for symptomatic relief. Which of these instructions for re-using the MDI is not correct?
   a. Wait for 1 minute between two puffs
   b. Shake the inhaler again before use
   c. Carefully rinse your mouth and throat
   d. Clean the inhaler before use

114. Which of the following is not true regarding iron supplementation in iron deficiency anemia?
   a. Administer a small diluted dose first prior to infusion to look for any allergy to iron preparation
   b. Oral iron therapy should be stopped once the patient achieves a hemoglobin of >12 mg/dL
   c. If gastric intolerance to oral iron therapy occurs, all patients should be administered parenteral forms
   d. Parenteral iron supplementation is required in a patient with Hb of less then 7 mg/dL

115. A patient presents to the emergency with altered sensorium. All of these tests should be done except:
   a. Complete blood counts
   b. Random blood sugar
   c. Lumbar puncture
   d. Non-contrast CT head

116. A patient diagnosed with carcinoma of lung presented with a serum calcium level of 16.4 mmol/L. What will be the first step in management?
   a. IV fluids and furosemide
   b. Immediate hemodialysis
   c. Bisphosphonates
   d. Chemotherapy with gemcitabine and carboplatin

117. About Transfusion Related Acute Lung Injury (TRALI), all of the following are true except:
   a. Signs and symptoms usually subsides within 2–3 weeks of onset
   b. Supportive care is the mainstay of treatment
   c. Steroids have a doubtful role in management
   d. Mortality is less than 10%

118. Which of the following infections causes a non-centrally distributed rash?
    a. Epidemic typhus
    b. Measles
    c. Secondary syphilis
    d. Typhoid

119. Cerebellar lesion can produce all of the following *except:*
    a. Nystagmus
    b. Past pointing
    c. Resting tremor
    d. Ataxic gait

120. A 40 years old female is diagnosed to have epilepsy and is started phenytoin and valproate. Four weeks later, she developed a diffuse rash all over her body, which gradually disappeared on stopping both the drugs. In how many weeks, will the rash reappear when she is re-challenged with phenytoin and valproate?
    a. 1 day
    b. 1 week
    c. 2 weeks
    d. 4 weeks

121. Which of the following is not true about the salivary gland output in Sjogren's syndrome?
    a. Increase in sodium concentration
    b. Increase in phosphate concentration
    c. Decreased output of salivary glands <0.5 ml/min
    d. Increase in IgA concentration

122. A patient was found to have splenomegaly anemia and jaundice all of the following are true about this condition *except*:
    a. Increased urobilinogen
    b. Increased LDH
    c. Decreased haptoglobin
    d. Low reticulocyte count

123. Which of the following is the best test for assessment of intestinal malabsorption?
    (AIIMS November 2016, May 2010)
    a. Fecal fat estimation
    b. Serum amylase levels
    c. D-xylose absorption test
    d. NBT-PABA test

SURGERY

124. Which of the following is a true diverticulum of esophagus?
    a. Parabronchial diverticulum
    b. Epiphrenic diverticulum
    c. Meckel's diverticulum
    d. Zenker's diverticulum

125. Which of the regions marked in the following picture represents the zone 4 of retroperitoneal hemorrhage?

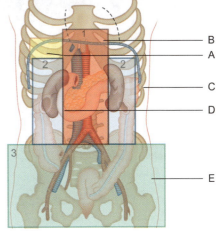

    a. A
    b. C and D
    c. B
    d. E

126. All of the following are signs of respiratory insufficiency *except:*
    a. Hypoxia
    b. Inability to speak
    c. Strider during inspiration
    d. All of the above

127. Which one of the following is a muscle splitting incision?
    a. Kocher's incision
    b. Rutherford-Morrison incision
    c. Pfannenstiel incision
    d. Lanz incision

128. After a midline laparotomy, you have been asked to suture the incision. What length of suture material will you choose?
    a. 2x incision length
    b. 4x incision length
    c. 6x incision length
    d. 8x incision length

129. A 30 years old young male met with a road traffic accident and came to the trauma center. On examination his BP is 90/56 mm Hg, pulse rate is 150/min, SpO_2 86% and a Glasgow coma score of 8. On examination the patient had multiple injuries and FAST reveals haemorrhage in all quadrants. He was operated upon and the postoperative pictures are shown below. Which of the following option correctly describe the two pictures?

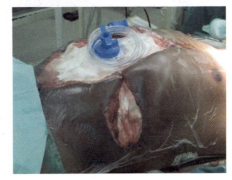

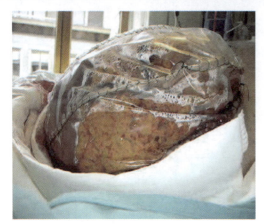

a. Midline laparotomy and meshplasty
b. Abdominothoracic surgery with abdominal zipping
c. Damage control surgery and mesh closure of abdomen
d. Abdominoplasty and primary closure of abdomen

130. Identify the instrument shown below:

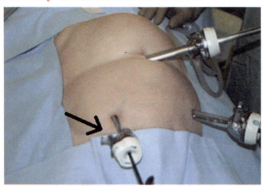

a. Laparoscopic port trocar
b. Peritoneal dialysis catheter
c. Endoscopic ultrasound probe
d. DPL catheter

131. A 60 years old male came with bleeding per rectum and was diagnosed to have carcinoma colon. The patient underwent extended right hemicolectomy as shown below. Identify the instrument that the surgeon is using:

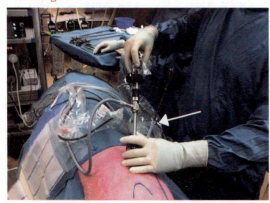

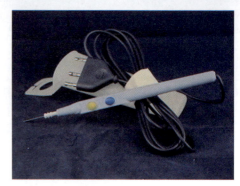

a. Monopolar cautery
b. LigaSure vessel ligating system
c. Harmonic scalpel
d. Hyfrecator

132. A 44 years old male underwent a VATS thymectomy for Myasthenia graves. During surgery, the pleura was accidentally injured. The surgeon decided to put a drain in the pleural cavity. Which of the following statements is correct about the timing of removal of intercostal chest tube?
   a. After partial expansion of lungs and <50 mL output from drain for 2 consecutive days
   b. After complete expansion of lungs and <30 mL output from drain for 2 consecutive days
   c. After complete expansion of lungs and <200 mL output from drain for 2 consecutive days
   d. On 4th day, irrespective of the output from the drain and lung expansion

133. The police has brought an unresponsive patient to you. What is the first thing you will do?
   a. Start chest compressions immediately
   b. Check carotid pulse
   c. Check for response and call help
   d. Start rescue breaths

134. A 45 years old patient presented to you with ongoing massive hematemesis. The patient is alert and hemodynamically stable. What will be the first step in management?
   a. Do an urgent upper GI endoscopy
   b. Put the patient in recovery position and secure airway
   c. Insert a cannula and start IV fluids
   d. Send for blood transfusion

135. Which of the following is the most common symptom of aortoiliac occlusive disease?
   a. Calf claudication   b. Gluteal claudication
   c. Impotence   d. Symptomless

136. In a patient with obstructive jaundice, what is the possible explanation for a bilirubin level of 40 mg/dL?
   a. Malignant obstruction
   b. Complete obstruction of common bile duct
   c. Renal failure
   d. Liver failure

137. All of the following are seen in MEN-1 syndrome *except:*
    a. Posterior pituitary tumors
    b. Pancreatic neuroendocrine tumors
    c. Foregut carcinoid
    d. Parathyroid hyperplasia

138. Fine needle aspiration cytology (FNAC) is not enough to diagnose:
    a. Papillary carcinoma of thyroid
    b. Follicular carcinoma of thyroid
    c. Carcinoma breast
    d. Adenocarcinoma lung

139. Which of these scoring systems is helpful in assessing severity of wound infection and is used for research and surveillance?
    a. Southampton grading scale
    b. ASA classification
    c. Glasgow score
    d. APGAR

140. After a laparotomy, a woman presents with burst abdomen. After treating the infection. The surgeon decides for resuturing. Which of the following suture material should be used?
    a.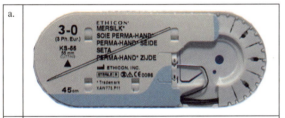
    b.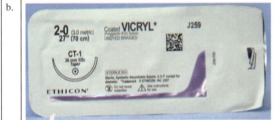
    c.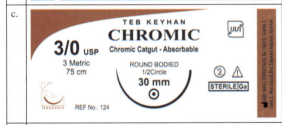
    d.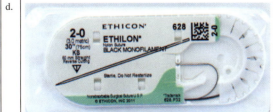

141. Non-visualization of gallbladder in hepatic scintigraphy is suggestive of:
    a. Chronic cholecystitis
    b. Carcinoma gallbladder
    c. Acute cholecystitis due to gallstones
    d. Gallstones obstructing CBD

OBSTETRICS & GYNECOLOGY

142. A 35 years old female presented with an adnexal mass. CA125 was slightly raised, CA199 was normal and LDH was elevated. Tumor was resected and the gross and microscopic image were as given below. What is the most likely diagnosis?

    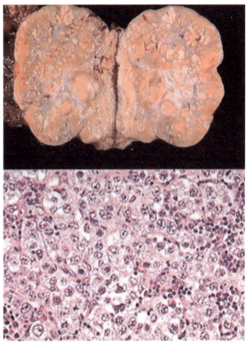

    a. Papillary serous cystadenocarcinoma
    b. Dysgerminoma
    c. Teratoma
    d. Choriocarcinoma

143. The following graph represents the stages of labor. Which of the following statements is true about the graph C?

    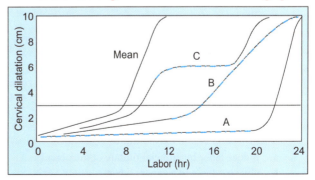

a. Secondary arrest after progression of labor
b. Prolonged active phase of labor
c. Prolonged latent phase/primary arrest of labor
d. Normal labor in a primigravida

144. **Which of the following is done for screening of Down's syndrome in first trimester?**
    a. Beta HCG and PAPP-A
    b. Unconjugated estradiol and PAPPA
    c. AFP and Inhibin A
    d. AFP and Beta HCG

145. **A patient presenting with an adnexal mass was operated and the following tumor was removed. What is the likely diagnosis?**

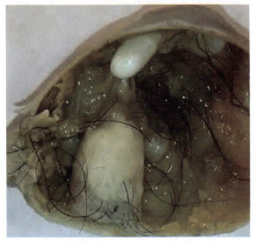

   a. Mature teratoma
   b. Dysgerminoma
   c. Granulosa cell tumor
   d. Mucinous adenocarcinoma

146. **What dose of misoprostol is used orally to control bleeding in post partum hemorrhage?** *(AIIMS November 2015)*
    a. 400 micrograms
    b. 600 micrograms
    c. 800 micrograms
    d. 1000 micrograms

147. **What is the maximum capacity of Bakri balloon which is used in post partum hemorrhage?**
    a. 200 mL
    b. 300 mL
    c. 500 mL
    d. 1000 mL

148. **A 38 weeks primigravida presented to the labor room with minimal labor pains and contraction. On examination, the cervix is 2 cm dilated and 50% effaced. The heart rate of the patient is 86/min and blood pressure is 126/76 mm Hg. What should be done next?**
    a. Induce labor by artificial rupture of membranes
    b. Give oxytocin to augment labor
    c. Sedate the patient by and give phenergan to decrease labor pains
    d. Observe the patient and wait for increase in uterine contractions

149. **What is the drug of choice for precocious puberty in girls?**
    a. GnRH analogues
    b. Cyproterone acetate
    c. Danazol
    d. Medroxyprogesterone acetate

150. **A young female presented to you with primary amenorrhea. Examination reveals normal breast development and absent axillary hairs. Pelvic examination shows a normally developed vagina with clitoromegaly. On ultrasound, gonads are visible in the inguinal region. What is the most likely diagnosis?**
    a. Complete androgen insensitivity syndrome
    b. Partial androgen insensitivity syndrome
    c. Mayer Rokitansky Kuster Hauser syndrome
    d. Gonadal dysgenesis

151. **Which of the following statements is not true about cervical cancer screening guidelines according to WHO?**
    a. Pap smear should be repeated yearly in women of reproductive age group
    b. HPV test should be done five yearly in women between age of 30 to 49 years
    c. Visual inspection with acetic acid is more reliable at older age as it becomes easier to identify the transformation zone with age
    d. Pap smear can be repeated less frequently if it comes out negative for 3 consecutive years

152. **Which of the following statements is true regarding medical abortion?**
    a. Ultrasound should be done in all cases
    b. If the patient has an IUCD in-situ, it doesn't need to be removed
    c. Can only be done up to 72 days
    d. Only a person certified under MTP act can perform medical termination of pregnancy

153. **Partograph represents various stages of labor with respect to time. True about partograph is all *except*:**
    a. Each small square represents one hour
    b. Alert and action lines are separated by a difference of 4 hours
    c. Partograph recording should be started at a cervical dilation of 4 cm
    d. Send the patient to first referral unit if the labor progression line crosses the alert line

154. **Which of the following is the correct representation of the normal oral glucose tolerance test?**

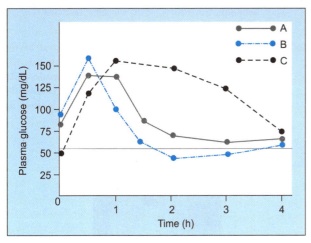

a. A
b. B
c. C
d. None of the above

PAEDIATRICS

155. A child presented at 2 years of age with delayed motor development, mental retardation and finger biting. He was normal at birth. He subsequently develops cerebral palsy arthritis and dies due to renal failure at age of 25 years. What is the likely enzyme deficiency implicated?
    a. Hexosaminidase deficiency
    b. Adenosine deaminase deficiency
    c. HGPRT deficiency
    d. Ornithine transcarbamoylase deficiency

156. A neonate on routine examination at birth was found to have hepatomegaly. Rest of the examination was essentially unremarkable. On investigations, Anti-HCMV antibodies were found to be positive. What sequelae in later life is the child at risk of?
    a. Renal failure
    b. Mental retardation
    c. Hepatic fibrosis
    d. Sensorineural hearing loss

157. Which of the following medicines taken during pregnancy is responsible for the defect seen in the child below?

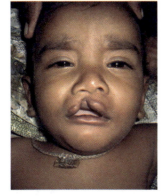

    a. Ferrous sulfate
    b. Isotretinoin
    c. Folic acid
    d. Metoclopramide

158. Palivizumab is a humanized monoclonal antibody. For which of the following conditions has it been approved for?
    a. Avian influenzae
    b. Parainfluenzae
    c. Respiratory syncytial virus
    d. Coxsackie virus

159. In which of the diseases is the following appearance of calves seen in a child?

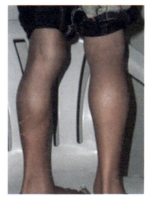

    a. Spinal muscular atrophy
    b. Myopathy
    c. Muscular dystrophy
    d. Peripheral neuropathy

160. A 2 months old child was brought to the subcenter by his mother with complaints of fever for two days. Weight of the child is 2 kg. On examination, the child is restless and irritable, skin pinch went back in 2 seconds, oral mucosa is dry and eyes were sunken. There were ten pustules on his forehead. What should be done at the subcenter?
    a. Refer to higher center with mother giving frequent sips of ORS
    b. Immediately admit the child, give IV fluids and then refer to higher center
    c. Give first dose of antibiotic and refer to higher center in an ambulance with sips of ORS along the way
    d. Send child home with few packets of ORS and call after 3 days.

161. A 6 days old neonate weighing 2800 gm (birth weight 3200 gm) was brought with the complaints of fever, poor feeding and poor activity. There was no history of vomiting or diarrhea. Axillary temperature was 39°C with depressed fontenalle, sunken eyes, decreased urine output and decreased skin turgor. Her mother has the history of decreased milk production. What is your diagnosis?
    a. Neonatal sepsis
    b. Galactosemia
    c. Fever & dehydration
    d. Acute renal failure

162. A neonate presented with cicatrizing skin lesions all over the body with hypoplasia of all limbs. An MRI of the brain revealed diffuse cerebral atrophy. An ophthalmologic evaluation reveals chorioretinitis. Which of these tests is most likely to show a positive result in this patient?
    a. Anti-HCMV antibodies
    b. Anti-toxoplasma antibodies
    c. Anti-VZV antibody
    d. Anti-rubella antibody

163. What should be the ideal temperature in delivery room for the neonates to be kept in warmer?
    a. 22-26°C
    b. 28-30°C
    c. 30-35°C
    d. 37°C

164. Ponderal index is:
    a. Square root of height in feet by weight in grams
    b. Weight in kilograms by cube of height in meters
    c. Mid-upper arm circumference to head circumference ratio
    d. Head circumference to abdominal circumference ratio

165. Ideal route of drug delivery in neonatal resuscitation is:
    a. Intraosseous
    b. Through umbilical vein
    c. Through peripheral vein
    d. Through umbilical artery

166. A neonate presented with jaundice on first day of life. His mother's blood group is 'O' positive. How will you manage this patient?
    a. Observe only as it is mostly physiological jaundice
    b. Exchange transfusion
    c. Liver function tests and liver biopsy as it is mostly due to cholestasis
    d. Phototherapy

167. What is the recommended dose of steroids for attaining fetal lung maturity?
    a. Inj. betamethasone 12 mg for 2 doses 12 hours apart
    b. Inj. betamethasone 12 mg for 2 doses 24 hours apart
    c. Inj. dexamethasone 6 mg for 4 doses 24 hours apart
    d. Inj. dexamethasone 12 mg for 2 doses 12 hours apart

ORTHOPAEDICS

168. What is the most likely cause of the abnormality seen in the wrist X-ray from a 12 years old boy as shown below?

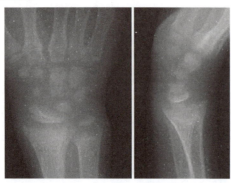

    a. Scaphoid fracture
    b. Colles' fracture
    c. Osteoporosis
    d. Rickets

169. A patient after a roadside trauma presented to the trauma centre. He has a severe pain in his left hip and, on examination the hip is exquisitely tender with restricted range of motion. The patient is lying in the posture seen below. Which of the following deformity is seen in the patient?

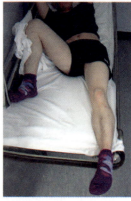

    a. Anterior dislocation of hip
    b. Posterior dislocation of hip
    c. Inferior dislocation of hip
    d. Central dislocation of hip

170. A 12 years old boy presented with pain in his right hip. A pelvic X-ray was taken and is shown below. What is the likely diagnosis?

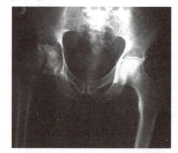

    a. Osteoporosis
    b. Osteopetrosis
    c. Osteogenesis imperfecta
    d. Osteopoikilocytosis

170b. A child comes with the history of pain in the right hip and difficulty in walking. X-ray hip was done as seen in the picture. Which of the following is the most likely diagnosis?

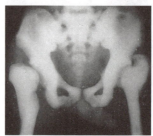

a. Osteopetrosis b. Osteoporosis
c. Osteopoikilocytosis d. Osteogenesis imperfecta

171. The following X-ray was taken of a 16 years old patient. What is the most likely pathology seen?

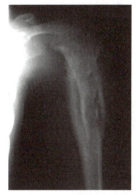

a. Ewing's sarcoma b. Osteosarcoma
c. Chronic osteomyelitis d. Acute osteomyelitis

172. An athlete suffers a fracture as shown in the Knee X-ray below. How is this fracture managed?

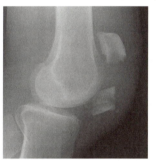

a. Tension band wiring b. Compression plating
c. Internal fixation d. K-wire fixation

173. The following deformity shown in the picture is likely to be a complication of which of these?
(AIIMS November 2015)

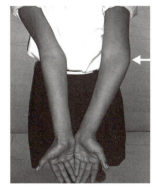

a. Lateral condylar fracture
b. Monteggia fracture dislocation
c. Radial head fracture
d. Supracondylar fracture

174. Which of the following increases callus formation?
a. Rigid immobilization b. Movement at fracture site
c. Compression plating d. Intraosseous nailing

OPHTHALMOLOGY

175. The following device shown in the figure is used for indirect ophthalmoscopy. What is the power of the lens that should be used with it to visualize the retina?

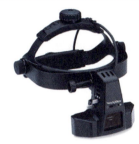

a. −58 D b. +20 D
c. +60 D d. +90 D

176. These days, a variety of eye surgeries including cataract surgeries are performed using lasers, with small incisions and fewer postoperative complications and early recovery. What is the pulse duration of laser used in cataract surgery as shown below?

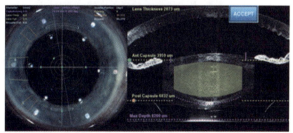

a. 10^{-15} seconds b. 10^{-12} seconds
c. 10^{-9} seconds d. 10^{-6} seconds

177. A farmer presented to the ophthalmological emergency with blurred vision, redness, tearing, photophobia, pain and foreign body sensation following a stick injury of the eye. Examination reveals a corneal ulcer with fuzzy margins and redness. A picture of the eye is shown below. How will you manage this patient?

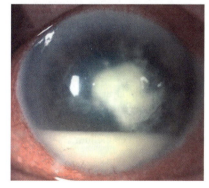

a. Topical antibiotics and drainage of hypopyon
b. Topical natamycin and drainage of hypopyon
c. Topical natamycin only, no need to drain the hypopyon
d. Topical Steroids

178. **Maximum contribution to the refractive power of the eye is by which part of the eye?**
    a. Anterior surface of cornea
    b. Posterior surface of cornea
    c. Anterior surface of lens
    d. Posterior surface of lens

179. **What is the usual weight of rabbit used in ophthalmological experiments?**
    a. 0.5-1 kg   b. 1.5-2.5 kg
    c. 5–7 kg   d. 10–12 kg

180. **A 26 years old male presented to the emergency with sudden diminution of vision in left eye. The fluorescein angiography revealed a picture as shown below. A diagnosis of retinal tear was made. The optical coherence tomography image is shown below. In which layers of retina, accumulation of fluid occurs?**

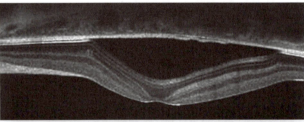

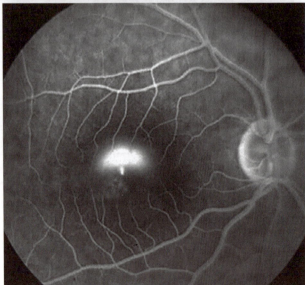

a. Outer plexiform layer
b. Inner nuclear layer
c. Nerve fibre layer
d. Retinal pigment epithelium

181. **The given picture represents which of the following condition?**

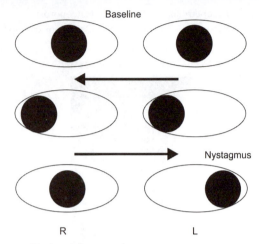

a. Horizontal gaze palsy
b. Internuclear ophthalmoplegia
c. 3rd nerve palsy
d. Duane retraction syndrome

182. **Which of these is not a correct definition of blindness as per NPCB?**
    a. Diminution of field vision to 20° or less in better eye
    b. Inability of a person to count fingers from a distance of 6 meters or 20 feet
    c. Vision 6/60 or less with the best possible spectacle correction in the better eye
    d. Vision 4/60 or less with the best possible spectacle correction in the better eye

ENT

183. **A construction worker met with an accident and presented to the trauma centre when a heavy concrete block fell over his face. He was found to have severe maxillofacial and laryngeal injury. He was not able to open his mouth and, on examination, he is found to have multiple fractures and obstruction in nasopharynx as well as oropharynx. In order to maintain a patent airway, the following procedure was done for him. Which of the following options define the procedure correctly?**

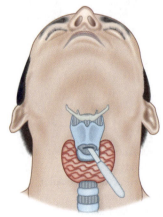

a. Submental endotracheal intubation
b. Emergency tracheostomy
c. Cricothyroidotomy
d. Subcutaneous tracheostomy

184. **According to the WHO definition of hearing loss, what is the value to classify as profound hearing loss?**
    a. 61-71 dB
    b. >81 dB
    c. >91 dB
    d. >101 dB

SKIN

185. **Postherpetic neuralgia is defined as pain lasting beyond how many weeks?**
    a. 1 week
    b. 2 weeks
    c. 3 weeks
    d. 4 weeks

186. **A 24 years old female presented with patchy hair loss in the right temporal and occipital region. Examination revealed non-scarring alopecia with multiple small broken hairs. Scrapings from scalp showed mild inflammation, peri-follicular hemorrhage and surrounding mild lymphocytic infiltration. What is the most likely diagnosis?**
    a. Alopecia areata
    b. Androgenic alopecia
    c. Loose anagen hair
    d. Trichotillomania

187. **A 35 years old female presented with painful blisters over oral mucosa and genital areas. She gave the history of similar lesions in the past. A biopsy from the lesion showed a suprabasal split on histopathology. Immunofluorescence microscopy revealed intercellular IgG deposits as shown below. What is the most likely diagnosis?**

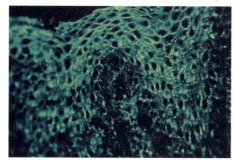

    a. Dermatitis herpetiformis
    b. Pemphigus vulgaris
    c. Behcet's disease
    d. Allergic dermatitis

188. **A sexually active male presented with warts on his penis as shown below. Which of these strains of HPV is most commonly the cause of these lesions?**

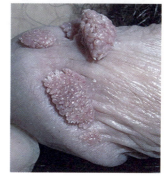

    a. HPV 1,2 and 3
    b. HPV 3, 5
    c. HPV 6 and 11
    d. HPV 16 and 18

189. **A 12 years old boy presented with gradually progressive annual plaque on his buttocks with central scarring. What is the most likely diagnosis?**
    a. Tinea cruris
    b. Annular psoriasis
    c. Granuloma annulare
    d. Lupus vulgaris

ANAESTHESIA

190. **A 40 years old chronic smoker was scheduled for cholecystectomy under general anesthesia. He was induced with propofol and vecuronium and started on isoflurane for maintenance of anesthesia. During the procedure, the following capnograph plot was observed. What is the possible cause?**

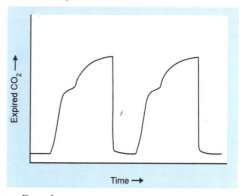

    a. Bronchospasm
    b. Entry into the right-sided bronchus
    c. Leak from expiratory valve
    d. Rebreathing

191. **During laryngoscopy and intubation procedure, all of these are true, *except:* (AIIMS November 2016, 2003)**
    a. A slight pressure may be applied at the cricoid cartilage
    b. The laryngoscope is held in the right hand introduced from the right side of the patient
    c. The neck is flexed with extension at the atlanto-occipital joint
    d. After insertion of laryngoscope, it is levered on the upper incisor to pull up the tongue and visualize the vocal cords

192. What is the ratio of chest compressions and breaths when a lone person is giving cardiopulmonary resuscitation?
    a. 10:1
    b. 15:1
    c. 30:1
    d. 30:2

193. Why 100% oxygen is administered after nitrous oxide is discontinued on emergence from anesthesia?
    a. Second gas effect
    b. Diffusion hypoxia
    c. For adequate analgesia
    d. As air is costlier then oxygen

194. A surgeon decides to operate a patient under epidural anesthesia. 3% Xylocaine with adrenaline is used for administering epidural anesthesia. The patient suddenly develops hypotension after 3 minutes of administration. What is the most likely cause for this?
    a. Systemic absorption of the drug
    b. Vasovagal effect
    c. Allergy to the drug preparation
    d. Penetration into the subarachnoid space

RADIOLOGY

195. A 12 years old male involved in a bike accident presents to emergency department with cough, dyspnea and chest discomfort. On evaluation, BP was 130/80 mm Hg, Pulse rate 88/min and respiratory rate 22/min. On auscultation, there was decreased air entry on one side with absent breath sounds. Pulse oximeter shows saturation of 98%. Chest X-ray is given below. Most probable diagnosis is:

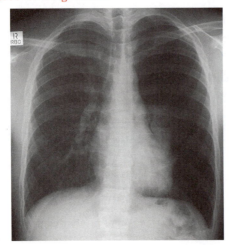

   a. Left sided pneumothorax with lung collapse
   b. Rupture of esophagus compressing the pericardium
   c. Flail chest due to fracture of ribs 5, 6, 7 & 8
   d. Normal chest X-ray

PSYCHIATRY

196. An elderly female had her house destroyed in an earthquake. Following this, she presented to your office with complaints of anxiety, sadness, lack of sleep, anger, palpitations and despair. Consider the following statements:
    a. The lady is suffering from acute stress reaction
    b. The defense mechanism involved is projection
    c. Drug of choice in this situation is risperidone
    d. She needs referral to a psychiatrist for psychotherapy

    Which of the following statements are true?
    a. a & c
    b. b & d
    c. a, b & c
    d. a & d

197. A 22 years old male comes to your office with complains of frequenting checking of doors even when they are locked. He is distressed about this fact. He is subsequently diagnosed to have obsessive compulsive disorder. Consider the following statements:
    a. Repression and reaction formation are the defense mechanisms involved
    b. SSRIs are the drug of choice
    c. Risperidone may be used in SSRI resistant cases to augment the response
    d. Systemic desensitization is the psychotherapy of choice

    Which of the above are correct statements?
    a. a & b
    b. b & c
    c. b, c & d
    d. a, b, c & d

198. Which of these is the correct sequence of Maslow's hierarchy of needs?
    a. Safety - Physiological needs - Self-actualization - Belonging - Self-esteem
    b. Physiological needs - Safety - Belonging - Self-esteem - Self- actualization
    c. Safety - Self-actualization - Belonging - Physiological needs - Self-esteem
    d. Self-actualization - Physiological needs - Safety - Belonging - Self-esteem

199. A person has been referred to you by the court. You find a discrepancy between the history and examination findings. Which of these conditions you should be aware of in this situation?
    a. Malingering
    b. Factitious disorder
    c. Somatization syndrome
    d. Dissociative fugue

200. Polysomnography contains all of the following tests except:
    a. Electroencephalography
    b. Pulse oximetry
    c. Electrooculography
    d. Arterial pCO_2 measurement

Explanations

ANATOMY

1. **Ans. d. Urinary bladder** *(Ref: Gray's 40/e p30, 1250)*
   The given image is of transitional epithelium, which is present in urinary tract (urinary bladder).

   "Urothelium is a specialized epithelium that lines much of the urinary tract and prevents its rather toxic contents from damaging surrounding structures. It extends from the ends of the collecting ducts of the kidneys, through the ureters and bladder, to the proximal portion of the urethra."- Gray's 40/e p30

   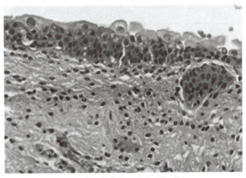

   Fig. 1: Transitional epithelium

   *"The **bladder** consists of **four layers**: a **lining epithelium (urothelium)**, lamina propria, muscularis propria and serosa."- Gray's 40/e p1250*

Urothelium (Urinary or Transitional Epithelium)
• **Urothelium lines urinary tract** (major portion) & **prevents** its rather **toxic contents from damaging surrounding structures**[Q].   • Also called transitional because of the apparent transition between a stratified cuboidal epithelium & a stratified squamous epithelium, which occurs as it is stretched to accommodate urine in bladder[Q].

   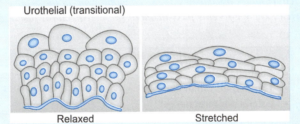

• It appears to be **4-6 cells thick, lines organs** that undergo **considerable distension & contraction**.   • It can **stretch greatly without losing its integrity.**   • In stretching, **cells become flattened** & are **firmly connected by numerous desmosomes**[Q].

Extent:
• Ends of **collecting ducts** of kidneys, **ureters, bladder** & **proximal portion of urethra**[Q].   • **Males:** It **covers urethra till ejaculatory ducts**, then becomes intermittent and is finally **replaced by stratified columnar epithelium in membranous urethra**[Q].   • **Females:** It extends **till urogenital membrane**[Q].

Development:
• Part of it is derived from **mesoderm** & part from **ectoderm & endoderm**[Q].

Urinary Bladder

• **Lining: Transitional epithelium**[Q]
• **Mean capacity** of bladder: **220 ml**[Q] (Filling can be tolerated up to **500 ml**[Q])
• **Micturition** takes place when the **bladder contains** about **280 ml** of urine[Q].
    • **Apex of bladder** is joined to **umbilicus by remains of urachus**, which form the **median umbilical ligament**[Q].
    • **Medial umbilical folds** are **remnants of obliterated umbilical arteries**[Q].

Blood supply: • **Superior** & **inferior vesical** arteries[Q] (Branch of **anterior trunk** of **internal iliac** artery)
Nerve supply: • **Sympathetic fibers (T11-L2)** are **inhibitory to detrusor** & **motor to sphincter vesicae**[Q]. • **Parasympathetic supply** is from **nervi erigentes (S2, S3, S4)**, which is **motor to detrusor muscle** but **inhibitor to sphincter vesicae**[Q].

2. **Ans. c. Thoracoacromial artery, cephalic vein, lateral pectoral nerve** *(Ref: Gray's 40/e p791)*

   Structures passing through clavipectoral fascia are lateral pectoral nerve, thoraco-acromial artery, cephalic vein & lymphatics.

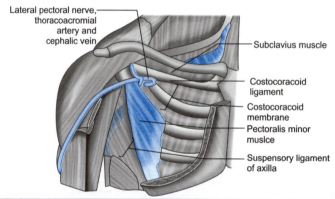

"The cephalic vein, thoraco-acromial artery and vein, and lateral pectoral nerve pass through the (clavipectoral) fascia."- Gray's 40/e p791

*"One or two **infraclavicular nodes** appear beside the cephalic vein, in the groove between pectoralis major and deltoid, just inferior to the clavicle. Their **efferents pass through the clavipectoral fascia to the apical axillary nodes**."- Gray's 40/e p818*

Clavipectoral fascia is traversed by	
• **Cephalic vein**[Q] • **Thoraco-acromial vessels**[Q] • **Lateral pectoral nerve**[Q]	• **Lymphatics**[Q]: Passing between infraclavicular & apical nodes of axilla

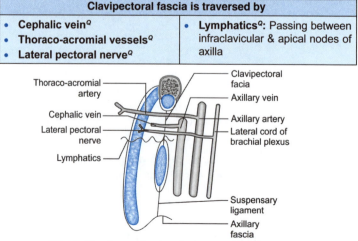

Fig. 2: Structures piercing clavipectoral fascia

Clavipectoral Fascia (CPF)

- **Strong fibrous sheet behind** the **clavicular part of pectoralis major**[Q].
- It **fills the gap between pectoralis minor & subclavius**, and **covers axillary vessels & nerves**[Q].
- Extends from **axillary fascia to enclose pectoralis minor & subclavian muscles** and **attaches to clavicle**[Q].
- **Costacoracoid membrane**: Part of CPF superior to pectoralis minor[Q]
- **Suspensory ligament of axilla**: Part of CPF inferior to pectoralis minor[Q]
    - It **splits around subclavius** and is **attached to clavicle** both anterior & posterior to the groove for subclavius.
    - **Posterior layer fuses with deep cervical fascia**, which connects omohyoid to clavicle & with sheath of the axillary vessels.
    - **Medially** it **blends with fascia** over **first two intercostal spaces** & is **attached to 1st rib**, medial to subclavius.
    - **Laterally**, it is **attached to coracoid process, blending with coracoclavicular ligament**.
- Between **1st rib & coracoid process**, fascia often thickens to form a band, the **costocoracoid ligament**.
- Below this, fascia becomes thin, splits around pectoralis minor and descends to blend with the axillary fascia and laterally with the fascia over the short head of biceps.
    - **Cephalic vein, thoraco-acromial artery & vein, lateral pectoral nerve & lymphatics** pass through the fascia[Q].

3. **Ans. b. Cranial nerves III, VII, IX, X and sacral nerves S2, S3, S4** *(Ref: Gray's 40/e p235; Ganong 25/e p257, 24/e p257)*
   Parasympathetic flow is cranio-sacral, carried by cranial nerves III, VII, IX, X & sacral nerves S2, S3, S4.

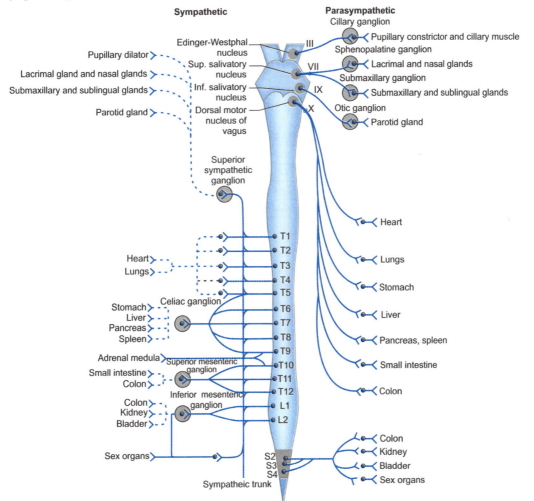

> *"Preganglionic parasympathetic neuron cell bodies are located in certain cranial nerve nuclei of the brain stem and in the grey matter of the second to fourth sacral segments of the spinal cord. Efferent fibres, which are myelinated, emerge from the CNS only in cranial nerves III, VII, IX and X and in the second to fourth sacral spinal nerves."- Gray's 40/e p235*

> *"The **parasympathetic nervous system** is sometimes called the **craniosacral division** of the ANS because of the location of its preganglionic neurons; preganglionic neurons are located in several cranial nerve nuclei (III, VII, IX, and X) and in the IML of the sacral spinal cord. The **parasympathetic sacral outflow (pelvic nerve)** supplies the pelvic viscera **via branches of the second to fourth sacral spinal nerves**."- Ganong 25/e p257*

Parasympathetic Nervous System

- **Preganglionic parasympathetic neuron cell bodies** are **located in** certain **cranial nerve nuclei of the brain stem** and in the grey matter of the **second to fourth sacral segments of the spinal cord**[Q].
- **Efferent fibres (myelinated**[Q]**)** emerge from CNS only in cranial nerves III, VII, IX & X and in **second to fourth sacral spinal nerves**[Q].
- Both preganglionic & postganglionic parasympathetic neurons are **cholinergic**[Q].
- Cell bodies of postganglionic parasympathetic neurons are mostly sited **distant from CNS**, either in **discrete ganglia located near the structures innervated**, or **dispersed in the walls of viscera**[Q].
    - **Four small peripheral ganglia in cranial part of parasympathetic system: Ciliary, pterygopalatine, submandibular & otic**[Q].
    - These are solely **efferent parasympathetic ganglia**, unlike the trigeminal, facial, glossopharyngeal and vagal ganglia, all of which are **concerned exclusively with afferent impulses** and **contain the cell bodies of sensory neurons**[Q].
- **Cranial parasympathetic ganglia** are also **traversed by afferent fibres, postganglionic sympathetic fibres**, and, in the case of the otic ganglion, even by branchial efferent fibres[Q].
- **Postganglionic parasympathetic fibres** are usually **unmyelinated & shorter** than their counterparts in the sympathetic system (**ganglia** in which parasympathetic fibres synapse are **in or near the viscera**[Q] they supply)

Feature	Sympathetic	Parasympathetic
Location of **preganglionic** neuron	**Thoracolumbar** segments of spinal cord[Q]	Nuclei of **III, VII, IX & X** cranial nerves and **S2, S3 & S4** segments of spinal cord[Q]
Location of **postganglionic** neuron	**Away** from target organ[Q]	**Near** or in the target organ
Length of **preganglionic** fibers	Relatively **short**[Q]	Relatively **long**[Q]
Length of **postganglionic** fibers	Relatively **long**[Q]	Relatively **short**[Q]
Preganglionic neurotransmitter	**Acetylcholine**[Q]	**Acetylcholine**[Q]
Postganglionic neurotransmitter	**Noradrenaline**[Q]	**Acetylcholine**[Q]

4. **Ans. c. C**   *(Ref: Gray's 40/e p439)*

   A-Prevertebral space; B-Retropharyngeal space; C-Danger space; D-Pretracheal space

> *"The **prevertebral fascia** is particularly prominent in front of the vertebral column, where there may be **two distinct layers of fascia**. The space created by the splitting of the anterior prevertebral fascia, the danger space, is a **part of the prevertebral space**."- Gray's 40/e p439*

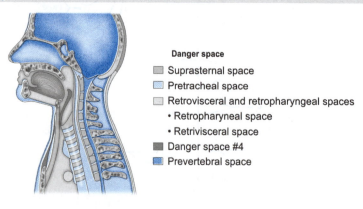

Danger space
- Suprasternal space
- Pretracheal space
- Retrovisceral and retropharyngeal spaces
  • Retropharyneal space
  • Retrivisceral space
- Danger space #4
- Prevertebral space

*"The **prevertebral tissue space** has been variously described as the **potential space lying between the prevertebral fascia and the vertebral column**, and as the **space between the two layers of the prevertebral fascia**, the so-called **danger space**. Infection usually spreads into the space via its fascial walls from the retrovisceral area because it is **closed superiorly and laterally. Inferiorly, it extends into the posterior mediastinum**. Clinically, however, the danger space and the retropharyngeal or retrovisceral space are often considered together because they cannot be differentiated radiologically."* - *Gray's 40/e p43*

Danger Space of Neck

- **Danger space of neck:** Potential space located **behind true retropharyngeal space**, which **connects deep cervical spaces to mediastinum**[Q].

Boundaries of Danger Space of Neck	
Anteriorly	**Alar fascia**[Q]
Posteriorly	**Prevertebral layer** of deep cervical fascia[Q]
Superiorly	**Clivus**[Q]
Inferiorly	**Posterior mediastinum** at the level of diaphragm[Q]

- It is **indistinguishable from retropharyngeal space** and **visible only when distended by fluid or pus**, below the level of **T1-T6**, since the retropharyngeal space variably ends at this level[Q].

  - It is a **potential path for spread of infections** (e.g. retropharyngeal abscess) from the **pharynx to mediastinum**[Q].
  - It is a **median space without a midline raphe** & infection can **spread easily to either side**[Q].

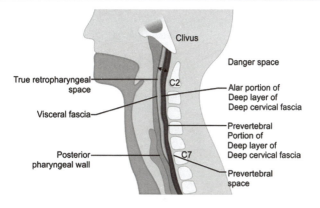

5. **Ans. c. 1-Medial cord of brachial plexus, 2-long thoracic nerve, 3-subscapularis** *(Ref: Gray's 41/e p833, 40/e p814)*

*"The **axilla contains** the **axillary vessels**, the **infraclavicular part** of the **brachial plexus** and **its branches**, lateral branches of some **intercostal nerves**, many **lymph nodes and vessels**, **loose adipose areolar tissue** and, in many instances, the **'axillary tail' of the breast**. The axillary vessels and brachial plexus run from the apex to the base along the lateral wall, nearer to the anterior wall: the axillary vein is anteromedial to the artery."* - *Gray's 40/e p814*

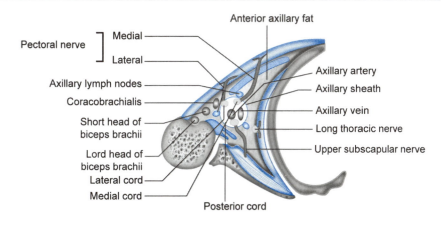

Axilla

- **Axilla** is a **pyramidal region** between **upper thoracic wall & arm**.

Boundaries of Axilla	
Anterior wall	Pectoralis major & minor, subclavius muscle, clavipectoral fascia[Q]
Posterior wall	Subscapularis (above), teres major & latissimus dorsi (below)[Q]
Medial wall	First 4 ribs & intercostal muscles with upper part of serratus anterior[Q]
Lateral wall	Intertubercular sulcus, coracobrachialis & short head of biceps muscles[Q]
Apex	Interval between clavicle, 1st rib & upper border of scapula[Q]
Base	Axillary fascia & skin[Q]

Contents of Axilla	
• Axillary artery, vein & lymphatics [Q]	• Long thoracic nerve, intercostobrachial nerve[Q]
• Brachial plexus[Q] (cords & branches)	• Axillary tail of Spence[Q]

6. **Ans. c. Aphasia** *(Ref: Gray's 40/e p229)*

   The arrow in the image is pointing towards the frontal lobe, which contains the Broca's area. Involvement of this area leads to aphasia.

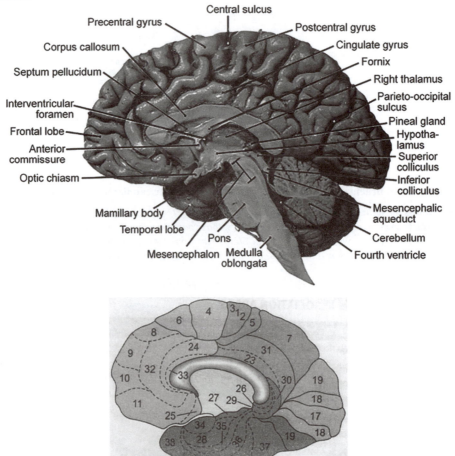

Brodmann Association Areas	
Vision	
Primary	17 [Q]
Secondary	18, 19, 20, 21, 37 [Q]
Audition	
Primary	41 [Q]
Secondary	22, 42 [Q]
Body Sensation	
Primary	1, 2, 3 [Q]
Secondary	5, 7 [Q]
Tertiary	7, 22, 37, 39, 40 [Q]
Motor	
Primary	4 [Q]
Secondary	6 [Q]
Eye movement	8 [Q]
Speech	44 [Q]

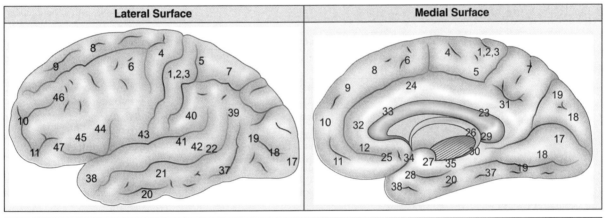

Brodmann Areas of Cerebral Cortex			
Area	Name	Location	Lesion
1, 2, 3	Primary sensory cortex[Q]	Lies in postcentral gyrus	Impairment of all somatic sensations of contralateral side of body[Q]
4	Primary motor cortex[Q]	Lies along posterior part of postcentral gyrus adjoining central sulcus	Spastic paresis of contralateral side of body[Q]
5	Somatosensory association cortex[Q]	Part of parietal cortex	Apraxia & astereognosis[Q]
6	Premotor cortex & supplementary motor cortex (Secondary Motor Cortex[Q])	Part of the frontal cortex, situated just anterior to primary motor cortex (BA4)	Apraxia[Q]
7	Visuo-motor coordination	Situated posterior to primary somatosensory cortex (BA 3, 1 & 2), & superior to occipital lobe	Contralateral astereognosis & sensory neglect
8	Frontal eye fields	Situated just anterior to premotor cortex (BA6)	Contralateral horizontal gaze palsy

Contd....

Contd....

Area	Name	Location	Lesion
9	Dorsolateral prefrontal cortex	Part of frontal cortex, contributes to dorsolateral & medial prefrontal cortex.	**Dysexecution syndrome** (problems with social judgment, executive memory, abstract thinking)
10	Anterior prefrontal cortex	Most rostral part of superior & middle frontal gyri	Similar to lesion of Area 9
11	Orbitofrontal area	Orbital & rectus gyri, plus part of rostral part of superior frontal gyrus	Deficits in general olfaction
12	Orbitofrontal area	Area between superior frontal gyrus & inferior rostral sulcus	Apathy, inappropriate behavior
13, 14, 16	Insular cortex	Anterior of the insular cortex	Deficit in perception, motor control, self-awareness, cognitive functioning,
15	Anterior Temporal lobe	Located in part of insula nearest the temporal lobe	Impaired baroreceptors & chemoreceptors response
17	**Primary visual cortex^Q (V1)**	Lies in **calcarine fissure** of occipital pole	**Unilateral lesion: Contralateral homonymous hemianopia** with macular sparing^Q **Bilateral lesion: Cortical blindness** with intact pupillary light reflex^Q
18	**Sensory visual cortex^Q (V2)**	Parastriate cortex	Deficit in perceiving visual motion
19	**Visual association areas^Q (V3, V4, V5)**	Peristriate region	Deficit in perceiving visual motion
20	**Inferior temporal gyrus^Q**	Inferotemporal cortex	**Visual agnosia, achromatopsia, prosopagnosia^Q**
21	**Middle temporal gyrus^Q**	Encompasses most of the lateral temporal cortex,	**Visual agnosia, achromatopsia, prosopagnosia^Q**
22	**Wernicke's speech area^Q** (includes part of 39 & 40 also)	Lies in the **posterior part** of **superior temporal lobe**	**Sensory or fluent or receptive aphasia^Q**
23	Ventral posterior cingulate cortex	Located on the medial wall of the **cingulate** gyrus	Inability to detect errors, emotional instability, inattention & akinetic mutism.
24	Ventral anterior cingulate cortex	In cingulate gyrus adjacent to area 6	Similar to lesion of area 23
25	Subgenual area	Part of ventromedial prefrontal cortex	Impairments in personal & social decision-making
26	**Ectosplenial area**	Retrosplenial region of cerebral cortex	Topographical disorientation
27	Piriform cortex	Rostral part of the parahippocampal gyrus	Impaired olfaction
28	Ventral entorhinal cortex	Hippocampal-uncal area	Olfactory & gustatory hallucinations
29	**Granular retrosplenial cortex**	Narrow band located in the isthmus of **cingulate** gyrus	Amnesia
30	Agranular retrolimbic area	Narrow band located in the isthmus of **cingulate** gyrus	Amnesia
31	Dorsal Posterior cingulate cortex	Near **posterior** cingulate gyrus	Impaired learning & spatial memory
32	Dorsal anterior cingulate cortex	Near **anterior** cingulate gyrus	Inability to detect errors, emotional instability, inattention & akinetic mutism
33	Pregenual area	Narrow band located in anterior cingulate gyrus	Inability to detect errors, emotional instability, inattention & akinetic mutism

Area	Name	Location	Lesion
34	Primary olfactory cortex	Hippocampal – entorhinal area	Ipsilateral anosmia
35	Perirhinal cortex	In the rhinal sulcus	Impairment of visual recognition memory
36	Ectorhinal area	In the fusiform gyrus	Impairment of visual recognition memory
37	Fusiform gyrus	Fusiform gyrus – occipitotemporal cortex	Prosopagnosia
38	Temporopolar area	Most rostral part of superior & middle temporal gyri	Impaired visceral emotional responses
39	Angular gyrus (considered to be part of Wernicke's area)	Near junction of temporal, occipital & parietal lobes.	Finger agnosia, dysgraphia, dyslexia, dyscalculia
40	**Supramarginal gyrus** (considered to be part of Wernicke's area)	Part of the parietal cortex	Aphasia & alexia.
41, 42	Primary auditory cortex	Lies on **cephalic border** of **superior temporal gyrus** in depths of lateral fissure	**Unilateral lesion: Contralateral slight hearing loss** & difficulty in localizing sounds **Bilateral lesion: Deafness**
43	Primary gustatory cortex	Just **below somatosensory cortex** in postcentral gyrus	Dysguesia
44, 45	**Broca's speech area**Q	Lies in the **posterior part** of **inferior frontal gyrus**	**Aphasia & agraphia**Q
46	Dorsolateral prefrontal cortex	Middle third of middle frontal gyrus	Deficits in concentration, orientation, abstracting ability, judgment
47	Pars orbitalis	Part of inferior frontal gyrus	Deficits in concentration, orientation, abstracting ability, judgement
48	Retrosubicular area	A small part of medial surface of temporal lobe	-
49	Parasubicular area in a rodent	Transitional zone between the presubiculum and the entorhinal area	-
52	Parainsular area	At the junction of temporal lobe & insula	-

7. **Ans. b. Lateral rectus**   *(Ref: Gray's 41/e p275, 40/e p240)*

The marked structure is facial colliculus. Abducent nerve nucleus is located deep to facial colliculus. Abducens nerve supplies lateral rectus.

"Facial colliculus is situated in the pons. It overlies the abducent nucleus. The facial nerve originates from its nucleus and goes around the abducent nerve. This is called as neurobiotaxis."- Gray's 40/e p240

*"Facial **colliculus** is **formed by the axons of facial nerve** (not by the abducens nucleus deep to it). Facial nerve supplies muscles of facial expression like **risorius".***

*"On each side of the median sulcus is a **longitudinal elevation, the medial eminence**, lateral to which lies sulcus limitans. Its **superior part is the locus ceruleus**, coloured bluish-grey from the patch of deeply pigmented nerve cells. Also **lateral to the upper part of the medial eminence is a slight depression**, the superior fovea, and **just below and medial in this fovea is a rounded swelling, the facial colliculus**, which **overlies the nucleus of the abducens (VI) nerve** and the facial (VII) nerve fibers encircling in the motor nucleus of the facial nerve lies more deeply in the pons. Inferolateral to the superior fovea is the upper part of the vestibular area, which overlies parts of the nuclei of the vestibulococchlear (VIII) nerve." -Netter Collection of Medical Illustrations 2013/Volume-7/178*

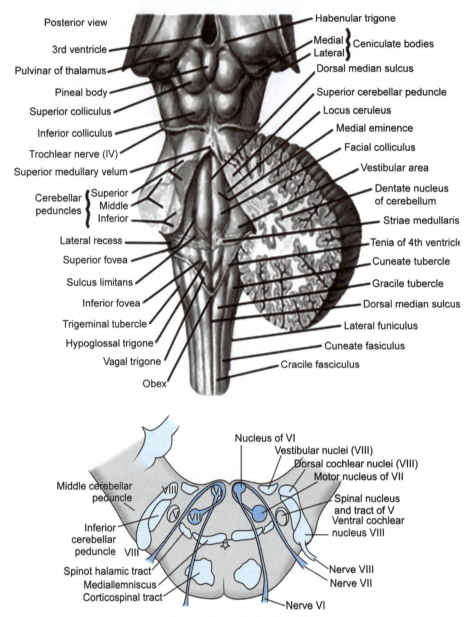

Fig. 3: Cut section at the level of mid pons

Functions of Extraocular Muscles		
Muscle	**Nerve Supply**	**Action**
Superior rectus	Oculomotor (Superior division)^Q	Elevation, Adduction, Intortion^Q
Inferior rectus	Oculomotor (Inferior division)^Q	Depression, Adduction, Extortion^Q
Medial rectus	Oculomotor (Inferior division)^Q	Abduction^Q
Lateral rectus	Abducens^Q	Adduction^Q
Superior oblique	Trochlear^Q	Depression, Abduction, Intortion^Q
Inferior oblique	Oculomotor (Inferior division)^Q	Elevation, Abduction, Extortion^Q

8. **Ans. b. Primary yolk sac** *(Ref: Gray's 41/e p169, 40/e p167, 173, 186-189; Langman's 13/e p45, 62, 9/e p54-55)*
Extra-embryonic mesoderm is derived from primary yolk sac.

"Extraembryonic mesoderm is formed by delamination of yolk sac cells and later by migration of cells through the primitive streak during gastrulation."-Langman

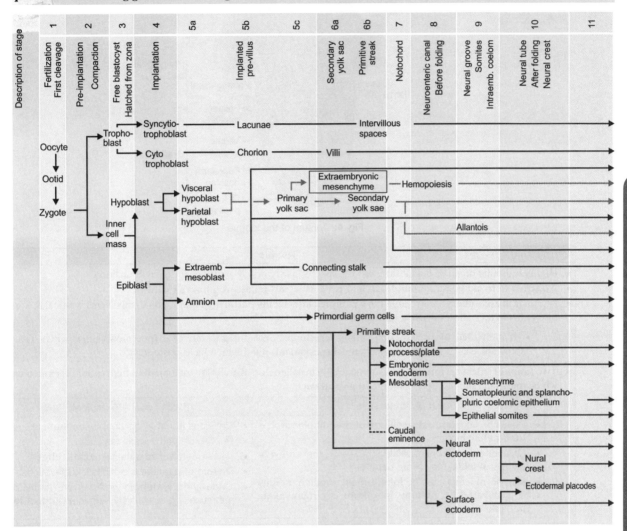

Extraembryonic Mesoderm

- A **new population of cells** appears **between inner surface of cytotrophoblast & outer surface of exocoelomic cavity**. These cells, **derived from yolk sac cells**, **form a fine, loose connective tissue**, the **extraembryonic mesoderm**, which eventually **fills all of the space between trophoblast externally & amnion and extracoelomic membrane internally**[Q].
- Soon **large cavities develop in extraembryonic mesoderm**, and when these become confluent, they form a new space known as the **extraembryonic coelom** or **chorionic cavity**[Q].
- **Extraembryonic mesoderm lining the cytotrophoblast & amnion** is called **extraembryonic somatopleuric** mesoderm; the **lining covering the yolk sac** is known as **extraembryonic splanchnopleuric mesoderm**[Q].

9. **Ans. c. Sulcus terminalis**   *(Ref: Gray's 41/e p511, 40/e p503)*

Anterior two third of the tongue is demarcated from the posterior one-third by sulcus terminalis.

"Tongue: It is divided by a V-shaped sulcus terminalis into an anterior, oral (presulcal) part which faces upwards, and a posterior, pharyngeal (postsulcal) part which faces posteriorly. The anterior part forms about two-thirds of the length of the tongue."- Gray's 41/e p511

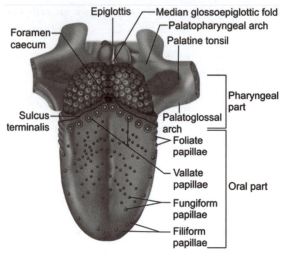

Fig. 4: Dorsum of the tongue

Tongue
- Highly muscular organ of deglutition, taste & speech; partly oral & partly pharyngeal in position
- **Attached to hyoid bone, mandible, styloid processes, soft palate & pharyngeal wall**[Q].
- **Intrinsic muscle fibers** are **arranged in a complex interlacing pattern** of longitudinal, transverse, vertical & horizontal fasciculi and this allows **great mobility**[Q].
• It is **divided by a V-shaped sulcus terminalis**[Q] into an **anterior, oral (presulcal) part,** which faces upwards, and a **posterior, pharyngeal (postsulcal) part,** which faces posteriorly[Q].
- **Two limbs of sulcus terminalis** run anterolaterally to palatoglossal arches **from a median depression, foramen caecum**, which marks the site of upper end of thyroglossal duct.

Oral (Presulcal) Part	Pharyngeal (Postsulcal) Part
• Develops from **lingual swellings of mandibular arch & tuberculum impar**[Q] • On each side, in front of palatoglossal arch, there are **4 or 5 vertical folds**, the **foliate papillae**[Q]. • Dorsal mucosa has a **longitudinal median sulcus & is covered by filiform, fungiform & circumvallate papillae**[Q].	• Develops from **hypobranchial eminence**[Q]. • Post sulcal part constitutes **base** • It lies **posterior to palatoglossal arches**[Q]. • **Devoid of papillae** & exhibits low elevations. • **Underlying lymphoid nodules** are embedded in submucosa & collectively termed as **lingual tonsil**[Q].

Development of Tongue	
Epithelium	Muscles
• **Anterior 2/3** from **lingual swelling of Ist arch and tuberculum impar**[Q] • **Posterior 1/3** from large dorsal part of **hypobranchial eminence**[Q] i.e. 3rd arch • **Posterior most part** from small dorsal part hypobranchial eminence i.e. 4th arch	• **Palatoglossal** from **6th arch**[Q] • Rest by **occipital myotomes**[Q]

Nerve supply of Tongue		
Part of Tongue	Taste	General
Anterior 2/3rd (except vallate papilla)[Q]	**Chorda tympani**[Q] (branch of facial nerve)	**Lingual nerve**[Q] (branch of trigeminal)
Posterior 1/3rd (including vallate papilla)[Q]	Glossopharyngeal nerve[Q]	Glossopharyngeal nerve[Q]
Posterior most or **vallecula**[Q]	Internal laryngeal branch of vagus[Q]	Internal laryngeal branch of vagus[Q]

Contd...

Contd...

Tongue
Lymphatic Drainage of Tongue
• **Tip of tongue** by **submental**[Q] lymph node • **Anterior two third** by **submandibular**[Q] lymph node • **Posterior 1/3rd** by **jugulo-omohyoid**[Q] lymph node
Remember
• All **extrinsic & intrinsic muscles** of tongue are supplied by **hypoglossal (12th)**[Q] nerve except **Palatoglossal** which is supplied by **cranial accessory nerve**[Q] through pharyngeal plexus. • **Genioglossus** is the **safety muscle of the tongue**[Q]. Its function can be used to test hypoglossal nerve.

10. **Ans. c. Quadratus lumborum** *(Ref: Gray's 41/e p1251, 40/e p1239)*
    Left ureter is related posteriorly to psoas major muscle (not quadratus lumborum).

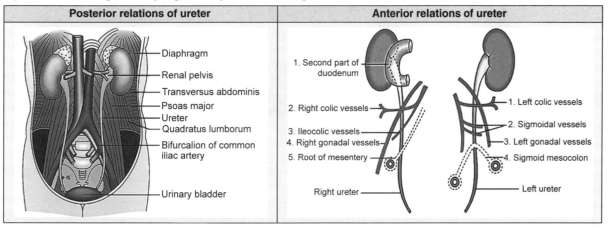

Ureter
• Develops from the **ureteric diverticula** arising from the **mesonephric duct**[Q] • **Length: 25–30 cm; Diameter: 3 mm**[Q] • Descends slightly medially, **anterior to psoas major** & enters pelvic cavity where it curves initially laterally, then medially, to open into base of urinary bladder. • **Narrowest part: Intravesical part**[Q]
Ureteric Constrictions
• **Pelviureteric junction**[Q] • **Brim of lesser pelvis near medial border of psoas major**[Q] • **Vesicoureteric junction**[Q] (Narrowest part)

Posterior Relations	Anterior Relations	
• Both ureters run **anterior to psoas major muscle & bifurcation of common iliac artery**[Q]	**Right Ureter**	**Left Ureter**
	• **Duodenum**[Q] (2nd part) • **Right colic** vessels[Q] • **Ileocolic** vessels[Q] • **Right gonadal** vessels[Q] • **Root of mesentery**[Q]	• **Left colic** vessels[Q] • **Sigmoidal** vessels[Q] • **Left testicular or ovarian** vessels[Q] • **Sigmoid mesocolon**[Q]

Ureter
Vascular Supply: • **Arterial supply**: Branches from **renal, gonadal, common iliac, internal iliac, vesical, uterine arteries** & abdominal aorta[Q] • Venous drainage of ureters follows arterial supply.
Lymphatic drainage: • Lymph drains to **lateral aortic nodes & iliac nodes**[Q]
Innervation: • **Lower three thoracic, first lumbar & 2nd to 4th sacral segments of spinal cord** by branches from **renal & aortic plexuses**, and **superior & inferior hypogastric plexuses**[Q]

11. **Ans. b. 1. Linea alba, 2- linea semilunaris, 3-inner lip of iliac crest, 4-outer lip of iliac crest, 5-inguinal ligament, 6-deep inguinal ring** (Ref: Gray's 41/e p1071, 1079, 1343, 40/e p1063)

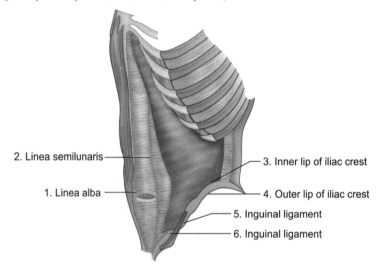

Fig. 5: Put the labels in the image

External Oblique

• **Largest & most superficial** of three lateral abdominal muscles.
• **Attached to external surfaces & inferior borders of lower 8 ribs**[Q].
  • Attachments rapidly become muscular & **interdigitate with lower attachment of serratus anterior & latissimus dorsi** along an oblique line that extends **downwards & backwards**[Q].
  • Upper attachments are **close to cartilages** of corresponding ribs, **middle ones** arise **from ribs** at some distance from their cartilages & **lowest** are **close to apex of cartilage of 12th rib**[Q].
• **Fibres diverge** as they pass to their lower attachments.
• Those **from the lower two ribs pass nearly vertically downwards & attached to anterior half or more of outer lip of anterior segment of iliac crest**[Q].
• **Middle & upper fibres** pass **downwards & forwards** and **end in anterior aponeurosis**, along a line drawn vertically from 9th costal cartilage to a little below the level of umbilicus[Q].
  • **Inguinal ligament** is formed by **margin of aponeurosis of external oblique extending between anterior superior iliac spine & pubic tubercle**[Q].
• **Deepest fibres** of aponeurosis **spread out posteromedially to insert into pectineal line**[Q].
Origin:
• **Anterior fibers:** Originate from **outer surface** of **5-8 ribs**[Q]
• **Lateral fibers:** Originate from **outer surface of 9th rib** interdigitates with **serratus anterior muscle**; fibers originating from ribs **10-12**, interdigitates with **latissimus dorsi**[Q].

Contd...

Contd...

External Oblique
Insertion: • **Anterior fibers:** Forms a broad aponeurosis, terminates at **linea alba**[Q] • **Lateral fibers:** Inserts to **anterior iliac spine & pubic tubercle, external lip of iliac crest**[Q]
• Vascular Supply: • Branches from **lower posterior intercostal & subcostal** arteries, **superior & inferior epigastric** arteries, **superficial & deep circumflex** arteries and **posterior lumbar** arteries[Q].
Innervation: • Ventral primary rami of thoracic nerves **T7-T12**[Q]
Actions: • Supports abdominal contents; compresses abdominal contents; assists in **flexing & rotation of trunk**[Q] • Assists in **forced expiration, micturition, defecation, parturition & vomiting**[Q]

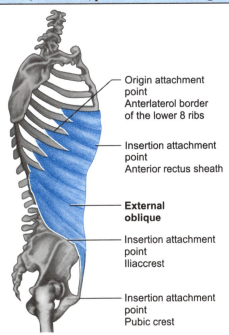

Fig. 6: External oblique origin & insertion

12. **Ans. d. Tibialis anterior**   *(Ref: Gray's 41/e p112, 40/e p104-105)*

The individual fibers of a muscle are arranged either parallel or oblique to the long axis of the muscle. Sartorius, rectus abdominis and sternohyoid have parallel oriented fibers while tibialis anterior muscle is a multipennate muscle with oblique fibers.

*"Where fibres are oblique to the line of pull, muscles may be **triangular** (e.g. **temporalis, adductor longus**) or **pennate** (feather-like) in construction. The latter vary in complexity from **unipennate** (e.g. flexor pollicis longus) and **bipennate** (e.g. **rectus femoris, dorsal interossei**) to **multipennate** (e.g. **deltoid**). Fibres may pass obliquely between deep and superficial aponeuroses, in a type of '**unipennate' form** (e.g. **soleus**), or muscle fibres may start from the walls of osteofascial compartments and converge obliquely on a central tendon in **circumpennate** fashion (e.g. **tibialis anterior**)." - Gray's 40/e p104*

*"Muscles whose **fibers run obliquely to the line of pull** are referred to as **pennate muscles** (they **resemble a feather**). A **unipennate muscle** is one in which the **tendon lies along one side of the muscle** and the **muscle fibers pass obliquely to it** (e.g., extensor digitorum longus). A **bipennate muscle** is one in which the **tendon lies in the center of the muscle** and the muscle fibers pass to it from two sides (e.g., rectus femoris). A **multipennate muscle** may be arranged as a **series of bipennate muscles lying alongside one another** (e.g., acromial fibers of the deltoid) or may have the **tendon lying within its center and the muscle fibers passing to it from all sides, converging as they go** (e.g., **tibialis anterior**)." - Snells 9/e p8*

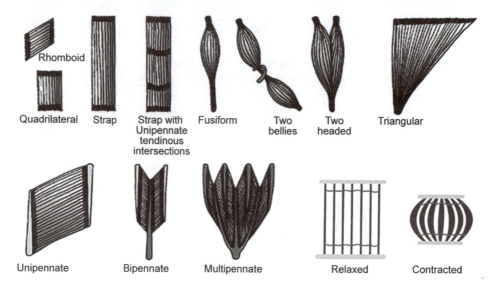

Fig. 7: Morphological types of muscle based on their general form and fascicular architecture

Skeletal Muscle	
• The **individual fibers of a muscle** are arranged either **parallel** or **oblique to the long axis of the muscle**[Q].	
Muscles with Parallel Fasciculi	**Muscles with Oblique Fasciculi**
• Muscles in which **fasciculi are parallel to the line of pull** & have **greater degree of movement**[Q]. • These muscles may be: • **Quadrilateral: Thyrohyoid**[Q] • **Strap-like: Sternohyoid & sartorius** [Q] • **Strap-like with tendinous intersections: Rectus abdominis**[Q] • **Fusiform: Biceps brachii, digastric**[Q]	• Muscles in which **fasciculi are oblique to the line of pull**, muscle may be **triangular, or pennate (feather-like)** in the construction[Q]. • This arrangement makes **muscle more powerful**, but the **range of movement is reduced**[Q]. • Oblique arrangements are of the following types: • **Triangular: Temporalis, adductor longus**[Q] • **Unipennate: Flexor pollicis longus, extensor digitorum longus**[Q] • **Bipennate: Rectus femoris, flexor hallucis longus**[Q] • **Multipennate: Tibialis anterior, submscapularis, deltoid (acromial fibers)**[Q].

PHYSIOLOGY

13. **Ans. a. Zona occludens**   *(Ref: Gray's 40/e p140; Ganong 25/e p41, 24/e p43)*
    The given diagram is showing intercalated discs of cardiac muscle, which contains all types of cellular junctions except occluding tight junction (Zona occludens).

    "Intercalated disc is a junctional complex between neighbouring cells in cardiac muscle cells. The **interdigitating transverse parts of the intercalated disc form a fascia adherens, with numerous desmosomes; gap junctions** are found in the longitudinal parts of the disc."- *Gray's 40/e p140*

    "Three types of cell junction make up an intercalated disc- fascia adherens, desmosomes & gap junctions."

    "The types of *junctions that tie cells together* and endow tissues with strength and stability include *tight junctions*, which are also known as the *zonula occludens*. The *desmosome* and *zonula adherens* also help to hold cells together, and the *hemidesmosome* and *focal adhesions* attach cells to their basal laminas. The *gap junction* forms a cytoplasmic "tunnel" for diffusion of small molecules (< 1000 Da) between two neighboring cells. *Tight junctions characteristically surround the apical margins of the cells in epithelia* such as the *intestinal mucosa*, the walls of the renal tubules, and the *choroid plexus*."- *Ganong 25/e p41*

    See Q. No. 14 AIIMS November 2017

14. **Ans. c.** C *(Ref: Ganong 25/e p201, 24/e p201-202)*
    The peripheral processes of spiral ganglia ends at inner hair cells (marked as C in the given image).

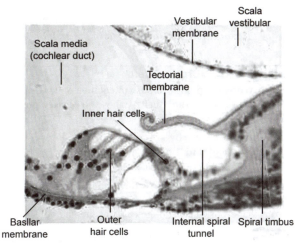

Fig. 8: (A: Basilar membrane; B: Outer hair cells; C: Inner hair cells; D: Vestibular membrane)

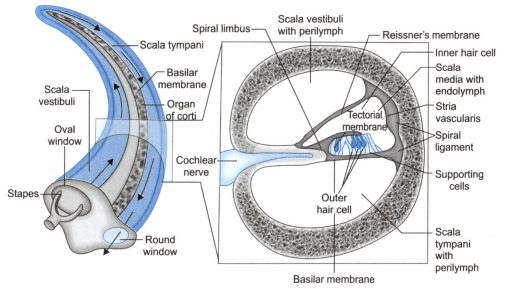

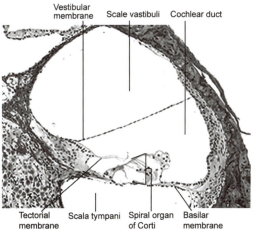

"The cell bodies of the sensory neurons that arborize around the bases of the hair cells are located in the spiral ganglion within the modiolus, the bony core around which the cochlea is wound. Ninety to 95% of these sensory neurons innervate the inner hair cells; only 5–10% innervates the more numerous outer hair cells, and each sensory neuron innervates several outer hair cells. By contrast, most of the efferent fibers in the auditory nerve terminate on the outer rather than inner hair cells. The axons of the afferent neurons that innervate the hair cells form the auditory (cochlear) division of the eighth cranial nerve."- Ganong 25/e p201

Organ of Corti

- **Organ of Corti** on basilar membrane **extends from apex to base of cochlea** & has a **spiral shape**.
- It **contains highly specialized auditory receptors (hair cells)** whose **processes pierce the tough, membrane like reticular lamina** that is supported by **pillar cells** or **rods of Corti**[Q].

  - **Hair cells** are **arranged in four rows**. **Three rows** of **outer hair cells lateral to tunnel** formed by **rods of Corti** & one row of **inner hair cells medial to tunnel**[Q].
  - There are **20,000 outer hair cells**[Q] & **3500 inner hair cells** in **each human cochlea**[Q].

- **Covering the rows of hair cells** is a thin, viscous, but elastic **tectorial membrane** in which the **tips of hairs of outer** but not the inner **hair cells are embedded.**
- The cell bodies of the sensory neurons that arborize around the bases of the hair cells are located in the **spiral ganglion** within the **modiolus,** the bony core around which the cochlea is wound.

  - **90-95%** of these **sensory neurons innervate the inner hair cells**; only 5–10% innervates the more numerous outer hair cells, and **each sensory neuron innervates several outer hair cells.** [Q]
  - By contrast, **most of efferent fibers in auditory nerve terminate on outer** rather than inner **hair cells.**
  - **Axons of afferent neurons** that **innervate the hair cells** form **auditory (cochlear) division** of **VIII cranial nerve**[Q].

15. Ans. d. +85 mV *(Ref: Ganong 25/e p204, 24/e p203; Guyton 13/e p677)*

Endocochlear potential is generated by continual secretion of positive potassium ions into the scala media by the stria vascularis & it is +85 mV.

"Cells in the stria vascularis have a high concentration of Na, K ATPase. In addition, it appears that a unique electrogenic K+ pump in the stria vascularis accounts for the fact that the scala media is electrically positive by 85 mV (endocochlear potential) relative to the scala vestibuli and scala tympani."- Ganong 25/e p204

"An electrical potential of about +80 millivolts exists all the time between endolymph and perilymph, with positivity inside the scala media and negativity outside. This is called the endocochlear potential, and it is generated by continual secretion of positive potassium ions into the scala media by the stria vascularis."- Guyton 13/e p677

Endocochlear Potential

- **Scala media** is **filled with endolymph** whereas **perilymph** is present **in scala vestibuli & scala tympani**[Q].
- **Scala vestibuli & scala tympani communicate directly** with subarachnoid space around the brain, so the **perilymph is almost identical to CSF**[Q].
- **Endolymph** (that fills the scala media) is an **entirely different fluid secreted by the stria vascularis**, a highly vascular area on the outer wall of scala media[Q].

  - **Endolymph** contains a **high concentration of K⁺ & low concentration of Na⁺**, which is **exactly opposite to** contents of **perilymph**[Q].
  - Electrical potential of **+80 millivolts**[Q] exists all the time **between endolymph & perilymph**, with **positivity inside scala media & negativity outside**. This is called **endocochlear potential**, and it is **generated by continual secretion of K⁺ ions into scala media** by **stria vascularis**[Q].

- **Tops of hair cells project through reticular lamina** & are **bathed by endolymph of scala media**, whereas **perilymph bathes the lower bodies of hair cells**[Q].

  - **Hair cells** have a **negative intracellular potential of −70 mV with respect to perilymph** but **−150 mV with respect to endolymph at their upper surfaces** where hairs project through reticular lamina & into endolymph[Q].
  - It is believed that **this high electrical potential at tips of stereocilia sensitizes the cell an extra amount**, thereby **increasing its ability to respond to the slightest sound**[Q].

16. Ans. a. 6000/mm³ *(Ref: Textbook of Practical Physiology by GK Pal 2/e pg57)*

Total leucocyte count is 6000/mm³.

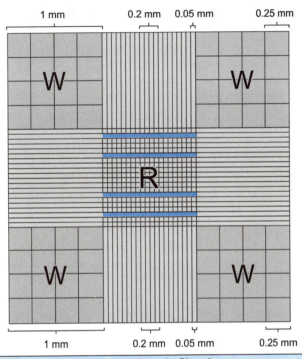

Neubauer's Chamber

- **Each of the square** has a dimension of 1mm x 1mm.
- When you keep coverslip over this chamber, the depth is **0.1 mm**.
- So the volume of one square = $(1 \times 1 \times 0.1)$ mm³ = **0.1 mm³**

  - Concentration of cells = n/V x d
  - (n= No. of cells, V= Volume of distribution, d= Dilution)

- **Cells counted** in 4 corner squares = **n** = (25 + 35 + 40 + 20) = **120**
- Total **Volume** of 4 squares = 4 x 0.1 = **0.4 mm³**
- Dilution factor = **20**
- WBC Count = n/V x d) = 120/0.4 x 20 = **6000 cells/mm³**

17. **Ans. b. I-band** *(Ref: Ganong 25/e p101, 24/e p99; Guyton 13/e p75)*

Abducent nerve nucleus is located deep to facial colliculus.

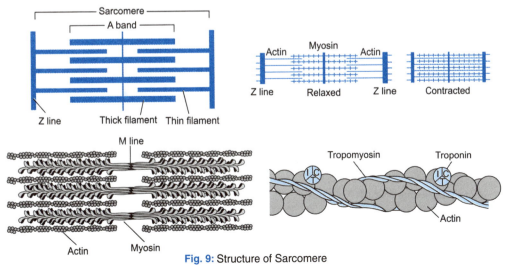

Fig. 9: Structure of Sarcomere

The area marked, as 'E' is the lighter and isotropic band, called as I-band. It contains a dark, Z-line at its center (A: A-band ; B: Actin filaments; C: Sarcomere width; D: H-zone).

"The parts of the cross-striations are frequently identified by letters. The **light I band is divided by the dark Z line**, and the **dark A band has the lighter H band in its center**. A transverse **M line is seen in the middle of the H band**, and this line plus the narrow light areas on either side of it are sometimes called the **pseudo-H zone**. The area between two adjacent Z lines is called a **sarcomere**." - Ganong25/e p101

Physiologic Anatomy of Muscle Fiber

- Each **muscle fiber** is a **single cell** that is **long multinucleated, cylindric** & surrounded by a cell membrane, sarcolemma.
- Muscle fibers are **made up of myofibrils** in turn are made up of individual filaments made up of contractile proteins.

Muscle contractile Proteins		
Actin	• Thin filaments are **polymers made up of two chains of actin** that form a long double helix[Q].	
Myosin	• **Thick filaments** are **made up of myosin**[Q] • **Heads of myosin** molecules **form cross-bridges with actin**[Q]	
Troponin (I, T, C)	• Troponin molecules are **small globular units located at intervals along** the **tropomyosin molecules.**	
	Troponin T	• **Binds the troponin** components to tropomyosin[Q]
	Troponin I	• **Inhibits the interaction of myosin with actin**[Q]
	Troponin C	• **Contains the binding sites for Ca^{2+}** that helps to initiate contraction[Q]
Tropomyosin	• **Tropomyosin molecules** are long filaments **located in groove between two chains in actin**[Q]	
Additional structural proteins (actinin, titin & desmin)	• **Actinin binds actin to Z lines**[Q] • **Titin (largest known protein) connects Z lines to M lines** & **provides scaffolding for sarcomere**[Q] • **Desmin binds Z lines to plasma membrane**[Q]	

- L**I**ght **I** band is **divided by dark Z line**; d**A**rk **A** band has **lighter H band in its center**[Q].
- A transverse **M line** is seen **in the middle of H band** & **this line plus narrow light areas on either side** of it are called **pseudo-H zone**[Q].
- **Area between two adjacent Z lines** is called a **sarcomere**[Q].

  - **Thick filaments** are **made up of myosin; thin filaments** are made up of **actin, tropomyosin & troponin**[Q].
  - **Thick filaments** are **lined up to form A bands**[Q]
  - **Array of thin filaments** extends out of A band & into less dense staining **I bands**[Q].

- **Lighter H bands** in center of A bands are the regions where, when the muscle is relaxed, thin filaments do not overlap thick filaments.
- **Z lines** allow for **anchoring of thin filaments**.

18. **Ans. c. Eye** *(Ref: Ganong 25/e p417, 420, 685, 24/e p687, 419, 422)*
    Countercurrent mechanism is not seen in eye.

"The **spermatic arteries to the testes are tortuous,** *and blood in them runs parallel but in the opposite direction to blood in the pampiniform plexus of spermatic veins. This anatomic arrangement may permit countercurrent exchange of heat and testosterone.*"- Ganong 25/e p417

"The **testes are normally maintained at a temperature of about 32°C.** *They are kept cool by air circulating around the scrotum and probably by heat exchange in a countercurrent fashion between the spermatic arteries and veins.*"- Ganong 25/e p420

*"A **countercurrent system** is a system in which **the inflow runs parallel to, counter to, and in close proximity to the outflow for some distance**. This **occurs for both the loops of Henle and the vasa recta in the renal medulla**."- Ganong 25/e p685*

"Counter current blood flow is seen in the intestinal villi where oxygen directly diffuses from arterioles to vein."

Countercurrent System

- **A countercurrent mechanism system** is a system that **expends energy to create a concentration gradient**.
- System in which **inflow runs parallel to, counter to & in close proximity to outflow for some distance**.
- Countercurrent system is seen in **kidney, limbs, testis & intestine**[Q].

Countercurrent System	
Locations	**Function**
Kidney (Loop of Henle & Vasa recta)	• **Concentration of urine, production of hyperosmotic urine**[Q]
Limbs	• **Hairpin arrangement of artery & vein**[Q] • **Heat** is **transferred from warm arterial blood** going to the limbs **to cold venous blood** coming from the extremities[Q]
Testis	• Between **spermatic arteries & pampiniform plexus of spermatic veins**[Q] • **Permit countercurrent exchange of heat & testosterone**[Q]
Intestine	• Counter current blood flow is seen in **intestinal villi** where **oxygen directly diffuses from arterioles to vein**[Q]. • **Materials** absorbed into the capillaries **diffuse directly from veins into arterioles**[Q]

19. Ans. a. Superior olivary complex   *(Ref: Gray's 40/e p628; Ganong 25/e 207, 24/e p207)*

Superior olivary complex is the control center for the stapedial reflex.

*"The **olivocochlear bundle** is a **prominent bundle of efferent fibers in each auditory nerve** that **arises from both ipsilateral and contralateral superior olivary complexes** and **ends primarily around the bases of the outer hair cells of the organ of Corti**. The activity in this nerve bundle modulates the sensitivity of these hair cells via the release of acetylcholine. The **effect is inhibitory**, and it may **function to block background noise** while allowing other sounds to be heard."- Ganong 25/e p207*

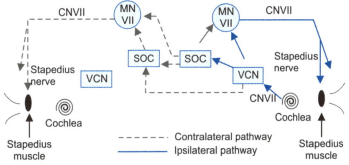

Fig. 10: Schematic diagram of the acoustic Reflex neural pathways

*"**Acoustic (stapedial) reflex:** Once a **high intensity auditory stimulus** is initiated and reaches the cochleae, **neural impulses from the auditory nerves (CN VIII) ascend from both cochleae to each ipsilateral ventral cochlear nucleus (VCN)**. From VCN the reflex has **two main neural pathways**: one passes from the VCN directly to the ipsilateral facial motor nucleus (CN VII) that directly innervates the stapedius muscle via the facial nerve and its stapedius branch; the other passes from the VCN to the superior olivary complex (SOC) before the impulses cross at the brainstem to innervate both ipsilateral and contralateral facial motor nuclei. Contraction of the stapedius muscle stiffens the middle ear ossicles and tilts the stapes in the oval window of the cochlea; this effectively **decreases the vibrational energy transmitted to the cochlea**. Stapedius muscle contraction is clinically apparent by a marked change in the impedance properties of the middle ear.*

AIIMS ESSENCE

20. Ans. c. Alkaline pH in gut   *(Ref: Ganong 25/e p483, 24/e p485; Harrison 19/e p2457)*

In alkaline medium Ca_2^+ forms insoluble tricalcium phosphate, which decreases its absorption in the gut. Phytates also decrease calcium absorption, but alkaline pH is a better answer in this context.

> *"**Active calcium transport** occurs **mainly in the proximal small bowel (duodenum and proximal jejunum)**, although some active calcium absorption occurs in most segments of the small intestine. **Optimal rates of calcium absorption require gastric acid.** This is especially true for weakly dissociable calcium supplements such as calcium carbonate. In fact, **large boluses of calcium carbonate are poorly absorbed because of their neutralizing effect on gastric acid. In achlorhydric subjects and for those taking drugs that inhibit gastric acid secretion, supplements should be taken with meals to optimize their absorption.** Use of calcium citrate may be preferable in these circumstances."*
> *- Harrison 19/e p2457*

Factors increasing Calcium Absorption		Factors decreasing Calcium Absorption	
• **Vitamin D**[Q]	• **Lactose**[Q]	• **Oxalates**[Q]	• **High Mg²⁺**
• **Parathormone**[Q]	• **Amino acids**[Q] (protein rich diet)	• **Phytates**[Q]	• **Caffeines**[Q]
• **Acidic pH**[Q]		• **Alkaline pH**[Q]	• **Dietary fibers**[Q]
		• **High phosphate**[Q]	

21. Ans. a. Cardiac rhythm generation   *(Ref: Ganong 25/e p224, 521, 24/e p224, 523)*

Hyperpolarizing Cycling Nucleotide (HCN) gated channels are present in the SA and AV nodes. The channel opens in hyperpolarization phase, which is essential for generating pacemaker potential in SA Node (cardiac rhythm generation).

Hyperpolarization-activated Cyclic Nucleotide-gated (HCN) channels
• **HCN channels** are **inter-membrane proteins** that serve as **nonselective ligand-gated cation channels** in the plasma membranes of **heart & brain cells**.
• **HCN channels** are sometimes referred to as "pacemaker channels" because they **help to generate rhythmic activity within groups of heart & brain cells**[Q].
• **HCN channels** are encoded by **four genes (HCN1, 2, 3, 4)** and are widely expressed throughout the **heart & CNS**.
• **HCN channels** are **activated by membrane hyperpolarization**[Q]
• Channels are permeable to Na^+ & K^+, and are open at voltages near the resting membrane potential
• **Activation of channels is facilitated by direct interaction with cyclic nucleotides**, and hence the name.
• The **cation current through HCN channels** is known as **I(h);** also known as **funny current.**
• **Opening of HCN channels elicits membrane depolarization toward threshold for action potential generation, & reduces membrane resistance & magnitude of excitatory & inhibitory postsynaptic potentials**[Q].

HCN–Nervous system	HCN–Cardiovascular system
• **Controls neuronal excitability, synaptic transmission & rhythmic oscillatory activity** in individual neurons & neuronal networks.	• **HCN4** is the **main isoform expressed in the SA node**, but low levels of HCN1 & HCN2 are also **seen.**
• Play an important **role in synaptic plasticity & memory,** thalamocortical rhythms & somatic sensation.	• **Current** through **HCN channels**, called the **funny current** or **pacemaker current I(f)**, plays a **key role in generation & modulation of cardiac rhythmicity**[Q].
• Some evidence indicates they also play a role in mechanisms of epilepsy & pain.	

22. Ans. a. Aldosterone   *(Ref: Ganong 25/e p353, 24/e p354; Guyton 13/e p966)*

Region marked as 'A' is zona glomerulosa, which secretes aldosterone.

A	Zona **Glomerulosa**	• Secretes **mineralocorticoid (Aldosterone)**
B	Zona **Fasciculata**	• Secretes **glucocorticoids (Cortisol & corticosterone)** mainly
C	Zona **Reticularis**	• Secretes **adrenal androgens (Dehydroepiandrosterone & androstenedione)**

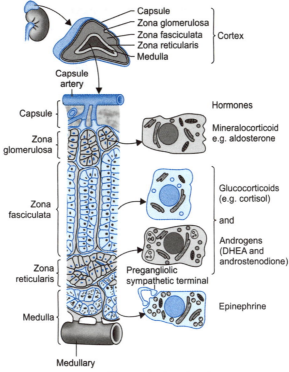

Fig. 11: Zones of adrenal cortex

*"In adult mammals, the **adrenal cortex is divided into three zones**. The outer **zona glomerulosa** is **made up of whorls of cells** that are continuous with the columns of cells that form the **zona fasciculata**. These columns are separated by venous sinuses. The **inner portion of the zona fasciculata merges** into the **zona reticularis**, where the **cell columns become interlaced in a network**. The **zona glomerulosa** makes up **15% of the mass of the adrenal gland**; the **zona fasciculata, 50%**; and the **zona reticularis, 7%**. The adrenocortical cells contain **abundant lipid, especially in the outer portion of the zona fasciculata**. All three cortical zones secrete corticosterone, but the **active enzymatic mechanism for aldosterone biosynthesis is limited to the zona glomerulosa**, whereas the **enzymatic mechanisms for forming cortisol and sex hormones are found in the two inner zones**. Furthermore, subspecialization occurs within the inner two zones, with the **zona fasciculata secreting mostly glucocorticoids** and the **zona reticularis secreting mainly sex hormones**."- Ganong 25/e p353*

23. **Ans. d. D**   *(Ref: Ganong 25/e p661; Guyton 13/e p542-544)*
    C and B: Progressive hypoxia without change in pH
    D: Only pH change without additional hypoxia
    E: Hypoxia as well as pH change.

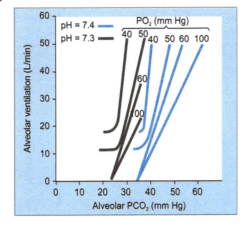

*"This graph gives a quick overview of the manner in which the **chemical factors pO₂, pCO₂, and pH—together affect alveolar ventilation.** To understand this diagram, first observe the **four lighter curves. These curves were recorded at different levels of arterial pO₂-40 mm Hg, 50 mm Hg, 60 mm Hg, and 100 mm Hg.** For each of these curves, the pCO₂ was changed from lower to higher levels. Thus, this "family" of lighter curves represents the combined effects of alveolar pCO₂ and pO₂ on ventilation. Now observe the darker curves. The lighter curves were measured at a blood pH of 7.4; the darker curves were measured at a pH of 7.3. We now have two families of curves representing the combined effects of pCO₂ and pO₂ on ventilation at two different pH values. Still other families of curves would be displaced to the right at higher pHs and displaced to the left at lower pHs. Thus, using this diagram, one can predict the level of alveolar ventilation for most combinations of alveolar pCO₂, alveolar pO₂, and arterial pH."- Guyton 13/e p544*

24. **Ans. d. Phosphocreatine** *(Ref: Guyton 13/e p1087, Ganong 25/e p108, 24/e p106)*
Phosphocreatine is the rapid source of energy by resynthesizing ATP for exercising muscles.

"During periods of high activity, cycling of phosphorylcreatine allows for quick release of ATP to sustain muscle activity."- Ganong 25/e p108

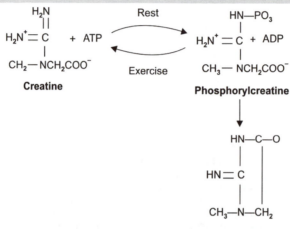

Fig. 12: Creatine, phosphorylcreatine & creatinine cycling in muscle

"ATP is resynthesized from ADP by the addition of a phosphate group. Some of the energy for this endothermic reaction is supplied by the breakdown of glucose to CO₂ and H₂O, but there also exists in muscle another energy-rich phosphate compound that can supply this energy for short periods. This compound is **phosphorylcreatine**, which is **hydrolyzed to creatine and phosphate groups with the release of considerable energy. At rest, some ATP in the mitochondria transfers its phosphate to creatine, so that a phosphorylcreatine store is built up. During exercise, the phosphorylcreatine is hydrolyzed at the junction between the myosin heads and actin, forming ATP from ADP and thus permitting contraction to continue."- Ganong 25/e p108*

25. **Ans. a. Testosterone** *(Ref: Ganong 25/e p 422, 24/e p424; Harper 30/e p 516, 517)*
Testosterone binds to SHBG with higher affinity than does estradiol. Therefore, a change in the level of SHBG causes a greater change in the free testosterone level than in the free estradiol level.

"Sex hormone binding globulin is a glycoprotein which binds sex steroids with high affinity as: DHT>Testosterone>>Esterone/ estradiol. Because of the higher affinity of SHBG for DHT and Testosterone, compared to E, variation in SHBG has profound effects on the levels of androgens."

Steroid	% Free	% Bound to		
		CBG	GBG	Albumin
Testosterone	2	0	65^Q	33^Q
Androstenedione	7^Q	0	8	85^Q
Estradiol	2	0	38^Q	60^Q
Progesterone	2	18^Q	0	80^Q
Cortisol	4	90^Q	0	6

CBG, corticosteroid-binding globulin; GBG, gonadal steroid-binding globulin

*"Most mammals, humans included, have a **plasma beta-globulin that binds testosterone with specificity, relatively high affinity, and limited capacity**. This protein, usually called **sex hormone-binding globulin (SHBG)** or testosterone-estrogen-binding globulin (TEBG), is **produced in the liver**. Its **production is increased by estrogens** (women have twice the serum concentration of SHBG as men), **certain types of liver disease, and hyperthyroidism**; it is **decreased by androgens, advancing age, and hypothyroidism**. Many of these conditions also affect the production of CBG and TBG. Since **SHBG and albumin bind 97–99% of circulating testosterone**, only a small fraction of the hormone in circulation is in the free (biologically active) form. The **primary function of SHBG** may be to **restrict the free concentration of testosterone in the serum**. Testosterone binds to SHBG with higher affinity than does estradiol. Therefore, a change in the level of SHBG causes a greater change in the free testosterone level than in the free estradiol level. Because the metabolic clearance rates of these steroids are inversely related to the affinity of their binding to SHBG, estrone is cleared more rapidly than estradiol, which in turn is cleared more rapidly than testosterone or DHT."*-Harper 30/e p517

26. **Ans. b. 90 minutes** *(Ref: Ganong 25/e p496, 24/e p498)*
Migrating motor complexes in the gut reappear after intervals of 90 minutes.

*"The **MMCs are initiated by motilin**. The circulating level of this hormone increases at intervals of approximately 100 min in the interdigestive state, coordinated with the contractile phases of the MMC. The **contractions migrate aborally at a rate of about 5 cm/ min, and also occur at intervals of approximately 100 min**."- Ganong 25/e p496*

Migrating Motor Complex

- **During fasting between periods of digestion, pattern of electrical & motor activity in gastrointestinal smooth muscle becomes modified** so that **cycles of motor activity migrate from stomach to distal ileum**[Q].
  - Each cycle, or **migrating motor complex (MMC)**, starts with a **quiescent period (phase I)**, continues with a period of **irregular electrical and mechanical activity (phase II)** & ends with a burst of **regular activity (phase III)**[Q].
- **MMCs are initiated by motilin**[Q]. Circulating level of motilin increases at intervals of approximately **100 min in interdigestive state,** coordinated with contractile phases of MMC.
  - **Contractions migrate aborally** at a rate of about **5 cm/ min** & occur at **intervals of approximately 100 min**[Q].
  - **Gastric secretion, bile flow & pancreatic secretion increase during each MMC**[Q]. They likely serve to **clear stomach & small intestine of luminal contents** in preparation for next meal.
- Conversely, when a **meal is ingested, secretion of motilin is suppressed** (ingestion of food suppresses motilin release via mechanisms that have not yet been elucidated) & **MMC is abolished, until digestion & absorption are complete**. Instead, there is a return to peristalsis & other forms of BER and spike potentials during this time.
  - **Erythromycin binds to motilin receptors,** and derivatives of this compound **may be of value in treating patients in whom gastrointestinal motility is decreased**[Q].

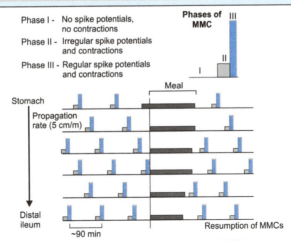

Fig. 13: Migrating motor complexes (MMCs).
(Complexes move down the GIT at a regular rate during fasting, that they are completely inhibited by a meal, and that they resume 90–120 min after the meal)

AIIMS ESSENCE

27. Ans. a. Polycythemia   *(Ref: Ganong 25/e p635, 24/e p635)*

Diffusion capacity of carbon monoxide is increased in polycythemia.

> *"The **diffusing capacity of the lung** for a given gas is **directly proportional to the surface area of the alveolo-capillary membrane** and **inversely proportional to its thickness**. The diffusing capacity for CO (DICO) is measured as an index of diffusing capacity because its uptake is diffusion-limited. **DICO is proportional to the amount of CO entering the blood (Vco) divided by the partial pressure of CO in the alveoli minus the partial pressure of CO in the blood entering the pulmonary capillaries.** Except in habitual cigarette smokers, this latter term is close to zero, so it can be ignored and the equation becomes: DLCO = VCO/ PACO."- Ganong 25/e p635*

> *"**DLCO decreases in diseases that thicken or destroy alveolar membranes** (e.g., **pulmonary fibrosis, emphysema), curtail the pulmonary vasculature** (e.g., **pulmonary hypertension**), or **reduce alveolar capillary hemoglobin** (e.g., **anemia**). Single-breath diffusing capacity may be elevated in acute congestive heart failure, asthma, polycythemia & pulmonary hemorrhage."*

Diffusing Capacity of the Lung for Carbon Monoxide (DLCO)

- **Diffusing capacity of lung** for a given gas is **directly proportional to the surface area of alveolo-capillary membrane** and **inversely proportional to its thickness**[Q].
- **Diffusing capacity for CO (DICO)** is measured as an **index of diffusing capacity** because **its uptake is diffusion-limited.**

  - DICO is proportional to the amount of CO entering the blood (VCO) divided by partial pressure of CO in alveoli minus the partial pressure of CO in the blood entering the pulmonary capillaries[Q].

- **Normal value of DICO** at rest is about **25 mL/min/mm Hg.** It **increases up to threefold during exercise** because of capillary dilation and an increase in the number of active capillaries.
- This test uses a **small (and safe) amount of carbon monoxide to measure gas exchange across the alveolar membrane** during a 10-second breath hold.
- Carbon monoxide in exhaled breath is analyzed to determine the **quantity of CO absorbed by crossing the alveolar membrane & combining with hemoglobin in RBCs.**

  - This **'single-breath diffusing capacity'** [diffusion capacity of the lung for carbon monoxide (DLCO)] value increases with surface area available for diffusion & amount of hemoglobin within the capillaries, & varies **inversely with alveolar membrane thickness**[Q].

Factors Affecting DLCO	
Increased DLCO	**Decreased DLCO**
• **Exercise**[Q]	• **Post-exercise**[Q]
• **Supine position**[Q]	• **Standing**[Q]
• **Muller maneuver**[Q] (inspiration against closed mouth & nose after forced expiration)	• **Valsalva maneuver**[Q]
	• **Lung resection**[Q]
• **Pulmonary hemorrhage**[Q]	• **Pulmonary emphysema**[Q]
• **Polycythemia**[Q]	• **Pulmonary vascular disease**[Q] (pulmonary arterial hypertension & chronic venous thromboembolism)
• **Left-to-right shunt** (e.g. **atrial septal defect**[Q])	
• **Obesity**[Q]	• **Interstitial lung diseases**[Q]
• **Asthma**[Q]	• **Anemia**[Q]
• **Chronic bronchitis** without major emphysema	• **Drugs: Amiodarone, bleomycin, methotrexate**[Q]
• **Pregnancy**[Q]	• Pulmonary lymphangitic carcinomatosis

28. Ans. a. Nernst equation   *(Ref: Ganong 25/e9, p24/e p9-10; Guyton 13/e p61*

Potential generated due to movement of freely diffusible ions across a semi-permeable membrane is calculated using Nernst equation.

> *"The Nernst equation describes the relation of diffusion potential to the ion concentration difference across a membrane."- Guyton 13/e p61*

- The Nernst equation is used to calculate the equilibrium potential at a given concentration difference of a permeable ion across a cell membrane.
- The potential develops due to free movement of ion through leaky channels. **Gibbs equation is used to govern the distribution of ions across a semi-permeable membrane.**
- The potential developed due to this distribution is governed by Nernst equation.

  - $E_{Cl} = RT/FZ_{Cl} \ln [Cl_o^-]/[Cl_i^-]$
  - where E_{Cl} = equilibrium potential for Cl^-
  - R = gas constant
  - T = absolute temperature
  - F = the Faraday of charge)
  - Z_{Cl} = valence of Cl^- (–1)
  - $[Cl_o^-]$ = Cl^- concentration outside the cell
  - $[Cl_i^-]$ = Cl^- concentration inside the cell
  - Converting from the natural log to the base 10 log and replacing some of the constants with numeric values holding temperature at 37°C, the equation becomes:
  - $E_{Cl} = 61.5 \log [Cl_i^-]/[Cl_o^-]$ at 37°C

29. **Ans. a. RT_3** *(Ref: Harper 30/e p510; Ganong 25/e p342-343, 24/e p345)*

The most pronounced effect of starvation on thyroid profile is a reduction in T_3 levels with a reciprocal rise in RT3. The changes, which conserve calories by reducing tissue metabolism, are reversed promptly by refeeding. Similar changes occur in wasting diseases.

"Much more RT_3 and much less T_3 are formed during fetal life, and the ratio shifts to that of adults about 6 weeks after birth. Various drugs inhibit deiodinases, producing a fall in plasma T_3 levels and a reciprocal rise in RT_3. Selenium deficiency has the same effect. A wide variety of nonthyroidal illnesses also suppress deiodinases. These include burns, trauma, advanced cancer, cirrhosis, chronic kidney disease, myocardial infarction, and febrile states. The low-T_3 state produced by these conditions disappears with recovery. It is difficult to decide whether individuals with the low-T_3 state produced by drugs and illness have mild hypothyroidism. Diet also has a clear-cut effect on conversion of T_4 to T_3. In fasted individuals, plasma T_3 is reduced by 10–20% within 24 h and by about 50% in 3–7 days, with a corresponding rise in RT_3. Free and bound T_4 levels remain essentially normal. During more prolonged starvation, RT_3 returns to normal but T_3 remains depressed. At the same time, the basal metabolic rate (BMR) falls and urinary nitrogen excretion, an index of protein breakdown, is decreased. Thus, the decline in T_3 conserves calories and protein. Conversely, over-feeding increases T_3 and reduces RT_3."- Ganong 25/e p342

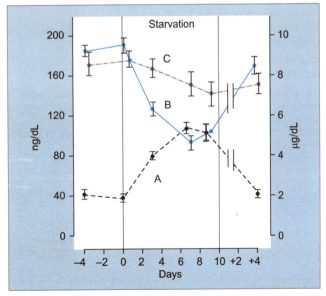

Fig. 14: Effect of starvation on plasma levels of T_4, T_3, and RT_3 in humans.

(The scale for T_3 and RT_3 is on the left and the scale for T_4 is on the right. **The most pronounced effect is a reduction in T_3 levels with a reciprocal rise in RT_3. The changes, which conserve calories by reducing tissue metabolism, are reversed promptly by refeeding.** Similar changes occur in wasting diseases.)

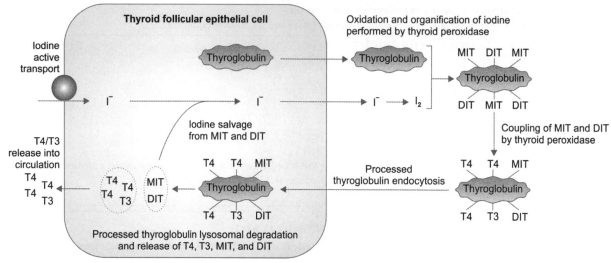

Fig. 15: Thyroid hormone synthesis

Thyroid Hormone Synthesis
• **Thyroid peroxidase generates reactive iodine species** that can **attack thyroglobulin**.
• **First product is monoiodotyrosine (MIT)**. MIT is **next iodinated on the carbon 5 position to form diiodotyrosine (DIT)**.
• **Two DIT** molecules then **undergo an oxidative condensation to form T_4** with elimination of alanine side chain from the molecule that forms the outer ring.
• **Thyroid peroxidase** is **involved in coupling as well as iodination**.
• T_3 is formed by condensation of **MIT with DIT**. A small amount of RT_3 is also formed, probably by **condensation of DIT with MIT**.
• In normal human thyroid, average distribution of iodinated compounds is **3% MIT, 33% DIT, 35% T_4 & 7% T_3**. Only traces of RT_3 and other components are present.
• **Much more RT_3 & much less T_3 are formed during fetal life & ratio shifts to that of adults about 6 weeks after birth**[Q].
• Various drugs inhibit deiodinases, producing a **fall in plasma T_3 levels & a reciprocal rise in RT_3**.
• **Selenium deficiency has the same effect**[Q].
• A wide variety of nonthyroidal illnesses also suppress deiodinases. These include **burns, trauma, advanced cancer, cirrhosis, renal failure, myocardial infarction & febrile states**[Q].
• The low-T_3 state produced by these conditions disappears with recovery.
• **Diet also has a clear-cut effect on conversion of T_4 to T_3**.
• In **fasted individuals, plasma T_3 is reduced by 10–20% within 24 hours and by about 50% in 3–7 days**, with a corresponding rise in RT_3. Free & bound T_4 levels remain essentially normal. During more prolonged starvation, RT_3 returns to normal but T_3 remains depressed[Q].
• At the same time, BMR falls & urinary nitrogen excretion, an index of protein breakdown, is decreased. Thus, **decline in T_3 conserves calories & protein**[Q].
• Conversely, **over feeding increases T_3 & reduces RT_3**.

Condition	Conc. of binding proteins	Total plasma T_4, T_3, RT_3	Free plasma T_4, T_3, RT_3	Plasma TSH	Clinical State
Hyperthyroidism	Normal	**High**[Q]	**High**[Q]	**Low**[Q]	Hyperthyroid
Hypothyroidism	Normal	**Low**[Q]	**Low**[Q]	**High**[Q]	Hypothyroid
Estrogens, methadone, heroin, major tranquilizers, clofibrate	**High**[Q]	**High**[Q]	Normal	Normal	Euthyroid
Glucocorticoids, androgens, danazol, asparaginase	**Low**[Q]	**Low**[Q]	Normal	Normal	Euthyroid

BIOCHEMISTY

30. Ans. a. Methylation *(Ref: Harper 30/e p438, 439; Harrison 19/e p102e-7)*

CG islands also known as CpG islands play a vital role in regulation of gene expression. Cytosine (C) residues in CG rich islands can undergo methylation by DNA methyl transferase.

"There is evidence that the **methylation of deoxycytidine residues (in the sequence 5'-^{m}CpG-3') in DNA may effect gross changes in chromatin so as to preclude its active transcription**."- Harper 30/e p438

"**Epigenetics is defined as changes that alter the pattern of gene expression that persist across at least one cell division** but are **not caused by changes in the DNA code. Epigenetic changes include alterations of chromatin structure mediated by methylation of cytosine residues in CpG dinucleotides, modification of histones by acetylation or methylation**, or changes in higher-order chromosome structure."- Harrison 19/e p102e-7

See Q. No. 54 AIIMS May 2017

31. Ans. b. 2.3 *(Ref: Harper 30/e p10)*

The pH of a solution containing 5 millimole/liter of H^+ ions is closest to 2.3.

> pH is the negative log of the hydrogen ion concentration
> Here, $pH = -\log[H^+]$
> $pH = -\log[5 \times 10^{-3}] = -\log(5) - \log(10^{-3})$
> $= -\log(10/2) + 3 = -1 + \log 2 + 3$
> $= 2 + 0.3010$
> $= 2.3$ (approx.)
> [log 2 = 0.3010, log 10 = 1]

32. Ans. c. Galactosemia *(Ref: Harper 30/e p205; Nelson 20/e p726; Harrison 19/e p433e-5)*

Apart from glucose, both fructose & galactose gives positive Benedict's test. If patient has fructosemia (Hereditary fructose intolerance), then patient must have hypoglycemia because in this situation fructose-1-phosphate accumulates, which inhibits glycogen phosphorylase leading to hypoglycemia. Fructosemia is less likely. Preferred option would be galactosemia.

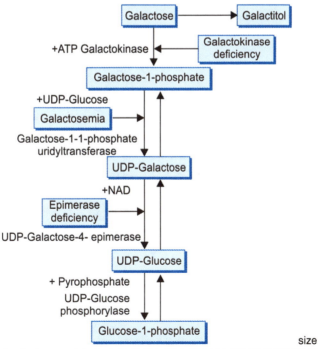

Fig. 16: Pathway of galactose metabolism depicting sites of metabolic block that lead to galactosemia.

Galactosemia
• Classic galactosemia is **caused by galactose 1-phosphate uridyl transferase (GALT) deficiency**[Q].   • **Deficiency of galactokinase** causes **cataracts**[Q].   • **Deficiency of uridine diphosphate galactose 4-epimerase** can be **benign**[Q] (enzyme deficiency is **limited to blood cells**) or severe (when the enzyme deficiency is **generalized**[Q])
Pathophysiology: • **Newborn** normally receives up to **40% of caloric intake as lactose**[Q] (glucose + galactose).   • **Without transferase**, infant is **unable to metabolize galactose 1-phosphate**, leading to accumulation, resulting in **injury to** parenchymal cells of **kidney, liver & brain**[Q].
Clinical Features: • **After first feeding**, infants can present with **vomiting, diarrhea, hypotonia, jaundice & hepatomegaly**[Q].   • **Increased risk for E. coli neonatal sepsis**[Q]   • Women with classic galactosemia: **Hyper gonadotropic hypogonadism**[Q] (80–90%)
Diagnosis: • **Urine** of patient shows **reducing sugar (galactose),** which can be **detected by Benedict's reagent**[Q].   • **Glucose oxidase test** is **negative** as it is **specific for glucose.**   • Presence of reducing sugar **(galactose) in urine** with a **negative glucose oxidase test** suggests the diagnosis of **galactosemia**[Q].
Treatment: • **Dietary restriction: Elimination of galactose from diet reverses growth failure** as well as **renal & hepatic dysfunction**, improving the prognosis[Q].

33. **Ans. d. Glutamine** *(Ref: Harper 30/e p292)*
Ammonia from brain is removed as glutamine.

"While ammonia, derived mainly from the alpha-amino nitrogen of amino acids, is highly toxic, tissues convert ammonia to the amide nitrogen of nontoxic glutamine. Subsequent deamination of glutamine in the liver releases ammonia, which is then converted to nontoxic urea."- Harper 30/e p292

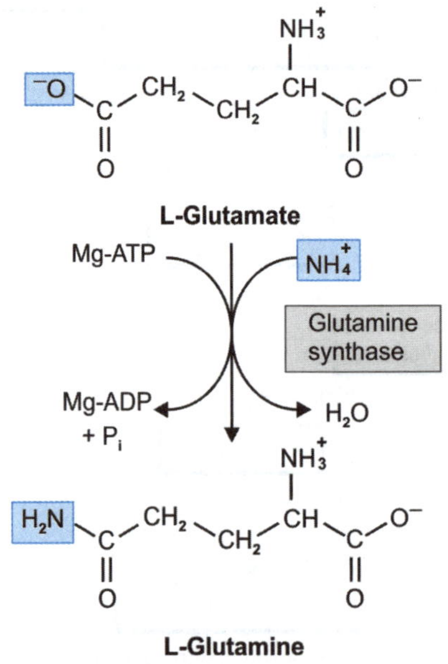

L-Glutamate

L-Glutamine

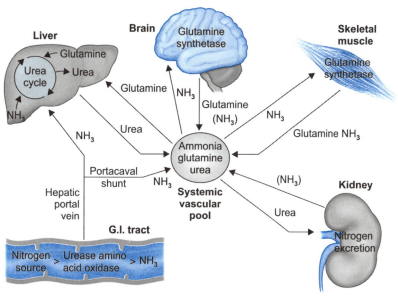

Fig. 17: Ammonia transport and metabolism

Ammonia Transport & Metabolism

- **Ammonia** is **produced by enteric bacteria** & **absorbed into portal venous blood**[Q]
- **Ammonia** produced by tissues are **rapidly removed from circulation by liver** & **converted to urea**[Q].

Ammonia Transport	
From most of the tissues (Including Brain)	**From Skeletal Muscle**
• **Glutamine** is the **ammonia transporter from most tissues including brain**[Q]. • **Ammonia** formed in most tissues including brain is **trapped by glutamate to form glutamine**[Q] (1st line trapping of ammonia) • In liver, glutaminase removes ammonia from glutamine[Q]. • Ammonia enters into urea cycle in the liver[Q].	• **Alanine** is the **ammonia transporter from muscles**[Q] • In skeletal muscles, **excess amino groups are transferred to pyruvate to form alanine**[Q].

- **Ammonia disposal:** Ammonia from all over body **reaches liver, detoxified to urea by liver cells & excreted through kidney**[Q].
- If **portal blood bypasses the liver**, systemic blood **ammonia levels** may **rise to toxic levels**. This occurs in **severely impaired hepatic function** or **development of collateral** links between **portal & systemic veins** in cirrhosis[Q].

  - **Ammonia** is **toxic to CNS** because it **reacts with α-ketoglutarate to form glutamate**.
  - The resulting **depleted levels of α-ketoglutarate impair function of TCA cycle in neurons**[Q].

- **Symptoms of ammonia intoxication:** Tremor, slurred speech, blurred vision, coma & ultimately **death**.

34. **Ans. b. 1** *(Ref: Harper 30/e p148)*

Respiratory Quotient (RQ) of a person on pure carbohydrate diet will be 1.

"*For several hours after a meal, while the products of digestion are being absorbed, there is an abundant supply of metabolic fuels. Under these conditions, **glucose is the major fuel for oxidation in most tissues; this is observed as an increase in the respiratory quotient (the ratio of carbon dioxide produced to oxygen consumed) from about 0.8 in the starved state to near 1.***"-*Harper 30/ep148*

	Energy Yield (kJ/g)	O_2 Consumed (L/g)	CO_2 Produced (L/g)	RQ (CO_2 Produced/ O_2 Consumed)	Oxygen (kJ/L)
Carbohydrate	16	0.829	0.829	1.00[Q]	20
Protein	17	0.966	0.782	0.81[Q]	20
Fat	37[Q]	2.016	1.427	0.71[Q]	20
Alcohol	29	1.429	0.966	0.66[Q]	20

AIIMS ESSENCE

35. Ans. d. Pregnenolone *(Ref: Harper 30/e p503)*

All mammalian steroid hormones are formed from cholesterol via pregnenolone through a series of reactions.

"All mammalian steroid hormones are formed from cholesterol via pregnenolone through a series of reactions that occur in either the mitochondria or endoplasmic reticulum of the adrenal cell. Hydroxylases that require molecular oxygen and NADPH are essential, and dehydrogenases, an isomerase, and a lyase reaction are also necessary for certain steps."-Harper 30/e p503

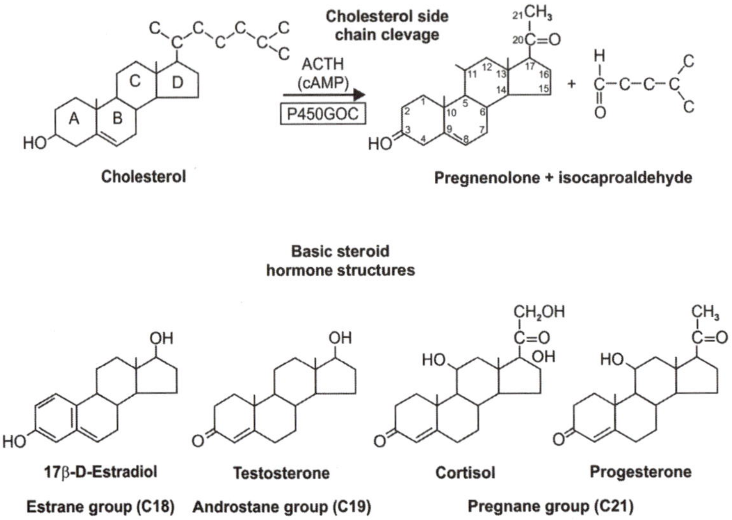

Fig. 18: Cholesterol side-chain cleavage and basic hormone structures

Adrenal Steroidogenesis

- **Adrenal steroid hormones** are **synthesized from cholesterol^Q**.
- **Cholesterol** is **mostly derived from plasma**, but a small portion is **synthesized in situ from acetyl-CoA** via mevalonate & squalene.
- Much of **cholesterol in adrenal is esterified & stored in cytoplasmic lipid droplets^Q**.

  - Upon stimulation of adrenal by ACTH, an **esterase is activated & free cholesterol** formed is **transported into mitochondrion**, where a **cytochrome P450 side chain cleavage enzyme (P450scc)** converts **cholesterol to pregnenolone^Q**.

- Cleavage of the side chain involves **sequential hydroxylations, first at C22 & then at C20**, followed by **side chain cleavage** (removal of the six-carbon fragment isocaproaldehyde) to give 21-carbon steroid.
- An ACTH-dependent **steroidogenic acute regulatory (StAR) protein** is **essential for transport of cholesterol to P450scc in inner mitochondrial membrane^Q**.

  - **All mammalian steroid hormones** are **formed from cholesterol via pregnenolone** through a series of reactions that **occur in** either **mitochondria** or **endoplasmic reticulum** of **adrenal cell^Q**.

- Hydroxylases that require molecular oxygen and **NADPH** are **essential & dehydrogenases, an isomerase, & a lyase reaction** is also **necessary for certain steps.**

  - There is **cellular specificity in adrenal steroidogenesis**.
  - **18- hydroxylase & 19-hydroxysteroid dehydrogenase** are **required for aldosterone synthesis, are found only in the zona glomerulosa cells^Q**.
  - **Biosynthesis of aldosterone is confined to zona glomerulosa^Q**.

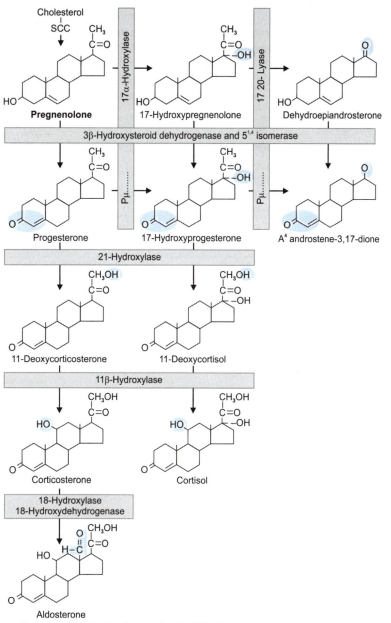

Fig. 19: Pathways involved in the synthesis of the three major classes of adrenal steroids (mineralocorticoids, glucocorticoids, and androgens)

36. **Ans. c. Arginine**   *(Ref: Harper 30/e p21)*

At physiological pH, arginine has a positive charge.

> "The acid strengths of weak acids are expressed as their pK_a. **The imidazole group of histidine and the guanidino group of arginine exist as resonance hybrids with positive charge distributed between both nitrogens (histidine) or all three nitrogens (arginine)."** - *Harper 30/e p21*

Chemistry of Amino Acids

- **Amino acids** may have **positive, negative,** or **zero net charge**
- In aqueous solution, charged & uncharged forms of ionizable weak acid **groups −COOH & −NH$_3^+$ exist in dynamic protonic equilibrium.**

Chemistry of Amino Acids

- While both $R'COOH^+$ & $R'NH_3^+$ are weak acids, $R'COOH$ is a far **stronger acid than** $R'NH_3^+$.
- At **physiologic pH (7.4), carboxyl groups exist** almost entirely **as** $R'COO^-$ & **amino groups** predominantly as $R'NH_3^+$.
- **Imidazole group** of **histidine** & **guanidino group** of **arginine** exist as **resonance hybrids** with **positive charge distributed** between **two nitrogens (histidine)** or **three nitrogens (arginine)**[Q].

Charge of the Amino Acid (AA) Side Chains

- When an **AA is incorporated** into a **polypeptide, charges on amino** & **carboxyl groups disappear.**
- Among the 20 common amino acids, **five** have a **side-chain, which can be charged.**

  - At pH7:
    - Negative charged: aspartic acid & glutamic acid (acidic side chains)
    - Positive charged: histidine, arginine & lysine[Q] (basic side chains-HALy).

- Charge on AA side chain depends on pK of AA & pH of solution.

Negative Charged (Acidic Side Chains)	Positive Charged (Basic Side Chains)
- **Aspartic acid & glutamic acid**[Q] - At a **pH superior to their pK**, carboxylic side chains **lose** an H^+ ion (proton) & are **negative charged**. They are therefore acid. - At a pH inferior to their pK, aspartic acid & glutamic acid side chains are uncharged.	- **Histidine, arginine & lysine**[Q] - At a pH superior to their pK, amine side chains are uncharged. - At a **pH inferior to their pK, histidine, arginine & lysine** side chains **accept** an H^+ ion (proton) & are **positive charged**. They are therefore **basic**[Q].

Amino Acids			
Hydrophobic (Non-polar) Amino Acid	Hydrophilic (Polar) Amino Acid	Aliphatic Amino Acid	Aromatic Amino Acid
(TT MILAP) - **T**yrosine - **T**ryptophan - **M**ethionine - **I**soleucine - **L**eucine - **A**lanine - **P**henylalanine, **P**roline	**Uncharged side chain** (TCS GT) - **T**hreonine - **C**ystine - **S**erine - **G**lycine - **T**yrosine **Acidic side chain** - Aspartic acid, asparagine - Glutamic acid, glutamine **Basic side chain (HALy)** - **H**istidine[Q] - **A**rginine (Most basic)[Q] - **Ly**sine[Q]	(VALIG) - **V**aline - **A**lanine - **L**eucine - **I**soleucine - **G**lycine	(PTH) - **P**henylalanine - **T**yrosine, **T**ryptophan - **H**istidine
		Imino Acid	**Sulphur** containing Amino acid
		- **Proline**[Q]	- **Cysteine**[Q] - **Methionine**[Q]

Essential Amino Acids (MP VITTHALL)[Q]	
- **M**ethionine[Q] - **P**henylalanine[Q] - **V**aline[Q] - **I**soleucine[Q] - **T**hreonine[Q]	- **T**ryptophan[Q] - **H**istidine (Semi essential amino acid)[Q] - **A**rginine (Semi essential amino acid[Q] - **L**eucine[Q] - **L**ysine[Q]

37. Ans. b. Apoproteins *(Ref: Harper 30/e p254)*

HDL contains the highest proportion of apoproteins as it has the highest density and migrates the least during electrophoresis. It also contains maximum phospholipids.

"The protein moiety of a lipoprotein is known as an apolipoprotein or apoprotein, constituting nearly 70% of some HDL and as little as 1% of chylomicrons." - Harper 30/e p254

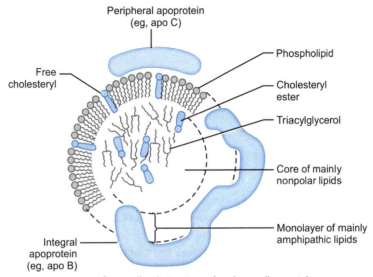

Fig. 20: Generalized structure of a plasma lipoprotein

*"One or more apolipoproteins (proteins or polypeptides) are present in each lipoprotein. **The major apolipoproteins of HDL (α-lipoprotein) are designated A. The main apolipoprotein of LDL (β-lipoprotein) is apolipoprotein B (B-100) and is found also in VLDL. Chylomicrons contain a truncated form of apo B (B-48) that is synthesized in the intestine, while B-100 is synthesized in the liver. Apo B-100 is one of the longest single polypeptide chains** known, having 4536 amino acids and a molecular mass of 550,000 Da. Apo B-48 (48% of B-100) is formed from the same mRNA as apo B-100 after the introduction of a stop signal by an RNA editing enzyme. Apo C-I, C-II, and C-III are smaller polypeptides (molecular mass 7000– 9000 Da) freely transferable between several different lipoproteins. Apo E is found in VLDL, HDL, chylomicrons, and chylomicron remnants; it accounts for 5– 10% of total VLDL apolipoproteins in normal subjects."*
- Harper 30/e p254

Composition of Lipoproteins in Plasma of Humans								
Lipoprotein	Source	Diameter (nm)	Density (g/mL)	Protein (%)	Lipid (%)	Main Lipid Components	Apolipoproteins
Chylomicrons	Intestine[Q]	90–1000[Q]	<0.95[Q]	1–2[Q]	98-99[Q]	Triacylglycerol[Q]	A-I, A-II, A-IV, B-48, C-I, C-II, C-III, E[Q]
Chylomicron remnants	Chylomicrons[Q]	45–150	<1.006	6–8	92–94	Triacylglycerol, phospholipids, cholesterol[Q]	B-48, E[Q]
VLDL	Liver[Q] (intestine)	30–90	0.95-1.006	7–10	90–93	Triacylglycerol[Q]	B-100, C-I, C-II, C-III[Q]
IDL	VLDL[Q]	25–35	1.006-1.019	11	89	Triacylglycerol, cholesterol[Q]	B-100, E[Q]
LDL	VLDL[Q]	20–25	1.019-1.063	21	79	Cholesterol[Q]	B-100[Q]

Contd...

Contd...

HDL	Liver, intestine, VLDL, chylomicrons[Q]					Phospholipids, cholesterol[Q]	A-I, A-II, A-IV, C-I, C-II, C-III, D, E[Q]
HDL$_1$		20–25	1.019-1.063	32	68		
HDL$_2$		10–20	1.063-1.125	33	67		
HDL$_3$		5–10[Q]	1.125-1.210[Q]	57[Q]	43[Q]		
Pre beta-HDL		<5[Q]	>1.210[Q]				A–I[Q]

Types of Cholesterol	Characteristic Feature
Chylomicrons	• **Maximum lipid content overall[Q]** • **Maximum triglyceride content overall[Q]** • **Maximum exogenous (dietary) triglyceride content[Q]** • **Transport of exogenous lipids[Q]** • Minimum cholesterol content • Minimum phospholipid content • **Lipoprotein with lowest density[Q]** • **Lipoprotein with largest size[Q]** • **Lipoprotein with minimum protein content[Q]** • **Dietary lipids (including triglyceride) are transported from intestine to liver by** Chylomicrons[Q] • **Least (no) electrophoretic mobility[Q]**
HDL	• Minimum lipid content overall • Minimum triglyceride content • **Maximum phospholipid content[Q]** • **Lipoprotein with maximum density[Q]** • **Lipoprotein with smallest size[Q]** • **Lipoprotein with maximum protein content[Q]** • **Maximum electrophoretic mobility[Q]**
VLDL	• **Maximum endogenous triglyceride content[Q]** • **Transport of endogenous triglycerides[Q]** • **Endogenous triglycerides are transported from liver to peripheral tissues by VLDL[Q]**
LDL	• **Maximum cholesterol[Q]** • **LDL is the major source of cholesterol for peripheral tissues,** i.e. cholesterol is transported to peripheral (extrahepatic) tissues by LDL[Q]
IDL	• **LDL is the immediate precursor for IDL[Q]**

38. Ans. b. Its components can be increased or decreased in the body as needed *(Ref: Harper 30/e p11; Ganong 25/e p6; Guyton 13/e p413, 415)*

HCO_3^-/H_2CO_3 *is the best buffer because its components can be increased or decreased in the body as needed.*

> *"The bicarbonate buffer system is the most powerful extracellular buffer in the body. This apparent paradox is due mainly to the fact that the two elements of the buffer system, HCO_3^- & CO_2 are regulated respectively by the kidneys and the lungs. As a result of this regulation, the pH of the extracellular fluid can be precisely controlled by the relative rate of removal and addition of HCO_3^- by the kidneys and the rate of removal of CO_2 by the lungs."*
> *- Guyton 13/e p413*

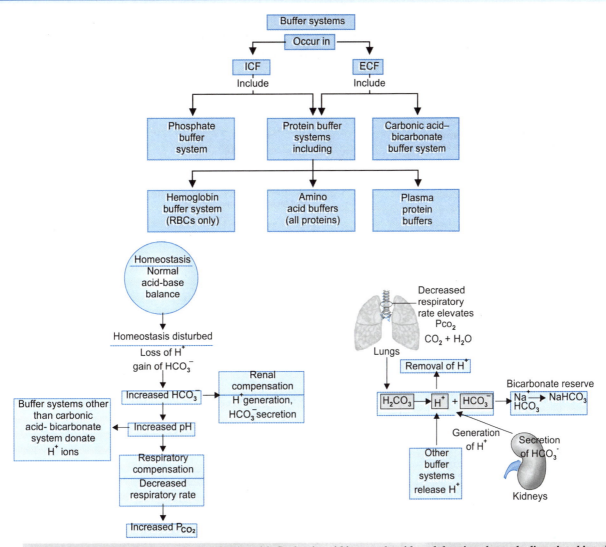

"*An important buffer in the body is carbonic acid. Carbonic acid is a weak acid, and thus is only partly dissociated into H^+ and HCO_3^-. If H^+ is added to a solution of carbonic acid, the equilibrium shifts to the left and most of the added H^+ is removed from solution. If OH^- is added, H^+ and OH^- combine, taking H^+ out of solution. However, the decrease is countered by more dissociation of HCO_3, and the decline in H^+ concentration is minimized. A unique feature of HCO_3^- is the linkage between its buffering ability and the ability for the lungs to remove CO_2 from the body. The overall mechanism by which the kidneys excrete acidic or basic urine is as follows: Large numbers of HCO_3^- are filtered continuously into the tubules, and if they are excreted into the urine, this removes base from the blood. Large numbers of H^+ are also secreted into the tubular lumen by the tubular epithelial cells, thus removing acid from the blood. If more H^+ is secreted than HCO_3^- is filtered, there will be a net loss of acid from the extracellular fluid. Conversely, if more HCO_3^- is filtered than H^+ is secreted, there will be a net loss of base.*" - *Guyton 13/e p415*

39. **Ans. c. Fatty acid synthesis** *(Ref: Harper 30/e p232)*
    Fatty acid synthesis takes place completely in the cytosol.

    "*Fatty acids are synthesized by an extra-mitochondrial system, which is responsible for the complete synthesis of palmitate from acetyl-CoA in the cytosol.*" - *Harper 30/e p232*

    "*The main pathway for de novo synthesis of fatty acids (lipogenesis) occurs in cytosol. This system is **present in many tissues, including liver, kidney, brain, lung, mammary gland, and adipose tissue**. Its cofactor requirements include NADPH, ATP, Mn^{2+}, biotin, and HCO_3^- (as a source of CO_2). Acetyl- CoA is the **immediate substrate**, and free palmitate is the **end product**.*" - *Harper 30/e p232*

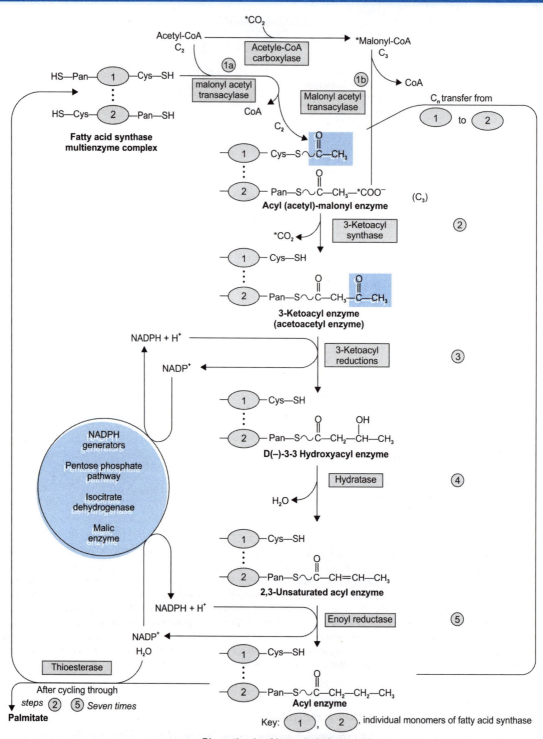

Fig. 21: Biosynthesis of long chain fatty acids

Fatty Acid Synthesis
• **Synthesis** takes place in **cytosol**[Q].
• Intermediates covalently linked to acyl carrier protein[Q].
• Acetyl CoA + $CO_2 \rightarrow$ Malonyl CoA[Q]

Contd...

Contd...

- **Four-step repeating cycle, extension by 2-carbons/cycle**- Condensation, reduction, dehydration, reduction.
- **Enzymes of fatty acid synthesis** are packaged together in a complex called as **fatty acid synthesis (FAS)**.
- **Product** of FAS action is **palmitic acid[Q]**.

> - **FA synthesis begins from methyl end & proceeds toward carboxylic acid end[Q]**.
> - **C16 & C15 are added first** and **C2 & C1 are added last[Q]**.
> - **C15 & C16 are derived directly from acetyl CoA[Q]**.

Fatty Acid Synthesis & Degradation		
	Degradation	**Synthesis**
Location	**Mitochondria[Q]**	**Cytosol[Q]**
Activated intermediates	**Thioesters CoA[Q]**	**Thioesters of ACP[Q]**
Enzymes	4 different enzymes[Q]	FAS multienzyme complex
Direction	Starts at **carboxyl end[Q]**	Starts from **methyl end[Q]**
Fatty acid size	**All sized FA[Q]**	**Only Palmitate is made[Q]**
Major tissue	**Muscle & liver[Q]**	**Liver[Q]**
Hormonal status	**Low insulin/glucagon[Q]**	**High insulin/glucagon ratio[Q]**
Inhibitor	**Malonyl CoA[Q]**	**Fatty acyl CoA[Q]**

Metabolic Pathways (Cycle or Reactions)	Site
- **Cholesterol** biosynthesis[Q] - **Glycolysis**[Q] - **HMP shunt**[Q] - **Glycogenesis & glycogenolysis**[Q] - **Fatty acid synthesis**[Q] **(Cholesterol GH GF)**	**Cytosol**[Q]
- **Beta oxidation**[Q] - **Ketone body utilization**[Q] - **Pyruvate dehydrogenase**[Q] - **Electron transport chain**[Q] - **TCA** cycle[Q] **(BK PET)**	**Mitochondria**[Q]
- **Oxidation of very long chain fatty acids**[Q]	**Peroxisomes**[Q]
- **Triglyceride** synthesis[Q] - **Cholesterol** synthesis[Q] - **Steroid** synthesis[Q] - **Phospholipid** synthesis[Q] **(TCS Phospholipid)**	**Smooth endoplasmic reticulum**[Q]
- **Protein** synthesis[Q]	**Rough endoplasmic reticulum**[Q]
- **DNA & RNA** synthesis[Q]	**Nucleus**[Q]

40. **Ans. a. Acetyl Co-A stimulation of pyruvate carboxylase** *(Ref: Harper 30/e p1880)*

Acetyl Co-A stimulation of pyruvate carboxylase is most effective for gluconeogenesis among the given options.

"In gluconeogenesis, pyruvate carboxylase, which catalyzes the synthesis of oxaloacetate from pyruvate, requires acetyl-CoA as an allosteric activator. The presence of acetyl-CoA results in a change in the tertiary structure of the protein, lowering the K_m value for bicarbonate. This means that as acetyl-CoA is formed from pyruvate, it automatically ensures the provision of oxaloacetate and, therefore, its further oxidation in the citric acid cycle. The activation of pyruvate carboxylase and the reciprocal inhibition of pyruvate dehydrogenase by acetyl-CoA derived from the oxidation of fatty acids explains the action of fatty acid oxidation in sparing the oxidation of pyruvate and in stimulating gluconeogenesis. The reciprocal relationship between these two enzymes in both liver and kidney alters the metabolic fate of pyruvate as the tissue changes from carbohydrate oxidation, via glycolysis, to gluconeogenesis during transition from a fed to a fasting state."- Harper 30/e p188

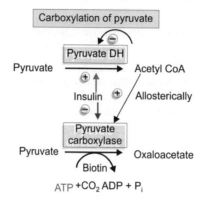

Regulation of Gluconeogenesis

- **Glucagon stimulates gluconeogenesis** by following three mechanisms:
  1. Decreasing level of fructose-2, 6-bisphosphate, which is inhibitor of fructose-1, 6-bisphosphatase enzyme, thus. In turn stimulating the gluconeogenesis[Q].
  2. Glucagon elevates the level of cAMP, which phosphorylates pyruvate kinase & thus inactivates it, shunting PEP to gluconeogenesis[Q].
  3. Glucagon increases the transcription of PEP carboxykinase gene & stimulates gluconeogenesis[Q].
- **Substrate availability**
- **Allosteric activation by acetyl Co-A**: Acetyl Co-A derived from fatty acid oxidation **inhibits pyruvate dehydrogenase (PDH) enzyme & stimulates pyruvate carboxylase, shunting pyruvate to gluconeogenesis**[Q].
- **Allosteric inhibition by AMP**[Q]

Gluconeogenesis

- **Gluconeogenesis prevent hypoglycemia** during **short & long term fasting**[Q].
- **Gluconeogenesis** occurs primarily in **liver; serves to maintain euglycemia during fasting**[Q].
- **Enzymes** also found in **kidney, intestinal epithelium**[Q].

  > - **Liver & kidneys** are the **major gluconeogenic tissues**[Q].
  > - **Glucogenic key enzymes** are **expressed in small intestine**[Q] but their role in fasting state is unclear.

- **Muscle cannot participate in gluconeogenesis** because **it lacks glucose-6-phosphatase**[Q].
- **Odd-chain fatty acids yield 1 propionyl-CoA during metabolism, which can enter the TCA cycle** (as succinyl-CoA), **undergo gluconeogenesis, and serve as a glucose source**[Q].
- **Even-chain fatty acids cannot produce new glucose**, since they yield only acetyl-CoA equivalents.

  > **Carbon skeletons** for gluconeogenesis are **derived primarily from glucogenic amino acids & lactate from muscle & glycerol** from **adipose tissues**[Q].

- Although the **lactate produced in muscle, is used by liver for gluconeogenesis**[Q].
- **Gluconeogenesis is stimulated by excess of acetyl Co-A & decrease in fructose 2, 6 biphosphate concentration**[Q].

Substrates for Gluconeogenesis

Glucogenic amino acids (all except **Leucine & lysine** which are **purely ketogenic**): Most important is alanine[Q]	Pyruvate[Q]
	Propionate[Q]
	Glycerol[Q]
Lactate[Q]	Fumarate[Q]

Regulatory and Adaptive Enzymes Associated with Gluconeogenesis

	Inducer	Repressor	Activator	Inhibitor
Pyruvate carboxylase	Glucocorticoids, glucagon, epinephrine[Q]	Insulin[Q]	Acetyl CoA	ADP[Q]
Phosphoenol pyruvate carboxykinase	Glucocorticoids, glucagon, epinephrine[Q]	Insulin[Q]	Glucagon	
Glucose 6-phosphatase	Glucocorticoids, **glucagon**, epinephrine[Q]	Insulin[Q]		

AIIMS November 2016   871

41. Ans. a. Niacin   *(Ref: Harper 30/e p547, 556)*

Niacin can be synthesized in the body from the essential amino acid tryptophan.

*"A vitamin is defined as an organic compound that is required in the diet in small amounts for the maintenance of normal metabolic integrity. Deficiency causes a specific disease, which is cured or prevented only by restoring the vitamin to the diet. However, **vitamin D,** which **can be made in the skin after exposure to sunlight,** and **niacin,** which **can be formed from the essential amino acid tryptophan,** do not strictly conform to this definition."- Harper 30/e p547*

*"**Niacin** was discovered as a nutrient during studies of **pellagra.** It is **not strictly a vitamin** since it can be synthesized in the body from the essential amino acid tryptophan. Two compounds, **nicotinic acid** and **nicotinamide,** have the biologic activity of niacin; its metabolic function is as the nicotinamide ring of the coenzymes **NAD** and **NADP** in oxidation-reduction reactions."- Harper 30/e p 556*

PATHOLOGY

42. Ans. c. Fat embolism   *(Ref: Robbins 9/e p128; Apley's 9/e p681, 8/e 535-536, Rockwood 6/e p553)*

The patient has a history of traffic accident with lower limb fracture, which is a risk factor for fat embolism. The histopathological image is showing clear fat globules, suggestive of fat embolism.

*"**Microscopic fat globules—sometimes with associated hematopoietic bone marrow—can be found in the pulmonary vasculature after fractures of long bones or,** rarely, in the setting of soft tissue trauma and burns. Presumably these injuries rupture vascular sinusoids in the marrow or small venules, allowing marrow or adipose tissue to herniate into the vascular space and travel to the lung. Fat and marrow emboli are very common incidental findings after vigorous cardiopulmonary resuscitation and are probably of no clinical consequence. **Indeed, fat embolism occurs in some 90% of individuals with severe skeletal injuries, but less than 10% of such patients have any clinical findings.**"- Robbins 9/e p128*

See Q. No. 122 AIIMS May 2017

43. Ans. b. Clumps of RBCs due to IgM mediated cold autoimmune hemolytic anemia   *(Ref: Robbins 9/e p643-644; Chandrasoma & Taylor 3/e p401)*

In the given peripheral smear spherocytes are seen. Spherocytes on peripheral smear are seen only in hereditary spherocytosis and autoimmune hemolytic anemia. The given history of cell lysis in winters is typical of autoimmune hemolytic anemia- cold antibody type.

Warm Antibody Hemolytic Anemia	Cold Antibody Hemolytic Anemia
• **Antibodies** here **bind with antigens (on RBC) at body temperature**[Q] (37°C) • These antibodies are called **warm antibodies** & are **nearly IgG**[Q]	• **Antibodies** here **bind with antigens (on RBC)** better at temperature **lower than 37°C**[Q] • These antibodies are called **reactive antibodies** & are **usually IgM**[Q] • **Rarely IgG antibodies** e.g. The Donath Landsteiner antibody of **Paroxysmal cold hemoglobinuria)**[Q]
Causes	**Causes**

1. Idiopathic
2. Lymphomas: **CLL**[Q]**, Non-Hodgkins** etc.
3. **SLE**[Q] and other **Collagen Vascular Diseases**[Q]
4. Drugs:
  – **Alpha-Methyldopa**[Q]
  – **Penicillin type (stable pattern)**
  – **Quinidine type (unstable pattern)**
	1. Acute: **Mycoplasma Infection**[Q]**, Infections mononucleosis**[Q]
	2. Chronic: **Idiopathic**[Q]**, Lymphoma**
	3. **Paroxysmal cold hemoglobinuria**[Q] **IgG**

Mechanism of Hemolysis	**Mechanism of Hemolysis**
• **Human red cells cooled with IgG** are **trapped by splenic macrophages** leading to **red cell destruction**[Q]	• **Antibodies of IgM type bind on red cell surface** and cause **agglutination**[Q]**.** • **Hemolytic effect** is **mediated through fixation of C3 to RBC surface**[Q]
Diagnosis	**Diagnosis**
• **Positive direct Coomb's test**, at 37°C for presence of warm antibodies **on surface of Red cell.** • **Positive Indirect Coomb's test** at 37°C for presence of large quantities of warm antibodies **in serum**[Q]	• Positive direct Coomb's test for detection of **C3 on the red cell surface**, but IgM responsible for coating on red cells is not found[Q]

44. Ans. c. C *(Ref: Wintrobes 13/e p303; Robbins 9/e p99)*
A: Lymphocyte; B: Neutrophil; C: Eosinophil; D: Basophil
Eosinophils are markedly raised in worm infestations.

> "**Most bacterial infections** induce an increase in the blood neutrophil count, called **neutrophilia**. Viral infections, such as **infectious mononucleosis, mumps, and German measles,** cause an absolute increase in the number of lymphocytes **(lymphocytosis)**. In some allergies and parasitic infestations, there is an increase in the absolute number of eosinophils, creating an **eosinophilia**. Certain infections **(typhoid fever and infections caused by some viruses, rickettsiae, and certain protozoa)** are associated with a decreased number of circulating white cells **(leukopenia).**" - *Robbins 9/e p99*

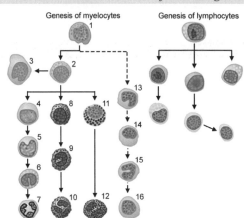

Genesis of white blood cells. The different cell of the myelocyte series are 1, myeloblast; 2, promyelocyte; 3, megakaryocyte; 4, neutrophil myelocyte; 5, young neutrophil metamyelocyte; 6, "band" neutrophil metamyelocyte; 7, polymorphonuclear neutrophil; 8, eosinophil myelocyte; 9, eosinophil metamyelocyte; 10, polymorphonuclear eosinophil; 11, basophil myelocyte; 12, poly-morphonuclear basophil; 13–16, stages of monocyte formation.

Peripheral Smear		
Cells	**Morphology**	**Image**
RBCs	• **Biconcave discs**, approx. **8 μm** in diameter with **no nucleus** or metabolic machinery[Q]	
Neutrophils	• **Granulocyte, most abundant**[Q] • Comprise **60–70%** of leukocytes[Q] • Diameter: **10–12 μm** • **2–5 lobes** in nucleus[Q]	
Eosinophil	• **2-4%** of leukocytes • Diameter: **12–15 μm** • Nucleus: Less lobed, **usually bilobed**[Q] • **Cytoplasm:** Numerous **brick red granules**[Q] • **Increased** in parasitic infection & in **hypersensitivity reactions**[Q]	
Basophil	• Accounts for **0.5-1%** of leukocytes • Diameter: **14 μm** • Nucleus: **Large & bilobed**[Q] • Chromatin is more finely textured • **Granules:** Dense basophilic granules[Q] obscuring the nucleus	

Lymphocyte	• Account for **20–25%** of leukocytes • Diameter: **6–8 μm** • **Nucleus: Spheroid or ovoid**[Q] • **Chromatin** is **dense & dark**[Q]	
Monocyte	• Account for **3–8%** of leukocytes • **Largest leukocyte**[Q] **(Diameter: 20 μm)** • Nucleus: **Indented or kidney shaped**[Q] with agranular slate grey cytoplasm	
Platelets	• Small cell fragments with many vesicles & no nucleus • Number: 1.5-4.0 lack • Diameter: **2–4 μm**	

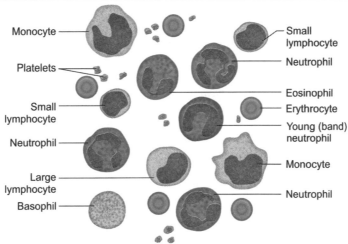

Fig. 22: Blood cells on peripheral smear

45. **Ans. d. Folic acid deficiency**   *(Ref: Robbins 9/e p631, 648)*

   A high MCV, high MCH and MCHC here are suggestive of macrocytic, hyperchromic anemia, typically seen in folic acid deficiency.

   "A deficiency of folic acid (more properly, pteroylmono- glutamic acid) results in a megaloblastic anemia having the same pathologic features as that caused by vitamin B12 deficiency."- Robbins 9/e p648

RBC Indices	Mean Cell Volume (MCV)	Mean Cell Hemoglobin (MCH)	Mean Cell Hemoglobin Concentration (MCHC)	Red Cell Distribution Width (RDW)
Definition	Average volume of a red cell expressed in **femto litres (fL)** MCV = PCV/RBC count[Q]	Average content of hemoglobin per red cell, expressed in **picograms** MCH = Hb/RBC count[Q]	Average concentration of hemoglobin in a given volume of packed red cells, expressed in **grams per dl** MCHC = Hb/MCV[Q]	**Coefficient of variation** of red cell volume[Q]
Normal Range	79–93.3 fL[Q]	26.7–31.9 pg/cell[Q]	32.3–35.9 gm/dL[Q]	<14.5%[Q]

- In the question, Hb= 9.5 mg/dL, PCV = 30, RBC count = 2 millions/mm³
- **Hematocrit** or **PCV = MCV x RBC concentration**
- MCV = PCV/RBC count = 30/0.2 = 150 (increased/**Macrocytic**)
- MCH = Hb/ RBC count =9.5/0.2 = 47.5 (increased/**Hyperchromic**)
- MCHC = Hb/MCV = 31 (normal)
- *Macrocytic, hyperchromic anemia is typically seen in folic acid deficiency.*

46. **Ans. c. Giardiasis**   *(Ref: Robbins 9/e p795; Harrison 19/e p1416)*

History of diarrhea, constipation and weight loss in a slum dweller with duodenal biopsy showing the characteristic pear shaped structures is highly suggestive of Giardiasis.

*"**Giardia trophozoites** can be identified in **duodenal biopsies** based on their **characteristic pear shape and the presence of two equally sized nuclei**. Despite large numbers of **trophozoites**, which are **tightly bound to the brush border of villous enterocytes**, there is **no invasion and small intestinal morphology may be normal**. However, **villous blunting with increased numbers of intraepithelial lymphocytes and mixed lamina propria inflammatory infiltrates can develop in patients with heavy infections**."- Robbins 9/e p795*

*"Disease manifestations of giardiasis range from asymptomatic carriage to **fulminant diarrhea and malabsorption**. Most infected persons are asymptomatic, but in epidemics the proportion of symptomatic cases may be higher. Symptoms may develop suddenly or gradually. In persons with acute giardiasis, symptoms develop after an incubation period that lasts at least 5–6 days and usually 1–3 weeks. **Prominent early symptoms include diarrhea, abdominal pain, bloating, belching, flatus, nausea, and vomiting**."- Harrison 19/e p1416*

See Q. No. 82 AIIMS November 2017

47. **Ans. b. Prussian blue**   *(Ref: Robbins 9/e p849; Netter's Essential Histology 2/e p479)*

Hemochromatosis (excess of iron in the from of hemosiderin) is accumulated in organs which can be demonstrated by Pearls stain (Prussian blue stain).

*"**Intracellular ferritin** is located in the cytosol and in lysosomes, in which partially degraded protein shells of ferritin aggregate into hemosiderin granules. Iron in hemosiderin is chemically reactive and turns blue-black when exposed to potassium ferrocyanide, which is the basis for the Prussian blue stain. With normal iron stores, only trace amounts of hemosiderin are found in the body, principally in macrophages in the bone marrow, spleen, and liver, most being stored as ferritin. In iron-overloaded cells, most iron is stored in hemosiderin."- Robbins 9/e p849*

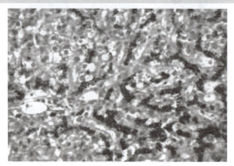

Fig. 23: Hereditary hemochromatosis
(Prussian blue-stained section: Hepatocellular iron appears blue)

For Minerals, pigments and miscellaneous	
Name of stain	Elements stained
Von Kossa's stain (MC used) **Alizarin red S** at pH 4.2 (specific for Calcium)	Calcium[Q]
Prussian blue	Iron[Q]
Fontana Masson Silver stain	Melanin[Q]
Modified Fouchet's	Bile pigments[Q]
Orcein Modified rhodamine (method of choice)	Copper[Q]

For Connective Tissue and Lipids	
Name of stain	**Elements stained**
Trichrome Stain	• **Collagen**[Q]
Verhoeff-Van Gieson stain (Best for Elastin)	• **Elastic fibers**[Q]
Luna stain	• Elastin & Mast cells
Silver Methenamine stain	• **Reticulin**[Q]
Oil red 'O' stain (on Fresh specimen) Sudan black (on fixed specimen)	• **Fat**[Q]
Mallory's PTAH stain	• Muscle striations
Martius scarlet blue (MSB)	• **Fibrin**[Q]
PAS, Silver Methenamine stain	• **Basement membrane**[Q]
Bielschowsky (silver stain)	• **Neurofibrillary tangles senile plaques**[Q]
Luxol fast blue	• **Myelin**[Q]

Hemochromatosis (AR)

- **Autosomal recessive**[Q] **disorder** of iron metabolism
- Characterized by **dysregulation of intestinal iron absorption** leading to **deposition of excessive iron** in **parenchymal cells** leading to **fibrosis & organ failure**[Q].
- **Genetic Defect: MC mutation is HFE (C282Y) gene mutation** on **chromosome 6**[Q]

Pathophysiology:
- **Mucosal absorption** is **greater than body requirements**[Q] (≥ 4 mg/d).
- **Tissue injury** results from **disruption of iron-laden lysosomes**, from **lipid peroxidation of subcellular organelles**, or from **stimulation of collagen synthesis** by activated stellate cells[Q].

> - **Deposition of hemosiderin** occurs in **liver, pancreas, myocardium, pituitary, adrenal, thyroid, parathyroid, joints & skin**[Q]

Clinical Features:
- **Major clinical manifestations: Cirrhosis, DM, arthritis, cardiomyopathy & hypogonadotropic hypogonadism**[Q]
- **Initial symptoms**: Lethargy, arthralgia, change in skin color, loss of libido & DM.

> - **Triad** seen in **advanced cases: Micronodular cirrhosis + Bronze diabetes + Skin pigmentation**[Q]

- **Features of advanced disease: Hepatomegaly, increased pigmentation (bronzing of skin**[Q]**), spider angiomas, splenomegaly, arthropathy, ascites, cardiac arrhythmias, CHF (MC CVS manifestation**[Q]**), loss of body hair, testicular atrophy** (impairment of hypothalamic-pituitary function) **& jaundice**[Q].

> - **First organ affected: Liver (hepatomegaly** in **>95%** of symptomatic patients)[Q]
> - **MC cause of death** in treated patients: **HCC**[Q]
> - **Adrenal insufficiency, hypothyroidism & hypoparathyroidism** are rare manifestations[Q].

Diagnosis:

Degree of increase in total body iron stores can be assessed by
- Measurement of **serum iron & percent saturation of transferrin**[Q]
- Measurement of serum **ferritin** concentration (**level >1000 µg/L is strongest predictor** of disease expression)
- **Liver biopsy**: Golden yellow hemosiderin granules in periportal hepatocytes, micronodular cirrhosis with absence of inflammation[Q]
- **MRI of liver** for determining hepatic iron concentration[Q]
- **Buccal mucosal biopsy** for **iron staining**[Q]
- *Iron in* **hemosiderin** *is* **chemically reactive & turns blue-black** *when* **exposed to potassium ferrocyanide**, *which is the* **basis for Prussian blue stain (used in hemochromatosis)**[Q].

Hemochromatosis (AR)

Treatment:
- **Principle: Removal of excess body iron** (weekly or twice-weekly **phlebotomy of 500 mL**) & **supportive treatment** of damaged organs[Q].
- Patients with advanced disease: Weekly phlebotomy for 1-2 years & should be continued until **serum ferritin level is <50 µg/L**[Q].
- **Abstinence** from **alcohol**[Q].

Chelating agents (deferoxamine)	In cases of **severe anemia or hypoproteinemia,** which preclude phlebotomy
Testosterone replacement or **gonadotropin therapy**	For **loss of libido** & **change in secondary sex characteristics**[Q]
Liver transplantation	For **end-stage liver disease**[Q]

Prognosis:
- **Principal causes of death: Cardiac failure, hepatocellular failure or portal hypertension & HCC**[Q].
- **Life expectancy** is **improved by removal of excessive stores of iron**[Q].

48. **Ans. a. Crescent formation**   *(Ref: Robbins 9/e p912)*
    Abducent nerve nucleus is located deep to facial colliculus.

> *"Rapidly Progressive (Crescentic) Glomerulonephritis: The most common histologic picture is the presence of crescents in most of the glomeruli (crescentic glomerulonephritis)."- Robbins 9/e p912*

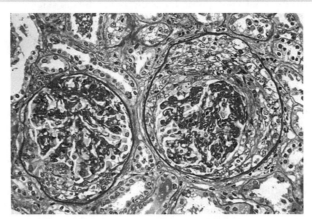

Fig. 24: Crescentic glomerulonephritis (collapsed glomerular tufts & crescent-shaped mass of proliferating parietal epithelial cells & leukocytes internal to Bowman capsule)

Rapidly Progressive (Crescentic) Glomerulonephritis (RPGN)

- RPGN is characterized by **severe glomerular injury** leading to **rapid & progressive loss of renal function**[Q]
- Associated with **severe oliguria** & signs of **nephritic syndrome**[Q]
- **If untreated, death from renal failure** occurs **within weeks to months**[Q]

  - **MC histologic picture: Presence of crescents** in most glomeruli[Q]
  - **Crescents**: Produced by **proliferation of parietal cells**[Q] & **infiltration** of **monocytes & macrophages**[Q]

Contd...

Contd...

Types of RPGN		
	Type I (20%)	**Type II (25%)**	**Type III (55%)**
Mechanism	• **Anti-GBM antibody-mediated**[Q]	• **Immune complex deposition**[Q]	• **Pauci-immune RPGN**[Q]
Etiology	• Renal limited • **Goodpasture syndrome**[Q]	**Post Infectious:** • **Post-streptococcal glomerulonephritis**[Q] • **Bacterial endocarditis**[Q] • Shunt nephritis[Q] **Non-infectious:** • **SLE**[Q] • **Henoch-Schonlein purpura**[Q] • **Mixed cryoglobulinemia**[Q] • Solid tumors[Q] **Primary Renal Disease:** • **MPGN & IgA nephropathy**[Q]	• **ANCA associated**[Q] • **Idiopathic** • **Wegner's granulomatosis**[Q] • **Microscopic polyangitis**[Q] • **Churg-Strauss syndrome**[Q]

RPGN: Morphology	
Gross	• Kidneys are **enlarged & pale**, with **petechial hemorrhages** on **cortical surfaces**[Q] (**Flea-Bitten Kidney**[Q])
Light microscopy	• **Crescent** are **histological hallmark of RPGN**[Q] • **Crescents obliterate urinary space**[Q] (more the **number of crescents, poorer** the **prognosis**[Q]) • **Fibrin strands** are prominent **between cellular layers in crescents**[Q] • **Focal & segmental necrosis, endothelial & mesangial proliferation**[Q] • **Pauci-immune RPGN: Most typical feature is segmental glomerular necrosis**[Q]
Immunofluorescence	• **Type I: Linear GBM fluorescence**[Q] • **Type II: Granular immune deposits**[Q] • **Type III: No deposition of immune reactants**[Q]
Electron microscopy	• **Ruptures in GBM**[Q] • **Immune complex deposition in type II**[Q]

Clinical Features:
• **Hematuria** with **RBC casts in urine, moderate proteinuria, hypertension & edema**[Q]
• **Progressive** over weeks & ends in severe oliguria or renal failure[Q]

49. Ans. d. Cryptococcus *(Ref: Robbins 9/e p387-388; Ananthanarayan 10/e p616, 8/e p611; Harrison 19/e p1340)*

On the basis of clinical features (Meningoencephalitis) and images (soap bubble lesions in brain parenchyma), most likely pathogen involved is Cryptococcus.

"The 5- to 10-µm cryptococcal yeast has a highly characteristic thick gelatinous capsule containing a poly- saccharide that stains intense red with periodic acid- Schiff and mucicarmine in tissues and can be detected with antibody-coated beads in an agglutination assay. India ink preparations create a negative image, visualizing the thick capsule as a clear halo within a dark background. The major lesions caused by Cryptococcus are in the CNS, involving the meninges, cortical gray matter, and basal nuclei. The host response to Cryptococci is extremely variable. In immunosuppressed people, organisms may evoke virtually no inflammatory reaction, so gelatinous masses of fungi grow in the meninges or expand the perivascular Virchow- Robin spaces within the gray matter, producing the so-called soap-bubble lesions."- Robbins 9/e p388

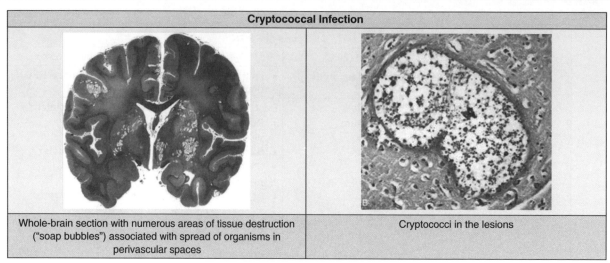

See Q. No. 81 AIIMs May 2017

Most Common in AIDS	
MC opportunistic infection	Pneumocystis carinii pneumonia (TB in India[Q])
MC pulmonary disease	Pneumonia[Q]
MC space occupying lesion	Toxoplasmosis[Q] >Primary CNS lymphoma[Q]
MC hematologic abnormality in HIV	Anemia[Q]
MC HIV drugs causing myopathy	Zidovudine[Q]
MC skin disease	Seborrheic dermatitis[Q]
MC endocrinologic abnormality in HIV-infected men	Hypogonadism[Q]
MC malignancy	Kaposi's sarcoma[Q]
MC electrolyte abnormality	Hyponatremia, SIADH[Q]
MC presentation of syphilis in HIV	Condyloma lata, a form of secondary syphilis[Q]
MC Fungal infection	Cryptococcosis[Q]
MC lymphoma	NHL, B cell immunoblastic lymphoma[Q] (CNS Lymphoma)
MC heart disease	Coronary heart disease[Q]
MC route of mother to child transmission of HIV	Perinatal/Intrapartum (during delivery)
MC cause of pancreatitis in HIV	Drug toxicity
MC ocular lesions	Cotton wool spots[Q]
MC cause of blindness	CMV retinitis[Q]

50. **Ans. a. Hyaline casts**   *(Ref: Robbins 9/e p929; Campbell 10/e p96)*
    The given image is urine cytology in samples obtained during clinical rejection showing numerous renal tubular cells, lymphocytes, and macrophages along with few hyaline casts.

    *"**Eosinophilic hyaline casts**, as well as pigmented granular casts, are common, **particularly in distal tubules and collecting ducts**. These casts consist **principally of Tamm-Horsfall protein** (a urinary glycoprotein normally secreted by the cells of ascending thick limb and distal tubules) **in conjunction with other plasma proteins**."- Robbins 9/e p929*

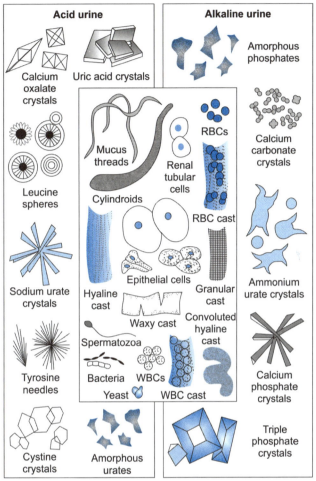

Types of Urinary Casts			
Type	Description	Image	Significance
Hyaline	Cylindrical & clear, with a low refractive index[Q]		• MC type of cast[Q] • Hyaline cast are solidified Tamm-Horsfall mucoprotein secreted from the tubular epithelial cells[Q] • Low urine flow, concentrated urine, or an acidic environment can contribute to formation of hyaline casts[Q] • Increased number is seen in: Renal disease, dehydration, fever, CHF & diuretic therapy[Q]
Waxy	Cylindrical with higher refractive index More rigid, with sharp edges, fractures & broken-off ends[Q].		• Most frequently observed in chronic renal failure[Q] • Larger than hyaline casts[Q] • Waxy casts are broad casts[Q]

Contd...

Contd...

Type	Description	Image	Significance
Epithelial cell	**Protein matrix with tubular cells** Distinguished by **large, round nuclei** & a **lower amount of cytoplasm**[Q]	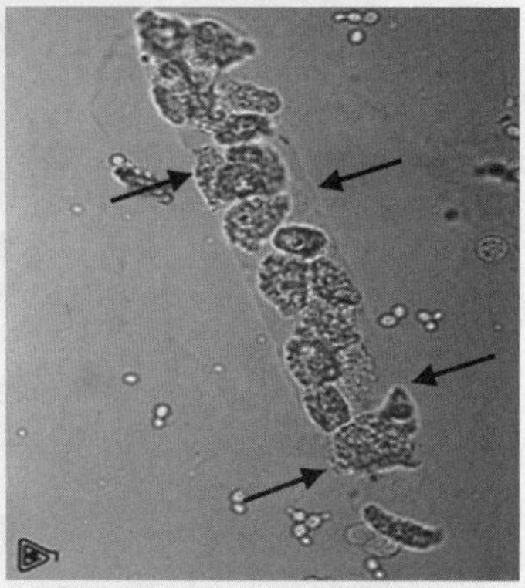	• Formed via **inclusion or adhering of desquamated epithelial cells** of tubule lining[Q]. • **Seen in acute tubular necrosis & toxic ingestion (mercury, diethylene glycol, or salicylate), CMV infection & viral hepatitis**[Q]
RBC	**Yellowish-brown in colour, generally cylindrical sometimes with ragged edges**[Q]	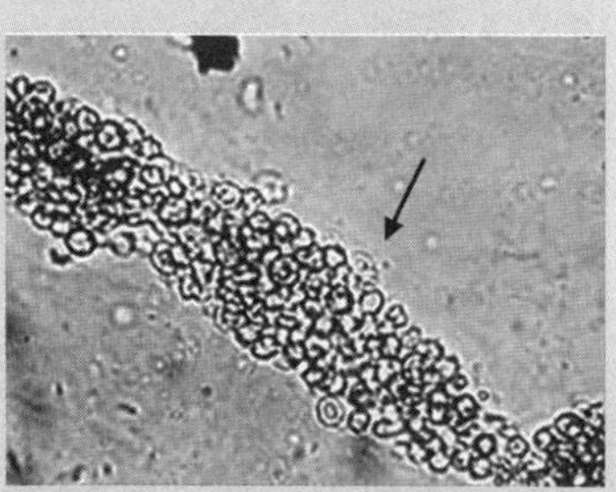	• **Pathognomonic of glomerulonephritis**[Q] **(RPGN)** • **Indicator of bleeding within nephrons**[Q] • Seen in **Wegener's granulomatosis, SLE, poststreptococcal glomerulonephritis, Goodpasture's syndrome, renal infarction & subacute bacterial endocarditis**[Q]
WBC	Presence of hyaline matrix with WBCs	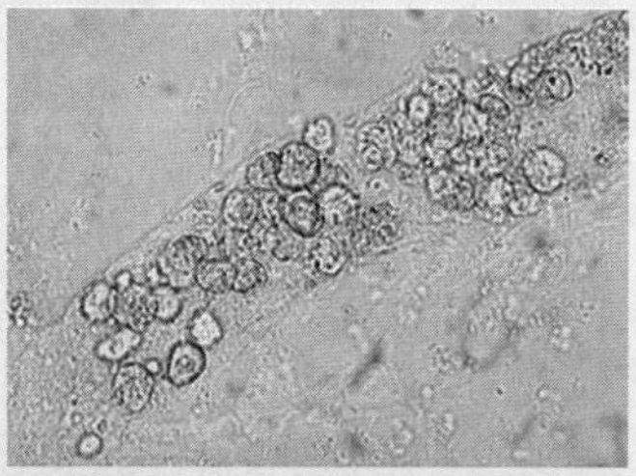	• Indicative of **inflammation or infection** • Seen in **pyelonephritis, interstitial nephritis, nephrotic syndrome, post-streptococcal glomerulonephritis, lupus nephritis**[Q]
Fatty	**Yellowish-tan in** appearance **"Maltese cross" sign**[Q] under polarized light	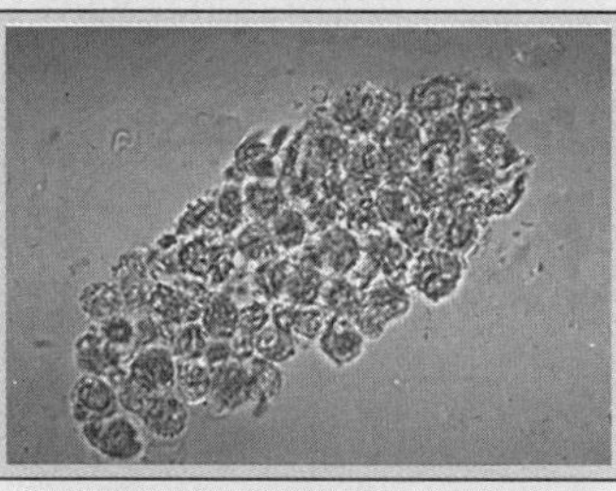	• Formed by **breakdown of lipid rich epithelial cells**[Q] • Hyaline casts with **fat globule inclusions**[Q] • Present in **high urinary protein nephrotic syndrome, diabetic or lupus nephropathy**[Q]
Granular	**Cigar-shaped** with **higher refractive index**[Q] than hyaline casts.	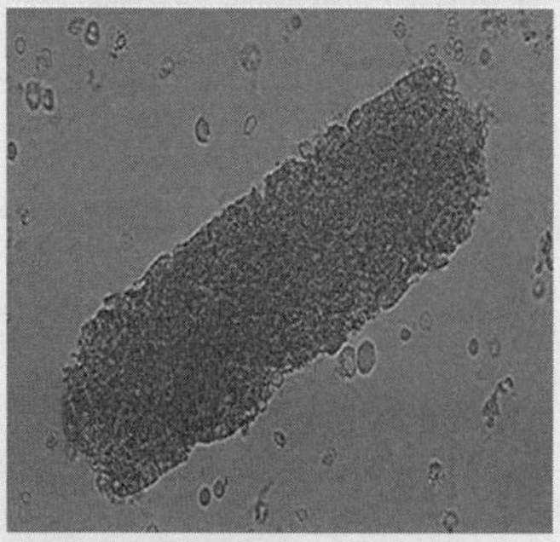	• Can result either from **break down of cellular casts** or **inclusion of aggregates of plasma proteins** or **immunoglobulin light chains**[Q] • **Muddy brown cast** seen in **acute tubular necrosis** is a type of granular cast[Q] • **Coarse** in **renal papillary necrosis**[Q] • **Fine: Hyperparathyroidism**[Q] (May be physiological)

Contd...

Contd...

Type	Description	Image	Significance
Pigment	Granular cast with pigment stain[Q]		• Formed by **adhesion of metabolic breakdown products** or **drug pigments**[Q] • Pigments include **hemoglobin in hemolytic anemia, myoglobin in rhabdomyolysis & bilirubin in liver disease**[Q] • Drug pigments **phenazopyridine** may cause **cast discoloration**[Q]
Broad	Diameter 2 to 6 times of normal cast[Q]		• Typically seen in chronic renal failure • Indicate poor prognosis[Q]

51. Ans. d. Dysarthria *(Ref: Hutchinson's Clinical Methods 23/e p304; Gray's 40/e p42, 309)*
The given micrographic image is that of the cerebellum, injury to which may cause dysarthria.

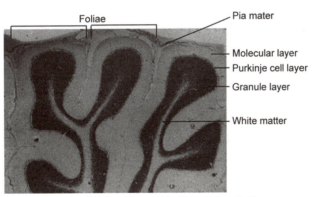

Fig. 25: Section through the human cerebellum

"Midline cerebellar lesions, e.g. tumours such as medulloblastoma and secondary carcinoma, lead to abnormalities of posture, so that the patient cannot sit or stand, without toppling, usually backwards. Unilateral lesions in the cerebellar hemispheres, e.g. stroke, produce ipsilateral symptoms and signs. Incoordination of eye movements leads to nystagmus, which is most marked when gaze is directed to the side of the lesion. Incoordination of the ipsilateral upper limb is manifested in the finger-nose test. The movements are inaccurate (dysmetria); the limb oscillates to and fro, the amplitude being greater as the target is reached (intention tremor); there is a breakdown of smooth co-operation between muscles controlling the joints of the upper limb (asynergia); alternating hand movements are clumsy (dysdiadochokinesia). When the arm is outstretched, there is a tendency for the limb to hyper-pronate and rise, and when pressure is applied to the extended arm and then released, there is a marked rebound of the limb. Unilateral incoordination of the lower limb is apparent because heel/shin testing is inaccurate.
Bilateral lesions of the cerebellar hemisphere lead to nystagmus and a form of dysarthria in which the syllables are extended and prosody is lost (scanning speech). The gait is wide based, reeling, and incoordinate (ataxia): the ataxia is not made significantly worse on eye closure (negative Romberg's sign)."- Gray's 40/e p309

AIIMS ESSENCE

Contd...

Cerebellum	
• **Cerebellum** consists of a **cortex of gray matter** & a **central core of white matter**.	
• Contains **three well-defined layers**: Granular layer, Purkinje cell layer & molecular layer (from inside to outside)	

	Granular layer	• Densely packed with granule cells, small neurons whose axons extend into the molecular layer.
	Purkinje cell layer	• Consists of a **single row of Purkinje cells**, **large neurons with a single axon** extending deep into cerebellum & multiple dendrites branching extensively in the molecular layer.
	Molecular layer	• Contains mostly **axons of granule cells** & **dendrites of Purkinje cells.** • Cells in molecular layer are **primarily glial cells.**

Cerebellar Lesions	
Deficit	**Manifestation**
Ataxia	• Reeling, wide-based gait
Decomposition of movement	• Inability to correctly sequence fine, coordinated acts
Dysarthria	• **Inability to articulate words correctly**, with slurring & inappropriate phrasing
Dysdiadochoki-nesia	• Inability to perform rapid alternating movements
Dysmetria	• Inability to control range of movement
Hypotonia	• Decreased muscle tone
Nystagmus	• **Fast component** maximal **toward the side of cerebellar lesion**
Scanning speech	• **Slow enunciation** with a tendency to hesitate at beginning of a word or syllable
Tremor	• Coarse, 2–4 Hz, classically intentional tremors

52. **Ans. b. Red** *(Ref: Robbins 9/e p544)*
Triphenyltetrazolium chloride (TTC) stain imparts a brick-red color to intact, non-infarcted myocardium where the dehydrogenase enzymes are preserved.

> *"Early morphologic recognition of acute MI can be difficult, particularly when death occurs within a few hours of the onset of symptoms. MIs less than 12 hours old are usually not apparent on gross examination. However, if the infarct preceded death by 2 to 3 hours, it is possible to highlight the area of necrosis by immersion of tissue slices in a solution of triphenyltetrazolium chloride. This gross histochemical stain imparts a brick-red color to intact, non-infarcted myocardium where lactate dehydrogenase activity is preserved. Because dehydrogenases leak out through the damaged membranes of dead cells, an infarct appears as an unstained pale zone. By 12 to 24 hours after infarction, an MI can usually be identified grossly as a reddish-blue area of discoloration caused by stagnated, trapped blood. Thereafter, the infarct becomes progressively more sharply defined, yellow-tan, and soft. By 10 days to 2 weeks, it is rimmed by a hyperemic zone of highly vascularized granulation tissue. Over the succeeding weeks, the injured region evolves to a fibrous scar."- Robbins 9/e p544*

See Q. No. 49 AIMS May 2017

53. **Ans. c. Thickness of the film** *(Ref: Bancroft Theory & Practice of Histochemical Techniques/p45-47)*
Resolving power of a microscope doesn't depend on the specimen nature or thickness. It is specific for a microscope.

> *"For microscopes, the resolving power is the inverse of the distance between two objects that can be just resolved."*

Contd...

Resolving Power of Microscope

- For microscopes, resolving power is inverse of distance between two objects that can be just resolved.[Q]

Abbe's Criterion

$\Delta d = \lambda/2 \, n \sin\theta$[Q]
Resolving power $= 1/\Delta d = 2n \sin\theta/\lambda$[Q]
n: refractive index of the medium separating object and aperture
n sin θ: Numerical aperture

- To achieve high resolution, n sin θ must be large. This is known as the numerical aperture.
- For good resolution:
  - Sin θ must be large: To achieve this, objective lens is kept as close to specimen as possible[Q]
  - A higher refractive index (n) medium must be used. Oil immersion microscopes use oil to increase the refractive index[Q]
  - Decreasing wavelength by using X-rays & gamma rays[Q]

54. Ans. b. Erythrocyte *(Ref: Ananthanarayan 10/e p141-143, 8/e p 132-135)*

MHC antigens are absent on erythrocytes.

"HLA class I antigens (A, B and C) are found on the surface of virtually all nucleated cells. They are the principal antigens **involved in graft rejection and cell-mediated cytolysis**. Class I molecules may function as components of hormone receptors. HLA class II antigens are more restricted in distribution, being found only on cells of the immune system- macrophages, dendritic cells, activated T cells, and particularly on B cells."- *Ananthanarayan 10/e p142*

See Q. No. 84 AIIMS May 2017

55. Ans. a. Toluidine blue *(Ref: Ballenger's Otorhinolaryngology/p 1018; J Oral Pathol Med (2011)40:300–304)*

Stain useful for identifying premalignant lesions of the lip is toluidine blue.

"There are **different methods of screening for oral cancer. Clinical Examination is the current most common method used to detect visible lesions.** For **clinically undetectable lesions**, there is need for an adjunctive method to visual examination to detect precancerous lesions. The current adjunctive methods are **toluidine blue, brush biopsy and fluorescence imaging**. Toluidine blue, a basic metachromatic dye, stains the nuclear material of malignant lesions, but not that of normal mucosa. The nuclei of cancer cells show increased DNA synthesis, resulting in increased pickup of toluidine blue. The use of toluidine blue (toluidine chloride) dye as a mouthwash is currently receiving much attention as an aid to the diagnosis of oral cancer and potentially malignant lesions. The method has good sensitivity with a very low false negative rate. It is **effective in demonstrating dysplasia and early malignant lesion**, which is not clinically recognizable."

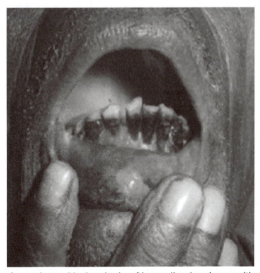

Fig. 26: Clinical picture of a patient with dysplasia of lower lip showing positive toluidine blue staining

PHARMACOLOGY

56. Ans. b. B is epinephrine *(Ref: Goodman Gilman 12/e p277, 283; KDT 7/e p130-131)*

According to the graph given in the question, it is evident that A: Norepinephrine, B: Adrenaline, C: Isoproterenol. Action of Isoproterenol is blocked by beta-blockers and not by muscarinic blockers.

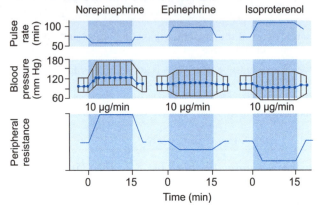

Fig. 27: Effects of intravenous infusion of norepinephrine, epinephrine or isoproterenol in humans

"Epinephrine is one of the most potent vasopressor drugs known. If a pharmacological dose is given rapidly by an intravenous route, it evokes a characteristic effect on blood pressure, which rises rapidly to a peak that is proportional to the dose. The increase in systolic pressure is greater than the increase in diastolic pressure, so that the pulse pressure increases. As the response wanes, the mean pressure may fall below normal before returning to control levels. The mechanism of the rise in blood pressure due to epinephrine is 3-fold: a direct myocardial stimulation that increases the strength of ventricular contraction (positive inotropic action); an increased heart rate (positive chronotropic action); vasoconstriction in many vascular beds—especially in the precapillary resistance vessels of skin, mucosa, and kidney—along with marked constriction of the veins. The pulse rate, at first accelerated, may be slowed markedly at the height of the rise of blood pressure by compensatory vagal discharge. Small doses of epinephrine (0.1 mg/kg) may cause the blood pressure to fall."- Goodman Gilman 12/e p283

Drug	Acts on	Relative Receptor Affinity
Adrenaline (Epinephrine)	Both **alpha** (alpha-1 & alpha-2) & **beta receptors**[Q] (beta-1, beta-2 & weak beta-3[Q] action)	alpha-1 = alpha-2[Q] beta-1 = beta-2[Q]
Noradrenaline	Alpha-1, alpha-2, beta-1, beta-3[Q] & no beta-3[Q] action	alpha-1 = alpha-2[Q] beta-1 >> beta-2[Q]
Isoprenaline (Isoproterenol)	Beta-1, beta-2, beta-3[Q] & no beta-3[Q] action	beta-1 = beta-2 >>>> alpha[Q]

Differences between Alpha & Beta Receptors		
	Alpha	**Beta**
Rank order of potency of agonists	Adr ≥NA >Iso[Q]	Iso >Adr >NA[Q]
Antagonist	**Phenoxybenzamine**[Q]	**Propranolol**[Q]
Effector pathway	IP$_3$/DAG↑, cAMP ↓, K$^+$ channel ↑	cAMP ↑, Ca^{2+} channel ↑

	Adrenaline	**Noradrenaline**	**Isoprenaline**
Heart rate	↑	↓	↑↑
Cardiac output	↑↑	-	↑↑
Blood Pressure			
Systolic	↑↑	↑↑	↓↑
Diastolic	↓↑	↑↑	↑↑

Contd...

Contd...

	Adrenaline	**Noradrenaline**	**Isoprenaline**
Mean	↑	↑↑	↓
Blood flow			
Skin	↓	↓	-
Muscle	↑↑	-, ↓	↑
Kidney	↑	↓	-
Liver	↑↑	-	↑
Coronary	↑	↑	↑
Bronchial muscle	↓↓	-	↓↓
Intestinal muscle	↓↓	↓	↓
Blood sugar	↑↑	-, ↑	↑

`57. Ans. is a Both A and B are full agonists* (Ref: Goodman Gilman 12/e p46; Katzung 13/e p22, 12/e p19; KDT 7/e p54, 58-60)*

In the given dose response curve, A and B are full agonists having maximum possible efficacy. Potency in this DRC is A>B>C and efficacy is A=B>C. C is a not a non-competitive antagonist as the starting point is different, hence the C is a partial agonist.

"The position of dose response curve on the dose axis (x-axis) is the index of drug potency, which refers to the minimum amount of drug needed to produce a certain response. A DRC positioned leftward indicates higher potency as the response can be produced with a lesser dose of the drug. The upper limit of DRC is the index of drug efficacy and refers to the maximal response that can be elicited by the drug. So, higher the upper limit, more potent is the drug. Noncompetitive antagonists may have same or different potencies but they always have lesser efficacy. Noncompetitive antagonists can bind on the same or different site as the main drug. A competitive antagonist will have lesser potency but will tend to reach the same efficacy as the dose increases."

*"An antagonist may dissociate so slowly from the receptor that its action is exceedingly prolonged, as with the opiate partial agonist buprenorphine and the Ca^{2+} channel blocker amlodipine. In the presence of a slowly dissociating antagonist, the maximal response to the agonist will be depressed at some antagonist concentrations. Operationally, this is referred to as **noncompetitive antagonism**, although the molecular mechanism of action really cannot be inferred unequivocally from the effect."- Goodman Gilman 12/e p46*

Dose Response Curve (DRC)

- Simple DRC is hyperbolic while log DRC is sigmoid in shape.

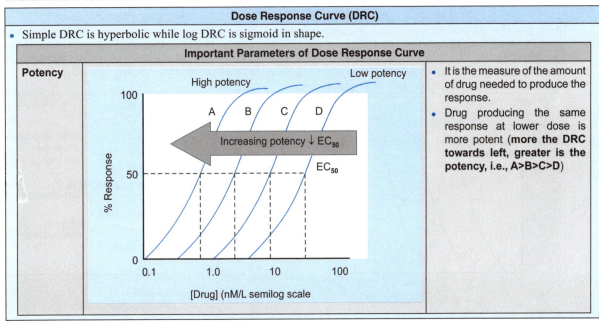

Important Parameters of Dose Response Curve

Potency
- It is the measure of the amount of drug needed to produce the response.
- Drug producing the same response at lower dose is more potent (**more the DRC towards left, greater is the potency, i.e., A>B>C>D**)

Efficacy	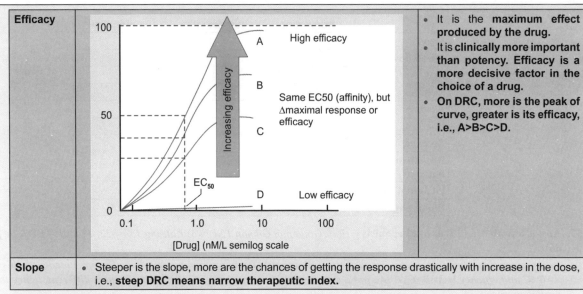 • It is the **maximum effect produced by the drug**. • It is **clinically more important than potency. Efficacy is a more decisive factor in the choice of a drug**. • On DRC, more is the peak of curve, greater is its efficacy, i.e., A>B>C>D.
Slope	• Steeper is the slope, more are the chances of getting the response drastically with increase in the dose, i.e., **steep DRC means narrow therapeutic index**.

Competitive Antagonism	Noncompetitive Antagonism	Irreversible or Non-equilibrium Antagonism
• Antagonist is **chemically similar to the agonist** & **competes with it**[Q]. • Has **affinity but no intrinsic activity**[Q]. • DRC of the agonist is **shifted to the right**[Q]. • A **parallel shift of the agonist DRC with no suppression of maximal response** is obtained[Q]. • Extent of shift depends on **concentration** & **affinity of antagonist**[Q].	• Drug binds to a **different allosteric site altering the receptor** in such a way that it is **unable to combine with agonist**[Q]. • Also called **allosteric antagonism**[Q]. • **Irreversible: Even with high agonist concentration**[Q]. • **Increasing concentrations of the antagonist progressively flatten the agonist DRC**[Q]	• Few **antagonists bind to receptor with strong (covalent) bonds** or **dissociate from it slowly (due to very high affinity)** so that agonist molecules are unable to reduce receptor occupancy of the agonist molecules- an irreversible antagonism is produced[Q].

Examples of Competitive & Noncompetitive Antagonism	
Competitive Antagonism	Noncompetitive Antagonism
Both the agonist (isoproterenol) and the antagonist (propranolol) bind reversibly to the same receptor subtype (beta-adrenoceptor). In the presence of the **competitive antagonist, the dose response curve is shifted to the right in a parallel manner**.	Phenoxybenzamine binds irreversibly (with covalent bonds) to alpha-adrenergic receptors. This **reduces the fraction of available receptors**, and **reduces the maximal effect that can be produced by the agonist**.

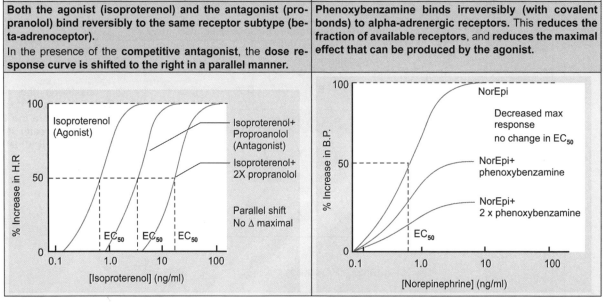

AIIMS November 2016

58. Ans. d. Multivitamins containing Vitamin K *(Ref: Goodman Gilman 12/e p1043, 1499; Katzung 13/e p1145)*
Routine use of multivitamins with Vitamin K doesn't cause thrombocytopenia. Vitamin K is used as an antidote to Warfarin (anticoagulant) excess.

"2% of theophylline user from thrombocytopenia. Mechanism under study is inhibition of transduction of message received at platelet surface."

Drug-induced Immune Thrombocytopenia (DITP)
• **Drug-induced immune thrombocytopenia (DITP)** is often suspected in patients with **acute thrombocytopenia unexplained by other causes.**

Most Common Causes of DITP	
Antiplatelet	• Abciximab, Eptifibatide, Tirofiban[Q]
Analgesics	• Acetaminophen, Ibuprofen, Naproxen[Q]
Antibiotic	• Ampicillin, Piperacillin, Ethambutol, Cephalosporins[Q]
Drugs acting on CNS	• Carbamazepine, Haloperidol, Phenytoin, Antidepressants[Q]
Anti-Cancer	• Irinotecan, Oxaliplatin[Q] (selective thrombocytopenia apart from pancytopenia)

Mechanism of DITP		
Designation	**Mechanism**	**Examples**
Hapten-dependent antibody	• **Drug (hapten) links covalently to membrane protein** & induces a drug-specific immune response.	• **Antibiotics: Penicillin, piperacillin, cephalosporin[Q]**
Drug-dependent antibody	• **Drug induces antibody** that binds to membrane protein only in the presence of soluble drug.	Antibiotics, Quinine, NSAIDS • **Anticonvulsants: Carbamazepine, Haloperidol, Phenytoin[Q]** • **Antidepressants: SSRI[Q]**
Glycoprotein IIb/IIIa Inhibitors	• **Drug (ligand) reacts with membrane glycoprotein IIb/IIIa** & induces conformational change recognized by naturally-occurring antibody	• **Anti-platelets: Abciximab, Eptifibatide, Tirofiban[Q]**

59. Ans. d. Flumazenil *(Ref: Goodman Gilman 12/e p468; Katzung 13/e p377-378, 12/e p381, 399; Harrison 19/e p2727, 18/e p2727)*
Flumazenil is a $GABA_A$ receptor antagonist primarily used intravenously to treat benzodiazepine overdoses or toxicity.

*"**Flumazenil**, the only member of this class, is an **imidazobenzodiazepine** that behaves as a **specific benzodiazepine receptor antagonist**. Flumazenil binds with high affinity to specific sites on the $GABA_A$ receptor, where it **competitively antagonizes the binding and allosteric effects of benzodiazepines** and other ligands. Flumazenil antagonizes both the electrophysiological and behavioral effects of agonist and inverse- agonist benzodiazepines and beta-carbolines. The drug is given intravenously."* - Goodman Gilman 12/e p468

Flumazenil
• Flumazenil is an **imidazobenzodiazepine** that behaves as a **specific benzodiazepine receptor antagonist[Q]**.
Mechanism of Action:
• Flumazenil **binds with high affinity to specific sites on GABA$_A$ receptor**, where it **competitively antagonizes binding & allosteric effects of benzodiazepines** & other ligands[Q].
• Flumazenil **antagonizes both electrophysiological & behavioral effects of agonist & inverse- agonist benzodiazepines & beta-carbolines[Q]**.
Therapeutic Uses:
• **Primary indication: Management of suspected benzodiazepine overdose** & reversal of sedative effects produced by benzodiazepines administered during various procedures[Q].
• A total of **1 mg flumazenil given over 1-3 minutes** usually is sufficient to abolish the effects of therapeutic doses of benzodiazepines[Q]
• Flumazenil is **not effective in single-drug overdoses with either barbiturates or tricyclic antidepressants.**

60. Ans. b. Linagliptin *(Ref: Goodman Gilman 12/e p1264; Katzung 13/e p740, 12/e p761; FDA website: http://www.fda.gov/ Safety/ MedWatch/SafetyInformation/ucm319215.htm)*

Linagliptin can be given safely in renal failure.

*"This suggests that **linagliptin has the ability to be safely dosed in chronic kidney disease patients**. **Chronic kidney disease is a major complication in type 2 diabetes** and presents one of the circumstances where using metformin can be challenging. The more severe the renal disease, the less likely one is to use metformin because of safety concerns. **Linagliptin is an option for these patients**."- http://www.medpagetoday.com/meetingcoverage/ada/27343*

See Q. No. 62 AIIMS May 2017

61. Ans. b. Smoking *(Ref: Goodman Gilman 12/e p1259; Katzung 13/e p736-737, 12/e p757)*

Smoking does not increase the risk of lactic acidosis in patients taking metformin.

*"**Many cases of lactic acidosis associated with the use of metformin** have been reported in patients with concurrent conditions that can cause **poor tissue perfusion such as sepsis, myocardial infarction,** and **congestive heart failure. Renal failure** is another common comorbidity reported in patients having lactic acidosis associated with metformin use, and decreased glomerular filtration rates are thought to increase plasma metformin levels by reducing clearance of drug from the circulation. Metformin should not be used in severe pulmonary disease, decompensated heart failure, severe liver disease, or chronic alcohol abuse."- Goodman Gilman 12/e p1259*

*"**Biguanides (metformin) are contraindicated in patients with renal disease, alcoholism, hepatic disease, or conditions predisposing to tissue anoxia (e.g., chronic cardiopulmonary dysfunction) because of the increased risk of lactic acidosis induced by these drugs**."- Katzung 12/e p757*

Risk of Lactic Acidosis due to Metformin is Increased in	
• Hypotensive states[Q]	• Hepatic failure[Q]
• Cardiovascular disease (MI & CHF) [Q]	• Renal failure[Q]
• Respiratory disease[Q]	• Alcoholics[Q]

See Q. No. 54 AIIMS November 2017

62. Ans. b. Date of expiry of the drug *(Ref: Goodman Gilman 12/e p1883; Manual of Experimental and Clinical Pharmacology/p 345)*

Date of expiry of the drug need not to be given in the drug advertisement letter.

"The Federal Food, Drug, and Cosmetic Act as amended (Food and Drug Administration Modernization Act of 1997) permits the use of print and television advertising of prescription drugs. The law requires that all drug advertisements contain (among other things) summary information relating to side effects, contraindications, and effectiveness. The current advertising regulations specify that this information disclosure needs to include all the risk information in a product's approved labeling or must direct consumers to healthcare professionals to obtain this information. Typically, print advertisements will include a reprinting of the risk-related sections of the product's approved labeling (package insert), while television advertising will not. In addition, advertisements cannot be false or misleading or omit material facts. They also must present a fair balance between effectiveness and risk information."- Goodman Gilman 12/e p1883

Drug Advertisement Protocol
All advertisement electronic or pamphlets for the promotion of a drug must include:
• **Name** of the product
• **Brand name** of the product
• **Active ingredients** of the product
• **Name & address** of **pharma company** or the person responsible for marketing
• **Date of production** of the advertisement
• **Most common** & **most serious side effects** documented
• **Abbreviated prescription information** which includes indications, dosage to be used for different ages, correction in dosage where required

63. Ans. d. Anaphylaxis *(Ref: Goodman Gilman 12/e p1149; Katzung 13/e p671, 12/e p688)*

Anaphylaxis is not associated with use of antithyroid drugs.

*"Adverse reactions to the thioamides occur in 3–12% of treated patients. **Most reactions occur early**, especially **nausea and gastrointestinal distress**. An **altered sense of taste or smell** may occur with methimazole. **The most common adverse effect is a maculopapular pruritic rash (4–6%)**, at times accompanied by systemic signs such as fever. Rare adverse effects include an **urticarial rash, vasculitis, a lupus-like reaction, lymphadenopathy, hypoprothrombinemia, exfoliative dermatitis, polyserositis, and acute arthralgia**. An **increased risk of severe hepatitis, sometimes resulting in death, has been reported with propylthiouracil (black box warning), so it should be avoided in children and adults** unless no other options are available. **Cholestatic jaundice is more common with methimazole than propylthiouracil. Asymptomatic elevations in transaminase levels** can also occur. **The most dangerous complication is agranulocytosis (granulocyte count <500 cells/mm³)**, an infrequent but **potentially fatal adverse reaction**."*- Katzung 13/e p671, 12/e p688

*"**Agranulocytosis usually occurs during the first few weeks or months of therapy** but may occur later. **Agranulocytosis is reversible upon discontinuation of the offending drug**, and the administration of recombinant human granulocyte colony-stimulating factor may hasten recovery. **The most common reaction is a mild, occasionally purpuric, urticarial papular rash. It often subsides spontaneously without interrupting treatment,** but it sometimes calls for the administration of an antihistamine, corticosteroids, and changing to another drug (cross- sensitivity between propylthiouracil and methimazole is uncommon). **Other less frequent complications are pain and stiffness in the joints, paresthesias, headache, nausea, skin pigmentation, and loss of hair. Drug fever, hepatitis, and nephritis** are rare, although abnormal liver function tests are not infrequent with higher doses of propylthiouracil. Although vasculitis was previously thought to be a rare complication, **antineutrophilic cytoplasmic antibodies (ANCAs) have been reported to occur in ~50% of patients receiving propylthiouracil and rarely with methimazole. Propylthiouracil-associated hepatic failure has been increasingly recognized, especially in children and pregnant women.**"*- Goodman Gilman 12/e p1149

Anti-Thyroid Drugs
• **Anti-thyroid drugs** that have clinical utility are **thioureylenes** belonging to **family of thionamides.** • Currently used drugs: **Propylthiouracil, methimazole & carbimazole (carbethoxy derivative** of methimazole)
Mechanism of Action: • **Inhibit formation of thyroid hormones** by **interfering with incorporation of iodine into tyrosyl residues** of thyroglobulin^Q • **Inhibit coupling of iodotyrosyl residues to form iodothyronines**^{Q} • **Inhibit peroxidase enzyme** preventing oxidation of iodide or iodotyrosyl groups to required active state^Q • **Propylthiouracil** partially **inhibits peripheral deiodination of T_4 to T_3.**^{Q}
Pharmacokinetics: • **Propylthiouracil & methimazole cross the placenta equally** and also can be found in milk^Q.

Untoward Reactions:
• **Most serious reaction: agranulocytosis**^{Q}
• **MC reaction**: Mild, purpuric, urticarial papular rash^Q.
• **Less frequent complications**: Pain & stiffness in joints, paresthesias, headache, skin pigmentation & loss of hair.
• **ANCAs** in ~50% of patients receiving **propylthiouracil**^{Q}
• **Cholestatic jaundice is more common with methimazole than propylthiouracil**^{Q}.
 	
    • **Propylthiouracil-associated hepatic failure** has been increasingly recognized, especially in **children & pregnant women**^{Q}.
    • **Propylthiouracil** should **not** be **used in children except** in the case of **methimazole allergy**^{Q}.

Therapeutic Uses:
• Used in **treatment of hyperthyroidism**^{Q}
• **Methimazole** is **DOC** for **Grave's disease (single daily dose, improved adherence, less toxic** than propylthiouracil)^Q
• **Thyrotoxicosis in pregnancy**: Anti-thyroid drugs (DOC: Carbimazole) are **treatment of choice (radioactive iodine is contraindicated)**^{Q}
 	
    • **Propylthiouracil** can cause **liver failure in pregnancy**^{Q}
    • **Methimazole** is very rarely **associated with aplasia cutis & choanal atresia**^{Q}
    • **Carbimazole** is **rarely associated with congenital gut abnormalities**^{Q}.
 	
• **Thyroid storm: DOC is propylthiouracil** (Preferred over methimazole because it **impairs peripheral conversion of $T_4 \rightarrow T_3$)**^{Q}

63b. Ans. d. Lung fibrosis *(Ref: Goodman Gilman 12/e p1149; Katzung 12/e p688)*

64. Ans. b. Postauricular skin > scrotum > scalp > dorsal aspect of hand > sole *(Ref: Goodman Gilman 12/e p22, 1803, 1806)*
Correct sequence of systemic absorption via transdermal application of the drug is: Postauricular skin > scrotum > scalp > dorsal aspect of hand > sole.

> *"The stratum corneum differs in thickness, with the palm and sole being the thickest (400-600 μm) followed by the general body stratum corneum (10-16 μm), and the scrotum (5 μm). Facial and post-auricular regions have the thinnest stratum corneum. Thickness is only one variable in determining regional differences in drug penetration. Cellular arrangement has a significant role as well."* - Goodman Gilman 12/e p 1803

> *"A hydrated stratum corneum allows more percutaneous absorption and often is achieved through the selection of drugs formulated in occlusion vehicles such as ointments and the use of plastic films, wraps, or bags for the hands and feet and shower or bathing caps for the scalp, or through the use of medications that are impregnated on patches or tapes. Occlusion may be associated with increased growth of bacteria with resultant infection (folliculitis) or maceration and breakdown of the epidermis. Transport of most drugs is a passive thermodynamic process, and heat generally increases penetration. Ultrasonic energy or laser-induced vibration also can be used to increase percutaneous absorption. The latter may function by the production of lacunae in the stratum corneum."* - Goodman Gilman 12/e p1806

Topical Drug Bioavailability and Penetration

- **Stratum corneum** differs in thickness, with the **palm & sole** being the **thickest (400-600 μm) followed by the general body stratum corneum (10-16 μm) & scrotum (5 μm)**. **Facial & post-auricular regions** have the **thinnest stratum corneum**.

Absorption of substances through the skin depends on a number of factors:	
• **Concentration**[Q] – **Molecular weight** of the molecule[Q] – **Duration of contact**[Q] – **Solubility of medication**[Q]	• **Physical condition** of the skin[Q] • **Part of the body exposed** including the amount of hair on skin[Q]

- **Rate of absorption** of chemicals through skin follows the following scheme from fastest to slowest: **Postauricular skin > Scrotum > Abdomen > Scalp > Forearm > Palm = under surface of foot**[Q].
- **Differences** are likely **due to** a combination of **skin thickness, hair follicles, density of capillaries** in the skin, **lipid content & degree of skin hydration**[Q].

65. Ans. b. Lateral thigh *(Ref: Goodman Gilman 12/e p1252)*
Insulin usually is injected into the subcutaneous tissues of the abdomen, buttock, anterior thigh, or dorsal arm. Absorption is usually most rapid from the abdominal wall, followed by the arm, buttock, and thigh.

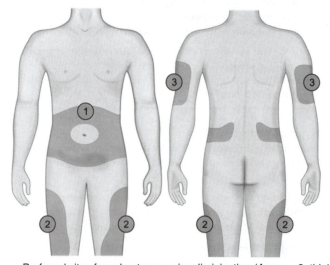

Fig. 28: Preferred sites for subcutaneous insulin injection (Arm no. 2, thigh 3)

AIIMS November 2016

891

"Insulin usually is injected into the subcutaneous tissues of the abdomen, buttock, anterior thigh, or dorsal arm. Absorption is usually most rapid from the abdominal wall, followed by the arm, buttock, and thigh. If a patient is willing to inject into the abdomen, injections can be rotated throughout the entire area, thereby eliminating the injection site as a cause of variability in the rate of absorption. The abdomen currently is the preferred site of injection in the morning because insulin is absorbed 20-30% faster from that site than from the arm. If the patient refuses to inject into the abdominal area, it is preferable to select a consistent injection site for each component of insulin treatment (e.g., before-breakfast dose into the thigh, evening dose into the arm). Rotation of insulin injection sites traditionally has been advocated to avoid lipohypertrophy or lipoatrophy, although these conditions are infrequent with current preparations of insulin. In a small group of patients, subcutaneous degradation of insulin has been observed, and this has necessitated the injection of large amounts of insulin for adequate metabolic control." - Goodman Gilman 12/e p1252

66. **Ans. d. Rifabutin is more efficacious for pulmonary TB as compared to rifampicin**   *(Ref: Goodman Gilman 12/e p1550, 1552, 1554, 1568; Katzung 12/e p845)*

Rifabutin has stronger activity against Mycobacterium avium complex as compared to rifampicin, but not against Mycobacterium tuberculosis.

	Rifabutin	Rifampicin (Rifampin)	Rifapentine
Protein binding (%)	71	85	97
Oral bioavailability (%)	20	**68**[Q]	-
t$_{max}$ (hours)	2.5-4.0	1.5-2.0	**5.0-6.0**[Q]
Half-life (hours)	**32-67**[Q]	**2-5**[Q]	14-18
Intracellular/extracellular penetration	9	5	**24-60**[Q]
Autoinduction	**40%**[Q]	38%	20%
CYP3A induction	Weak	Pronounced	Moderate
CYP3A substrate	**Yes**[Q]	No	No

"After oral administration, the rifamycins are absorbed to variable extents. Food decreases the rifampin C_{Pmax} by one third; a high-fat meal increases the area under the curve (AUC) of rifapentine by 50%. Food has no effect on rifabutin absorption. Thus rifampin should be taken on an empty stomach, whereas rifapentine should be taken with food, if possible." - Goodman Gilman 12/e p1550

"Rifabutin concentrations are substantially higher in tissue than in plasma due to its lipophilic properties, leading to the very high apparent volumes of distribution. The consequence is that C_{Pmax} values for rifabutin are lower than one would predict by comparison with other rifamycins." - Goodman Gilman 12/e p1552

*"Because **rifampin potently induces CYPs 1A2, 2C9, 2C19, and 3A4**, its administration results in a decreased $t_{1/2}$ for a number of compounds, including HIV protease and non-nucleoside reverse transcriptase inhibitors, digitoxin, digoxin, quinidine, disopyramide, mexiletine, tocainide, ketoconazole, propranolol, metoprolol, clofibrate, verapamil, methadone, cyclosporine, corticosteroids, coumarin anticoagulants, theophylline, barbiturates, oral contraceptives, halothane, fluconazole, and the sulfonylureas. It leads to therapeutic failure of these agents, with potentially catastrophic consequences. Rifabutin is a less potent inducer of CYPs than rifampin, both in terms of potency and number of CYP enzymes involved; however, rifabutin does induce hepatic microsomal enzymes and decreases the $t_{1/2}$ of zidovudine, prednisone, digitoxin, quinidine, ketoconazole, propranolol, phenytoin, sulfonylureas, and warfarin. It has less effect than rifampin on serum levels of indinavir and nelfinavir. Compared to rifabutin and rifampin, the CYP-inducing effects of rifapentine are intermediate."* - Goodman Gilman 12/e p1554

"In HIV-infected patients, the substitution of rifabutin for rifampin minimizes drug interactions with the HIV protease inhibitors and non-nucleoside reverse transcriptase inhibitors." - Goodman Gilman 12/e p1568

Rifabutin
• Rifabutin is **derived from rifamycin** and is related to rifampin.
• It has **significant activity against M. tuberculosis, MAC, and Mycobacterium fortuitum**[Q].
• Rifabutin is **both substrate & inducer of cytochrome P450** enzymes[Q].

Rifabutin
Mechanism of Action:
• Rifampin derivative with same mechanism of action (**DNA dependent RNA polymerase inhibition**)[Q]
Pharmacokinetics:
• **Rifabutin** is **more lipid soluble** than is rifampicin, resulting in **more-extensive tissue uptake**, a **larger volume of distribution**, **lower maximum plasma concentrations**, **lower trough concentrations**, a **longer terminal half-life** & higher tissue-to-plasma drug concentration ratios[Q].
• **Oral bioavailability** of rifabutin is **low**.
Drug Interactions:
• **Lesser drug interactions** than rifampicin because rifabutin is a **less potent inducer of CYPs**[Q]
Therapeutic Uses:
• **Effective against** *Gram-positive,* some *Gram-negative* bacteria & highly resistant *mycobacteria*, e.g. ***Mycobacterium tuberculosis, M. leprae, and M. avium intracellulare***[Q].
• **Rifabutin is indicated** in place of rifampin **for treatment of TB in patients with HIV patients** receiving ART[Q].   • **Rifabutin** is effective in **prevention & treatment of disseminated atypical mycobacterial infection in AIDS** patients with CD4 counts below 50/μL[Q].
Side-Effects:
• Unique side effects are **polymyalgia & anterior uveitis**[Q].

67. Ans. a. Milnacipran *(Ref: Goodman Gilman 12/e p1299; Katzung 13/e p761-762, 12/e p775; Harrison 19/e p2493, 18/e p3120; Apley 9/e p131-133)*
Milnacipran is a serotonin–norepinephrine reuptake inhibitor (SNRI), approved for treatment of pain in fibromyalgia, not in osteoporosis.

Drugs useful in Osteoporosis		
Inhibit Bone Resorption	**Stimulates Bone Formation**	**Both action**
• **Bisphosphonates:** Alendronate, risedronate, **etidronate**[Q] • Calcium receptor agonist: **Cinacalcet**[Q] • **Calcitonin**[Q] • SERMs: Tamoxifen, raloxifene • **Gallium nitrate**[Q] • **RANKL inhibitors: Donesumab**[Q]	• **Teriparatide**[Q] • Calcium • **Calcitriol**[Q] • Fluoride	• **Strontium ranelate**[Q]

68. Ans. d. Amiodarone *(Ref: Goodman Gilman 12/e p1405, 837; KDT 7/e p534)*
Amiodarone can cause corneal deposits but doesn't cause nail pigmentation.

"Chloroquine may cause discoloration of nail beds and mucous membranes." -Goodman Gilman 12/e p1405

"Cyclophosphamide: Apart from systemic toxicity such as anaphylaxis, bone marrow suppression, and hemorrhagic cystitis, cyclophosphamide can cause a variety of mucocutaneous side effects including anagen effluvium, stomatitis, and hyperpigmentation involving the skin, mucous membranes, nails, palms, and soles and teeth."

Causes of Melanonychia or Nail Pigmentation		
• **Phenothiazines like chlorpromazine**[Q] • **Chloroquine**[Q] • **Minocycline**[Q] • **Arsenic**[Q] • **Clofazimine**[Q] • **Clomipramine**[Q] • **Cyclophosphamide**[Q]	• Fluconazole • Fluoride • Gold salts • Ibuprofen • Ketoconazole • **Lamivudine**[Q] • **Mercury**[Q] • **Phenytoin**[Q]	• Psoralen • **Roxithromycin**[Q] • Steroids • **Sulfonamide**[Q] • **Tetracycline**[Q] • **Thallium**[Q] • **Timolol**[Q] • **Zidovudine**[Q]

Nail	Nail Area Affected	Potential Causes
Onycholysis	Nail bed	Docetaxel, paclitaxel, doxorubicin, bleomycin, tetracycline
Paronychia and pyogenic granuloma	Periungual folds	Retinoids, indinavir, EGFR inhibitors, capecitabine
Hemorrhage	Nail vasculature	Taxanes, sirolimus, sunitinib, sorafenib, aspirin, retinoids
Melanic pigmentation	Entire nail	Infliximab, zidovudine, chlorpromazine, chloroquine
Non-melanic pigmentation	Entire nail	Minocycline, amodiaquine, chloroquine, mepacrine
Irritant or allergic reactions	Nail plate or surrounding tissues	Antifungal drugs

69. **Ans. a. To adjust maintenance dose of digoxin required to keep the blood levels within therapeutic range** *(Ref: Goodman Gilman 12/e p33, 37; KDT 7/e p31, 515)*

The loading dose of digoxin is governed by volume of distribution and maintenance dose is determined by $t_{1/2}$ and creatinine clearance. The given half-life determines the daily maintenance dosing to maintain therapeutic plasma levels. The half-life of digoxin is 36 to 48 hours in patients with normal renal function and 3.5 to 5 days in anuric patients. In patients with normal renal function, an oral daily maintenance dose without a loading dose results in a steady-state blood concentration in approximately 7 days. Hence, the daily maintenance dose is decided based on the half-life of the drug. The usual digoxin therapeutic serum concentrations range is 0.8 to 2 ng/mL.

"The appreciation of longer terminal $t_{1/2}$ values for some medications may relate to their accumulation in tissues during chronic dosing or shorter periods of high-dose treatment. Such is the case for gentamicin, where the terminal $t_{1/2}$ is associated with renal and ototoxicities. The relevance of a particular $t_{1/2}$ may be defined in terms of the fraction of the clearance and volume of distribution that is related to each $t_{1/2}$ and whether plasma concentrations or amounts of drug in the body are best related to measures of response." - Goodman Gilman 12/e p33

"Although it can be a poor index of drug elimination from the body per se (disappearance of drug may be the result of formation of undetected metabolites that have therapeutic or unwanted effects), the $t_{1/2}$ defined in Equation 2–14 provides an approximation of the time required to reach steady state after a dosage regimen is initiated or changed (e.g., four half-lives to reach ~94% of a new steady state) and a means to estimate the appropriate dosing interval." - Goodman Gilman 12/e p33

"A loading dose may be desirable if the time required to attain steady state by the administration of drug at a constant rate (4 elimination $t_{1/2}$ values) is long relative to the temporal demands of the condition being treated." - Goodman Gilman 12/e p37

	Digitoxin	Digoxin
Oral absorption	V. good[Q] (90–100%)	Good (60–80%)
Plasma protein binding	95%	25%
Time course of action: • Onset • Peak • Duration	½–2 hours[Q] 6–12 hours[Q] 2–3 weeks[Q]	15–30 min 2–5 hours 2–6 days
Plasma $t_{1/2}$	5–7 days[Q]	40 hours[Q]
Plasma concentration: • Therapeutic • Toxic	15–30 ng/mL[Q] > 35 ng/mL[Q]	0.5–1.4 ng/mL[Q] >2 ng/mL[Q]
Daily maintenance dose	0.05–0.2 mg	0.125–0.5 mg
Daily elimination	10–15%	35%[Q]
Route of elimination (predominant)	Hepatic metabolism[Q]	Renal excretion[Q]
Administration	Oral[Q]	Oral, IV[Q]
Generally used for	Maintenance[Q]	Routine treatment & emergency[Q]

MICROBIOLOGY

70. Ans. d. Neisseria gonorrhoeae *(Ref: Ananthanarayan 8/e p50, 10/e p13, 234)*

Pink coloured paired cocci are seen in the given image. This is a Gram-negative cocci, most likely to be Neisseria meningitidis or N. gonorrhoeae.

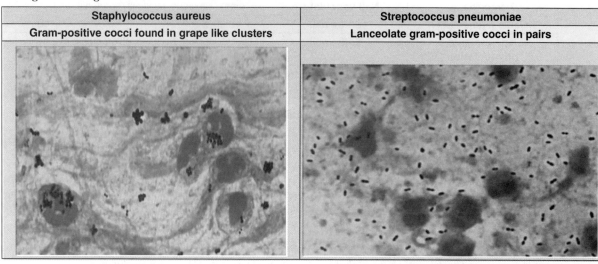

Gram's Staining

Principle:
- Dependent on **permeability of bacterial cell wall & cytoplasmic membrane**[Q], to dye-iodine complex.

Gram's Staining Procedure
- Application of **primary stain crystal violet** to a heat-fixed smear of bacterial culture for **1 minute**.
- **Crystal violet** interacts with negatively charged bacterial components & **stains bacterial cells purple**[Q].
- **Addition of Gram's Iodine:** Iodine acts as a **mordant** and as a trapping agent[Q].
- **Decolorization** with **acetone** or **95% ethyl alcohol** for 5 seconds[Q]
- **Counterstain with Safranin** for 1 minute[Q]
  - **Gram negative (red) & Gram positive (blue)**[Q]
  - Assess Gram reaction & morphology

Contd...

Gram's Staining	
Gram Positive Bacteria	**Gram Negative Bacteria**
• Crystal violet dye-iodine complex combines to form a larger molecule, which precipitates in the cell. • **Alcohol/acetone mixture, which acts as decolorizing agent, cause dehydration of multi-layered peptidoglycan of the cell wall[Q].** • This causes **decreasing of the space** between molecules causing **cell wall to trap crystal violet iodine complex within the cell[Q].** • Hence **Gram-positive bacteria do not get decolorized** & retain primary dye appearing violet.	• **Alcohol**, being a lipid solvent, **dissolves outer Lipopolysaccharide membrane of cell wall[Q]** & also damage cytoplasmic membrane to which peptidoglycan is attached. • As a result, **dye-iodine complex is not retained[Q]** within the cell & permeates out of it during process of decolorization. • Hence when a counter stain is added, they **take up the colour of stain & appear pink.**

Neisseria Gonorrhoeae
• **Gonococci** is **non-encapsulated, Gram-negative, kidney shaped diplococci[Q]** • **Gonococci oxidize only glucose** & differ antigenically from the other neisseriae[Q]. • Usually **produce smaller colonies** than those of other neisseriae[Q].

Antigenic Structure:

• N. gonorrhoeae is antigenically heterogeneous & capable of changing its surface structures in vitro & in vivo to avoid host defenses.

Virulence Factors of Neisseria Gonorrhoeae	
Pili (Fimbriae)	• **Enhance attachment to host cells & resistance to phagocytosis[Q]** • Made up of **stacked pilin proteins[Q]** • **Pilins of almost all strains of N. gonorrhoeae are antigenically different[Q]**
Por	• Form pores in surface through which some nutrients enter the cell. • Por proteins **may impact intracellular killing of gonococci within neutrophils by preventing phagosome-lysosome fusion[Q].**
Opa Proteins	• Function in **adhesion of gonococci within colonies** & in **attachment of gonococci to host cell** receptors[Q]
Rmp (Protein III)	• Antigenically conserved in all gonococci • It associates **with Por in formation of pores in the cell surface[Q].**
Lipooligosaccharide	• Gonococcal lipopolysaccharide **does not have long O-antigen side chains** & is called a **lipooligosaccharide[Q] (LOS).** • Can **express >1 antigenically different LOS** chain simultaneously. • **Toxicity** in gonococcal infections **is largely attributable to endotoxic effects of LOS[Q].**
Other Proteins	• **Lip (H8):** Heat modifiable surface-exposed protein • **Fbp (ferric-binding protein):** Expressed when the available iron supply is limited. • **IgA1 protease: Splits and inactivates mucosal IgA1 (Meningococci, H. influenzae & Streptococcus pneumoniae elaborate similar IgA1 proteases)[Q]**

Typing of Gonococci:

• **Serotyping** is **based on protein-I (porin)[Q]**
• **Auxotyping:** Typing is **based on nutritional requirements** of strains, e.g. AHU auxotype that require **arginine, hypoxanthine and uracil** as growth factors[Q].

Pathology:

• **Gonococci attack mucous membranes** of genitourinary tract, eye, rectum & throat, producing **acute suppuration** that may lead to **tissue invasion** followed by **chronic inflammation & fibrosis[Q].**

Cond...

Neisseria Gonorrhoeae

Clinical Features:
- **Men: MC manifestation** is **acute urethritis**, with **yellow, creamy pus & painful urination**; can lead to **urethral strictures** in untreated cases[Q].
- Infection may spread to **periurethral tissues** leading to **abscess & sinus formation (water-can perineum)**[Q]
- **Urethral infection in men** can be **asymptomatic**[Q].

> - **Women: Primary infection** is in **endocervix** & extends to **urethra & vagina**, giving rise to **mucopurulent discharge**[Q].
> - It may **progress to uterine tubes, causing salpingitis, fibrosis & obliteration of the tubes**[Q].
> - **Infertility** occurs in **20%** of women with **gonococcal salpingitis**[Q].
> - **Chronic gonococcal cervicitis & proctitis** are often **asymptomatic**.
> - **Fitz-Hugh-Curtis syndrome: Peritonitis & associated perihepatitis**[Q]

- **Gonococcal bacteremia** leads to **skin lesions (hemorrhagic papules & pustules)** on hands, forearms, feet & legs and to **tenosynovitis & suppurative arthritis**, usually of **knees, ankles & wrists**[Q].
- Gonococci can be cultured from **blood or joint fluid** of only 30% of patients with **gonococcal arthritis**.
- **Gonococcal endocarditis** is an uncommon but severe infection.
- **Gonococci** can cause **meningitis & eye infections** in adults.

> - **Complement deficiency** is **frequently found in patients with gonococcal bacteremia**. Patients with **recurrent bacteremia** should be **tested for total hemolytic complement activity**[Q].

- **Gonococcal ophthalmia neonatorum** is acquired during **passage through an infected birth canal** (initial conjunctivitis rapidly progresses & if **untreated, results in blindness**)[Q]

Laboratory Diagnosis:

Specimens	• **Pus & secretions** from urethra, cervix, rectum, conjunctiva, throat, or synovial fluid for culture & smear. • **Blood culture** is necessary in systemic illness
Transport media	• **Charcoal impregnated swabs/medium (Stuart/Amies media)**[Q] • **For longer holding period: CO$_2$ generated system (JEMBEC system)**[Q]
Smears	• **Gram-stained smears of urethral or endocervical exudates** reveal **diplococci within pus cells**[Q]. • **Stained smears of conjunctival exudates** can also be **diagnostic**[Q]
Culture	• **Culture media** in **acute** gonorrhoeae: **Chocolate agar & Mueller-Hinton agar**[Q] • **Selective media** useful in **chronic** cases: **Thayer-Martin medium, modified New York city medium, Martin-Lewis media**[Q]
Nucleic Acid Amplification Tests	• **NAATs** are available for **direct detection of *N. gonorrhoeae* in genitourinary specimens** with **excellent sensitivity & specificity** in symptomatic, high-prevalence populations[Q].
Serology	• **Serum & genital fluid** contain **IgG & IgA antibodies against** gonococcal **pili, outer membrane proteins & LPS**[Q]. • Detected by **immunoblotting, radioimmunoassay & ELISA**[Q]. • **Not useful as diagnostic aids** because of **delay in development of antibodies** in acute infection & **high level of antibodies** in sexually active population[Q].

Treatment
- **DOC: Ceftriaxone (IM) single dose**[Q]
- **Gonococcal ophthalmia neonatorum:** Prevented by **0.5% erythromycin** or **1% tetracycline ointment** to the conjunctiva of newborns[Q].

71. Ans. b. Due to adherence to the capillary endothelium, they are not seen in peripheral blood *(Ref: Harrison 19/e p1371; Jawetz 27/e p719)*

Schizonts and late trophozoite stages of Plasmodium falciparum not seen in peripheral blood smear because due to adherence to the capillary endothelium, they are not seen in peripheral blood.

"Ordinarily, only ring stages or gametocytes are seen in peripheral blood infected with P. falciparum; parasites make red cells sticky, and they tend to be retained in deep capillary beds, except in overwhelming, usually fatal, infections."- Jawetz 27/e p719

"P. vivax, P. malariae, and P. ovale parasitemias are relatively low grade, primarily because the parasites favor either young or old red cells but not both; P. falciparum invades red cells of all ages, including the erythropoietic stem cells in bone marrow, so parasitemia may be very high. P. falciparum also causes parasitized red cells to adhere to the endothelial lining of blood vessels, with resulting obstruction, thrombosis, and local ischemia. P. falciparum infections are therefore far more serious than the others, with a much higher rate of severe and frequently fatal complications (cerebral malaria, malarial hyperpyrexia, gastrointestinal disorders, algid malaria, blackwater fever)."- Jawetz 27/e p719

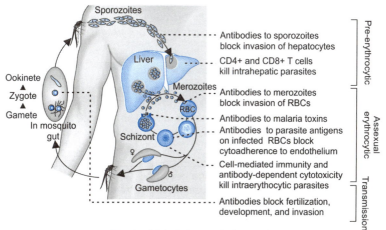

Fig. 29: Malaria transmission cycle

*"In P. falciparum infections, membrane protuberances appear on the erythrocyte's surface 12–15 h after the cell's invasion. These "knobs" extrude a high-molecular-weight, antigenically variant, strain-specific erythrocyte membrane adhesive protein (PfEMP1) that mediates attachment to receptors on venular and capillary endothelium—an event termed **cytoadherence**. Several vascular receptors have been identified, of which intercellular adhesion molecule 1 is probably the most important in the brain, chondroitin sulfate B in the placenta, and CD36 in most other organs. **Thus, the infected erythrocytes stick inside and eventually block capillaries and venules. At the same stage, these P. falciparum–infected RBCs may also adhere to uninfected RBCs (to form rosettes) and to other parasitized erythrocytes (agglutination). The processes of cytoadherence, rosetting, and agglutination are central to the pathogenesis of falciparum malaria. They result in the sequestration of RBCs containing mature forms of the parasite in vital organs (particularly the brain),** where they interfere with microcirculatory flow and metabolism. Sequestered parasites continue to develop out of reach of the principal host defense mechanism: splenic processing and filtration. As a consequence, only the younger ring forms of the asexual parasites are seen circulating in the peripheral blood in falciparum malaria, and the level of peripheral parasitemia underestimates the true number of parasites within the body. Severe malaria is also associated with reduced deformability of the uninfected erythrocytes, which compromises their passage through the partially obstructed capillaries and venules and shortens RBC survival."- Harrison 19/e p1371*

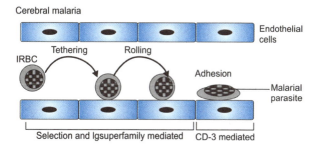

"In the other human malarias, sequestration does not occur, and all stages of the parasite's development are evident on peripheral-blood smears. Whereas P. vivax, P. ovale, and P. malariae show a marked predilection for either young RBCs (P. vivax, P. ovale) or old cells (P. malariae) and produce a level of parasitemia that is seldom >2%, P. falciparum can invade erythrocytes of all ages and may be associated with very high levels of parasitemia."- Harrison 19/e p1371

72. **Ans. a. Asymptomatic**   *(Ref: Paniker's 7/e p162, 6/e pg180, 219)*

Larvae of Ascaris, Hookworm and Strongyloides migrate through the lung and various other tissues during their lifecycle. They may cause local alveolar hemorrhages but clinical pneumonitis is seen only in massive infections. Hence, they are mostly asymptomatic.

Ascaris: The pathogenic effects of larval migration due to allergic reaction and not the presence of larvae as such. Therefore, the initial exposure to larvae is usually asymptomatic, except when the larval load is very heavy."- Paniker's 7/e p198

"Symptomatic visceral larvae migrans is produced by infection with non-human nematodes, i.e. nematodes which frequently infect dogs and cats. Symptoms during migration are produced only due to allergic reaction and are significant only in massive infections."

Larva Migrans
• Life cycles of most nematodes parasitising humans include **larval migration through various tissues & organs of body[Q]**.
• Sometimes the **larvae appear to lose their way & wander around aimlessly**. This condition is known as **larva migrans**.
• This is generally seen when **human infection occurs with nonhuman species of nematodes[Q]**.

Cutaneous Larva Migrans	Visceral Larva Migrans

• **Creeping eruption** caused by **nematode larvae** that **infect by skin penetration**, most commonly by the **non-human species of hookworms Ancylostoma braziliense & A. caninum[Q]**.
  – Larvae produce **itching papules**, which develop into serpiginous tunnels in epidermis.
  – With the **movements of larva in skin, lesion also shifts (creeping eruption)[Q]**.
  – **Thiabendazole** is useful in treatment[Q].
 	
Larva Currens
• A **rapidly moving lesion** is produced by **Strongyloides stercoralis** particularly in immune persons[Q].
	• Caused by **migration of larvae of non-human species** of nematodes that **infect by oral route**.
	• **MC cause**: Dog ascarid **Toxocara canis** & less often the cat ascarid **T. cati**.
	  – These nematodes **can infect** but not mature in humans and **after migrating through intestinal wall, travel with blood stream to various organs** where they cause inflammation & damage[Q].
	  – **Affected organs: Liver, heart** (causing myocarditis) & **CNS** (causing dysfunction, seizures & coma).
	• A special variant is **ocular larva migrans** where usually **T. canis larvae travel to the eye[Q]**.

73. **Ans. c. Plasmodium falciparum**   *(Ref: Paniker's 7/e p69, 6/e p79; Jawetz 27/e p721)*

The given clinical presentation is suggestive of malaria. Double rings in erythrocytes on peripheral blood smear are typically seen in P. falciparum infections.

"Double rings and banana-shaped gametocytes are typically seen in P. falciparum infections."- Jawetz 27/e p721

Examination of Blood Films for Malaria Parasite
• Malaria parasites pass through a number of developmental stages. In all stages, however, the specific parts of the parasite will stain a specific colour.

Parts of parasite	Staining characteristic
Chromatin (parasite nucleus)	Usually **round in shape & stains a deep red[Q]**.
Cytoplasm	**Blue**, although shade of blue may vary between malaria species[Q].

Examination of Blood Films for Malaria Parasite

Recognition of a Malarial Parasite
- Malaria parasite takes up Giemsa stain in a special way in both thick & thin blood films.

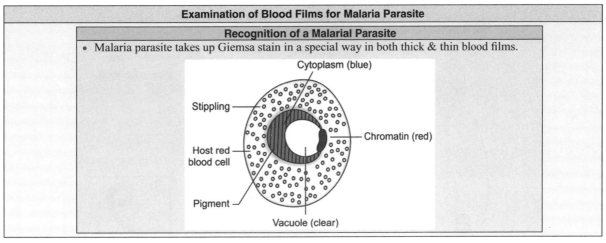

See Q. No. 84 AIIMS November 2017

74. Ans. b. Embryonated egg is the infectious stage for this worm   *(Ref: Paniker's 7/e p172, 6/e p166; Jawetz 27/e p724; Harrison 19/e p1416)*

The pictorial representation of adults (anterior end is slender & posterior end is thicker, giving it a "buggy whip" appearance, hence the name whipworm) above is suggestive of Trichuris trichura. Embryonated egg is the infectious stage for this worm. It is transmitted through oral route. The adult worm usually lives in the large intestine & appendix. The drug of choice is Thiabendazole.

> "Adult female **whipworms** are approximately 30–50 mm in length; adult male worms are smaller. **The anterior end of the worms is slender, and the posterior end is thicker, giving it a "buggy whip" appearance, hence the name whipworm.** Adult whipworms inhabit the colon, where male and female worms mate. Females release eggs that are passed in the feces, and eggs become infective after about 3 weeks of incubation in moist and shady soil. Humans acquire the infection by eating foods contaminated with infective eggs. Once eggs are swallowed, the larvae hatch in the small intestine, where they mature and migrate to the colon." - Jawetz 27/e p724

Trichuris trichiura (Whipworm)
• Adult **female whipworms** are approximately **30–50 mm** in length; adult male worms are smaller. • **Anterior end** of worms **is slender** & **posterior end is thicker**, giving it a **"buggy whip" appearance**, hence the **name whipworm**[Q].
Life cycle: • **Adult Trichuris** worms reside in **colon & cecum**, the **anterior portions threaded into superficial mucosa**[Q]. • **Thousands of eggs** laid daily by adult female worms **pass with feces** & mature in the soil. • **Infective stage: Embryonated eggs**[Q] • After ingestion, **infective eggs hatch in duodenum**, **releasing larvae** that **mature before migrating to large** bowel[Q]. • Entire cycle takes ~3 months & adult worms may live for several years.
Clinical features: • Most infected individuals have **no symptoms or eosinophilia**. • **Heavy infections** may result in **anemia, abdominal pain, anorexia & bloody or mucoid diarrhea** resembling inflammatory bowel disease. • **Rectal prolapse** can result from **massive infections in children**, who often suffer from **malnourishment** & other diarrheal illnesses.

Diagnosis:
• Characteristic **50-20-μm lemon-shaped Trichuris eggs** are readily detected **on stool examination**[Q].
    • Barrel shaped structure seen with lightly stained mucus plugs at each pole[Q]
    • Egg-shell is stained brown & encloses light yellow stained unsegmented ovum[Q]

Treatment: • **Mebendazole or albendazole**[Q] is safe & moderately **effective for treatment**, with **cure rates of 70–90%**.

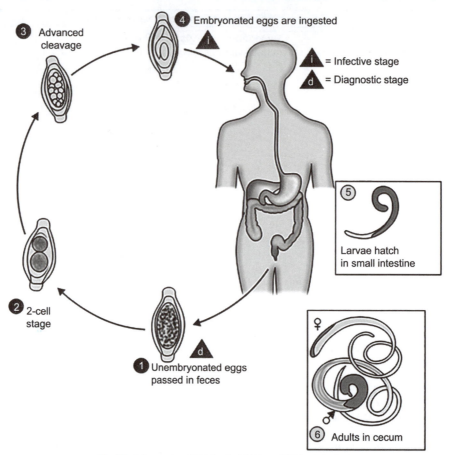

Fig. 30: Life-cycle of Trichuris trichiura (Whipworm)

	Parasitic Nematodes				
Feature	Ascaris lumbricoides (Roundworm)	Necator Americanus, Ancylostoma duodenale (Hookworm)	Strongyloides stercoralis	Trichuris trichiura (Whipworm)	Enterobius vermicularis (Pinworm)
Infective stage	Egg^Q	Filariform larva^Q	Filariform larva^Q	Egg^Q	Egg^Q
Route of infection	Oral^Q	Percutaneous^Q	Percutaneous or autoinfection^Q	Oral^Q	Oral^Q
Gastro- intestinal location of worms	Jejunal lumen^Q	Jejunal mucosa^Q	Small bowel mucosa^Q	Cecum, colonic mucosa^Q	Cecum, appendix^Q
Pulmonary passage of larvae	Yes^Q	Yes^Q	Yes^Q	No^Q	No^Q
Principal symptoms	Rarely gastro-intestinal or biliary obstruction	Iron deficiency anemia in heavy infection^Q	Gastrointestinal symptoms; malabsorption or sepsis in hyperinfection	Gastro-intestinal symptoms, anemia^Q	Perianal pruritus^Q
Feature	Ascaris lumbricoides (Roundworm)	Necator Americanus, Ancylostoma duodenale (Hookworm)	Strongyloides stercoralis	Trichuris trichiura (Whipworm)	Enterobius vermicularis (Pinworm)
Diagnostic stage	Eggs in stool^Q	Eggs in fresh stool, larvae in old stool^Q	Larvae in stool or duodenal aspirate; sputum in hyperinfection	Eggs in stool^Q	Eggs from perianal skin on cellulose acetate tape^Q
Treatment	Mebendazole, Albendazole	Mebendazole, Albendazole	Ivermectin, Albendazole	Mebendazole, Albendazole	Mebendazole Albendazole

75. Ans. c. Proteus mirabilis *(Ref: Ananthanarayan 10/e p288, 8/e p280; Jawetz 27/e p233)*
The given blood agar shows concentric swarming, which is seen in Proteus infections.

"Proteus species move very actively by means of peritrichous flagella, resulting in "swarming" on solid media unless the swarming is inhibited by chemicals, such as phenylethyl alcohol or CLED (cystine-lactose-electrolyte-deficient) medium."- Jawetz 27/e p233

"Proteus species show concentric swarming on the blood agar while Clostridium species show non-concentric swarming."

Motility of Organisms	
Motility	**Organism**
Falling leaf motility	Giardia lamblia trophozoites[Q]
Darting motility or swarm of gnats	Vibrio cholerae[Q]
	Campylobacter[Q]
	Gardnerella[Q]
Stately motility	Clostridium[Q]
Swarming motility	Proteus[Q]
	Bacillus cereus[Q]
	Clostridium tetani[Q]
Spinning motility	Fusobacterium gyrans[Q]
Tumbling motility	Listeria[Q]
Gliding motility	Mycoplasma[Q]
Cork-screw motility	Treponema pallidum[Q]
Lashing motility	Borrelia[Q]

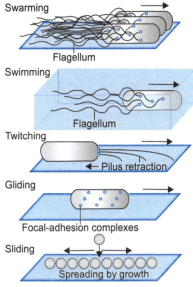

Fig. 31: Types of motility

Swarming motility
• **Swarming motility** is a **rapid (2–10 μm/s) & coordinated translocation of a bacterial population** across solid or semi-solid surfaces[Q].
• It is an example of **bacterial multicellularity & swarm behavior**[Q].
• It has been mostly studied in **genus Serratia, Salmonella, Aeromonas, Bacillus, Yersinia, Pseudomonas, Proteus, Vibrio & Escherichia**[Q].
• This multicellular behavior has been mostly observed in controlled laboratory conditions and relies on two critical elements: **nutrient composition & viscosity of culture medium** (i.e. % agar).

Cond...

Swarming motility

- **Increase of concentration from 2 to 6% agar inhibits swarming[Q].**
- One particular feature of this type of motility is the formation of **dendritic fractal-like patterns formed by migrating swarms moving away from an initial location[Q].**
  - Although the majority of species can produce tendrils when swarming, some species like **Proteus mirabilis do form concentric circles motif instead of dendritic patterns[Q].**
  - **Slow form of swarming (stately motility) is seen in Clostridium species also[Q].**

Proteus

- **Proteus is Gram negative, urease positive, pleomorphic bacilli[Q]**
- **Opportunistic pathogen** responsible for **UTI (MC by P. mirabilis[Q])** & nosocomial infections
- **Associated with staghorn calculi[Q]**
- **Species: Proteus mirabilis (indole negative[Q]), Proteus vulgaris (indole positive[Q])**

Culture:
- Cultures have characteristic **putrefactive odour (fishy or seminal odour)[Q]**
- **Swarming motility with peritrichous flagella[Q]**
- **Swarming can be inhibited by: Increasing conc. of agar (6%); Incorporation of chloral hydrate, sodium azide, alcohol, sulfonamides, surface active agents, boric acid[Q]**
- **Swarming does not occur on MacConkey's medium[Q]**
- **Characteristic feature of Proteus bacilli: PPA reaction[Q]**

Diene's Phenomenon

- Used to **detect swarming growth[Q]**
- When two different strains of swarming Proteus mirabilis encounter one another on an agar plate, swarming ceases and a **visible line of demarcation forms-Diene's line** & is **associated with formation of rounded cells[Q]**

76. **Ans. a. Leptospira interrogans** *(Ref: Ananthanarayan 10/e p3287, 8/e p372; Jawetz 27/e p330)*

Hook like appearance of the spirochetes in this dark field microscopy image is suggestive of Leptospira infection.

"Leptospirae are tightly coiled, thin, flexible spirochetes 5–15 μm long, with very fine spirals 0.1–0.2 μm wide; one end is often bent, forming a hook. They are actively motile, which is best seen using a dark-field microscope. Electron micrographs show a thin axial filament and a delicate membrane. The spirochete is so delicate that in the dark-field view, it may appear only as a chain of minute cocci. It does not stain readily but can be impregnated with silver."- Jawetz 27/e p330

Spirochaetes

- Species in the phylum Spirochaetes (order: Spirochaetales) are **thin, spiral-shaped or wave-like, highly motile bacteria** that are **best visualized by dark field microscopy[Q].**
- Spirochaetes are **Gram-negative-like**, in that they **possess inner & outer membranes separated by a peptidoglycan containing periplasmic space[Q].**

Morphology		
Borrelia burgdorferi	**Leptospira**	**Treponema**
• **Spiral organism** 20–30 μm long and 0.2–0.3 μm wide. • Distance between turns varies from 2-4 μm. • Organisms have variable numbers **(7–11) of endoflagella** & are **highly motile[Q].** • **Stains** readily with **acid' & aniline dyes** & by **silver impregnation** techniques[Q].	• **Tightly coiled, thin, flexible** spirochetes 5–15 μm long, with very fine spirals 0.1–0.2 μm wide; **one end is often bent, forming a hook[Q].** • **Actively motile**, best seen using a **dark-field microscope[Q]** • Electron micrographs show a **thin axial filament & a delicate membrane[Q].**	• Slender spirals measuring about 0.2 μm in width and 5–15 μm in length. • Spiral coils are regularly spaced at a distance of 1 μm from one another. • **Actively motile, rotating steadily around their endoflagella** even after attaching to cells by their tapered ends[Q]. • **Long axis** of the spiral is generally **straight[Q].** • Seen in tissues when stained by a **silver impregnation method[Q].**

AIIMS November 2016

77. Ans. b. ELISA for antibody against dengue virus *(Ref: Ananthanarayan 10/e p529, 8/e p519; Harrison 19/e p1319)*
ELISA for antibody detection against dengue virus usually yields diagnostic results only after 5 days, i.e. acute phase of infection.

"ELISA for antibody detection against Dengue virus usually yields diagnostic results only after 5 days, i.e. acute phase of infection. The diagnosis is made by IgM ELISA or paired serology during recovery or by antigen-detection ELISA or RT-PCR during the acute phase. Virus is readily isolated from blood in the acute phase if mosquito inoculation or mosquito cell culture is used."

"Laboratory findings in dengue include leukopenia, thrombocytopenia, and, in many cases, serum aminotransferase elevations. Before day 5 of illness, during the febrile period, dengue infections may be diagnosed by virus isolation in cell culture, by detection of viral RNA by nucleic acid amplification tests (NAAT), or by detection of viral antigens by ELISA or rapid tests. Virus isolation in cell culture is usually performed only in laboratories with the necessary infrastructure and technical expertise. For virus culture, it is important to keep blood samples cooled or frozen to preserve the viability of the virus during transport from the patient to the laboratory. The isolation and identification of dengue viruses in cell cultures usually takes several days."

"Nucleic acid detection assays with excellent performance characteristics may identify dengue viral RNA within 24–48 hours. However, these tests require expensive equipment and reagents and, in order to avoid contamination, tests must observe quality control procedures and must be performed by experienced technicians. NS1 antigen detection kits now becoming commercially available can be used in laboratories with limited equipment and yield results within a few hours."

"Rapid dengue antigen detection tests can be used in field settings and provide results in less than an hour. Currently, these assays are not type-specific, are expensive and are under evaluation for diagnostic accuracy and cost effectiveness in multiple settings."

"After day 5, dengue viruses and antigens disappear from the blood coincident with the appearance of specific antibodies. NS1 antigen may be detected in some patients for a few days after defervescence. Dengue serologic tests are more available in dengue-endemic countries than are virological tests. Specimen transport is not a problem as immunoglobulins are stable at tropical room temperatures. For serology, the time of specimen collection is more flexible than that for virus isolation or RNA detection because an antibody response can be measured by comparing a sample collected during the acute stage of illness with samples collected weeks or months later."

"Low levels of a detectable dengue IgM response – or the absence of it – in some secondary infections reduces the diagnostic accuracy of IgM ELISA tests. A four-fold or greater increase in antibody levels measured by IgG ELISA or by haemagglutination inhibition (HI) test in paired sera indicates an acute or recent Flavivirus infection. However, waiting for the convalescent serum collected at the time of patient discharge is not very useful for diagnosis and clinical management and provides only a retrospective result."

Dengue Fever and Related Syndromes
• Dengue viruses are arboviruses which may result in: **Asymptomatic infection, Dengue, Dengue hemorrhagic fever (DHF) & Dengue shock syndrome** (DSS)
• Dengue viruses have **4 serotypes^Q (Den 1, 2, 3, 4)**

Vector for dengue	Aedes aegypti^Q
Reservoir	Man, Mosquito^Q
Incubation period	5-6 days^Q

High-risk Patients for Dengue	
• Infants, elderly^Q	• Hemolytic disorders^Q (G6PD, Thalassemias)
• Obesity^Q	
• Pregnancy^Q	• Congenital heart disease^Q
• Peptic ulcer disease^Q	• Chronic disease
• Menstruating females	• Steroids/NSAIDs treatment

Dengue Fever and Related Syndromes		
Classical dengue fever (DF)	**Dengue hemorrhagic fever (DHF)**	**Dengue shock syndrome (DSS)**

• Also known as **'break bone fever'**[Q]
 • **Clinical features**[Q]: **High grade fever** (biphasic curve) with **chills, intense headache, muscle** and **joint pains, retro-orbital pain, photophobia, colicky pain, abdominal tenderness, skin rash**[Q]
	• Severe form of DF, caused by infection with more than one dengue virus type
	 • **Incubation period: 4-6 days**[Q]
	 • *Clinical features*[Q]: Features of DF plus:
	   – **Rash** less common
	   – **Rising hematocrit value (> 20% of baseline**[Q]**)**
	   – **Moderate-to-marked thrombocytopenia (<1 lac/mm³)**
	   – *Positive tourniquet test*[Q]: **>20 petechiae per sq. inch**
	 • **Diagnosis of DHF: Fever + hemorrhagic manifestations + thrombocytopenia + hemoconcentration or rising hematocrit**[Q]
		• **Diagnosis of DSS**[Q]: **DHF + shock [rapid & weak pulse, narrow pulse pressure (<20 mm Hg)/ hypotension, cold clammy skin, restlessness]**

Laboratory tests for Dengue

- Virus isolation within six days: Serum, plasma, autopsy tissue
- Viral nucleic acid detection (RT-PCR assay)

Diagnostic Method	Time to Results	Specimen	Time of collection after onset of symptoms
Viral isolation & serotype identification	**1–2 weeks**	Whole blood, serum, tissues	**1–5 days**[Q]
Nucleic acid detection	**1 or 2 days**	Tissues, whole blood, serum, plasma	**1–5 days**[Q]
Antigen detection	**1 day**	Serum	**1–6 days**[Q]
	>1 day	Tissue for immunochemistry	NA
IgM ELISA	**1–2 days**	Serum, plasma, whole blood	**After 5 days**[Q]
IgM rapid test	**30 minutes**		
IgG (paired sera) by **ELISA, HI** or **neutralization test**	**7 days or more**	Serum, plasma, whole blood	**Acute sera, 1–5 days**[Q]**; convalescent after 15 days**

WHO classification and Grading of Dengue Fevers

DHF Grade **I**	**Dengue fever + Hemorrhagic manifestations + Positive tourniquet test**
DHF Grade **II**	Grade I + Spontaneous bleeding
DHF Grade **III**	Grade II + Circulatory failure
DHF Grade **IV**	Grade III + Profound shock

- **DHF Grades III, IV** are **Dengue shock syndrome (DSS)**

Management of Dengue:
- DHF Grade I, II: Oral rehydration, Antipyretics
- DHF Grade III, IV: Colloidal solution, Fresh whole blood transfusion

Indications for Red cell transfusion	Indications for Platelets transfusion
• Loss of overt blood (>10% blood volume)[Q] • Refractory shock[Q]	• Prophylactic transfusion at count <10,000/mm[3Q] • Prolonged shock with coagulopathy[Q]

Criteria for discharge	
• Absence of fever >24 hours • Return of appetite • Visible clinical improvement • Good urine output	• Minimum 2-3 days after recovery from shock • No respiratory distress form pleural effusion/ ascites • Platelet count >50,000/cu.mm.

78. Ans. c. RT-PCR for rabies virus   *(Ref: Ananthanarayan 10/e p536, 8/e p529; Harrison 19/e p1302; Jawetz 27/e p610)*
RT-PCR techniques can accurately identify rabies genome in CSF, saliva, corneal scrapings or urine.

"Detection of rabies virus RNA by RT-PCR is highly sensitive and specific. This technique can detect virus in fresh saliva samples, skin, CSF, and brain tissues. In addition, RT-PCR with genetic sequencing can distinguish among rabies virus variants, permitting identification of the probable source of an infection."-Harrison 19/e p1302

"Reverse transcription-polymerase chain reaction testing can be used to amplify parts of a rabies virus genome from fixed or unfixed brain tissue or saliva. Sequencing of amplified products can allow identification of the infecting virus strain."- Jawetz 27/e p610

See Q. No. 79 AIIMS May 2017

79. Ans. a. Coxiella burnetii   *(Ref: Harrison 19/e p 1161; Ananthanarayan 10/e p418, 8/e p409; Jawetz 27/e p346)*
Coxiella burnetii is a small obligate intracellular organism having a membrane similar to Gram-negative bacteria.

"The agent of Q fever is Coxiella burnetii, a small intracellular prokaryote that only recently was grown in cell-free medium. C. burnetii, a pleomorphic coccobacillus with a Gram-negative cell wall, survives in harsh environments; it escapes intracellular killing in macrophages by inhibiting the final step in phagosome maturation (cathepsin fusion) and has adapted to the acidic phagolysosome by producing superoxide dismutase. Infection with C. burnetii induces a range of immunomodulatory responses, from immunosuppression in chronic Q fever to the production of autoantibodies, particularly those to smooth muscle and cardiac muscle."- Harrison 19/e p 1161

Obligate Intracellular Parasites (CRV CM PTL)		Facultative Intracellular Parasites (MBBS CRY For NHL)	
• Chlamydia[Q] • Rickettsia[Q] • (Ehrlichia & Anaplasma) • Viruses[Q] • Coxiella burnetii[Q] • Cryptosporidium parvum[Q]	• Mycobacterium leprae[Q] • Plasmodium species[Q] • Pneumocystis jiroveci[Q] • Toxoplasma gondii[Q] • Trypanosoma cruzi[Q] • Leishmania species[Q]	• Mycobacterium[Q] • Bartonella henselae[Q] • Brucella[Q] • Salmonella typhi[Q] • Cryptococcus neoformans[Q] • Rhodococcus equi[Q] • Yersinia[Q]	• Francisella tularensis[Q] • Nocardia[Q] • Neisseria meningitidis[Q] • Histoplasma capsulatum[Q] • Listeria monocytogenes[Q] • Legionella[Q]

Coxiella Burnetti

• **C. burnetii** is a **small obligate intracellular organism** having a **membrane similar to Gram-negative bacteria**[Q].
 • **Does not stain with Gram stain** but does **stain with Gimenez**[Q].
      • **Resistant to drying**, may **survive pasteurization at 60°C for 30 minutes**[Q]
      • Can **survive for months in dried feces or milk** because of **formation of endospore-like structures**[Q]
      • **Grow only in cytoplasmic vacuoles**[Q].

Antigens and Antigenic Variation:
- When grown in cell culture, C. burnetii exhibits various phases.

Phase I	Phase II
Phase I is **virulent form**, found in humans with[Q] **fever** & is **infectious form**[Q] **Key virulence factor: Lipopolysaccharide** expressed during phase I[Q]	Phase II forms are **not infectious**[Q] **Occur only** by serial passage **in cell cultures**[Q].

Epidemiology:
- C. burnetii is **found in ticks**, which **transmit the agent to sheep, goats & cattle**[Q]
- **Transmission by ticks to humans is uncommon.**
- **Transmitted by respiratory pathway** in workers of **slaughterhouses**[Q]
  - **Transmission** results **from inhalation of dust contaminated** with organism from **placenta, dried feces, urine, or milk or from aerosols** in slaughterhouses[Q].

Clinical Features:
- **Acute Q fever resembles influenza, nonbacterial (atypical) pneumonia & hepatitis**[Q].
- **Chronic Q fever** is infection that lasts **>6 months**. **Infective endocarditis** is **MC form** of disease **in this phase**[Q].

Laboratory Findings
- C. burnetii can be **cultivated in cell cultures**
- **Serology** is **diagnostic method of choice & (Best method: indirect immunofluorescence)**[Q]
- **PCR:** Useful in **diagnosis of culture-negative endocarditis** caused by C. burnetii[Q].

Treatment:
- **DOC for acute Q fever: Doxycycline**[Q]
- **Chronic Q fever: Prolonged treatment (≥18 months)** with a **doxycycline & hydroxychloroquine**[Q]

FORENSIC MEDICINE

80. **Ans. a. Ergot alkaloids** *(Ref: Reddy 34/e p517, 33/e p556; Parikh 6/e p9.32)*

After an overdose of medications derived from ergot or after eating flour milled from ergot-infected rye, humans and livestock may develop ergotism, a condition sometimes called St. Anthony's Fire.

*"Ergotism is the effect of long-term ergot poisoning, traditionally due to the ingestion of the **alkaloids produced by the Claviceps purpurea fungus** that infects rye and other cereals, and more recently by the action of a number of **ergoline-based drugs**. It is also known as **ergotoxicosis, ergot poisoning** and **Saint Anthony's Fire**. In the Middle Ages, the gangrenous poisoning was known as "holy fire" or "Saint Anthony's fire", named after monks of the Order of Saint Anthony who were particularly successful at treating this ailment."*

Ergot
• Ergot is **dried sclerotinum of** fungus **Claviceps purpurea** that **grow on rye, barley, wheat, oats**, etc[Q].   • **Active principles of ergot: Ergotoxin, ergotamine & ergometrine**[Q]   • **Fatal dose: 2-10 gm**[Q]   • **Fatal period: One to several days**[Q]

Mechanism of Action:
- Ergot alkaloids exert their primary effects by **stimulating adrenergic receptors**, both **peripherally & centrally**[Q].

Clinical Features:

Acute Poisoning	Chronic Poisoning (Ergotism)
• **Gastrointestinal effects:** Nausea, vomiting & diarrhoea • **CNS effects: Headache**, giddiness • **Respiratory: Chest tightness**, difficulty in breathing[Q] • **Musculoskeletal:** Marked muscular weakness & exhaustion, **tingling & numbness** in hands & feet, paraesthesias[Q] • **Hematological: Bleeding** from nose & other mucous surface	• **Tingling & numbness** of skin[Q] • Vasomotor disturbances leading to **dry gangrene** of fingers[Q] • Sensation of insects creeping under skin (**tactile hallucination/formication**)[Q] • Associated with **St. Anthony's Fire**[Q] (Consumption of Rye bread contaminated with Ergot causing **burning sensation of limbs**[Q])

Contd...

Contd...

Ergot
Treatment: • Gastric lavage, activated charcoal & cathartics   • **Nitroprusside** for **hypertension & severe ischemic changes**^{Q} • **IV diazepam for convulsions**^{Q}

81. Ans. d. Section 92 *(Ref: Reddy 34/e p51, 33/e p51; Parikh 6/e p1.36)*

Under Sections 92 of Indian Penal Code (IPC), neurosurgeon can perform the procedure without obtaining an informed consent from a guardian.

Laws Related to Consent	
Section 53 (1) CrPC	• In **criminal cases** when examination of an **arrested person** can lead to vital evidence related with the commission of crime, he can be **examined by the doctor without his consent and even using force**, if the application for examination is from a person not below the rank of sub Inspector.
Section 54 CrPC	• An **arrested person can also request to be examined by a doctor to detect any evidence,** which he feels is good for him.
Section 87 IPC	• A person >18 years of age can give consent to suffer any harm if the act is not intended & not known to cause death or grievous hurt.
Section 89 IPC	• A **child <12 years of age** or **a person of unsound mind cannot give consent to suffer any harm** for an act which may cause grievous hurt or death even if done in good faith, but the consent has to be obtained from the guardian of the child or a sane person.
Section 90 IPC	• **Consent given by an insane person** or **given under fear of injury, death** etc. or **due to misconception of a fact** is **invalid.**
Section 92 IPC	• **Any harm caused to a person in good faith even without the person's consent is not an offence if the circumstances were such that it was impossible to obtain consent of the person** or **his lawful guardian at that material time for that thing to be done for the benefit of the person**. However the act should not extend to intentionally causing hurt other than for preventing death, grievous hurt or curing of disease or infirmity.

Exceptions to the Informed Consent	
Doctrine of Therapeutic Procedure	• Certain **procedural details** (especially **invasive tests** or **complicated surgery**) may be **difficult to explain to the patient**^{Q}. • Often **patients** themselves **do not want to know about it.** • It is better to **explain to family members**
Doctrine of Emergency	• Under Section **92 of IPC, treating without consent of patient** is permissible **if patient is unconscious, mentally ill** or **gravely sick & no attendant with the patient**^{Q}. • It is implied that the **procedure/surgery is done to save the life** or **limb of the patient**. • If possible, surrogate/proxy consent should be taken.
Doctrine of Loco Parentis	• In **children in an emergency,** when **parents/guardians are not available,** consent can be obtained **from the person bringing the child**^{Q} (school teacher etc).
Incompetence	• **Incompetent patients** such as **delirious, unconscious, senile, psychotic natures** etc. are **unable to make rational decision.** In these cases they can be **treated without informed consent** involving the "Emergency" doctrine^Q.
Therapeutic Privilege	• If doctor suspects that **passing full information could have detrimental effect on the health of the patient** than **he need not follow "Doctrine of Full Disclosure"** and can be **excused of obtaining consent from the patient**^{Q}. • However, to take the privilege of the doctrine, he should **disclose full information to the competent relative of the patient**^{Q}.

82. Ans. c. Sulfhemoglobin *(Ref: Reddy 34/e p157, 33/e p166)*

The given picture is of marbling of skin, caused by deposition of sulfhemoglobin.

"Marbling of skin: The superficial veins especially over the roots of the limbs, thigh, sides of the abdomen, shoulders, chest and neck are stained greenish-brown or purplish-red depending on the total amount of sulfhemoglobin formation within the affected vessels (linear branching pattern) due to the hemolysis of red cells, which stains the wall of the vessel and infiltrates into the tissue, giving a marbled appearance (red, then greenish pattern in skin resembling the branches of tree)."- Reddy 33/e p166

Marbling of skin

- **Superficial veins** especially over the **roots of limbs, thigh, sides of abdomen, shoulders, chest & neck** are **stained greenish-brown** or **purplish-red** depending on the **total amount of sulfhemoglobin formation**^{Q} within the **affected vessels (linear branching pattern**^{Q}**)** due to **hemolysis of red cells**, which stains the wall of the vessel and infiltrates into the tissue, **giving a marbled appearance**^{Q} **(red, then greenish pattern in skin resembling the branches of tree)**.
- This **starts in 24 hours,** but is **prominent in 36–48 hours**^{Q}.
- Clotted blood becomes fluid & position of postmortem staining is altered & fluid blood collects in serous cavities.
- **Reddish-green colour of the skin** may become **dark green** or almost **black in 3–4 days**^{Q}.

83. **Ans. d. Section 269** *(Ref: Reddy 34/e p53, 33/e p44; Parikh 6/e p1.10; Textbook on the Indian Penal Code by Krishna Deo Gaur 4th/594; the-indian-penal-code-pdf-d74214920)*

The doctor here has done a negligent act, which has caused HIV to a patient. This is punishable under Section 269 of IPC.

269 IPC	• **Negligent act** likely to **spread infection** or **disease dangerous to life**^{Q}
270 IPC	• **Malignant act** likely to **spread infection** or **disease dangerous to life**^{Q}

Important Criminal Procedure Codes (CrPC)

CrPC	Description
39	**Doctor is duty bound to provide information about enlisted offences to the police**^{Q}
53	Examination of **accused by medical practitioner at request of police**^{Q}
53A	Examination of **accused of rape**^{Q}
54	Examination of **arrested person by medical officer at request of arrested person**^{Q}
61	**Format of summons**^{Q}
62	**Summons how served**^{Q}
70	**Form of warrant of arrest and duration**^{Q}
174	**Police inquest**^{Q}
176	**Magistrates inquest**^{Q}
238-265	**Magistrates trial**^{Q}
293	**Exception to oral evidence**^{Q}
327	**Open trial-closed room In camera trial-rape cases**^{Q}
416	**Postponement of capital sentence pregnant woman**^{Q}

Important Indian Evidence Acts (IEA)

IEA	Description
114A	• **Doctrine of adverse inference**^{Q} (presume absence of consent)
137	• **Recording of evidence**^{Q}
139	• **Cross-examination of a person called to produce a document**^{Q}
141	• **Leading questions**^{Q}
152	• **Question intending to insult or annoy**^{Q}
159	• **Refreshing memory**^{Q}
162	• **Production of documents**^{Q}

Section	Deals with
44 IPC	• **Definition of injury** (any harm caused to a person in body, mind, reputation or property)
53 IPC	• An **accused** can be **examined** by a medical practitioner **at the request of police**, even without his consent and by use of force^Q
84 IPC	• **Insanity & criminal responsibility**^{Q}
85 IPC	• **Criminal responsibility** of a person **incapable of judgment** by reasons **intoxication** caused **against his will**
191 IPC	• Defines **perjury** or **hostile witness**^{Q}
193 IPC	• **Punishment for perjury**^{Q}
197 IPC	• Punishment for **doctors** for submitting **false medical certificates**

AIIMS November 2016

Section	Deals with
202 IPC	• Intentional omission to give information of offence by person bound to inform
228A IPC	• **Disclosure of identity of victim** of certain offences **under Section 376 (rape)**[Q]
269 IPC	• **Negligent act** likely to **spread infection** or **disease dangerous to life**[Q]
270 IPC	• **Malignant act** likely to **spread infection** or **disease dangerous to life**[Q]
299 IPC	• **Culpable homicide**[Q]
300 IPC	• **Definition of murder**[Q]
302 IPC	• **Punishment for murder**[Q]
304A IPC	• Causing death by negligence, punishment up to 2 years (medical negligence)
304B IPC	• **Dowry death**[Q], **punishment 7 years to life imprisonment**
306 IPC	• **Abetment of suicide**[Q]
307 IPC	• **Attempt to murder**[Q]
308 IPC	• Abetment to **commit culpable homicide**[Q]
312 IPC	• Causing **illegal miscarriage with woman's consent**[Q]
313 IPC	• Causing **illegal miscarriage without woman's consent**[Q]
314 IPC	**Death of mother** caused by **act done with intent to cause miscarriage**[Q]
315 IPC	Act done with **intent to prevent child being born alive** or to **cause it to die after birth**[Q]
316 IPC	Causing **death of quick unborn child** by act amounting to culpable homicide[Q]
317 IPC	Exposure & abandonment of child under 12 years
318 IPC	Concealment of birth by secret disposal of dead body
319 IPC	Definition of Hurt (whoever causes bodily pain, disease, or infirmity to any person is said to cause hurt)
320 IPC	**Grievous hurt**[Q] definition
321 IPC	**Voluntarily causing hurt**[Q]
322 IPC	**Voluntarily causing Grievous hurt**[Q]
323 IPC	Punishment for **voluntarily causing hurt**
324 IPC	Voluntarily causing hurt by dangerous weapons or means
325 IPC	Punishment for voluntarily causing grievous hurt
326 IPC	Voluntarily causing **grievous hurt by dangerous weapons or means**
330 IPC	Voluntarily causing hurt to extort confession or to compel restoration of property
331 IPC	Voluntarily causing grievous hurt to extort confession or to compel restoration of property
351 IPC	**Deals with assault**[Q]
354 IPC	Assault or criminal force to woman with intent to outrage her modesty
375 IPC	**Defines rape**[Q]
376 IPC	**Punishment of rape**[Q]
377 IPC	**Unnatural sexual offences**[Q]
497 IPC	Adultery

84. **Ans. a. Yellow colored sputum** *(Ref: Reddy 33/e p325-326; Parikh 6/e p4.160)*

In the question, patient presented in emergency with grade 3 burn which points towards acute burn injury. Yellow sputum/ phlegm is mostly a sign of bacterial infection, and takes time to develop. In grade 3 burns, sputum will be carbonaceous colored. Singeing of facial hair seen in acute burns inhalation injury, burns on face, soot marks & singed eyebrows or facial hair are indicative of inhalational injury.

"Smoke inhalation is the leading cause of death due to fires. It produces injury through several mechanisms, including thermal injury to the upper airway, irritation or chemical injury to the airways from soot, asphyxiation, and toxicity from carbon monoxide (CO) and other gases such as cyanide."

"Features characteristic of inhalation injury include history of fire in an enclosed space, burns of the face, singed nasal and facial hair, inflamed pharyngeal mucosa, carbonaceous sputum, and evidence of edematous glottis (e.g., hoarseness)."

'Clinical indicators' of existence of smoke inhalation
1. **Facial burns**[Q]
2. **Singeing of nasal hair or eyebrows**[Q]
3. **Oropharyngeal acute inflammatory changes**[Q] (swelling, ulceration of oral mucosa, or tongue)
4. **Soot** (carbonaceous materials) in the **oropharynx or sputum**[Q]
5. **Airway obstruction, hoarseness, stridor or wheezing**[Q]
6. A history of impaired mentation (or unconsciousness) and/or being trapped in a burning location.
7. **Carboxyhemoglobin level** >10% if the patient is involved in a fire[Q]

85. **Ans. a. Wormian bones**   *(Ref: Reddy 34/e p417; Parikh 6/e p4.187)*

Wormian bones are seen in Osteogenesis imperfecta and not child abuse.

"With severe and varied changes in the metaphyses, periosteal new bone formation or epiphyseal separation, always consider the possibility of non-accidental injuries – the 'battered baby' syndrome."-Apley 9/e p155

"The histopathology of the classic metaphyseal lesion (CML) shows "a subepiphyseal planar series of microfractures through the most immature portion of metaphyseal bone. The fracture involves disruption of the priomary spongiosa and calcified cartilage core at the metaphysis of long bones, the site where maximum bone growth and turnover is occurring. Radiographically, the CML often appears as a "corner" or "bucket handle" fracture."- Child Abuse and Neglect: Diagnosis, Treatment, and Evidence By Carole Jenny (2010)/p277

"Of all the injuries observed in child physical abuse, none is more specific than the metaphyseal fracture. First described in 1957 by the eminent pediatric radiologist John Caffey, metaphyseal fracture is virtually pathognomonic of abuse. Kleinman et al coined the term classic metaphyseal lesion (CML) to describe the injury. CMLs are relatively common in abused infants and are discovered in 39%–50% of abused children less than 18 months of age. Thus, CMLs are highly specific for abuse, although they are observed in half or fewer of cases. Overall, CMLs most often occur in the distal femur, proximal tibia, distal tibia, and proximal humerus. They are seen almost exclusively in children less than 2 years of age for reasons detailed in the following biomechanical discussion. The elegant work of Kleinman and colleagues in the 1980s established the histologic definition of the CML as a series of microfractures in the subepiphyseal region of bone."- http://pubs.rsna.org/doi/full/10.1148/rg.234035030

"Osteogenesis imperfecta: There is generalized osteopenia, thinning of the long bones, fractures in various stages of healing, vertebral compression and spinal deformity. The type of abnormality varies with the severity of the disease. The skull may be enlarged and shows the presence of Wormian bones– areas of vicarious ossification in the calvarium. After puberty, fractures occur less frequently, but in those who survive the incidence rise again after the climacteric. It is thought that very mild ('subclinical') forms of OI may account for some cases of recurrent fractures in adults."- Apley 9/e p173

Battered Baby Syndrome (Caffey's Syndrome/Infantile Whiplash Syndrome)
• **Battered child:** Child who has received **repetitive physical injuries** as a result of **non-accidental violence, produced by a parent or guardian**[Q].
• **Age of child:** <3 years; often **unwanted or illegitimate**[Q]
• **Violence included:** Physical abuse, sexual abuse, emotional abuse, nutritional deprivation, intentional drugging or neglect of medical care[Q]
Classical Features:
• **Discrepancy between the nature of injuries & explanation offered by the parents**[Q]
• **Delay between injury & medical attention**[Q]
• **Repetition of injuries at different dates**, progressing from minor to more severe[Q]
Injuries Type & Pattern:
• **MC method of injury: Direct manual violence**[Q]
• **Most characteristic lesion: Laceration of mucosa inside the upper lip with tear of frenulum & alveolar margins of gums**[Q]
• Bruises of varying age, burns, lacerations, **retinal & subhyaloid hemorrhage**, rib fractures, **spiral fractures of long bones & displaced epiphysis**, subperiosteal hematoma[Q]
• **Major cause of subdural hematoma & intraocular bleeding: Effects of violent shaking (Infantile whiplash syndrome)**[Q]
• **MC cause of death: Head injury (Fracture skull or subdural hematoma) >Rupture of abdominal organs (Ruptured liver & mesenteric hemorrhage)**[Q]

Contd...

Contd...

Battered Baby Syndrome (Caffey's Syndrome/Infantile Whiplash Syndrome)
• **Chest is compressed resulting in rib fractures. Rib fractures are very common & highly specific for abuse in young children <2 years[Q].**
• **Arms & legs move about in a whiplash movement** resulting in the typical **'corner' or 'bucket-handle'-fractures in metaphyseal region[Q].**
• **Classical metaphyseal corner[Q]** or bucket handle fracture is **virtually pathognomonic for abuse[Q].**
• **Fractures of acromion, sternum & spinous processes** are having **high specificity** for abuse[Q].
• **Occipital impression** & other skull fractures occur when the head strikes a solid object[Q].
• **Patterns of skull fracture that suggest child abuse are: Multiple 'eggshell' fractures[Q]**, occipital impression fractures[Q] & fractures crossing sutures[Q]

86. Ans. c. 7 months *(Ref: Reddy 34/e p81, 33/e p84; Parikh 6/e p5.67; Modi 22/e p602)*

Estimated age of the fetus is 7 months as pupillary membrane disappears at 7 months. The testes reach the level of superficial inguinal ring at 7 months. At 7 months, weight is 900-1200 gm.

• **Hasse rule is most commonly used criteria to estimate fetal age,** which states that square root of the length of the fetus in cm gives the approx. age in months in the first five months. After the fifth month, the length in cm divided by five gives the age in months. Head to feet length is not same as CHL (crown-heel length).

• Crown-Rump length, CRL=2/3 CHL
                         • CHL= 3/2 CRL
                         • CHL= $3/2 \times 23 = 34.5 \approx 35$ cm
                         • Now, applying Hasse rule
                         • Age= 35/5 = 7 months

• **Pupillary membrane disappears at 7 months.**
• **The testes reach at the level of superficial inguinal ring at 7 months.**
• Weight at **7 months** is 900-1200 gm (**1000 gm**).

Rule of Hasse
• Rule of Hasse is used to determine the age of fetus from crown to heel length in cm.
• During first five months, **Length in cm = (Age in months)^2**
• **After age of >5 months, Age in months = (Length in cm)/5[Q]**

Age of the Fetus	
End of **first** month	• Length 1 cm, weight two and half gram • Eyes are seen as two dark spots & mouth as a cleft
End of **second** month	• **Length 4 cm**, weight 10 gms • **Hands & feet are webbed[Q]** • Anus is seen as a dark spot
End of **third** month	• Length 9 cm, weight 30 gms • **Eyes are closed[Q]**, pupillary membrane appears • Nails appear and neck is formed
End of **fourth** month	• **Length 16 cm, weight 120 gms[Q]** • **Sex can be recognized[Q]**
End of **fifth** month	• Length 25 cm, weight 400 gms • **Nails are distinct & soft[Q]** • **Light hairs appear on head[Q]**
End of **sixth** month	• Length 30 cm, weight 700 gms • **Eyebrow and eyelashes appear[Q]** • **Subcutaneous fat begins to be deposited[Q]** • Testes are seen close to kidney
End of **seventh** month	• **Length 35 cm, weight 900-1200 gms[Q]** • Nails are thick • **Eyelids open & pupillary membrane disappears[Q]** • **Testes found at external inguinal ring[Q]**

Contd...

AIIMS ESSENCE

Contd...

Age of the Fetus	
End of **eighth** month	• Length 40 cm, weight one & half to two kg • **Nails reach the tips of fingers**[Q] • **Left testes in scrotum**[Q]
End of **ninth** month	• Length 45 cm, weight two & half to three kg • **Scalp hair is dark & 4 cm long**[Q] • **Scrotum is wrinkled & contains both testes**[Q]
End of **tenth** month	• Length 50-53 cm, weight 2.5-5 kg • **Nails project beyond the end of fingers** but **reach only the tip of toes**[Q]

87. Ans. b. 1-ii, 2-iii, 3-iv, 4-i   *(Ref: Reddy 34/e p278, 600, 33/e p26, 400, 647; Parikh 6/e p1.26)*

Declaration of **Geneva (1948)**	• **Modernized version of Hippocratic oath**[Q]
Declaration of **London (1949)**	• International code of **medical ethics**
Declaration of **Helsinki (1964)**	• **Human experimentation & clinical trials**[Q]
Declaration of **Sydney (1968)**	• Definition of **death & recovery of organs**
Declaration of **Oslo (1970)**	• **Therapeutic (legalized) abortion**[Q]
Declaration of **Munich (1973)**	• Discrimination in medicine
Declaration of **Tokyo (1975)**	• **Torture & medicine**[Q]
Declaration of **Lisbon (1981)**	• Rights of patients
Declaration of **Venice (1983)**	• Terminal illness
Declaration of **Malta (1992)**	• Role of doctors in hunger strikes
Declaration of **Istanbul (2008)**	• Organ trafficking & transplant tourism

88. Ans. c. Conium maculatum   *(Ref: Reddy 34/e p371, 33/e p614; Parikh 6/e p10.57-10.60)*

Typical ascending paralysis as described in the question is seen in poisoning with Conium or hemlock.

> *"**Conium Maculatum**: The odour of dried leaves is strong and narcotic. **Ingestion causes burning in mouth and throat, gastric inflammation, vomiting, diarrhea, slow respiration**, increased and later slow pulse, mental confusion, tremors, ataxia, sometimes blindness, **progressive motor paralysis extending upwards from the extremities, come and death from respiratory paralysis.**"- Reddy 34/e p371*

Conium Maculatum (Hemlock)
• **Conium maculatum contains coniine & seven other alkaloids.** • **Coniine content** is **highest** in the **unripe fruit** & in the **seeds,** in the **leaves** especially at flowering time & in the **root** particularly during summer[Q]. • **Toxic properties** are due to alkaloids **coniine & methyl coniine**[Q] • **Hemlock** was **administered to Socrates** as a form of **execution**[Q].
Mechanism of Action: • **Coniine & methyl coniine** cause **paralysis of motor nerve terminals in muscles,** gradually **spreading to motor cells of cord & brain**[Q].
• **Fatal dose: 60 mg of coniine**[Q] • **Fatal period: Few hours**[Q]

Symptoms & Signs:
• Odour of dried leaves is **strong & narcotic**. Breath may have a **mousy odor**[Q].
      • There may be some **gastric irritation**, which causes **pain & vomiting**[Q].
      • This is **followed by muscular weakness & gradually increasing paralysis due to depression of motor nerves**[Q].
      • **Lower limbs are first affected & paralysis ascends till the muscles of respiration are affected**[Q].
• Delirium, convulsions or coma may supervene & **patient dies of asphyxia due to respiratory paralysis**[Q].

Conium Maculatum (Hemlock)
Treatment:
• **Gastric lavage** with a dilute solution of **tannic acid, artificial respiration, oxygen inhalations & stimulants**[Q].

89. **Ans. c. Vasopressors should be administered intravenously** *(Ref: Reddy 34/e p487, 33/e p; Parikh 6/e p10.41-10.45)*
The signs and symptoms are suggestive of organophosphorus poisoning. The antidote of choice is atropine and it is used to revert the bradycardia and hypotension. Blood pressure of the patient (90/53) is not too low. Vasopressors are not indicated, as it is due to cholinergic effect and is combated by atropine.

Organophosphorus Poisoning
• The effect of **acute intoxication by one anti-choninesterase agents** are manifested by **muscarinic** and **nicotinic signs & symptoms.**
• Systemic effects appear within minutes after inhalation of vapors or aerosols.
• In contrast, the onset of symptoms is delayed after GI & percutaneous absorption.
• **Typical smell of organophosphorus compounds**, which is a **pungent garlic-like odour**[Q].
• **Organophosphorus irreversibly inhibits acetyl cholinesterase decreasing its activity**[Q].

Severity of poisoning	Acetyl cholinesterase activity
Mild poisoning	**20–50%** of normal
Moderate poisoning	**10–20%** of normal
Severe poisoning	**<10%** of normal

Manifestation:
- Nicotinic action at NMJ of skeletal muscle consists of **fatigability & generalized weakness, involuntary twitchings, scattered fasciculations & eventually severe weakness & paralysis**[Q].

> - **Most serious consequence** is **paralysis of respiratory muscle**[Q].
> - **Ocular manifestations: Miosis**[Q], pain, conjunctival congestion, diminished vision, ciliary spasm

- **Respiratory effects: Tightness in the chest, wheezing respiration**[Q]
- **GI effects:** Anorexia, nausea, vomiting, cramps
- Others: **Extreme salivation, involuntary defecation, lacrimation, bradycardia, hypotension, penile erection**[Q]

Red Tears or Chromolacryorrhea
• **Shedding of red tears due to accumulation of porphyrin pigments in lacrimal glands**[Q]
• **Very rare phenomenon, seen in organophosphorus poisoning**[Q]

Treatment:
- Termination of further exposure to the poison
- **Maintain patent airway**[Q], positive pressure ventilation if it is failing
- **Supportive measures:** Maintain BP, hydration, control of **convulsions** with judicious use of **diazepam**[Q]

> - Specific antidote:
>   – Atropine: It is highly effective in counteracting the muscarinic symptoms but higher doses are required to antagonize the central effects. It doesn't reverse peripheral muscular paralysis[Q].
> - Pralidoxime:
>   – Reactivate inhibited cholinesterase, remove the block at NM junction, prevent formation of phosphorylated enzyme & directly detoxify organophosphates[Q].
>   – Decrease the amount of atropine required & potentiates the action of atropine[Q].

- **Gastric lavage**: Consider for presentations **within one or two hours**[Q], when the airway is protected. A single aspiration of the gastric contents may be as useful as lavage.
- **Activated charcoal without cathartic:** In **cooperative or intubated patients**[Q], particularly if they are admitted within one or two hours or have severe toxicity.
- **Vasopressors: Severe hypotension**[Q] might benefit from vasopressors.

Characteristic Odours produced by Toxins	
Odour	**Toxins**
Acrid (Pear smell)	• **Paraldehyde**[Q]**, Chloral hydrate**[Q]
Bitter almonds	• **Cyanide**[Q]
Burnt rope	• **Marijuana (Cannabis)**[Q]
Disinfectant	• **Phenol** (Carbolic acid), Creosote
Garlic	• **Phosphorus**[Q], Tellurium, Thallium • Dimethyl sulfoxide (DMSO)
Fish or raw liver (Musty)	• **Zinc phosphide**[Q]**, Aluminum phosphide**[Q]
Kerosene like	• **Organophosphate**[Q]
Mint	• Methylsalicylate (Oil of Wintergreen), Menthol
Mothballs	• Naphthalene, Camphor, p-dichlorobenzene
Pepper	• o-chlorobenzylidene malonitrile (Tear gas)
Rotten eggs	• **Hydrogen sulphide**[Q]**, Carbon disulphide**[Q] • **Mercaptans· Disulfiram**[Q]**, N-acetylcysteine**[Q]
Shoe polish	• **Nitrobenzene**[Q]
Vinegar	• **Acetic acid**[Q]**; Hydrofluoric acid**[Q]

90. **Ans. a. Osmium blue**   *(Ref: Reddy 34/e p89, 33/e p92)*

Osmin blue is not used for tattooing.

> *"Tattoo marks are design made in the skin by multiple puncture wounds with needles or an electric vibrator dipped in colouring matter. The dyes commonly used are Indian ink, carbon (black), cinnabar or vermilion (mercuric sulphide) red, chromic acid (green), indigo, cobalt, Prussian blue (ferric ferrocyanide), ultramarine (blue)."- Reddy 34/e p89, 33/e p92*

> *"Osmium tetroxide is used in optical microscopy to stain lipids. It dissolves in fats, and is reduced by organic materials to elemental osmium, an easily visible black substance."*

Tattoos

- Tattoos are a characteristic pattern or design **made by multiple puncture wound using a needle or an electric vibrator dipped in ink**
- **Dyes commonly used are Indian ink**[Q]**, carbon**[Q] **(black), cinnabar**[Q] **or vermilion (mercuric sulphide) red, chromic acid (green), indigo, cobalt, Prussian blue (ferric ferrocyanide), ultramarine (blue)**[Q]**.**

> - **Faded tattoo mark** become **visible by ultraviolet lamp**[Q]**.**
> - **Infrared photography** makes old tattoo visible[Q]**.**
> - **Cannot be used as identification mark in burnt & decomposed dead bodies**[Q]**.**

Pathology of tattoo:
- **Dye injected into dermis** is **phagocytized by macrophages**, which are **permanent**
- After several weeks, they localize around vessels in upper & mid dermis in macrophages & fibroblasts
- **Extracellular deposits of pigment** are also found between **collagen bundles**; pigment is generally refractile

Different Dyes used to Impart Different Colors	
Dye	**Color**
• **Indian ink, Carbon, China ink, Soot**	**Black**
• **Cinnabar, Vermilion**	**Red**
• **Ochre**	**Brown**
• **Chromic oxide**	**Green**
• **Prussian blue (Ferric ferrocyanide)** • **Indigo, Cobalt, Ultramarine**	**Blue**

Methods to Erase Tattoo:
- Burning & scarring, laser, corrosives & caustic chemicals (Glycerin + papain),
- Dry ice, electrolysis, excision & graft

AIIMS November 2016

PSM

91. Ans. d. 80/100   *(Ref: Park 24/e p149-151, 23/e p125; 22/e p131)*

Assessment & Value of a Diagnostic Test		
	Condition Present	**Condition Absent**
Positive Test	a (True positive)	b (False positive)
Negative Test	c (False negative)	d (True negative)

Sensitivity	Proportion of persons with the condition who test positive: $a/(a + c)$[Q]
Specificity	Proportion of persons without the condition who test negative: $d/(b + d)$[Q]
Positive predictive value (PPV)	Proportion of persons with a positive test who have the condition: $a/(a + b)$[Q]
Negative predictive value (NPV)	Proportion of persons with a negative test who do not have the condition: $d/(c + d)$[Q]

Predictive Value
• **Prevalence, sensitivity, and specificity determine predictive value**[Q]
• **PPV = Prevalence × Sensitivity /(Prevalence × Sensitivity) + (1 − Prevalence)(1 − Specificity)**[Q]
• **NPV = (1 − Prevalence)(Specificity) /(1 − Prevalence)(Specificity) + (1 − Sensitivity)(Prevalence)**[Q]

- According to the data presented here, the following 2×2 contingency table can be made, considering CA-125 as the test and histopathology as definite evidence of the disease.

	Disease present	Disease absent
Test Positive	60 (a: TP)	40 (b: FP)
Test Negative	20 (c: FN)	80 (d: TN)
Total	80	120

- **Negative Predictive Value (NPV) = Number of true negatives/(Number of true negatives + number of false negative)**
- **True negatives = 80**
- **Total negatives = 100**
- **Negative predictive value = 80/100 = 80%**

92. Ans. a. There is positive correlation between two groups   *(Ref: Evaluation of pulse-oximetry oxygen saturation taken through skin protective covering: Jyotsna James, Lokesh Tiwari, Pramod Upadhyay, Vishnubhatla Sreenivas, Vikas Bhambhani and Jacob M Puliyel; BMC Pediatrics, 2006, 6:14)*

The figure and the case is taken directly from a study "Evaluation of pulse-oximetry oxygen saturation taken through skin protective covering" done at St, Stephen's Hospital, New Delhi. The conclusion drawn from the given plot is that there is positive correlation between two groups.

Correlation	Agreement
• Correlation studies the **relationship between two variables** not the difference	• **Agreement studies the difference between the two variables**
• **Calculated by regression analysis plot**	• **Calculated by Bland Altman plot**
• **Perfect correlation if the points lie along any straight line.**	• **Perfect agreement only if the points in Fig. 1 lie along the line of equality**
• **Change in scale of measurement does not affect the correlation,** if we were to plot calipers measurement against half calipers measurement, for skin fold thickness the correlation would be 1.0	• Change in scale of measurement affects the agreement. If we were to plot calipers measurement against half calipers measurement the two measurements would not agree. Since one is twice the other
• **Test of significance (P value) may show that the two methods are correlated**	• The test of significance is irrelevant to the question of agreement

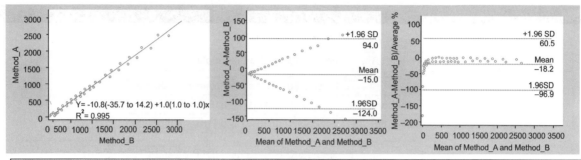

Bland and Altman Analysis

- **Bland-Altman analysis** is a statistical method, which **allows the clinician to compare two different measurement techniques**[Q].
- **Bland-Altman graph plots the difference between two techniques against their averages**[Q].
- Typically **used to compare measurement techniques against a reference value**, especially when the reference value may not have a true gold standard.
  - Bland and Altman suggest that **when a new technology has bias and precision comparable with the previous technology, then it may be accepted in the clinical setting**[Q].
  - **Focus exclusively on differences**[Q].

	Evaluation of Pulse-Oximetry Oxygen Saturation Taken Through Skin Protective Covering
Back-ground	• The hard edges of adult finger clip probes of the pulse oximetry oxygen saturation (POOS) monitor can cause skin damage if used for prolonged periods in a neonate. • Covering the skin under the probe with Micropore surgical tape or a gauze piece might prevent such injury. • The study was done to see if the protective covering would affect the accuracy of the readings.
Methods	• POOS was studied in 50 full-term neonates in the first week of life. After obtaining consent from their parents the neonates had POOS readings taken directly (standard technique) and through the protective covering. • Bland-Altman plots were used to compare the new method with the standard technique. A test of repeatability for each method was also performed.
Results	• The Bland-Altman plots suggest that there is no significant loss of accuracy when readings are taken through the protective covering. • The mean difference was 0.06 (SD of 1.39) and 0.04 (SD 1.3) with Micropore and gauze respectively compared to the standard method. The mean difference was 0.22 (SD 0.23) on testing repeatability with the standard method.
Conclu-sion	• Interposing Micropore or gauze does not significantly affect the accuracy of the POOS reading. The difference between the standard method and the new method was less than the difference seen on testing repeatability of the standard method.

93. **Ans. a. A: Mode; B: Median; C: Mean** *(Ref: Park 23/e p847, 24/e p884)*

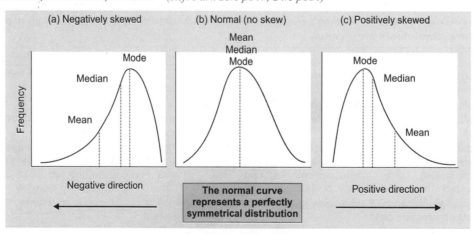

Measures of Central Tendency

- An **average or central tendency of a data** set refers to a **measure of the middle or expected value of the data set**. It gives a **mental picture of the central value**[Q].
- Commonly used statistical averages: **Mean, Median & Mode**

Mean	Median	Mode
- **Most commonly used**[Q] statistical average. - Obtained as sum of all values divided by no. of values - **Advantage:** Easy to calculate & understand[Q]. - **Disadvantage:** Sometimes it may be **unduly influenced by abnormal values**[Q] (either very high or very low) in the distribution	- **Middle most value**[Q] in the distribution arranged in an ascending or descending order of values - It **does not depend on the total & number of items**[Q]. - If there are two values in the middle instead of one, the median is worked out by taking the average of the two middle values. - **Advantage:** The value of median is **not affected by abnormal very high or very low value**[Q]. - Median is used when distribution of values is skewed with some small number of very high values[Q].	- **Most frequent** or **most commonly occurring value**[Q] in a distribution - Mode = Average of 2 modes in Bimodal distribution (If there are **2 most frequent value in the distribution**[Q]) - **Advantage:** Not affected by extreme items[Q] (skewed deviation). - **Disadvantage:** Exact location is often uncertain and is often not clearly defined[Q].

Distribution	Central Tendency
Normal (Gaussian) Distribution	Mean = Median = Mode[Q]
Right (Positive) Skew Distribution	Mean > Median > Mode[Q]
Left (Negative) Skew Distribution	Mean < Median < Mode[Q]

In Distribution with Extreme Values (Outliers)	
- **Most affected** measure of central tendency	Mean[Q]
- **Least affected** measure of central tendency	Mode[Q]
- **Most preferable** measure of central tendency	Median[Q]

94. **Ans. c. Receiver-operating characteristic curve** *(Ref: http://www.lexjansen.com/nesug/nesug10/hl/hl07.pdf)*
    Receiver-operating characteristic (ROC) curve is the best for determining the threshold for diagnosis of a positive test.

    "The receiver operating characteristic (ROC) curve, which is defined as a plot of test sensitivity as the y coordinate versus its 1-specificity or false positive rate (FPR) as the x coordinate, is an effective method of evaluating the performance of diagnostic tests."-https://www.ncbi.nlm.nih.gov/pmc/articles/PMC2698108/

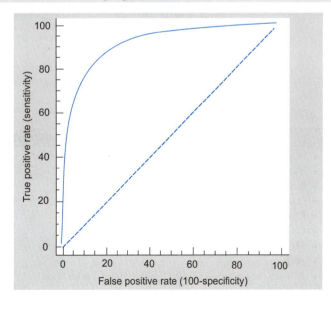

"Receiver-operating characteristic (ROC) curves are an excellent way to compare diagnostic tests." - http://ebp.uga.edu/courses/Chapter%204%20-%20Diagnosis%20I/8%20-%20ROC%20curves.html

*"ROC curve is a **graphic presentation of the relationship between both sensitivity and specificity** and it helps to decide the optimal model through determining the best threshold for the diagnostic test. Accuracy measures how correct a diagnostic test identifies and excludes a given condition. Accuracy of a diagnostic test can be determined from sensitivity and specificity with the presence of prevalence."* - http://www.lexjansen.com/nesug/nesug10/hl/hl07.pdf

95. **Ans. b. Cross-sectional study** *(Ref: Park 24/e p74, 23/e p69; 22/e p76)*

The study design in which a type of observational study is done that analyzes data collected from a population, or a representative subset, at a specific point in time, just like in the questions is known as cross-sectional study.

*"**Cross-sectional study** is the **simplest form of an observational study**. It is **based on a single examination of a cross-section of population at one point of time**- the results of which can be projected on the whole population provided the sampling has been done correctly. **Cross sectional study** is also known as **prevalence study.**"- Park 23/e p69*

Cross-sectional Study	• **Simplest form** of an **observational study**[Q]. • Based on a **single examination of a cross-section of population at one point of time**[Q] • **More useful for chronic rather than short-lived diseases**[Q] • Provides **information about prevalence** (Also known as **prevalence study**[Q]) • It provides **little information about incidence** or **natural history of disease**[Q].
Field Trial	• Type of **interventional trial**[Q] • Deals with **disease-free subjects**[Q] • **Conducted in the 'field'** rather than in hospitals or clinics[Q] • **Main objective**: To evaluate whether an **agent or procedure reduces the risk of developing disease**[Q] among those free from the condition at enrolment. • **Conducted at an individual level**[Q], if the unit of allocation is the individual, or at an **aggregated level**[Q], if the unit is a group of people. • **Example: Community trials** (carried out at an aggregated level, where communities are the unit of allocation)

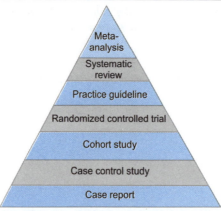

Evidence-Pyramid in Research (From top to bottom)[Q]
• Meta-analysis (Highest clinical relevance: Gold standard[Q]) • Systematic review[Q] • Cohort study[Q] • Case control study[Q] • Case series[Q] • Case report[Q] • Ideas, Editorials, Opinions[Q] • Animal research • In-vitro (test-tube) research (Lowest clinical relevance[Q])

Types of Epidemiological Studies

Observational studies[Q]	Experimental studies (Hypothesis confirmation)[Q]
• **Descriptive studies** (Hypothesis formulation[Q]) • **Analytical studies** (Hypothesis testing[Q])	

Analytical studies

Types	Unit
Cohort study	Individual[Q]
Case control study	Individual[Q]
Cross sectional study	Individual[Q]
Ecological study	Population[Q]

Experimental studies

Types	Unit
Randomized controlled trial	Patients[Q]
Field trial	Healthy people[Q]
Community trial	Community[Q]
Clinical trial	Patients[Q]

Cohort Study

- A **study design** where **one or more samples (called cohorts) are followed prospectively & subsequent status evaluations with respect to a disease or outcome are conducted to determine which initial participants exposure characteristics (risk factors) are associated with it**[Q].
- As the study is conducted, **outcome from participants in each cohort is measured** and **relationships with specific characteristics determined**[Q].

Cohort Study

Advantages	Disadvantages
• **Subjects in cohorts can be matched**, which **limits the influence of confounding variables**[Q] • **Standardization of criteria/outcome is possible**[Q] • **Easier & cheaper than** a randomized controlled trial (**RCT**).	• Cohorts can be **difficult to identify due to confounding variables**[Q] • **No randomization**, which means that **imbalances in patient characteristics could exist**[Q] • **Blinding/masking is difficult**[Q] • **Outcome of interest could take time to occur** • The cohorts need to be chosen from separate, but similar, populations.

Cohort Study can be used to calculate Relative risk (RR):

- RR = Risk of disease in exposed/ Risk of disease in non-exposed
- **RR< 1: Exposure/incidence is protective. It lowers the risk for expressing the outcome**[Q].
- **RR = 1: No association between an exposure** that delineates the cohorts **and the outcome**[Q].
- **RR > 1: Association between an exposure** that delineates the cohorts **and the outcome**[Q].

- In medicine, a **cohort study is often undertaken to obtain evidence to try to refute the existence of a suspected association between cause and effect**; failure to refute a hypothesis often strengthens confidence in it.
- Crucially, cohort is identified before appearance of disease under investigation.
- Study groups follow a group of people who do not have the disease for a period of time and see who develops the disease (new incidence).
- Cohort cannot be defined as a group of people who already have the disease.

  - **Prospective (longitudinal) cohort studies between exposure and disease strongly aid in studying causal associations**[Q], though distinguishing true causality usually requires further corroboration from further experimental trials.
  - **Advantage of prospective cohort study data** is that it can **help determine risk factors for contracting a new disease**[Q] because it is a longitudinal observation of the individual through time, and the collection of data at regular intervals, so recall error is reduced.

- **Cohort studies are expensive to conduct**, are **sensitive to** *attrition* & **take a long follow-up time to generate useful data**[Q].
- **Results that are obtained from long-term cohort studies are of substantially superior quality to those obtained from retrospective/cross-sectional studies**[Q].
- **Prospective cohort studies** are considered to **yield the most reliable results in observational epidemiology**. They **enable a wide range of exposure-disease associations to be studied**[Q].

Case control study	Cohort study
• **Proceeds from 'effect to cause'**[Q]	• **Proceeds from 'cause to effect'**[Q]
• **Starts with the disease**[Q]	• **Starts with people exposed to risk factor** or suspected cause[Q]
• **Tests** whether the **suspected cause occurs more frequently in those with the disease than among those without the disease**[Q].	• **Tests** whether **disease occurs more frequently in those exposed, than in those not similarly exposed**[Q].
• Usually the **first approach to the testing of a hypothesis**[Q], but also useful for exploratory studies.	• **Reserved for testing of precisely formulated hypothesis**[Q].
• Involves **fewer number of subjects**[Q].	• Involves **larger number of subjects**[Q].
• Yields relatively **quick results**[Q].	• **Long follow-up period often needed**, involving **delayed results**[Q].
• **Suitable for the study of rare diseases**[Q].	• Inappropriate when the **disease or exposure under investigation is rare.**
• Generally **yields only estimate of RR (odds ratio)**[Q].	• **Yields incidence rates, RR as well as AR**[Q].
• **Cannot yield information about diseases other than that selected for study**[Q].	• **Can yield information about more than one disease outcome**[Q].
• **Relatively inexpensive**[Q]	• **Expensive**[Q]

96. **Ans. d. Lathyrus sativus** *(Ref: Park 24/e p682, 23/e p644, 657)*

The signs and symptoms mentioned above along with history of origin from a dry state are suggestive of food adulteration and neurolathyrism, caused by Lathyrus sativus.

"Neurolathyrism is a crippling disease of the nervous system characterized by gradually developing spastic paralysis of lower limbs, occurring mostly in adults consuming the pulse, Lathyrus sativus."- Park 23/e p644

Disease	Food	Toxic Agents
Neurolathyrism	**Lathyrus sativus (Kheshari dal)**[Q]	**Beta-oxalyl amino alanine**[Q]
Epidemic dropsy	**Mustard oil containing argemone oil**[Q]	**Sanguinarine**[Q]
Endemic ascites	**Millets contaminated with seeds of Crotolaria (jhunjhunia)**[Q]	**Pyrrolizidine**[Q]
Fusarium Toxins	**Sorghum contaminated with fungus fusarium**[Q]	-
Hepatotoxicity	**Food grains**[Q]	**Aflatoxins**[Q]
Ergotism	**Food grains contaminated with Claviceps purpurea**[Q]	**Ergotoxin, ergotamine & ergometrine**[Q]

Lathyrism or Neurolathyrism
• Lathyrism is **paralyzing disease** of humans & animals • Caused by **consumption** of pulse **Lathyrus sativus**[Q] • **Toxin: Beta Oxalyl Amino Alanine (BOAA)**[Q]

Humans	Animals
• Known as **neurolathyrism** as it affects **nervous system**[Q] in human beings.	• Known as **osteolathyrism**[Q] **(odoratism)** as it **affects bones** in animals leading to **skeletal deformities**[Q].

• **Neurolathyrism: Crippling disease** of nervous system characterized by **gradually developing spastic paralysis** of lower limbs[Q]
Prevalence: • Neurolathyrism is prevalent in parts of **Madhya Pradesh, Uttar Pradesh, Bihar & Orissa**[Q].
Clinical Features: • Affects **young males**, age **15-45 years** • Withdrawal of pulse from diet leads to complete remission of disease

Contd...

Contd...

Lathyrism or Neurolathyrism		
Successive Stages in Untreated Cases		
Latent stage	• Individual displays only **unsteadiness of gait**[Q] and is otherwise normal	
No-stick stage	• Person walks with **short jerky steps without help of stick**[Q]	
One-stick	• Person walks with **crossed gait with tendency to walk on toes**. Stick is necessary **to maintain balance**[Q].	
Two-stick	• Gait is **slow & clumsy**, patient needs **two crutches for support**[Q].	
Crawler stages	• **Erect posture** is **impossible** because knee joint cannot support the weight of body. • **Atrophy of thigh & calf muscles** occur[Q]	

Interventions:
Interventions for prevention & control of lathyrism:
- **Vitamin C prophylaxis**[Q]
- **Banning the crop**[Q]
- **Removal of toxin by steeping** method or **parboiling**[Q]

97. Ans. c. There is no correlation between the two variables (Ref: Park 24/e p889, 23/e p852)
In the given graph, there is no correlation between the two variables.

"In the first half of the graph, slope is close to +1 while it is close to –1 in the second half of the graph. Hence, although there is some relation between the two variables, there is no overall definite positive or negative correlation between the two variables."

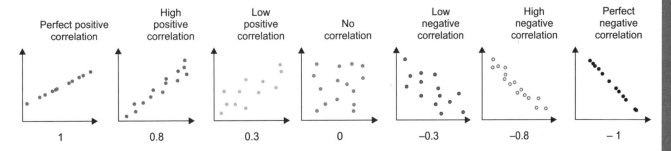

Correlation Coefficient (*r*)
• The quantity **r**, called the **linear correlation coefficient, measures the strength and the direction of a linear relationship between two variables**[Q]. • The **linear correlation coefficient** is sometimes referred to as the **Pearson product moment correlation coefficient** in honor of its developer Karl Pearson[Q].
Formula of Correlation Coefficient (*r*) $$r = \frac{n(\Sigma xy) - (\Sigma x)(\Sigma y)}{\sqrt{[n\Sigma x^2 - (\Sigma x)^2][n\Sigma y^2 - (\Sigma y)^2]}}$$

Advantage:
- It does not depend on the units of X & Y[Q]
- Can be used to compare any two variables regardless of their units[Q].

How to calculate?
- An essential first step in calculating a correlation coefficient is **to plot the observations in a "scattergram" or "scatter plot"** to visually evaluate the data for a potential relationship or the presence of outlying values.
- It is frequently possible to visualize a smooth curve through the data and thereby identify the type of relationship present.
- **Independent variable** is plotted **on X-axis**, dependent variable is plotted **on Y-axis.**

Correlation Coefficient (*r*)

Range of values:

- Pearson's Correlation Coefficient (r) has a value of between –1 & +1.

Interpretation	
–1	+1
• **Strong negative correlation**[Q]	• **Strong positive correlation**[Q]

Positive correlation	No correlation	Negative correlation
• If **x & y have a strong positive linear correlation**, **r is close to + 1**[Q]. • **An r value of exactly +1 indicates a perfect positive fit**[Q]. • Positive values indicate a relationship between x and y variables such that as values for x increases, values for y also increase.	• If there is **no linear correlation** or a **weak linear correlation, r is close to 0**[Q]. • A value near zero means that there is a random, nonlinear relationship between the two variables.	• If **x & y have a strong negative linear correlation, r is close to –1**[Q]. • **An r value of exactly –1 indicates a perfect negative fit**[Q]. • Negative values indicate a relationship between x and y such that as values for x increase, values for y decrease.

98. **Ans. a. Confirmed extra-pulmonary tuberculosis patient with cough of 2 weeks or more**   *(Ref: Park 24/e p188-189, 23/e p178; 22/e p168; http://tbcindia.nic.in)*

A contact of confirmed extra-pulmonary tuberculosis patient is a suspect of TB if he has cough of any duration (2 weeks is not required).

Pulmonary TB Suspect	MDR-TB Suspect
A pulmonary TB suspect is defined as: • Any individual having **cough of ≥2 weeks**[Q] • **Contacts of smear positive TB patients** having **cough of any duration**[Q] • **Suspected/confirmed extra-pulmonary TB** having **cough of any duration**[Q] • **HIV-positive patient** having **cough of any duration**[Q]	**MDR-TB suspect can be any of the following:** • Any **TB patient** who **fails an RNTCP Category I or III treatment regimen**[Q] • Any **RNTCP Category II patient** who is **sputum smear positive** at the **end of 4th month of treatment or later**[Q] • **Close contacts of MDR-TB** patients who are found to have **smear positive pulmonary TB**[Q]

99. **Ans. c. 24-26 mm Hg**   *(Ref: Park 24/e p887)*

Confidence Intervals

The lower limit & upper limit estimates for the statistic are given as:

- **Lower limit: Statistic – C x SE (statistic)**
- **Upper limit: Statistic + C x SE (statistic)**

Cond...

Confidence Intervals

- Standard error, SE = {standard deviation / $\sqrt{n}$)}
- n = sample size
- C = Confidence coefficient = **1.96 for 95% confidence interval**
  - = 2.58 for 99% confidence interval
  - = 3.29 for 99.9% confidence interval

Hence in this question, **n = 400**
- **SD = 10**
- **SE = 10/$\sqrt{400}$ = 10/20 = 0.5**
- **Mean statistic = 25 mm Hg**
- Now for 95% confidence interval, C = 2 approximately 95%
- **CI = 25 – 2x0.5 to 25 + 2x0.5 = 24-26 mm Hg**
- **Hence, 95% CI of IOP will be 24 to 26 mm Hg.**

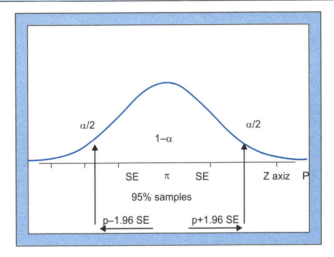

100. **Ans. a. There is no association present between the factor and the disease** *(Ref: Park 24/e p83, 23/e p78; 22/e p75)*

*"Estimation of relative risk (RR) is important in etiological enquiries. It is a **direct measure (or index) of the strength of association between suspected cause and effect**. A relative risk of one indicates no association; relative risk greater than one suggest positive association between exposure and the disease under study. A relative risk of two indicates that the incidence rate of disease is 2 times higher in exposed group as compared with the unexposed."- Park 24/e p83, 23/e p78*

Cohort Study can be used to calculate Relative risk (RR)

RR = Risk of disease in exposed/Risk of disease in non-exposed
- **RR< 1: Exposure/incidence is protective. It lowers the risk for expressing the outcome**[Q]
- **RR = 1: No association between an exposure** that delineates the cohorts **and the outcome**[Q]
- **RR > 1: Association between an exposure** that delineates the cohorts **and the outcome**[Q]

MEDICINE

101. **Ans. c. Intravenous clindamycin and fluids** *(Ref: Harrison 19/e p814-815, 18/e p2145-2146)*

Clinical features with history of smoking & binge drinking (increases risk of aspiration) and chest X-ray findings showing cavitation & necrosis are suggestive of lung abscess. Most common cause of primary lung abscess is anaerobes. Next step in management is intravenous clindamycin and fluids.

*"Primary lung abscesses is thought to originate when chiefly anaerobic bacteria (as well as microaerophilic streptococci) in the gingival crevices are aspirated into the lung parenchyma in a susceptible host. Thus, patients who develop primary lung abscesses usually carry an overwhelming burden of aspirated material or are unable to clear the bacterial load. Pneumonitis develops initially (exacerbated in part by tissue damage caused by gastric acid); then, **over a period of 7–14***

days, the anaerobic bacteria produce parenchymal necrosis and cavitation whose extent depends on the host–pathogen interaction. Anaerobes are thought to produce more extensive tissue necrosis in polymicrobial infections in which virulence factors of the various bacteria can act synergistically to cause more significant tissue destruction."- Harrison 19/e p814

"For primary lung abscesses, the recommended regimens are (1) clindamycin (600 mg IV three times daily; then, with the disappearance of fever and clinical improvement, 300 mg PO four times daily) or (2) an IV-administered β-lactam/β-lactamase combination, followed—once the patient's condition is stable—by orally administered amoxicillin-clavulanate. This therapy should be continued until imaging demonstrates that the lung abscess has cleared or regressed to a small scar. Treatment duration may range from 3–4 weeks to as long as 14 weeks."- Harrison 19/e p815

Lung Abscess
• **Lung abscess** refers to a **microbial infection** of the **lung** that results in necrosis of pulmonary parenchyma.
• **MC cause** of **primary lung abscess: Anaerobic bacteria**[Q]
• **Etiology** of anaerobic lung abscess: **Aspiration**[Q]

Routes of Infection:
- **Aspiration of organisms** that colonize oropharynx (**MC**)[Q]
- **Inhalation** of infection or aerosols[Q]
- **Hematogenous** dissemination from extra-pulmonary site
- **Direct inoculation** (as in tracheal intubation or stab wounds)
- **Contiguous spread** from an adjacent site of infection

Clinical Features:
- **Classic presentation**: An **indolent infection** that **evolves over several days or weeks**, usually in a host who has a **predisposition to aspiration**[Q].
- A **common feature** is **periodontal infection** with **pyorrhea** or **gingivitis**[Q].
- **Symptoms**: **Fatigue, cough, sputum production** & **fever**[Q]. Chills are uncommon.

Diagnosis:
- Lung abscess can be detected by **chest X-ray** & **CT**
- **CT scan**: **Investigation of choice** for **lung abscess**[Q]

Treatment:
- **Treatment** depends on **presumed** or **established etiology**.
- Infections caused by **anaerobic bacteria: Clindamycin**[Q]

> - **Persistence of fever beyond 5–7 days** or **progression of infiltrate** suggests **failure of therapy** & a need to **exclude** factors such as **obstruction, complicating empyema** & **involvement of antibiotic-resistant bacteria**[Q].

- Lung abscess due to **S. aureus: Vancomycin**[Q]

Causes of Failures of Medical Management	
• **Failure to drain** pleural collections[Q]	• **Giant abscess**[Q]
• **Inappropriate antimicrobial therapy**[Q]	• **Resistant pathogen**[Q]
• **Obstructed bronchus**[Q]	• **Refractory lesions**[Q]

- **Indications for surgery: Failure to respond** to medical management, **suspected neoplasm**, and **hemorrhage**[Q].

> - Patients who **do not respond to initial regimen** & who **do not have surgical indications, early percutaneous drainage** is done[Q].
> - When surgery is indicated, **lobectomy** is **preferred choice**[Q].
> - **Tube thoracotomy** & **open pleural drainage** is **also done for lung abscess**[Q].

102. Ans. a. 2:1 heart-block *(Ref: Harrison 19/e p1472, 1473 18/e p1835)*
The ECG given in the question is typically seen in a 2:1 heart block, which is a type of 2nd degree AV nodal block.

"Second-degree AV block is sub classified as Mobitz type I (Wenckebach) or Mobitz type II. The periodic failure of conduction in Mobitz type I block is characterized by a progressively lengthening PR interval, shortening of the RR interval, and a pause that is less than two times the immediately preceding RR interval on the electrocardiogram (ECG). The ECG complex after the pause exhibits a shorter PR interval than that immediately preceding the pause. This ECG pattern most often arises because of decremental conduction of electrical impulses in the AV node."- Harrison 19/e p1472

"Type II second-degree AV block is characterized by intermittent failure of conduction of the P wave without changes in the preceding PR or RR intervals. When AV block is 2:1, it may be difficult to distinguish type I from type II block. Type II second-degree AV block typically occurs in the distal or infra-His conduction system, is often associated with intraventricular conduction delays (e.g., bundle branch block), and is more likely to proceed to higher grades of AV block than is type I second-degree AV block. Second-degree AV block (particularly type II) may be associated with a series of non conducted P waves, referred to as paroxysmal AV block, and implies significant conduction system disease and is an indication for permanent pacing."- Harrison 19/e p1473

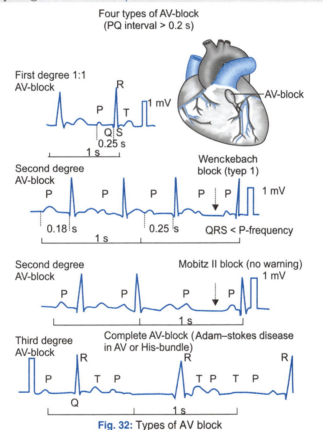

Fig. 32: Types of AV block

Cardiac Conduction Blocks		
First degree AV blocks	• First degree AV block is characterized by a **delay in conduction across the conducting tissue (prolonged PR interval)**[Q]	
	Features of First degree AV blocks	
	Rhythm	• Regular[Q]
	Rate (beats/minute)	• That of underlying **single rhythm**; both **atrial & ventricular rates will be same**[Q]
	P waves (lead II)	• Sinus origin; one P wave to each QRS complex[Q]
	PR interval	• PR interval is prolonged (>0.20 seconds)[Q] • PR interval is constant (at the prolonged duration)[Q]
	QRS complex	• QRS complex morphology/duration is normal[Q]

Contd...

Contd...

Second degree AV blocks	Second degree AV blocks is characterized by **intermittent failure of conduction from atria to ventricles.**

Mobitz I (Wenckebach Phenomenon)	Mobitz II
• This is characterized by **progressive prolongation of PR interval prior to a non-conducted P wave**[Q]	• This is characterized by **constant PR interval prior to a non-conducted P wave**[Q]
Features	**Features**
• Atrial rhythm regular[Q] • Ventricular rhythm irregular[Q] • Atrial rate exceeds ventricular rate[Q] • PR internal varies[Q] • PR progressively gets longer until a QRS is dropped[Q] • QRS morphology is often normal[Q]	• Atrial rhythm regular[Q] • Ventricular rhythm irregular (unless conduction rations vary)[Q] • Atrial rate exceeds ventricular rate[Q] • PR interval is constant[Q] • PR interval does not get progressively longer & a QRS is dropped suddenly • QRS morphology is usually abnormal[Q] (rarely normal)

Third degree AV blocks	Third degree AV blocks or **complete AV block** is characterized by **complete failure of conduction from atria to ventricles (Atria & ventricles are under the control of separate pacemakers)**[Q]

Features of Third degree AV blocks	
Rhythm	• Atrial rhythm regular[Q]; Ventricular rhythm irregular[Q]
Rate (beats/minute)	• Atrial rate exceeds ventricular rate[Q] (ventricular rate of ventricular pacemaker is slower)
P waves (lead II)	• P waves have no constant relationship to QRS complexes[Q] (AV dissociation)
PR interval	• PR interval varies[Q]
QRS complex	• QRS complex morphology may be abnormal[Q]

103. **Ans. a. Due to occlusion of right posterior inferior cerebellar artery** *(Ref: Gray's 40/e p251; Harrison 19/e p2577)*
Complaints of right-sided facial weakness and loss of sensation on right side of the face with left sided hemiparesis with Horner's syndrome, nystagmus, vertigo, ataxia and dysphagia is highly suggestive of lateral medullary syndrome, which can be caused by occlusion of any of five vessels i.e. vertebral, posterior inferior cerebellar, superior, middle, or inferior lateral medullary arteries.

> "Embolic occlusion or thrombosis of a V4 (4th segment of vertebral artery) segment causes ischemia of the lateral medulla. The constellation of vertigo, numbness of the ipsilateral face and contralateral limbs, diplopia, hoarseness, dysarthria, dysphagia, and ipsilateral Horner's syndrome is called the lateral medullary (or Wallenberg's) syndrome. Most cases result from ipsilateral vertebral artery occlusion; in the remainder, PICA occlusion is responsible. Occlusion of the medullary penetrating branches of the vertebral artery or PICA results in partial syndromes. Hemiparesis is not a feature of vertebral artery occlusion; however, quadriparesis may result from occlusion of the anterior spinal artery."- *Harrison 19/e p2577*

Characteristic features of Wallenberg syndrome (Lateral medullary syndrome):
- **Spinothalamic tract involvement:** Impaired pain & thermal sense over half of the body, sometimes face
- **Vestibular nucleus involvement:** Nystagmus, diplopia, oscillopsia, vertigo, nausea, vomiting\
- Issuing fibers **IX & X nerves:** Dysphagia, hoarseness, paralysis of palate, paralysis of vocal cord, diminished gag reflex

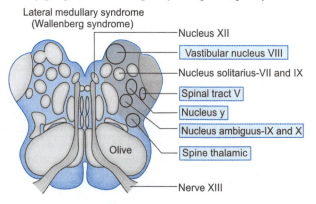

Wallenberg syndrome (Lateral medullary syndrome)	

- **Lateral medullary syndrome (occlusion of any of five vessels** may be responsible i.e. **vertebral, posterior inferior cerebellar, superior, middle, or inferior lateral medullary arteries**[Q])
- Most cases result from **ipsilateral vertebral artery occlusion (Embolic occlusion** or **thrombosis of 4th segment of vertebral artery**[Q]); in the remainder, **occlusion of posterior inferior cerebellar artery** is responsible.

Component of Lateral medullary syndrome	
Structure Involved	**Clinical Features**
On the side of the lesion	
Descending tract & nucleus of **V nerve**	**Pain, numbness, impaired sensation** over **one-half the face**[Q]
Cerebellar hemisphere, cerebellar fibers, spinocerebellar tract (?)	**Ataxia of limbs, falling to side of lesion**[Q]
Vestibular nucleus	**Nystagmus**[Q], diplopia, oscillopsia, vertigo, nausea, vomiting
Descending sympathetic tract	**Horner's syndrome**[Q]
Issuing fibers of **IX & X nerves**	**Dysphagia, hoarseness, paralysis of palate, paralysis of vocal cord, diminished gag reflex**[Q]
Nucleus & tractus solitarius	**Loss of taste**[Q]
Cuneate & gracile nuclei	**Numbness of ipsilateral arm, trunk, or leg**[Q]
Genuflected upper motor neuron fibers to ipsilateral facial nucleus	Weakness of lower face
On the opposite side of the lesion	
Spinothalamic tract	**Impaired pain and thermal sense over half the body, sometimes face**[Q]

104. Ans. c. >1500/ mm³   *(Ref: Harrison 19/e p1686, 135e-8, 18/e p481e-21.5)*

Eosinophil count for the diagnosis of hypereosinophilia syndrome should be ≥1.5 × 10⁹/L (≥1500/mm³).

*"Blood eosinophilia that is neither secondary nor clonal is operationally labeled as being idiopathic. **Hypereosinophilic Syndrome (HES)** is a subcategory of idiopathic eosinophilia **with persistent increase of the AEC to ≥1.5 × 10⁹/L (≥1500/ mm³)** and **presence of eosinophil-mediated organ damage, including cardiomyopathy, gastroenteritis, cutaneous lesions, sinusitis, pneumonitis, neuritis, and vasculitis.** In addition, some patients manifest thromboembolic complications, hepatosplenomegaly, and either cytopenia or cytosis."*-Harrison 19/e p135e-8

Diagnosis of Chronic Eosinophilic Leukemia & Hypereosinophilic Syndrome	
Required: Persistent eosinophilia >1500/μL in blood, increased marrow eosinophils & myeloblasts <20% in blood or marrow[Q].	
1.	**Exclude all causes of reactive eosinophilia:** allergy, parasites, infection, pulmonary disease (e.g. hypersensitivity pneumonitis, Loeffler's), and collagen vascular diseases
2.	**Exclude primary neoplasms associated with secondary eosinophilia:** T cell lymphomas, Hodgkin's disease, acute lymphoid leukemia, mastocytosis
3.	**Exclude other primary myeloid neoplasms that may involve eosinophils:** chronic myeloid leukemia, acute myeloid leukemia with inv(16) or t(16;16) (p13;q22), other myeloproliferative syndromes & myelodysplasia
4.	Exclude T cell reaction with increased IL-5 or other cytokine production

- **If these entities have been excluded** & no evidence documents a clonal myeloid disorder, the diagnosis is **hypereosinophilic syndrome**.
- **If these entities have been excluded & myeloid cells show a clonal chromosome abnormality** or some other **evidence of clonality** & blast cells are present in the peripheral blood (>2%) or are **increased in marrow (but <20%),** the diagnosis is **chronic eosinophilic leukemia.**

Hypereosinophilic Syndrome (HES)	

- HES is a **subcategory of idiopathic eosinophilia** with **persistent increase of the AEC to ≥1.5 × 10⁹/L & presence of eosinophil-mediated organ damage** (cardiomyopathy, gastroenteritis, cutaneous lesions, sinusitis, pneumonitis, neuritis & vasculitis)[Q]

AIIMS ESSENCE

Clinical Features:
- **Cardiomyopathy, gastroenteritis**, cutaneous lesions, **sinusitis, pneumonitis, neuritis & vasculitis.**
- **Thromboembolic complications, hepatosplenomegaly** & either cytopenia or cytosis in some patients

Diagnosis:
- **Bone marrow histologic & cytogenetic/molecular studies** examination
- Serum **tryptase**, T-cell **immunophenotyping** & T-cell receptor antigen gene rearrangement analysis.
- **Typical echocardiographic findings in HES:** Ventricular apical thrombus, posterior mitral leaflet or tricuspid valve abnormality, endocardial thickening, dilated left ventricle & pericardial effusion.

Treatment:
- **Cornerstone of therapy: Glucocorticoids^Q**
- **Alternatives: Mepolizumab** (targets IL-5) & **Alemtuzumab** (targets CD52)^Q

105. Ans. a. Metabolic acidosis *(Ref: Harrison 19/e p317, 18/e p365)*

Acid Base Disorders
pH < 7.35 is acidosis; pH >7.45 is alkalosis
• 1° change in HCO_3^- is termed as Metabolic (Normal HCO_3^- = 22-30 mEq/L)
• **If change in HCO_3^- is in keeping with the pH** (i.e. if there is acidosis and HCO_3^- is decreased) the problem is **metabolic** one.   • **If change in HCO_3^- is opposite with the pH** (i.e. if there is acidosis and HCO_3^- is increased or normal) the problem is **compensatory metabolic.**
• 1° change in CO_2 is termed as Respiratory (Normal CO_2 = 35-45 mEq/L)
• **If change in CO_2 is in keeping with the pH** (i.e. if there is acidosis and CO_2 is increased) the problem is **respiratory.**   • **If change in CO_2 is in opposite with the pH** (i.e. if there is acidosis and CO_2 is decreased or normal) the problem is termed as **compensatory respiratory.**

Acid Base Disorders
Acidosis as pH = 7.22
• HCO_3^- = 9 mEq/L (1° change in HCO_3^- is termed as Metabolic)
• Here the change in **HCO_3^- is in keeping with the pH** (i.e. **acidosis and HCO_3^- is decreased**) this problem is **metabolic** one.   • **The expected compensation for metabolic acidosis is respiratory alkalosis and the low pCO_2 indicates that the compensation is going on.**   • **Expected change in pCO_2 = (1.5 x HCO_3^-) + 8 ± 2**   • Expected change in pCO_2 = (1.5 x 9) + 8 ± 2 = 21.5 ± 2 (19.5-23.5)   • In this case, **pCO_2 is 30 mm Hg**, which suggest **coexistent respiratory acidosis.**

106. Ans. c. 500 mEq *(Ref: Harrison 19/e p317, 18/e p368)*

Base deficit in the given question is 400 mEq.

Base Deficit
• **Base excess** and **base deficit** refer to an **excess or deficit**, respectively, in the **amount of base present in the blood.**   • **Total bicarbonate deficit** = 0.3 × weight (kg) × base deficit   • **Total bicarbonate deficit is calculated as:** 0.3 × weight (kg) × base deficit (Standard Base deficit, as described below)   • **Alternatively:** Base deficit in mEq = 0.4 × weight (kg) × [24 – serum HCO_3 (mEq/L)]   • Total Base Deficit = (24–6) × 0.4 × 75 = **540 mEq = 500 mEq (approx.)**   • To obtain deficit in grams, divide mEq by 12.

Base Deficit & Base Excess
• **Base excess** is the **quantity of base (HCO_3^-, in mEq/L) that is above or below the normal range of buffer base in the body (22–28 mEq/L).** This cannot be calculated from PCO_2 and pH as the hemoglobin also contributes to the buffer base.   • The value is usually **reported as a concentration in units of mEq/L**, with positive numbers indicating an excess of base and negative a deficit.   • A **typical reference range** for base excess is **−2 to +2 mEq/L.**

Base Deficit & Base Excess

- Comparison of the base excess with the reference range assists in determining whether an acid/base disturbance is **caused by a respiratory, metabolic, or mixed metabolic/respiratory problem.**
- While CO_2 **defines the respiratory component** of acid-base balance, **base excess defines the metabolic component.**
- Accordingly, measurement of **base excess** is defined under a **standardized pressure of carbon dioxide, by titrating back to a standardized blood pH of 7.40.**
- **Predominant base contributing to base excess is bicarbonate.** Thus, a deviation of serum bicarbonate from the reference range is ordinarily mirrored by a deviation in base excess. However, base excess is a more comprehensive measurement, encompassing all metabolic contributions.
- Base excess can be estimated from the serum bicarbonate concentration $[(HCO_3^-)]$ and pH by the equation:
  - Base excess = $0.93 \times [(HCO_3^-) - 24.4 + 14.8 \times (pH - 7.4)]$ with units of mEq/L.
  - The same can be alternatively expressed as Base excess = $0.93 \times (HCO_3^-) + 13.77 \times pH - 124.58$

107. Ans. b. 2 *(Ref: Harrison 19/e p2552, 18/e p3262; Goodman Gillman 11/e p605)*

In typical absence seizures, carbamazepine and phenytoin are contraindicated, while ethosuximide is given as a first line drug.

"Ethosuximide and valproate are considered equally effective in the treatment of absence seizures. Between 50% and 75% of newly diagnosed patients are free of seizures following therapy with either drug. If tonic-clonic seizures are present or emerge during therapy, valproate is the agent of first choice."- Goodman Gillman 11/e p605

Selection of Anti-Epileptic Drugs			
Generalized- Onset Tonic- Clonic	**Focal**	**Typical Absence**	**Atypical Absence, Myoclonic, Atonic**
First-Line			
• **Lamotrigine[Q]** • **Valproic acid[Q]**	• **Lamotrigine[Q]** • **Carbamazepine[Q]** • **Oxcarbazepine[Q]** • **Phenytoin[Q]** • **Levetiracetam[Q]**	• **Valproic acid[Q]** • **Ethosuximide[Q]** • **Lamotrigine[Q]**	• **Valproic acid[Q]** • **Lamotrigine[Q]** • **Topiramate[Q]**
Alternatives			
• Zonisamide • Phenytoin • Carbamazepine • Oxcarbazepine • Topiramate • Phenobarbital • Primidone • Felbamate	• Topiramate • Zonisamide • Valproic acid • Tiagabine • Gabapentin • Lacosamide • Exogabine • Phenobarbital • Primidone • Felbamate	• Lamotrigine • Clonazepam	• Clonazepam • Felbamate • Clobazam • Rufinamide

Drug of Choice for Various Types of Seizures	
Type of Seizures	**Drug of Choice**
• Absence seizures • GTCS (Grand mal) • Tonic seizures • Clonic seizures • Myoclonic seizures • Atonic (Akinetic) seizures	• **Valproate[Q]**
• Partial seizures	• **Carbamazepine[Q]**
• Infantile spasm	• **ACTH[Q]**
• Infantile spasm with tuberous sclerosis	• **Vigabatrin[Q]**
• Febrile seizures	• **Diazepam[Q] (per rectal)**
• Status epilepticus	• **Lorazepam[Q] (IV)**
• Seizures in eclampsia	• **Magnesium sulphate[Q]**

108. Ans. b. 8 drops/min

- A dosing of 10 mgm/kg/min of the drug is required
- Weight = 80 kg
- **Total dose required** = 10×80 = 800 mgm/min = **0.8 mg/min**
- Now two 5 mL vials each containing 200 mg is diluted to a 250 mL solution i.e. 400 mg is mixed in 250 mL
- Concentration of solution: 1 mL = 400/250 = 1.6 mg/mL
- **Now, 1 mL = 16 drops = 1.6 mg** i.e. 16 drops contain 1.6 mg
- Hence, 0.8 mg/min = **8 drops/min** = 0.5 mL/min

109. Ans. b. Change imipramine and haloperidol to fluoxetine and risperidone and add bisacodyl for constipation *(Ref: Harrison 19/e p1623-1624, 18/e p3531; Goodman Gilman 12/e p410, 1333)*

In this question, the patient is having postural hypotension, probably because of alpha blockade by Imipramine and it's interaction with thiazides. She is also having anti-cholinergic side-effect of Imipramine. Hence, Imipramine (TCA), must be discontinued and she should be started on an SSRI, fluoxetine along with a laxative for existing constipation. Also, typical anti-psychotics like haloperidol have anti-cholinergic side effects, she should be started on atypical antipsychotic Risperidone. Thiazides need to changed to CCBs/ACE inhibitors to avoid postural hypotension. She is also having bradycardia, which is a side effect of beta-blocker, atenolol, so it must be changed.

*"Tricyclic antidepressants have **anticholinergic side-effects, acts on muscarinic receptors**, manifested as **dry mouth**, bad taste, **constipation**, epigastric distress, **urinary retention** (specially in males with enlarged prostate), blurred vision, palpitation."*

"The SSRIs (Fluoxetine), unlike the TCAs, do not cause major cardiovascular side effects. The SSRIs are generally free of antimuscarinic side effects (dry mouth, urinary retention, confusion), do not block histamine or α adrenergic receptors, and are not sedating. The favorable side effect profile of the SSRIs may lead to better patient compliance compared to that for the TCAs."- Goodman Gilman 12/e p410

Side Effects of Tricyclic anti-depressants
- **Anticholinergic:**   – Acts on muscarinic receptors, manifested as dry mouth, bad taste, constipation, epigastric distress, urinary retention (specially in males with enlarged prostate), blurred vision, palpitation.   - **Sedation, mental confusion** and **weakness** especially with amitriptyline and more sedative congeners.   - **Increased appetite** and **weight gain** is noted with most TCAs and trazadone, but not with SSRIs and bupropion.   - Some patients receiving any antidepressants may abruptly switch over to a **dysphoric-agitated state** or to **mania.**   - **Sweating** and **fine tremors** are relatively common.   - **Seizure threshold** is lowered—fits may be precipitated, **especially in children.**   - **Postural hypotension**, especially in **older patients**   - **Cardiac arrhythmias**, especially in patients with **ischemic heart disease**—may be responsible for sudden death in these patients.   - Rashes and jaundice due to hypersensitivity are rare.

Bisacodyl (Dulcolax)
- An organic compound that is used as a **stimulant laxative drug.**
Mechanism of Action: - Bisacodyl works by **stimulating enteric nerves to cause colonic contractions.**   - It is also a **contact laxative**; it **increases fluid & salt secretion**.   - **Action of bisacodyl on small intestine is negligible**; stimulant laxatives **mainly promote evacuation of the colon**
Uses: - It is typically **prescribed for relief of constipation** & for **management of neurogenic bowel dysfunction** as well as part of **bowel preparation** before medical examinations, such as for a colonoscopy.

110. Ans. c. RT-PCR for hepatitis C virus *(Ref: Harrison 19/e p2017, 2018, 18/e p2551)*

This patient has positive Anti-HCV antibody along with positive Anti-HBcAg IgG. Anti-HBcAg IgG positivity here is a mere indicator of hepatitis B infection in the past. Presence of Anti-HCV antibody points to a hepatitis C infection, and thus HCV-RNA levels should be determined to establish a diagnosis of chronic hepatitis C before starting Interferon therapy.

"A proportion of patients with hepatitis C have isolated anti-HBc in their blood, a reflection of a common risk in certain populations of exposure to multiple blood borne hepatitis agents. The anti-HBc in such cases is almost invariably of the IgG class and usually represents HBV infection in the remote past (HBV DNA undetectable); it rarely represents current HBV infection with low-level virus carriage. "-Harrison 19/e p2017

"The presence of anti-HCV supports a diagnosis of acute hepatitis C. Occasionally, testing for HCV RNA or repeat anti-HCV testing later during the illness is necessary to establish the diagnosis."- Harrison 19/e p2018

"The most sensitive indicator of HCV infection is the presence of HCV RNA, which requires molecular amplification by PCR. Occasionally, testing for HCV RNA or repeat anti-HCV testing later during the illness is necessary to establish the diagnosis."

"Liver biopsy is rarely necessary or indicated in acute viral hepatitis, except when the diagnosis is questionable or when clinical evidence suggests a diagnosis of chronic hepatitis."-Harrison 19/e p2017

"In patients with chronic hepatitis, initial testing should consist of HBsAg and anti-HCV. Anti-HCV supports and HCV RNA testing establishes the diagnosis of chronic hepatitis C. If a serologic diagnosis of chronic hepatitis B is made, testing for HBeAg and anti-HBe is indicated to evaluate relative infectivity. Testing for HBV DNA in such patients provides a more quantitative and sensitive measure of the level of virus replication and, therefore, is very helpful during antiviral therapy"- Harrison 19/e p2018

Hepatitis C Virus Infection

- In patients with hepatitis C, an episodic pattern of aminotransferase elevation is common.
- A **specific serologic diagnosis of hepatitis C** can be made by **demonstrating presence of anti-HCV^Q**.
- When contemporary immunoassays are used, **anti-HCV** can be **detected in acute hepatitis C during the initial phase of elevated aminotransferase activity** & remains detectable after recovery (rare) and during chronic infection (common).

  - **Assays for HCV RNA are most sensitive tests for HCV infection** & represent **"gold standard"** in establishing a **diagnosis of hepatitis C^Q**.

- **HCV RNA** can be **detected even before acute elevation of aminotransferase activity** & **before appearance of anti-HCV** in patients with acute hepatitis C^Q.
- **HCV RNA remains detectable indefinitely,** continuously in most but intermittently in some, in patients with chronic hepatitis C^Q.
- In the very small minority of **patients with hepatitis C who lack anti-HCV, a diagnosis can be supported by detection of HCV RNA^Q.**

  - **Amplification techniques are required to detect HCV RNA^Q.**
  - **Branched-chain complementary DNA (bDNA) assay: Detection signal** (a colorimetrically detectable enzyme bound to a complementary DNA probe) **is amplified^Q.**
  - **Target amplification by PCR or TMA: Viral RNA is reverse transcribed** to complementary DNA & **amplified by repeated cycles of DNA synthesis^Q.**

Simplified Diagnostic Approach in Patients Presenting with Acute Hepatitis
Serologic Tests of Patient's Serum

HBsAg	IgM Anti-HAV	IgM Anti-Hbc	Anti-HCV	Diagnostic Interpretation
+	–	+	–	**Acute hepatitis B**
+	–	–	–	**Chronic hepatitis B**
+	+	–	–	**Acute hepatitis A superimposed on chronic hepatitis B**
+	+	+	–	**Acute hepatitis A and B**
–	+	–	–	**Acute hepatitis A**
–	+	+	–	**Acute hepatitis A and B** (HBsAg below detection threshold)
–	–	+	–	**Acute hepatitis B** (HBsAg below detection threshold)
–	–	–	+	Acute hepatitis C

Commonly Encountered Serologic Patterns of Hepatitis B Infection

HBsAg	Anti-HBs	Anti-HBc	HBeAg	Anti-HBe	Interpretation
+	–	IgM	+	–	• Acute hepatitis B, high infectivity
+	–	IgG	+	–	• **Chronic hepatitis B, high infectivity**[Q]
+	–	IgG	–	+	• **Late acute** or **chronic hepatitis B, low infectivity**[Q] • **HBeAg-negative** ('precore–mutant') hepatitis B (chronic or rarely acute)
+	+	+	+/–	+/–	• HBsAg of one subtype and heterotypic anti-HBs (common) • Process of seroconversion from HBsAg to anti-HBs (rare)
–	–	IgM	+/–	+/–	• **Acute hepatitis B**[Q] • **Anti–HBc 'window'**[Q]
–	–	IgG	–	+/–	• **Low-level hepatitis B carrier**[Q] • **Hepatitis B in remote past**[Q]
–	+	IgG	–	+/–	• **Recovery from hepatitis B**[Q]
–	+	–	–	–	• **Immunization with HBsAg** (after vaccination) • **Hepatitis B in the remote past** (?) • False-positive

111. Ans. d. Opioid poisoning *(Ref: Harrison 19/e p1774, 2583, 18/e p3295)*

In the given question, patient is having pin-point pupils (miosis) along with hypotension and tachycardia with a slightly decreased respiratory rate. Miosis, hypotension in combination with depressed respiration is the hallmark sign of opiate overdose.

"Unilateral miosis in coma has been attributed to dysfunction of sympathetic efferents originating in the posterior hypothalamus and descending in the tegmentum of the brainstem to the cervical cord. It is therefore of limited localizing value but is an occasional finding in patients with a large cerebral hemorrhage that affects the thalamus. Reactive and bilaterally small (1–2.5 mm) but not pinpoint pupils are seen in metabolic encephalopathies or in deep bilateral hemispherical lesions such as hydrocephalus or thalamic hemorrhage. Even smaller reactive pupils (<1 mm) characterize narcotic or barbiturate overdoses but also occur with extensive pontine hemorrhage. The response to naloxone and the presence of reflex eye movements (see below) assist in distinguishing between these."- Harrison 19/e p1774

"In pontine hemorrhages, deep coma with quadriplegia often occurs over a few minutes. Typically, there is prominent decerebrate rigidity and "pinpoint" (1 mm) pupils that react to light. There is impairment of reflex horizontal eye movements evoked by head turning (doll's-head or oculocephalic maneuver) or by irrigation of the ears with ice water. Hyperpnea, severe hypertension, and hyperhidrosis are common. Most patients with deep coma from pontine hemorrhage ultimately die, but small hemorrhages are compatible with survival."- Harrison 19/e p2583

Pupillary reaction

Miosis (Constricted pupil)	Mydriasis (Dilated pupil)
• **Carbolic acid**[Q]	• **Viper venom**[Q]
• **Chloral hydrate**[Q]	• **Dhatura**[Q]
• **Morphine (opium)**[Q]	• **Alcohol**[Q]
• **Organophosphorus poisoning**[Q]	• **Aconite**[Q]
• **Barbiturates**[Q]	• **Nux vomica**[Q]
• **Pontine hemorrhage**[Q]	• **Cyanide, cocaine, CO**[Q]
• Muscarine	• Chloroform, Ether
• Nicotine	• Pethidine

Opioid Overdose	Pontine Hemorrhage
• **Opioid overdose triad: Decreased level of consciousness + Pinpoint pupils + Respiratory depression**[Q]. • Other Signs & symptoms: **Hypotension, Seizures** & muscle spasms[Q] • **All secretions are suspended except sweat**[Q] • **Naloxone: Specific opioid antagonist**[Q] (**Effective at reversing the cause**, rather than just the symptoms, of an opioid overdose)	• **Deep coma with quadriplegia** usually occurs over a few minutes[Q]. • **Prominent decerebrate rigidity** & **"pinpoint" (1 mm) pupils that react to light**[Q]. • **Impairment of reflex horizontal eye movements evoked by head turning** (doll's-head or oculocephalic maneuver) or **by irrigation of the ears with ice water**[Q]. • **Hyperpnea, severe hypertension** & **hyperhidrosis** are common. • **Death often occurs within a few hours**, but small hemorrhages are compatible with survival. • Patients often exhibit **rebound nystagmus**[Q], which is a variant of gaze-evoked nystagmus.

112. **Ans. a. VSD with aortic regurgitation**   *(Ref: Harrison 19/e p51e-2, 1449, 18/e p1829)*

VSD with aortic regurgitation produces pansystolic and early diastolic murmur, not continuous.

"The classic example of a continuous murmur is that associated with a PDA, which usually is heard in the second or third interspace at a slight distance from the sternal border. Other causes of a continuous murmur include a ruptured sinus of Valsalva aneurysm with creation of an aortic–right atrial or right ventricular fistula, a coronary or great vessel arteriovenous fistula, and an arteriovenous fistula constructed to provide dialysis access."- *Harrison 19/e p1449*

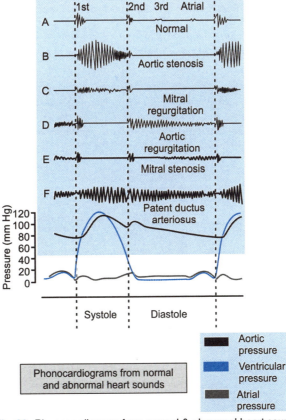

Fig. 33: Phonocardiogram from normal & abnormal heart sounds

Continuous Murmurs
• Continuous murmurs **begin in systole, peak near 2nd heart sound** & **continue into all or part of diastole**[Q]. • **Continuous murmur** implies a **pressure gradient between two chambers or vessels during both systole & diastole**[Q]. • **Not all continuous murmurs are pathologic**[Q].
Mechanism:
• It results due to **pressure gradient between two cardiac chambers** or **blood vessels across systole & diastole**[Q].

Contd...

Contd...

Causes of Continuous Murmurs			
Continuous murmur caused by blood flow	Continuous murmurs caused by high-to-low pressure shunts		Continuous murmurs secondary to localized arterial obstruction
Venous hum Mammary souffle Hemangioma Hyperthyroidism Acute alcoholic hepatitis Hyperemia of neoplasm Hepatoma RCC Paget's disease	Systemic artery to pulmonary artery **Patient ductus arteriosus**[Q] Aortopulmonary window **Truncus arteriosus**[Q] **Pulmonary atresia**[Q] Anomalous left coronary artery Sequestration of the lung Systemic artery to right heart **Ruptured sinus of Valsalva**[Q] **AV fistula (systemic or pulmonic)**[Q]	**Coronary AV fistula** Left-to-right atrial shunting Lutembacher syndrome Mitral atresia plus atrial septal defect Venovenous shunts Anomalous pulmonary veins Portosystemic shunts Bronchiectasis	Coarctation of aorta Branch pulmonary artery stenosis Carotid artery occlusion Celiac mesenteric occlusion Renal artery occlusion Femoral artery occlusion Coronary artery occlusion

Complications:
- Large, uncorrected shunts may lead to **pulmonary hypertension, attenuation or obliteration of diastolic component of the murmur**, reversal of shunt flow & differential cyanosis of the lower extremities.

113. **Ans. d. Clean the inhaler before use**   *(Ref: Ghai 8/e p387; GINA Guidelines-Asthma Prevention & Management (2016))*
Between two uses, the mouth has to rinsed, but the inhaler doesn't need to be cleaned. The inhaler can be cleaned on a weekly basis.

> *"When finished with all of the doses, rinse the mouth with water and spit the water out (Especially if it is a steroid inhaler). Clean the inhaler mouthpiece at least once a week with warm running water for 30 seconds, and dry it completely. If there is a need to use the inhaler before it is completely dry, shake off the excess water, replace the canister, and spray it 2 times in the air away from the face. Use regular dose. After using the inhaler, wash the mouthpiece again and dry it completely. If the mouthpiece becomes blocked, washing it will help."*

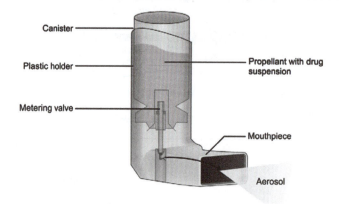

Correct Usage of Metered Dose Inhaler
To use an MDI
• **Shake the inhaler** well before use (3 or 4 shakes) for about 5 seconds • Remove the cap • Breathe out, away from your inhaler • Bring the inhaler to your mouth. Place it in your mouth between your teeth & close your mouth around it. • Start to breathe in slowly. Press the top of your inhaler once and keep breathing in slowly until you have taken a full breath. • Remove the inhaler from your mouth & hold your breath for about 10 seconds, then breathe out.

> - **If you are using a corticosteroid MDI, rinse your mouth & gargle using water or mouthwash after each use.** You should always use a chamber with a steroid MDI[Q].
> - **If you need a second puff,** wait 30 seconds to 1 minute, shake your inhaler again, and repeat steps 3-6.
> - After you've used your MDI, rinse out your mouth & record the number of doses taken.
> - Store all puffers at room temperature

Cleaning Your MDI
- **Remove the metal canister by pulling it out and clean it once a week.** Clean the plastic parts of the device using mild soap and water. (Never wash the metal canister or put it in water.) - **Let the plastic parts dry in the air** (for example, leave them out overnight). - Put the MDI back together. - Test the MDI by releasing a puff into the air.

114. **Ans. b. Oral iron therapy should be stopped once the patient achieves a hemoglobin of >12 mg/dL** *(Ref: Harrison 19/e p629, 18/e p849)*

The goal of therapy in individuals with iron-deficiency anemia is not only to repair the anemia, but also to provide stores of at least 0.5–1 g of iron. Sustained treatment for a period of 6–12 months after correction of the anemia will be necessary to achieve this.

> *"The goal of therapy in individuals with iron-deficiency anemia is not only to repair the anemia, but also to provide stores of at least 0.5–1 g of iron. Sustained treatment for a period of 6–12 months after correction of the anemia will be necessary to achieve this."- Harrison 19/e p629*

> *"In administering intravenous iron dextran, anaphylaxis is a concern. Anaphylaxis is much rarer with the newer preparations. The factors that have correlated with an anaphylactic-like reaction include a **history of multiple allergies or a prior allergic reaction to dextran** (in the case of iron dextran). If a large dose of iron dextran is to be given (>100 mg), the iron preparation should be diluted in 5% dextrose in water or 0.9% NaCl solution."- Harrison 19/e p629*

Treatment of Iron-Deficiency Anemia (IDA)	
- **Severity & cause of IDA** will **determine the** appropriate **approach** to treatment. - **Symptomatic elderly patients with severe IDA & cardiovascular instability** may require **red cell transfusions**. - **Younger patients** who have compensated for their anemia can be treated more conservatively with **iron replacement.** - **Oral iron therapy: For majority of cases of IDA** (pregnant women, growing children & adolescents, patients with infrequent episodes of bleeding, those with inadequate dietary intake of iron)	

Therapeutic approaches based on diagnosis & cause of IDA	
Red Cell Transfusion	- Reserved for individuals with **symptoms of anemia, cardiovascular instability, continued & excessive blood loss requiring immediate intervention**[Q].
Oral Iron Therapy	- **Asymptomatic patient with established IDA**, treatment with **oral iron** is usually adequate. - For **iron replacement therapy**, up to **200 mg of elemental iron per day** is given - **Oral iron preparations** should be **taken on an empty stomach** (food may inhibit iron absorption)[Q] - A dose of **200 mg of elemental iron per day** should **result in absorption of iron up to 50 mg/d**[Q]. - **Goal of therapy** in individuals with IDA: **Repair the anemia** & **provide stores of at least 0.5–1 g of iron. Sustained treatment for a period of 6–12 months after correction of anemia** will be necessary to achieve this[Q]. - **Complications: GI distress** (in 15–20%), abdominal pain, nausea, vomiting, or constipation (**GI side effects** are a **major impediment to effective treatment**)[Q]

Parenteral Iron Therapy	- **IV iron** can be given to patients **who are unable to tolerate oral iron; whose needs are relatively acute;** or **who need iron on an ongoing basis, usually due to persistent gastrointestinal blood loss**[Q].
	- **Parenteral iron** is used in two ways:
	  – Administer total dose of iron required to correct hemoglobin deficit & provide at least 500 mg of iron stores[Q]
	  – Give repeated small doses over a protracted period.

Contd...

Contd...

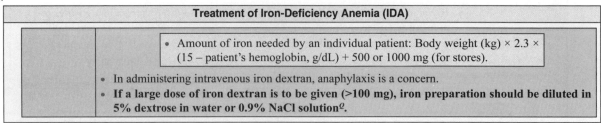

Treatment of Iron-Deficiency Anemia (IDA)
• Amount of iron needed by an individual patient: Body weight (kg) × 2.3 × (15 – patient's hemoglobin, g/dL) + 500 or 1000 mg (for stores).
• In administering intravenous iron dextran, anaphylaxis is a concern.
• If a large dose of iron dextran is to be given (>100 mg), iron preparation should be diluted in 5% dextrose in water or 0.9% NaCl solution^Q.

115. **Ans. c. Lumbar puncture**   *(Ref: Harrison 19/e p1773, 18/e p2251)*

For patients with altered sensorium, it is generally recommended that an imaging study be performed prior to lumbar puncture to exclude the causes of raised ICP (large intracranial mass lesion) and to prevent herniation.

"Lumbar puncture is performed less frequently than in the past for coma diagnosis because neuroimaging effectively excludes intracerebral & extensive subarachnoid hemorrhage. For patients with an altered level of consciousness, it is generally recommended that an imaging study be performed prior to lumbar puncture to exclude a large intracranial mass lesion and prevent herniation."

Work-up in a Coma Patient
• **Studies most useful in the diagnosis of coma: chemical- toxicologic analysis of blood & urine, cranial CT** or **MRI, EEG & CSF examination**.
• Arterial blood gas analysis including **electrolytes, glucose, calcium, osmolarity, renal (blood urea nitrogen) & hepatic (NH$_3$) function**
• **Plasma glucose should be the first test & if the test is not immediately available, empirical glucose should be given** .
• **Toxicologic analysis** may be necessary in any case of acute coma where the **diagnosis is not immediately clear**.
• **Presence of exogenous drugs or toxins**, especially **alcohol**, **does not exclude the possibility** that other factors, particularly **head trauma**, are also contributing to the clinical state.
• **CT & MRI for causes of coma** that are detectable by imaging (e.g. **hemorrhage, tumor, or hydrocephalus**).
• **EEG** is **useful in metabolic or drug-induced states** but is **rarely diagnostic**, except when **coma is due to clinically unrecognized seizure, to herpes virus encephalitis, or to prion** (Creutzfeldt-Jakob) **disease**.
• The most important use of **EEG recordings in coma** is to **reveal clinically inapparent epileptic discharges**.
• Lumbar puncture is performed less frequently than in the past for coma diagnosis because neuroimaging effectively excludes intracerebral & extensive subarachnoid hemorrhage.
• For patients with an altered level of consciousness, it is generally recommended that an imaging study be performed prior to lumbar puncture to exclude a large intracranial mass lesion and prevent herniation.
• Blood culture and antibiotic administration usually precede the imaging study if meningitis is suspected
• **Urgent brain imaging** is needed in the presence of **rapid deterioration of mental status**, and may be done simultaneously with or even before some laboratory tests under certain circumstances (e.g. suspected stroke or intracranial hemorrhage).
• A Non-contrast CT can be performed easily to rule out features of raised ICP, risk of herniation and a cerebral hemorrhage.

116. **Ans. a. IV fluids and furosemide**   *(Ref: Harrison 19/e p314; 18/e p361)*

Initial therapy of significant hypercalcemia begins with volume expansion because hypercalcemia invariably leads to dehydration; 4–6 L of intravenous saline may be required over the first 24 h, keeping in mind that underlying comorbidities (e.g., congestive heart failure) may require the use of loop diuretics to enhance sodium and calcium excretion.

*"Mild, asymptomatic hypercalcemia does not require immediate therapy, and management should be dictated by the underlying diagnosis. By contrast, **significant, symptomatic hypercalcemia usually requires therapeutic intervention independent of the etiology of hypercalcemia. Initial therapy of significant hypercalcemia begins with volume expansion because hypercalcemia invariably leads to dehydration; 4–6 L of intravenous saline may be required over the first 24 h, keeping in mind that underlying comorbidities (e.g., congestive heart failure) may require the use of loop diuretics to enhance sodium and calcium excretion. However, loop diuretics should not be initiated until the volume status has been restored to normal. If there is increased calcium mobilization from bone (as in malignancy or severe hyperparathyroidism), drugs that inhibit bone resorption should be considered.**"- Harrison 19/e p314*

"Zoledronic acid, pamidronate, and ibandronate are bisphosphonates that are commonly used for the treatment of hypercalcemia of malignancy in adults. Onset of action is within 1–3 days, with normalization of serum calcium levels occurring in 60–90% of patients." - Harrison 19/e p314

Hypercalcemia

- **Calcium ion** plays a **critical role in normal cellular function** & signaling, **regulating neuromuscular signaling, cardiac contractility, hormone secretion & blood coagulation**[Q].
- Hypercalcemia is relatively common & serves as a harbinger of underlying disease.

Causes of Hypercalcemia	
Excessive PTH production	- **Primary hyperparathyroidism**[Q] (adenoma, hyperplasia, rarely carcinoma) - **Tertiary hyperparathyroidism**[Q] (long-term stimulation of PTH secretion in renal insufficiency) - **Ectopic PTH secretion**[Q] (very rare) - **Inactivating mutations in the CaSR or in G proteins (FHH)**[Q] - **Alterations in CaSR function (lithium therapy)**[Q]
Hypercalcemia of malignancy	- **Overproduction of PTH-rP (many solid tumors)**[Q] - **Lytic skeletal metastases** (breast, myeloma)[Q]
Excessive 1,25(OH)$_2$D production	- **Granulomatous diseases (sarcoidosis, tuberculosis, silicosis)**[Q] - **Lymphomas , Vitamin D intoxication**[Q]
Primary increase in bone resorption	- **Hyperthyroidism**[Q] - **Immobilization**[Q]
Excessive calcium intake	- **Milk-alkali syndrome & total parenteral nutrition**[Q]
Other causes	- Endocrine disorders (**adrenal insufficiency, pheochromocytoma, VIPoma**)[Q] - Medications (**thiazides, vitamin A, antiestrogens**)[Q]

Clinical Features:

Mild hypercalcemia (up to 11–11.5 mg/dL)	Severe hypercalcemia (>12–13 mg/dL)
- Usually **asymptomatic**, recognized on routine calcium measurements; - **Neuropsychiatric symptoms, peptic ulcer disease, nephrolithiasis & increased fracture risk** in some patients.	- If develops acutely, result in **lethargy, stupor, coma** - GI symptoms (**nausea, anorexia, constipation, pancreatitis**)[Q] - **Polyuria & polydipsia: Hypercalcemia decreases renal concentrating ability**[Q] - **Bone pain & pathologic fractures** in long-standing hyperparathyroidism[Q] - **ECG changes: Bradycardia, AV block & short QT interval**[Q]

Treatment:
- **Mild, asymptomatic hypercalcemia does not require immediate therapy** & management should be dictated by underlying diagnosis.
- **Significant, symptomatic hypercalcemia requires therapeutic intervention independent of etiology**[Q].

Management of Significant, Symptomatic Hypercalcemia

- **Initial therapy: Volume expansion** (hypercalcemia leads to dehydration) **with 4–6 L of IV saline** over the first 24 h, keeping in mind that underlying comorbidities (e.g., congestive heart failure) may require **use of loop diuretics to enhance Na$^+$ & Ca^{2+} excretion**[Q].
- **Increased calcium mobilization from bone** (in **malignancy** or **severe hyperparathyroidism**): -
- **Drugs that inhibit bone resorption should be considered**[Q].
 	
    - **Zoledronic acid, pamidronate & ibandronate** are used for **treatment of hypercalcemia of malignancy in adults**[Q].
    - **Onset of action is within 1–3 days**, with **normalization of serum calcium** levels occurring in **60–90%** of patients.

Contd...

Hypercalcemia
• **Gallium nitrate:** Alternative to bisphosphonates, effective but **nephrotoxic**[Q]
• **Dialysis** may be necessary in rare instances

$1,25(OH)_2$ D-mediated Hypercalcemia
• **Preferred therapy: Glucocorticoids (IV hydrocortisone** or **oral prednisone)**[Q]
• **Glucocorticoids decrease $1,25(OH)_2D$ production**[Q].

117. **Ans. a. Signs and symptoms usually subsides within 2–3 weeks of onset:**   *(Ref: Harrison 19/e p138e-5, 18/e p1217; Wintrobes 14/e p575)*

The patient usually recovers from TRALI within 2–3 days instead of 2–3 weeks.

"No definitive treatment is available for TRALI, but with supportive care the patient's oxygenation often improves and return to normal in 2-3 days."- Anesthesia Student Survival Guide: A Case-Based Approach by Jesse M. Ehrenfeld, Richard D. Urman/p 284

"TRALI is associated with a high morbidity with the majority of patients requiring ventilatory support. However, the lung injury is generally transient with PO_2 levels returning to pre-transfusion levels within 48–96 hours and CXR returning to normal within 96 hours."- https://professionaleducation.blood.ca/en/transfusion/publications/transfusion-related-acute-lung-injury-trali

Transfusion-Related Acute Lung Injury (TRALI)
• **TRALI is MC cause of transfusion related fatalities**[Q]
• **Implicated donors** are **frequently multiparous women**.
• **Transfusion of plasma from male & nulliparous women donors reduces the risk of TRALI.**

Recipient factors associated with increased risk of TRALI	
• **Smoking**[Q]	• **Mechanical ventilation** with **>30 cm** H_2O **pressure support**[Q]
• **Chronic alcohol use**[Q]	
• **Shock**[Q]	• **Positive fluid balance**[Q]
• **Liver surgery (transplantation)**[Q]	

Etiopathogenesis:
• TRALI usually **results from transfusion of donor plasma** that **contains high-titer anti-HLA class II antibodies** that **bind recipient leukocytes**[Q].
• **Leukocytes aggregate in pulmonary vasculature & release mediators** that **increase capillary permeability**[Q].

Clinical Features:
• Recipient develops **symptoms of hypoxia (PaO_2/FIO_2 <300 mm Hg) & signs of non-cardiogenic pulmonary edema,** including **bilateral interstitial infiltrates on chest X-ray, either during or within 6 hours of transfusion**[Q].

Diagnosis:
• Testing the **donor's plasma for anti-HLA antibodies can support this diagnosis**[Q].

Treatment:
• Treatment is **supportive** & patients usually **recover without sequelae**.
  • **No definitive treatment is available for TRALI, but with supportive care the patient's oxygenation often improves and return to normal in 2-3 days**[Q].

118. **Ans. is a Epidemic typhus**   *(Ref: CMDT (2018)/p1445; Harrison 19/e p1158, 1051, 1297, 1135)*

Centrifugal rash starts from face or trunk centrally and moves to extremities peripherally whereas centripetal rash starts from extremities peripherally and moves to trunk and face centrally. Non-centripetally distributed (centrifugal) rash is seen in epidemic typhus.

"Epidemic typhus: A rash begins on the upper trunk, usually on the fifth day, and then becomes generalized, involving the entire body except the face, palms, and soles. Initially, this rash is macular; without treatment, it becomes maculopapular, petechial, and confluent."-Harrison 19/e p1158

*"Jaundice, bradycardia, and the absence of a headache are correlated with a delayed defervescence (in both epidemic and endemic typhus). The illness may be associated with maternal death, miscarriage, preterm birth, and low birth weight if acquired early during pregnancy. **The most common entity in the differential diagnosis is Rocky Mountain spotted fever, usually occurring after rural exposure and with a different rash (centripetal versus centrifugal for epidemic or endemic endemic typhus)."-CMDT (2018)/p1445***

"Typhoid: Early physical findings of enteric fever include rash ("rose spots"; 30%), hepatosplenomegaly (3–6%), epistaxis, and relative bradycardia at the peak of high fever (<50%). Rose spots make up a faint, salmon-colored, blanching, maculopapular rash located primarily on the trunk and chest. The rash is evident in ~30% of patients at the end of the first week and resolves without a trace after 2–5 days. Patients can have two or three crops of lesions, and Salmonella can be cultured from punch biopsies of these lesions. The faintness of the rash makes it difficult to detect in highly pigmented patients."- Harrison 19/e p1051

"The rash of measles begins as erythematous macules behind the ears and on the neck and hairline. The rash progresses to involve the face, trunk, and arms, with involvement of the legs and feet by the end of the second day. Areas of confluent rash appear on the trunk and extremities, and petechiae may be present. The rash fades slowly in the same order of progression as it appeared, usually beginning on the third or fourth day after onset. Resolution of the rash may be followed by desquamation, particularly in undernourished children."- Harrison 19/e p1297

*"Secondary Syphilis: **The skin rash consists of macular, papular, papulosquamous, and occasionally pustular syphilides; often more than one form is present simultaneously.** The eruption may be very subtle, and 25% of patients with a discernible rash may be unaware that they have dermatologic manifestations. **Initial lesions are pale red or pink, nonpruritic, discrete macules distributed on the trunk and proximal extremities; these macules progress to papular lesions that are distributed widely and that frequently involve the palms and soles**."- Harrison 19/e p1135*

*"Secondary Syphilis: This stage is characterised by sore throat, anaemia, skin rashes, lymphadenitis, and swelling in bones and joints. Arthralgia may be worse at night. Systemic symptoms like headache, fever, and malaise may be present. **Cutaneous lesions are symmetrically distributed, polymorphic, non-pruritic and are abundant on the central part of the body, as compared to the extremities (called "centripetal distribution"). These skin lesions may manifest as rose-coloured macules, coppery papules, pustules or ulcers.**"-HIV and AIDS:: Basic Elements and Priorities By S. Kartikeyan, R.N. Bharmal, R.P. Tiwari, P.S. Bisen/p204*

119. **Ans. c. Resting tremor** *(Ref: Harrison 19/e p2618, 18/e p3238)*

Cerebellar lesions produce intention tremors. Resting tremors are seen in basal ganglia diseases like Parkinsonism.

"Parkinson disease is characterized by a resting tremor, essential tremor (ET) by a postural tremor (trying to sustain a posture), and cerebellar disease by an intention or kinetic tremor (on reaching to touch a target)."- Harrison 19/e p2618

Clinical Features of Cerebellar Lesions	
Of Localizing Value	
Disorders of postural fixation (Paleocerebellum)	• **Hypotonia[Q], Weakness[Q]** • **Pendular knee jerk[Q]: Series of jerky to and free movements of the leg** before the leg finally comes to rest. • **Past pointing[Q]**
Disorders of movement (Neocerebellum)	• **Intention tremors[Q]: Increased irregularity of the movements** as the finger approaches the nose in the finger nose test. • **Dysmetria[Q]: Inability to arrest the movements at desired points** due to **loss of ability to gauge the distance, speed** and **power of movement.** • **Dyssynergy[Q]: Defective co-ordination of various muscles** and muscle groups participating in a movement. • **Dysdiadochokinesia[Q]: Disturbance in the reciprocal innervations of agonists & antagonists (loss of ability to stop one act** and **follow it immediately by a diametrically opposite act)** • **Rebound phenomenon: Failure of antagonist to counter overshoot movements totally.**
Disorders of gait	• **Broad-based gait[Q], Reeling gait[Q], Deviation to the side of lesion[Q]** • **Truncal ataxia[Q], Titubation[Q]**

Clinical Features of Cerebellar Lesions
Of no Localizing Value
• Static tremors: Tremors at rest due to hypotonia[Q]
• Skew deviation: Ipsilateral eye turns downwards & inwards and contralateral eye turns upwards & outwards[Q]
• Nystagmus & Vertigo
• Speech disturbance: Staccato, scanning or explosive speech, sometimes dysarthria[Q]

120. Ans. a. 1 day *(Ref: Harrison 19/e p382, 18/e p3263; Goodman Gillman 12/e p592; Andrews' Diseases of the Skin: Clinical Dermatology By William D. James, Timothy Berger, Dirk Elston/p 113)*

Hypersensitivity to anti-epileptic drugs is a Type 4 Hypersensitivity reaction (Steven-Johnson Syndrome), which comes in about 3–4 weeks. When the drug is re-challenged, the mediators are already pre-formed and are released much quicker (on the day of starting the treatment), causing the rash.

Phenytoin Hypersensitivity Syndrome (PHS)
• Reaction **typically develops within 3 weeks** to **3 months after initiation of treatment** with phenytoin
• Characterized by **fever, exanthemas** that range from **acneiform to erythema multiforme major, lymphadenopathy & eosinophilia.**
• Re-exposure to the drug, or exposure to phenobarbital or carbamazepine, will result in reactivation of the syndrome with a potentially fatal outcome.
Mechanism:
• It is a result of **an allergic hypersensitivity reaction.**
• **Phenytoin** may **act directly as antigen** or **indirectly as a hapten to trigger antibody production**.
• Some individuals may lack the **enzyme epoxide hydrolase,** which is **needed to detoxify arene oxides.**
• These oxides, which are **very highly reactive & potentially cytotoxic**, are formed as a **result of oxidative metabolism of phenytoin.**
• **Phenobarbital & carbamazepine share the same metabolic pathway** as phenytoin and consequently **cross-sensitivity to these drugs** is found in most patients with a history of PHS.
Clinical Features:
• **Skin rashes, hepatitis** (Hepatomegaly with raised serum aminotransferase values) **& lymphadenopathy**.
• A generalized **macular papular eruption with follicles & pustules on face & upper trunk** is **characteristic**.
• **Localized or generalized lymphadenopathy** usually **resolves following discontinuation of phenytoin.**
• **Additional findings:** Interstitial nephritis, myopathy, Coomb's negative hemolytic anemia & interstitial pulmonary infiltrates.
• **Laboratory evaluation: Leukocytosis with eosinophilia & atypical lymphocytosis; mild Coomb-negative hemolytic anemia.**
Treatment:
• **Immediate discontinuation of phenytoin & supportive care**.
• **No specific therapy for phenytoin hypersensitivity syndrome**
• **Positive response to corticosteroids when initiated early** in the course of illness

121. Ans. b. Increase in phosphate concentration *(Ref: Harrison 19/e p2166; Oxford Textbook of Rheumatology 4/e p1049; Textbook of Oral & Maxillofacial Surgery (Elsevier)/402)*

Phosphate concentration of saliva is decreased in Sjögren's syndrome.

"Sjögren's syndrome: Increased concentration of sodium and chloride and decreased concentrations of phosphate. IgA is increased. Rate of salivary flow is reduced. In addition, there are changes in the relative concentration of some minor salivary proteins."- Textbook of Oral & Maxillofacial Surgery (Elsevier)/402

Salivary Analysis of Patients of Sjögren's syndrome	
Salivary **sodium**	**Increased**[Q]
Salivary **chloride**	**Increased**[Q]
Salivary **IgA**	**Increased**[Q]
Salivary **phosphate**	**Decreased**[Q]
Unstimulated salivary flow rate	**Decreased** (<0.1 mL/min)[Q]
Stimulated salivary flow rate	**Decreased** (<0.5 mL/min)[Q]

Sjögren's Syndrome
• Chronic disease characterized by **dry eyes (keratoconjunctivitis sicca)** & **dry mouth (xerostomia)** resulting from **immunologically mediated destruction** of **lacrimal & salivary glands**[Q].
• It occurs as an **isolated disorder (primary form)**, also known as **sicca syndrome** or more often **in association with another autoimmune disease (secondary form)**[Q].
• **MC** associated disorder: **Rheumatoid arthritis**[Q]

Pathology:
- Characterized by **lymphocytic infiltration** & **fibrosis** of lacrimal & salivary glands[Q].
- **Earliest histologic finding** in both major & minor salivary glands: **Periductal** & **perivascular lymphocytic infiltration**[Q].

- **Most important antibodies**: Directed against **SS-A (Ro)** & **SS-B (La)**[Q], detected in 90% of patients (**serologic markers**[Q] of disease)
- Patients with **high titers of antibodies to SS-A** are **more likely to have early disease onset, longer disease duration** & **extra-glandular manifestations**[Q].

Clinical Features:
- Occurs **most commonly in women**[Q] between the ages of **50 & 60**.
- **Characteristic symptoms: Keratoconjunctivitis & xerostomia**[Q]
- **Parotid gland enlargement** is present in **half of** the **patients**[Q]
- **Extra-glandular disease** are seen **in one third** of patients

- **Glandular manifestations: Dry eye, dry mouth & parotid enlargement**[Q]
- **Extra-glandular manifestations: Arthritis, Raynaud's phenomenon, vasculitis, lymphoma, renal tubular acidosis**[Q]

Diagnosis:
- **Biopsy of lip (to examine minor salivary glands)** is **essential for** the **diagnosis of Sjögren's syndrome**[Q].

Treatment:
- **Symptom treatment** for relief & limitation of damaging effects of chronic xerostomia & keratoconjunctivitis sicca **through substitution** for or **stimulation of missing secretions**[Q]

122. **Ans. d. Low reticulocyte count** *(Ref: Robbins 9/e p631, 632)*

A reactive increase in reticulocyte count occurs in hemolytic anemias due to increased erythropoiesis.

"Certain changes are seen in hemolytic anemias regardless of cause or type. Anemia and lowered tissue oxygen tension trigger the production of erythropoietin, which stimulates erythroid differentiation and leads to the appearance of increased numbers of erythroid precursors (normoblasts) in the marrow. Compensatory increases in erythropoiesis result in a prominent reticulocytosis in the peripheral blood."- Robbins 9th/e p631, 632

Hemolytic Anemia
Characteristic Features of Hemolytic anemias:
• A **shortened RBC life span** <120 days (**premature destruction**)[Q]
• **Elevated erythropoietin levels** & **increased erythropoiesis** in marrow & other sites, to compensate for loss of RBCs[Q]
• **Accumulation of products of hemoglobin catabolism**, due to an **increased rate of red cell destruction**[Q]
Morphology:
• **Anemia & lowered tissue oxygen tension** → **Increased production of erythropoietin** → Stimulates erythroid differentiation → Appearance of **increased numbers of erythroid precursors (normoblasts)** in the marrow[Q].

Contd...

Contd...

Hemolytic Anemia
• **Compensatory increases in erythropoiesis** result in a **prominent reticulocytosis**[Q].
• **Phagocytosis of RBCs** leads to accumulation of **hemosiderin** in spleen, liver & bone marrow (Hemosiderosis).
• If the **anemia is severe, extramedullary hematopoiesis** can appear in **liver, spleen & lymph nodes**[Q].
• With **chronic hemolysis, elevated biliary excretion of bilirubin** promotes the formation of **pigment gallstones**[Q].

Types of Hemolysis		
	Extravascular hemolysis	**Intravascular hemolysis**
Site of hemolysis	Mononuclear phagocytes[Q] of RE system (Spleen[Q], bone marrow[Q])	Within the circulation[Q]
Diseases causing hemolysis	Thalassemia[Q], sickle cell anemia[Q]	PNH[Q], G-6-PD deficiency[Q]
Serum haptoglobin	Normal	Decreased[Q]
Hemoglobinuria	Not seen	Positive[Q]
Methhemoglobinuria	Not seen	Positive[Q]
Hemosiderinuria	Not seen	Positive[Q]
Unconjugated bilirubin	Moderately elevated	Mildly elevated
Splenomegaly	Usual[Q]	Uncommon

123. Ans. c. D-xylose absorption test *(Ref: Harrison 19/e p1938)*

Fecal fat estimation is the gold standard test for diagnosis of malabsorption. Best test though, for diagnosis of intestinal malabsorption is D-xylose test as it tests for absorption of xylose in the intestinal villi and can distinguish intestinal from pancreatic malabsorption. NBT-PABA & serum amylase are the tests for pancreatic malabsorption.

Malabsorption
• **Gold standard** for diagnosis of **steatorrhea: Quantitative stool fat determination**[Q].
• **Sudan III stain (qualitative test):** Used to establish the **presence of increased stool fat**, rapid & inexpensive, does not establish the degree of fat malabsorption, used as a **preliminary screening study**[Q].
• **Fecal fat excretion** in healthy individuals should be **<7 gm/day**[Q].
• Presence of steatorrhea requires further assessment to establish the pathophysiologic process(es) responsible for the defect in dietary lipid digestion-absorption.
• Other studies used: **Schilling test, D-xylose test, duodenal mucosal biopsy, small-intestinal radiologic examination & tests of pancreatic exocrine function**[Q].

D-xylose Test	• If the 72-hour fecal fat collection results demonstrate fat malabsorption, **D-xylose test is used to document the integrity of intestinal mucosa**[Q]. • Facilitated diffusion in the proximal intestine primarily absorbs D-xylose. • Approximately **half of absorbed D-xylose is excreted in urine, unmetabolized.** If the **absorption of D-xylose** is **impaired due to** either a **luminal factor** (e.g. bacterial overgrowth) or a **reduced** or **damaged mucosal surface area** (e.g. surgical resection, celiac disease), **urinary excretion is lower than normal**[Q]. • **Cases of pancreatic insufficiency** result in **normal urinary excretion** because **absorption of D-xylose is intact**[Q].
Schilling Test	• **Malabsorption of vitamin B12** may occur as a consequence of **deficiency of intrinsic factor** (e.g. pernicious anemia, gastric resection), **pancreatic insufficiency, bacterial overgrowth, ileal resection, or disease**[Q]. • The **3-stage Schilling test** results can help **differentiate these conditions**[Q].
Pancreatic Function Tests	• A tube is placed through the nose or mouth so that its tip is lying next to the opening of pancreatic duct into duodenum. • Secretions are collected & content of bicarbonate & enzymes are measured after the **pancreas** has been **stimulated with secretin** or **with a test meal**[Q]. • **Pancreatic insufficiency** is indicated if the **bicarbonate & enzyme concentrations** are **very low.** • **Bentiromide test** (Pancreatic function test): Involves ingestion of a chemical called **bentiromide**, which is **broken by pancreatic enzymes** & one constituent (para aminobenzoic acid, **PABA**) is **absorbed & excreted in urine. Pancreatic insufficiency** is suspected when **urinary PABA levels are low**[Q].

Results of Diagnostic Studies in Different Causes of Steatorrhea			
	D-Xylose Test	**Schilling Test**	**Duodenal Mucosal Biopsy**
Chronic pancreatitis	Normal	**50% abnormal; if abnormal, normal with pancreatic enzymes**[Q]	Normal
Bacterial overgrowth syndrome	Normal or only modestly abnormal	**Often abnormal; if abnormal, normal after antibiotics**[Q]	Usually normal
Ileal disease	Normal	**Abnormal**[Q]	Normal
Celiac disease	**Decreased**[Q]	Normal	**Abnormal: probably "flat"**
Intestinal lymphangiectasia	Normal	Normal	**Abnormal: "dilated lymphatics"** [Q]

SURGERY

124. Ans. a. Parabronchial diverticulum *(Ref: Bailey 27/e p1102, 26/e p1018; Sabiston 20/e p1019; Schwartz 10/e p994)*

Traction diverticula (parabronchial or midesophageal diverticula) are true diverticula, which occur secondary to scarring, fibrosis and inflammatory processes in the mediastinum pulling on the esophageal wall.

"Traction, or true, diverticula result from external inflammatory mediastinal lymph nodes adhering to the esophagus as they heal and contract, pulling the esophagus during the process. Over time, the esophageal wall herniates, forming an outpouching, and a diverticulum ensues. These are more common in the midesophageal region around the carinal lymph nodes."- Sabiston 20/e p1019

Esophageal Diverticula	
True diverticula	• Include **all esophageal layers**[Q]
False diverticula	• Contain **only mucosa & submucosa**[Q] herniating through the muscular layer (**Zenker's & Epiphrenic** diverticulum)[Q]
Traction diverticula	• Occurs **secondary to pulling forces** on the outer aspect of the esophagus[Q]
Pulsion diverticula	• Occurs **secondary to increased intraluminal pressure** (**Zenker's & Epiphrenic** diverticulum)[Q]

Types of Esophageal Diverticula Based on Location		
Upper Esophageal	**Mid-Esophageal** (Parabronchial)	Lower Esophageal
• **Zenker's diverticulum**[Q] • **Killian-Jamieson diverticulum**[Q]	• **Traction, or true diverticula**[Q]	• **Epiphrenic diverticula**[Q]

Mid-esophageal or Traction Diverticula
• **Inflammation** of **lymph nodes** exerts **traction** on the wall of esophagus leading to formation of a **true diverticulum** in mid-esophagus[Q].   • **More common on right & wide mouthed**[Q].
Etiology: • Caused by **inflamed mediastinal lymph nodes** from **tuberculosis, histoplasmosis**[Q] & resultant **fibrosing mediastinitis**[Q].
Clinical Features: • **Most patients** are **asymptomatic** (**incidentally detected** during radiological investigations)   • **Dysphagia, chest pain & regurgitation** can be present & are usually indicative of an **underlying primary motility disorder**[Q].
Diagnosis: • **IOC for diagnosis: Barium swallow**[Q] (**lateral views** to determine side)   • **CT scan**: To identify any **mediastinal lymphadenopathy** & to **lateralize the sac**.   • **Manometry: Done** in **all patients**, symptomatic or not, **to identify** a **primary motor disorder**.
Treatment: • **Asymptomatic patients** with inflamed mediastinal LNs from **tuberculosis** or **histoplasmosis**: **ATT** or **antifungal agents**[Q]   • **Diverticulopexy** for **symptomatic** or **2 cm or larger** diverticulum   • **Esophagomyotomy** in **severe chest pain** or **dysphagia** & a documented **motor abnormality**[Q]

Zenker's or Pharyngo-esophageal diverticula

- **MC esophageal diverticula[Q]**
- **Mucosal outpouching (pulsion diverticulum)** occurring **through** triangular bare area (**Killian's triangle**)[Q], between **upper oblique fibers (thyropharyngeus muscle)** & **lower horizontal fibers (cricopharyngeus muscle)** of **inferior constrictor muscle[Q]**
- It is **not a true esophageal diverticula[Q]**, as it arises above upper esophageal sphincter (cricopharyngeus sphincter)
  - **Increased intraluminal pressures** (secondary to **abnormal esophageal motility**)[Q] pushes **mucosa & submucosa** through a muscular defect in the wall of the esophagus creating a **pulsion diverticulum[Q]**
  - It is a **pseudodiverticula[Q]**
  - It **arises posteriorly** in midline of neck, **mouth is in midline** but **sac projects laterally[Q]** (usually **left laterally**)

Pathology
- **Neuromuscular incordination[Q]** in this region
- May be due to **different nerve supply** of the **two parts of inferior constrictor muscle[Q]**
  - Thyropharyngeus (oblique fibers) supplied by pharyngeal plexus
  - Cricopharyngeus (horizontal fibers) by recurrent laryngeal nerve

Clinical features
- Usually seen in patients over **50 years[Q]**
- **MC symptom** is **dysphagia[Q]**
- **Undigested food** is **regurgitated into the mouth**, especially when the patient is in **recumbent position[Q]**
- **Swelling of neck, gurgling noise** after eating, **halitosis** & a sour metallic taste in mouth are common symptoms
- **Cervical webs** are seen **associated in 50%[Q]** of patients with Zenker's diverticula, can cause dysphagia post-operatively if not treated

Diagnosis:
- **IOC for diagnosis: Barium swallow[Q]**

Complications
- **Pneumonia** & **lung abscess** due to **aspiration[Q]** (**MC**)
- Perforation, Bleeding
- Carcinoma

Management:
- Surgical therapy (**Cricopharyngeal myotomy + Diverticulopexy**) is **treatment of choice[Q]**

Treatment options for Zenker's diverticula

- **Cricopharyngeal myotomy**—a myotomy alone is sufficient for small diverticula
- **Myotomy with excision of sac**—done for large (>4 cm) diverticula
- **Diverticulopexy**
- **Diverticulo-esophagostomy** using a linear cutting staple gun
- The septum between the esophagus and the diverticula is divided
- Also known as **Dohlman procedure[Q]**

Epiphrenic diverticula

- Epiphrenic diverticula are found **adjacent to diaphragm** in the **distal third** of esophagus, within 10 cm of GE junction.
- Most often related to **thickened distal esophageal musculature** or **increased intraluminal pressure**.
- **Pulsion** or **false diverticula**, often **associated with DES, achalasia,** and **most commonly NEM** (non-specific esophageal motility) **disorders.**
- In patients in whom a motility abnormality cannot be identified, a congenital (**Ehlers-Danlos syndrome**) or **traumatic cause** is considered.
- More common on **right side** & **wide-mouthed[Q]**.

Clinical Features:
- Most patients are **asymptomatic**.
- **Dysphagia** or **chest pain** indicative of a **motility disturbance**.
- The diagnosis is often made during the workup for a motility disorder, and the diverticulum is **found incidentally.**

Epiphrenic diverticula
Diagnosis: • **IOC for diagnosis: Barium swallow**[Q] (**lateral views** to determine side) • **Manometry** to identify a **primary motor disorder**.
Treatment: • **Diverticulopexy** • **Long esophagomyotomy** in severe chest pain, dysphagia, or a **documented motor abnormality**[Q]

Killian-Jamieson Diverticula
• **Lateral cervical** esophageal diverticula • Located **just below cricopharyngeus** • Mostly **asymptomatic**

125. Ans. a. A *(Ref: Bailey 27/e p964-965, 25/e p339-340, Oxford Textbook of Vascular Surgery/ p202; Trauma 7/e p623)*
Marked region 'A' represents the zone 4 of retroperitoneal hemorrhage.

*The **retroperitoneum** is usually **divided into three parts** based on site of injury. Some authors also describe a **4th zone**, i.e. the portal and retro hepatic area. Zone 1 (central) extends from the **esophageal hiatus to the sacral promontory**. Zone 2 (lateral) extends from the **lateral diaphragm to the iliac crest**. Zone 3 (pelvic) is confined to the **retroperitoneal space of the pelvic bowl**.*

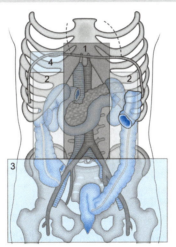

Zones of Retroperitoneal Hematoma		
Zone	**Extent**	**Management**
Zone 1 (central)	• Extends from **esophageal hiatus to sacral promontory**[Q] • Hematoma or hemorrhage in the **midline** associated with **injuries** to **abdominal aorta, IVC**, their proximal **branches & tributaries**[Q]. • Zone 1 is divided into **supramesocolic & inframesocolic zone** depending on **origin of vascular structure in relation to transverse mesocolon**[Q]. | **Supramesocolic Zone 1**	**Inframesocolic Zone 1**
---	---
• **Suprarenal aorta, IVC, coeliac axis, proximal SMA & vein**, and **proximal renal arteries & veins**[Q].	• **Infrarenal aorta & IVC** including their **bifurcations**[Q].		**Central hematoma** should **always be explored** with **proximal & distal vascular control**[Q]
Zone 2 (lateral)	• Extends from **lateral diaphragm to iliac crest**[Q] • Include distal renal arteries & veins[Q]	**Lateral hematomas** are **usually renal** in origin & can be **managed non-operatively**[Q], sometimes with **angioembolization**.

Contd...

Contd...

Zone	Extent	Management
Zone 3 (pelvic)	• Confined to **retroperitoneal space of pelvic bowl**[Q] • **Include iliac arteries & veins**[Q]	**Pelvic hematomas** are **exceptionally difficult to control** and should, whenever possible, **not be opened**[Q] Should be **controlled with packing** (intra- or extrapelvic) & **angioembolization**[Q]
Zone 4	• **Include portal & retrohepatic area**[Q]	

126. **Ans. d. All of the above**   *(Ref: Bailey 27/e p929-925, 26/e p303; Sabiston 20/e p557; Harrison 19/e p1661, 1731, 1732)*
Hypoxia, inability to speak & stridor during inspiration, all are signs of respiratory insufficiency.

*"Respiratory Insufficiency: A condition where the **lungs are unable to function properly and maintain the normal processes of oxygen uptake and carbon dioxide removal**. Sign & symptoms of respiratory insufficiency are **fatigue, shortness of breath, heavy breathing, rapid breathing, exercise intolerance, hypoxia.**"*

Airway obstruction
• Any **upper or lower airway obstruction** generates a **pathological respiratory sound** resulting from the **rapid, turbulent flow of air** through the **narrowed segment of respiratory tract**[Q]. • **MC symptoms: Cough, dyspnoea & voice change**[Q] • **Dyspnea if progressive** imminent **complete upper airway obstruction**[Q]

Signs of Airway obstruction	
• **Stridor** is noisy breathing resulting from **narrowing of larynx or trachea** (Noise tends to be high pitched) • **Obstruction or collapse of pharyngeal airway** causes **stertor**[Q]. • **Inspiratory stridor:** Obstruction at or above the level of **glottis**[Q] • **Expiratory stridor: obstruction of intrathoracic airway**[Q] • **Biphasic stridor: tracheal lesions**[Q] • **Hoarseness:** Greater the degree of hoarseness the greater the severity of **laryngeal damage**[Q].	• **Suprasternal retraction:** It is **to overcome the airflow obstruction**, so the **accessory muscles of respiration are used**, which causes **suprasternal retraction, intercostal recession & flaring of the nostrils**[Q]. • **Restlessness:** The result of anxiety or may be indicative of hypoxia. • **Drooling & bleeding**[Q] • **Fracture & subcutaneous emphysema**[Q]

127. **Ans. d. Lanz incision**   *(Ref: Bailey 27/e p1309, 26/e p1208, 25/e p1212)*
Lanz incision is an oblique, muscle splitting incision used for appendectomy. It is a modification of McBurney's (Grid Iron) incision and is considered cosmetically better.

*"In recent years, a **transverse skin crease (Lanz) incision** has become **more popular, as the exposure is better and extension, when needed, is easier**. The incision, appropriate in length to the size and obesity of the patient, is made approximately 2 cm below the umbilicus centered on the midclavicular–midinguinal line. When necessary, the incision may be extended medially, with retraction or suitable division of the rectus abdominis muscle."- Bailey 27/e p1309*

Incisions used for Abdominal Cavity Exploration

• **Vertical incision:** Midline incision & Paramedian incisions
Transverse and oblique incisions:
   – Kocher's subcostal incision (Chevron-Roof top modification & Mercedes Benz modification)
   – Transverse muscle dividing incision
   – McBurney's (grid iron) or muscle splitting incision[Q]
   – Oblique muscle cutting incision (Rutherford-Morrison)[Q]
   – Pfannenstiel incision
   – Maylard transverse muscle cutting incision[Q]
• Abdominothoracic incisions

AIIMS November 2016 947

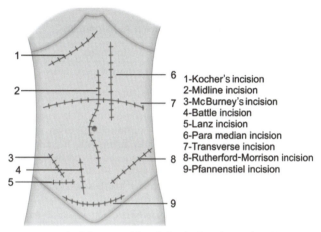

Fig. 34: Incisions used for abdominal cavity exploration

1-Kocher's incision
2-Midline incision
3-McBurney's incision
4-Battle incision
5-Lanz incision
6-Para median incision
7-Transverse incision
8-Rutherford-Morrison incision
9-Pfannenstiel incision

Name of Incision	Used for
Lazy 'S'; Sistrunk; Modified Blair's	• Parotidectomy[Q]
McBurney's, Grid-Iron or McArthur Lanz	• Appendectomy[Q]
Pfannenstiel incision	• Caesarean section & abdominal hysterectomy[Q]
Chevron incision	• Whipple's procedure & upper abdominal malignancies[Q]
Cherney incision	• Pelvic surgery (excellent surgical exposure to the space of Retzius and pelvic side walls)
Kocher's incision	• Open cholecystectomy[Q]
Kustner's incision	• Transverse incision made 5 cm above the symphysis pubis but below the anterior superior iliac spine
Maylard incision	• A variation of Pfannenstiel incision[Q] • Rectus abdominis muscles are sectioned transversely to permit wider access to the pelvis.
McEvedy's incision	• Lateral paramedian incision[Q]
Turner-Warwick's incision	• Placed 2 cm above the symphysis pubis and within the lateral borders of the rectus muscle. • Good for exposure of retropubic space[Q]

128. **Ans. b. 4x incision length** *(Ref: Bailey 27/e p1041, 26/e p965, 25/e p234)*
 According to Jenkins' rule, optimal ratio of suture length to wound length is 4:1.

"There is no evidence that interrupted sutures are better or worse than continuous. However, if continuous suturing is used, the tissue bites must not be too near the fascial edge nor pulled too tight or they may cut out. **It has also been confirmed that the optimal ratio of suture length to wound length is 4:1 (Jenkins' rule). If less length than this is used, the suture bites are too far apart or too tight and the converse applies if more length than this is used.***"- Bailey 27/e p1041*

Wound Closure & Anastomoses

- As a general rule, **each suture** should be **separated by a gap** that is **twice** the **thickness of skin**[Q].
- When **knots are cut short**, **free ends** or 'ears' should be left **at least 1-2 mm** long[Q]. This is particularly important with **monofilament non-absorbables**[Q].
  - It has been suggested by **Jenkins** that a **suture length to wound length ratio** of **4:1** indicates the **optimum size of tissue bites** and of **suture spacing**[Q].
- **Anastomosis of vessels** was **pioneered by Carrel**[Q].

Contd...

Contd...

Wound Closure & Anastomoses
Bowel Anastomoses
• **Lembert** described **seromuscular suture technique** for **bowel anastomosis** in 1826[Q]. • **Senn** advocated a **two-layer technique for closure**[Q]. • **Halsted** favored a **one-layer extramucosal closure**[Q]. • **Connell** used a **single layer of interrupted sutures** incorporating all layers of the bowel[Q]. • **Kocher's method**, a **two layer anastomosis**, first a **continuous all-layer suture using catgut**, then an **inverting continuous** (or interrupted) **seromuscular layer** suture **using silk**, became the standard. There is evidence that **inversion is safest in bowel** (least likely to leak), although end-to-end staplers give an everted anastomosis without complication. • **Single-layer extramucosal anastomosis**, advocated by **Matheson**[Q], causes the least tissue necrosis or luminal narrowing. • **Cheatle split** (making a **cut into** the **anti-mesenteric border**) may help to **enlarge** the **lumen of distal, collapsed bowel**[Q]. • **Bowel anastomotic leaks** are generally occurs **on day 7**[Q].

129. **Ans. c. Damage control surgery and mesh closure of abdomen** *(Ref: Schwartz 10/e p192-195; Bailey 27/e p318-319, 26/e p362-363)*

The pictures above are showing minimal abbreviated laparotomy i.e. damage control surgery in a setting of trauma, and closure of abdomen using meshplasty so as to prevent abdominal compartment syndrome.

> *"Damage control surgery is minimal intervention done to stabilize the patient and do the definitive surgery later. Damage control includes an abbreviated laparotomy, temporary packing, and closure of the abdomen in an effort to blunt the physiologic response to prolonged shock and massive hemorrhage."*

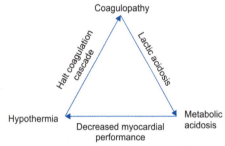

Fig. 43: Trauma triad of death

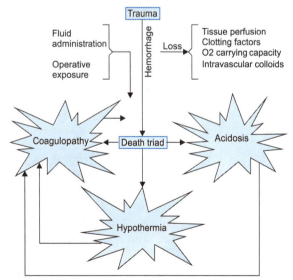

Fig. 35: Components involved in trauma triad of death

Damage Control Surgery (DCS)

- **DCS** centers on coordinating **staged operative interventions** with periods of **aggressive resuscitation** to salvage trauma patients sustaining major injuries[Q].
- **Damage control includes** an **abbreviated laparotomy, temporary packing**, and **closure of the abdomen** in an effort to **blunt the physiologic response to prolonged shock & massive hemorrhage**[Q].
  - These patients are often **at limits of their physiological reserve** when they present to operating room & **persistent operative efforts** result in exacerbation of their **underlying hypothermia, coagulopathy & acidosis**, initiating a **vicious cycle** that **culminates in death**[Q].
- In these situations, **abrupt termination of** the **procedure** after **control of surgical hemorrhage & contamination**, followed by **ICU resuscitation & staged reconstruction**, can be life saving[Q].

Phases of Damage Control Surgery

Phase I (Initial Exploration)	Phase II (Secondary Resuscitation)	Phase III (Definitive Operation)
• Consists of an **initial operative exploration** to attain rapid **control of active hemorrhage & contamination**[Q] • Abdomen is entered via **midline incision** & if exsanguinating hemorrhage is encountered **four quadrant packing** should be performed • **Any violations of GI tract** should be treated with **suture closure** or **segmental stapled resection**[Q] • **External drains**[Q] are placed to control any major pancreatic or biliary injuries	• Following completion of initial exploration, **critically ill patient** is **transferred to ICU**[Q]. • **Invasive monitoring & complete ventilator support** are often needed[Q]. • This phase focuses on **secondary resuscitation** to **correct hypothermia, coagulopathy & acidosis**[Q]	• It consists of **planned re-exploration & definitive repair** of injuries • This phase typically occurs **48 to 72 hours following initial & after successful secondary resuscitation**[Q] • The abdomen should be closed primarily if possible • **Risky GI anastomoses** or **complex reconstruction** should be **avoided**[Q]

130. **Ans. a. Laparoscopic port trocar** *(Ref: Jaypee Manual of Surgical Equipments/267)*

The instrument marked in the laparoscopy image above is the port containing the trocar. It is used for creating pneumoperitoneum and inserting the instruments for the procedure.

Laparoscopic Port Trocar

Laparoscopic port trocars are required to **access the peritoneal cavity during surgery** and for **maintaining pneumoperitoneum when instruments are exchanged.**

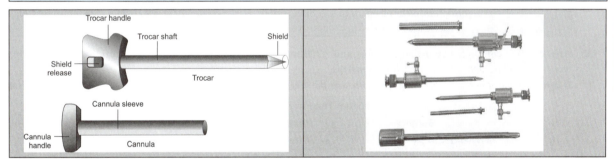

131. **Ans. a. Monopolar cautery** *(Ref: Sabiston 20/e p235-236)*

The instrument being used by surgeon is monopolar cautery.

Monopolar Electrocautery	Bipolar Electrocautery	LigaSure	Hyfrecators

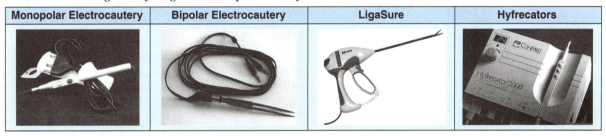

Surgical Devices & Energy Sources		
Monopolar Electrocautery	<ul><li>Monopolar electrocautery is used for **cutting, blending, desiccation** & **fulguration.**</li><li>Using a pencil instrument, active electrode is placed in the entry site and can be **used to cut tissue** & **coagulate bleeding.**</li></ul>	
	Cutting	<ul><li>Cautery **activated** with a **constant waveform**[Q]</li><li>**Heat** is **generated relatively quickly** over the target with **minimal lateral thermal spread**[Q].</li></ul>
	Coagulation	<ul><li>Cautery activated with an **intermittent waveform**[Q]</li><li>**Less heat** is **generated** on a **slower frequency, with** the potential for **large lateral thermal spread**, resulting in **tissue dehydration** & **vessel thrombosis**[Q].</li></ul>
	<ul><li>**Blended waveform** have the **advantage of both cutting** & **coagulation** modes.</li><li>**Grounding pad** is placed securely on the patient **for monopolar cautery** device **to function properly** & **to prevent thermal burn injury** at the current reentry electrode site.</li><li>**MC used** because of **versatility** & **effectiveness**[Q].</li></ul>	
Bipolar Electrocautery	<ul><li>**Bipolar electrocautery** establishes a **short circuit between the tips of instrument** (forceps)[Q]</li><li>**Grounding pad** is **not required**[Q]</li><li>**Grasped tissue** between the **tips of instrument completes** the **circuit**[Q]<ul><li>It provides **precise thermal coagulation** (generating **heat affects only the tissue within short circuit**)[Q]</li><li>**More effective than the monopolar instrument in coagulating vessels** due to **mechanical advantage of compression of tissue between the tips** of the instrument to the thermal coagulation**[Q].</li></ul></li><li>Particularly useful for procedures in which **lateral thermal injury** or an **arcing phenomenon needs to be avoided**[Q].</li></ul>	
LigaSure	<ul><li>**LigaSure** is a **new electrothermal bipolar tissue sealing system**[Q]</li><li>Applied in **abdominal** & **pelvic surgery**, mostly **through laparoscopy**[Q].</li><li>**Advantage:** It improves **vessel sealing** with **minimal lateral thermal spread**[Q].</li></ul>	
Hyfrecators	<ul><li>Hyfrecator functions by sending electrical impulses into body with the use of a probe[Q].<ul><li>It **works by emitting low-power high-frequency AC** (alternating current) **electrical pulses via a probe**, directly to the affected area of the body[Q].</li></ul></li><li>Hyfrecator is used for removal of warts, pearly penile papules, desiccation of sebaceous gland disorders, electrocautery of bleeding, epilation, destruction of small cosmetically unwanted superficial veins, destruction of skin cancers (basal cell carcinoma).</li></ul>	

132. **Ans. c. After complete expansion of lungs and <200 mL output from drain for 2 consecutive days** (*Ref: http://www. modernmedicine.com/content/chest-tube-removal*)

It is recommended to remove the drain after checking the lung for full expansion & drain output is <200 mL for 2 consecutive days.

Ideal Time to Remove Drain	
Surgery	**Postoperative Time to Remove the Drain**
Thyroidectomy	<ul><li>**24 hours**[Q]</li></ul>
ICD drain	<ul><li>**<200 mL in 24 hours**[Q]</li></ul>
Mastectomy	<ul><li>**5 days**[Q]</li></ul>
Colorectal anastomosis	<ul><li>**5-7 days**[Q]</li></ul>
T-Tube Drain	<ul><li>**10 days**[Q]</li></ul>

Chest Tube Removal
<ul><li>No matter what's the reason for insertion, a **chest tube must be removed within a week**[Q]. Leaving it in place for >7 days raises the risk for infection along the chest tube tract.</li><li>**An improvement in respiratory status is one of the first signs**[Q]. The patient will no longer be short of breath, and his breathing won't be labored. You will hear bilateral breath sounds and see a symmetrical rise of the chest on inspiration.</li><li>A **respiratory rate <24 breaths/minute** is another indication that the tube can come out[Q].</li></ul>

Contd...

AIIMS November 2016

Contd...

Chest Tube Removal
• If the chest tube was inserted because of excess fluid, it can be safely removed when the **drainage is <200 mL in 24 hours**[Q].

- If blood precipitated tube insertion, minimal output & a **change in drainage from bloody to serous or serosanguinous is also a key indicator.** In the case of **pneumothorax**, tube can **safely be removed when bubbling or fluctuation in the water-seal chamber ceases during expiration or during a cough**[Q].
- A **chest X-ray** should be done **prior to tube removal to confirm re- expansion of the affected lung** and **to assure that the timing is right**[Q].

133. **Ans. b. Check carotid pulse** *(Ref: BLS/ACLS Guidelines: https://www.resus.org.uk/resuscitation guidelines /adult-advanced-life-support; Harrison 19/e p1768; Braunwald's 10/e p844-845)*

   According to Adult Basic Life Support (BLS) algorithm in an unresponsive patient, next step is to check carotid pulse.
   See Q. No. 122 AIIMS November 2017

134. **Ans. b. Put the patient in recovery position and secure airway** *(Ref: BLS/ACLS Guidelines: https://www.resus.org.uk/resuscitation guidelines /adult- advanced-life-support; Harrison 19/e p1768; Braunwald's 10/e p844-845)*

   As a part of the BLS algorithm, start the airway management in any patient who is collapsed/expected to collapse. Since the patient is hemodynamically stable, the airway is the most important component at risk in this patient and requires immediate attention. The patient should be put in a recovery position i.e. left lateral decubitus position to prevent the risk of aspiration.

135. **Ans. b. Gluteal claudication** *(Ref Bailey 27/e p943-944, 26/e p837, 879, 25/e p901; Sabiston 20/e p1739; Schwartz 10/e p874; Harrison 19/e p1643)*

   Most common symptom of aortoiliac disease is gluteal claudication.

   "The site of claudication is distal to the location of the occlusive lesion. For example, buttock, hip, thigh, and calf discomfort occurs in patients with aortoiliac disease, whereas calf claudication develops in patients with femoral-popliteal disease."- Harrison 19/e p1643

   "Aortoiliac disease (30 per cent of cases) may cause thigh or buttock claudication. Buttock claudication in association with sexual impotence resulting from arterial insufficiency is eponymously called Leriche's syndrome. It is very rare."- Bailey 27/e p943

Site of Block	Clinical Presentation
Aortoiliac disease	• **Buttock, thigh & calf** claudication[Q] • **Leriche syndrome**[Q]
Common femoral disease	• **Thigh & calf** claudication[Q]
Superficial femoral disease	• Calf claudication[Q]
Popliteal artery disease	• Calf claudication[Q]
Crural artery disease	• Calf claudication[Q]

Aortoiliac Occlusive Disease

• **Distal abdominal aorta & iliac arteries** are **common sites affected by atherosclerosis**[Q].
• **Symptoms & natural history** of the atherosclerotic process are influenced by the **disease distribution & extent.**
   • Presence of **pelvic & groin collaterals** is important in **providing crucial collateral flow** in **maintaining lower limb viability**[Q].
   • It is **rarely limb threatening**[Q] (Opposite to femoropopliteal disease[Q])

Clinical Features: • **Bilateral thigh** or **buttock claudication**[Q] • **Erectile dysfunction** or **impotence (Leriche syndrome**[Q]) • **Pulses distal to occlusion** are **absent or diminished** • Rest pain & gangrene are unusual with isolated segment of aortoiliac disease. • **Examination: Weakened femoral pulses & reduced ABI**[Q].

Contd...

952   AIIMS ESSENCE

Contd...

Aortoiliac Occlusive Disease
Diagnosis: • **Duplex ultrasound** make the diagnosis of iliac occlusive disease   • **Angiography** is indicated if symptoms warrant **surgical intervention**[Q].
Treatment: • **Failure to respond to exercise** and/or **drug therapy** should prompt consideration for **limb revascularization**[Q].   • **Limb revascularization options**: Aortobifemoral bypass, aortic endarterectomy, axillofemoral bypass, iliofemoral bypass, femorofemoral bypass

136. Ans. c. Renal failure   *(Ref: Zakim and Boyer's Hepatology (2016)/p109; Bailey 25/e p1128, Textbook of hepatology 6/e p206)*

All causes of cholestatic jaundice i.e. malignant obstruction, complete CBD obstruction can cause high jaundice but presence of concomitant renal failure leads to increase in bilirubin beyond 30 mg/dL.

> *"Conjugated hyperbilirubinemia results from impaired intrahepatic bilirubin excretion or extrahepatic obstruction. However, because of continued urinary excretion, maximum serum bilirubin levels plateau at approximately 500 mmol/L (30 mg/dL) even with complete bile duct obstruction. Extreme hyperbilirubinemia, with levels higher than 500 mmol/L (30 mg/dL), commonly indicates severe parenchymal liver disease in association with hemolysis (as in sickle cell anemia) or renal failure."- Zakim and Boyer's Hepatology (2016)/p109*

> *All causes of **cholestatic jaundice** i.e. malignant obstruction, complete CBD obstruction **can cause high jaundice** but presence of concomitant **renal failure leads to increase in bilirubin beyond 30 mg/dL.** This is because **conjugated bilirubin is soluble and can be excreted in urine.** But in renal failure, this mechanism is absent and the **serum bilirubin can rise up to very high levels.** Usually even in the **presence of total absence of bile flow the bilirubin levels reach a plateau of around 25-30 mg/dL** as there is continuous excretion of conjugated bilirubin the bile. When there is such **high bilirubin (>30/40 mg/dL)** in obstructive jaundice, then suspect associated **renal failure** or ongoing hemolysis (Sepsis with DIC which may be the case in **ascending cholangitis, sickle cell anemia, etc.)**

137. Ans. a. Posterior pituitary tumors   *(Ref: Bailey 27/e p856-858, 26/e p795-797; Sabiston 20/e p993, 1003; Harrison 19/e p2335)*

MEN type 1 (MEN 1) is characterized by the triad of tumors involving the parathyroids, pancreatic islets, and anterior pituitary (not the posterior pituitary tumors).

> *"MEN type 1 (MEN 1), which is also referred to as Wermer's syndrome, is characterized by the **triad of tumors involving the parathyroids, pancreatic islets, and anterior pituitary.** In addition, adrenal cortical tumors, carcinoid tumors usually of the foregut, meningiomas, facial angiofibromas, collagenomas, and lipomas may also occur in some patients with MEN 1. The disorder **affects all age groups,** with a reported age range of **5 to 81 years,** with **clinical and biochemical manifestations developing in the vast majority by the fifth decade.** In the absence of treatment, endocrine tumors are associated with an **earlier mortality in patients with MEN 1,** with a **50% probability of death by the age of 50 years.** The cause of death is usually a malignant tumor, often from a pancreatic neuroendocrine tumor (NET) or foregut carcinoid. In addition, the treatment outcomes of patients with MEN 1–associated tumors are not as successful as those in patients with non–MEN 1 tumors. This is because **MEN 1–associated tumors, with the exception of pituitary NETs, are usually multiple, making it difficult to achieve a successful surgical cure."- Harrison 19/e p2335*

MEN-1 (WerMer's Syndrome)		
Parathyroid Adenoma	**Pancreatic NET (PGI)**	**Pituitary Adenoma**
• **MC endocrine abnormality (>98%** of affected individuals) in MEN-1 is **multiglandular parathyroid tumors**[Q]. • **Hyperparathyroidism** is **MC manifestation** (**cardinal sign** of MEN-1 is **parathyroid adenoma** of **multicentricity**)[Q]. • **Hypercalcemia** is **1st biochemical abnormality**[Q] detected in MEN-1 and may precede the clinical onset of a pancreatic NET or pituitary neoplasm by several years.	• Pancreatic NET is **2nd MC manifestation**[Q]. • **Nonfunctioning** or that secrete **pancreatic polypeptide**[Q] are **MC** pancreatic NET in MEN-1. • **MC functional NET** in patients with MEN-1: **Gastrinoma**[Q] > Insulinoma • **MC increased pancreatic hormone: P**ancreatic polypeptides >**G**astrin >**I**nsulin[Q] **(PGI)**	• **Prolactinoma** is **most common**[Q]. • Diagnosed by increased prolactin (>200 µg/L) & MRI.

	MEN-1	MEN-2 (MEN-2A or Sipple syndrome)	MEN-3 (MEN-2B)	MEN-4 (MEN-X)
Components	Parathyroid hyperplasia or adenoma[Q] Pancreatic NET[Q] Pituitary adenoma[Q] Bronchial & thymic carcinoids[Q] Adrenocortical tumors Subcutaneous or visceral lipomas[Q] Facial cutaneous angiofibromas[Q] Collagenomas[Q]	Medullary carcinoma thyroid[Q] Pheochromocytoma[Q] Parathyroid hyperplasia or adenoma[Q] Hirschsprung's disease[Q] Cutaneous lichen amyloidosis[Q]	Medullary carcinoma thyroid[Q] Pheo-chromocytoma[Q] Intestinal ganglioneuroma[Q] Mucosal neuromas[Q] Megacolon[Q] Marfanoid features[Q]	Hyper-parathyroidism Pituitary adenoma[Q] Pancreatic NET Gonadal, adrenal, renal & thyroid tumors (MEN-1 not having mutation of MEN-1 gene is known as MEN-4)[Q]
Gene/Defect	MEN-1 gene[Q]	RET oncogene (cysteine[Q] codon)	RET oncogene (tyrosine kinase[Q] domain)	Cyclin dependent kinase inhibitor (CDNKIB) gene[Q]
Chromosome	11[Q]	10[Q]	10[Q]	12[Q]
Transmission	Autosomal dominant[Q]	Autosomal dominant[Q]	Autosomal dominant[Q]	Autosomal dominant[Q]

138. Ans. b. Follicular carcinoma of thyroid (Ref: Bailey 27/e p808, 26/e p765, 25/e p775; Sabiston 20/e p905; Schwartz 10/e p1544; Robbins 9/e p1094, 8/e p1123)

FNAC is not enough to diagnose follicular carcinoma, because follicular carcinoma is differentiated from follicular adenoma based on capsular invasion and vascular invasion, which is not diagnosed by FNAC.

"Although FNA cytology is important in the workup of thyroid nodules, it is of limited value in the preoperative diagnosis of FTC. Diagnosis of FTC requires demonstration of cellular invasion of the capsule or vascular or lym-phatic channels. These structural characteristics cannot be determined with FNA. Additionally, intraoperative frozen section has been notoriously ineffective in making a definitive diagnosis of FTC."- Sabiston 20/e p905

"The hallmark of all follicular adenomas is the presence of an intact, well-formed capsule encircling the tumor. Careful evaluation of the integrity of the capsule is therefore critical in distinguishing follicular adenomas from follicular carcinomas, which demonstrate capsular and/or vascular invasion. This cannot be done by cytology of aspirate alone obtained by a fine needle. Because of the need for evaluating capsular integrity, the definitive diagnosis of adenomas can be made only after careful histologic examination of the resected specimen."- Robbins 9/e p1094

Limitations of FNAC in Thyroid Diseases

- **Not able** to **distinguish follicular adenoma** from **follicular carcinoma**[Q]
- Not able to distinguish **Hurthle cell adenoma** from **Hurthle cell carcinoma**[Q]
- **Useless** in **Reidel's thyroiditis**[Q] (Biopsy is preferred)[Q]
- FNAC is **less reliable** in patients who have **history** of **head & neck irradiation** or **family history** of **thyroid cancer** due to higher likelihood of **multifocal lesions & occult cancer**[Q]

Follicular carcinoma of Thyroid

- FTC account for **10%** of **thyroid cancers**
- Occurs more commonly in **iodine-deficient areas**[Q]; **MC malignancy seen in long standing goiter**[Q]
- **More common** in **women** with mean age of **50 years**
- **Genes** implicated in **FCT: p53**[Q], **PTEN**[Q], **Ras**[Q] , **PAX8/PPAR1**

Pathology:
- Usually **solitary lesion** surrounded by **capsule**[Q].
- Histologically, **follicles** are present, but the **lumen** may be **devoid of colloid**[Q].

  - **Malignancy** is defined by the presence of **capsular & vascular invasion**[Q].
  - **Tumor infiltration & invasion**, as well as **tumor thrombus** within **middle thyroid** or **jugular veins**, may be apparent at operation[Q].

Follicular carcinoma of Thyroid

Clinical Features:
- Usually present as **solitary thyroid nodules**, occasionally with a history of **rapid size increase**, and **long-standing goiter**[Q].
- Pain is uncommon, unless hemorrhage into the nodule has occurred.
- Preoperative clinical diagnosis of cancer is difficult unless distant metastases are present.
- Large follicular tumors (>4 cm) in **older men** are **more likely** to be **malignant**[Q].

  - **MC route of spread: Hematogenous**
  - **Lymphatic spread is not seen (Cervical lymphadenopathy** is **uncommon)**
  - **MC site** of metastasis: bone (Osteolytic metastasis with **pulsating secondaries** in **flat bones)**[Q]
  - **MC site** of metastasis: **Vertebra**[Q] **>Ribs >Pelvic bones > Skull**

Diagnosis:
- **FNAC** is **unable to distinguish benign** follicular lesions **from follicular carcinomas**[Q].

  - Diagnosis of FTC requires demonstration of cellular invasion of the capsule or vascular or lymphatic channels.

- **Intraoperative frozen-section** examination usually is **not helpful**, but should be **performed** when there is evidence of **capsular** or **vascular invasion**, or when **adjacent lymphadenopathy** is present[Q].

Treatment:
- **Follicular lesion: Hemithyroidectomy**[Q] (**80%** of these patients will have **benign** adenomas)
- **Thyroid cancer: Total thyroidectomy**[Q]
- **Total thyroidectomy** in **older patients** with follicular lesions **>4 cm** because of the **higher risk of cancer** in this setting **(50%)**[Q].
- **Prophylactic nodal dissection** is **unwarranted**[Q] because LN involvement is infrequent

Prognosis:
- **Cumulative mortality: 15% at 10 years & 30% at 20 years**.
- **Most important prognostic factor: Age & distant metastasis**.

Poor long-term prognosis	
• Age >50 years[Q]	• Marked vascular invasion[Q]
• Tumor size >4 cm[Q]	• Extrathyroidal invasion[Q]
• Higher tumor grade[Q]	• Distant metastases[Q]

139. **Ans. a. Southampton grading scale** *(Ref: Bailey 27/e p48, 26/e p53-54, 25/e p35-36)*
Southampton grading is used for surgical site infections.

*"The differentiation between major and minor and the definition of **surgical site infection (SSI)** is important in audit or trials of antibiotic prophylaxis. **There are scoring systems for the severity of wound infection, which are particularly useful in surveillance and research. Examples are the Southampton and ASEPSIS systems.**"- Bailey 26/e p53*

Surgical Site Infections

- A **major SSI** is defined as a **wound** that either **discharges significant quantities of pus spontaneously** or **needs a secondary procedure to drain it**.
- The patient may have **systemic signs** such as **tachycardia, pyrexia** and a **raised WBC count [systemic inflammatory response syndrome (SIRS)]**[Q]
- Minor wound infections may discharge pus or infected serous fluid but should not be associated with excessive discomfort, systemic signs or delay in return home.

  - **Differentiation between major & minor and definition of SSI is important in audit or trials of antibiotic prophylaxis.**
  - There are **scoring systems for the severity of wound infection**, which are particularly **useful in surveillance & research**. Examples are **Southampton & ASEPSIS systems**[Q].

Southampton Wound Grading System	
Grade/Appearance	**Subtype/Appearance**
0: Normal healing[Q]	
I: Normal healing with mild bruising or erythema[Q]	• **Ia:** Some **bruising** • **Ib: Considerable bruising** • **Ic: Mild erythema**
II: Erythema plus other signs of inflammation[Q]	• **IIa:** At **one point** • **IIb: Around sutures** • **IIc: Along** wound • **IId: Around** wound
III: Clear or hemoserous discharge[Q]	• **IIIa:** At **one point** only (<2 cm) • **IIIb: Along** wound (>2 cm) • **IIIc: Large volume** • **IIId: Prolonged** (>3 days)
IV: Pus[Q]	• **IVa:** At **one point** only (<2 cm) • **IVb: Along** wound (>2 cm)
V: Deep or severe wound infection with or without tissue breakdown; Hematoma requiring aspiration[Q]	

140. Ans. d. Ethilon   *(Ref: Bailey 27/e p90, 26/e p37-38, 25/e p236-239)*

For abdominal wall closure with evidence of infection, monofilament non-absorbable sutures (Prolene or Ethilon) should be used.

> *"Multifilament or braided sutures are much easier to knot, but have a surface area of several thousand times that of monofilament sutures and thus have a capillary action and interstices where bacteria may lodge and be responsible for persistent infection or sinuses. In order to overcome some of these problems, certain materials are produced as a braided suture which is coated with silicone in order to make it smooth."- Bailey 26/e p35*

Suture Materials	
Absorbable	**Non-absorbable**
• These sutures **get absorbed** in the tissues either **by enzymatic digestion** or by **phagocytosis**[Q]. • **Natural absorbable:** • Plain & chromic **catgut**[Q] • **Synthetic absorbable:** (PVD) • **Polydioxanone (PDS)**[Q] • **P**olyglycaprone • Polyglactin (**V**icryl)[Q] • Polyglycollic acid (**D**exon)[Q]	• These sutures **remain in** the **tissues for indefinite period.** • Natural non-absorbable: • **Linen**[Q] & **Silk**[Q] • **Synthetic non-absorbable:** (PEN) • **P**olypropylene (**Prolene**)[Q] • **Polyester**[Q] (ethibond) • Monofilament polyamide (**Ethilon**)[Q] • **Nylon**[Q]

Depending upon Number of Strands	
Monofilament	**Polyfilament**
• Consist of **single strand**[Q] of fiber • Sutures are **smooth & strong**[Q] • Chances of **bacterial contamination is less**[Q] • **Knot tied** may become **loose**[Q] • **Prolene, polyamide (Ethilon), catgut**[Q]	• Consist of **multiple strands**[Q] braided together • **Easier to handle & knot tied doesn't slip**[Q] • Bacteria may lodge in the crevices of the suture, so **not suitable in presence of infection**[Q] • **S**ilk, **Li**nen, **P**olyglycollic acid (SLiP)[Q]

Suture	Types	Raw material	Tensile strength	Absorption rate
Silk	Braided or twisted **multifilament;** Coated (with wax or silicone) or uncoated	Natural protein Raw silk from silkworm	Loses 20% when wet; 80-100% lost by 6 months	Fibrous encapsulation in body at 2-3 weeks; **Absorbed** slowly over **1-2 year**[Q]

Contd...

Contd...

Suture	Types	Raw material	Tensile strength	Absorption rate
Catgut	Plain	Collagen derived from **submucosa** of healthy **sheep**[Q] or cattle	Lost within 7-10 days	**Phagocytosis & enzymatic degradation** within **7-10 days**[Q]
Catgut	Chromic	Tanned with **chromium salts** to **improve handling & resist degradation** in tissue[Q]	Lost within 21-28 days	Phagocytosis & enzymatic degradation **within 90 days**[Q]
Polyglactin (Vicryl)	Braided multifilament	Copolymer of **lactide & glycolide**[Q] in a ratio of 90:10, coated with **polyglactin** & calcium stearate	Approx, 60% remains at 2 weeks; 30% remains at 3 weeks	Hydrolysis minimal until 5-6 weeks; Complete absorption 60-90 days[Q]
Polyglyconate	Monofilament Dyed or undyed	Copolymer of **glycolic acid & trimethylene carbonate**[Q]	Approx, 70% remains at 2 weeks; 55% remains at 3 weeks	Hydrolysis minimal until 8-9 weeks; Complete absorption 180 days[Q]
Polyglycaprone	Monofilament	Copolymer of **glycolite & caprolactone**[Q]	21 days maximum	90-120 days[Q]
Polyglycolic acid (Dexon)	Braided multifilament Dyed or undyed Coated or Uncoated	Polymer of **polyglycollic acid**[Q]	Approx, 40% remains at 1 weeks; 20% remains at 3 weeks	**Hydrolysis**[Q] minimal at 2 weeks; significant at 4 weeks; Complete absorption 60-90 days[Q]
Polydioxanone (PDS)	Monofilament dyed or undyed	**Polyester polymer**[Q]	Approx, 70% remains at 2 weeks; 50% remains at 4 weeks; 14% remains at 8 weeks	**Hydrolysis** minimal at 90 days; Complete absorption **180 days**[Q]

141. Ans. c. Acute cholecystitis due to gallstones *(Ref: Sabiston 20/e p1488, 19/e p1482; Schwartz 10/e p1315, 1320; Bailey 27/e p1192, 26/e p1101; Blumgart 5/e p254-270; Shackelford 7/e p1306)*
Non-visualization of gallbladder in hepatic scintigraphy is suggestive of Acute cholecystitis.

*"Ultrasonography is the most useful radiologic test for diagnosing acute cholecystitis. It has a sensitivity and specificity of 95%. In addition to being a sensitive test for documenting the presence or absence of stones, it will **show the thickening of the gallbladder wall and the pericholecystic fluid**. Focal tenderness over the gallbladder when compressed by the sonographic probe (sonographic Murphy's sign) also is suggestive of acute cholecystitis. Biliary radionuclide scanning (HIDA scan) may be of help in the atypical case. Lack of filling of the gallbladder after 4 hours indicates an obstructed cystic duct and, in the clinical setting of acute cholecystitis, is highly sensitive and specific for acute cholecystitis. A normal HIDA scan excludes acute cholecystitis."*- Schwartz 10/e p1320

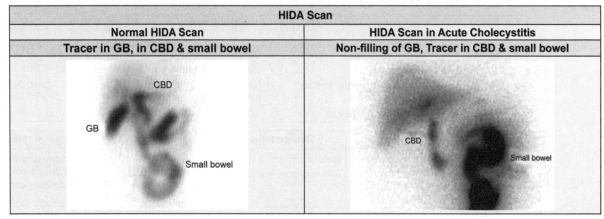

Contd...

Contd...

Biliary Radionuclide Scanning (HIDA Scan)

- **Biliary scintigraphy** provides a **noninvasive evaluation of liver, gallbladder, bile ducts & duodenum** with both **anatomic & functional information**[Q].
- **Technetium-99m labelled derivatives** of iminodiacetic acid (**HIDA**, IODIDA) are, when injected IV, **selectively taken up** by **reticuloendothelial cells** of liver & **excreted into bile**[Q].

HIDA Scan

- Allows **visualization** of the **biliary tree & gall bladder**[Q].
- **GB** is **visualized within 30 min** of **isotope injection** in **90%** of normal individuals and within 1 hour in the remainder[Q].
- **Bowel** is usually **seen within 1 hour** in majority of patients[Q].
- **Non-visualization** of the **GB** is suggestive of **acute cholecystitis**[Q] (Sensitivity & specificity-95%)
- If the patient has **contracted gall bladder**, as often occurs in **chronic cholecystitis, GB visualization** may be **reduced** or **delayed**[Q].

- **Biliary scintigraphy** may also be **helpful in diagnosing bile leaks** and **iatrogenic biliary obstruction**[Q].
- **Scintigraphy can confirm** the **presence** and **quantify the leak**[Q].

OBSTETRICS AND GYNECOLOGY

142. Ans. b. Dysgerminoma   *(Ref: Shaw's 16/e p441-442, 15/e p378; Novak's 15/e p1506-1508; Robbins 9/e p1031)*

Tumor given in the question is soft and fleshy, has solid yellow-white to gray-pink appearance. On microscopic examination, there are large vesicular cells having a clear cytoplasm, well-defined cell boundaries, and centrally placed regular nuclei suggestive of dysgerminoma.

"Most dysgerminomas (80% to 90%) are unilateral tumors ranging in size from barely visible nodules to masses that virtually fill the entire abdomen. On cut surface they have a solid yellow-white to gray-pink appearance and are often soft and fleshy. Like seminoma, it is composed of large vesicular cells having a clear cytoplasm, well-defined cell boundaries, and centrally placed regular nuclei. The tumor cells grow in sheets or cords separated by scant fibrous stroma, which is infiltrated by mature lymphocytes and may contain occasional granulomas."- Robbins 9/e p1031

See Q. No. 142 AIIMS November 2017

143. Ans. a. Secondary arrest after progression of labor   *(Ref: Management of Labor by Arul Kumaran 3/e p39)*

Graph A: Prolonged Latent phase; Graph B: Prolonged active phase ; Graph C: Arrest in Active phase (Secondary arrest)

Friedman's original research in 1955 defined the following three stages of labor:
- **First stage starts with uterine contractions leading to complete cervical dilation** and is divided into **latent & active phases**.
- In **latent phase, irregular uterine contractions** occur with **slow & gradual cervical effacement & dilation**.
- **Active phase** is demonstrated by an **increased rate of cervical dilation & fetal descent**.
- **Active phase** usually starts at **3-4 cm cervical dilation** and is subdivided into **acceleration, maximum slope & deceleration phases**[Q].
- **Second stage** of labor is defined as **complete dilation of cervix to delivery of infant**[Q].
- **Third stage of labor involves delivery of placenta.** He established the following definitions of labor progression:
  - Active phase at rest: No dilation for 2 hours[Q]
  - Protracted descent: >1 cm/hour[Q]
  - Arrested descent: No descent for 1 hour[Q]

Abnormal labor is the problems with one of the following 'P'

- **Passenger: Infant size, fetal presentation** (occiput anterior, posterior, or transverse) [Q]
- **Pelvis or passage:** Size**, shape & adequacy of the pelvis**[Q]
- **Power: Uterine contractility**[Q]

Abnormal Labor Patterns, Diagnostic Criteria & Methods of Treatment				
Labor Pattern	**Diagnostic Criteria**		**Preferred Treatment**	**Exceptional**
	Nullipara	**Multipara**		
Prolongation disorder				
Prolonged latent phase	> 20 hours[Q]	>14 hours[Q]	Bed rest	Oxytocin or cesarean delivery for urgent problems

Contd...

Contd...

Protraction disorders				
Protracted active-phase dilatation	<1.2 cm/hour[Q]	1.5 cm/hour[Q]	Expectant & support	Cesarean delivery for CPD
Protracted descent	<1 cm/hour[Q]	<2 cm/hour[Q]		
Arrest disorders				
Prolonged deceleration phase	>1 hour[Q]	>1 hour[Q]	**Evaluate for CPD**[Q]	Rest if exhausted Cesarean delivery
Secondary arrest of dilation	>2 hour[Q]	>2 hour[Q]	CPD: cesarean	
Arrest of descent	>1 hour[Q]	>1 hour[Q]	No CPD: Oxytocin	
Failure of descent	No descent in deceleration phase or second stage[Q]			

144. Ans. a. Beta HCG and PAPP-A   *(Ref: Williams 24/e p289, 290)*

Two analytes used for first-trimester aneuploidy screening are human chorionic gonadotropin—either intact or free β-hCG— and pregnancy-associated plasma protein A (PAPP-A).

"Two analytes used for first-trimester aneuploidy screening are human chorionic gonadotropin—either intact or free β-hCG— and pregnancy-associated plasma protein A (PAPP-A). In cases of fetal Down syndrome, the first-trimester serum free β-hCG level is higher, approximately 2.0 MoM, and the PAPP-A level is lower, approximately 0.5 MoM. With trisomy 18 and trisomy 13, levels of both analytes are lower. If gestational age is correct, the use of these serum markers— without NT measurement—results in detection rates for fetal Down syndrome up to 67% at a false-positive rate of 5%. Aneuploidy detection is significantly greater if these first-trimester analytes are either: (1) combined with the sonographic NT measurement or (2) combined with second-trimester analytes, which is termed serum integrated screening."- Williams 24/e p290

"Combined First-Trimester Screening: The most commonly used screening protocol combines the NT measurement with serum hCG and PAPP-A. Using this protocol, Down syndrome detection rates in large prospective trials range from 79 to 87%, at a false-positive rate of 5 percent. The detection rate is approximately 5% higher if performed at 11 compared with 13 weeks. The detection rate for trisomies 18 and 13 is approximately 90 percent, at a 2% false-positive rate."- Williams 24/e p290

See Q. No. 151 AIIMS November 2017

145. Ans. a. Mature teratoma   *(Ref: Shaw 16/e p439, 15/e p377, Robbins 9/e p1029, 8/e p478)*

The gross specimen is showing hair cells, teeth as well as ovarian tissue, which is typical of a benign teratoma or dermoid cyst of ovary.

"Benign teratomas are bilateral in 10% to 15% of cases. Characteristically they are unilocular cysts containing hair and sebaceous material. Sectioning reveals a thin wall lined by an opaque, gray-white, wrinkled epidermis, frequently with protruding hair shafts. Within the wall, it is common to find grossly evident tooth structures and areas of calcification."- Robbins 9/e p1029

Teratomas
• Teratomas are divided into: Mature (benign), Immature (malignant) & Monodermal or highly specialized.

Mature (Benign) Teratoma	
• Most benign teratomas are **cystic**[Q] • Referred as **dermoid cysts**, almost always **lined by skin-like structures**[Q]. • Found in **young women** during **active reproductive years**[Q]. • **Karyotype: 46,XX**[Q] • **Majority of teratomas** arise from an ovum **after 1st meiotic division**[Q]; minority arises before 1st division. • **Malignant transformation** (1%) most commonly to **squamous cell carcinoma**[Q]	**Morphology:** • **Bilateral in 10-15%; Unilocular cysts** containing **hair & sebaceous material**[Q]. • Thin wall lined by an opaque, gray-white, wrinkled epidermis, with protruding hair shafts. • Within the wall, **grossly evident tooth structures & areas of calcification**[Q]. • Cyst wall is composed of **stratified squamous epithelium** with underlying **sebaceous glands, hair shafts & other skin adnexal structures**[Q]. • Tissues from other germ layers **cartilage, bone, thyroid & neural tissue** are present[Q]

Contd...

Contd...

Teratomas
Monodermal (Highly Specialized) Teratoma
• **MC** are **struma ovarii & carcinoid; Always unilateral**[Q] • Struma ovarii is composed of **mature thyroid tissue**, which may be **functional** & cause **hyperthyroidism**[Q]. • **Ovarian carcinoid** arises **from intestinal tissue** found in teratomas; **functional** if large (>7 cm), **produce 5-hydroxytryptamine** to cause **carcinoid syndrome even in absence of hepatic metastases** (ovarian veins are directly connected to systemic circulation)[Q]

Immature (Malignant) Teratoma	
• Component tissues resemble **embryonal & immature fetal tissue**[Q]. • Mainly seen in **prepubertal adolescents & young women**[Q] (mean age: 18 years). • **Grow rapidly**, frequently **penetrate capsule & spread either locally or distantly**[Q]. • **Stage I tumors** with **low-grade (grade 1) histology**, have **excellent prognosis**[Q]. • **Higher-grade tumors confined to ovary** are generally **treated with prophylactic chemotherapy**[Q]. • **Most recurrences** develop **in first 2 years**[Q]	**Morphology:** • Tumors are **bulky** with **smooth external surface**, solid on sectioning. • **Hair, sebaceous material, cartilage, bone & calcification** may be present, along with areas of **necrosis & hemorrhage**[Q]. • **Microscopic examination:** Varying amounts of **immature neuroepithelium, cartilage, bone, muscle** & other elements[Q]. • **Risk for extraovarian spread:** Histologic grade of tumor (based on proportion of tissue containing immature neuroepithelium)[Q].

146. **Ans. b. 600 micrograms** *(Ref: Williams 24/e p785)*
The approved dose of misoprostol in emergent management of postpartum hemorrhage is 600 µg.

*"**Misoprostol**: Derman (2006) compared a **600 µg oral dose given at delivery against placebo** and found that the **drug decreased hemorrhage incidence from 12 to 6 percent** and that of **severe hemorrhage from 1.2 to 0.2 percent.**"- Williams 24/e p785*

Misoprostol
• **Misoprostol** (*Cytotec*) is a **synthetic prostaglandin E1 analogue** has been **found to be effective in prevention & treatment of atony & postpartum hemorrhage**[Q]. • Derman (2006) compared a **600 µg oral dose given at delivery against placebo** and found that the **drug decreased hemorrhage incidence from 12 to 6 percent** and that of **severe hemorrhage from 1.2 to 0.2 percent**[Q]. • In another study, however, 400 microgram misoprostol administered rectally was not more effective than intravenous oxytocin in preventing postpartum hemorrhage.

147. **Ans. c. 500 mL** *(Ref: Williams 24/e p786)*
Bakri balloon has a maximum capacity of 500 mL.

*"Enthusiasm has developed for specially constructed intra-uterine balloons to treat hemorrhage from uterine atony and other causes. A **Bakri Postpartum Balloon or BT-Cath may be inserted and inflated to tamponade the endometrial cavity and stop bleeding**. Insertion requires two or three team members. The first performs abdominal sonography during the procedure. The second places the deflated balloon into the uterus and stabilizes it. The third member **instills fluid to inflate the balloon, rapidly infusing at least 150 mL followed by further instillation over a few minutes for a total of 300 to 500 mL to arrest hemorrhage**."- Williams 24/e p786*

Bakri Balloon for PPH	
• **Bakri balloon** can be **inserted and inflated to tamponade the endometrial cavity to stop bleeding.** • **Initially started by rapidly infusing at least 150 mL** followed by further instillation over a few minutes for a **total of 500 mL to arrest hemorrhage**[Q].	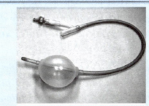

148. Ans. d. Observe the patient and wait for increase in uterine contractions   *(Ref: Williams 24/e p523, 525; Dutta 7/e p722)*
In a primigravida, the progress of labor is often slow. Since the patient is at term and the vitals are stable, the best option is to observe for the normal progress of labor and frequently monitor the vitals.

"One quantifiable method used to predict labor induction outcomes is the score described by Bishop. As favorability or Bishop score decreases, the rate of induction to effect vaginal delivery also declines. A Bishop score of 9 conveys a high likelihood for a successful induction. Put another way, most practitioners would consider that a woman whose cervix is 2-cm dilated, 80% effaced, soft, and mid- position and with the fetal occiput at –1 station would have a successful labor induction. For research purposes, a Bishop score of 4 or less identifies an unfavorable cervix and may be an indication for cervical ripening."- Williams 24/e p525

Score	Cervical Factor				
	Dilatation (cm)	Effacement (%)	Station (-3 to +2)	Consistency	Position
0	Closed	0-30	–3	Firm	Posterior
1	1-2	40-50	–2	Medium	Midposition
2	3-4	60-70	–1	Soft	Anterior
3	≥ 5	≥ 80	+1, +2	–	–

Induction of Labor

- **Induction** implies **stimulation of contractions before the spontaneous onset of labor**, with or without ruptured membranes. When the **cervix is closed & uneffaced**, labor induction will commence with cervical ripening.
- **Augmentation** refers to **enhancement of spontaneous contractions** that are **considered inadequate** because of **failed cervical dilation & fetal descent.**

Indications for Induction of Labor	
Maternal (CAMP)	**Fetal (PRULI Fetus)**
• **C**horioamnionitis[Q] • **C**hronic hydramnios /Oligohydramnios[Q] • **A**bruptio placenta[Q] • **M**edical complications (DM, chronic renal disease)[Q] • **P**remature rupture of membranes[Q] • **P**reeclampsia/Eclampsia[Q]	• **P**rolonged pregnancy[Q] • **R**h-incompatibility[Q] • **U**nstable lie after correction into longitudinal lie[Q] • **L**ethal malformation[Q] • **I**UGR[Q] • **I**ntrauterine fetal death[Q] • **Fetus** with major congenital anomaly[Q]

Contraindications for Induction of Labor	
Maternal (CAP)	**Fetal (MANS)**
• **C**ontracted or distorted pelvic anatomy[Q] • **C**ervical cancer[Q] • **A**bnormally implanted placentas[Q] • **A**ctive genital herpes infection[Q] • **P**rior uterine incision type[Q]	• **M**alpresentation[Q] • **A**ppreciable macrosomia[Q] • **N**onreassuring fetal status[Q] • **S**evere hydrocephalus[Q]

- **Indications for Augmentation of Labor: Dystocia & uterine hypocontractility[Q]**
- **Uterine hypocontractility** should be **augmented only after both maternal pelvis & fetal presentation have been assessed[Q].**

149. Ans. a. GnRH analogues   *(Ref: Shaw 16/e p59, 15/e p56; Nelson 20/e 2658; Ghai 8/e p533)*
Treatment for precocious puberty depends on the cause. The primary goal of treatment is to enable the child to grow to a normal adult height. GnRH and Medroxy progesterone acetate have both been used with good results but GnRH analogues are preferred.

"Regardless of the cause, therapy with GnRH agonists is as effective in children with organic brain lesions causing central precocious puberty, and these analogs are the therapy of choice to halt premature sexual development. This includes patients with a hypothalamic hamartoma, if precocious puberty is its only manifestation." - Nelson 20/e 2658

Precocious Puberty

- **Definition: Onset of secondary sexual characters before 8 years in girls & 9 years in boys.**
- **Types: Central** (also known as **gonadotropin dependent,** or **true**) or **peripheral** (also known as **gonadotropin independent** or **precocious pseudopuberty**).

Central Precocious Puberty	Peripheral Precocious Puberty
• Caused by **premature hypothalamic-pituitary-gonadal activation** with **sex hormone secretion & progressive sexual maturation**[Q]. • **MC form** of precocious puberty[Q] • More common in **girls**[Q] • **MC cause: Idiopathic in girls; CNS pathology in boys**[Q] • **MC brain lesion** causing central precocious puberty: **Hypothalamic hamartoma**[Q] • **Breast development, pubic hair development & cyclical vaginal bleeding** are **seen**[Q]. • **Treatment: GnRH analogues** are **DOC**[Q]	• Caused by **excessive sex steroid secretion** from **adrenal gland** or **gonads**; it is **independent of hypothalamic-pituitary-gonadal axis**[Q] • **More common in boys**[Q] • **MC cause: CAH in boys; ovarian causes in girls**[Q] • It can lead to **breast development & pubic hair development** but **not the cyclical vaginal bleeding**[Q] as **menarche requires** not only **production of estrogen** but its **withdrawal** also. • **Treatment: Treat the cause**[Q]

150. Ans. b. Partial androgen insensitivity syndrome *(Ref: Williams 24/e p149; Shaw's 16/e p141, 15/e p111-112; Novak's 14/1037-1038; Dutta Gynae 6/e p424)*

Most likely diagnosis in young female girl who presents with primary amenorrhea, normal breasts development, absent axillary hair with normally developed vagina and is androgen insensitivity syndrome. Clitoromegaly points towards partial androgen insensitivity syndrome.

"Androgen Insensitivity Syndrome: Because the testes produce normal amounts of Mullerian-inhibiting factor (MIF), also known as Mullerian-inhibiting substance (MIS) or anti-Mullerian hormone/factor (AMH/AMF), affected individuals do not have fallopian tubes, a uterus, or a proximal (upper) vagina. Most cases are identified in the newborn period by the presence of inguinal masses, which later are identified as testes during surgery. Some patients are first seen in the teenage years for evaluation of primary amenorrhea. In addition, adolescent patients have no pubic and axillary hair, with otherwise scanty body hair, and lack acne, although breast is normal as a result of conversion of testosterone to estradiol."

"Individuals with incomplete androgen insensitivity are slightly responsive to androgen. They usually have modest clitoral hypertrophy at birth. These patients also develop feminine breasts, presumably through the same endocrine mechanisms as in those with the complete form of the disorder."-Williams 24/e p149

Feature	Mullerian Agenesis	Turner's syndrome (Gonadal Dysgenesis)	Androgen Insensitivity Syndrome
Presentation	**Amenorrhea**[Q]	**Amenorrhea**[Q]	**Amenorrhea**[Q]
Breasts	Normally developed	**Poorly developed**[Q]	**Enhanced (Tanner Stage 5)**[Q]
Pubic/Axillary Hair	Present	Present	**Absent**[Q]
Stature	Normal	**Short**[Q]	Normal
Uterus	**Absent**[Q]	Present	**Absent**[Q]
Vagina	**Blind**[Q]	**Present/Ambiguous**[Q]	**Absent proximal (upper) vagina**[Q]
Ovaries	Present	**Streak gonads**[Q]	**Abdominal testis present**[Q]

Androgen insensitivity syndrome (AIS)

- **Androgen insensitivity syndrome** formerly known as **testicular feminization**[Q]
- **X-linked recessive condition**[Q]
- Results in a **failure of normal masculinization of external genitalia** in **chromosomally male individuals**[Q].
- **Failure of virilisation** can be either **complete androgen insensitivity syndrome** (CAIS) or **partial androgen insensitivity syndrome** (PAIS), depending on amount of residual receptor function.

Contd...

Contd...

| Androgen insensitivity syndrome (AIS) ||
Complete Androgen Insensitivity Syndrome	**Partial Androgen Insensitivity Syndrome**
• **Karyotype: 46, XY**[Q] • **Female external genitalia** with **normal labia, clitoris & vaginal introitus**[Q].	• **Karyotype: 46, XY**[Q] • Range from **mildly virilised female external genitalia** (**clitorimegaly** without other external anomalies) **to mildly undervirilized male external genitalia**[Q] (hypospadias and/or diminished penile size).

- Affected individuals have **normal testes with normal production of testosterone & normal conversion to dihydrotestosterone (DHT),** which differentiates this condition from 5-alpha reductase deficiency.
  - Because **testes produce normal amounts of Mullerian-inhibiting factor** (MIF), also known as **Mullerian-inhibiting substance** (MIS) or anti-mullerian hormone/factor (AMH/AMF), affected individuals **do not have fallopian tubes, a uterus, or a proximal (upper) vagina**[Q]

Characteristic Features:
- **Most cases** are **identified in newborn period by presence of inguinal masses**, which later are identified as **testes** during surgery[Q].
  - Some patients are **first seen** in teenage years for **evaluation of primary amenorrhea.**
  - Many of patients have a **history of surgery for hernias** and/or **presence of gonads in inguinal canals,** which were considered ovaries & returned to abdomen[Q].
  - **Adolescent patients have no pubic & axillary hair**, with otherwise **scanty body hair & lack acne,** although **breast** is **normal** as a result of **conversion of testosterone to estradiol**[Q].

Management:
- Management of AIS is currently limited to **symptomatic management; no method is currently available to correct the malfunctioning androgen receptor proteins produced by AR gene mutations**[Q].
- Areas of management include **sex assignment, genitoplasty, gonadectomy** in relation to tumor risk, hormone replacement therapy, genetic counseling, and psychological counseling.

Rokitansky-Kuster-Hauser syndrome

- **Mullerian agenesis** is the cause of **primary amenorrhea,** which is characterized by **absence of uterus /vagina,** also known as **Rokitansky-Kuster- Hauser syndrome**[Q].
- **Rare** disorder; Prevalence: 1:4000-5000 female births
- Patients have a **46,XX karyotype** and **normal secondary sex characteristics**[Q].

Characteristic Features of Rokitansky-Kuster-Hauser Syndrome
• **External genitalia appear normal**, but only a **shallow vaginal pouch** is present[Q].   • **Ovarian function is normal**[Q].   • **Absence of both the vagina & uterus**[Q].   • **Only symmetric uterine remnants** (the muscular buds), **normal fallopian tubes**, and **normal ovaries are present**[Q].

151. **Ans. a. Pap smear should be repeated yearly in women of reproductive age group** *(Ref: Harrison 19/e p481, 18/e p662)*
Pap smear should be repeated three yearly, not yearly. There are 2 types of tests used for cervical cancer screening.

"VIA (Visual inspection with acetic acid) is appropriate to use in women whose transformation zone is visible (typically in those younger than 50). This is because once menopause occurs, the transformation zone, where most precancerous lesions occur, frequently recedes into the endocervical canal and prevents it from being visible."

Latest Screening Guidelines (ASCCP/ACOG)

- All women should begin **cervical cancer screening at age 21**
  - Women between ages of **21-29 years** should have a **Pap test every 3 years**. They **should not be tested for HPV unless it is needed after an abnormal Pap test result**[Q].
  - Women between the ages of **30-65 years** should have **both Pap test & HPV test every 5 years**[Q]. This is the **preferred approach**, but it is also ok to have a Pap test alone every 3 years.

Contd...

Contd...

Latest Screening Guidelines (ASCCP/ACOG)
• Women **>65 years** who have had **regular screenings with normal results should not be screened for cervical cancer**[Q]. Women who have been diagnosed with cervical pre-cancer should continue to be screened. • Women who have had their **uterus & cervix removed in a hysterectomy** & have **no history of cervical cancer or pre-cancer should not be screened.** • Women who have had the HPV vaccine should still follow the screening recommendations for their age group. <ul><li>**Women who are at high risk for cervical cancer may need to be screened more often.** Women at high risk might include those with **HIV infection, organ transplant, or exposure to the drug DES.**</li><li>**American Cancer Society no longer recommends that women get a Pap test every year**, because it generally takes much longer than that, 10 to 20 years, for cervical cancer to develop & overly frequent screening could lead to procedures that are not needed.</li></ul>

Screening Recommendations for Asymptomatic Subjects		
Cancer Type	**Test or Procedure**	**ACS: American Cancer Society**
Breast	**Self-examination**	Women ≥20 years: Breast self-exam is an option[Q]
	Clinical examination	Women 20–39 years: Perform every 3 years[Q] Women ≥40 years: Perform annually[Q]
	Mammography	Women **≥40 years: Screen annually for as long as the woman is in good health**[Q]
	Magnetic resonance imaging (MRI)	Women with **>20% lifetime risk** of breast cancer: Screen with **MRI plus mammography annually**[Q] Women with **15–20% lifetime risk** of breast cancer: Discuss option of **MRI plus mammography annually**[Q] Women with **<15% lifetime risk** of breast cancer: **Do not screen annually with MRI**[Q]
Cervical	**Pap test (cytology)**	Women **21–29 years**: Screen **every 3 years**[Q] Women **30–65 years**: Acceptable approach to screen with cytology **every 3 years**[Q] Women **<21 years: No screening**[Q] Women **>65 years: No screening following adequate negative prior screening**[Q]
	HPV test	Women **30–65 years**: Preferred approach to screen with **HPV and cytology co-testing every 5 years**[Q] Women **<30 years: Do not use HPV testing**[Q] Women **>65 years: No screening following adequate**[Q] **negative prior screening** Women **after total hysterectomy** for noncancerous causes: **Do not screen**[Q]
Colorectal	**Sigmoidoscopy**	Adults **≥50 years**: Screen every **5 years**[Q]
	Fecal occult blood testing (FOBT)	Adults **≥50 years**: Screen every **5 years**[Q]
	Colonoscopy	Adults **≥50 years**: Screen every **10 years**[Q]
	Fecal DNA testing	Adults ≥50 years: Screen, but interval uncertain
	Fecal immunochemical testing (FIT)	Adults **≥50 years**: Screen **every year**[Q]
	CT colonography	Adults **≥50 years**: Screen **every 5 years**[Q]
Lung	**Low-dose computed tomography (CT) scan**	Men & women, 55–74 years, with ≥30 pack-year smoking history, still smoking or have quit within past 15 years: Discuss benefits, limitations & potential harms of screening; only perform screening in facilities with right type of CT scanner & with high expertise/specialists

Contd...

Contd...

Cancer Type	Test or Procedure	ACS: American Cancer Society
Ovarian	CA-125 Transvaginal ultrasound	There is **no sufficiently accurate test proven effective in the early detection of ovarian cancer**[Q]. For women at high risk of ovarian cancer and/or who have unexplained, persistent symptoms, combination of CA-125 & transvaginal ultrasound with pelvic exam may be offered.
Prostate	Prostate-specific anti-gen (PSA)	**Starting at age 50**[Q], men should talk to a doctor about pros & cons of testing so they can decide if testing is the right choice for them. If African American or have a father or brother who had prostate cancer before age 65, men should have this talk starting at age 45. How often they are tested will depend on their PSA level.
	Digital rectal examination (DRE)	As for PSA; if men decide to be tested, they should have the PSA blood test with or without a rectal exam
Skin	Complete skin examination	**Self-examination monthly**; clinical exam as part of routine cancer-related checkup

152. **Ans. d. Only a person certified under MTP act can perform medical termination of pregnancy** *(Ref: Shaw 16/e p287-289, 15/e p244-245, Williams 24/e p368)*
   MTP can be performed upto 20 weeks according to MTP act. Ultrasound is not needed in all the cases. Only a person certified under MTP act can perform medical termination of pregnancy.
   See Q. No. 87 AIIMS Novmeber 2017

153. **Ans. c. Partograph recording should be started at a cervical dilation of 4 cm** *(Ref: Williams 24/e p452)*
   Partograph recording is usually started after a cervical dilation of 3 cm (not the 4 cm), i.e. the active stage of labor.

   "A partograph was designed by the World Health Organization (WHO) for use in developing countries. According to Orji (2008), the partograph is similar for nulliparas and multiparas. Labor is divided into a latent phase, which should last no longer than 8 hours, and an active phase. The active phase starts at 3 cm dilatation, and progress should be no slower than 1 cm/hr. A 4-hour wait is recommended before intervention when the active phase is slow. Labor is graphed, and analysis includes use of alert and action lines."- Williams 24/e p452

   See Q. No. 139 AIIMS November 2017

154. **Ans. a. A** *(Ref: Ganong 25/e p435; 24/e p448; Williams 24/e p1137)*
   Graph A is the correct representation of the normal oral glucose tolerance test.
   Graph B: Excessively rapid carbohydrate absorption
   Graph C: Liver disease

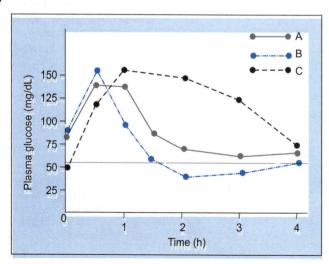

Glucose Tolerance Test (GTT)
• GTT is a test in which glucose is given & blood samples taken afterward to determine how quickly it is cleared from the blood. • **Used to test for diabetes, insulin resistance, impaired beta cell function & sometimes reactive hypoglycemia and acromegaly, or rarer disorders of carbohydrate metabolism.** • In the most commonly performed version of the test, an **oral glucose tolerance test (OGTT)**, a **standard dose of glucose is ingested by mouth & blood levels are checked two hours later.**

Procedure:

- A zero time (baseline) blood sample is drawn.
- The patient is then given a measured dose (below) of glucose solution to drink within a 5-minute time frame.
- Blood is drawn at intervals for measurement of glucose (blood sugar), and sometimes insulin levels.
- Intervals & number of samples vary according to the purpose of test.
- **For simple diabetes screening, the most important sample is the 2 hours sample and the 0 and 2-hour samples may be the only ones collected.**
- A laboratory may continue to collect blood for up to 6 hours depending on the protocol requested by the physician.

> - **75g of oral dose is the recommendation of the WHO to be used in all adults, the dose should be drunk within 5 minutes.**
> - A variant is often **used in pregnancy to screen for gestational diabetes**, with a **screening test of 50 grams over one hour. If elevated, this is followed with a test of 100 grams over three hours.**

Substances Measured and Variations:

- If **renal glycosuria** (sugar excreted in the urine despite normal levels in the blood) **is suspected, urine samples** may also be **collected for testing along with fasting & 2 hours blood tests.**

Results:

Oral Glucose Tolerance Testing		
Time	75-gm Glucose	Interpretation
Fasting	<110 mg/dL[Q] <6.1 mmol/L	Normal[Q]
	110-125 mg/dL[Q] 6.1-7.0 mmol/L	Impaired fasting glycemia[Q]
	≥126 mg/dL >7.0 mmol/L	diabetes[Q]
1-hour	180 mg/dL[Q] 10.0 mmol/L	Normal[Q]
2-hours	<140 mg/dL[Q] <7.8 mmol/L	Normal[Q]
	140-200 mg/dL[Q] 7.8-11.1 mmol/L	Impaired glucose tolerance[Q]
	>200 mg/dL[Q] >11.1 mmol/L	Diabetes[Q]

- **For gestational diabetes**, the American College of Obstetricians and Gynecologists (**ACOG**) recommends a two-step procedure, wherein the first step is a 50 g glucose dose. If it results in a blood glucose level of more than 7.8 mmol/L (140 mg/dL), it is followed by a 100-gram glucose dose.

The **diagnosis of gestational diabetes** is then defined by a **blood glucose level exceeding the cutoff value on at least two intervals, with cutoffs as follows:**		
Before glucose intake (fasting)	95 mg/dL[Q]	5.3 mmol/L
1 hour (after drinking the glucose solution)	180 mg/dL[Q]	10 mmol/L
2 hours (after drinking the glucose solution)	155 mg/dL[Q]	8.6 mmol/L
3 hours (after drinking the glucose solution)	140 mg/dL[Q]	7.8 mmol/L

PAEDIATRICS

155. **Ans. c. HGPRT deficiency** *(Ref: Harrison 19/e p431e-5; Nelson 20/e p746-747)*

A complete deficiency of HGPRT, the Lesch-Nyhan syndrome, is characterized by hyperuricemia, self-mutilative behavior, choreoathetosis, spasticity, and mental retardation.

> *"The **HPRT gene is located on the X chromosome**. Affected males are hemizygous for the mutant gene; carrier females are asymptomatic. A complete deficiency of HPRT, the Lesch-Nyhan syndrome, is characterized by hyperuricemia, self-mutilative behavior, choreoathetosis, spasticity, and mental retardation. A partial deficiency of HPRT, the Kelley-Seegmiller syndrome, is associated with hyperuricemia but no central nervous system manifestations. In both disorders, the hyperuricemia results from urate overproduction and can cause uric acid crystalluria, nephrolithiasis, obstructive uropathy, and gouty arthritis. Early diagnosis and appropriate therapy with allopurinol can prevent or eliminate all the problems attributable to hyperuricemia without affecting behavioral or neurologic abnormalities." - Harrison 19/e p431e-5*

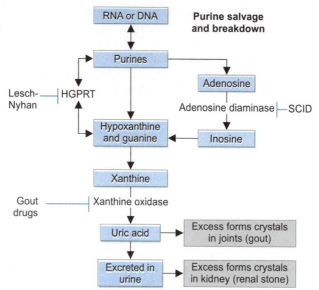

Fig. 36: Purine Salvage & breakdown

Lesch-Nyhan Syndrome
• Rare **disorder of purine metabolism** that **results from HPRTase (hypoxanthine phosphor ribosyl transferase) deficiency**[Q]. • **HPRTase enzyme** is normally present in each cell in the body but **highest concentration** is **in brain, especially in basal ganglia**[Q].
Genetics: • X-linked recessive inheritance[Q]
Biochemical defect: • **Complete deficiency of HPRTase** leading to **purine accumulation**[Q] • **Purine degrades to uric acid** leading to **hyperuricemia**[Q]
Clinical Features: • **Hyperuricemia, mental retardation, cerebral palsy** with early choreoathetosis & later spasticity & dystonia, dysarthric speech, **compulsive self-biting, usually beginning with eruption of teeth (self-mutilative behavior**[Q]**)**
Diagnosis: • **Definitive diagnosis requires analysis of HPRTase enzyme**[Q]. • **Hyperuricemia** with **deficient HPRTase enzyme in RBCs**[Q] • **MRI: Reductions in volume of basal ganglia nuclei**[Q] (primarily involved areas: caudate nucleus, putamen & nucleus accumbens)
Treatment: • **Hyperuricemia** is treated with **high fluid intake with alkalinization & allopurinol**[Q]. • Efforts to reduce **self-mutilation** through **behavior management & psychosocial support**[Q].
Prognosis: • Patients with classic disease **rarely survive 3rd decade** because of **renal or respiratory compromise**[Q].

156. Ans. d. Sensorineural hearing loss *(Ref: Ghai 8/e p272; Nelson 20/e p1592-1594)*

Positive human cytomegalovirus (HCMV) antibodies at birth are suggestive of congenital asymptomatic CMV infection. The child with symptomatic CMV infection is at an increased risk to develop mental retardation, but an asymptomatic child is at as high as 7% risk to develop sensorineural hearing loss.

> "*Congenital CMV Infection*: The characteristic signs and symptoms of clinically manifested infections include **intrauterine growth restriction, prematurity, hepatosplenomegaly and jaundice, blueberry muffin–like rash, thrombocytopenia and purpura, and microcephaly and intracranial calcifications**. Other neurologic problems include **chorioretinitis, sensorineural hearing loss,** and mild increases in cerebrospinal fluid protein." - *Nelson 20/e p1592*

AIIMS November 2016

"Asymptomatic congenital CMV infection is likely a leading cause of sensorineural hearing loss, which occurs in approximately 7-10% of all infants with congenital CMV infection, whether symptomatic at birth or not."- Nelson 20/e p1592

See Q. No. 161 AIIMS November 2017

157. Ans. b. Isotretinoin *(Ref: Goodman Gillman 12/e p1812; Nelson 20/e 812-813)*

The facial defects including cleft lip seen in the child are characteristic of teratogenic effect of Isotretinoin. This drug is usually used for treatment of acne and should never be started in a girl of reproductive age without ruling out pregnancy.

"Systemic retinoids are highly teratogenic. There is no safe dose during pregnancy. Common malformations include craniofacial, cardiovascular, thymic, and central nervous system (CNS) abnormalities."- Goodman Gillman 12/e p1812

"Fetal Retinoid Syndrome: Affected infants often display small, low-set ears (microtia) with narrowing (stenosis) of the ear canals. Abnormalities of the middle and inner ears may also be present. Additional craniofacial findings include widely spaced eyes (hypertelorism), incomplete closure of the roof of the mouth (cleft palate), an abnormal groove in the upper lip (cleft lip), and/or underdevelopment of the middle area of the face (midface hypoplasia)."

See Q. No. 160 AIIMS May 2017

158. Ans. c. Respiratory syncytial virus *(Ref: Nelson 20/e p1608)*

Palivizumab is a monoclonal antibody used in the prevention and treatment of respiratory syncytial virus (RSV) infections. It is recommended for infants that are high-risk because of prematurity or other medical problems such as congenital heart disease.

"A major monoclonal antibody used in infectious diseases is palivizumab, which can prevent severe disease from respiratory syncytial virus (RSV) among children 24 months of age with chronic lung disease (CLD, also called bronchopulmonary dysplasia), with a history of premature birth or with congenital heart lesions or with neuromuscular diseases."- Nelson 20/e p1608

Acute Bronchiolitis
• Common serious **acute lower respiratory infection of infants**[Q], mainly affecting **1-6 months**[Q] old
• More common in **boys**; Usually occurs in **winter & spring**[Q]
• **Respiratory syncytial virus**[Q] is implicated in most cases
• Protection against RSV is mediated by antibodies of **IgG$_3$ subclass**[Q]. These antibodies have **shorter half-life & do not cross the placenta** in substantial amount so as to offer protection to the infant.
Pathogenesis:
• **Resistance** to the airflow is **increased** both during **inspiration & expiration**[Q]
• Trapping of air inside the alveoli causes **emphysematous changes**[Q]
• Presence of eosinophils in blood & respiratory secretions suggest that virus infection initiates **wheezing attack** in a child who is already sensitized.
• Characterized by **bronchiolar mucosal inflammation, edema, thickening, formation of mucus plugs & cellular debris**[Q]
Clinical Features:
• **Respiratory distress**[Q] is out of proportion to the physical signs in the lung.
• Air is trapped in the lung leading to **emphysema**[Q].
• **Chest X-ray: Hyperinflation & infiltrates**[Q]
Treatment:
• **Essentially symptomatic treatment**[Q]
• **Mainstay of treatment: Oxygen (administered continuously even in absence of cyanosis**[Q])
• **Antibiotics have no role**[Q].
• **Ribavirin (an antiviral agent)** has **no role in infants who were previously healthy**[Q].
• **Ribavirin shortens the course of illness** in infants with underlying **congenital heart disease, chronic lung disease and immunodeficiency**[Q].

Contd...

Contd...

Acute Bronchiolitis
• **Beta-2 adrenergic drugs** & **ipratropium** are **not recommended** for infants **<6 months**[Q].
• **Palivizumab** (monoclonal antibody): Used in **prevention & treatment of RSV infection** in **high-risk infants** (in cases of **prematurity, chronic lung disease or congenital heart disease**)[Q]
Prognosis: • **Self-limiting illness**, symptoms **subside in 3-7 days**[Q].

Monoclonal antibodies marketed for therapeutic use		
Antibody	**Isotype/structure**	**Primary indication**
Abciximab	**Chimeric mouse/human Fab**[Q]	**Prevention of cardiac ischemic complications**[Q]
Adalimumab	**Human IgG1**[Q]	**Rheumatoid arthritis**[Q]
Alemtuzumab	**CDR-grafted rat/human IgG1**[Q]	**B-cell chronic lymphocytic leukemia**[Q]
Basiliximab	**Chimeric mouse/human IgG1**[Q]	**Prophylaxis of acute organ rejection**[Q]
Bevacizumab	**CDR-grafted mouse/human IgG1**[Q]	**Colorectal, lung & breast cancer**[Q]
Certolizumab pegol	PEGylated Fab	Crohn's disease
Cetuximab	**Chimeric mouse/human IgG1**[Q]	**Head & neck cancer, colorectal cancer**[Q]
Daclizumab	CDR-grafted mouse/human IgG1	Prophylaxis of acute organ rejection
Eculizumab	CDR-grafted mouse/human IgG2/IgG4	Paroxysmal nocturnal hemoglobinuria
Efalizumab	**CDR-grafted mouse/human IgG1**[Q]	**Psoriasis**[Q]
Gemtuzumab ozogamicin	**CDR-grafted mouse/human IgG4**[Q]	**Acute myeloid leukemia**[Q]
Ibritumomab tiuxetan	Murine IgG1	Non-Hodgkin's lymphoma
Infliximab	**Chimeric mouse/human IgG1**[Q]	**Rheumatoid arthritis, Crohn's disease**[Q]
Muromonab-CD3	**Murine IgG2a**[Q]	**Acute organ rejection**[Q]
Natalizumab	**CDR-grafted mouse/human IgG4**[Q]	**Multiple sclerosis**[Q]
Omalizumab	**CDR-grafted mouse/human IgG1**[Q]	**Asthma**[Q]
Palivizumab	CDR-grafted mouse/human IgG1	Prevention of respiratory tract disease
Panitumumab	**Human IgG2**[Q]	**Colorectal cancer**[Q]
Ranibizumab	**CDR-grafted human IgG1 Fab**[Q]	**Macular degeneration**[Q]
Rituximab	**Chimeric mouse/human IgG1**[Q]	**Non-Hodgkin's lymphoma, rheumatoid arthritis**[Q]
Tositumomab	Murine IgG2a	Non-Hodgkin's lymphoma
Trastuzumab	**CDR-grafted mouse/human IgG1**[Q]	**Breast cancer**[Q]

(CDR) complementarity determining region; IgG, Immunoglobulin G.

159. Ans. c. Muscular dystrophy   *(Ref: Harrison 19/e p462e-6, 18/e p3490-3491; Nelson 20/e p2976-2977)*

In the given picture, enlargement of the calves (pseudohypertrophy) are seen along with wasting of thigh muscles, which is a classic feature of Duchenne muscular dystrophy, the most common form of muscular dystrophy.

"Duchenne muscular dystrophy: Enlargement of the calves (pseudohypertrophy) and wasting of thigh muscles are classic features. The enlargement is caused by hypertrophy of some muscle fibers, infiltration of muscle by fat, and proliferation of collagen. After the calves, the next most common site of muscular hypertrophy is the tongue, followed by muscles of the forearm. Fasciculations of the tongue do not occur. The voluntary sphincter muscles rarely become involved."- Nelson 20/e p2976

Duchenne Muscular Dystrophy (Pseudohypertrophic Muscular Dystrophy)

- **DMD** is **MC hereditary neuromuscular disease** affecting **all races & ethnic groups**.
- **Inheritance: X-linked recessive; Abnormal gene lies on chromosome 21 (Xp21)**[Q]
- **Age on onset: 2-5 years**[Q] (**Doesn't present at birth** or during **infancy**[Q])

Pathogenesis:

- Caused by **mutation** in **gene** responsible for producing **dystrophin**[Q]
- **Dystrophin** is **subsarcolemmal protein** localized to **inner surface** of sarcolemma of muscle fiber.
  - **Dystrophin** is part of **Dystrophin-Glycoprotein sarcolemmal complex & this protein deficiency** leads to **secondary loss of sarcoglycans** & dystroglycans resulting in **weakness of sarcolemma**, causing **membrane tears** and **muscle fiber necrosis**[Q].

Clinical Features:

- **Early development** of child is **normal**, disease begins to **manifest** when **child starts walking**[Q].
- Child **walks clumsily**, has **difficulty in climbing stairs** & gait is **waddling**[Q].
  - **Hypertrophy of calf muscle** is a **characteristic sign** & is visible by age of **4-5 years**, called **pseudohypertrophy**[Q] (not true hypertrophy because **muscle is replaced by fat & connective tissue**)
  - **Pelvic girdle involvement** is very common & elicited by **Gower's sign**[Q]
- **Gower's sign: Patient using his arms to climb up the legs in attempting to get up from the floor**[Q].

Hypertrophied Muscles	Atrophied Muscles
- **Calf, Glutei & Deltoid**[Q] - **Brachioradialis**[Q] - Tongue muscles	- **Sternal head of pectoralis major**[Q] - **Supraspinatus**[Q]

- **Loss of muscle strength** is **progressive; Proximal muscles & neck** are **involved more**[Q]
- **Leg involvement is more severe than arm involvement**[Q]
  - **Contracture of heel cords & iliotibial band occurs**[Q] (by age of 6 years)
  - **Eventually all muscles are atrophied**[Q]

Complications of Duchenne Muscular Dystrophy

Chest Deformity	Cardiac	Intellectual Impairment
- **Progressive scoliosis**[Q] develops - **Impairs pulmonary function**[Q] - By **16–18 years** of age, patients are predisposed to **serious fatal pulmonary infections**[Q].	- **Cardiomyopathy & CHF** may be seen[Q] - **Cardiac cause of death** is **uncommon**	- Intellectual impairment is common - **Intelligence** is usually **subnormal**

Diagnosis:

- **Elevation of creatinine phosphokinase (20-200 times)**[Q]
- **EMG: Features of myopathy**[Q]

Muscle Biopsy

- **Definitive diagnosis is established on the basis of dystrophin deficiency in biopsied muscle tissue**[Q]
- Diffuse changes of **degeneration & muscle fibers of varying size**[Q]
- **Group of necrotic & regenerating muscle fibers are seen**[Q]

Treatment:

- Significant **alteration in the progression of disease** has been seen with **prednisolone**[Q].

Contd...

Contd...

Duchenne Muscular Dystrophy (Pseudohypertrophic Muscular Dystrophy)

Prognosis:

- Patients **die in** the **second decade** of life because of **respiratory failure** or due to **associated cardiomyopathy**[Q].

Age on onset	• **Before 5 years**[Q]
Confined to wheel chair Inability to walk	• **After age 12 years**[Q]
Respiratory failure	• **In 2nd or 3rd decade (After 16-18 years**[Q])

160. **Ans. c. Give first dose of antibiotic and refer to higher center in an ambulance with sips of ORS along the way**   *(Ref: Ghai 8th/e p752-753; IMNCI Guidelines)*

The patient has multiple signs of possible serious bacterial infection (10 skin pustules, diarrhea with severe dehydration & weight = 2 kg which is <-3SD). Hence, the child should be immediately given first dose of injectable antibiotic, kept warm and referred to hospital with sips of ORS along the way.

IMNCI Guidelines for Young Infants (<2 months)		
Signs	**Classify as**	**Identify Treatment**
• **Convulsions**[Q] or • Fast breathing **≥ 60 breaths/minute**[Q] or more or • **Severe chest indrawing**[Q] or • **Nasal flaring**[Q] or • **Grunting**[Q] or • **Bulging fontanel**[Q] or • **≥ 10 or more skin pustules or a big boil**[Q] or • Axillary temperature **37.5°C or above**[Q] [or 35.5°(or feels **cold to touch**)] or • **Lethargic or unconscious**[Q] or • **Less than normal movements**[Q]	• Possible serious bacterial infection	• **Give first dose of intra-muscular ampicillin & gentamicin**[Q] • Treat to **prevent low blood sugar**[Q] • **Warm the young infant by skin to skin contact**[Q] if temperature less than 36.5°C (or feels cold to touch) **while arranging referral** • Advise mother how to keep the young infant warm on the way to the hospital • **Refer urgently to hospital**[Q]

161. **Ans. a. Neonatal sepsis**   *(Ref: Nelson 20/e p832, 915; Ghai 8/e p163)*

In this situation, sepsis should be ruled out where the baby has excessive weight loss (>10% of birth weight) with features of dehydration (depressed tontanella, sunken eyes, decreased urine output and decreased skin turgor), along with poor activity. Failure to feed properly is seen in most sick newborn infants and should lead to a careful search for infection, a central or peripheral nervous system disorder, intestinal obstruction, and other abnormal conditions.

"Neonatal sepsis often manifests with vague and ill-defined symptoms and requires high index of suspicion for early diagnosis. An early but non-specific manifestation is alteration in the established feeding behavior. The baby, who has been active and sucking normally, refuses to suck and becomes lethargic, or unresponsive. Poor cry, hypothermia, abdominal distention, vomiting and apneic spells are other common manifestations. Diarrhea is uncommon. Fast breathing, chest retractions, and grunt indicate pneumonia Most cases of meningitis do not have any distinct clinical picture per se, making it mandatory to suspect meningitis in all cases of sepsis. Though the presence of excessive or high pitched crying, fever, seizures, blank look, neck retraction or bulging anterior tontanel are suggestive of meningitis. Shock, bleeding, sclerema and renal failure are indicators of overwhelming sepsis."- Ghai 8/e p163

Initial Signs & Symptoms of Infection in Newborn Infants	
General	**Cardiovascular System**
• **Fever, temperature instability**[Q] • **Not doing well, poor feeding**[Q] • **Edema**[Q]	• **Pallor, mottling, cold clammy skin**[Q] • **Hypotension, tachycardia**[Q] • Bradycardia
Gastrointestinal System	**Central Nervous System**
• **Abdominal distention**[Q] • **Vomiting, diarrhea**[Q] • Hepatomegaly	• **Irritability, lethargy, high pitched cry**[Q] • **Tremors, seizures**[Q] • **Hyporeflexia, hypotonia, abnormal Moro's reflex**[Q]

Respiratory System	Hematological System
• Apnea, dyspnea, tachypnea[Q]	• Pallor, jaundice, splenomegaly[Q]
• Retractions, flaring, grunting[Q]	• Bleeding
• Cyanosis[Q]	• Petechiae, purpura

162. Ans. c. Anti-VZV antibody   *(Ref: Ghai 8/e p215; Nelson 20/e p1581-1583)*

Clinical picture of cicatrizing skin lesions and limb hypoplasia with evidence of chorioretinitis and diffuse cerebral atrophy on MRI brain is suggestive of congenital varicella infections, which are detected using Anti-VZV antibodies.

"The congenital varicella syndrome is characterized by cicatrial skin scarring in a zoster-like distribution, limb hypoplasia, and neurologic (e.g., microcephaly, cortical atrophy, seizures, and mental retardation), eye (e.g., chorioretinitis, microphthalmia, and cataracts), renal (e.g., hydroureter and hydronephrosis) and autonomic nervous system abnormalities (neurogenic bladder, swallowing dysfunction, and aspiration pneumonia)." -Nelson 20/e p1581

Congenital Varicella Syndrome (Varicella Embryopathy)
• **Causative agent:** Varicella Zoster virus (VZV); a **double stranded DNA virus**[Q]
• **Maximum risk: 8-20 weeks of gestation**[Q]

Cause:
• **Virus-induced injury to CNS** with **predilection for tissues in a rapid developmental stage** like **limb buds**[Q].

Clinical Manifestations	
Scarring of Skin (Cicatricial skin lesions)	• **Characteristic cutaneous lesion: 'Cicatrix'**[Q] • **Cicatrix** presenting as a **zigzag scarring**[Q] in a dermatomal distribution • **Hypopigmentation**[Q]
Limb reduction defects (Limb hypoplasia)	• **Fetus infected at 6-12 weeks** of gestation appears to have **maximal interruption with limb development**, resulting in **1 or more shortened & malformed extremities**[Q] • The **remaining of torso** may be **entirely normal in appearance.**
Brain	• Aplasia, **microcephaly,** hydrocephaly & **calcification**[Q]
Spinal cord	• Motor/sensory deficit, **absent deep tendon reflexes**[Q] • Anisocoria, Horner syndrome, anal & urinary sphincter dysfunction
Eye	• **Microphthalmia, cataracts, optic atrophy & chorioretinitis**[Q]

Diagnosis:
• **Diagnosis of VZV fetopathy** is based mainly on **history of gestational chickenpox** with **stigmata** seen **in fetus**[Q].
• **Rapid method: Direct immunofluorescence**[Q]
• **Confirmatory test: VZV DNA detection by PCR**[Q] (anti-VZV IgM antibody is **not the method of choice)**

Treatment:
• **Antiviral treatment is not indicated**[Q] (**Damage** caused by **fetal VZV infection does not progress postpartum)**

163. Ans. a. 22-26°C   *(Ref: Ghai 8/e p133; Nelson 20/e p800; https://www3.nd.edu/~nicudes/stan%20delivery.html)*

The ideal temperature in delivery room for the neonates to be kept in warmer should be 22-26°C.

"The temperature of delivery room should be 25°C and it should be free from drift of air." - Ghai 8/e p133

"The nursery temperature should be kept between 22-26°C (72-78°F)." - Nelson 20/e p800

"The ventilation system for each delivery and resuscitation room shall be designed to control the ambient temperature between 72-78 degrees Fahrenheit (22-26 degrees Centigrade) during the delivery, resuscitation, and stabilization of a newborn." - https://www3.nd.edu/~nicudes/stan%20delivery.html

164. Ans. b. Weight in kilograms by cube of height in meters   *(Ref: Daftary Manual of Obstetrics 3/e p199)*

Ponderal Index is calculated by multiplying weight in grams by hundred and then dividing by cube of length in cm. This parameter is usually less than 2 in asymmetric growth retardation and 2 or more in babies with normal growth or symmetric growth retardation.

Ponderal index = Birth weight (gm)/ Length (cm)³ x 100

Intrauterine Growth Restriction (IUGR)
• Definition: **IUGR** refers to all babies with **clinical features of malnutrition**, like **3 or more loose skin folds in buttock region, decreased subcutaneous fat, peeling of skin**[Q].
• **IUGR** is a **clinical definition, irrespective of birth weight**, while **small for gestational age (SGA)** is a **statistical definition** that includes **babies with birth weight <10th centile of expected**[Q].

Types of IUGR		
	Symmetric IUGR (20%)	**Asymmetric IUGR (80%)**
Timing of insult	Insult in **1st & early 2nd trimester**	Problem in **late 2nd or 3rd trimester**
Etiology	TORCH infection Chromosomal anomaly Genetic causes	**Medical/Obstetric problem** of mother in late trimesters like **poor maternal nutrition, maternal hypertension, placental insufficiency**[Q]
Effect on cells	**Fetal cell number mainly decreased**[Q]	**Size of cells more affected than number of cells**[Q]
Anthropometric parameters	**Head circumference, length & weight equally affected**[Q]	**Brain growth (head circumference) spared**[Q]
Ponderal index	≥ 2[Q]	<2[Q]
Brain/Liver size Ratio	<5[Q]	>5[Q]
Prognosis	**Poorer**[Q]	**Better outcome**[Q]

165. **Ans. b. Through umbilical vein**   *(Ref: Ghai 8/e p132)*

Umbilical vein is the preferred route for drug delivery during resuscitation.

"Since veins in scalp or extremities are difficult to access during resuscitation, umbilical vein is the preferred route. No intracardiac injection is recommended. For umbilical vein catheterization, 3.5 Fr or 5 Fr umbilical catheter, is inserted into the umbilical vein such that its tip is just inside the skin surface and there is free flow of blood. Direct injection into umbilical cord is not desirable."- Ghai 8/e p132

166. **Ans. d. Phototherapy**   *(Ref: Ghai 8/e p173; Nelson 20/e p873-874)*

Jaundice on day 1 of life is usually due to some hemolytic disease or congenital infections and must be treated using phototherapy. Possibility of Rh incompatibility is ruled out as mother blood group is O+. Ideally basic investigations for hemolytic anemia should be sent simultaneously (not given in the option). Best option would be phototherapy.

See Q. No. 157 AIIMS November 2017

Phototherapy
• **Phototherapy** has been found to be **effective in treating jaundice in neonates**[Q].
• **Unconjugated bilirubin in skin converted into water-soluble photoproducts on exposure to light** of a particular wavelength (**425-475 mm**)[Q].
• These photoproducts are water soluble, nontoxic and excreted in intestine & urine[Q].
• For **phototherapy to be effective, bilirubin needs to be present in skin** so there is **no role for prophylactic phototherapy**[Q].

Phototherapy Acts by		
Configurational isomerization	**Structural Isomerization**	**Photo oxidation**
• The **Z-isomers of bilirubin** are **converted into E-isomers**[Q]. • The **reaction is instantaneous** upon exposure to light but **reversible** as bilirubin reaches into the bile duct. • After exposure of 8-12 hours of phototherapy, this constitutes about **25% of STB**, which is **non-toxic**. • Since this is **excreted slowly** from body, this is **not a major mechanism for decrease of STB**[Q].	• This is an **irreversible reaction** where the **bilirubin is converted into lumirubin.** • The reaction is **directly proportional to dose of phototherapy**[Q]. • These products forms **2-6% of STB, which is rapidly excrete from body, mainly responsible for phototherapy induced decline in STB**[Q].	• This is a **minor reaction**, where photo products are excreted in urine[Q].

Phototherapy
Types of Light:
• **Most effective lights** are those with **high energy output near the maximum adsorption peak of bilirubin (450-460 nm)**[Q].
• **Special blue lamps** with a **peak output at 425-475 nm are the most efficient**[Q].
• **Cool daylight lamps** with a **principal peak at 550 to 600 nm are most commonly used but not very effective phototherapy units** in our country[Q].
• The **lamps should be changed every 3 months** or **earlier if irradiance is monitored**[Q].
• **Double surface phototherapy is more effective** than the single surface[Q].
• **Double surface phototherapy** can be provided either by **double surface special blue lights** or by **conventional blue light & undersurface fiberoptic phototherapy**.

Factors affecting efficacy of phototherapy	
• Irradiance[Q]	• Initial serum total bilirubin[Q]
• Surface area exposed[Q]	• Adequacy of breast feeding[Q]
• Distance from phototherapy unit[Q]	

167. Ans. b. Inj. betamethasone 12 mg for 2 doses 24 hours apart   *(Ref: Williams 24/e p850; Goodman Gillman 12/e p1231)*

For attaining lung maturity betamethasone (12 mg intramuscularly every 24 hours for two doses) or dexamethasone (6 mg intramuscularly every 12 hours for four doses) is administered to women with definitive signs of premature labor between 26 and 34 weeks of gestation.

"Antenatal glucocorticoids are used frequently in the setting of premature labor, decreasing the incidence of respiratory distress syndrome, intraventricular hemorrhage, and death in infants delivered prematurely. Betamethasone (12 mg intramuscularly every 24 hours for two doses) or dexamethasone (6 mg intramuscularly every 12 hours for four doses) is administered to women with definitive signs of premature labor between 26 and 34 weeks of gestation. Due to evidence of decreased birth weight and adrenal suppression in infants whose mothers were given repeated courses of glucocorticoids, only a single course of glucocorticoids should be administered."-Goodman Gillman 12/e p1231

Antenatal Corticosteroids in Preterm Labor
• **Antenatal glucocorticoids** are used frequently in the setting of **premature labor, decreasing the incidence of RDS, intraventricular hemorrhage (IVH) & death in infants delivered prematurely**[Q].
Drug regimens: • **Inj. Betamethasone 12 mg IM every 24 hours, 2 doses (preferred)**[Q] • **Inj. Dexamethasone 6 mg IM every 12 hours, 4 doses (only if betamethasone cannot be arranged)**[Q]
Indication: • All women with **preterm labor** who are **likely to deliver within the next 1 week**[Q]
Contraindications: • **Clinical chorioamnionitis & Eclampsia** [Q]
Advantages: • **50% reduction** in incidence of **RDS, 50% reduction** in incidence of **IVH & 40% reduction** in **mortality**[Q]
• **Maximum effect** is seen **between 24 hours & 7 days of administration of antenatal steroids**[Q].   • **Corticosteroid therapy** is effective in lowering the incidence of RDS & neonatal mortality rates in preterms if birth was delayed for at least 24 hours after initiation of betamethasone[Q].

ORTHOPAEDICS

168. Ans. d. Rickets   *(Ref: Apley 9/e p136)*

The radiological image above shows cupping and fraying of the metaphyses, typically seen in rickets.

"In active rickets there is thickening and widening of the growth plate, cupping of the metaphysis and, sometimes, bowing of the diaphysis. The metaphysis may remain abnormally wide even after healing has occurred."-Apley 9/e p136

Rickets
• Characterized by **inadequate mineralization of bone** with **effects on physeal growth & ossification**, resulting in **deformities of the endochondral skeleton**[Q].

Etiology of Rickets	
• Nutritional lack • Underexposure to sunlight • **Intestinal malabsorption**[Q] • **Decreased 25-hydroxylation (liver disease, anticonvulsants)**[Q]	• **Reduced 1alpha-hydroxylation (renal disease, nephrectomy, 1alpha-hydroxylase deficiency)**[Q] • **Calcium deficiency**[Q] • **Hypophosphatemia**[Q]

Pathology:
- **Inability to calcify intercellular matrix in deeper layers of physis**[Q].

  - **Entire physeal plate increases in thickness, zone of calcification is poorly mineralized & bone formation is sparse in zone of ossification**[Q].
  - **New trabeculae are thin & weak with broad & cup-shaped juxta-epiphyseal metaphysis**[Q].

Clinical features:
- Infant may present with **tetany or convulsions**; Failure to thrive, listlessness & muscular flaccidity

Bone changes in Rickets
• **Deformity of skull (craniotabes**[Q]**) & thickening of knees, ankles & wrists** from **physeal overgrowth.** • **Enlargement of costochondral junctions ('rickety rosary'**[Q]**) & lateral indentation of chest (Harrison's sulcus**[Q]**), distal tibial bowing**[Q] • **Spinal curvature, coxa vara & bending or fractures of long bones** in severe rickets[Q]

X-rays:
- **Thickening & widening of growth plate, cupping of metaphysis** & sometimes, **bowing of diaphysis**[Q]
- **Abnormally wide metaphysis**[Q]

Biochemistry:
- **Diminished** levels of **serum calcium & phosphate, low 25-OH D**[Q]
- **Increased ALP & diminished urinary excretion of calcium**[Q]

  - **Calcium phosphate product** (derived by **multiplying calcium & phosphorus levels** expressed in mmol/L), **normally about 3**, is **diminished; values of <2.4 are diagnostic**[Q].

Treatment:
- Treatment with **vitamin D (400–1000 IU per day) & calcium supplements** is usually effective[Q]

169. **Ans. a. Anterior dislocation of hip**   *(Ref: Apley 9/e p846)*

The limb of the patient is seen lying in a flexed, abducted and slightly externally rotated posture, classically seen in anterior hip dislocation.

"Anterior Dislocation of Hip: The leg lies externally rotated, abducted and slightly flexed. It is not short, because the attachment of rectus femoris prevents the head from displacing upwards. Occasionally the leg is abducted almost to a right angle. Seen from the side, the anterior bulge of the dislocated head is unmistakable, especially when the head has moved anteriorly and superiorly. The prominent head is easy to feel, either anteriorly (superior type) or in the groin (inferior type). Hip movements are impossible."- Apley 9/e p846

Anterior Dislocation of Hip
• **Rare** as compared to posterior dislocation • **Cause: Road accident or air crash**[Q]
Mechanism: • Occur when a **weight falls onto the back of a miner** or **building laborer** who is **working with his legs wide apart, knees straight & back bent forwards**[Q].
Types: • **Type I: Pubic** (femoral **head** lies **superiorly**[Q]); **Type II: Obturator** (femoral **head** lies **inferiorly**[Q])
Clinical Features: • **Leg lies externally rotated, abducted & slightly flexed.** It is **not short**, because **attachment of rectus femoris prevents the head from displacing upwards. Occasionally** the **leg is abducted** almost to a right angle. [Q]

Contd...

Anterior Dislocation of Hip
• **Prominent head** is easy to feel, **either anteriorly (superior type^Q) or in the groin (inferior type^Q).**   • **Hip movements** are **impossible.**
X-ray: • **AP view: Dislocation** is **usually obvious** (occasionally **head** is almost directly **in front of its normal position**; any doubt is **resolved by a lateral film^Q**)
Treatment: • Dislocation must be **reduced as soon as possible under GA^Q.**
Complications: • **Avascular necrosis^Q** (<10%)

170. **Ans. c. Osteogenesis imperfecta** *(Ref: Apley 9/e p173, 166, 167, 132)*

In the X-ray, a subcapital femoral neck fracture can be seen, and suspected multiple fractures in the greater trochanter also. The finding is suggestive of osteogenesis imperfecta among the options here. Femoral neck fractures in adolescents are caused mostly due to domestic abuse or in setting of osteopenia of bones due to osteogenesis imperfecta.

*"Osteogenesis imperfecta: There is **generalized osteopenia, thinning of the long bones, fractures in various stages of healing, vertebral compression and spinal deformity.** The type of abnormality varies with the severity of the disease. The skull may be enlarged and shows the presence of Wormian bones– areas of vicarious ossification in the calvarium. After puberty, fractures occur less frequently, but in those who survive the incidence rise again after the climacteric. It is thought that **very mild ('subclinical') forms of OI may account for some cases of recurrent fractures in adults."*- Apley 9/e p173*

*"Osteopetrosis is one of several conditions which are **characterized by sclerosis and thickening of the bones which appear with increased radiographic density.** This is the **result of an imbalance between bone formation and bone resorption;** in the most common form, osteopetrosis, there is failed bone resorption due to a defect in osteoclast production and/or function."- Apley 9/e p166*

*"Spotted bones (osteopoikilosis): Routine X-rays sometimes show (quite incidentally) **numerous white spots distributed throughout the skeleton.** Closer examination occasionally reveals **whitish spots in the skin (disseminated lenticular dermatofibrosis).** The condition is inherited as an autosomal dominant trait."- Apley 9/e p167*

*"The term osteopaenia is sometimes used to describe bone which appears to be **less 'dense' than normal on x-ray,** without defining whether the **loss of density is due to osteoporosis** or osteomalacia, or indeed whether it is sufficiently marked to be regarded as at all pathological. **More characteristic signs of osteoporosis are loss of trabecular definition, thinning of the cortices and insufficiency fractures."- Apley 9/e p132*

Osteogenesis imperfecta	Osteopetrosis
• Characterized by **generalized osteopenia, thinning of the long bones, fractures in various stages of healing, vertebral compression & spinal deformity^Q.** • In the X-ray, a subcapital femoral neck fracture can be seen, and suspected multiple fractures in the greater trochanter also.	• Characterized by **sclerosis & thickening of the bones** which appear with **increased radiographic density^Q.**

Osteoporosis	Osteopoikilocytosis
• Bone appears to be less 'dense' than normal on X-ray[Q] • More characteristic signs of osteoporosis are loss of trabecular definition, thinning of cortices & insufficiency fractures[Q]	• Routine X-rays show (quite incidentally) numerous white spots distributed throughout the skeleton[Q]. • Multiple punctate sclerotic bone islands or foci of compact bone located in cancellous bone around the joint[Q].
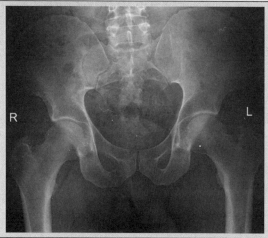	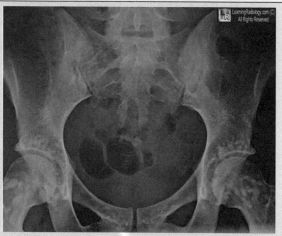

Osteogenesis Imperfecta (Brittle Bones)

- Characterized by **abnormal synthesis & structural defects of type I collagen** result in **abnormalities of bones, teeth, ligaments, sclera & skin**[Q].

  - **Defining clinical features**: Osteopenia, liability to fracture, laxity of ligaments, blue coloration of sclera & dentinogenesis imperfecta ('crumbling teeth')[Q].

Pathology:
- **Alteration in structural integrity**, or a **reduction in total amount of type I collagen**[Q]
- It leads to **immature woven bone, thinning of dermis, laxity of ligaments, increased corneal translucency & loss of dentin** leading to tooth decay[Q].

- Classification:
- Most widely used: **Sillence classification**[Q]
- MC type: **Type I**[Q]

Clinical Features:
- **Most striking abnormality: Propensity to fracture after minor trauma** without much pain or swelling[Q].
- **Fractures** are **discovered during infancy & recur frequently** throughout childhood[Q].
- **Florid callus formation** leads to lump formation[Q]

  - **Severe deformities of long bones & vertebral compression fractures** often lead to **kyphoscoliosis**[Q].
  - Thin & loose skin, hypermobile joints, blue or grey sclera, discolored & carious tooth[Q]

X-rays:
- **Generalized osteopenia, thinning of long bones, fractures** in various stages of healing, **vertebral compression & spinal deformity**[Q].
- **Enlarged skull** with **presence of Wormian bones**[Q] (areas of **vicarious ossification in calvarium**[Q])

Diagnosis:
- Diagnosis is made by **clinical & radiological features**[Q]

Management:
- **No medical treatment available**[Q] to counteract the effects of this abnormality
- **Conservative treatment** is directed at preventing fractures[Q]
- **Fractures are treated conservatively**[Q], but immobilization must be kept to a minimum.

170b. Ans. a. Osteopetrosis   *(Ref: Apley 9/e p166)*

History of pain in the right hip and difficulty in walking in a child with X-ray hip showing sclerosis & thickening of the bones (appear as increased radiographic density) is highly suggestive of osteopetrosis.

> *"Osteopetrosis (Marble Bones, Albers–Schonberg Disease): Osteopetrosis is one of several conditions which are characterized by sclerosis and thickening of the bones which appear with increased radiographic density. This is the result of an imbalance between bone formation and bone resorption; in the most common form, osteopetrosis, there is failed bone resorption due to a defect in osteoclast production and/or function."- Apley 9/e p166*

171. Ans. c. Chronic osteomyelitis   *(Ref: Apley 9/e p33, 36, 39)*

In this X-ray of humerus head, a faint patch with loss of density and a sequestrum is seen within the bone. This radiological feature along with the young age of patient is suggestive of chronic osteomyelitis.

> *"Chronic osteomyelitis: Weeks or months after the onset of acute infection a sequestrum appears in the follow-up x-ray and the patient is left with a chronic infection and a draining sinus."- Apley 9/e p36*

> *"Chronic osteomyelitis: X-ray examination will usually show bone resorption – either as a patchy loss of density or as frank excavation around an implant – with thickening and sclerosis of the surrounding bone. However, there are marked variations: there may be no more than **localized loss of trabeculation**, or an **area of osteoporosis**, or **periosteal thickening**; **sequestra show up as unnaturally dense fragments**, in contrast to the surrounding osteopaenic bone; sometimes the bone is crudely thickened and misshapen, resembling a tumour."- Apley 9/e p39*

Acute osteomyelitis	Ewing sarcomas	Osteosarcoma
• **No abnormality of bone during 1st week** after the onset of symptoms **on plain X-ray**[Q] • **Displacement of fat planes** signifies soft-tissue swelling[Q] • **2nd week**: Faint extra-cortical outline due to **periosteal new bone formation (classic X-ray sign of early pyogenic osteomyelitis)**[Q] • **Periosteal thickening** becomes more obvious later & **patchy rarefaction of metaphysis**[Q] • **Regional osteoporosis** with **localized segment of apparently increased density** is important **late sign**[Q]	• Area of **bone destruction** predominantly **in mid-diaphysis** on X-rays • **New bone formation** may extend **along shaft** & appears as **fusiform layers of bone around the lesion (Onion-peel effect**[Q]**)** • **Tumour extends into surrounding soft tissues**, with radiating streaks of ossification **(Sunray appearance**[Q]**)** & reactive periosteal bone at proximal & distal margins **(Codman's triangles**[Q]**)**	• **Hazy osteolytic areas** alternate with **dense osteoblastic areas**[Q]. • **Endosteal margin** is **poorly defined**[Q]. • **Cortex is breached & tumour extends into adjacent tissues**; when this happens, **streaks of new bone appear, radiating outwards from cortex ('sunburst' effect**[Q]**)** • Tumour emerges from cortex, reactive new bone forms at angles of periosteal elevation **(Codman's triangle**[Q]**)**. • **Sunburst appearance & Codman's triangle are typical of osteosarcoma**[Q] (occasionally seen in other rapidly growing tumours)

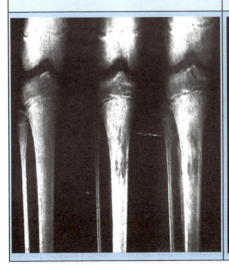
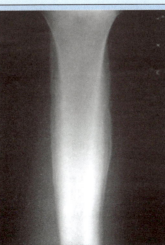
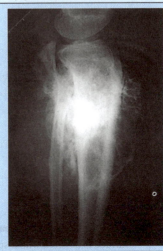

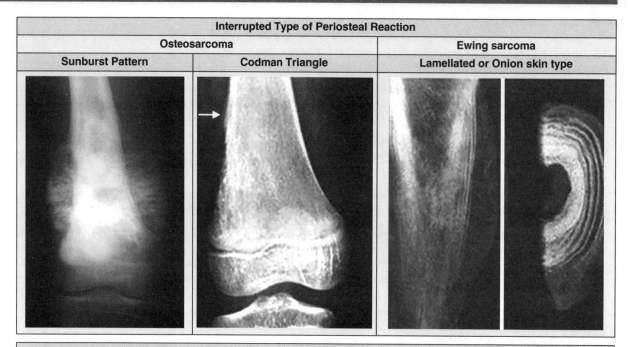

Chronic Osteomyelitis
• Dreaded complication of acute hematogenous osteomyelitis • **MC organisms** responsible for chronic osteomyelitis: **Staphylococcus aureus**[Q] • **MC organisms** responsible for chronic osteomyelitis **in presence of foreign implants: Staph. epidermidis**[Q]
Predisposing factors: • **MC predisposing factor: Local trauma**[Q] (**open fracture** or a **prolonged bone operation** with use of a **foreign implant**) • Inadequately treated acute osteomyelitis; old or debilitated, substance abuse, diabetes, peripheral vascular disease, skin infections, malnutrition, lupus erythematosus or immune deficiency.
Pathology: • Bone is **destroyed or devitalized, cavities containing pus & pieces of dead bone (sequestra**[Q]**)** are surrounded by vascular tissue & beyond that by **areas of sclerosis** (due to **chronic reactive new bone formation**[Q]), which may take the form of a distinct bony sheath (**involucrum**[Q]). • Sequestra act as **substrates for bacterial adhesion** leading to **persistence of infection**[Q] • Bone destruction & increasingly brittle sclerosis results in a **pathological fracture**[Q]
Clinical Features: • **Pain, fever, redness & tenderness** have recurred **with a discharging sinus**[Q]. • **Longstanding cases: Tissues are thickened & puckered or folded inwards** where a **scar or sinus** adheres to underlying bone; **seropurulent discharge & excoriation** of surrounding skin[Q].
Investigations: • **X-ray:** Bone resorption with **thickening & sclerosis, pieces of dead bone (sequestra) &** form of a distinct bony sheath (**involucrum**)[Q] • **Radioisotope scintigraphy** is **sensitive but not specific**, useful for showing up **hidden foci of infection**[Q].
Treatment: • **Antibiotics:** Chronic infection is **seldom eradicated by antibiotics alone**. Antibiotics are given for **4–6 weeks before considering operative treatment**[Q]. • Surface is covered with a split-skin graft or by transferring a myocutaneous island flap on a long vascular pedicle.

Contd...

Chronic Osteomyelitis
• **Radical excision of all avascular & infected tissue** followed by **closed irrigation & suction drainage & appropriate antibiotic solution** in high concentration[Q].

Chronic Osteomyelitis

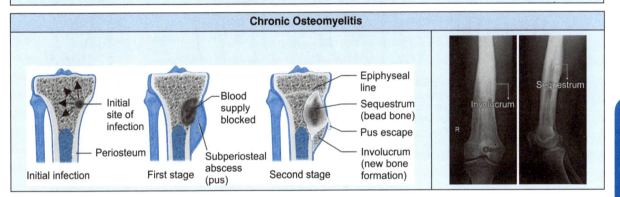

172. **Ans. a. Tension band wiring**   *(Ref: Apley 9/e p887-888)*

 The given X-ray shows displaced transverse fracture of patella, which is treated by tension band wiring.

 *"Displaced transverse fracture: The lateral expansions are torn and the entire extensor mechanism is disrupted. **Operation is essential**. Through a longitudinal incision the fracture is exposed and the **patella repaired by the tension-band principle**. The fragments are reduced and transfixed with two stiff K-wires; flexible wire is then looped tightly around the protruding K-wires and over the front of the patella. The tears in the extensor expansions are then repaired. A plaster back-slab or hinged brace is worn until active extension of the knee is regained; either may be removed every day to permit active knee-flexion exercises."- Apley 9/e p888*

 See Q. No. 173 AIIMS May 2017

173. **Ans. d. Supracondylar fracture**   *(Ref: Apley 9/e p371, 760)*

 The given picture shows cubitus varus or gun-stock deformity. The most common cause is malunion of a supracondylar fracture.

 "Cubitus Varus ('Gun-Stock' Deformity): The deformity is most obvious when the elbow is extended and the arms are elevated. The most common cause is malunion of a supracondylar fracture. The deformity can be corrected by a wedge osteotomy of the lower humerus but this is best left until skeletal maturity."- Apley's 9/e p371

 *"Cubitus Valgus: The normal carrying angle of the elbow is 5–15 degrees of valgus; anything more than this is regarded as a valgus deformity, which is usually quite obvious when the patient stands with arms to the sides and palms facing forwards. The commonest cause is longstanding non-union of a fractured lateral condyle; the deformity may be associated with marked prominence of the medial condylar outline. The importance of cubitus valgus is the **liability to delayed ulnar palsy**; years after the causal injury the patient notices weakness of the hand, with numbness and tingling of the ulnar fingers. The deformity itself needs no treatment, but for delayed ulnar palsy the nerve should be transposed to the front of the elbow. Great care is needed in performing the operation. Excessive dissection of the nerve or rough handling can impair nerve function."- Apley's 9/e p371*

 See Q. No. 168 AIIMS May 2017

174. **Ans. b. Movement at fracture site**   *(Ref: Apley 9/e p689, 700, 704)*

 Micro movements at fracture site increases callus formation.

 "The small amount of movement that occurs at the fracture site through using the limb encourages vascular proliferation and callus formation."- Apley 9/e p700

"Depending on the stability of fixation and the underlying fracture pattern, weight bearing is started as early as possible to 'stimulate' fracture healing. Some fixators incorporate a telescopic unit that allows 'dynamization'; this will convert the forces of weight- bearing into axial micro movement at the fracture site, thus promoting callus formation and accelerating bone union." - Apley 9/e p704

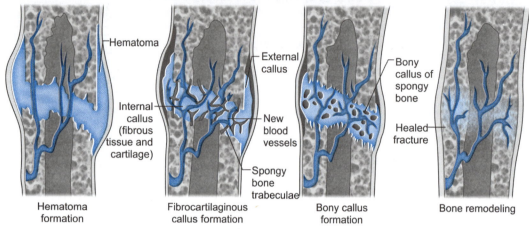

Fig. 37: Stages of fracture healing

Fracture Healing

- Bone is a unique tissue as **fractures of bone heals by formation of normal bone**, not the scar.
- **Immobilization of fracture is not mandatory** for healing as fractures unite whether they are splinted or not.
- **Most fractures are splinted**, not to ensure union but to: **Alleviate pain, ensure that union takes place in good position & permit early movement of limb & return of function**[Q].
- Process of **fracture repair varies** according to **type of bone involved & amount of movement at fracture site**[Q].
- Most fractures heal by callous formation; **Intramembranous ossification** (hard callous formation) & **endochondral ossification** (soft callous formation)[Q].

Stages of Fracture Healing by Callus

Tissue destruction & hematoma formation	• Hematoma forms around & within fracture. • Bone at fracture surfaces, **deprived of a blood supply, dies back for 1-2 mm**.
Inflammation & cellular proliferation	• Within **8 hours of fracture**, acute inflammatory reaction with **migration of inflammatory cells & initiation of proliferation & differentiation of mesenchymal stem cells** from periosteum, breached medullary canal & surrounding muscle. • Fragment ends are **surrounded by cellular tissue**, which **creates a scaffold across the fracture site**[Q]. • **Clotted hematoma** is slowly absorbed & fine new capillaries grow[Q]
Callus formation	• **Micro movements at fracture site increases callus formation**. • Cell population changes to osteoblasts & osteoclasts; dead bone is mopped up & woven bone appears in the fracture callus[Q]. • As the **immature fibre bone (or 'woven' bone) becomes more densely**[Q] mineralized, movement at fracture site decreases progressively & **at about 4 weeks after injury the fracture 'unites'**[Q].

Cond...

Cond...

Fracture Healing	
Consolidation	• With continuing osteoclastic & osteoblastic activity, **woven bone** is **replaced by lamellar bone & fracture is solidly united**[Q].
Remodelling	• Newly formed bone is **remodelled to resemble the normal structure**[Q].

OPHTHALMOLOGY

175. **Ans. b. +20 D**   *(Ref: Yanoff and Duker 4/e p69; Khurana 6/e p586-587, 5/e p600; Parson's 22/e p136, 21/e p134*
With indirect ophthalmoscope, most commonly a lens of +20 D is used which gives a magnification of about 3x (Magnification = power of eye (+60D)/ power of lens).

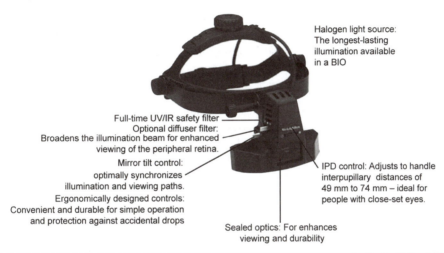

*"Examination by indirect ophthalmoscopy: The binocular indirect ophthalmoscope is applicable to all refractive errors and, as its beam penetrates opacities in most media and there is **a reduced image size**, it is possible to obtain a wide view of the retina and its defects. Binocular indirect ophthalmoscopy has the **advantages of a large field of view, brighter illumination, and decreased distortion** while examining the peripheral retina. Disadvantages of indirect ophthalmoscopy are that the image is inverted both vertically and laterally, a fact that needs to be remembered while drawing retinal diagrams and during surgery. A wide convex lens is held between the thumb and forefinger of the left hand with the curved surface towards the examiner, and with the lens itself in a plane parallel to the plane of the iris of the patient. The strength of the lens may be +28 D, +20 D or +14 D, the weaker powered lenses giving images of increasing size, narrower fields of view and lesser stereopsis. The periphery of the retina may be brought into view by scleral depression and it is best seen with the patient recumbent."*- Parson's 22/e p136

Features	Direct ophthalmoscopy	Indirect ophthalmoscopy
Condensing lens	Not required[Q]	Required (Convex lens)[Q]
Examination distance	As close to patient's eye as possible	At an arm's length
Image	Virtual, erect[Q]	Real, inverted[Q]
Magnification	About 15 times[Q]	4-5 times[Q]
Illumination	Not so bright, so not useful in hazy media	**Bright**, so useful for **hazy media**[Q]
Area of field in focus	About 2 disc diopters[Q]	About 8 disc diopters[Q]
Stereopsis	Absent	Present[Q]

Features	Direct ophthalmoscopy	Indirect ophthalmoscopy
Accessible fundus view	Slightly beyond equator	**Up to Ora serrata i.e. Peripheral retina**[Q]
Examination through hazy media	Not possible	**Possible**[Q]
Patient position	**Sitting**[Q]	**Supine**[Q]
Ease	**Easy procedure for visualization of posterior pole of retina**[Q]	**Difficult,** require training[Q]

176. Ans. a. 10^{-15} seconds *(Ref: Yanoff and Duker 4/e p304; Parson's 22/e p608, 21/e p584)*

In the given image for cataract surgery, Femtosecond laser is used. The pulse duration of femtosecond laser is 10^{-15} seconds.

*"**Femtosecond (FS) laser is an infrared laser with a wavelength of 1053 nm.** FS laser is like Nd:YAG laser, **works by producing photodisruption or photoionization of the optically transparent tissue such as the cornea.** Application of either FS laser or Nd:YAG laser **results in the generation of a rapidly expanding cloud of free electrons and ionized molecules. The acoustic shock wave so generated results in disruption of the treated tissue.** However, the two lasers differ significantly in the amount of collateral damage they cause. **Nd:YAG laser has a pulse duration in the nanosecond range (10^{-9} seconds) where as FS laser has pulse duration in the femtosecond range (10^{-15} seconds)."*

Femtosecond Laser
• **Femtosecond (FS) laser** is an **infrared laser** with a **wavelength of 1053 nm.**
• Works by producing **photodisruption or photoionization** of **optically transparent tissue** such as cornea.
• **Application** of either FS laser results in **generation of a rapidly expanding cloud of free electrons & ionized molecules.** **Acoustic shock wave** generated results in **disruption of treated tissue**[Q].
• **Nd:YAG laser** has a **pulse duration** in the **nanosecond range (10^{-9} seconds)** where as **FS laser** has **pulse duration** in the **femtosecond range (10^{-15} seconds)**[Q].   • **Reducing** the **pulse duration reduces** the **amount of collateral tissue damage**[Q].
• **Collateral damage** with FS laser is **106 times less than with the Nd:YAG laser.**
• **FS laser is safe for use in corneal surgeries,** which **require exquisite precision.**

Applications of FS Laser	
• **Corneal refractive surgery:** • **LASIK flap creation** • **Astigmatic keratotomy** (AK) • Channel creation for implantation of intrastromal corneal ring segments (ICRS) • **Presbyopia correction,** femtosecond lenticule extraction (FLEx) • Small-incision lenticule extraction (SMILE) & intrastromal presbyopia correction (INTRACOR)	• **Laser-assisted anterior & posterior lamellar keratoplasty** • Cutting of donor buttons in **endothelial keratoplasty** • Customized trephination in **penetrating keratoplasty** • Wound construction, capsulorhexis & nuclear fragmentation in **cataract surgery.**

Lasers used in ophthalmology		
Laser	Wavelength (nanometer)	Clinical Applications
Nd:YAG (Neodymium-Yttrium-Aluminium-Garnet)	1064	• **Posterior capsulotomy, iridotomy, vitreolysis**[Q]
Frequency-doubled Nd:YAG	532	• **Retinal photocoagulation, cyclophotocoagulation**[Q]

Cond...

Contd...

Laser	Wavelength (nanometer)	Clinical Applications
Argon green	**514**	• Trabeculoplasty, iridoplasty, pupillomydriasis, retinal photocoagulation[Q]
Diode laser	**800**	• Retinal photocoagulation[Q]
Krypton red	**714**	• Retinal photocoagulation[Q]
Excimer (argon fluoride)	**193**	• Photorefractive keratectomy (**PRK**), phototherapeutic keratectomy (**PTK**), **LASIK, LASEK**[Q]
Femtosecond laser (neodymium-glass)	**1053**	• Femtosecond laser assisted refractive surgery, lamellar & full thickness corneal transplants[Q]

177. **Ans. c. Topical natamycin only, no need to drain the hypopyon** *(Ref: Khurana 6/e p106, 5/e p101, 4/e p100; Parson 22/e p203-204, 21/e p199-200; Kanski 7/e p180-82; Yanoff and Duker 4/e p219)*
Clinical features and examination findings showing big hypopyon suggests the diagnosis of fungal corneal ulcer, which should be treated by topical natamycin without draining the hypopyon.

*"It is important to remember that a **hypopyon is sterile, since the leucocytosis is due to toxins, not to actual invasion by bacteria which, indeed, are as incapable of passing through the intact Descemet's membrane as are leucocytes**. This accounts for the ease and rapidity with which the hypopyon is often absorbed. It may develop in an hour or two, rapidly disappear, and as readily reappear. Such hypopyons are fluid, always moving to the lowest part of the anterior chamber depending on the position of the patient's head. **The fact that the hypopyon is sterile has great practical importance—it is unnecessary to remove the pus, as is the rule in other parts of the body; if the ulcerative process is controlled, the hypopyon will be absorbed."*-Parson 22/e p201*

*"**Fungal Corneal Ulcer: Treatment is by means of local natamycin and amphotericin B drops, and miconazole ointment; these are effective against Aspergillus and Fusarium. Nystatin is effective against Candida.** Oral antifungal agents may be needed if the ulcers are severe and there is a suspicion of endophthalmitis."*-Parson 22/e p203*

178. **Ans. a. Anterior surface of cornea** *(Ref: Yanoff and Duker 4/e p38)*
Maximum contribution to the refractive power of the eye is by anterior surface of cornea.

"The cornea's anterior surface is approximately spherical with a radius of curvature that is typically 8 mm. This surface is responsible for about two-thirds of the eye's refractive power."- Yanoff and Duker 4/e p38*

Cornea
• **Cornea (the anterior surface)** is **most important refractive surface of eye**[Q]
• **Power: 45 diopter**[Q] (3/4th of total power of eye)
• **Refractive index: 1.376**[Q]

	Corneal diameter		
	Horizontal	**Vertical**	**Radius of curvature**
Anterior surface	**11.7 mm**[Q]	**10.6 mm**[Q]	**7.8 mm**[Q]
Posterior surface	**11.7 mm**[Q]	**11.7 mm**[Q]	**6.5 mm**[Q]

• **Corneal thickness (pachymetry): Central** (thinner) = **0.5-0.6 mm**; **Periphery** (thicker) = **1.2 mm**
• **Microcornea ≤10 mm; Megalocornea >13 mm**

> • **Critical angle is 46° at cornea tear interface**[Q]
> • Healthy cornea is **avascular** & **devoid of lymphatic channels**[Q].
> • Corneal cell derives **nourishment by diffusion from aqueous, capillaries at limbus & oxygen dissolved in tear film**[Q].

Cornea

Layers of Cornea

- Stratified squamous epithelium[Q]
- Bowman's layer (once eroded, it does not regenerate)[Q]
- Substantia propria (stroma-90% thickness of cornea): Contains **uniformly spaced collagen lamellae (mainly type I collagen[Q]) lying parallel[Q] (responsible for corneal transparency[Q])**; keratocytes are present in stroma
- Descemet's membrane: Readily regenerates after injury, very **resistant to chemicals, trauma, infection[Q]**
- Endothelium: Most metabolically active layer, maintains deturgescence of cornea[Q]; endothelial Na^+/K^+ ATPase pump limits fluid entering the cornea from aqueous
  - Dua's layer: Newly discovered 15 micron thick layer of cornea, located **between stroma & Descemet's membrane (pre-Descemet's)[Q]**

- Metabolic active cells are endothelium, epithelium & stromal keratocytes[Q].

Factors Responsible for Corneal Transparency

Anatomical	Physiological (Factors maintaining corneal hydration)
- Avascular[Q]	- Endothelial pump[Q]
- Unmyelinated nerve fibers[Q]	- Barrier function of limiting layers[Q]
- Uniform spacing of collagen fibrils in stroma[Q]	- Stromal swelling pressure[Q]
- Uniform refractive index of all layers[Q]	- Normal IOP[Q]
- Epithelium with high mitotic figures[Q] (ensures rapid wound repair of epithelium & maintain barrier function)	- Evaporation from corneal surface[Q]

Corneal Metabolism	Blood Supply	Nerve Supply
Preferentially aerobic[Q] **Can function anaerobically for 6-7 hours[Q]** O_2 is mostly derived **from tear film[Q]** **Glucose supply mainly (90%) from aqueous[Q]** & supplemented (10%) by limbal capillaries. **Hypoxic corneal stromal edema** results **from osmotic changes** produced by **lactate[Q] accumulation[Q].**	Cornea is **avascular** but the **limbus** is supplied by conjunctival branches of **anterior ciliary arteries[Q]**	Cornea is **richly supplied by nerves[Q] (without myelin sheaths & Schwann cell sheath)**, which originate from **small ophthalmic division of trigeminal nerve,** mainly by **long ciliary nerve[Q].**

Refraction: Important Points

Refractive index of aqueous	1.34[Q]
Refractive index of cornea	1.376[Q]
Refractive index of lens	1.39[Q]
Power of cornea	+43-45 D[Q]
Power of lens	+15-17 D[Q]
Power of eye (Total)	+58-60 D[Q]
Power of eye at birth (eye is hypermetropic)	+2.5 D[Q]

179. Ans. b. 1.5-2.5 kg *(Ref: Animal Models in Eye Research/ p188)*
The usual weight of rabbit used in ophthalmological experiments is between 1.5-2.5 Kg.

Laboratory Animals

Animal	Weight
Rat	180-200 gm
Guinea Pig	400-600 gm
Mouse	20-25 gm
Rabbit	**1.5-2.5 Kg[Q]**
Hamster	80-90 gm

180. **Ans. d. Retinal pigment epithelium** *(Ref: Khurana 6/e p292, 5/e p290; Yanoff and Duker 4/e p607)*
On the basis of clinical features and images of optical coherence tomography and fluorescein angiography, most probable diagnosis is Central serous retinopathy, in which fluid accumulates in the subretinal space and there is detachment of retinal pigment epithelium from the neurosensory retina.

> "**Central Serous Retinopathy:** It is well known, however, that the **subneural retinal fluid originates from choroid**. The leakage of dye through an abnormal focal defect at the level of retinal pigment epithelium (RPE) and its accumulation in the subneural retinal space are seen clearly on fluorescein angiography."- *Yanoff and Duker 4/e p607*

Central Serous Retinopathy

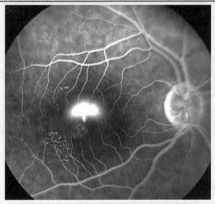
Fig. 38: Fluorescein angiography demonstrates pooling of dye within the subneural retinal space

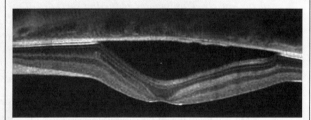
Fig. 39: Optical coherence tomography showing subretinal fluid

Central Serous Retinopathy (CSR)

- Characterized by **spontaneous detachment of neurosensory retina in macular region, with or without retinal pigment epithelium detachment**[Q].
- When the disorder is **active** it is characterized by **leakage of fluid under the retina**[Q] (subretinal space) that has a propensity to accumulate under the central macula.

Etiology:
- **Stress** appears to play an important role
- **Associated with cortisol & corticosteroids**[Q].
  - "There is **extensive evidence** to the effect that **corticosteroids** (e.g. cortisone), commonly used to treat inflammations, allergies, skin conditions and even certain eye conditions, can **trigger central serous retinopathy, aggravate it and cause relapses**."

Clinical features:
- **Typically affects males**[Q] between **20 to 40 years** of age.
- Patients present with a **sudden onset of painless loss of vision** (usually unilateral, in the involved eye).
- It is also **associated with scotoma, micropsia & metamorphopsia**[Q].
- **Other eye** is **usually normal.**

Diagnosis:
- **Fundus-fluorescein angiography** helps in **confirming the diagnosis**. Two patterns are seen:
- **Ink-blot pattern**[Q]: It consists of a small hyperfluorescent spot which gradually increases in size.
- **Smoke-stack pattern**[Q]: It consists of a small hyperflourescent spot which ascends vertically like a smoke stack and gradually spreads laterally to take a mushroom or umbrella configuration.

Treatment:
- **Spontaneous resorption of subretinal fluid within 3-4 months, recovery of visual acuity usually follows**[Q].
- Any ongoing **corticosteroid treatment** should be **tapered and stopped**, where possible[Q].
- **Laser photocoagulation:** In cases where there is **little improvement in a 3-4 months duration** & leakage is confined to a single or a few sources of leakage at a safe distance from fovea[Q].
- **Photodynamic therapy** (PDT) with **verteporfin** has shown promise as an effective treatment with minimal complications.

Cond...

Cond...

Central Serous Retinopathy (CSR)
Prognosis: • **Excellent**   • **Complications**: **Subretinal neovascularization** & **pigment epitheliopathy**.

181. **Ans. b. Internuclear ophthalmoplegia** *(Ref: Yanoff & Ducker 4/e p919; Parson's 22/e p534, 21/e p511)*

In the given image, on attempted lateral gaze, away from the side of lesion, the abducting eye overshoots the target leading to appearance of dissociated nystagmus, which is characteristically seen in internuclear ophthalmoplegia.

*"**Internuclear ophthalmoplegia**: Demonstrating **poor adduction left eye on dextroversion but normal adduction on convergence.**"- Parson's 21/e p511*

Internuclear Ophthalmoplegia: Injury to medial longitudinal fasciculus, between the abducens nucleus and contralateral medial rectus subnucleus of the oculomotor nerve, interrupts transmission of neural impulses to the ipsilateral medial rectus muscle. This impairs adducting saccades of the ipsilateral eye, which become either slow or absent. On attempted lateral gaze, away from the side of lesion, the abducting eye overshoots the target (Dysmetria) leading to appearance of dissociated (disconjugate) nystagmus. If the internuclear ophthalmoplegia is bilateral, abduction saccades also may be slow because of impaired inhibition of resting tone in the medial rectus muscle. Upward beating and torsional nystagmus are frequently present, particularly if both MLFs are affected. A subtle INO may be demonstrated when the patient makes repetitive horizontal saccades, which disclose slow adduction of the ipsilateral eye. Convergence may be preserved."

Internuclear Ophthalmoplegia (INO)

• **INO** is a **disorder of conjugate lateral gaze** in which **affected eye shows impairment of adduction**[Q].
 • When **an attempt is made to gaze contralaterally** (relative to the affected eye), the **affected eye adducts minimally, if at all**. The **contralateral eye abducts, however with nystagmus**[Q].
 • Additionally, **divergence of the eyes leads to horizontal diplopia**.
 • That is, **if the right eye is affected the patient will "see double" when looking to the left, seeing two images side-by-side**[Q].
 • **Convergence is generally preserved.**
      • **INO** is **caused by injury** or **dysfunction in medial longitudinal fasciculus**[Q] **(MLF)**, a heavily-myelinated tract that allows conjugate eye movement by connecting the paramedian pontine reticular formation (PPRF)- abducens nucleus complex of contralateral side to oculomotor nucleus of ipsilateral side.
 • **If the lesion affects the PPRF** (or the abducens nucleus) & **MLF on the same side** (the MLF having crossed from the opposite side), then the **"one and a half syndrome"** occurs which, simply put, **involves paralysis of all conjugate horizontal eye movements other than abduction of eye on the opposite side to the lesion**[Q].
      • A **rostral lesion within the midbrain** may **affect the convergence center** thus causing **bilateral divergence of the eyes,** which is known as the **WEBINO syndrome**[Q] **(Wall Eyed Bilateral INO)** as each eye looks at the opposite "wall".
 • **INO** also may occur with a **variety of disorders that affect the brainstem (vascular, demyelinating & metastatic)** and must be differentiated from the pseudo-INO of myasthenia or a long-standing exotropia.

Duane Retraction Syndrome
• Duane retraction syndrome is a **congenital strabismus syndrome** occurring in **isolated or syndromic forms**.   • It presents with a variety of **clinical features** including **diplopia, anisometropia & amblyopia**[Q].

Types of Duane Retraction Syndrome		
Type1	**Type 2**	**Type 3**
• Comprises **75–80%** of patients • Presents with **anesotropia in primary gaze** with a **compensatory head tilt to the involved side**[Q].	• Comprises **5–10%** of patients • Presents with an **exotropia in primary gaze** with a **compensatory head tilt to the uninvolved side**[Q]	• Comprises **10–20%** of patients • Present with either an **esotropia or exotropia in primary gaze**, & have a **compensatory head tilt to involved side.** • The **ability to adduct** in this type is **absent to restricted** as compared to normal to mildly restricted in types 1 & 2.

AIIMS November 2016

182. Ans. d. Vision 4/60 or less with the best possible spectacle correction in the better eye *(Ref: National Programme for Control of Blindness - http://npcb.nic.in/index1.asp?linkid=55)*

Vision 4/60 or less with the best possible spectacle correction in the better eye is not included in the NPCB definition of blindness.

National Programme for Control of Blindness (NPCB) Definition of Blindness
• **Inability of a person to count fingers from a distance of 6 meters or 20 feet**[Q] (technical definition).
• **Vision 6/60 or less with the best possible spectacle correction**[Q].
• **Diminution of field vision to 20 feet or less in better eye**[Q].

According to WHO, (Vision 2020)
• **'Low vision'** is defined as **visual acuity of less than 6/18 but equal to or better than 3/60**, or a **corresponding visual field loss to less than 20°**, in the **better eye with the best possible correction**[Q].
• **'Blindness'** is defined as **visual acuity of less than 3/60**, or a **corresponding visual field loss to less than 10°, in the better eye with the best possible correction**[Q].
• **'Visual impairment'** includes both **low vision & blindness**[Q].

Types of Blindness	
Economic blindness	• **Inability of a person to count fingers** from a **distance of 6 meters or 20 feet** technical definition.
Social blindness	• **Vision 3/60** or **diminution** of field of vision **to 10°**
Manifest blindness	• Vision 1/60 to just perception of light.
Absolute blindness	• No perception of light
Curable blindness	• That stage of blindness where the **damage is reversible** by prompt management, e.g. cataract.
Preventable blindness	• Blindness that could have been **completely prevented** by institution of effective preventive or prophylactic measures, e.g. xerophthalmia, trachoma and glaucoma.
Avoidable blindness	• Sum total of **preventable and curable blindness**

ENT

183. Ans. c. Cricothyroidotomy *(Ref: Scott-Brown's 7/e p476; Bailey 27/e p749, 26/e p695)*

The given image is of cricothyroidotomy, a life-saving procedure performed in extreme circumstances intended to be a temporizing measure until a definitive airway can be established.

*"**Cricothyroidotomy:** The patient's neck is extended and the area between the prominence of the thyroid cartilage and the cricoid cartilage below is palpated with the index finger of the free hand. **In the emergency situation, a vertical skin incision is recommended with dissection rapidly carried down to the cricothyroid membrane. A 1-cm transverse incision is made through the membrane immediately above the cricoid cartilage and the scalpel twisted through a right angle to gain access to the airway.** If available, artery forceps, dilator or tracheal hook will improve the aperture and insertion of an available tube. "- Bailey 26/e p695*

Cricothyrotomy (Cricothyroidotomy, Inferior laryngotomy)
• **Cricothyrotomy** is an **incision made through the skin & cricothyroid membrane**
• **Establish a patent airway** during certain **life-threatening situations** (airway obstruction by a **foreign body, angioedema, or massive facial trauma**) or the conditions in which **orotracheal & nasotracheal intubation** are **contraindicated**[Q].
• Cricothyrotomy is **easier & quicker to perform than tracheotomy**
• **Does not require manipulation of cervical spine** & associated with fewer complications.

Contd...

Cricothyrotomy	
Indications	**Contraindications**
• Inability to intubate or ventilate[Q] • Trauma causing oral, pharyngeal, or nasal hemorrhage[Q] • Facial muscle spasms or laryngospasm[Q] • Uncontrollable emesis[Q] • Upper airway stenosis or congenital deformities[Q] • Foreign body obstruction[Q] • Clenched teeth[Q] • Tumor or trauma causing mass effect • Oropharyngeal edema (anaphylaxis)	• Inability to identify landmarks (cricothyroid membrane) • Underlying anatomical abnormality (tumor) • Tracheal transection • Acute laryngeal disease due to infection or trauma • Children <10 years of age

184. Ans. b. >81 dB *(Ref: http://www.who.int/pbd/deafness/hearing_impairment_grades/en/)*

According to the WHO (2008) definition of hearing loss, hearing threshold in better ear >81 dB is classified as profound hearing loss.

WHO (2008) Classification of Degree of Hearing Loss	
• **Hearing threshold in better ear** (average of 500, 1000, 2000 Hz)	• Grade of Impairment
• 0-25	• No impairment
• 26-40	• **Mild**[Q] impairment
• 41-60	• **Moderate**[Q] impairment
• 61-80	• **Severe**[Q] impairment
• >81	• **Profound**[Q] impairment including deafness

SKIN

185. Ans. d. 4 weeks *(Ref: Fitzpatrick 6/e p2302, 7/e p490-493, 1873-1898; Rooks 8/e p33.14-33.22; Roxburgh 18/e p52-54)*

PHN has been defined as pain after the rash has healed or pain 1 month or 3 months after rash onset. So best answer would be 4 weeks.

"Herpes zoster may be attended by a variety of neurologic complications, of which post-herpetic neuralgia (PHN) is the most common and important. PHN has been defined as pain after the rash has healed or pain 1 month or 3 months after rash onset. In clinic and community studies using the first two definitions, the overall incidence of PHN is 8 to 15 percent. Age is the most significant risk factor for PHN. In a recent study, patients aged 50 years or older had a 14.7-fold higher prevalence of pain 30 days after rash onset than patients younger than 50 years of age. Other risk factors for PHN include the presence of prodromal pain, severe pain during the acute phase of herpes zoster, greater rash severity, more extensive sensory abnormalities in the affected dermatome and, possibly, ophthalmic (as opposed to thoracic or abdominal) herpes zoster." - Fitzpatrick 6/e p2302

Post-Herpetic Neuralgia (PHN)	
• **PHN is MC & important neurologic complication of Herpes zoster**[Q] • PHN has been defined as **pain after the rash has healed or pain 1 month** or **3 months after rash onset**[Q].	
Risk Factors for Post-Herpetic Neuralgia	
• **Age: Most significant risk factor;** seen in patients ≥ 50 years[Q] • Presence of **prodromal pain** • **Severe pain during acute phase** of herpes zoster	• **Greater rash severity**, more extensive sensory abnormalities in affected dermatome • **Ophthalmic** (as opposed to thoracic or abdominal) **herpes zoster**[Q].

Clinical Features:
• **Risk of long-lasting PHN increases with increasing age**.
  - **Constant pain** (described as **"burning, aching, throbbing"**), intermittent pain (**"stabbing, shooting"**), and/or stimulus-evoked pain, including **allodynia ("tender, burning, stabbing")**[Q].
  - **Allodynia** (experience of pain elicited by stimuli that are normally not painful) is a **particularly disabling component** of the disease[Q].

Contd...

Contd...

Post-Herpetic Neuralgia (PHN)
• These subtypes of pain may produce **disordered sleep, depression, anorexia, weight loss, chronic fatigue, & social isolation**[Q].
Treatment: • **First-line treatment: Tricyclic antidepressants (amitriptyline**[Q]**), gabapentin**[Q] **& pregabalin**[Q] **& topical lidocaine 5% patch**[Q]. • **Opioids, tramadol, capsaicin cream**[Q] **& capsaicin 8% patch**[Q] are recommended as either 2nd or 3rd line therapies in different guidelines.

Herpes Zoster
• Caused by reactivation of **Varicella Zoster (chicken pox) virus**[Q] lying latent in **posterior root ganglion of a spinal nerve; one attack gives life long immunity**[Q] • **Thoracic nerves (intercostal nerves)**[Q], **ophthalmic division of trigeminal nerve** & other **spinal nerves** are **most commonly affected**[Q]
Pathology: • **Ballooning** is **characteristic**[Q] • **Tzanck smear: Multinucleated giant cells**[Q]

Clinical Features:
• Prodrome of segmental **pain** begins **1-4 days before the eruption**[Q], erythema & edema is rapidly followed by appearance of **grouped vesicles unilateral & in a segmental distribution (MC thoracic dermatome)**[Q], mucous membrane within the affected dermatome may be involved
• **Unilateral vesicular eruption within a dermatome** associated with **severe pain**[Q]
 	
      • **MC involved dermatome: T3 to L3**[Q]
      • **HIV positive patients are 2o times more likely to develop herpes zoster**[Q]

Complications: • **Post-herpetic neuralgia**[Q] (persistent neuralgic pain): **MC after involvement of trigeminal region**[Q], **treated by capsaicin patch, oral amitriptyline, gabapentin or duloxetine**[Q]. • **Corneal ulcer & scarring** (zoster of ophthalmic division of trigeminal nerve), eye involvement is indicated when **vesicles are present on the side of nose- Hutchinson's sign**[Q]

Variants of Herpes Zoster	
Ramsay Hunt Syndrome (Herpes zoster oticus)	**Herpes Zoster Ophthalmicus**
• H. zoster involving **geniculate ganglion of sensory branch** of **facial nerve**[Q]	• H. zoster involving **ophthalmic division of trigeminal nerve**[Q]

186. Ans. d. Trichotillomania *(Ref: Rooks 8/e p55.4, Fitzpatrick 6/e p735)*

Patchy hair loss in the right temporal and occipital region in A 24-years-old female non- scarring alopecia with multiple small broken hairs and mild (sparsity) of a perifollicular inflammatory infiltrate is highly suggestive of trichotillomania. See Q. No. 189 AIIMS May 2017

187. Ans. b. Pemphigus vulgaris *(Ref: Harrison 19/e p370, 18/e p426-428; Fitzpatrick 7/e p432-441; Rooks 8/e p40.27, 13.19, 10.12-10.28)*

On immunofluorescence, suprabasal split and intercellular IgG deposits with fish net appearance in the given image is suggestive of pemphigus vulgaris.

Immunologically Mediated Blistering Disease				
Disease	**Pemphigus vulgaris**	**Bullous pemphigoid**	**Linear IgA disease**	**Dermatitis herpetiformis**
Auto antigen	**Desmoglein 3**[Q]	BP230 > BP180	BPAG 2	Epidermal & tissue transglutaminase

Contd...

Contd...

Disease	Pemphigus vulgaris	Bullous pemphigoid	Linear IgA disease	Dermatitis herpetiformis
Histology	Epidermal **Acantholytic** blister in **suprabasal spinous cell layer**	**Subepidermal** blister with **eosinophil rich infiltrate**[Q] in perivascular & vesicular sites.	**Subepidermal** blister with **neutrophils in dermal papillae**[Q]	**Subepidermal** blister with **neutrophils in Dermal papillae**[Q]
Direct Immuno-fluorescence Microscopy	Cells surface **deposits of IgG on keratinocytes in fishnet pattern**	**Linear band of IgG** and/or **C3 in epidermal BMZ**	**Linear band of IgA, in epidermal BMZ**	**Granular deposits of IgA in dermal papillae**[Q]
Associations	HLA- DR4 **& DRW6**[Q]	HLA-DQ β1 * 0301	- HLA-B8 (+) - TNF2 allele	**Subclinical gluten sensitive enteropathy (100%)** HLA-B8 (60%) / DRW3 (95%) & HLA-DQW2 haplotype (95-100%)
Clinical features	**Flaccid blisters, denuded skin, oro-mucosal lesions**[Q]	**Large tense blisters on flexor surfaces & trunk**[Q]	Pruritic small papules on extensor surfaces occasionally larger, acneiform blisters in adults	**Extremely pruritic small vesicles on elbows, knees, buttocks & posterior neck**[Q]

See Q. No. 185 AIIMS May 2017

188. Ans. c. HPV 6 and 11 *(Ref: Harrison 19/e p1198, 351)*

The given image is of anogenital warts on penis. Anogenital warts are caused by HPV 6 and 11.

> *"Genital warts are caused primarily by HPV-6 or HPV-11; their surface is either smooth or rough. Penile genital warts are usually 2–5 mm in diameter and often occur in groups. A second type of penile lesion, keratotic plaques, is slightly raised above the normal epithelium and has a rough, often pigmented surface. Vulvar warts are soft, whitish papules that either are sessile or have multiple fine, finger-like projections."- Harrison 19/e p1198*

Type of Wart	HPV Type
Verruca vulgaris	**2, 4, 27**[Q]
Palmoplantar warts	**1, 2, 4**[Q]
Myrmecia wart	**1**[Q]
Verruca plana	**3, 10**[Q]
Epidermodysplasia verruciformis	**3, 5, 8, 9**[Q]
Anogenital warts	**6, 11**[Q] (low oncogenic potential) **16, 18, 31, 33**[Q] (high oncogenic potential)
Butchers wart	**7**[Q]
Mosaic wart	**2**[Q]

Genital Warts
• **Wars are MC virus induced tumors, caused by HPV**[Q] • **Genital warts** are **contagious HPV related lesion**, transmitted by skin to skin contact during oral, genital or anal sex. • Most commonly affects **young males**
Etiology: • **MC sites: Glans, foreskin, meatus & shaft**[Q] • **Caused by HPV type: 6, 11**[Q] (low oncogenic potential); **16, 18, 31, 33**[Q] (high oncogenic potential)
Gross appearance: • **Papillary, fungating, wart-like**, often multiple lesions & 1 mm or larger. • Cut surface of a condyloma has **tiny finger like projections**[Q].

Contd...

Contd...

Microscopy:
• **Arborescent spiky papillae** with **prominent central fibrovascular cores**^{Q}.
• **Acanthotic & hyperkeratotic epidermis with pappilomatosis & parakeratosis**^{Q}
 	
      • **Koilocytes**^{Q} (epidermal cells with **hyperchromatic irregular nuclei** with **perinuclear halo**): **Characteristic of HPV papilloma**^{Q}
      • **Perinuclear vacuolization**^{Q}

Treatment: • **Podophyllin**^{Q} **(15%)** or **podophyllotoxin**^{Q} **(0.5%)** • **Imiquimod**^{Q}, **5-fluorouracil & Cryotherapy**^{Q}
Quadrivalent Vaccine (Gardasil) • The quadrivalent vaccine is approved for: • Vaccination of **girls & women 9–26 years of age** to **prevent genital warts & cervical cancer** caused by **HPV 6, 11, 16 & 18**^{Q} • Vaccination of the same population **to prevent precancerous or dysplastic lesions**, including cervical adenocarcinoma in situ, CIN 2/3, VIN 2/3, VaIN 2/3 & CIN 1 • Vaccination of **boys & men 9–26 years** of age to prevent genital warts caused by **HPV 6 & 11** • Vaccination of individuals **9–26 years of age** to **prevent anal cancer & associated precancerous lesions** due to HPV 6, 11, 16 & 18.

189. **Ans. d. Lupus vulgaris** *(Ref: Harrison 19/e p367; Rooks 8/e p31.11, Fitzpatrick 6/e p2152)*

Annular plaque with central scarring is typically seen in Lupus vulgaris. In the western countries, Lupus vulgaris rarely occurs on the buttocks but most common sites in India are buttocks and face. Although Tinea cruris is far more common annular plaque-like lesion seen on buttocks, central scarring is never seen in these lesions.

"Lupus vulgaris originates from an underlying focus of TB, typically in a bone, joint or lymph node, and arises by either contiguous extension of the disease from underlying affected tissue or by hematogenous or lymphatic spread. It can also arise after exogenous inoculation or as a complication of BCG vaccination. In west, over 80% of lesions are on the head and neck, particularly around the nose. Next in frequency are the arms and legs, but involvement of the trunk is uncommon. In India, cutaneous TB more commonly affects the buttocks and extremities rather than the face. Such a pattern is usually due to reinoculation and may relate to playing without clothing or shoes."

"Lesions may become flat plaques with a serpiginous or polycyclic outline and a smooth surface or psoriasiform scaling; there may be erosions, ulceration, and scarring. Hypertrophic forms appear as a soft mass with a nodular, hyperkeratotic surface."- Fitzpatrick 6/e p21520

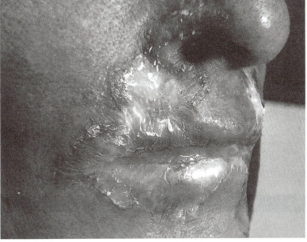

Fig. 40: Lupus Vulgaris

Lupus Vulgaris
• Lupus vulgaris is an extremely **chronic & progressive form of skin TB**
• Occurs in individuals with **moderate immunity & high degree of tuberculin sensitivity**[Q].
• More common in **females**

Pathogenesis:

• It originates by **hematogenous, lymphatic, or contiguous spread from tuberculosis elsewhere in body**, most often from **cervical adenitis or pulmonary TB**[Q].

Clinical Features:

• **Painful cutaneous skin lesions with nodular appearance**, most often on face around nose, eyelids, lips, cheeks, ears & neck[Q].

• A single or several, unilateral, **well-defined** reddish-brown papules/ **annular plaques**[Q] first appear on the face, neck or arms, coalescing into erythematous plaques.

> • **Surface of papules exfoliates & centers scar**[Q]. **Center is depigmented with paper-thin scar with nodules**[Q].
> • **On diascopy: Typical apple-jelly nodules**[Q] (Highly **characteristic lesion** of Lupus vulgaris)

• Papules recur on the scarred areas, gradually and repeatedly enlarging and coalescing. This leads to the formation of large, firm, elevated plaques. At the periphery are **small reddish-yellow or brown nodules**[Q].

> • **In west, over 80% of lesions are on head & neck, particularly around the nose**[Q]. Next in frequency are the arms and legs, but involvement of the trunk is uncommon.
> • **In India, cutaneous TB more commonly affects buttocks & extremities rather than the face**[Q]. Such a pattern is usually due to reinoculation and may relate to playing without clothing or shoes.

Diagnosis:

• **Histologic examination** & a **positive culture for M. tuberculosis/bovis confirm the diagnosis**[Q].
• **Most prominent histopathologic feature: Formation of typical tubercles**[Q]

Complication:

• **Secondary scarring & squamous cell carcinomas** can develop within the plaques[Q].

Cutaneous Tuberculosis	
Lupus vulgaris	• **Painful cutaneous TB seen** in individuals with **moderate immunity & high degree of tuberculin sensitivity**[Q]. • It originates by **hematogenous, lymphatic, or contiguous spread from tuberculosis elsewhere in body**, most often from **cervical adenitis or pulmonary TB**[Q].
Scrofuloderma	• Scrofuloderma is a **subcutaneous TB leading to cold abscess formation** & a **secondary breakdown of overlying skin**[Q]. • Results from **contiguous involvement of skin overlying another tuberculous process**, most commonly **tuberculous lymphadenitis, TB of bones** and joints, or **tuberculous epididymitis**[Q].
Tuberculosis verrucosa cutis	• Caused by **accidental inoculation** of TB bacilli **in previously sensitized individuals with high immunity**[Q]
Tuberculosis cutis orificialis	• **Cutaneous TB involving skin & mucosa**[Q] • **Oral mucosa** in pulmonary TB, **anal region** in GI TB & **urogenital mucosa** in renal TB[Q]
Lichen scrofulosorum	• **Lichen scrofulosorum** is usually **associated with chronic tuberculous disease of LNs & bones** or **with specific pleurisy**[Q] • It has been observed **after BCG vaccination** & in association with **M. avium-intracellulare infections**[Q].

ANESTHESIA

190. Ans. c. Leak from expiratory valve *(Ref: Miller 7/e p1427; Hemodynamic Monitoring: Evolving Technologies and Clinical Practice By Mary E. Lough/p240)*

The biphasic pattern of capnograph is usually seen in cases of leak from the expiratory valve, which adds to the CO_2 output. It is more likely in a chronic smoker with emphysema because of hyper expanded lung.

"A biphasic capnogram is seen in a patient that has had single lung transplantation. The initial peak in the waveform represents the transplanted, the healthy lung, which has normal compliance and ventilation/perfusion (V/Q) ratio. The delayed, second peak of the waveform represents the native, diseased lung, which has poor compliance and significantly greater V/Q mismatch. The native lung takes longer to expel CO_2 and mimics a capnogram from a patient with COPD. The differing capnograms produced by each lung produces a dual peak capnogram. A similar capnogram may be seen when a partial disconnection or leak occurs within apparatus."-*Hemodynamic Monitoring: Evolving Technologies and Clinical Practice By Mary E. Lough/p240*

Capnography

• **Capnography** is the **continuous measurement** of **end tidal carbon dioxide** ($ETCO_2$) and its waveform.
• **Normal: 32 to 42 mmHg** (3 to 4 mmHg less than arterial pCO_2 which is 35 to 45 mmHg)
• **Principle**: Infrared light is **absorbed by carbon dioxide**
    • **Alpha angle**: Angle between phases II & III (normally **100-110°**)
    • **Beta angle**: Angle between **end of phase III** & descending limb of capnogram (normally **90°**)

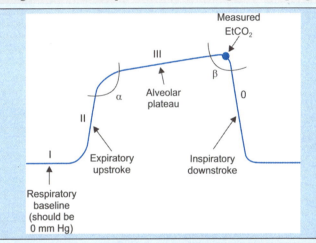

Phases of Capnography			
Phase I (Inspiratory baseline)	**Phase II** (Expiratory upstroke)	**Phase III** (Alveolar plateau)	**Phase 0** (Inspiratory downstroke)
• It represents beginning of expiration. • Capnograph register zero.	• **Sharply rising** expiratory upstroke front • Represents **mixing of dead space with alveolar gas**	• **End expiratory slowly rising** plateau representing mostly alveolar gas exhalation. • PCO_2 value at the end of exhalation is referred to as end tidal PCO_2 ($P_{ET}CO_2$)	• **Inspiratory phase** • It is a **sharp downward return** of traces towards zero at the onset of inspiration

Causes of decreased $ETCO_2$	No Change of $ETCO_2$	Causes of increased $ETCO_2$
• **Pulmonary embolism** by air, fat or thrombus • It may become **zero** if embolus is large enough to block total pulmonary circulation	• **Bronchospasm**: CO_2 has got very high diffusibility therefore $ETCO_2$ remains normal even in severe bronchospasm	• **Exhausted sodalime** or **defective valves of closed circuit**, which impairs the absorption CO_2 of by sodalime. • **Increased production** in hypermetabolic states like fever, malignant hyperthermia ($ETCO_2$ may even rise to >100 mm Hg), thyrotoxicosis, neuroleptic malignant syndrome.

Capnography

Uses of Capnography

- It is the **surest confirmatory sign of correct intubation**[Q] (**esophageal intubation** will yield $ETCO_2 = 0$)
- **Intraoperative displacement of endotracheal tube**[Q] ($ETCO_2$ will become **zero**)
- **Diagnosis of malignant hyperthermia**[Q] ($ETCO_2$ may rise to **>100 mm Hg**)
- For **detecting obstructions** and **disconnections of endotracheal tubes** ($ETCO_2$ **will fall**)
- **Diagnosing pulmonary embolism** by air, fat or thrombus (**sudden fall of $ETCO_2$** occurs. It may become zero if embolus is large enough to block total pulmonary circulation)
- **Exhausted sodalime or defective valves** of closed circuit will show high $ETCO_2$ values.
- **To control level of hypocapnia during hyperventilation in neurosurgery**[Q].
- **Indicator of cardiac output. In cardiac arrest $ETCO_2$ is zero**[Q].

Deviations from Normal Capnogram

Type of Deviation	Features	Capnograph
Curare Notch/Cleft	• Patient on **controlled ventilation showing some spontaneous respiration activities** during respiratory cycle of controlled ventilation. • It is usually present in the **later third part of capnogram**. • It indicated that the **muscle relaxant is wearing off**.	
Biphasic capnogram (Two peaks)	**Causes:** • **Unilateral hypoventilation or unilateral high airway pressure** • **Single lung transplantation**[Q] • **Endobronchial intubation**[Q] • **Severe Kyphoscoliosis**[Q] • **Air-leak**[Q] (**Loose connection** between sampling tube & capnograph / **broken connection** or **filter**)	
Capnogram not touching the baseline	**Causes:** • **Breathing of expired CO_2**[Q] • **Exhausted CO_2 absorber**[Q] • Malfunctioning expiratory valve • Extremely low flow of fresh gas	
Capnogram with increased alpha angle	**Causes:** • **Mechanical airway obstruction: Kinking**, blockade by **secretions or foreign body**[Q] • **Pathological airway obstruction: Bronchial asthma, COPD**[Q]	
Capnogram with increased beta angle	**Causes:** • **Rebreathing**[Q] • **Inefficient respiratory valve**[Q]	

191. **Ans. d. After insertion of laryngoscope, it is levered on the upper incisor to pull up the tongue and visualize the vocal cords** *(Ref: Miller 8/e p1666-1667, 7/e p1587)*

The laryngoscope should never be hinged on the teeth to lift up the epiglottis. The patient is aligned in a "sniffing" position, i.e. neck (atlanto-axial joint) flexion and face extension (atlanto-occipital joint), at around 35° and 15° respectively.

Laryngoscope
• **Laryngoscope** is an instrument **used to visualize the larynx & surrounding structures** either **by displacing the soft tissue away from the line of vision or by optical aids**[Q].
• The **main purpose** of a laryngoscope is **to aid the intubation**[Q].
• **Laryngoscopes**, by bringing the esophagus and larynx under view, are helpful in passing the nasogastric tube, oral suctioning, throat packing and removing oral foreign body[Q].

Laryngoscope Blades:
- **Commonly used straight blade: Magill Blade**[Q] **(used in infants)**
- **Commonly used curved blade: Macintosh blade**[Q]

Head & Neck Position for Laryngoscopy:
- **Extension at atlanto-occipital joint & flexion at cervical spine**[Q]

> • Teeth most vulnerable to damage during laryngoscopy: Upper incisor[Q]

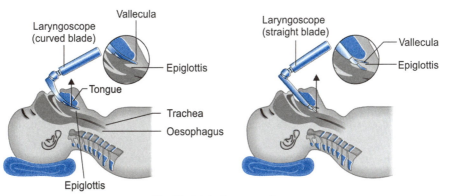

Fig. 41: Intubation procedure

Procedure of Intubation

- **Direct laryngoscopy** is used **to facilitate tracheal intubation under vision.**
- During intubation, there should be **extension at atlanto-occipital joint & flexion** at **cervical spine**[Q] **(Sniffing the morning air position)**
- Patients **mouth** should be **fully opened with index finger & thumb of right hand** in a **scissor action**
- **Laryngoscope** should be **held in the left hand (by both right and left handed people) & blade** should be **introduced along the right side** of the patient's mouth **displacing the tongue to the left.**
- The direct **laryngoscope** is used to **displace the tongue & epiglottis out of the line of sight.**

> - **Tongue is displaced horizontally** (normally to the left) from the line of sight, **hyoid bone & attached tissues** are **moved anteriorly & epiglottis is elevated directly** or indirectly to reveal the larynx.
> - **Force applied to laryngoscope handle** should **lift the hyoid bone & attached tissues parallel to the line of sight. The laryngoscope should never be hinged on teeth.**
> - **Adequate lifting force**, which may **cause considerable tissue distortion**, is a **key factor in successful direct laryngoscopy.**

- It is important to achieve the best possible view of the larynx without causing tissue trauma.
- **Hold tube with right hand** & remove laryngoscope & stylet.
- Inflate cuff with 5-10 mL of air & ventilate with bag. Assess tube position: Auscultation of chest and epigastrium, capnometry; Stabilize the tube & confirm placement by chest X-ray.

996 AIIMS ESSENCE

192. Ans. d. 30:2 *(Ref: AHA 2015 CPR Guidelines "http://eccguidelines.heart.org/ wp-content/uploads/2015/10/2015-AHA-Guidelines-Highlights-English.pdf")*

Ratio of chest compressions to rescue breath in all adults, weather there are 1 or 2 rescuers, is 30:2.

Cardiopulmonary Resuscitation (AHA 2015 Guidelines)
• **"CAB"[Q]** is followed (**not ABC**): **Circulation, Airway, Breathing**[Q] (**Immediately start chest compressions rather than airway opening**[Q]).
• To allow **full chest wall recoil** after each compression, **rescuer must avoid leaning on the chest** between compressions[Q].
• **Rescuer should not interrupt compressions for >10 seconds**[Q].   • For patients with **ongoing CPR and an advanced airway in place**, a simplified **ventilation rate of 1 breath every 6 seconds**[Q] (**10 breaths per minute**[Q]) is recommended.
• **Routine use of impedance threshold device** (ITD) as an adjunct to conventional CPR is **not recommended**[Q].
• In **ACLS** (Advanced Cardiac Life Support), **vasopressin does not offer an advantage over the use of epinephrine alone**[Q]. Therefore, **vasopressin has been removed from the Adult Cardiac Arrest Algorithm-2015 Update. In 2010 update, atropine was removed**[Q] (earlier vasopressin was recommended as an alternative to epinephrine).
• **Low end-tidal carbon dioxide** (ETCO$_2$) in intubated patients **after 20 minutes of CPR** is associated with a **very low likelihood of resuscitation**[Q].
• **Emergency coronary angiography** is recommended for **all patients with ST elevation** and for **hemodynamically or electrically unstable patients without ST elevation** for whom a **cardiovascular lesion is suspected**[Q].
• During **adult CPR tidal volume of 600 ml (6-7 ml/kg)** should be **adequate to cause the chest to rise**[Q].
• During airway management in an **unconscious trauma patient with possible cervical injury, neck hyperextension** should be **avoided**.
• The **most widely used waveform** in the automated electrical defibrillators (AEDs) now is the **biphasic truncated exponential (BTE) waveform**.
• The following **drugs** may be **given through the endotracheal tube during CPR**: **L**ignocaine[Q], **E**pinephrine[Q], **V**asopressin[Q], **A**tropine[Q], **N**aloxone[Q] (**LEVAN**); (Amiodarone & sodium bicarbonate are not given endotracheally[Q])   • **Atropine is not recommended for routine use** in the management of **Pulseless Electrical Activity/asystole** and has been **removed from the ACLS Cardiac Arrest Algorithm**[Q] (Epinephrine, vasopressin & amiodarone are used[Q])

	Adult (>12 years)	Child (1-12 years)	Infant (<1 year)
Compression Depth	At least **2 inches**[Q] (5 cm, but not >2.4 inches/6 cm[Q])	About **2 inches**[Q] (5 cm; 1/3rd of chest depth[Q])	About **1.5 inches**[Q] (4 cm; 1/3rd of chest depth[Q])
Compression: Ventilation ratio	**30:2**[Q] (one or two rescuer CPR)	30:2[Q] (single rescuer) or 15:2[Q] (two rescuer)	
Compression rate	100-120/min[Q]		

193. Ans. b. Diffusion hypoxia *(Ref: Goodman Gillman 12/e p546, Miller 8/e p656, 3401)*

On discontinuation of N$_2$O administration, nitrous oxide gas can diffuse from blood to the alveoli, diluting O$_2$ in the lung. This can produce an effect called diffusional hypoxia. To avoid hypoxia, 100% O$_2$ rather than air should be administered when N$_2$O is discontinued.

"The rapid uptake of N$_2$O from alveolar gas serves to concentrate co-administered halogenated anesthetics; this effect (the "second gas effect") speeds induction of anesthesia. On discontinuation of N$_2$O administration, nitrous oxide gas can diffuse from blood to the alveoli, diluting O$_2$ in the lung. This can produce an effect called diffusional hypoxia. To avoid hypoxia, 100% O$_2$ rather than air should be administered when N$_2$O is discontinued."- Goodman Gillman 12/e p546

Nitrous Oxide (Dinitrogen monoxide/N_2O)

- N_2O is a **colorless, odorless gas** at room temperature, **heavier than air**[Q]
- **First prepared** by **Joseph Priestley** in **1774**[Q]
- **Neither flammable nor explosive**, but **supports combustion** as actively as oxygen does when it is **present in proper concentration with a flammable anesthetic or material**[Q].
- Also called **laughing gas, MAC is 105% (least potent)**[Q]
- **Can cause bone marrow depression & B_{12} deficiency**[Q]

Entonox

- **Entonox is mixture of 50% N_2O & 50% O_2**[Q]
- **Used for labour analgesia**[Q], painful dressing & changing thoracotomy drains

Anesthetic Properties:

- N_2O is **very insoluble in blood & other tissues** resulting in **rapid equilibration between delivered & alveolar anesthetic concentrations** & provides for **rapid induction & rapid emergence**[Q].

Second Gas Effect	Diffusion Hypoxia (Fink effect)	Poynting Effect
Rapid uptake of N_2O from alveolar gas concentrate co-administered halogenated anesthetics; this effect ("second gas effect") speeds induction of anesthesia[Q].	On discontinuation of N_2O, **N_2O gas can diffuse from blood to the alveoli, diluting O_2 in the lung** leading to diffusional hypoxia[Q]. **To avoid hypoxia, 100% O_2 rather than air should be administered when N_2O is discontinued**[Q].	Certain **mixture of N_2O & O_2** will remain in the gaseous phase at pressures & temperatures at which, **N_2O** by itself would **normally be liquid**[Q].

- N_2O is almost completely eliminated by the lungs (minimal diffusion through the skin), **99.9% of absorbed nitrous oxide is eliminated unchanged**[Q].

- N_2O can **oxidize the cobalt I (Co^+) form of vitamin B_{12} to Co^{3+}, preventing vitamin B_{12} from acting as a co-factor for methionine synthetase**[Q].
- **Methionine synthetase** is important in the **synthesis of DNA, RNA & myelin**[Q].
- **Methionine synthetase activity** is dramatically **reduced** after 24 hours of N_2O exposure
- **Inactivation of methionine synthetase** can produce **signs of vitamin B_{12} deficiency**, including **megaloblastic anemia & peripheral neuropathy** especially in patients with **malnutrition, vitamin B_{12} deficiency, or alcoholism**[Q].
- N_2O: Only anesthetic agent reported to have **hematological & neurotoxicity**[Q]
- N_2O is **not used as a chronic analgesic** or as a **sedative in critical care settings**[Q].

Clinical Use:

- **Weak anesthetic agent, poor muscle relaxant activity** with **significant analgesic effects with** significant sedation (in doses approaching 70-80%)
- Frequently used in **conc. of ~50%** to provide **analgesia & mild sedation** in outpatient dentistry.
- **Reduces requirement for inhalational anesthetics**, allowing for lower concentrations of halogenated anesthetics

- **N_2O exchange with N_2 in any air-containing cavity in the body.** Because of differential blood:gas partition coefficients, **nitrous oxide enters the cavity faster than nitrogen escapes, increasing** the **volume** and/or **pressure** in the **cavity**[Q].
- **Air collections (pneumothorax**[Q], **obstructed middle ear**[Q], **air embolus**[Q], **obstructed loop**[Q] of bowel, **intraocular air bubble**[Q], **pulmonary bulla**[Q] & **intracranial air**[Q]) can be **expanded by N_2O, so N_2O should be avoided in these conditions**[Q].

Nitrous Oxide (Dinitrogen monoxide/N_2O)	
Systemic Effects of Nitrous Oxide	
CVS	• **Negative inotropic effect on heart muscle** *in vitro*, but depressant effects on cardiac function are not observed in patients because of stimulatory effects of on the sympathetic nervous system. • When N_2O is **co-administered with halogenated inhalational anesthetics**, it produces an **increase in HR, BP & cardiac output.** • When N_2O is **co-administered with an opioid**, it **decreases BP & cardiac output.** • **Increases venous tone** in peripheral & pulmonary vasculature (**not used in** patients with **pre-existing pulmonary hypertension** because the **effects on pulmonary vascular resistance can be exaggerated**[Q])
Respiratory System	• **Increases RR & decreases tidal volume** (minute ventilation is not significantly changed & $PaCO_2$ remains normal) • **Markedly depress the ventilatory response to hypoxia**[Q]
CNS	• **Increase cerebral blood flow & ICP**[Q] • **Cerebral vasodilatory capacity** is significantly **attenuated by** the simultaneous administration of **opiates & propofol.** • **Combination with inhaled agents results in greater vasodilation**[Q]
Muscle	• **Does not relax skeletal muscle** • **Does not enhance** the effects of **neuromuscular blocking drugs.** • **Does not trigger malignant hyperthermia**
Kidney, Liver & GIT	• Neither nephrotoxic nor hepatotoxic.

Contraindications of N_2O
• **Air collections (pneumothorax**[Q], **obstructed middle ear**[Q], **tympanoplasty**[Q], **air embolus**[Q], **obstructed loop**[Q] of bowel, **intraocular air bubble**[Q], **pulmonary bulla**[Q] & **intracranial air**[Q]) can be **expanded by N_2O**   • **Microlaryngeal surgeries**[Q] (Cuff pressure may increase & aggravate laryngeal edema)   • **Vitreoretinal surgery**[Q]: Intravitreal air bubble is injected to tamponade the retina against globe. **Sulphur hexafluoride or perfluoropropane**[Q] are used to prolong the resorption of intravitreal air bubbles. **N_2O can diffuse & cause bubble expansion.**   • **Laparoscopic & posterior fossa surgeries**[Q]: Air embolism can occur

194. Ans. d. Penetration into the subarachnoid space *(Ref: Miller 7/e p1895; Barash 5/e p1478, 2405)*

Penetration of drug into the subarachnoid space shortly causes cardiovascular symptoms like hypotension. Systemic absorption of drugs causes neurological symptoms before hypotension. Vasovagal shock occurs immediately, i.e. even before the needle for epidural anesthesia is injected.

> *"**High or total spinal anesthesia is a rare complication of intrathecal injection that occurs after excessive cephalad spread of local anesthetic in the subarachnoid space.** Unintentional intrathecal administration of epidural medication as a result of dural puncture or catheter migration may also result in this complication. Left uterine displacement, placement in the Trendelenburg position, and **continued fluid and vasopressor administration may be necessary to achieve hemodynamic stability. Rapid control of the airway is essential, and endotracheal intubation may be necessary to ensure oxygenation without aspiration."- Barash 5/e p2405*

Total Spinal Anesthesia
• **Sensory block that rises above the cervical region** leads to total spinal anesthesia[Q]   • Total spinal anesthesia occurs when **local anesthetic spreads high enough to block the entire spinal cord** & **occasionally the brainstem** during either **spinal or epidural anesthesia**[Q].

Contd...

AIIMS November 2016

Contd...

Total Spinal Anesthesia
Causes:
• **Intrathecal injection after excessive cephalad spread of local anesthetic in subarachnoid space**[Q].
• **Unintentional intrathecal administration** of **epidural medication** as a result of **dural puncture or catheter migration** may also result in this complication[Q].
Clinical Features:
• **It manifest as bradycardia, profound hypotension, dyspnea, inability to speak & cough, difficulty in swallowing & loss of consciousness**[Q]
• **Respiratory arrest** may occur as a result of **respiratory muscle paralysis** or **dysfunction of brainstem respiratory control centers**[Q].
Management:
• Supportive treatment with **oxygenation & ventilation, maintain circulation with IV fluids & vasopressors**[Q]
• If the cardiovascular & respiratory consequences are managed appropriately, **total spinal block** will **resolve without sequelae**[Q].

RADIOLOGY

195. Ans. a. Left sided pneumothorax with lung collapse *(Ref: Bailey 26/e p304, 27/e p919, 25/e p341; Sabiston 20/e p230-231; Schwartz 10/e p164; Harrison 19/e p308e-13-14f)*

On the basis of clinical features and chest X-ray findings showing black left sided fields without vascular markings and slightly deviated trachea towards right side, most probable diagnosis is left sided pneumothorax with lung collapse.

Traumatic Pneumothorax
• Traumatic pneumothoraxes can result **from penetrating & non-penetrating chest trauma**.
• It should be **treated with tube thoracostomy** unless it's very small.
• **Iatrogenic pneumothorax** is a **type of traumatic pneumothorax** that is becoming more common.
• **Leading causes** are **transthoracic needle aspiration, thoracentesis**, and the **insertion of central intravenous catheters**[Q].
• **Most** can be **managed with supplemental oxygen** or **aspiration**[Q], but if these measures are unsuccessful, a tube thoracostomy should be performed.

PSYCHIATRY

196. Ans. d. a & d *(Ref: Kaplan & Sadock 11/e p421; Niraj Ahuja 7/e p111)*

Acute stress reaction is a normal experience, usually short lasting and resolves in a few days. Denial is the main defense mechanism. Projection is defense mechanism seen in hallucination and delusion. After acute trauma, psychological intervention can help improving the outcome. When a clinician is faced with a patient who has experienced a significant trauma, the major approaches are: support, encouragement to discuss the event, and education about a variety of coping mechanisms (e.g., relaxation) and requires a psychiatric consultation. Hence, referral to psychiatrist is more important than anti-psychotics like risperidone, though risperidone may be prescribed if the patient is having significant psychosomatic symptoms like palpitations and interference with sleep and appetite.

In DSM-IV, diagnosis of Acute Stress Disorder requires marked symptoms of anxiety or increased arousal, re-experiencing of the event, and three of the following five 'dissociative' symptoms;	
• A sense of **numbing or detachment**[Q]	• **Dissociative amnesia**[Q]
• **Reduced awareness of the surroundings**[Q]	• (**Avoidance of stimuli** that arouse recollections of trauma & significant distress or impaired social functioning[Q])
• **Derealization**[Q]	
• **Depersonalization**[Q]	

Acute Stress Reaction
• It is a **psychological condition arising in response to a terrifying or traumatic event**, or **witnessing a traumatic event** that **arises a strong emotional response** within the individual[Q].
• It may **develop into delayed stress reaction** or better known as **PTSD if stress is not correctly managed**[Q].

Contd...

Contd...

Risk factors:
- **Physical exhaustion** and in **extremes of age, female gender**[Q].

Symptoms:
- **Anxiety, depression, anger, despair, over-activity or withdrawal & constriction of field of consciousness**[Q].
- **Resolves rapidly on removal of stressful environment**[Q]
- If the stress continues or cannot be reversed, the **resolution of symptoms begins after 1-2 days**[Q]
  - Symptoms last for a minimum of 2 days & maximum of 4 weeks, after which point continued symptoms may result in a diagnosis of PTSD[Q].

Diagnosis:
- There must be a **clear temporal connection between the impact of an exceptional stressor (such as death of loved one, natural catastrophe, accident, rape) & onset of symptoms; onset is usually within a few minutes or days** but may occur up to one month after the stressor.
- Symptoms show a **mixed & usually changing picture**
- **Symptoms** usually **resolve rapidly** in those cases where **removal from stressful environment** is possible
  - **Avoidance** is the **most frequent coping strategy,** where the **person avoids talking or thinking about the stressful events & avoids reminders of them. The most frequent defense mechanism is denial**[Q].

Treatment:
- This disorder **may resolve itself with time** or may **develop into** a more severe disorder such as **PTSD.**
- **Removal of patient from stressful environment &** helping the patient pass through.
- **Medication** (benzodiazepines/anti-psychotics) can be used for a **short duration**.
- Combination of **relaxation, cognitive restructuring, imaginal exposure** is useful

Post traumatic Stress Disorder (PTSD)

- **Intense, prolonged & protracted or delayed response** to **exceptionally intense stressful events**[Q].

Etiology:
- Events involving **actual or threatened serious injury** or **death** of the person or other
- **Natural disasters, man made calamities & serious physical assault** or **rape**[Q]

Predisposing Factors for PTSD	
• **Female gender**[Q], neuroticism	• Previous history of trauma
• **Lower intelligence & lack of support**[Q]	• **Personal history of mood & anxiety disorder**[Q]

Neurobiological Factors:
- Monoamine neurotransmitters and HPA axis mediate defensive response to stressful events
- **Small hippocampus** leads to dysfunctional & inadequate memory processing while **increased noradrenergic activity of amygdala**, increases arousal & facilitates automatic recall & encoding of traumatic events.

Clinical Presentation:
- May begin **very soon after stressors** or **after an interval of days (usually),** months (occasionally) or rarely >6 months.
- Symptoms must be present for **at least 1 month**, until then it is called acute stress disorder.
- Must leads to **significant distress** or **impaired social functioning**.
  - **Flash backs, nightmares & intrusive images** collectively known, as **painful re-experiencing symptoms** along with **avoidance, emotional numbing & fairly constant hyper arousal** are most characteristic feature[Q].

Treatment:
- **Structured psychotherapy** is **more effective than drug treatment**[Q].
- **Counseling** is TOC for **short term PTSD**[Q]
- **Cognitive behaviour therapy** is TOC for **severe long standing PTSD**[Q]
- **Drug treatment: Antidepressants & benzodiazepines** (in low doses for short periods) are useful in treatment, if anxiety and/or depression are important components of the clinical picture.

Rational and Emotive Therapy	• It is a specialized type of CBT, proved to be useful for PTSD.
Eye movement desensitization and reprocessing (EMDR)	• Relatively new treatment, found to **reduce the symptoms of PTSD.**
	• EMDR involves **making side- to-side eye movements, usually by following the movement of** therapist's finger, while recalling the traumatic incident.

Contd...

197. **Ans. b, b & c**   *(Ref: Kaplan & Sadock 11/e p406; Niraj Ahuja 7/e 95-98)*

Frequent checking of door locks is suggestive of OCD. Three major psychological defensive mechanisms that determine the form and quality of obsessive-compulsive symptoms and character traits: Isolation, undoing, and reaction formation. Repression is a primary mechanism and is not involved in OCD. Drug of choice for OCD is SSRI (Fluoxetine, fluvoxamine, paroxetine, sertraline, citalopram). Psychotherapy of choice in OCD is exposure and response prevention rather than systemic desensitization.

> *"Behavior Therapy: Although few head-to-head comparisons have been made, **behavior therapy is as effective as pharmacotherapies in OCD**, and some data indicate that the **beneficial effects are longer lasting with behavior therapy**. Many clinicians, therefore, consider **behavior therapy the treatment of choice for OCD**. Behavior therapy can be conducted in both outpatient and inpatient settings. **The principal behavioral approaches in OCD are exposure and response prevention**. Desensitization, thought stopping, flooding, implosion therapy, and aversive conditioning have also been used in patients with OCD. In behavior therapy, patients must be truly committed to improvement."- Kaplan & Sadock 11/e p406*

198. **Ans. b. Physiological needs-Safety-Belonging-Self-esteem-Self-actualization**   *(Ref: Kaplan & Sadock 11/e p174)*

   According *to Maslow Hierarchy of Needs, order of increasing priority: Physiological needs-Safety - Belonging-Self-esteem-Self-actualization.*

> *"Abraham Maslow was born in Brooklyn, New York, and completed both his undergraduate and graduate work at the University of Wisconsin. Along with Goldstein, **Maslow believed in self-actualization theory—the need to understand the totality of a person**. A leader in humanistic psychology, **Maslow described a hierarchical organization of needs present in everyone**. As the more primitive needs, such as hunger and thirst, are satisfied, more advanced psychological needs, such as affection and self-esteem, become the primary motivators. **Self-actualization is the highest need**."- Kaplan & Sadock 11/e p174*

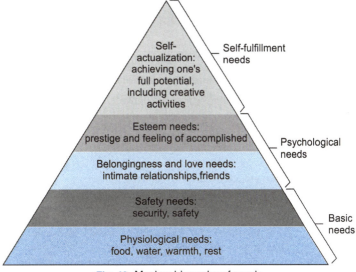

Fig. 42: Maslow hierarchy of needs

Maslow Hierarchy of Needs (Humanistic Theory of Personality)
• **Maslow's hierarchy of needs** is a theory in psychology proposed by **Abraham Maslow**.
• Maslow subsequently extended the idea to include his observations of humans' innate curiosity.
• Maslow used the terms **"physiological", "safety", "belongingness" and "love", "esteem", "self-actualization", and "self-transcendence" to describe the pattern that human motivations generally move through.**
• **Lowermost need in the hierarchy (Physiological)** must be at least partially fulfilled before going to the next level of hierarchy.

Contd...

Contd...

Maslow Hierarchy of Needs (Humanistic Theory of Personality)
• For the highest motive of self-actualization all other needs have to be fulfilled.
• So, though the **motive is self-actualization**, the **physiological is the most important** as one cannot proceed up in the pyramid without the base.   • In order of increasing priority: **Self-actualization < esteem < love < safety < physiological**[Q].

199. **Ans. a. Malingering** *(Ref: Kaplan & Sadock 11/e p812; Niraj Ahuja 7/e Pg119)*

Malingering is fabricating or **exaggerating** *the* **symptoms of** *mental* or **physical** *disorders for* a variety of **"secondary gain"** *motives*, which may include **financial compensation** (often tied to *fraud*); **avoiding school, work** or military service; **obtaining drugs**; getting **lighter** **criminal sentences**; or simply to **attract attention** or **sympathy**.

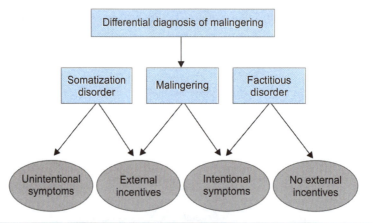

Malingering
• **Fabricating** or **exaggerating** the **symptoms of mental** or **physical disorders for** a variety of **"secondary gain"** motives, which may include **financial compensation** (often tied to fraud); **avoiding school, work** or military service; **obtaining drugs**; getting **lighter criminal sentences**; or simply to **attract attention** or **sympathy**. • Malingering can **lead to abuse of** the **medical system**, with **unnecessary tests being performed** & **time being wasted** **by** the **clinician** as opposed to those with legitimate health problems.
Treatment:
• Treatment lies in the **clinician being able to detect the disorder.**

Cues for the clinician include
• If the **patient has legal problems**
• **Potential for financial reward, antisocial personality disorder**
• If the patient's **story is incongruent** with known facts or other informant accounts
• If the patient will **not cooperate while being evaluated**

• **Psychological evaluation** is also recommended as a way **to diagnose malingering**, in particular, the **Minnesota Multiphasic Personality Inventory (MMPI-2)** as this measure has validity scales of value for this purpose.

200. **Ans. d. Arterial pCO₂ measurement** *(Ref: Kaplan & Sadock 11/e p264, 535)*

Polysomnography is used to assess disorders of sleep by concurrently assessing the EEG, ECG, blood oxygen saturation, respirations, body temperature, electromyogram, and electro-oculogram, not the arterial pCO₂ measurement.

"Polysomnography is used to assess disorders of sleep by concurrently assessing the EEG, ECG, blood oxygen saturation, respirations, body temperature, electromyogram, and electro-oculogram."-Kaplan & Sadock 11/e p264

Polysomnography

- Polysomnography is the **continuous, attended, comprehensive recording of biophysiological changes** occurring during sleep.
- A polysomnogram is **typically recorded at night** and lasts between **6 & 8 hours**.

> - **Brain wave activity, eye movements, submental electromyography activity, nasal-oral air flow, respiratory effort, oxyhemoglobin saturation, heart rhythm & leg movements during sleep are measured**[Q].
> - **Body position** is usually **noted & snoring sounds** may be **recorded.**

- **Brain wave activity, eye movements & submental electromyogram** are important for **identifying sleep stages.**
- **Muscle tension** & movements subside with **deeper sleep** & can also be useful in the **diagnosis of periodic limb movement disorder** & restless legs syndrome.
- **Nasal airflow, respiratory effort & oxyhemoglobin saturation** are **instrumental in diagnosing sleep apnea** & other sleep-related breathing disorders.

Indications for Polysomnography	
- Diagnosis of **sleep-related breathing disorders** - **Positive airway pressure titration & assessment of treatment efficacy**	- **Evaluation of sleep-related behaviors** that are violent or may potentially harm the patient or bed partner

Note

Note

Note

AIIMS MAY 2016

Multiple Choice Questions

ANATOMY

1. Portal vein develops from which of the following structures?
   a. A
   b. B
   c. C
   d. D

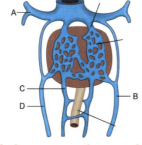

2. In this diagram, identify the structure whose paralysis causes decrease in respiratory movements?
   a. A
   b. B
   c. C
   d. D

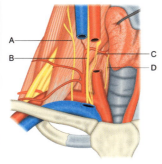

3. As shown in the figure, abnormal subclavian artery develops as a result of:

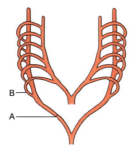

   a. Persistence of B
   b. Persistence of A
   c. Obliteration of A with persistence of B
   d. Obliteration of B with persistence of A

4. The following diagram depicts the various parts from which the diaphragm develops. Defects in which part most commonly lead to congenital diaphragmatic hernia?
   a. A
   b. B
   c. C
   d. D

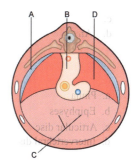

5. Which of the cells labeled below secretes hydrochloric acid?

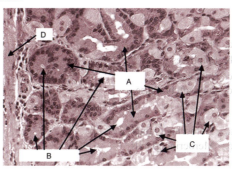

   a. A
   c. C
   b. B
   d. D

6. The area marked in the image below is responsible for various motor functions of the body. It receives afferents from all except:
   a. Spinal cord
   b. Cerebral cortex
   c. Substantia nigra
   d. Thalamus

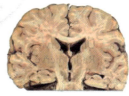

7. The following hematoxylin and eosin-stained biopsy is from which tissue?
   a. Tonsils
   b. Spleen
   c. Lymph Node
   d. Peyer's patches

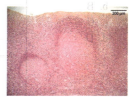

8. What is the artery labeled with black arrow in the given diagram called?

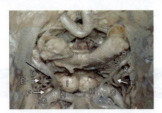

a. Superior cerebellar artery
b. Basilar artery
c. Posterior communicating artery
d. Anterior inferior cerebellar artery

9. The lower two-thirds of the following hematoxylin and eosin-stained specimen are similar in appearance to which of the following structures?

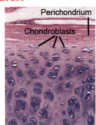

a. Pinna
b. Epiphyses
c. Articular disc
d. Intervertebral disc

10. Which type of gland is depicted here?
a. Pinna
b. Epiphyses
c. Articular disc
d. Intervertebral disc

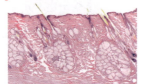

a. Holocrine glands   b. Endocrine glands
c. Merocrine glands   d. Apocrine glands

11. The deformity shown below can be due to involvement of which nerve?

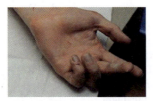

a. Ulnar nerve   b. Median nerve
c. Radial nerve   d. Musculocutaneous nerve

12. The following are the superior and side views of the larynx. Which letter denotes the abductor of the vocal cords?

a. A
b. B
c. C
d. D

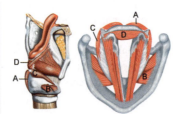

13. Which of the alphabets denotes insula in the cross-section of the brain?

a. A
b. B
c. C
d. D

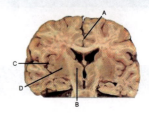

14. What is the nerve supply of the angle of the jaw?
a. Mandibular nerve   b. Maxillary nerve
c. Lesser occipital nerve   d. Greater auricular nerve

15. All of the following are true about venous drainage of esophagus except:
a. Thoracic esophagus drains into the azygos vein
b. Esophageal veins drain into a submucosal plexus
c. The cervical esophagus drains directly into the right brachiocephalic vein
d. Lower esophageal veins anastomose with the left gastric vein

PHYSIOLOGY

16. In this electron micrograph, what is the structure marked with arrow?

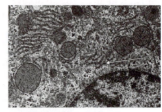

a. Smooth endoplasmic reticulum
b. Trans-Golgi network
c. cis-Golgi network
d. Medial Golgi network

17. All the statements are true about the titration curve of protein except:

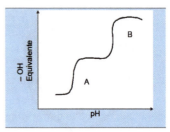

a. A and B represent ionization of amino and carboxyl ends of protein
b. The protein has 3 ionizable sites
c. The protein has 1 functional ion
d. Points A and B represent points of maximal buffering capacity

18. The following graph shows the transport kinetics of a solute transferred across cell membrane. What is the likely nature of the solute?

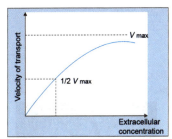

　　a. Glucose　　　　b. CO_2
　　c. O_2　　　　　　d. Na^+

19. Localization of the receptor of a hormone X is found to be in the nucleus. What is likely to be X?
    a. Adrenaline　　　b. Insulin
    c. Thyroxine　　　　d. FSH

20. Which of the following hormones has a permissive action at the onset of puberty?
    a. Insulin　　　　　b. Leptin
    c. GnRH　　　　　　d. Growth hormone

21. A couple comes for evaluation of infertility. The HSG was normal but semen analysis revealed azoospermia. What is the diagnostic test to differentiate between testicular failure and vas deferens obstruction?
    a. Serum FSH　　　　b. Karyotyping
    c. Testosterone levels　d. Testicular FNAC

22. Respiratory rhythm generation center is located at:
    a. Dorsal respiratory group
    b. Pre-Botzinger complex
    c. Ventral respiratory neurons
    d. Pneumotaxic center

23. In relaxed state, chest wall and lung recoil are balanced at:
    a. Minute volume　　b. TLC
    c. Residual volume　　d. FRC

24. According to Weber-Fechner's law, strength of stimulus perceived is directly proportional to:
    (AIIMS May 2016, November 2008)
    a. Intensity of stimulus
    b. Amplitude of action potential
    c. Number of neurons stimulated
    d. Number of receptors stimulated

25. Maximum alveolar arterial oxygen difference is seen in:
    a. Pulmonary embolism　b. Severe asthma
    c. Interstitial lung disease
    d. Foreign body in upper airway

26. During voluntary movements, Golgi tendon organ has an important role to play because it continuously relays to the efferent neurons:
    a. Length of the muscle at rest
    b. Change in angle of joint during motion
    c. Change in length of muscle before and after the movement
    d. Tension in the muscle

27. Best index to measure cardiac afterload is:
    a. Mean arterial pressure　b. LV end diastolic pressure
    c. LV mean systolic pressure
    d. Total peripheral resistance

28. On standing from sitting position, a person has a fall in BP of 10 mm Hg. After correction, the baroreceptor sets back the BP by 8 mm Hg with an error of 2 mm Hg. What is the gain of the system?
    a. 2　　　　　　　b. 4
    c. 6　　　　　　　d. 8

29. The concentration of a negative ion is 100 mMol/L extracellular and 10 mMol/l intracellular. What will be the Nernst potential for this ion?
    (AIIMS May 2013 November 2015)
    a. −10 mV　　　　b. +10 mV
    c. −61 mV　　　　d. +61 mV

30. In the formula for urea clearance, $C = U \times V/P$, U denotes: *(AIIMS May 2016, November 2015)*
    a. Urinary concentration in gm/24 hours
    b. Urine osmolarity
    c. Urinary concentration in mg/ml
    d. Urine volume per minute

BIOCHEMISTY

31. Which of the following is not glucogenic?
    a. Pyruvate　　　　b. Oxaloacetate
    c. Acetyl-CoA　　　d. Lactate

32. Which of these amino acids does not enter the Krebs cycle by forming Acetyl-CoA via pyruvate?
    a. Glycine　　　　　b. Tyrosine
    c. Hydroxyproline　　d. Alanine

33. A child to emergency with accidental ingestion of cyanide. It blocks citric acid cycle by blocking:
    a. Aconitase　　　　b. Acetyl-CoA production
    c. NAD^+　　　　　d. Citrate

34. Which of the following types of lipase is controlled by glucagon?
    a. Lipoprotein lipase　b. Hormone-sensitive lipase
    c. Gastric lipase　　　d. Pancreatic lipase

35. Second messenger for smooth muscle relaxation mediated by NO is:
    a. Ca^{2+}　　　　　b. cAMP
    c. cGMP　　　　　　d. Magnesium

36. Precipitation of proteins is done by all of these except:
    a. Adding trichloroacetic acid
    b. Adding acetyl alcohol and acetone
    c. Adjusting pH to other than the isoelectric point
    d. Salts of heavy metals

37. About the following Michaelis-Menten curve, true statement is:

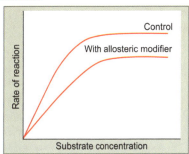

a. Modifier can affect the catalytic site by binding to the allosteric site
b. Allosteric modifiers changes the binding constant of the enzyme but not the velocity of reaction
c. Allosteric modifier binds in a concentration dependent manner
d. Adding more substrate to the enzyme can displace the allosteric modifier

38. In the mammalian genome, maximum number of genes code for the receptors of:
   a. Immunoglobulin receptors
   b. Interleukins
   c. Growth factors
   d. Odorants

PATHOLOGY

39. In this hematoxylin- and eosin-stained slide of inflammation, identify the cell marked with an arrow:

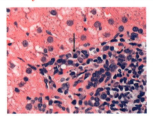

   a. Macrophage
   b. Lymphocyte
   c. Eosinophil
   d. Plasma cell

40. The following is the hematoxylin- and eosin-stained section from the heart of a patient after myocardial infarction. What can you say about the age of infarction?

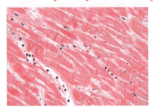

   a. 6 hours
   b. 1–2 days
   c. 1 week
   d. 3 weeks

41. A patient presented with a 4 months' history of cough with diarrheal episodes. Bronchoscopy revealed an intrabronchial polyp. Biopsy from the polyp showed atypical cells with microscopic necrosis and 5 mitotic figures per 10 high-power fields as shown below. Chromogranin staining was positive. What is the diagnosis and grade of the lesion?

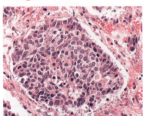

   a. Carcinoid grade 1
   b. Atypical carcinoid grade 2
   c. Small cell carcinoma grade IV
   d. Large cell neuroendocrine carcinoma Grade IV

42. The following is the FITC for IgG-stained kidney specimen. What is this suggestive of?

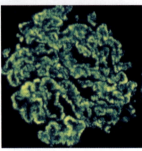

   a. Buerger's disease
   b. Goodpasture's syndrome
   c. Membranous glomerulonephritis
   d. Systemic lupus erythematosus

43. The resected specimen of a kidney is seen below. What is the diagnosis?

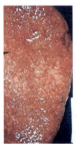

   a. Acute post-streptococcal glomerulonephritis
   b. Flea-bitten kidney of malignant hypertension
   c. Chronic glomerulonephritis
   d. Amyloidosis

44. In a patient, mitral valve vegetations are seen along the lines of closure along with fusion of commissures. What is the likely diagnosis?

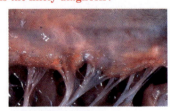

   a. Bacterial endocarditis
   b. Libman-Sacks endocarditis
   c. Rheumatic endocarditis
   d. Marantic endocarditis

45. Agarose gel electrophoresis from DNA of a population of cells as seen under ultraviolet light is shown below. What is the correct explanation for the finding as seen in the band labelled as "C"?

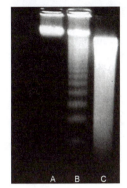

a. Apoptotic cells
b. A population of viable cells
c. Mixed population of normal and apoptotic cells
d. Predominantly necrotic cells

46. The surgical registrar successfully performs a testicular biopsy and hands over the specimen to the attending nurse. The sister asks you how to send the specimen to the pathologist. What fluid will you tell the sister to put the specimen in?
    a. 95% ethanol
    b. Zenker's solution
    c. Bouin's solution
    d. 10% formalin

47. Complement complex that attacks cell membrane is:
    a. C12345
    b. C23456
    c. C34567
    d. C56789

48. Which of the following complement factors is a marker of humoral rejection?
    a. C3d
    b. C3b
    c. C4d
    d. C5a

49. Antigen-presenting cells are all except:
    a. M-cells
    b. Macrophages
    c. Langerhans cells
    d. Thymocytes

50. RBCs are stored at what temperature?
    a. –2 to –4 °C
    b. 2–6 °C
    c. 20–25 °C
    d. 37 °C

51. RBC should be transfused:
    a. With a 18–20 G needle within 4 hours of receiving at the patient's side
    b. With a 18–20 G needle within 4 hours of issue from the blood bank
    c. With a 20–22 G needle within 4 hours of issue from the blood bank
    d. With a 20–22 G needle within 4 hours of receiving at the patient's side

52. Direct Coombs test is positive in all the following except:
    a. Hemolytic anemia due to transfusion
    b. Hemorrhagic disease of newborn
    c. Aplastic anemia
    d. Drug-induced AIHA

53. Serum sickness is:
    a. Type 1 hypersensitivity reaction
    b. Type 2 hypersensitivity reaction
    c. Type 3 hypersensitivity reaction
    d. Type 4 hypersensitivity reaction

54. Most reactive free radical is:
    a. Peroxide
    b. Carboxyl
    c. Hydroxyl
    d. Superoxide

55. Epstein-Barr virus-associated lymphomas are all of these except:
    a. NK T-cell lymphoma
    b. Nodular lymphocyte-predominant Hodgkin's lymphoma
    c. Plasmablastic lymphoma
    d. Lymphomatoid granulomatosis

PHARMACOLOGY

56. CYP450 inhibition is least by:
    a. Pantoprazole
    b. Rabeprazole
    c. Lansoprazole
    d. Omeprazole

57. Black deposits on conjunctiva in a patient with glaucoma are seen with the use of:
    a. Prostaglandins
    b. Carbonic anhydrase inhibitors
    c. Epinephrine
    d. Beta blocker

58. All of these are G2 phase blockers except:
    a. Etoposide
    b. Topotecan
    c. Paclitaxel
    d. Daunorubicin

59. L-asparaginase is used in the treatment of:
    a. AML
    b. ALL
    c. CML
    d. CLL

60. All are Gp IIb/IIIa inhibitors except:
    a. Prasugrel
    b. Abciximab
    c. Tirofiban
    d. Eptifibatide

61. Angiotensin receptor blocker (ARB) with PPAR-gamma function as well is:
    a. Olmesartan
    b. Candesartan
    c. Telmisartan
    d. Eprosartan

62. Ganglionic transmission is mediated by:
    a. Presynaptic alpha-receptors
    b. Postsynaptic beta-receptors
    c. Postsynaptic dopaminergic receptors
    d. Postsynaptic nicotinic receptors

63. Among the following properties of dopamine, which of them is not helpful in acute shock?
    a. Alpha-1 agonist action leading to peripheral vasoconstriction
    b. Increase in renal perfusion due to agonist action on D1 receptors
    c. Releases noradrenaline and causes positive inotropic effect
    d. Direct action on heart via beta-1 receptors

64. Antiemetic action is due to which property of metoclopramide?
    a. 5-HT3 antagonist
    b. D_2 antagonist
    c. 5-HT4 agonist
    d. M3 antagonist

65. In the management of anaphylaxis, which action of adrenaline is not observed?
    a. Bronchodilation by beta-receptors
    b. Cardiovascular effects of beta-receptors
    c. Action on blood vessels by alpha-receptors
    d. Action on presynaptic alpha-receptors

66. Which of these statements depicts vasomotor reversal of Dale?
    a. Propranolol followed by adrenaline
    b. Propranolol followed by noradrenaline
    c. Decrease in heart rate on adrenaline administration after phentolamine has been given
    d. Noradrenaline followed by propranolol

67. Post-marketing surveillance is a part of which phase of clinical trial?
    a. Phase I   b. Phase II
    c. Phase III   d. Phase IV

MICROBIOLOGY

68. A 23 years old female presents with fever and altered sensorium for two days with the following rash on legs. Her BP is 70/50 mm Hg and neck stiffness is present. Lumbar puncture reveals cloudy CSF with 4200 cells/µL, protein level 198 and glucose of 21 mg/dL. Which of the following correctly describes the organism causing this condition?

    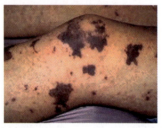

    a. Gram-positive cocci catalase negative, bacitracin-sensitive
    b. Gram-positive diplococci (lanceolate), catalase negative, optochin sensitive
    c. Gram-negative diplococci, ferments glucose and maltose
    d. Gram-negative diplococci (kidney-shaped), oxidase positive

69. A 26 years old male presented with fever and headache for 3 days. His BP is 90/60 mm Hg and examination revealed the following rash on the legs. What is the likely diagnosis?

    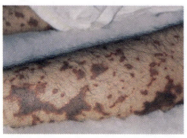

    a. Dengue hemorrhagic fever
    b. Enteric fever
    c. Meningococcus
    d. Scrub typhus

70. Gram-stain shows most likely which organism:

    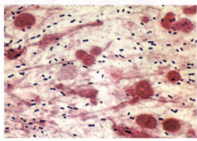

    a. Neisseria meningitidis
    b. Staphylococcus aureus
    c. Streptococcus pneumoniae
    d. Streptococcus pyogenes

71. A 23 years old male presented with abdominal pain and bloody diarrhea of one-week duration. The following colonoscopic biopsy is diagnostic of infection with:

    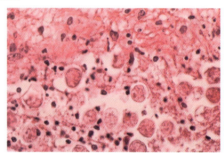

    a. Amoebiasis   b. Enterobius
    c. Giardiasis   d. Severe bacterial infection

72. The following pap smear shows infestation by:

    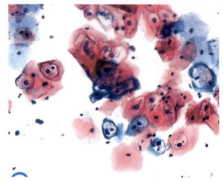

    a. Candida
    b. Herpes simplex virus type II
    c. Trichomonas
    d. Actinomyces

73. The following is the ovum of a helminth. What is true about the helminth?

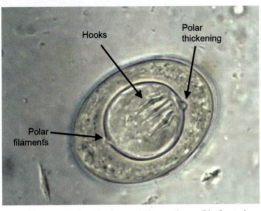

a. Transmission is through ingestion of infected pork
b. Both adult and larval stages are seen in humans
c. The helminth causes a transient self-resolving infection in humans
d. Drug of choice for this condition is albendazole

74. A 40 years old HIV positive male patient comes with odynophagia and watery diarrhea. An endoscopy reveals esophageal and gastric candidiasis. A wet mount of the stool of the patient reveals the following picture. What is true about this helminth?

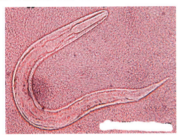

a. Filariform larva is infective for humans as shown in the diagram
b. Transmitted through contaminated food and water usually
c. Females of these species show parthenogenesis
d. Drug of choice is triclabendazole

75. Autoinfection can be caused by all the following helminths except:
a. Enterobius vermicularis   b. Hymenolepis nana
c. Taenia solium   d. Ascaris lumbricoides

76. Helminth implicated in causing pernicious anemia is:
a. Diphyllobothrium latum   b. Ascaris
c. Taenia solium   d. Hymenolepis nana

77. In which of the following ways is CLED medium better than MacConkey agar?
(AIIMS May 2016, November 2001)
a. It prevents proteus swarming
b. Inhibits growth of other commensals
c. It allows Staphylococcus and Candida to grow
d. It differentiates lactose fermenters from non-fermenters

78. Which of the following is an obligate intracellular parasite?
a. Tropheryma whippelii
b. Bartonella henselae
c. Ehrlichia chaffeensis
d. Coxiella burnetii

79. Transfusion-associated malaria has a shorter incubation period because of the presence in blood of:
a. Trophozoites   b. Sporozoites
c. Female gametocyte   d. Merozoites

FORENSIC MEDICINE

80. The following patient has what type of injury in the left anterior part of chest?

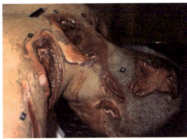

a. Laceration   b. Abrasion
c. Incised wound d. Chop wound

81. The following is a victim of a firearm injury. What is the suspected distance of the shot?

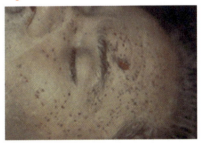

a. Close range   b. Intermediate range
c. Point-blank range   d. Distant shot

82. What is the predicted bone age from the wrist radiograph given below?

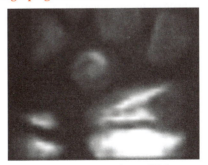

a. <15 years   b. <17.5 years
c. 18–19 years   d. 20–22 years

83. What does this picture depict?

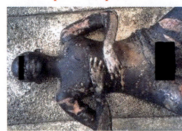

   a. Pugilistic attitude b. Postmortem caloricity
   c. Cadaveric spasm d. Rigor mortis

84. In an examination of a victim of sexual assault, toluidine blue dye test is done to identify:
   a. Healed microinjuries b. Dried seminal stains
   c. Recent microinjuries d. Clotted blood

85. Fingerprinting (FINDER) involves recording prints of 8 fingers. Which finger pair is excluded?
   a. Ring finger b. Thumb
   c. Little finger d. Middle finger

86. In assessing infant deaths, Ploucquet's test involves:
   a. Change in specific gravity of lungs
   b. Presence of air in stomach and duodenum
   c. Change in partial weight of lungs
   d. Air in middle ear

87. After a building collapse, among remnants, a person's length of humerus is 24.5 cm. What is the predicted height of this person?
   a. 90 cm b. 110 cm
   c. 130 cm d. 146 cm

88. Which of the following principles governs biomedical research in human subjects?
   a. Geneva declaration b. Helsinki declaration
   c. Hippocratic oath
   d. International code of medical ethics

89. According to Transplantation of Human Organs Act, which of the following doctors is/are not authorized to declare brainstem death?
   a. RMP incharge of the hospital
   b. Treating physician
   c. Neurosurgeon
   d. Surgeon doing liver transplant

90. The following system of depiction of 32 teeth is in accordance with which system?

Permanent Teeth																
Upper Right								Upper Left								
1	2	3	4	5	6	7	8	9	10	11	12	13	14	15	16	
32	31	30	29	28	27	26	25	24	23	22	21	20	19	18	17	
Lower Right								Lower Left								

   a. Universal system
   b. Palmer's system
   c. Haderup system
   d. Diagrammatic depiction

PREVENTIVE SOCIAL MEDICINE

91. Which of the following is true about antigenic drift?
   a. It is seen only in influenza virus type A
   b. It is a result of frameshift mutation
   c. It mostly affects the matrix protein
   d. It is responsible for seasonal epidemics of influenza

92. Which of these is the correct dosing schedule according to the Nation Iron Plus Program made to tackle iron-deficiency anemia?
   a. 20 mg of elemental iron to all 2–5-year-old children biweekly for an entire year
   b. 100 mg of elemental iron and 500 micrograms of folic acid to pregnant women weekly for an entire year
   c. 100 mg of elemental iron and 500 micrograms of folic acid to pregnant women biweekly for an entire year
   d. 20 mg of elemental iron and 100 micrograms of folic acid to 2–5-year-old children weekly for an entire year

93. According to RNTCP, sputum samples for testing of TB are packed in two containers, which are labelled as:
   a. Alpha and Beta b. 1 and 2
   c. A and B d. Y and Z

94. All of the following are duties of an ASHA worker except:
   a. Assisting and accompanying pregnant women to hospital for delivery
   b. Primary screening for prevalence of non-communicable diseases
   c. Administering zero dose of DPT and OPV
   d. Assessing the success of national programs under ANM

95. A psychiatrist is not posted at:
   a. PHC b. Military hospitals
   c. District hospitals
   d. Hospitals with medical colleges

96. ABC and VED analysis at PHC are done for:
   a. Drug inventory
   b. Staff management
   c. Vaccination coverage
   d. National Programs implementation

97. True about Total Goitre Rate (TGR) is:
   a. It is an indicator of iron deficiency in the community
   b. Community survey of TGR does not require doctors in the team
   c. Goitres are classified as not visible, palpable and visible
   d. The criteria of endemicity is a total goitre rate of >10%

98. Which of the following is the best study design to assess in quick time the strength of association between smoking and lung cancer?
   a. Cross-sectional study b. Case control study
   c. Randomized controlled trial
   d. Cohort study

99. All of these are continuous variables except:
   a. Height in cms b. Weight in kgs
   c. Blood groups A, B, ABO d. Age in years and months

100. Which of the following is used for selecting patients with respect to potential factors that will affect the results?
    a. Systematic random sampling
    b. Simple random sampling
    c. Stratified random sampling
    d. Cluster sampling

101. Which of these indicators is used at anganwadi centers for growth monitoring in children?
    a. Height for age
    b. Weight for age
    c. Weight for height
    d. Mid-arm circumference

102. A study finds no significant association between two variables but truly there exists a difference. What type of error is this?
    a. Type I error
    b. Type II error
    c. Random error
    d. Systematic error

103. The strength of association between the risk factor and disease is measured by:
    a. Attributable risk
    b. Absolute risk of the variable
    c. Odds ratio/Relative risk
    d. p-value

104. What will be the 95% confidence interval (CI) for an estimated prevalence of 10% and a sample size of 100?
    a. 2–18
    b. 4–16
    c. 7–13
    d. Given data inadequate for calculation of class intervals

105. Which of the following statements is not true about incidence?
    a. Incidence decreases when a programme is effective
    b. Vaccination strategies decrease the incidence of a disease
    c. Newer and effective treatment modalities decrease the incidence
    d. Incidence implies number of new cases detected over a fixed time

106. APGAR scores of 30 children are recorded in a hospital and most of the readings are found to be 7 or above. What can you make out about this data distribution?
    a. Positively skewed data
    b. Negatively skewed data
    c. Normal distribution
    d. Symmetrically skewed data

107. You have been asked to design a study for a disease whose prevalence in the community is 10%. The alpha error has to be kept at 5% with a relative precision of 20% and a power of 20%. What will be the accurate sample size for this study?
    a. 400
    b. 900
    c. 1800
    d. 3600

MEDICINE

108. All these are true about the procedure in which this needle is used except:

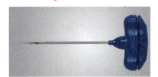

    a. No breath-holding is required for the procedure
    b. Platelet count of less than 40,000 is a contraindication
    c. It is useful is diagnosis of infiltrative and granulomatous disorders
    d. It can be done in both prone and lateral positions

109. A 52 years old diabetic male presents with palpitations to the AIIMS emergency. On examination, the systolic blood pressure was 70 mm Hg. The following was his ECG recorded in emergency. What is the immediate next step in management?

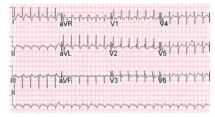

    a. Electrical cardioversion
    b. Amiodarone
    c. Adenosine
    d. Immediate PCI

110. A 76 years old male patient presents to the AIIMS emergency with retrosternal chest pain for 6 hours. The following EKG was taken. What will be your primary management?

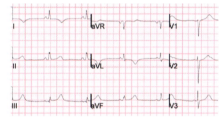

    a. Primary PCI
    b. Thrombolysis
    c. Abciximab
    d. Low molecular weight heparin

111. The following person is performing deep tendon reflex in a patient. Which of these is the correct statement?

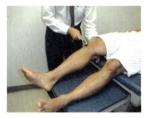

    a. The root value for this reflex is L1, L2 and L3
    b. Always absent in peripheral neuropathy
    c. The guy is performing it in the wrong way
    d. Deep tendon reflexes are always brisk in motor neuron disease

112. All are true about isolated aortic stenoses except:
    a. Pulsus bisferiens
    b. Cardiac apex is displaced laterally to left
    c. Thrill in carotid artery
    d. Blood pressure maintained in initial phase

113. **Tourniquet test is used in daily follow-up of patients with:**
    a. Zika virus
    b. Dengue virus
    c. Chikungunya
    d. Swine flu

114. **In a patient with dengue hemorrhagic fever, which of the following is most important to monitor?**
    a. Hemoglobin
    b. TLC
    c. Platelet count
    d. Hematocrit

115. **In a patient with post-tuberculosis bronchiectasis, which of the following will you observe on auscultation?**
    a. Late inspiratory crackles
    b. Bibasilar crepts
    c. Both early and late inspiratory crackles
    d. Tubular breath sounds

116. **You have performed a pleural tap in a patient with suspected TB. You will send the sample for all of the following studies except:**
    a. Gene Xpert
    b. ADA
    c. LDH
    d. Albumin

117. **All of the following are indications for thrombolysis in a patient with stroke except:**
    a. Age <18 years
    b. Sustained BP >185/110 mm Hg despite treatment
    c. On CT scan, edema less than 1/3rd of middle cerebral artery territory
    d. Acute ischemic stroke within 3 hours of onset

118. **A 40 years old female presented with acute onset shortness of breath. She has a history of nephrotic syndrome 1 year back and recent prolonged air travel. She has a BP of 90/60 mm Hg, heart rate of 115 per minute and sinus tachycardia on ECG. A 2-D echocardiogram revealed dilation of right ventricle with bulging of the interventricular septum to the left. What will be the primary treatment modality?**
    a. Thrombectomy
    b. Intravenous tissue plasminogen activator
    c. Unfractionated heparin
    d. IVC filter

119. **A patient with suspected cardiac tamponade presents to the AIIMS emergency. You are asked to monitor BP of this patient. All the following precautions should be taken except:**
    a. Patient should be asked to take deep breaths
    b. The cuff pressure should be increased to 20 mm over systolic pressure
    c. The cuff should be slowly deflated until the first Korotkoff sound is heard only during expiration
    d. Pulses paradoxus may not be present

120. **A 27 years old pregnant lady comes with severe jaundice and altered sensorium. On examination, the patient is deeply icteric, not responding to commands and pelvic sonogram reveals intrauterine fetal death. Serum bilirubin levels are 28.8 mg/dL (direct = 18.6 mg/dL), AST levels are 1063 and ALT levels are 1191. The viral markers are as follows. What is the likely diagnosis?**

Anti-HAV IgG	Reactive
Anti-HAV IgM	Nonreactive
HbSAg	Nonreactive
Anti-HbSAg	Nonreactive
Anti-HBc IgM	Nonreactive
Anti-HBc IgG	Reactive
Anti-HCV IgG	Nonreactive
Anti-HEV IgM	Reactive
Anti-HEV IgG	Nonreactive

    a. Acute hepatitis E superimposed on chronic liver failure due to hepatitis B
    b. Fulminant hepatitis due to hepatitis B infection
    c. Acute hepatitis E with chronic hepatitis A
    d. Fulminant hepatitis due to hepatitis E infection

121. **A patient of disseminated malignancy comes to the palliative care clinic with nausea, vomiting and altered sensorium. Hypercalcemia is detected on investigations. What will be the first line of management?**
    a. Intravenous steroids
    b. Thiazides
    c. Intravenous fluids
    d. Intravenous bisphosphonates

122. **A 50 years old lady, who has a known diagnosis of bronchial asthma, presented to the AIIMS emergency with complaints of severe breathlessness, diaphoresis and wheezing. On examination, you find that the patient is conscious with a respiratory rate of 30 per minute, blood pressure of 96/64 mm Hg and a pulse rate of 144 per minute. An arterial blood gas analysis showed a pH of 7.2, pO_2 of 50 mm Hg and pCO_2 of 70 mm Hg. How will you manage the patient?**
    a. Ventilation with continuous positive airway pressure
    b. Oxygen supplementation by nasal mask
    c. Mechanical ventilation with controlled ventilation
    d. Intubation

123. **A glass factory worker presented with complaints of numbness in hands and feet, generalized weakness and constipation. Radiograph showed linear lines on metaphyses of knee and wrist joints. How will you diagnose this patient?**
    a. Serum mercury levels
    b. Vitamin D levels
    c. RBC cholinesterase levels
    d. Amino levulinic acid levels in urine

124. **A second-year PG resident tells you to perform an ABG of a patient. All the following are true about performing an ABG except:**
    a. Before performing the ABG, syringe should be loaded with 0.3 cc of heparin
    b. Normal pH, HCO_3 and PCO_2 levels may not indicate absence of an acid-base imbalance
    c. A different site should be tried if modified Allen's test is negative
    d. Radial artery is the preferred site

125. **On laboratory investigations in a patient, pH = 7.3, pCO_2 = 35 mm Hg. What is the likely acid base imbalance?**
    a. Respiratory acidosis
    b. Metabolic acidosis
    c. Metabolic alkalosis
    d. Respiratory alkalosis

SURGERY

126. A 76 years old male presents to the emergency with abdominal pain and an episode of binge drinking in shock with a BP of 70/50 mm Hg and HR of 115/min. The oxygen saturation of the patient is 70 mm Hg. Serum creatinine level was 2.4 mg/dl. The patient had raised transaminases. What is the likely diagnosis based on the CT image shown below?

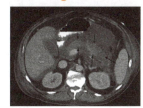

a. Liver abscess
b. Acute pancreatitis
c. Acute pyelonephritis
d. Severe acute pancreatitis

127. A 30 years old male patient presented with abdominal pain, fever, nausea, vomiting and respiratory distress. His BP was found to be 80/40 mm Hg and pulse rate of 115/min. The following chest X-ray was recorded in ER. What is the immediate management?

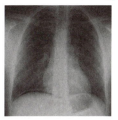

a. IV fluids and antibiotics followed by laparotomy
b. Immediate laparotomy
c. Intravenous fluids
d. Intravenous potassium

128. Following a laparoscopic hernia surgery, the attending surgeon asks you to the suture the skin wound with 3-0 nylon. Which is the correct set of instruments you will use for suturing?

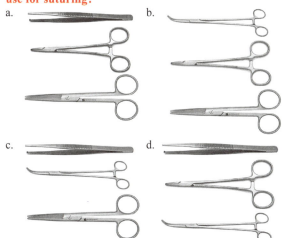

129. A 56 years old lady came to you with a diagnosis of carcinoma breast. The following was revealed in her immunohistochemistry staining. What can you say about the prognosis in this patient?

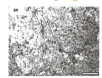 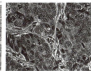

a. Good prognosis
b. Poor prognosis
c. Good outcome with trastuzumab
d. Good outcome without trastuzumab

130. A surgical attending has completed a modified radical mastectomy for a carcinoma breast patient. You have to suture the wound using subcuticular sutures. Which of these sutures will you choose?

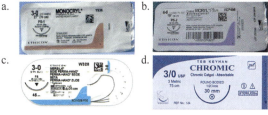

131. A pregnant lady was stabbed in the right side of the chest. She is shouting and yelling for help on entering the casualty. On examination, she has tachycardia and BP was 90/60 mm Hg, breath sounds are decreased on the right side. What is the first consideration for her?
a. Intercostal chest tube insertion
b. Emergent tracheostomy
c. Establish an intravenous line and start normal saline infusion
d. Immediate needle thoracostomy

132. Urobilinogen levels in obstructed jaundice due to gallstones will be:
a. Markedly raised
b. Slightly increased
c. Normal
d. Completely absent

133. A 70 years old patient presents with a lesion on the cheek with raised, pearly borders and with telangiectasias on surface of the lesion. What is the likely diagnosis?
a. Basal cell carcinoma
b. Squamous cell carcinoma
c. Warts
d. Actinic keratosis

134. A 2 years old child suffers flame burns involving face, bilateral upper limbs and front of chest and abdomen. What is the body surface area involved?
a. 40%
b. 45%
c. 54%
d. 60%

135. A surgeon decides to operate a patient of carcinoma cecum and perform a right hemicolectomy through a midline laparotomy approach. You have been instructed to prepare the parts of the patient for surgery. What will you do?
a. Clean and drape from the level of nipple to mid-thigh
b. Clean and drape from chin to knee
c. Clean and drape from umbilicus to mid-thigh
d. Clean and drape from rib cage to inguinal regions

136. In a patient with dehydration, which of the following color intravenous cannula will you place for rapid fluid resuscitation?
    a. Grey
    b. Blue
    c. Pink
    d. Green

137. After a surgery, the surgeon asked the intern to remove the Foley's catheter but he could not do it. The surgeon himself tried to remove the Foley's catheter but he was unsuccessful. What should be done next?
    a. CT-guided rupture of bulb of Foley's
    b. Inject ether to dissolve the balloon and pull it out
    c. Inject water to overdistend the balloon until it bursts and Foley's can be removed
    d. Use ultrasound guidance to locate and prick the balloon and then remove the catheter

138. In a 40 years old patient with head injury, which of the following is the best strategy to decrease the intracerebral pressure?
    a. Limiting pCO_2 of the patient
    b. Administer sedatives
    c. Oxygen supplementation by mechanical ventilation
    d. Administer nimodipine

139. Nimodipine is approved for use in:
    a. Subdural hemorrhage
    b. Extradural hemorrhage
    c. Intracerebral hemorrhage
    d. Subarachnoid hemorrhage

OBSTETRICS AND GYNECOLOGY

140. The following is the picture of the Pap smear of a 45 years old female with left ovarian tumor in her late menstrual phase showing squamous cells. What is the likely histology of the tumor?

    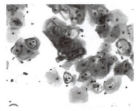

    a. Serous papillary carcinoma
    b. Granulosa cell tumor
    c. Mucinous adenocarcinoma
    d. Dysgerminoma

141. A 30 years old primigravida presented at 10 weeks gestation with painless, bright red bleeding per vaginum. On examination, the uterus is 12 weeks' size. Ultrasonography revealed the following picture. What is the most likely diagnosis?

    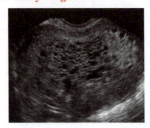

    a. Missed abortion
    b. Blighted ovum
    c. Placental polyp
    d. Hydatidiform mole

142. A routine ultrasound done at 20 weeks period of gestation done in a 31 years old gravida 1 para 0 revealed an anomaly. The patient comes to you with the following ultrasound film for a second opinion. What congenital anomaly would you explain to the couple?

    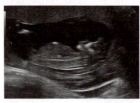

    a. Omphalocele
    b. Encephalocele
    c. Cystic hygroma
    d. Anencephaly

143. The instrument shown below is used for what procedure?

    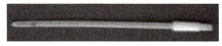

    a. Dye instillation in hysterosalpingography
    b. Fractional curettage
    c. Dilatation and curettage
    d. Endometrial biopsy

144. Double bleb signs in USG are depictive of:
    a. Intrauterine two gestations sac
    b. Amniotic sac and yolk sac
    c. Ectopic pregnancy
    d. Heterotopic pregnancy

145. All of the following increase at full term in pregnancy except:
    a. Minute volume
    b. GFR
    c. Blood volume
    d. Cardiac output

146. A mother brings her 19 years old daughter to your clinic with complaint that she has not started having menses. General examination reveals normally developed breasts and pubic hair. On pelvic examination, vaginal ending is blind and uterus is not palpable. Which of the following do you suspect?
    a. Mullerian agenesis
    b. Asherman syndrome
    c. Gonadal dysgenesis
    d. Turner's syndrome

147. A 25 years old female comes to your clinic for evaluation of infertility. A hysterosalpingogram reveals Asherman's syndrome. What symptoms will the patient have?
    a. Menorrhagia
    b. Oligomenorrhea
    c. Polymenorrhea
    d. Hypomenorrhea

148. A 26 years old female presented with mild pain in lower abdomen. She has had 2 full-term normal delivery earlier. Her last menstrual period was 3 weeks back. On pelvic examination, you find a palpable mass in the adnexa. On USG pelvis, you find a 5 cm ovarian cyst. What should be your next step?
    a. Observation and follow-up for cyst after 2–3 months
    b. CA-125 levels

c. Diagnostic exploratory laparotomy
d. CECT of pelvis

149. **An episiotomy is to be performed in a primigravida in labor. Which of these is an advantage of mediolateral episiotomy over midline episiotomy?**
    a. Less chance of extension
    b. Can be repaired at ease
    c. Fewer breakdown
    d. Lesser blood loss

150. **A 22 years old gravida 3 para 2 lady delivers a normal child followed by delivery of an intact placenta. Following delivery, the lady develops severe per vaginal bleeding after 30 minutes. On table sonogram revealed retained placental tissue. What is the suspected type of placenta?**
    a. Membranous placenta
    b. Placenta fenestrae
    c. Placenta accreta
    d. Placenta succenturiata

151. **A 30 years old G3P2 with 10 weeks of amenorrhea comes with an intrauterine pregnancy with intra uterine contraceptive device in situ. On pelvic examination, the string of the IUCD was visible at the cervical os. Patient wishes to continue pregnancy. What will you do?**
    a. Leave IUCD and continue pregnancy
    b. Terminate pregnancy because of high risk of infections
    c. Continue pregnancy with use of antibiotics throughout pregnancy
    d. Remove intrauterine contraceptive device

152. **A primigravida came to the labor room at 40 weeks + 5 days gestation for induction of labor. On per vaginal examination, the cervix is 1 cm dilated and 30% effaced. The vertex is at –1 station and the cervix is soft and posterior. What will be the modified bishop score for this lady?**
    a. 0
    b. 3
    c. 5
    d. 8

153. **A 45 years old patient presented with complaints of pain in abdomen and menorrhagia. Endometrial biopsy was normal and sonogram of uterus showed diffusely enlarged uterus with no adnexal mass. What is the diagnosis?**
    a. Fibroid uterus
    b. Endometritis
    c. Endometriosis
    d. Adenomyosis

154. **Which is the most common congenital abnormality in a baby of a diabetic woman?**
    a. Ventricular septal defect
    b. Anencephaly
    c. Meningomyelocele
    d. Sacral agenesis

PEDIATRICS

155. **A 4 years old child is admitted in the ward with pneumonia. He develops sudden respiratory distress. The following chest X-ray was recorded. What will you do next?**

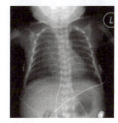

   a. Decrease mechanical ventilation
   b. Increase mechanical ventilation
   c. Intercostal chest drainage tube insertion
   d. Immediate needle thoracostomy

156. **A 5 years old male comes with complaints of pain in neck and right shoulder with restricted range of motion. What is the likely diagnosis?**

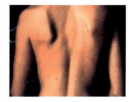

   a. Klippel-Fleil syndrome
   b. Facioscapulohumeral dystrophy
   c. Ankylosing spondylitis
   d. Long thoracic nerve palsy

157. **A 16 years old male presents with rapidly developing bilateral pleural effusion. The following chest radiograph was taken in the emergency. All are correct interpretations about this radiograph except:**

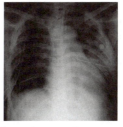

   a. Pneumothorax is present
   b. Bilateral intercostal chest tubes are present in correct place
   c. Mediastinum is shifted
   d. Left sided pleural effusion is present

158. **In a child with tetralogy of Fallot with fever and diarrhea, which of the following is the surest sign of a cyanotic spell?**
   a. Hepatomegaly
   b. Absence of murmur
   c. S3 gallop rhythm
   d. Arterial oxygen saturation of less than 75%

159. **A mother comes with her 3 months' child asking the physician if she can give cereals to her child. What problem can this lead to her child?**
   a. Allergy due to the food content
   b. Risk of gastrointestinal infection
   c. Retarded oro-motor development
   d. Contaminated food leading to reflux

160. A child who was normal at birth develops chronic liver failure and muscle weakness at 3 months of age. On investigations, serum glucose is low, along with ketoacidosis and decreased pH. ALT and AST are raised. Blood lactate and uric acid levels are normal. Intravenous glucagon given after meals raises the blood glucose levels, but does not raise glucose when given after an overnight fast. Liver biopsy shows increased glycogen in liver. Which is the enzyme likely to be defective in this child?
    a. Glucose-6-phosphatase b. Muscle phosphorylase
    c. Branching enzyme d. Debranching enzyme

161. A 5 years old child presented with continuous fever and features of sepsis with a BP of 90/60 mm Hg, Pulse rate 144/min and respiratory rate of 30/min. What is the initial fluid of choice for management?
    a. 10 mL/kg of 10% dextrose
    b. 10 mL/kg of hydroxyethyl starch
    c. 20 mL/kg of 0.45% normal saline
    d. 20 mL/kg of 0.9% normal saline

162. A 6 years male child comes with complaints of bedwetting. The child is continent during the day and problem is only at night. Growth and development of the child were normal. Urine microscopy is normal and urine specific gravity was 1.020. How will you manage?
    a. Reassure the parents and follow up after 6 months
    b. Refer to psychiatrist
    c. Complete blood counts d. Ultrasound-KUB

ORTHOPEDICS

163. What is the eponym for the fracture shown below?
    (AIIMS November 2015, May 2016)

    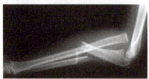

    a. Galeazzi's fracture b. Monteggia fracture
    c. Smith's fracture d. Colle's fracture

164. A 24 years old male presents with a humerus fracture as shown in the figure below. Which is the nerve likely to be involved by the fracture?

    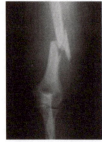

    a. Radial nerve b. Ulnar nerve
    c. Median nerve d. Musculocutaneous nerve

165. The following pelvic X-ray was seen in a patient. All the following signs will be present except:

    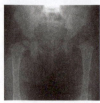

    a. Narath b. Ortolani
    c. Barlow d. Gaenslen's

166. The following deformity is seen in a child. What is the likely cause?

    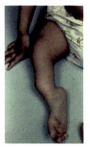

    a. Tibial hemimelia b. Fibula hemimelia
    c. Congenital pseudoarthrosis of tibia
    d. Congenital posteromedial angulation of tibia

167. The following sets of X-rays are suggestive of:

    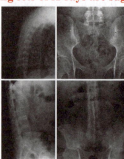

    a. Ankylosing spondylitis b. Paget's disease
    c. Rheumatoid arthritis d. Hyperparathyroidism

168. A 30 years old male presented with hip pain for the last 6 months. Hip X-ray is as shown below. What is the most likely diagnosis?

    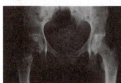

    a. Giant cell tumor b. Simple bone cyst
    c. Multiple myeloma d. Adamantinoma

169. About giant cell tumor, all are true except:
    a. Commonly presents in the 20–40 year age group
    b. Matrix consists of proliferating mononuclear cells
    c. Osteoclast giant cells constitute the proliferative component of the tumor
    d. It is a benign tumor which may have lung metastasis

OPHTHALMOLOGY

170. Corneal ulcer resembling fungal ulcer is seen in infection with which of the agents?
    a. Nocardia asteroides   b. Mycobacterium
    c. Klebsiella pneumoniae d. Chlamydia trachomatis

171. A 33 years old male came with pain and watering in the right eye for 36 hours. On examination, a 3 × 2 cm corneal ulcer is seen with elevated margins, feathery hyphae, finger like projections and minimal hypopyon in cornea. What is the likely causative organism?
    a. Aspergillosis   b. Pseudomonas
    c. Acanthamoeba   d. HSV-1

172. Phenol red thread test is used for dry eye:
    a. In the test, volume of tears is measured as it changes color on contact with tears
    b. If the color changes to blue, it depicts surface mucin deficiency
    c. Requires pH meter for reading the result
    d. Requires topical anesthetic agent

173. Immediately after photodynamic therapy, color of the lesion becomes:
    a. Unchanged   b. Grey
    c. Yellow   d. White

174. What is the angle subtended by the largest letter in the Snellen chart on a person's eye who is reading it from a distance of 6 meters?
    a. 1 minute   b. 10 minutes
    c. 50 minutes   d. 60 minutes

ENT

175. A 45 years old lady presented with complaints of nasal congestion, stuffiness, discharge and anosmia. CT scan of para-nasal sinus was done as shown below. What is the diagnosis?

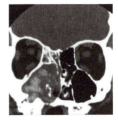

    a. Ethmoidal polyp   b. Antrochoanal polyp
    c. Allergic fungal sinusitis d. Nasoethmoidal carcinoma

176. Identify the encircled structure in middle-ear cavity:

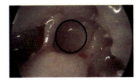

    a. Fossa incudis   b. Sinus tympani
    c. Facial recess   d. Pyramidal fossa

177. A 5 years old child presents with voice change and stridor. Identify the abnormality marked on the fiberoptic laryngoscopy:

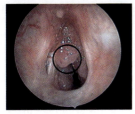

    a. Respiratory papillomatosis
    b. Respiratory nodules
    c. Carcinoma larynx   d. Hemangioma

178. A patient presented with decreased hearing in right ear. Interpret the following audiometric tracing:

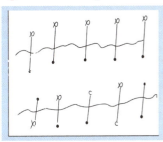

    a. Conductive hearing loss of left ear
    b. Conductive hearing loss of right ear
    c. Sensorineural hearing loss of left ear
    d. Sensorineural hearing loss of right ear

179. All the following instruments are required for tonsillectomy except:
    a. Coblation wand   b. Bipolar cautery
    c. Microdebrider   d. Harmonic scalpel

SKIN

180. A 5 years old girl presented with lesion on the face for the last 3 months. A skin biopsy was performed and the findings are shown below. What is the diagnosis?

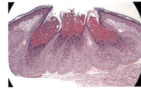

    a. Squamous cell carcinoma
    b. Squamous papilloma with central crater
    c. Molluscum contagiosum
    d. Herpes zoster

181. A 35 years old male comes with complain of baldness. On examination, well-defined bald patches were seen with no scarring. Small broken hairs were seen in the surrounding area. What is the likely diagnosis?
    a. Androgenetic alopecia   b. Alopecia areata
    c. Anagen effluvium   d. Telogen Effluvium

182. Treatment of choice for erythrodermic psoriasis:
    a. Methotrexate   b. Corticosteroids
    c. Coal tar topical d. Topical steroids

183. A 45 years old male presents with itchy papules over face, neck and V area of chest for the last three years, which are exacerbated in summers and improved in winters. What test will you do to confirm diagnosis?
   a. Patch test
   b. Prick test
   c. IgE levels
   d. Skin biopsy

184. A factory worker comes to you with itchy, annular scaly plaques in the groin. On prescribing corticosteroid ointment, there is significant relief in pruritus but the lesion continues to extend peripherally. What is the likely diagnosis?
   a. Tinea cruris
   b. Annular lichen planus
   c. Granuloma annulare
   d. Erythema annulare centrifugum

185. A 45 years old patient presented with multiple hypoaesthetic patches over trunk and extremities. On examination, ulnar and lateral popliteal nerves are enlarged bilaterally. What is the diagnosis?
   a. Lepromatous leprosy
   b. Borderline leprosy
   c. Borderline lepromatous leprosy
   d. Borderline tuberculoid leprosy

186. A 24 years old female presented with complaints of rash on exposure to sun, after exercise, when she gets angry or on eating spicy food. What is the likely diagnosis?
   a. Atopic dermatitis *(AIIMS May 2016, November 2012)*
   b. Chronic idiopathic urticaria
   c. Solar keratosis
   d. Cholinergic urticaria

ANESTHESIA

187. Which of the following drugs undergoes Hoffman elimination?
   a. Atracurium
   b. Mivacurium
   c. Pancuronium
   d. Tubocurare

188. All are drugs acting on neuromuscular junction except:
   a. Mivacurium
   b. Succinylcholine
   c. Dantrolene
   d. Pancuronium

189. All of the following are true about lumbar puncture except:
   a. Level of needle insertion should be L1-L2 vertebral junction
   b. The bevel end of needle should face up
   c. Needle should be inserted in a slightly cephalad direction
   d. Legs should be straightened for CSF pressure measurement

190. A sevoflurane vaporizer can accurately deliver the dose of an anesthetic agent. It resembles it in which of the following properties?
   a. Molecular weight
   b. Oil gas partition coefficient
   c. Blood gas partition coefficient
   d. Vapor pressure

191. All are true about rapid sequence induction done in a cardiac patient in emergency except:
   a. Inducing agent and neuromuscular relaxant are administered together
   b. The patient is pre-oxygenated for 3 minutes before the procedure
   c. Cricoid pressure has to be applied till the endotracheal tube has been secured with a cuff
   d. Induction should be done with thiopentone sodium and succinylcholine for muscle relaxation

192. Correct sequence of age and MAC required is:
   a. Adults > Infants > Neonates
   b. Infants > Neonates > Adults
   c. Neonates > Adults > Infants
   d. Neonates > Infants > Adults

193. Allergy in immediate perioperative period is due to:
   a. Opioids
   b. LA agents
   c. Induction agents
   d. Neuromuscular blockers

194. A 46 years old male patient was given subarachnoid block with bupivacaine (heavy) by the anesthetist. After 10 minutes he was found to have a BP of 72/44 mm Hg and heart rate of 52/min. On checking the level of block it was found to be T6. What is the likely explanation for the bradycardia?
   a. Bezold-Jarisch reflex
   b. Bainbridge reflex
   c. Block of Cardio-accelerator fibers of synthetic origin
   d. Reverse Bainbridge reflex

RADIOLOGY

195. Patient with carcinoma endometrium treated with pelvic external beam irradiation to whole pelvis. Which of the following organs is most radiosensitive in the pelvic region?
   a. Ovary
   b. Vagina
   c. Bladder
   d. Rectum

PSYCHIATRY

196. A 41 years old female patient comes to AIIMS emergency with complains of flurry, palpitations, profuse sweating and sense of impending doom. The following test should be done in emergency to rule out organic causes:
   a. Hemoglobin
   b. Blood sugar level
   c. ECG
   d. T3/T4/TSH

197. In psychiatry, personal history does not include:
   a. Food preference
   b. Academic history
   c. Occupational history
   d. Marital history

198. All of the following are true about obsession except:
   a. May be present in schizophrenia
   b. Ego-dystonic
   c. Persists on resistance and causes depression and anxiety
   d. Disorder of content of thought

199. MMSE evaluates which of the following:
   a. Thought
   b. Cognition
   c. Insight
   d. Mood and effect

200. Semantic memory includes all except memory of:
   a. Words
   b. Rules
   c. Events
   d. Language

Explanations

ANATOMY

1. **Ans. c. C** *(Ref: Langman 11/e p193)*
   Portal vein develops from right vitelline vein (c), left vitelline vein regresses.
   A: Carinal veins; B: Left umbilical vein; C: Right vitelline vein; D: Right umbilical vein

Development of Venous System	
Embryonic Structure	**Adult Structure**
Vitelline Veins	
Right & Left	• **Hepatic vein** & sinusoids, **ductus venosus, inferior hepatic** part of **IVC, portal vein, superior & inferior mesenteric vein, splenic vein**[Q] • **Most portion of left vitelline vein disappears**[Q]
Umbilical Veins	
Right	• **Regress early in development**[Q]
Left	• **Ligamentum teres**[Q]
Cardinal Veins	• **Internal jugular vein, SVC, part of IVC, common iliac veins, renal veins, gonadal veins,** intercostal veins, **hemiazygous & azygous vein**[Q]

Structure	Remnant/Fate
Right umbilical vein	• **Disappears**[Q]
Left umbilical vein	• **Ligamentum teres**[Q]
Proximal part of umbilical artery	• **Superior vesical artery**[Q]
Distal part of umbilical artery	• **Lateral umbilical ligament**[Q]
Ductus arteriosus	• **Ligamentum arteriosum**[Q]
Ductus venosus	• **Ligamentum venosum**[Q]
Urachus	• **Media<u>n</u> (not medial) umbilical ligament**[Q]
Obliterated umbilical artery	• **Media<u>l</u> umbilical fold**[Q]
Inferior epigastric artery	• **Lateral umbilical fold**[Q]
Left common cardinal vein	• **Oblique vein of left atrium**[Q]

Development of Vitelline and Umbilical veins	
Fourth & Fifth Week (Formation of hepatic sinusoids & initiation of left-to-right shunts between vitelline veins)	**Second & Third Month**

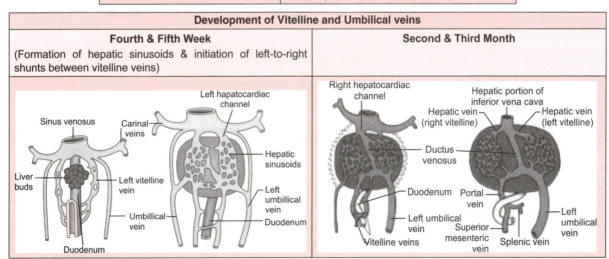

Venous System
– In the 5th week, three pairs of major veins can be distinguished: – **Vitelline veins (omphalomesenteric veins):** Carrying blood from yolk sac to sinus venosus[Q] – **Umbilical veins:** Originating in the chorionic villi, carrying oxygenated blood to embryo[Q] – **Cardinal veins:** Draining the body of embryo proper[Q]

Vitelline veins
• Before entering the sinus venosus, **vitelline veins form a plexus around duodenum & pass through the septum transversum**[Q] • Liver cords growing into septum interrupt the course of veins & an extensive vascular network, hepatic sinusoids, forms. • With reduction of left sinus horn, **blood from left side of liver is rechanneled toward right**, resulting in an **enlargement of right vitelline vein (right hepatocardiac channel)**[Q] • **Right hepatocardiac channel forms** the **hepatocardiac portion of IVC**[Q]<ul><li>**Proximal part of left vitelline vein disappears**[Q]</li><li>**Anastomotic network around duodenum develops into a single vessel, the portal vein**[Q]</li><li>**Superior mesenteric vein** derives from **right vitelline vein**[Q]</li><li>**Distal portion of left vitelline vein also disappears**[Q]</li></ul>

2. **Ans. a. A** *(Ref: Gray's 41/e p970, 40/e p218)*

   Phrenic nerve (A) paralysis causes decrease in respiratory movements.
   A: Phrenic nerve; **B:** Vagus nerve; **C:** Vertebral artery; **D:** Recurrent laryngeal nerve

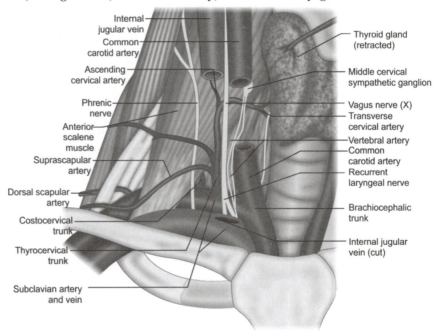

Fig. 1: Posterior Triangle of Neck

Phrenic Nerve
• **Phrenic nerve** originates in the neck (**C3-C5**) & passes down between lung & heart to reach diaphragm[Q]. • It is **important for breathing**, as it passes **motor information to diaphragm** & receives sensory information from it[Q].
Root Value:
• Phrenic nerve **originates mainly from 4th cervical nerve**, but also **receives contributions from 5th & 3rd cervical nerves (C3 & C5) in humans**[Q] • Receives innervation from **parts of both cervical plexus & brachial plexus**[Q] • Contain **motor, sensory & sympathetic nerve fibers**[Q].

Contd...

Contd...

Phrenic Nerve
Course:
• Found in **middle mediastinum**, both phrenic nerves **run from C3, C4 & C5 along anterior scalene muscle deep to the carotid sheath**[Q].
• **Phrenic nerve descends obliquely with internal jugular vein across anterior scalene, deep to prevertebral layer of deep cervical fascia & transverse cervical & suprascapular arteries**[Q].

Right Side	Left Side
• **Crosses anterior to 1st part of subclavian artery**[Q]	• It **lies on anterior scalene muscle & crosses anterior to 2nd part of subclavian artery**[Q].
• **Passes over brachiocephalic artery, posterior to subclavian vein & crosses root of right lung anteriorly**[Q]	• **Passes over pericardium of left ventricle & pierces diaphragm separately**[Q].
• **Leaves thorax by passing through vena cava hiatus** opening in diaphragm at **T8**[Q].	
• **Passes over the right atrium**[Q]	

• On **both sides, phrenic nerve runs posterior to subclavian vein as it enters the thorax** where it **runs anterior to root of lung** & between fibrous pericardium & mediastinal face of parietal pleura[Q].
Supply:
• **Motor: Diaphragm**[Q] (most important muscle of respiration)
• **Sensory: Pericardium, mediastinal parietal pleura,** and **pleura & peritoneum covering central diaphragm**[Q]

3. **Ans. d. Obliteration of B with persistence of A**   *(Ref: Langman's 13/e p206)*

Abnormal subclavian artery develops as a result of obliteration of B (4th arch) with persistence of A (distal portion of right dorsal aorta & 7th intersegmental artery).

Abnormal Origin of the Right Subclavian Artery (ARSCA)
• Occurs when the **artery is formed by distal portion of right dorsal aorta & 7th intersegmental artery**[Q].
• **Right IV aortic arch & proximal part of right dorsal aorta are obliterated**[Q].
• With shortening of aorta between left common carotid & left subclavian arteries, **origin of abnormal right subclavian artery** finally settles **just below** that of **left subclavian artery**[Q].
• **Left aortic arch** with an aberrant right subclavian artery is MC congenital anomaly of aortic arch[Q].
• Normally, **proximal part of right subclavian artery arises from right 4th aortic arch & distal part from right dorsal aorta** present **between IV aortic arch & right 7th intersegmental artery**[Q].
• **ARSCA** develops as a result of **abnormal involution of right IV aortic arch & abnormal persistence of right dorsal aorta** distal to right 7th intersegmental artery[Q].
• ARSCA typically travels in a **retro esophageal course in 80% of patients**, between trachea & esophagus in 10–15% **of patients** & anterior to both structures in 5% of patients[Q].

Aortic Arches and their Derivatives
• **Six pairs of aortic arches**, develop in a cephalo-caudal direction & **interconnect ventral aortic roots & dorsal aorta**[Q]
• **Most of 1st & 2nd arches disappear, 5th totally disappears**Q.

Fates of Aortic Arches	
Aortic Arch	**Derivatives & Fate**
I	• **Mainly disappears**, remaining part forms **inferior alveolar artery**[Q], branch of maxillary artery
II	• Mainly disappears, remaining part forms **hyoid & stapedial arteries**[Q]
III	• Proximal part forms **common carotid arteries**[Q] • Distal part join dorsal aorta to form **internal carotid arteries (1st part)** [Q]
IV (right)	• Proximal part of right subclavian artery & brachiocephalic artery
V	• Does not develop in human embryo
VI	• Also known as **pulmonary arch**[Q]

Left	Right
• Left proximal part forms **left pulmonary artery** & distal part persists as **ductus arteriosus**[Q]	• Right proximal part forms **right pulmonary artery** & distal part degenerates[Q]

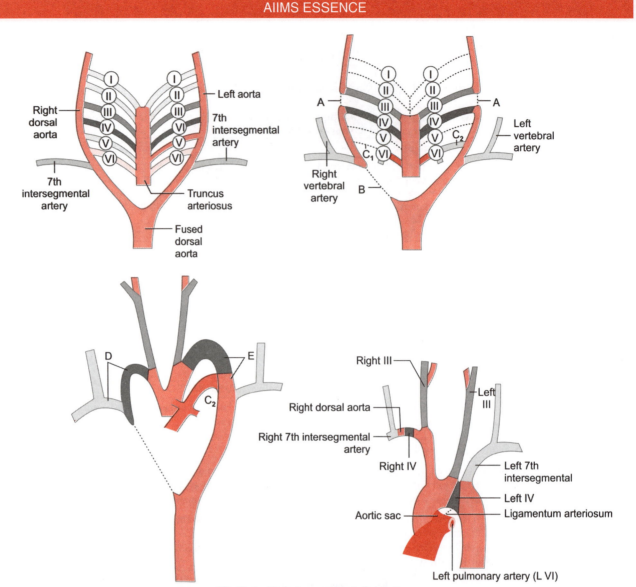

Fig. 2: Aortic Arches and their Derivatives

Anomalies of great arteries
• **Aberrant subclavian artery:** With **regression of right IV aortic arch & right dorsal aorta, right subclavian artery has an abnormal origin on left side, just below left subclavian artery**. To supply blood to right arm, this forces the **right subclavian artery to cross midline behind trachea & esophagus**, which **may constrict these organs**, although usually with no clinical symptoms[Q].
• **A double aortic arch:** Occurs with **development of an abnormal right aortic arch in addition to left aortic arch**, forming a **vascular ring around trachea & esophagus**, which causes **dyspnea & dysphagia**. Occasionally, **entire right dorsal aorta** abnormally **persists** & **left dorsal aorta regresses** in which case **right aorta** will have to arch **across from esophagus** causing **dyspnea or dysphagia**[Q].
• **Right-sided aortic arch**
• **Patent ductus arteriosus**
• **Coarctation of the aorta**

4. **Ans. d. D** *(Ref: Gray's 40/e p1015; Langman 11/e p161)*
Congenital diaphragmatic hernia is most frequently caused by failure of one or both of the pleuroperitoneal membranes (D) to close the pericardioperitoneal canals.

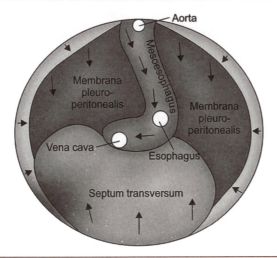

Development of Diaphragm

- **Septum transversum** →**Central tendon**[Q]
- **Pleuroperitoneal membranes** →Small **intermediate muscular portion**[Q]
- **Mesentery** of **esophagus** →**Crura**[Q]
- **Body wall** →**Peripheral muscular diaphragm**[Q]
- **Cervical myotomes** (muscular input)[Q]

Diaphragm

- Diaphragm is a **musculo tendinous, dome-shaped partition** between the thoracic & abdominal cavities
- **Develops from 4 major structures:** Septum transversum, pleuroperitoneal membranes, dorsal esophageal mesentery & body wall

Septum Transversum	Pleuroperitoneal Membranes	Dorsal Esophageal Mesentery	Body Wall
• **Septum transversum (most important component)** forms central tendon[Q] • First seen as a **thick mesodermal plate cranial to pericardial cavity**[Q] between base of thoracic cavity & stalk of yolk sac. • Septum **does not separate thoracic & abdominal cavities entirely**, but after the head fold forms (**week 4**), it becomes a **thick incomplete partition between the cavities**[Q] with an opening on each side of the gut, the pleural canals. • Septum fuses dorsally with **primitive mediastinal mesenchyme** below esophagus & later with pleuroperitoneal membranes[Q].	• Pleuroperitoneal membranes fuse with dorsal mesentery of esophagus & with dorsal part of septum transversum to complete the partition between thoracic & abdominopelvic cavities to form **primitive diaphragm**[Q]. • They represent only a **small portion of final adult structure**[Q].	• Dorsal esophageal mesentery (mesoesophagus) fuses with both & this mesentery forms median portion of diaphragm[Q]. • Crura of diaphragm develop from muscle fibers[Q], which grow into esophageal mesentery.	• The body wall: During **weeks 9-12**, pleural cavities enlarge & invade lateral body walls. Body wall tissue, at this time, splits off medially to form peripheral parts of diaphragm[Q] outside that formed by membranes. • Extensions of pleural cavities into body walls form costo-diaphragmatic recesses[Q].

Congenital Diaphragmatic Hernia (Bochdalek Hernia or Posterolateral Hernia)

- **CDH** term is used for **Bochdalek hernia**[Q]
  - **Incidence**: 1 in 2000 to 5000[Q] live births.
  - **Most CDH defects** are on the **left side (80%)**; up to **20%** on **right side**[Q].

Contd...

Contd...

Congenital Diaphragmatic Hernia (Bochdalek Hernia or Posterolateral Hernia)
• Exact **survival rate for CDH** is in the range of **70-90%**[Q].   • **Bag & Mask ventilation** is **contraindicated** in **CDH**[Q].

Pathogenesis:
 • **Caused by failure of one or both of pleuroperitoneal membranes to close pericardioperitoneal canals**[Q].
 • As a result, **abdominal contents herniate** through the resultant defect in the **posterolateral diaphragm** & **compress** the **ipsilateral developing lung**[Q].
      • **Posterolateral location** of this hernia is known as **Bochdalek hernia**[Q] and is distinguished from the congenital hernia of the **anteromedial, retrosternal** diaphragm, which is known as **Morgagni hernia**[Q].
 • **Compression** of lung results in **pulmonary hypoplasia** involving both lungs, with the **ipsilateral lung** being **most affected**[Q].
 • **Pulmonary vasculature** is distinctly **abnormal** in that the **medial muscular thickness** of **arterioles** is **excessive** & **extremely sensitive** to **multiple local & systemic factors** known to **trigger vasospasm**[Q].
      • **Main factors** affecting morbidity & mortality: **Pulmonary hypoplasia** >**pulmonary hypertension**[Q].

Clinical Features: • **Classic triad: Respiratory distress + Dextrocardia + Scaphoid abdomen**[Q]   • **MC presentation** is **respiratory distress** due to severe hypoxemia[Q].   • Infant appears dyspneic, tachypneic & cyanotic, with severe retractions.   • **Anteroposterior diameter** of chest may be **large** & **abdomen** may be **scaphoid**[Q].
Diagnosis: • **Diagnosis** is made at the time of a **prenatal ultrasound** during pregnancy.   • **Postnatal diagnosis** by a **plain chest radiograph** demonstrates **gastric air bubble** or **loops of bowel** within the **chest**[Q].   • There may also be a **mediastinal shift away** from the **side of hernia** or **polyhydramnios**[Q] from the obstructed stomach.   • **Pneumothorax** always occurs on **contralateral** to the **side of CDH**[Q].
Treatment: • **Physiologic stress** associated with **early repair** probably **adds more insult** and that **survival is not improved**[Q] when compared with delayed repair.   • A variable period of time (**24-72 hours**) to allow **for stabilization** before **surgical repair**[Q].   **Viscera are reduced into abdominal cavity & posterolateral defect in diaphragm is closed using interrupted, non-absorbable sutures**[Q].   • In **most cases (80%-90%)**, a **hernia sac** is **not present**. If **identified**, it is **excised** at the time of repair[Q].   • Advantage of a **prosthetic patch** is that a **tension-free repair** can be frequently obtained in **large defects**[Q].

Morgagni hernias (Retrosternal hernias or Larrey's hernia[Q]**)**

• **Congenital hernia** of **anteromedial, retrosternal diaphragm**[Q]
 • Occur in **triangular space** between the muscle fibers that make up the diaphragm
 • They extend from **xiphisternum** & **costal margin** to the central tendon of diaphragm[Q].
      • **Ninety percent** are **right sided**[Q] because pericardium itself prevents left-sided hernias
      • **Superior epigastric vessels** may **pass through Morgagni space**[Q]
      • **Most commonly involved viscus: Transverse colon**[Q]

Clinical Features: • Patients are **usually asymptomatic**[Q]
Diagnosis: • **Anterior mediastinal masses** are found incidentally on **chest radiographs**[Q].
Treatment: • **Prompt surgical repair** after diagnosis is prudent **to avoid incarceration** or **strangulation** of abdominal organs.   • A **transabdominal route**[Q] is the **preferred choice**.   • **Prosthetic mesh** is generally required **to repair the defect**[Q].

5. **Ans. c. C** *(Ref: Gray's 40/e p1121)*
   Parietal cell (C) secretes hydrochloric acid.

   "Parietal cells have copious pink cytoplasm and a central nucleus, giving them a "fried egg" appearance. In contrast, peptic cells have granular purple cytoplasm and basal nuclei."

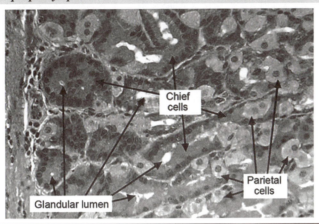

Types of Gastric gland

- **Gastric glands** are located in different regions of stomach (**fundic glands, cardiac glands & pyloric glands**).
- **Glands & gastric pits** are **located in stomach lining**.
- **Glands** are in lamina propria of mucous membrane & **open into bases of gastric pits** formed by epithelium.

Types of Gastric gland		
Cardiac glands	**Fundic or oxyntic glands**	**Pyloric glands**
• Found in **cardia of stomach**[Q] • Primarily **secrete mucus**[Q]. • **Fewer in number**[Q] than other gastric glands • More **shallowly positioned** in the mucosa.	• Found in **fundus & body**[Q] of stomach. • **Simple almost straight tubes**[Q], two or more of which open into a single duct. • **Secrete hydrochloric acid & intrinsic factor**[Q].	• Located in **antrum** • **Secrete gastrin** produced by **G cells**[Q].

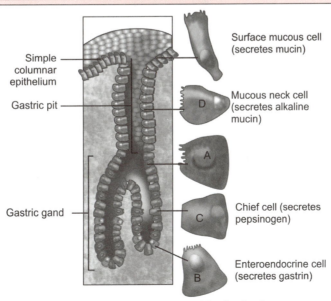

Fig. 3: Transverse section of fundic gland

Types of Gastric cells			
Chief cells	**Parietal cells**	**Entero chromaffin-like cells**	**G cells**
• Found in **basal**[Q] regions of gland • Release **pepsinogen**[Q] (precursor of pepsin).	• Found in walls of the tubes. • Secrete **hydrochloric acid & intrinsic factor**[Q]. • **Produce & release bicarbonate ions**[Q] in response to **histamine release from ECL cells**[Q], serve a **crucial role in the pH buffering system**[Q].	• **Store & release histamine**[Q] when the acidity of stomach becomes too high. • Release of histamine is stimulated by secretion of gastrin from G cells. • **Histamine promotes the production & release of bicarbonate ions from parietal cells** to the blood & **protons to stomach lumen**[Q]. • When stomach pH increases, ECL cells stop releasing histamine[Q].	• Mostly found in pyloric glands in antrum[Q] • G cells secrete gastrin[Q]. • Gastric pits of glands are much deeper than the others, hence, gastrin is secreted into bloodstream[Q] not the lumen.

6. **Ans. a. Spinal cord** *(Ref: Gray's 41/e p230, 40/e329-330)*

Marked area is caudate lobe (Part of basal ganglia), which receives afferents from all other areas of basal ganglia, thalamus as well as higher centres i.e. cerebral cortex, but not from the spinal cord.

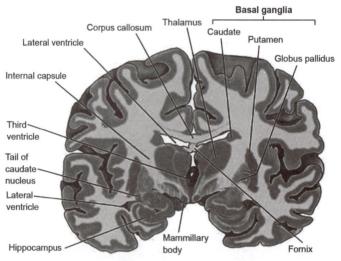

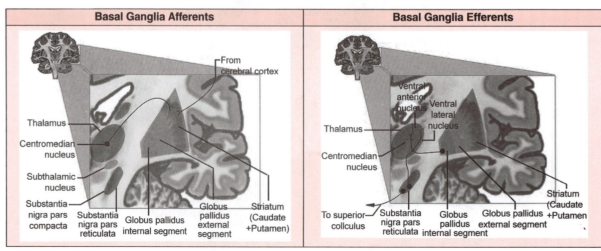

Basal Ganglia Afferents

- The **striatum** is **main recipient of afferents to the basal ganglia**[Q].
- These **excitatory afferents arise from entire cerebral cortex** & **from intralaminar nuclei of thalamus** (primarily the **centromedian nucleus & parafascicularis nucleus**)[Q].
  - **Frontal lobe projects predominantly to the caudate head & putamen**[Q]
  - **Parietal & occipital lobes project to caudate body; temporal lobe projects to caudate tail**[Q].
  - **Primary motor cortex & primary somatosensory cortex project mainly to putamen**[Q]
  - **Premotor cortex & supplementary motor areas project to caudate head**[Q].
- Other cortical areas project primarily to the caudate.
- **Along C-shaped extent of caudate nucleus, caudate cells receive their input from cortical regions** that are close by[Q].
- **Enlarged head of caudate** reflects the **large projection from frontal cortex to caudate**[Q].
- **Nucleus accumbens** (ventral striatum) **receives a large input from limbic cortex**[Q].
  - In the **motor regions of basal ganglia**, there is a **motor homunculus** similar to that **seen in the primary motor cortex**[Q].
  - **Projections from medial wall of the anterior paracentral lobule** (part of M1 that **contains a representation of legs & torso**) **innervate regions of striatum** that are next to the recipient zones from **dorsal surface of precentral gyrus** (part of M1 that contains a **representation of arms & hands**)[Q].
- **Projections from lateral surface of precentral gyrus** (part of M1 that contains a **representation of face**) **innervate regions that are next to arm & hand representation**[Q]. This topography of projections is maintained in the intrinsic circuitry of the basal ganglia.

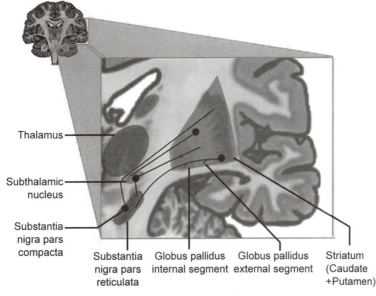

Fig. 4: Basal Ganglia Intrinsic Connections

7. **Ans. a. Tonsil** *(Ref: Gray's 40/e p567; Ross Histology 6/e p589)*

The given hematoxylin and eosin stained biopsy showing non-keratinized stratified squamous epithelium with lymphoid nodules in centre suggest that tissue is taken from tonsil.

Tonsil	Spleen
• **Lymphoid structures** located in **mucosa of tongue, palate & pharynx**[Q] • Provide sites where **immune surveillance cells**[Q] (lymphocytes) can **encounter foreign antigens** enter the body through the mouth or nose.	• **Largest lymphatic organ**[Q] • Capsule of **dense irregular connective tissue with trabeculae** dividing pulp incompletely[Q] • **White pulp with lymphoid nodules**[Q]

Tonsil	Spleen
• Each tonsil **consists of an epithelial crypt (invaginated pocket) surrounded by dense clusters of lymph nodules**, each **with a germinal center** where lymphocytes proliferate[Q] • **Nodules** are **embedded in a mass of diffuse lymphoid tissue** that consists of lymphocytes migrating to & from germinal centers[Q].	• **Red pulp** found **between sinusoids** has **reticular fibers, reticular epithelial cells & macrophages**[Q]

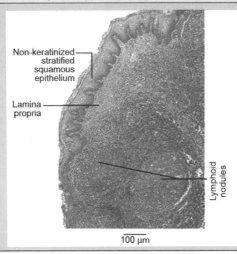

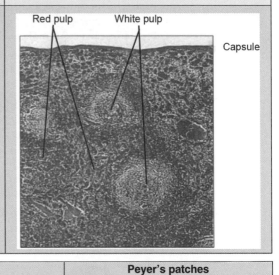

Lymph node	Peyer's patches
• **LNs** are **kidney or oval shaped** • Range from a **few millimeters to 1–2 cm** • **LN is surrounded by a fibrous capsule** • Inside LN, **fibrous capsule extends to form trabeculae.** • Divided into **outer cortex & inner medulla.**	• **Peyer's patches: Isolated clusters of lymphoid tissue**[Q] • **Found in wall of distal portion of the small intestine**[Q]
• **Cortex** is **continuous around medulla** except at **hilum**, where the **medulla comes in direct contact with hilum**[Q]. • **Thin reticular fibers & elastin form a supporting meshwork** called a reticular network inside the node[Q]. • **WBCs** are tightly packed in **follicles (B cells) & cortex (T cells).** • As part of reticular network there are **follicular dendritic cells in B cell follicle & fibroblastic reticular cells in T cell cortex.**	• Peyer's patches **destroy bacteria**, preventing them from breaching the intestinal wall • Generate **"memory" lymphocytes for long-term immunity**

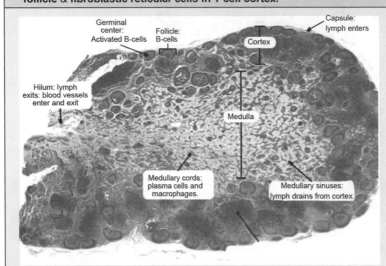

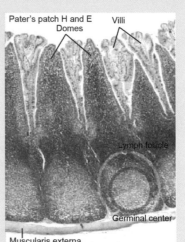

8. **Ans. c. Posterior Communicating Artery** *(Ref: Gray's 41/e p285, 40/e p248)*
Artery labeled with black arrow in the given diagram is posterior communicating artery.

Circle of Willis

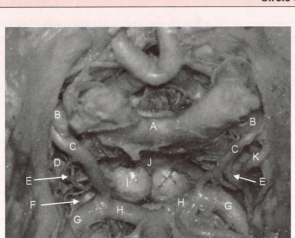
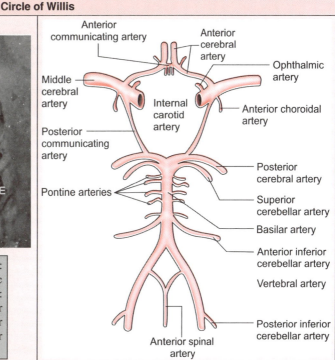

A: Optic chiasm, B: Internal carotid artery, C: **Posterior communicating artery,** D: Optic tract, E: Anterior thalamoperforating arteries, F: Cerebral peduncle, G: P2 segment of posterior cerebral artery, H: P1 segment of posterior cerebral artery, I: Mammillary body, J: Tuber cinereum, K: Anterior choroidal artery

Circle of Willis

Circle of Willis is the part of cerebral circulation & composed of

- Anterior cerebral artery[Q] (left & right)
- Anterior communicating artery[Q]
- Internal carotid artery[Q] (left & right)
- Posterior cerebral artery[Q] (left & right)
- Posterior communicating artery[Q] (left & right)
- Basilar artery[Q]

- Middle cerebral arteries are not considered part of the circle[Q].

Origin of arteries
- **Left & right internal carotid arteries** arise from **left & right common carotid arteries**[Q].
- **Posterior communicating artery** is given off as a **branch of internal carotid artery** just before it divides into its terminal branches, anterior & middle cerebral arteries.

- **Anterior cerebral artery** forms **anterolateral portion of circle of Willis**[Q]
- **Middle cerebral artery does not contribute** to the circle.

- Right & left posterior cerebral arteries arise **from basilar artery**, formed by left & right vertebral arteries.
- Vertebral arteries arise **from subclavian arteries**.
- **Anterior communicating artery connects** the **two anterior cerebral arteries** and could be said to arise from either the left or right side.

- **All arteries** involved give off **cortical & central branches**.
- **Central branches** supply the **interior of the circle of Willis**, more specifically, the **Interpeduncular fossa**.
- **Cortical branches** are named for the area they supply.

9. **Ans. b. Epiphyses** *(Ref: Ross Histology 6/e p203; Gray's 40/e p82)*
Image of hyaline cartilage is given. Epiphyseal plate is a layer of hyaline cartilage.

"Hyaline cartilage has a homogeneous glassy, bluish opalescent appearance. It has a firm consistency and some elasticity. Costal, nasal, some laryngeal, tracheobronchial, all temporary (developmental) and most articular, cartilages are hyaline." - Gray's 40/e p82

"Hyaline cartilage consists of cells (chondrocytes) of a rounded or bluntly angular form, lying in groups of two or more in a granular or almost homogeneous matrix. Chondrocytes are cartilage cells that produce the matrix. When arranged in groups of two or more, chondrocytes have generally straight outlines where they are in contact with each other, and in the rest of their circumference are rounded. They consist of clear translucent protoplasm in which fine interlacing filaments and minute granules are sometimes present; embedded in this are one or two round nuclei, having the usual intranuclear network."

"Articular disc is a type of fibrocartilage although articular cartilage is a type of hyaline cartilage."

"Cartilage is composed of specialized cells called chondrocytes that produce a large amount of collagenous extracellular matrix, abundant ground substance that is rich in proteoglycan and elastin fibers. Cartilage is classified in three types, elastic cartilage, hyaline cartilage and fibrocartilage, which differ in relative amounts of cartilage. Chondroblasts that get caught in the matrix are called chondrocytes."

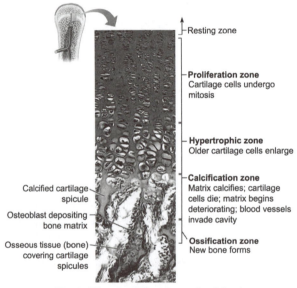

Fig. 5: Microscopic anatomy of epiphysis

Types of Cartilage		
Elastic cartilage	Fibrocartilage	Hyaline cartilage
• Highly flexible due to elastic fibres[Q] • Provides support, tolerates distortion without damage[Q] • Returns to original shape[Q]	• Cartilage matrix with type 1 collagen fibres to withstand stress[Q] • Resist compression • Prevent bone to bone contact • Limits relative movement	• Most abundant & common • All long bones (except clavicle) are preformed in hyaline cartilage (endochondral ossification) • Tendency to calcify > 40 years (except articular cartilage) • All hyaline cartilages are covered by perichondrium except articular cartilages
• Auricle[Q] • Auditory tube[Q] • Corniculate[Q] laryngeal cartilage[Q]	• Articular disc[Q] • Symphysis pubis[Q] • Glenoid labrum[Q] (shoulder joint)	• Arytenoid • Articular cartilage[Q] (most synovial joints)

Contd...

Contd...

Locations	Locations	Locations
• Cuneiform laryngeal cartilage[Q] • External auditory meatus (lateral part) • Epiglottis[Q] • Apex of arytenoid cartilage[Q] • Inlet of larynx[Q]	• Acetabular labrum[Q] (hip joint) • Menisci[Q] • Sternoclavicular joint[Q] • Temporomandibular joint[Q] • Inferior radio-ulnar joint[Q]	• Larynx (arytenoid lower end & cricoid cartilage)[Q] • Costal cartilage[Q] • Thyroid cartilage[Q] • Tracheobronchial cartilage[Q] • Nose (septum & lateral wall)[Q] • Epiphyseal plate[Q] • Embryonic cartilage[Q]

10. **Ans. a. Holocrine glands**   *(Ref: Gray's 40/e p153; Ross Histology 6/e p147)*
    The given histologic image is of sebaceous glands, which is a type of holocrine gland.

    "Sebaceous glands are small saccular structures lying in the dermis; together with the hair follicle and arrector pili muscle, they constitute the pilosebaceous unit. They are present over the whole body except the thick hairless skin of the palm, soles and flexor surfaces of digits. Typically, they consist of a cluster of secretory acini, which open by a short common duct into the dermal pilary canal of the hair follicle. They release their lipid secretory product, sebum, into the canal by a holocrine mechanism. In some areas of thin skin which lack hair follicles, their ducts open instead directly on to the skin surface, e.g. on the lips and corners of the mouth, the buccal mucosa, nipples, female breast areolae, penis, inner surface of the prepuce, clitoris and labia minora. At the margins of the eyelids, the large complex palpebral tarsal glands (Meibomian glands) are of this type. They are also present in the external auditory meatus." - Gray's 40/e p153

Sebaceous Glands

• Sebaceous glands **empty their secretory product into upper parts of hair follicles**.
• Found in **parts of the skin where hair is present (Exception: Lips, oral surfaces of cheeks & external genitalia**, sebaceous glands are present without hair)[Q]
• Pilosebaceous unit: **Hair follicle** & its **associated sebaceous gland**
• Sebaceous glands are **simple & branched**
• Secretory portion consists of **alveoli**.
   • **Basal cells** in outermost layer of alveolus **are flattened. Basal cells are mitotically active**.
   • Some of the **new cells** will **replenish the pool of basal cells**, while the remaining cells are displaced towards the centre of alveolus as more cells are generated by basal cells.
   • **Secretory cells** will gradually **accumulate lipids & grow in size**[Q].
   • Finally their **nuclei disintegrate & cells rupture**.
   • **Resulting secretory product of lipids & constituents of the disintegrating cell is a holocrine secretion**.

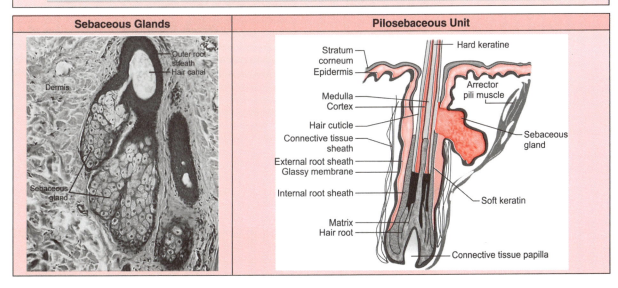

"*Exocrine glands* secrete their products through a duct onto an outer surface of the body, such as the skin or the human gastrointestinal tract. Secretion is directly onto the apical surface. The glands in this group can be divided into three groups: Apocrine glands, holocrine glands & merocrine glands."

Types of Glands		
Apocrine glands	**Holocrine glands**	**Eccrine (Merocrine) glands**

• **Apical part of cell is shed off to discharge secretion** (decapitation[Q] secretion).
 • **Responds** mainly **to sympathetic adrenergic stimuli**[Q]
 • **Becomes functional at puberty**[Q]
 • **Example:** Apocrine **sweat glands in axilla & groin, mammary glands; external auditory canal (ceruminous gland)**[Q] **& eyelids (gland of Moll)**[Q]
	• **Whole cell disintegrates**[Q] discharging secretion.
	 • **Found throughout skin except palms & soles.**
	 • **Sebaceous glands** are **usually associated with hair follicles** except in following locations:
	  – **Gland of Zeis & Meibomian gland**[Q] in eyelids
	  – **Montgomery tubercle**[Q]: Nipple & areola
	  – **Tyson's**[Q] **gland:** External fold of prepuce
	  – **Fordyce**[Q] spot: vermillion border of lips & mucosa
		• Cell is intact & **secretions are thrown out by exocytosis**[Q].
		 • **Example:** Sweat gland on palms & soles[Q].
		 • Found everywhere except clitoris, gland penis, labia minora, external auditory canal & lips[Q].

(a) Merocrine secretion	(b) Apocrine secretion	(c) Holocrine secretion

11. **Ans. a. Ulnar nerve** *(Ref: Gray's 40/e p837, 888)*

    Hyperextension of 4th and 5th metacarpophalangeal joint with flexion at proximal interphalangeal joint is suggestive of claw hand. This deformity is due to injury of deep branch of ulnar nerve.

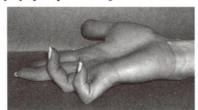

Fig. 6: Ulnar claw hand

"Division of the nerve at the elbow paralyses flexor carpi ulnaris, flexor digitorum profundus to the ring and little fingers and all the intrinsic muscles of the hand (apart from the radial two lumbricals). The clawing of the hand is less intense than occurs after division of the ulnar nerve at the wrist, reflecting the imbalance in action between the long flexors and extensors to the ring and little fingers when finger flexion is produced only by superficialis. In addition there is sensory loss over the little finger and the ulnar half of the ring finger." - *Gray's 40/e p837*

Claw Hand

• Hand shows hyperextension of metacarpophalangeal joints (MCP) & flexion of distal & proximal interphalangeal (IP) joints of 4th & 5th digits (ring & little finger)[Q].
 • Clawing becomes most obvious when the person is asked to flex the digits from an extended position as the 4th & 5th digits cannot flex due to injury to ulnar nerve[Q].
   ○ **1st, 2nd & 3rd digits will partially flex giving them a 'claw-like' appearance.** This happens because **thenar muscles (Abductor pollicis brevis, flexor pollicis brevis & opponens pollicis)** are **innervated by median nerve** as **first two lumbricals of digits 2 & 3 are**[Q].
   ○ An **ulnar claw may follow an ulnar nerve lesion**, which results in **partial or complete denervation of ulnar (medial) two lumbricals of hand**[Q].

Contd...

Contd...

Claw Hand

- Since the ulnar nerve also supplies 3rd & 4th lumbricals, which flex MCP joints, their denervation causes these joints to become extended by the now unopposed action of the long finger extensors[Q] (namely extensor digitorum & extensor digiti minimi).
  - **Lumbricals & interossei** also **extend interphalangeal joints of the fingers** by insertion into the extensor hood; their **paralysis results in weakened extension**[Q].
  - **Combination of hyperextension at MCP & flexion at IP joints** gives the hand its **claw-like appearance**[Q].

Ulnar Paradox

- The **ulnar nerve also innervates the ulnar (medial) half of the** flexor digitorum profundus **(FDP) muscle**[Q].
- If the **ulnar nerve lesion occurs more proximal (closer to the elbow), the flexor digitorum profundus muscle may also be denervated**[Q].
  - As a result, **flexion of the IP joints is weakened, which reduces the claw-like appearance of the hand**[Q].
  - Instead, **4th & 5th fingers** are **simply paralyzed in their fully extended position**.
  - This is called the **'ulnar paradox'** because **one would normally expect a more proximal**, and thus, **debilitating injury to result in a more deformed appearance**[Q].

	Ulnar claw hand	Median claw hand (Hand of benediction)
Nerve involved	Lesion of ulnar nerve at wrist[Q]	Lesion of median nerve at elbow or wrist[Q]
Typical presentation	Appears in long-standing cases of nerve damage[Q]	Appears when the patient attempts to make a fist[Q]
Digits affected	Little & ring fingers[Q]	Middle & index fingers[Q]
Muscles paralyzed	Medial two lumbricals[Q]	Lateral half of flexor digitorum profundus Lateral two lumbricals[Q]
Movements involved	Unopposed extension at MCP joints[Q] Unopposed flexion at IP joints[Q]	Inability to perform flexion at MCP & IP joints of middle & index fingers[Q]

12. **Ans. a. A** *(Ref: Gray's 41/e p571, 40/e p585)*

The only abductor of the larynx is posterior cricoarytenoid muscle, which is the posterior most muscle. All other muscles are adductors of the vocal cords.

A: Posterior cricoarytenoid muscle; B: Cricothyroid muscle; C: Lateral cricoarytenoid muscle; D: Oblique & transverse arytenoid muscle

> "The posterior cricoarytenoids are the only laryngeal muscles that open (abduct) the glottis. They rotate the arytenoid cartilages laterally around an axis that passes through the cricoarytenoid joints, producing separation of the vocal processes and the attached vocal cords. They also pull the arytenoids backwards, assisting the cricothyroids to lengthen the vocal cords. The most lateral fibres draw the arytenoid cartilages laterally, and so the rima glottidis becomes triangular when the posterior cricoarytenoid muscles contract. The posterior cricoarytenoids are active in the production of unvoiced sounds." - *Gray's 40/e p585*

Anatomy of Larynx

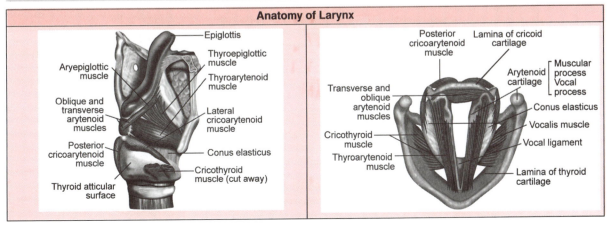

Posterior Cricoarytenoid Muscle

- Arises from posterior surface of cricoid lamina[Q].
- Its fibres **ascend laterally & converge to insert on the upper & posterior surfaces of muscular process of the ipsilateral arytenoid cartilage**[Q].
- Highest fibres run almost horizontally, middle obliquely & lowest are almost vertical[Q]

Vascular supply:
- Laryngeal branches of superior & inferior thyroid arteries[Q].

Innervation:
- Recurrent laryngeal nerve[Q]

Actions:
- Posterior cricoarytenoids are the **only laryngeal muscles that open (abductors of) the glottis**.
- Pull the arytenoids backwards, assisting the cricothyroids to lengthen the vocal cords.

Larynx Anatomy

- **Extent: From C3 to lower border of C6** where it is continuous with the trachea[Q].
- **Rima glottidis: Narrowest part of larynx in adults**[Q]; **Subglottis: Narrowest part of larynx in children**[Q]
- **Inlet of larynx** is formed by **free edge of epiglottis (anteriorly), aryepiglottic folds (sides)** & **mucus membrane over the interarytenoid fold (posteriorly)**[Q].

> - **Superior laryngeal vessels & internal laryngeal nerve pierce thyrohyoid membrane**[Q].
> - **Cricoarytenoid & cricothyroid joints are synovial joints**[Q].
> - **Delphian nodes: Prelaryngeal LN**[Q]

Laryngeal Skeleton (Consist of 9 cartilages)

Three single	Three paired
- **Thyroid cartilage: Largest laryngeal cartilage**[Q] - **Cricoid cartilage: Ring of hyaline cartilage; only incomplete ring of cartilage around trachea; "signet ring" shaped**[Q]. - **Epiglottis: Elastic cartilage**[Q]	- **Arytenoid**[Q] - **Corniculate**[Q] - **Cuneiform**[Q]

> - **Hyaline cartilage: Thyroid, cricoid & basal part of arytenoid cartilages**[Q] (may **ossify after 25 years**)
> - **Other cartilages of larynx** are made of **elastic cartilage (do not ossify**[Q])

Intrinsic Muscles of Larynx

Action	Intrinsic muscles
- Abductor of vocal cords (opens the glottis)	- **Posterior cricoarytenoid**[Q]
- **Adductor of vocal cords (close the glottis)**	- **Thyroarytenoid**[Q] - **Transverse arytenoid**[Q] - **Lateral cricoarytenoid**[Q]
- Tensors of vocal cords	- **Cricothyroid**[Q] - **Thyroarytenoid**[Q]
- Openers of laryngeal inlet	- **Thyroepiglottic**[Q] (part of thyroarytenoid)
- Closers of laryngeal inlet	- **Interarytenoid**[Q] (oblique & posterior oblique part)

Nerve Supply of Larynx

Motor	Sensory
- **All intrinsic muscles of larynx are supplied by the recurrent laryngeal nerve (RLN) except cricothyroid**[Q] - **Cricothyroid** is supplied by **external laryngeal branch of the superior laryngeal nerve**[Q] (SLN).	- **Up to vocal fold: Internal laryngeal nerve**[Q] - **Below vocal fold: Recurrent laryngeal nerve**[Q]

> - **Galen anastomosis** is a **connection between RLN & internal branch of SLN**[Q].
> - **Human communicating nerve** is an **anastomosis between external branch of SLN & distal RLN**[Q].

AIIMS May 2016   **1039**

13. **Ans. c.** C   *(Ref: Gray's 41/e p383, 40/e p346)*

Insula is located deep in lateral sulcus of cerebral cortex.

> *"The insula lies deep in the floor of the lateral fissure, almost surrounded by a circular sulcus, and overlapped by adjacent cortical areas, the opercula. The frontal operculum is between the anterior and ascending rami of the lateral fissure, forming a triangular division of the inferior frontal gyrus. The frontoparietal operculum, between ascending and posterior rami of the lateral fissure, consists of the posterior part of the inferior frontal gyrus, the lower ends of the precentral and postcentral gyri, and the lower end of the anterior part of the inferior parietal lobule. The temporal operculum, below the posterior ramus of the lateral fissure, is formed by superior temporal and transverse temporal gyri. Anteriorly, the inferior region of the insula adjoins the orbital part of the inferior frontal gyrus."*
> *- Gray's 40/e p346*

Insular cortex
• **Portion of cerebral cortex folded deep within the lateral sulcus** (fissure separating temporal lobe from parietal & frontal lobes).
• Insulae are believed to be involved in consciousness & play a role in diverse functions usually linked to **emotion** or **regulation of body's homeostasis**.
• Functions include perception, motor control, self-awareness, cognitive functioning & interpersonal experience.
• Cortical area overlying the insula toward the lateral surface of brain is the operculum. **Opercula** are formed **from parts of enclosing frontal, temporal & parietal lobes.**

Insular Cortex Connections
• **Anterior part of insula** is **subdivided by shallow sulci** into three or four **short gyri**.
• Anterior insula **receives a direct projection from basal part of ventral medial nucleus** of **thalamus** & a particularly large input from **central nucleus of amygdala**.
• Anterior insula itself projects to the amygdala.
• Posterior part of the insula is formed by a **long gyrus**.
• **Posterior insula connects** reciprocally **with secondary somatosensory cortex & receives input from spinothalamically activated ventral posterior inferior thalamic nuclei.** This region also **receives inputs from ventromedial nucleus** of thalamus that are highly specialized to convey homeostatic information such as pain, temperature, itch, local oxygen status & sensual touch[Q].
• **'Circular sulcus of insula'** (or **sulcus of Reil**) is a **semi-circular sulcus or fissure** that **separates insula from neighboring gyri of operculum in the front, above & behind**[Q].

14. **Ans. d.** Greater auricular nerve   *(Ref: Gray's 41/e p407, 413, 40/e p435)*

The skin over the angle of mandible is supplied by the greater auricular nerve, which carries branches from anterior ramus of C2 and C3.

> *"The great auricular nerve is the largest ascending branch of the cervical plexus. It arises from the second and third cervical rami, encircles the posterior border of sternocleidomastoid, perforates the deep fascia and ascends on the muscle beneath platysma with the external jugular vein. On reaching the parotid gland, it divides into anterior and posterior branches. The anterior branch is distributed to the facial skin over the parotid gland and connects in the gland with the facial nerve. This cross innervation between somatic sensory supply (great auricular) and para-sympathetic secretomotor fibres to the parotid is considered to be part of the anatomical basis for the phenomenon of gustatory sweating (Frey's syndrome) seen after parotid surgery, when the nerve is at risk of injury. The posterior branch supplies the skin over the mastoid process and on the back of the auricle (except its upper part); a filament pierces the auricle to reach the lateral surface where it is distributed to the lobule and concha. The posterior branch communicates with the lesser occipital nerve, the auricular branch of the vagus and the posterior auricular branch of the facial nerve."*
> *- Gray's 40/e p435*

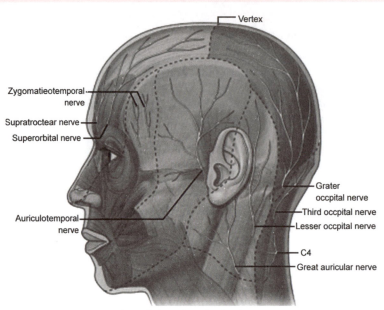

Fig. 7: Sensory supply of face

Sensory Supply of Face

- **Ophthalmic nerve (V_1)** carries **sensory information from scalp & forehead, upper eyelid, conjunctiva & cornea, nose** (including **tip of nose, except alae nasi**), **nasal mucosa, frontal sinuses & parts of meninges (dura & blood vessels)**[Q].

Branches of Ophthalmic Nerve	
Supraorbital nerve	• This nerve **branches from frontal nerve**[Q] (largest branch of ophthalmic nerve) • **Innervates frontal sinus, upper eyelid & anterolateral part of forehead & scalp**[Q].
Supratrochlear nerve	• Branching from **frontal nerve**[Q] • **Innervates medial superior eyelid & anteromedial forehead**[Q].
Lacrimal nerve	• Branches from **ophthalmic nerve**[Q] • **Innervates lacrimal gland & lateral part of superior eyelid**[Q].
Infratrochlear nerve	• Branching off the **nasociliary nerve**[Q] • **Innervates skin just lateral to nose, medial-most parts of eyelids, lacrimal sac & lacrimal caruncle**[Q].
External nasal nerve	• Branches from **anterior ethmoidal nerve**[Q] • **Innervates the skin of nose**[Q].

- **Maxillary nerve (V_2)** carries **sensory information from lower eyelid & cheek, nares & upper lip, upper teeth & gums, nasal mucosa, palate & roof of pharynx, maxillary, ethmoid & sphenoid sinuses & parts of meninges**[Q].

Branches of Maxillary Nerve	
Infraorbital nerve	• Comes from **maxillary nerve**[Q] & runs through orbit • **Innervates maxillary sinus, maxillary teeth, inferior eyelid, skin of cheek, lateral nose, nasal septum & upper lip**[Q].
Zygomaticofacial nerve	• Branching from **zygomatic nerve**[Q] • **Innervates skin on cheek**[Q]
Zygomaticotemporal nerve	• Branches off the **zygomatic nerve**[Q] • **Innervates the skin over temple**[Q].

- **Mandibular nerve (V_3)** carries sensory information from **lower lip, lower teeth & gums, chin & jaw (except angle of jaw, which is supplied by C2-C3), parts of external ear & parts of meninges**[Q].
- Mandibular nerve carries **touch-position & pain-temperature sensations from mouth**[Q].
- One of its branches, **lingual nerve carries sensation from tongue**[Q].

Contd...

Contd...

Sensory Supply of Face		
Branches of Mandibular Nerve		
Auriculotemporal nerve	• Branching off the **mandibular nerve**[Q] near middle meningeal artery • Innervates the skin in posterior part of temporal region, skin of auricle, external acoustic meatus & external surface of tympanic membrane[Q].	
Buccal nerve	• Branches from **mandibular nerve**[Q] • Innervates skin & mucosa of cheek & part of gums[Q].	
Mental nerve	• Branches from **inferior alveolar nerve**[Q] • Innervates skin of chin & inside of lower lip[Q].	
Branches of Upper Cervical Spinal Nerves		
Great auricular nerve	• Branches from anterior rami of **2nd & 3rd cervical spinal nerves**[Q] • Innervates skin over the angle of mandible, parotid gland & earlobe[Q].	
Lesser occipital nerve	• Branches from anterior rami of **2nd & 3rd cervical spinal nerves**[Q] • Innervates scalp behind the ear[Q].	
Greater occipital nerve	• Branching off the posterior ramus of the **2nd cervical spinal nerves**[Q] • Innervates scalp of occipital area[Q].	
3rd occipital nerve:	• Branches off the posterior ramus of **3rd cervical nerve**[Q] • Innervates scalp in occipital & sub occipital areas[Q].	

15. **Ans. c. The cervical esophagus drains directly into the right brachiocephalic vein** *(Ref: Gray's 41/e p1111, 40/e p950)*
    Cervical part of esophagus is drained into inferior thyroid vein, not the right brachiocephalic vein.

    *"**Venous** blood from the esophagus drains into a submucosal plexus. From the **cervical esophagus**, veins drain into the **inferior thyroid vein**. From **the thoracic esophagus**, veins drain into **the azygos veins, hemiazygos**, intercostal, and bronchial veins. From the **abdominal portion**, esophagus veins drain into the **left gastric vein**."- Esophagus Anatomy by B. Viswanatha*

    *"**Venous drainage of esophagus: Cervical part is drained by inferior thyroid vein. Thoracic part is drained by azygous and hemiazygous veins. Abdominal part is drained by two venous channels, hemiazygous vein and left gastric vein."- Textbook of Anatomy by Vishram Singh (2014)/298*

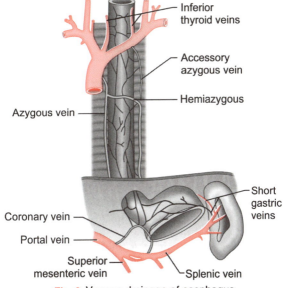

Fig. 8: Venous drainage of esophagus

AIIMS ESSENCE

Blood supply of the esophagus		
Part of esophagus	Arterial supply	Venous drainage
Cervical part	• Inferior thyroid artery[Q]	• Inferior thyroid veins[Q]
Thoracic part	• Branches from **descending thoracic aorta**[Q]	• Azygous vein[Q] • Hemiazygous vein[Q]
Abdominal part	• Branches from **left gastric artery**[Q]	• Hemiazygous vein[Q] • Left gastric vein[Q]

PHYSIOLOGY

16. Ans. c. Cis Golgi network   *(Ref: Ganong 25/e p44, 24/e p46)*

The arrow on the electron micrograph is pointing on the Golgi Network. In all eukaryotes, each Golgi cisternal stack has a cis entry face and a trans exit face. These faces are characterized by unique morphology and biochemistry. The end marked is towards the side of the Nucleus, hence the cis-side of the Golgi. Medial cisterna is a part of cis-Golgi network, seen only in some Protistans.

*"The Golgi apparatus is a polarized structure, with cis and trans sides. Membranous vesicles containing newly synthesized proteins bud off from the granular endoplasmic reticulum and fuse with the cistern on the cis side of the apparatus. The proteins are then passed via other vesicles to the middle cisterns and finally to the cistern on the trans side, from which vesicles branch off into the cytoplasm. From the trans Golgi, vesicles shuttle to the lysosomes and to the cell exterior via constitutive and non-constitutive pathways, both involving exocytosis. Conversely, vesicles are pinched off from the cell membrane by **endocytosis** and pass to endosomes. From there, they are recycled." - Ganong 25/e p44*

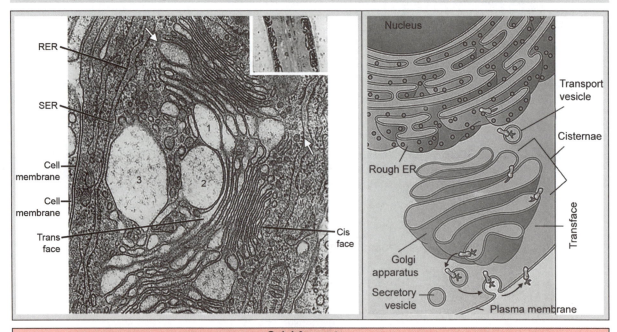

Golgi Apparatus

- **Golgi apparatus** is a **collection of membrane-enclosed sacs (cisternae)** that are **stacked like dinner plates**[Q].
- **Present in all eukaryotic cells**, usually **near the nucleus**[Q].
- Much of the organization of the Golgi is **directed at proper glycosylation of proteins & lipids**[Q].

  - **Golgi apparatus** is a **polarized structure**, with **cis & trans sides**[Q].
  - **Membranous vesicles containing newly synthesized proteins** bud off from granular endoplasmic reticulum & **fuse with cistern on the cis side of apparatus**[Q].
  - **Proteins** are then **passed via other vesicles to middle cisterns & finally to the cistern on the trans side, from which vesicles branch off into cytoplasm**[Q].

Contd...

Contd...

Golgi Apparatus

- From the **trans Golgi**, **vesicles shuttle to the lysosomes** & to the cell exterior via constitutive & non-constitutive pathways, both involving **exocytosis**. Conversely, vesicles are pinched off from cell membrane by **endocytosis** & pass to endosomes. From there, they are recycled.

  - Enzymes catalyzing early modifications are gathered in the cis face cisternae & enzymes catalyzing later modifications are found in trans face cisternae of the Golgi stacks[Q].

Functions of Golgi Complex

  - **Post-translational modification** of proteins; **Protein sorting & packaging**; Membrane recycling[Q]

17. **Ans. c. The protein has 1 functional ion**   (Ref: http://vlab.amrita.edu/?sub=3&brch=63&sim=1336&cnt=1)

The given titration curve is of a typical amino acid, either a biprotic or triprotic one, but certainly not a monoprotic amino acid. All amino acids are at least biprotic.

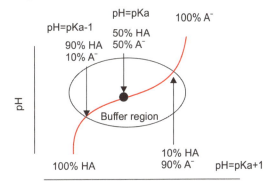

Titration Curve of Amino Acids

- Titration curves are obtained when the pH of given volume of a sample solution varies after successive addition of acid or alkali.
- The curves are usually **plots of pH against the volume of titrant added** or more correctly against the number of equivalents added per mole of the sample.
- Precise number of each characteristic depends on the nature of acid being titrated: Number of ionizing groups, pKa of ionizing group & buffer region.
- Amino acids are weak polyprotic acids. They are **present as Zwitter ions at neutral pH** and are **amphoteric molecules** that can be **titrated with both acid & alkali**.
- All amino acids have an acidic group (COOH) & a basic group (NH_2) attached to α carbon & contain **ionizable groups** that act as weak acids or bases, giving off or taking on protons when the pH is altered.

  - **Strong positive charge on amino group induces a tendency for carboxylic acid group to lose a proton**, so amino acids are considered to be strong acids.
  - When an **amino acid is dissolved in water** it exists predominantly in the **isoelectric form**.
  - **Isoelectric point (pI): pH of an aqueous solution of an amino acid at which the molecules have no net charge**.

- When the **dissolved amino acid is titrated with acid, it acts as a base** & with base, it acts as an acid which makes them an amphoteric molecule.
- These ionizations follow the Henderson-Hasselbalch equation:

Contd...

Contd...

Titration Curve of Amino Acids

$$pH = pKa + \log \frac{[Unprotonated\ form\ (base)]}{[Protonated\ form\ (acid)]}$$
• **When the concentration of unprotonated form equals that of unprotonated form, ratio of their concentrations equals 1, and log 1=0.**
   • **pKa:** pH at which **concentrations of protonated & unprotonated forms of ionizable species are equal** (pH at which ionizable group is at its best buffering capacity)
   • **pK:** pH at the midpoint of buffering region (pK is the pH corresponding to inflection point in titration curve)
   • **For a simple diprotic amino acid**, pI falls halfway between two pK values.
• For **acidic amino acids, pI is given by ½(pK1 + pK2)** & for **basic amino acids pI is ½(pK2 + pK3)**.
• In this experiment we are finding out the **titration curve of amino acid Glycine**.
 	
$$H_3N^+ - \underset{R}{\overset{H}{C_\alpha}} - COOH$$
 	
• **Glycine is a diprotic amino acid** (two dissociable protons, one on α amino group & other on carboxyl group). **In Glycine, R group does not contribute a dissociable proton.**
 	
Dissociation 1:
$$H_3N^+ - \underset{R}{\overset{H}{C_\alpha}} - COOH \rightleftharpoons H_3N^+ - \underset{R}{\overset{H}{C_\alpha}} - COO^- + H^+$$
 	
Dissociation 2:
$$H_3N^+ - \underset{R}{\overset{H}{C_\alpha}} - COO^- \rightleftharpoons H_2N - \underset{R}{\overset{H}{C_\alpha}} - COO^- - H^+$$
 	
• Dissociation of proton proceeds in a certain order, which depends on acidity of proton: **one which is most acidic & having a lower pKa will dissociate first**. So, the H+ on the **α-COOH group (pKa1) will dissociate before that on the α-NH₃ group (pKa2)**.

18. **Ans. a. Glucose** *(Ref: Harper 30/e p486)*
 The given graph is similar to the Michealis-Menton Curve for enzyme kinetics, hence describes carrier-mediated transport with saturation kinetics. Among the options, only Glucose shows facilitated diffusion via carriers (SGLT & GLUT). Others are transported by simple diffusion showing a straight line without saturation.

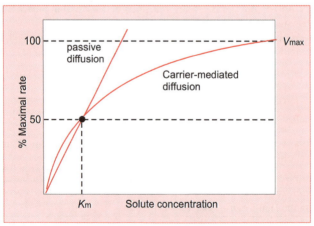

Fig. 9: Kinetics of carrier-mediated (facilitated) diffusion with passive diffusion

Contd...

Simple diffusion	Flow of solute from a higher to a lower concentration due to random thermal movement[Q].
Facilitated diffusion	• **Passive transport** of a solute from a higher concentration to a lower concentration, **mediated by a specific protein transporter**[Q]. • **Rate** of transport is **not always proportionate to** the **concentration gradient** because it is **mediated through carrier proteins**[Q].
Active transport	• **Transport of a solute** across a membrane **in the direction of increasing concentration & requires energy** (frequently derived from the **hydrolysis of ATP**); a **specific transporter or pump** is involved[Q].

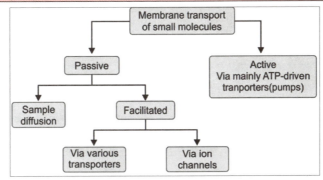

Feature	Simple diffusion	Facilitated diffusion	Active transport
Concentration/ Electrochemical gradient	**Along** the concentration gradient[Q]	**Along** the concentration gradient[Q]	**Against the concentration gradient**[Q]
Direction	**Bidirectional**[Q]	**Bidirectional**[Q]	**Unidirectional**[Q]
Transport protein	Not required	**Required**[Q]	**Required**[Q]
Energy (ATP) expenditure	Not required	Not required	**Required**[Q]
Saturation	No	Yes[Q]	Yes[Q]
Specificity	No	Yes[Q]	Yes[Q]
Rate of transport	**Proportionate** to concentration gradient[Q]	**Proportionate** only **at low concentrations** before carrier proteins become saturated[Q]	**Not proportionate** to concentration gradient[Q]
Competitive inhibition	Not inhibited[Q]	**Inhibited**[Q]	**Inhibited**[Q]
Example	Diffusion of O_2 & CO_2 in lungs[Q]	**Glucose uptake by muscles**[Q]	Na^+/K^+ ATPase[Q] H^+/K^+ ATPase[Q]

19. **Ans. c. Thyroxine** *(Ref: Ganong 25/e p300, 24/e p300; Harper 30/e p501)*
Thyroxine is a lipophilic hormone that acts on nuclear receptor.

"Steroids and thyroid hormones are distinguished by their predominantly intracellular sites of action, since they can diffuse freely through the cell membrane. They bind to a family of largely cytoplasmic proteins known as nuclear receptors. Upon ligand binding, the receptor–ligand complex translocates to the nucleus where it either homodimerizes, or associates with a distinct liganded nuclear receptor to form a heterodimer. In either case, the **dimer binds to DNA to either increase or decrease gene transcription in the target tissue.**"- *Ganong 25/e p300*

Classification of Hormones by Mechanism of Action					
Bind to intracellular receptor	**Bind to cell surface receptor**				
	Second messenger				
Cytoplasmic Receptors	c-AMP	c-GMP	Ca^{2+}/Phosphatidyl inositol	Kinase/ Phosphatase	
• Glucocorticoids[Q] • Mineralocorticoids[Q] • Androgens, estrogen & progestins[Q]	• Calcitonin[Q] • Glucagon[Q] • LH & FSH[Q] • Norepinephrine[Q]	• ANF[Q] • NO[Q]	• α_1 adrenergic • Angiotensin II • Oxytocin • GnRH	• Insulin[Q] • GH[Q] • EGF, FGF • IGF I & II	

Contd...

Contd...

Classification of Hormones by Mechanism of Action				
• Retinoic acid (retinoids)[Q] • Vitamin D₃ (1, 25-(OH)₂ D₃)[Q] **Nuclear Receptors** • Thyroid hormones[Q] • Retinoic acid[Q]	• HCG • ADH • CRH • PTH • TSH		• Substance P • Gastrin • Cholecystokinin • Muscarinic (Acetylcholine) • Vasopressin[Q] • TRH	• Nerve growth factor (NGF) • PDGF • Erythropoietin • Prolactin[Q] • Adiponectin & leptin

20. **Ans. b. Leptin** *(Ref: Ganong 25/e p397, 24/e p399; Knobil and Neill's Physiology of Reproduction 2014/p1607; Novaks 13/e p410)*
    Leptin has a permissive action at the onset of puberty.

Puberty	
Initiation of puberty	**Permissive action**
• **Pulsatile release of GnRH** is one of the **main hormones for initiation of puberty**[Q].	• For one hormone to exert effect, some **other hormone must have to prepare the tissue for this effect**[Q]. • **Leptin accelerates GnRH pulsatility in hypothalamic neurons, fastening puberty**[Q]. • **Other permissive factors**: Neuropeptide Y, serotonin, norepinephrine, melatonin • Although **GH level increase during puberty, it has no permissive action**[Q].

*"It now appears that **leptin, the satiety-producing hormone secreted by fat cells**, may be the link between body weight and puberty. Obese ob/ob mice that cannot make leptin are infertile, and their fertility is restored by injections of leptin. **Leptin treatment also induces precocious puberty in immature female mice.** However, the way that leptin fits into the overall control of puberty remains to be determined."- Ganong 25/e p397*

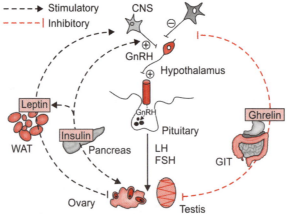

Fig. 10: Regulatory Roles of Key Hormone Signals, originating from different metabolic tissues involved in the integrative control of food intake, energy balance & reproductive function including puberty (Leptin: An inhibitory signal for food intake and a stimulatory or permissive signal for puberty and reproduction; Insulin: The same profile as leptin in terms of actions on food intake and reproduction; Ghrelin: A stimulatory signal for food intake and an inhibitory signal for the reproductive axis); WAT: White Adipose Tissues

*"Among the numerous endocrine regulators involved in the integrative control of reproduction and metabolism, leptin, a hormone identified in 1994 as a major secretory product of the white adipose tissue, is universally recognized as an essential neuroendocrine integrator linking the magnitude of body fat stores with several neuroendocrine axes, including that regulating the reproductive system. Leptin is secreted by the white adipose tissue in proportion to the size of body fat stores and acts as an anorexigenic and thermogenic factor at the hypothalamic level, thus contributing to dynamically adjusting energy requirements, fat reserves, and food intake. Regarding reproductive control, numerous studies have settled the concept that **leptin plays a central role in the metabolic control f puberty and fertility**."- Knobil and Neill's Physiology of Reproduction (2014)/p 1607*

*"**There** is now increasing evidence for **genetic and physiologic mechanisms linking the regulation of body fat content, caloric intake, and hypothalamic control of reproduction**. For instance, leptin and its receptor have recently been demonstrated*

Contd...

to have critical functions in body mass regulation, glucose homeostasis, and reproductive function at the hypothalamic level. Among other characteristic metabolic abnormalities, gene-targeted mice lacking leptin or leptin receptor were infertile secondary to hypogonadotropic hypogonadism. Homozygous mutation in the human leptin receptor gene also has been identified. In humans, abnormalities in leptin receptor function lead to early-onset morbid obesity and absent pubertal development, presumably secondary to defective hypothalamic function."-Novaks 13/e p410

21. **Ans. a. Serum FSH**   (Ref: Ganong 25/e p419, 425, 24/e p427)

    Prior to initiating treatment for a couple, in whom the man has azoospermia, it is important to distinguish whether the lack of sperm in the ejaculate is from an obstructive or non-obstructive process. The presence of normal volume testes with bilaterally indurated epididymis and/or absent vas deferens will point to an obstructive etiology for azoospermia. A history of cryptorchidism in the presence of small or soft testes suggests non-obstructive azoospermia, especially if associated with an elevated serum (FSH) level. A decreased spermatogenesis leads to decrease in production of inhibin, which causes an elevation in FSH.

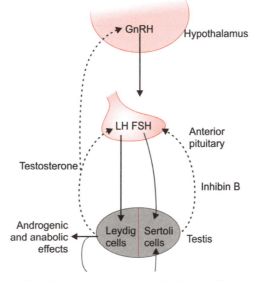

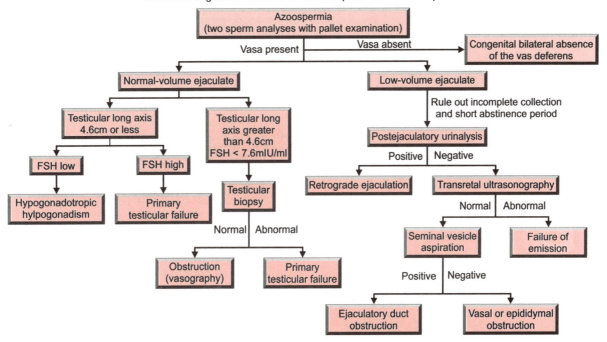

Flowchart: Algorithm for the evaluation of patients with azoospermia

"FSH and androgens maintain the gametogenic function of the testis. After hypophysectomy, injection of luteinizing hormone (LH) produces a high local concentration of androgen in the testes, and this maintains spermatogenesis. The stages from spermatogonia to spermatids appear to be androgen- independent. However, the maturation from spermatids to spermatozoa depends on androgen acting on the Sertoli cells in which the developing spermatozoa are embedded. FSH acts on the Sertoli cells to facilitate the last stages of spermatid maturation. In addition, it promotes the production of ABP."- Ganong 25/e p419*

"FSH is tropic for Sertoli cells, and FSH and androgens maintain the gametogenic function of the testes. FSH also stimulates the secretion of ABP and inhibin. Inhibin feeds back to inhibit FSH secretion. LH is tropic for Leydig cells and stimulates the secretion of testosterone, which in turn feeds back to inhibit LH secretion."- Ganong 25/e p425*

"Testosterone inhibits LH secretion by acting directly on the anterior pituitary and by inhibiting the secretion of gonadotropin-releasing hormone (GnRH) from the hypothalamus. Inhibin acts directly on the anterior pituitary to inhibit FSH secretion. In response to LH, some of the testosterone secreted from the Leydig cells bathes the seminiferous epithelium and provides the high local concentration of androgen to the Sertoli cells that is necessary for normal spermatogenesis.'- Ganong 25/e p425*

22. Ans. b. Prebotzinger complex   *(Ref: Ganong 25/e p656, 24/e p658)*

Rhythmic respiration is initiated by a small group of synaptically coupled pacemaker cells in the pre-Bötzinger complex (pre-BÖTC) on either side of the medulla between the nucleus ambiguus and the lateral reticular nucleus.

"The main components of the respiratory control pattern generator responsible for automatic respiration are located in the medulla. Rhythmic respiration is initiated by a small group of synaptically coupled pacemaker cells in the pre-Bötzinger complex (pre-BÖTC) on either side of the medulla between the nucleus ambiguus and the lateral reticular nucleus. These neurons discharge rhythmically, and they produce rhythmic discharges in phrenic motor neurons that are abolished by sections between the pre-BÖTC complex and these motor neurons. They also contact the hypoglossal nuclei, and the tongue is involved in the regulation of airway resistance."- Ganong 25/e p656*

Neural Control of Breathing		

Control System:
- **Two separate neural mechanisms regulate respiration**.
- **One** is responsible **for voluntary control** & other for **automatic control.**

Voluntary control	• **Voluntary system** is **located in cerebral cortex** • **Sends impulses to respiratory motor neurons via corticospinal tracts.**	
Automatic control	• **Automatic system** is driven by a group of **pacemaker cells in medulla**. • **Impulses** from these cells **activate motor neurons in cervical & thoracic spinal cord** that innervate inspiratory muscles. • **Those in cervical cord activate the diaphragm via phrenic nerves & those in thoracic spinal cord activate external intercostal muscles.** • **Impulses also reach innervation of internal intercostal muscles & other expiratory muscles.**	

Regulation of Respiration		
Medullary Respiratory Center	Dorsal Respiratory Group (DRG)	• **Primarily responsible for inspiration**[Q] • **Cause rhythmic inspiratory discharge** • Constitute initial **intracranial processing station for afferent inputs from 9th & 10th cranial nerve** originating from peripheral chemoreceptors & baroreceptors
	Ventral Respiratory Group (VRG)	• **Primarily responsible for active expiration during forceful breathing** • **Not active during normal breathing** when **expiration is passive.**
	Pre-Bötzinger Complex	• Initiate spontaneous automatic rhythmic respiration

AIMS May 2016

Neural Control of Breathing

Pontine Respiratory Center	Pneumotaxic center	• Located in **medial parabrachial & Kölliker-Fuse nuclei of upper dorsolateral pons** • **Contains neurons, active during inspiration** • May play a **role in switching between inspiration & expiration**. • **Inhibits inspiration**[Q] • **Regulates inspiratory volume & respiratory rate**.
	Apneustic center	• Located in the lower pons • Excitatory effect on inspiratory area of DRG • Stimulates inspiration producing deep & prolonged inspiratory gasp.
Cerebral cortex		• Controls the voluntary component of breathing[Q]

23. **Ans. d. FRC** *(Ref: Ganong 25/e p629, 24/e p629; Guyton 13/e p502)*

In relaxed state, chest wall and lung recoil are balanced at functional residual capacity (FRC).

> *"Compliance is developed due to the tendency for tissue to resume its original position after an applied force has been removed. After an expiration during quiet breathing (e.g., at the FRC), the lungs have a tendency to collapse and the chest wall has a tendency to expand."* - *Ganong 25/e p629*

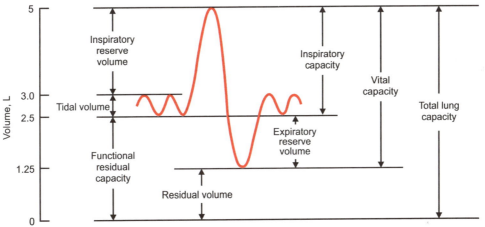

Fig. 11: Lung Volumes and Capacity Measurements

Lung volume		Lung capacities	
Tidal volume (TV): • Air that **moves into the lung with each normal inspiration** or **volume of air** that **moves out of lung with each expiration**	500 ml[Q]	**Inspiratory capacity: IC = TV + IRV** • **Total amount of air** that can be **breathed in**.	3800 ml[Q]
Inspiratory reserve volume (IRV): • Air inspired with a maximal Inspiratory effort in excess of tidal volume.	3300 ml[Q]	**Vital capacity: VC = TV + IRV + ERV** • Maximal amount of air that can be expelled out forcefully after a maximal (deep) inspiration.	4800 ml[Q]
Expiratory reserve volume (ERV): • Air expelled with a maximal expiratory effort in excess of tidal volume.	1000 ml[Q]	**Functional residual capacity:** **FRC = ERV + RV** • Volume of air remaining in the lung after normal expiration.	2200 ml[Q]
Residual volume (RV): • Amount of **air remaining in the lungs even after forced expiration**.	1200 ml[Q]	**Total lung capacity:** **TLC = TV + IRV + ERV + RV** • Amount of **air** present **in the lung after a maximal inspiration**. • This is **maximum volume to which the lungs can be expanded**.	6000 ml[Q]

AIIMS ESSENCE

24. Ans. a. Intensity of stimulus *(Ref: Guyton 13/e p615)*

According to Weber-Fechner's Law, strength of stimulus perceived is directly proportional to intensity of stimulus.

"Weber-Fechner Principle—Detection of "Ratio" of Stimulus Strength: In the mid1800s, Weber first and Fechner later proposed the principle that gradations of stimulus strength are discriminated approximately in proportion to the logarithm of stimulus strength."- Guyton 13/e p615

Weber-Fechner Principle
• Gradations of stimulus strength are discriminated approximately in proportion to the logarithm of stimulus strength[Q].
• That is, a person already holding 30 grams weight in his or her hand can barely detect an additional 1gram increase in weight, and, when already holding 300 grams, he or she can barely detect a 10 gram increase in weight.
• Thus, in this instance, the ratio of the change in stimulus strength required for detection remains essentially constant, about 1 to 30, which is what the logarithmic principle means.

To express this principle mathematically
• **Interpreted signal strength = Log (Stimulus) + Constant**[Q]

• Weber Fechner principle is quantitatively accurate only for higher intensities of visual, auditory & cutaneous sensory experience & applies only poorly to most other types of sensory experience[Q].

> • **Weber Fechner principle** emphasizes that the **greater the background sensory intensity**, the **greater an additional change must be for the psyche to detect the change**[Q].

25. Ans. a. Pulmonary embolism *(Ref: Ganong 25/e p634, 24/e p634)*

In pulmonary embolism gradient increases to very high level (10 to 83 mm Hg from normal level of 5 mm Hg). But normal PaO₂ level on arterial blood gas analysis does not exclude the diagnosis of acute pulmonary embolism. It is also increased in ILD.

"The Alveolar–arterial gradient is a measure of the difference between the alveolar concentration (A) and the arterial (a) concentration of oxygen. It helps to assess the integrity of alveolar capillary unit. In high altitude, the arterial oxygen [PaO₂] is low but only because the alveolar oxygen (PAO₂) is also low. In states of ventilation-perfusion mismatch, such as pulmonary embolism or right-to-left shunt, oxygen is not effectively transferred from the alveoli to the blood which results in elevated A-a gradient."

Alveolar–arterial (A-a) Gradient
• A–a gradient is useful in determining the source of hypoxemia[Q].
• It helps to **isolate the location of problem** as either **intrapulmonary or extrapulmonary**[Q].
• **Normal A–a gradient** for a **young adult non-smoker breathing air** is between **5–10 mm Hg.**
• Normally, A–a gradient increases with age.
• An **abnormally increased A–a gradient suggests a defect in diffusion, V/Q (ventilation/perfusion ratio) mismatch, or right-to-left shunt**[Q].

Increased A–a gradient	Normal A–a gradient
• **Right-to-left intrapulmonary shunt** (due to fluid filled alveoli): **CHF, ARDS & lobar pneumonia**[Q]	• **Hypoventilation:** Neuromuscular disorders, CNS disorders[Q]
• **V/Q mismatch** (due to lung dead space): **Pulmonary embolism, atelectasis, pneumonia, obstructive lung disease (asthma, COPD), pneumothorax**[Q]	• **Low inspired FIO₂: High altitude**[Q]
• **Alveolar hypoventilation: Interstitial lung disease**[Q]	

26. Ans. d. Tension in the muscle *(Ref: Ganong 25/e p232; Guyton 13/e p697, 701)*

Golgi tendon organ senses muscle tension.

"The Golgi organ (also called Golgi tendon organ, GTO, tendon organ, neurotendinous organ or neurotendinous spindle) senses changes in muscle tension. It is a proprioceptive sensory receptor organ that is at the origins and insertion of skeletal muscle fibers into the tendons of skeletal muscle. It provides the sensory component of the Golgi tendon reflex."

"Golgi tendon organs, which are located in the muscle tendons and transmit information about tendon tension or rate of change of tension."- Guyton 13/e p697

"However, discharge is regularly produced by contraction of the muscle, and the Golgi tendon organ thus functions as a transducer in a feedback circuit that regulates muscle force in a manner analogous to the spindle feedback circuit that regulates muscle length."- Ganong 25/e p232

Golgi tendon organ

- **Golgi tendon organ** is an **encapsulated sensory receptor**, consisting of a net like collection of knobby nerve endings among the fasicles of a tendon.
- There are **3–25 (usually 10-15) muscle fibers connected to each golgi tendon**[Q].
- **Golgi tendon organ** functions as a **transducer in a feedback circuit** that **regulates muscle force in a fashion analogous to the spindle feedback circuit** that **regulates muscle length**[Q].

  - Unlike muscle spindles, golgi tendon organs are in series with the muscle fibers, so they are **stimulated by both passive stretch and active contraction of muscle**[Q].
  - It is important to note that **spindle detects muscle length and changes in muscle length, whereas golgi tendon detects muscle tension**[Q].
  - So it is **stimulated when muscle fiber is tensed by contracting or stretching muscle**[Q].

- Like primary receptor of muscle spindle, tendon organ has both a **dynamic (intense response to sudden increase in tension)** and **static response (steady state firing of lesser degree almost directly proportional to muscle tension)**.
- Impulses from tendon organ are transmitted through **large, myelinated rapidly conducting sensory Ib nerve fibers**[Q].
- This Ib fibers end in the spinal cord on **inhibitory interneuron,** which in turn terminate on alpha-motor neuron supplying the muscle from which Ib originated. They also make excitatory connections with motor neurons supplying antagonist muscles.
- **Stimulation of tendon organ causes inhibition of alpha-motor neuron whereas muscle spindle stimulation excites alpha motor neuron.**

  - The **threshold of golgi tendon is low**[Q].
  - Since more elastic muscle fibers take up much of the stretch, **degree of stimulation by passive stretch is not great & strong stretch is required to produce relaxation**[Q].
  - Contraction of muscle regularly stimulate golgi tendon. It is responsible for **inverse stretch reflex.**

Intense stretch of a skeletal muscle result in:
1. Golgi tendon organs detect tension applied to a tendon.
2. Sensory neurons conduct action potentials to the spinal cord.
3. Sensory neurons synapse with inhibitory interneurons that synapse with alpha motor neurons.
4. Inhibition of the alpha motor neurons causes muscle relaxation, relieving the tension applied to the tendon. Note: The muscle that relaxes is attached to the tendon to which tension is applied.

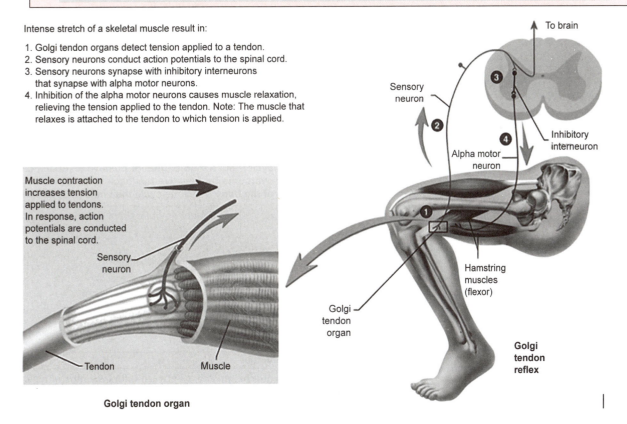

Golgi tendon organ

27. **Ans. d. Total peripheral resistance**   *(Ref: Ganong 25/e p544, 24/e p546)*
Cardiac output depends on both preload & afterload. The preload is defined by the venous return & left ventricular end-diastolic volume while the afterload is defined by the mean arterial pressure, which then further depends on total peripheral resistance.

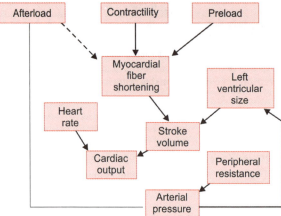

Fig. 12: Interactions between the components that regulate cardiac output & arterial pressure
(Solid arrows indicate increases & dashed arrow indicates a decrease)

*"**The force of contraction of cardiac muscle depends on its preloading and its after loading.** The initial phase of contraction is isometric; the elastic component in series with the contractile element is stretched, and tension increases until it is sufficient to lift the load. **The tension at which the load is lifted is the afterload.** The muscle then contracts isotonically without developing further tension. **In vivo, preload is the degree to which the myocardium is stretched before it contracts and the afterload is the resistance against which blood is expelled.** For cardiac contraction, preload is usually considered to be the end-diastolic pressure when the ventricle has become filled. **The afterload of the ventricle is the pressure in the artery leading from the ventricle.** (Sometimes the afterload is loosely considered to be the resistance in the circulation rather than the pressure.)"*

28. **Ans. b. 4**   *(Ref: Guyton 13/e p8-9)*

- **Gain = Correction/Error**
- Correction = 8 mm Hg
- Persisting error after correction = 10–8 = 2 mm Hg
- Hence, Gain = 8/2 = 4

Negative feedback	Positive feedback
Most control systems of the body act by negative feedback (e.g. In the arterial pressure-regulating mechanisms, a high pressure causes a series of reactions that promote a lowered pressure)[Q].	**Positive feedback** is better known as a **"vicious cycle,"** but a **mild degree of positive feedback can be overcome by negative feedback control mechanisms of the body & vicious cycle then fails to develop**[Q].
"Gain" of a Control System	**Examples of Positive Feedback Control (CLAPS)**
• Degree of effectiveness with which a control system maintains constant conditions. • Correction = Final—Uncorrected Pressure • Error = Final—Normal Pressure • **Gain = Correction/Error** • **Higher the gain, better is the feedback system.**	• **C**lotting[Q] • **L**H surge for ovulation[Q] • **A**ction potential generation[Q] • **P**arturition[Q] (Cervical dilation) • **S**hock[Q] (destabilizing)

29. **Ans. c. –61 mV**   *(Ref: Ganong 25/e p9, p24/e p9-10; Guyton 13/e p61)*

Equilibrium Potential
• **Equilibrium potential** is the **membrane potential at which equilibrium exists between influx & efflux of ions.** • The **Nernst equation** has a physiological application when **used to calculate the potential of an ion of charge z across a membrane.** This potential is **determined using the concentration of the ion both inside and outside the cell:**

Equilibrium Potential

- E= RT ln [ion outside the cell] = 2.3026 – RT $\log_{10}$ [ion outside the cell]
- zF [ion inside the cell] zF [ion inside the cell]

- When the membrane is in thermodynamic equilibrium (i.e. no net flux of ions), the membrane potential must be equal to the Nernst potential.
- E_m = The membrane potential
- P_{ion} = The permeability for that ion (in meters per second)
- $[ion]_{out}$ = The extracellular concentration of that ion
- $[ion]_{in}$ = The intracellular concentration of that ion
- R = The ideal gas constant
- T = The temperature in kelvin
- F = Faraday's constant (coulombs per mole)
- z is the number of moles of electrons transferred in the cell reaction (Valence of K^+).
- Hence, $E_k = 61.5 \log C_i/C_e$
- **Intracellular concentration C_i = 100**
- **Extracellular concentration C_e = 10**
- $E_k = –61.5 \log 100/10 = –61$ mV

Concentration (mmol/L of H_2O) of some ions inside and outside mammalian motor neurons			
Ion	Inside cell	Outside cell	Equilibrium potential (mv)
Na^+	15.0[Q]	150.0[Q]	+60[Q]
K^+	150.0[Q]	5.5[Q]	–90[Q]
Cl^-	9.0[Q]	125.0[Q]	–70[Q]
Resting membrane potential = –70 mV[Q]			

30. Ans. c. Urinary concentration in mg/ml *(Ref: Ganong 25/e p676, 24/e p678)*

In the Given Formula:
- C = Clearance of the substance
- U = Urinary concentration of the substance in mg/ml
- P = Plasma concentration of the substance in mg/ml
- V = Volume of urine

Measuring Glomerular filtration rate (GFR)

- **GFR** is **amount of plasma ultrafiltrate formed each minute** & can be measured in intact experimental animals & humans by measuring plasma level of a substance & amount of the substance that is excreted.

  - A **substance to be used to measure GFR must be freely filtered through the glomeruli & must be neither secreted nor reabsorbed by the tubules; should be nontoxic & not metabolized by the body**[Q].
  - **Inulin**, a polymer of fructose with a molecular weight of 5200, **meets these criteria in humans & most animals** and **can be used to measure GFR**[Q].

- **Renal plasma clearance** is the **volume of plasma from which a substance is completely removed by the kidney in a given amount of time** (usually minutes)[Q].
- The amount of that substance that appears in the urine per unit of time is the result of the renal filtering of a certain number of milliliters of plasma that contained this amount.
- **GFR & clearance are measured in mL/min.**

  - Therefore, if the substance is designated by the letter X, the **GFR is equal to the concentration of X in urine (U_x) times the urine flow per unit of time (V) divided by the arterial plasma level of X (P_x), or $U_x V/P_x$.**
  - **This value is called the clearance of X (C_x).**

Contd...

1054   AIIMS ESSENCE

Contd...

Measuring Glomerular filtration rate (GFR)
• In practice, a loading dose of inulin is administered intravenously, followed by a sustaining infusion to keep the arterial plasma level constant. After the inulin has equilibrated with body fluids, an accurately timed urine specimen is collected and a plasma sample obtained halfway through the collection.
• Plasma and urinary inulin concentrations are determined and the clearance is calculated:

- U_{IN} = 35 mg/mL
- V = 0.9 mL/min
- P_{IN} = 0.25 mg/mL
- C_{IN} = U_{IN} V/P_{IN} = 35 × 0.9/0.25 = 126 mL/min

- **Clearance of creatinine** can also be **used to determine GFR**, however **some creatinine is secreted by the tubules thus the clearance of creatinine will be slightly higher than inulin**[Q].

BIOCHEMISTY

31. Ans. c. Acetyl CoA   *(Ref: Harper 30/e p185, 29/e p187)*

Acetyl CoA is not a substrate for gluconeogenesis (not glucogenic) and cannot be converted back to glucose.

*"Acetyl CoA is **not a substrate for gluconeogenesis and cannot be converted back to glucose**[Q]. This is because **acetyl CoA cannot be converted back to pyruvate**[Q] since its carbon backbone is lost in citric acid cycle as CO_2."*

Gluconeogenesis
• **Gluconeogenesis prevent hypoglycemia** during **short & long term fasting**[Q].
• **Gluconeogenesis** occurs primarily in **liver; serves to maintain euglycemia during fasting**[Q].
• **Enzymes** also found in **kidney, intestinal epithelium**[Q].

- **Liver & kidneys** are the **major gluconeogenic tissues**[Q].
- **Glucogenic key enzymes** are **expressed in small intestine**[Q] but their role in fasting state is unclear.

- **Muscle cannot participate in gluconeogenesis** because **it lacks glucose-6-phosphatase**[Q].
- **Odd-chain fatty acids yield 1 propionyl-CoA during metabolism, which can enter the TCA cycle** (as succinyl-CoA), **undergo gluconeogenesis,** and serve as a glucose source[Q].
- **Even-chain fatty acids cannot produce new glucose**, since they yield only acetyl-CoA equivalents.

- **Carbon skeletons** for gluconeogenesis are **derived primarily from glucogenic amino acids & lactate from muscle & glycerol** from **adipose tissues**[Q].

- Although the **lactate produced in muscle, is used by liver for gluconeogenesis**[Q].
- **Gluconeogenesis is stimulated by excess of acetyl Co-A & decrease in fructose 2, 6 biphosphate concentration**[Q].

Substrates for Gluconeogenesis	
• **Glucogenic amino acids** (all except **leucine & lysine** which are **purely ketogenic**): Most **important is alanine**[Q] • **Lactate**[Q]	• **Pyruvate**[Q] • **Propionate**[Q] • **Glycerol**[Q] • **Fumarate**[Q]

Regulatory and Adaptive Enzymes Associated with Gluconeogenesis				
	Inducer	**Repressor**	**Activator**	**Inhibitor**
Pyruvate carboxylase	Glucocorticoids, glucagon, epinephrine[Q]	**Insulin**[Q]	**Acetyl CoA**[Q]	**ADP**[Q]
Phosphoenol pyruvate carboxykinase	Glucocorticoids, glucagon, epinephrine[Q]	**Insulin**[Q]	Glucagon?	
Glucose 6-phosphatase	Glucocorticoids, **glucagon,** epinephrine[Q0]	**Insulin**[Q]		

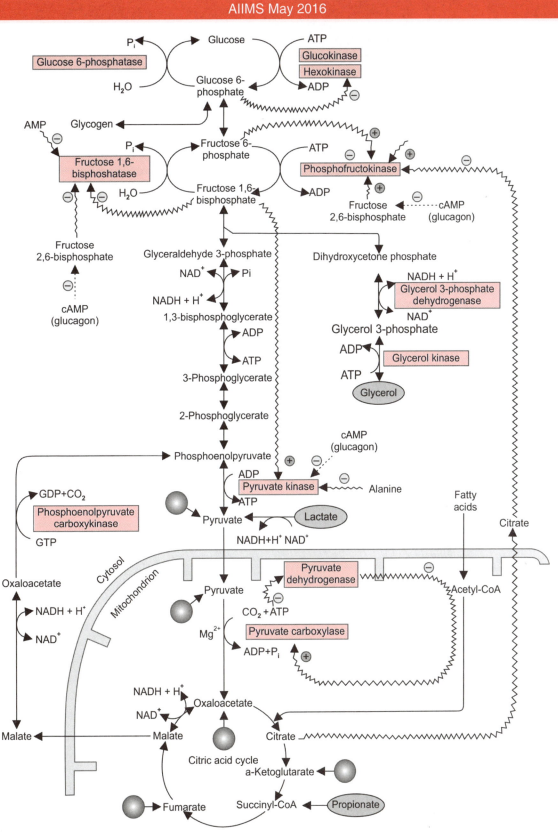

Fig. 13: Regulation of gluconeogenesis & glycolysis

32. **Ans. b. Tyrosine** *(Ref: Harper 30/e p165)*
Tyrosine enters Krebs cycle via fumarate, while all others form pyruvate to enter the Krebs cycle.

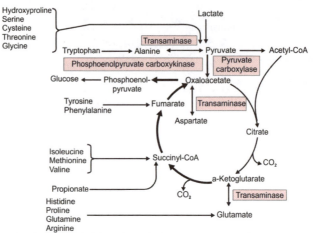

Fig. 14: Involvement of citric acid cycle in transamination & gluconeogenesis

"Aminotransferase (transaminase) reactions form pyruvate from alanine, oxaloacetate from aspartate, and α-ketoglutarate from glutamate. Because these reactions are reversible, the cycle also serves as a source of carbon skeletons for the synthesis of these amino acids. Other amino acids contribute to gluconeogenesis because their carbon skeletons give rise to citric acid cycle intermediates: Alanine, cysteine, glycine, hydroxyproline, serine, threonine, and tryptophan yield pyruvate; Arginine, histidine, glutamine, and proline yield α-ketoglutarate; Isoleucine, methionine, and valine yield succinyl-CoA; Tyrosine and phenylalanine yield fumarate."

33. **Ans. c. NAD$^+$** *(Ref: Harper 30/e p132)*
Cyanide blocks citric acid cycle by blocking NAD$^+$.

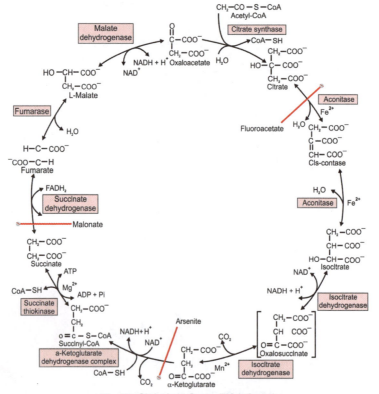

Fig. 15: Citric Acid Cycle (TCA Cycle)

"*Cyanide blocks complex IV (Cytochrome c reductase) of electron transport Chain. It has no direct effect on any component of Citric acid cycle. If the electron transport chain is blocked, then the electron carriers NADH and FADH$_2$ cannot unload their electrons into it, which means NAD+ and FAD are not regenerated. Since Glycolysis and the Krebs cycle both require NAD+ (and the Krebs cycle requires FAD), NAD+ will get depleted as NADH level is raised both of these processes will stop running.*"

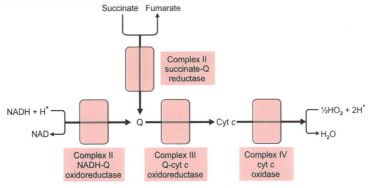

Fig. 16: Components of electron transport chain

Electron Transport Chain (ETC)/Respiratory Chain

- Electrons flow through the respiratory chain through a redox span of 1.1 V from NAD+/NADH to $O_2/2H_2O$.
- Passing through three large protein complexes:
  - NADH-Q oxidoreductase (Complex I), where electrons are transferred from NADH to coenzyme^Q (Q) (also called ubiquinone)^Q.
  - Q-cytochrome c oxidoreductase (Complex III), which passes the electrons to cytochrome c^Q
  - Cytochrome c oxidase (Complex IV), which completes the chain, passing the electrons to O_2 & causing it to be reduced to H_2O^Q.
- Some substrates with more positive redox potentials than NAD+/ NADH (e.g. succinate) pass electrons to Q via a fourth complex, **succinate-^{Q} reductase (Complex II)**, rather than Complex I^Q.

  - Four complexes are embedded in **inner mitochondrial membrane**, but **Q & cytochrome c are mobile**^{Q}.
  - **Q diffuses rapidly within the membrane**, while **cytochrome c is a soluble protein**^{Q}.
  - Flow of electrons through Complexes I, III & IV results in pumping of protons from matrix across the inner mitochondrial membrane into intermembrane space^Q.

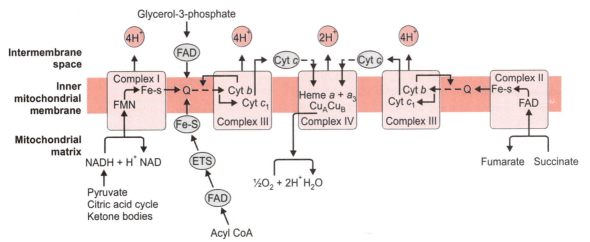

Fig. 17: Flow of Electrons in Electron Transport Chain

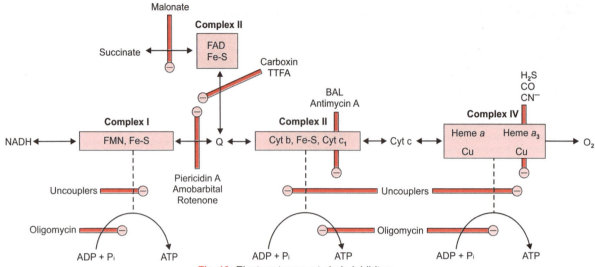

Fig. 18: Electron transport chain inhibitors

Inhibitors of Electron Transport Chain		
Inhibitors of Electron Transfer	Between NADH & Co^Q (At Complex I)	• Piercidin A^Q • Amobarbital^Q • Rotenone^Q (insecticide & fish poison)
	Inhibitors of Complex II	• Carboxin^Q • Malonate^Q • TTFA^Q (Trienoyl Trifluoro Acetone): Iron chelating agent
	Between Cyt b & Cyt c (At Complex III)	• BAL^Q (British antileviste or dimercaprol) • Antimycin A^Q
	Inhibitors at Cytochrome c oxidase (At Complex IV)	• Hydrogen sulphide^Q • Carbon monoxide^Q • Cyanide^Q • Sodium azide^Q
Inhibitors of oxidative phosphorylation	• **Atractyloside: Inhibits oxidative phosphorylation** by inhibiting transporter of ADP into & ATP out of mitochondrion^Q • **Oligomycin** (antibiotic): **Completely blocks oxidation & phosphorylation** by blocking flow of protons through ATP synthase^Q.	
Uncouplers of oxidative phosphorylation	• **Mechanism of Action: Disruption of proton gradient** across the **inner mitochondrial membrane**^Q • **Uncouplers: 2,4-dinitrophenol, dinitrocresol**^Q • **Physiological Uncouplers: Thermogenin**^Q (found in brown adipose tissue, functions to generate body heat), thyroxine, long chain free fatty acid	
Ionophores	• **Mechanism of Action: Permit specifications to penetrate membranes & dissipate proton gradient**^Q • **Ionophores: Valinomycin, Gramicidin, Nigericin**^Q	

34. **Ans. b. Hormone-sensitive lipase**   *(Ref: Harper 30/e p262)*

Hormone sensitive lipase is controlled by glucagon.

"Hormone-sensitive lipase is activated by ACTH, TSH, glucagon, epinephrine, norepinephrine, and vasopressin and inhibited by insulin, prostaglandin E$_p$, and nicotinic acid."- Harper 30/e p262

> *"Triacylglycerol undergoes hydrolysis by a hormone-sensitive lipase to form free fatty acids and glycerol. This lipase is distinct from lipoprotein lipase that catalyzes lipoprotein triacylglycerol hydrolysis before its uptake into extrahepatic tissues. Since glycerol cannot be utilized, it diffuses into the blood, whence it is utilized by tissues such as those of the liver and kidney, which possess an active glycerol kinase. The free fatty acids formed by lipolysis can be reconverted in the tissue to acyl-CoA by acyl-CoA synthetase and reesterified with glycerol 3-phosphate to form triacylglycerol. Thus, there is a continuous cycle of lipolysis and reesterification within the tissue. However, when the rate of reesterification is not sufficient to match the rate of lipolysis, free fatty acids accumulate and diffuse into the plasma, where they bind to albumin and raise the concentration of plasma free fatty acids."- Harper 30/e p262*

Hormone-Sensitive Lipase (Cholesteryl Ester Hydrolase)

- **HSL** is an **intracellular neutral lipase** that is capable of hydrolyzing a variety of esters.
- The enzyme has a long & a short form.

Long form	• Expressed in steroidogenic tissues[Q] (testis) • Converts cholesteryl esters to free cholesterol[Q] for steroid hormone production.
Short form	• Expressed in adipose tissue[Q] • Hydrolyzes stored triglycerides to free fatty acids[Q]

- During fasting-state, increased FFA secretion by adipocyte cells was attributed to adrenaline hormone. Hence the name **"hormone-sensitive lipase"**.
- **Main function** of hormone-sensitive lipase is **to mobilize the stored fats.**
- Hormone-sensitive lipase is **activated by ACTH, TSH, glucagon, epinephrine, norepinephrine, & vasopressin** and **inhibited by insulin, prostaglandin E_1 & nicotinic acid**[Q].

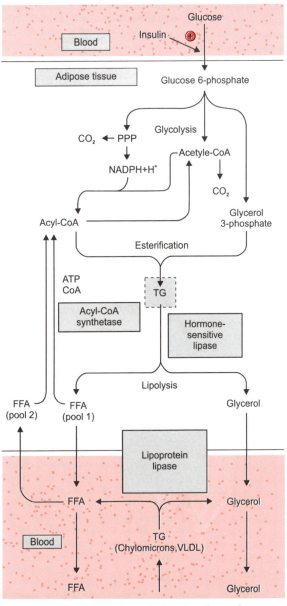

Fig. 19: Triacylglycerol metabolism in adipose tissue

	Lipoprotein Lipase (LPL)	Hormone Sensitive Lipase (HSL)
Location	• **Extracellular**[Q]: Attached to **luminal surface capillary endothelium** of **adipose tissue, heart skeletal muscle & lactating mammary gland**[Q]	• **Intracellular: Present inside adipocyte**[Q]
Acts on	• **Triacylglycerol** present in chylomicron & VLDL[Q]	• **Diacylglycerol** derived from ATGL[Q]
Activators	• **Insulin**[Q]	• **Glucagon, Epinephrine, ACTH**[Q]

Lipase	Description
Lingual lipase	• Secreted from **lingual serous glands; activated in stomach by HCl**[Q] • Its action starts mainly in stomach.
Gastric lipase	• Secreted by **chief cells** in stomach[Q]
Pancreatic lipase	• **Requires co-lipase** for action; Produces **2-mono acyl glycerol**[Q]
Adipose triglyceride lipase (ATGL)	• **Present in adipose tissues**[Q] • **Breaks TAG in adipose tissue to DAG** which is further acted upon by **HSL**[Q]
Endothelial lipase	• Synthesized & located in **vascular endothelial cells**[Q]. • Has **phospholipase A₁ activity**[Q]
Hepatic lipase	• **Hydrolyses triglycerides & phospholipids** in chylomicron remnants, VLDL & HDL[Q]

35. Ans. c. cGMP   *(Ref: Harper 30/e p290, 437)*
Second messenger for smooth muscle relaxation mediated by NO is cGMP.

> *"GTP serves as an allosteric regulator and as an energy source for protein synthesis, and cGMP serves as a second messenger in response to nitric oxide (NO) during relaxation of smooth muscle."- Harper 30/e p290*

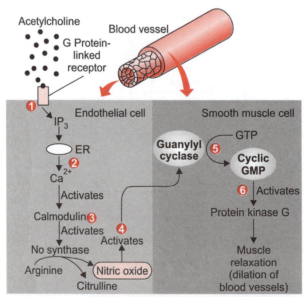

Fig. 20: Nitric oxide couples G protein-linked receptor stimulation in endothelial cells to relaxation of smooth muscle cells in blood vessels.

36. Ans. c. Adjusting pH to other than the isoelectric point   *(Ref: Harper 30/e p26)*
Protein precipitation is widely used to concentrate proteins and purify them from various contaminants. Protein precipitation occurs at the isoelectric point of the protein and not at any other pH.

AIIMS May 2016

*"**Highly purified protein** is essential for the detailed examination of its physical and functional properties. Cells contain thousands of different proteins, each in widely varying amounts. The **isolation of a specific protein in quantities sufficient for analysis** thus presents a formidable challenge that may **require multiple successive purification techniques**. Classic approaches exploit **differences in relative solubility of individual proteins as a function of pH (isoelectric precipitation), polarity (precipitation with ethanol or acetone), or salt concentration (salting out with ammonium sulfate).** Chromatographic separations partition molecules between two phases, one mobile and the other stationary. For separation of amino acids or sugars, the stationary phase, or matrix, may be a sheet of filter paper (paper chromatography) or a thin layer of cellulose, silica, or alumina (thin-layer chromatography [TLC])."- Harper 30th/e p26*

Isoelectric Precipitation

- **Proteins are less soluble at their isoelectric point** where they have **zero net charge** & can **most easily approach each other with minimal charge repulsion**[Q].
- Since proteins are also less soluble at very low ionic strength, **isoelectric precipitation is usually done at very low or no salt**[Q].
- **Isoelectric point (pI)** is the **pH of a solution at which the net primary charge of a protein becomes zero.**
- At a solution, **pH that is above the pI, surface of protein is predominantly negatively charged** & like- charged molecules will exhibit repulsive forces[Q].
- Likewise, at a solution **pH that is below pI, surface of protein is predominantly positively charged** and repulsion between proteins occur. However, at the pI the negative and positive charges cancel, repulsive electrostatic forces are reduced and the **attraction forces predominate. The attraction forces will cause aggregation & precipitation**[Q].
- **pI of most proteins** is in the pH range of **4–6.**
- Mineral acids, such as **hydrochloric & sulfuric acid** are **used as precipitants.**

Disadvantage of Isoelectric Precipitation

- **Greatest disadvantage to isoelectric point precipitation: Irreversible denaturation caused by mineral acids**[Q].
- For this reason **isoelectric point precipitation is most often used to precipitate contaminant proteins,** rather than the target protein.

Methods of Separation & Purification of Proteins

Technique	Property used
SDS-PAGE (Polyacrylamide gel electrophoresis)	• Mass[Q]
Gel filtration (size exclusion) chromatography Dialysis/Ultrafiltration	• Size[Q]
Ultracentrifugation	• Mass/density[Q]
High performance liquid chromatography (HPLC)	• Charge, size, affinity[Q]
Ion-exchange chromatography	• Charge[Q]
Chromato-focussing chromatography Isoelectric electrophoresis	• pI[Q]
Native gel electrophoresis	• Mass/charge[Q]
2D gel electrophoresis	• Molecular weight & pI[Q]
Ammonium sulfate precipitation Partition chromatography	• Solubility[Q]
Reversed phase chromatography Hydrophobic interaction chromatography	• Hydrophobicity[Q]
Affinity (absorption) chromatography	• Affinity binding[Q]

37. **Ans. a. Modifier can affect the catalytic site by binding to the allosteric site**   *(Ref: Harper 30/e p82, 91)*
In allosteric modification, the modifier binds to the allosteric site and changes the rate of enzymatic action at the catalytic site. Since it is not a type of competitive inhibition, the modifier does not bind in a concentration dependent manner and adding substrate doesn't overcome the inhibitory effect. Allosteric inhibition usually decreases the velocity of the reaction without any change in Km.

Allosteric Regulation	
Allosteric activation	**Allosteric deactivation**
• **Active site becomes available** to the substrates when a **regulatory molecule binds to a different site** on the enzyme[Q]	• **Active site becomes unavailable** to the substrates when a **regulatory molecule binds to a different site** on the enzyme[Q]

Allosteric inhibition

- **Allosteric enzymes** are those for which **catalysis at the active site** may be **modulated by presence of effectors at an allosteric site**[Q].
- **Inhibitor binds at an allosteric site,** one **spatially distinct from the catalytic site** of the target enzyme[Q].
- **Feedback inhibitors** typically bear **little or no structural similarity** to the substrates of the enzymes they inhibit[Q].
- **Kinetics of feedback inhibition** may be **competitive, noncompetitive, partially competitive, or mixed**[Q].
- **Binding of allosteric regulator influences catalysis** by **inducing a conformational change** that encompasses the active site[Q].
- **Allosteric effects may be on Km or on V_{max}.**
- Two classes of allosterically regulated enzymes: **K-series & V-series enzymes**.

K-series enzymes	V-series enzymes
• **Substrate saturation kinetics** is **competitive** • **Km is raised without an effect on V_{max}.** • **Conformational change** may **weaken the bonds** between substrate & substrate-binding residues[Q].	• Allosteric inhibitor **lowers V_{max} without affecting the Km**[Q]. • Primary effect may be to **alter the orientation** or **charge of catalytic residues, lowering V_{max}.**

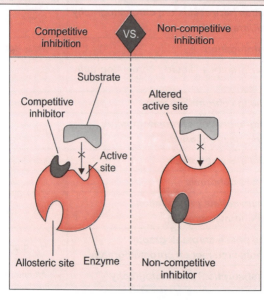

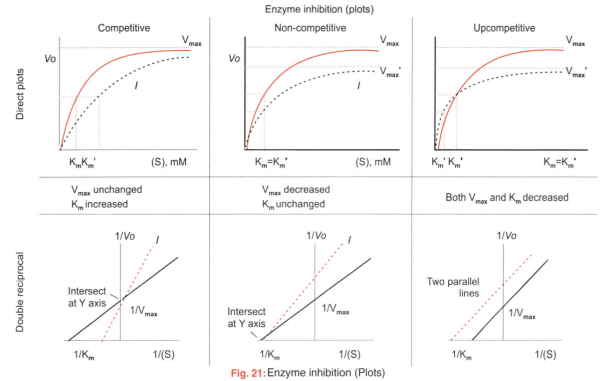

Fig. 21: Enzyme inhibition (Plots)

Inhibitor Type		
Competitive inhibitor	**Noncompetitive inhibitor**	**Uncompetitive inhibitor**
• Inhibitor is **structural analog** of substrate • Inhibitor **binds** specifically at the **catalytic site**[Q]	• Inhibitor is **not structural analog** of substrate • **Binds enzyme or enzyme-substrate complex** other that at the catalytic site[Q]. • **Substrate binding unaltered**, but **ESI complex cannot be reversed by substrate**[Q].	• Inhibitor is **not structural analog** of substrate • **Inhibitor binds only to enzyme-substrate complexes**[Q] at locations other than the catalytic site. • **Inhibition cannot be reversed by substrate**[Q].
• **Reversible**[Q]	• Irreversible	• Irreversible
• **Excess substrate abolishes inhibition**[Q]	• Excess substrate do not abolish inhibition.	• High substrate cannot overcome inhibition because presence of substrate is required to provide the site for binding the inhibitor[Q]
• Km increases[Q]	• Km remains the same[Q]	• Km decreases[Q]
• V$_{max}$ remains the **same**[Q]	• V$_{max}$ decreases[Q]	• V$_{max}$ decreases[Q]
Examples (Mostly drugs): • **Statins** inhibiting **HMG CoA reductase**[Q] • **Dicumarol** inhibiting Vitamin K epoxide[Q]	**Examples (Mostly poisons):** • Inhibition of cytochrome oxidase by cyanide[Q] • Inhibition of enolase by fluoride[Q]	• Examples: • Use of **lithium to prevent inositol monophosphatase** that causes **manic-depressive psychosis**[Q].

38. **Ans. d. Odorants**   *(Ref: http://hmg.oxfordjournals.org/content/11/10/1153.full)*
    In the mammalian genome, maximum number of genes code for the receptors of odorants.

"The olfactory receptor (OR) genes constitute the largest gene family in mammalian genomes. Humans have >1,000 OR genes, of which only ~40% have an intact coding region and are therefore putatively functional. Odorant receptor genes form the largest gene family in the genome of many animals: for example, the mouse genome contains approximately 1200 of these genes. These genes are distributed across 40 gene clusters in the mouse genome, and clusters contain varying numbers of receptor genes. Immunoglobulin receptors are coded by only 3 genes which undergoes V, D, J recombinations to form large number of receptors." - http://hmg.oxfordjournals.org/content/11/10/1153.full

PATHOLOGY

39. Ans. d. Plasma cell *(Ref: Wintrobes 13/e p303; Robbins 9/e p99)*

The cell marked with an arrow is plasma cell.

> *"Plasma cells are large lymphocytes with a considerable nucleus-to- cytoplasm ratio and a characteristic appearance on light microscopy. They have basophilic cytoplasm and an eccentric nucleus with heterochromatin in a characteristic cartwheel or clock face arrangement."*

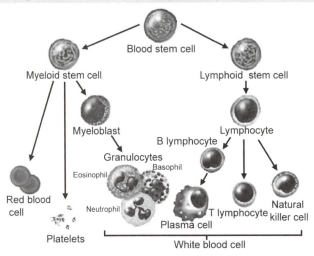

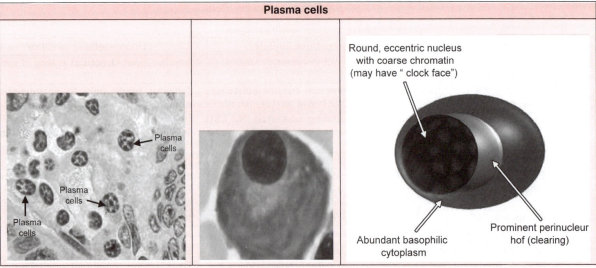

Plasma cells

- WBCs that secrete large volumes of antibodies[Q].
- Activated B cell begins to differentiate into more specialized cells.
- Germinal center B cells may differentiate into memory B cells or plasma cells[Q].
- Most of these B cells will become plasma blasts (or "immature plasma cells") & eventually plasma cells.
- Plasma cells can only produce a single kind of antibody in a single class of immunoglobulin[Q].

  - Plasma cells are **large lymphocytes** with a considerable nucleus-to-cytoplasm ratio & **basophilic cytoplasm & an eccentric nucleus with heterochromatin in a characteristic cartwheel or clock face arrangement**[Q] (on light microscopy)
  - Their **cytoplasm contains a pale zone** that on electron microscopy **contains an extensive Golgi apparatus & centrioles**[Q].

Plasma cells
• Do not express common pan-B cell markers, such as CD19 & CD20[Q].
• Plasma cells are identified by expression of CD138, CD78 & Interleukin-6 receptor & lack of expression of CD45[Q].
• In humans, **CD27** is a **good marker for plasma cells**, naive B cells are CD27-, memory B-cells are CD27+ & plasma cells are CD27++[Q].

40. **Ans. a. 6 hours**   (Ref: Robbins 9/e p544)

The myocardial biopsy is showing some coagulative necrosis along with wavy fibers with widened spaces between the dead fibers, which contain edema fluid and scattered neutrophils. No dense neutrophilic infiltrate is seen. These are typical early changes after MI, seen within 6 hours of infarction.

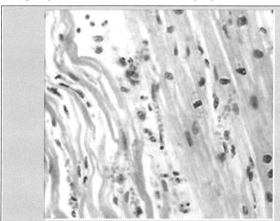

Morphological Changes in MI: Coagulative necrosis, edema & hemorrhage seen in 4-12 hours after myocardial infarction.

Evolution of Morphological Changes in MI		
Time	Gross	Light Microscopy
Reversible injury		
0-30 min	None	None
Irreversible injury		
30 min to 4 hour	None	**Waviness of fibers at border (earliest change)[Q]**
4-12 hour	None	Beginning of coagulative necrosis, edema and hemorrhage
12-24 hour	Dark mottling	On going coagulative necrosis, marginal contraction band necrosis, **beginning of neutrophilic infiltration[Q]**
1-3 days	Mottling with yellow tan infarct centre	**Coagulation necrosis, interstitial neutrophilic infiltrate[Q]**
3-7 days	Hyperemic borders, central yellow tan softening	Beginning of **disintegration with dying neutrophils, early phagocytosis by macrophages[Q]**
7-10 days	Maximum yellow tan and soft depressed red-tan margin	**Early formation of fibrovascular granulation tissue at margins[Q]**
10-14 days	Red grey depressed infarct borders	**Well established granulation tissue & collagen deposition[Q]**
2-8 weeks	Grey-white scar progressive from border towards infarct core	**Collagen deposition, ↓ Cellularity[Q]**
> 2 months	Scarring complete	**Dense collagenous scar[Q]**

41. **Ans. b. Atypical carcinoid grade 2**   (Ref: Robbins 9/e p719-720)

History of diarrhea with cough and associated findings are suggestive of carcinoid syndrome. Positivity for chromogranin confirms the neuroendocrine origin of the tumor. Typical carcinoids have <2 mitoses per 10 high-power fields & lack necrosis, while atypical carcinoids have between 2 & 10 mitoses per 10 high-power fields and/or foci of necrosis. These are traditionally classified as grade 2 carcinoids. Hence the patient is having a grade 2 atypical carcinoid.

*"Typical carcinoids have fewer than two mitoses per 10 high-power fields and lack necrosis, while atypical carcinoids have between two and 10 mitoses per 10 high-power fields and/or foci of necrosis. Atypical carcinoids also show increased pleomorphism, have more prominent nucleoli, and are more likely to grow in a disorganized fashion and invade lymphatics. On electron microscopy the **cells exhibit the dense-core granules characteristic of other neuroendocrine tumors** and, by immunohistochemistry, are found to **contain serotonin, neuron-specific enolase, bombesin, calcitonin, or other peptides.**"* - Robbins 9/e p720

Bronchial Carcinoid

- Represent 1-5% of all lung tumors.
- **Bronchial carcinoids (least malignant)** are the **most indolent** of the spectrum of pulmonary **neuroendocrine tumors**[Q]
- Most patients are **<40 years; Not related to smoking**[Q]
  - **Lower respiratory tract (Bronchus, lung, trachea)** is the **MC site of carcinoid tumor**[Q]
  - **Carcinoid syndrome** is **uncommon**[Q]

Pathology:
- **Most tumors** are **confined to main stem bronchus**, commonly **projects into** the **lumen**[Q]
- Some tumors penetrate the bronchial wall to fan out in the peri-bronchial tissue producing the **collar-button lesion**[Q]

Histology

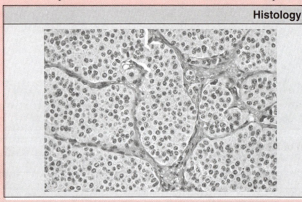

- Tumor is composed of **organoid, trabecular, palisading, ribbon, or rosette-like arrangements of cells separated by a delicate fibrovascular stroma**[Q].
- **Individual cells** are quite regular & have **uniform round nuclei** and a **moderate amount of eosinophilic cytoplasm**[Q].

Clinical Features:
- **Clinical manifestations** emanate from **intraluminal growth, capacity to metastasize & ability** of some of the lesions to elaborate vasoactive amines.[Q]
- **Persistent cough, hemoptysis, impairment of drainage of respiratory passages** with secondary infections, **bronchiectasis, emphysema & atelectasis** are all by-products of the **intraluminal growth** of these lesions[Q].
- **Classic carcinoid syndrome** characterized by **intermittent attacks of diarrhea, flushing & cyanosis** is seen in 10% of bronchial carcinoids[Q].

Treatment:
- **Most bronchial carcinoids do not have secretory activity & do not metastasize to distant sites** but **follow a relatively benign course for long periods** & are **amenable to resection**[Q].

Prognosis:
- **5-year survival rates** are **95% for typical carcinoids, 70% for atypical carcinoids, 30% for large cell neuroendocrine carcinoma & 5% for small cell carcinoma**, respectively.

42. **Ans. c. Membranous glomerulonephritis** *(Ref: Robbins 9/e p915-917; Harrison 19/e p1843)*
The immunofluorescence above is showing granular IgG deposits along the glomerular basement membrane seen in membranous glomerulonephritis.

*"**Membranous Glomerulonephritis:** By light microscopy the glomeruli either appear normal in the early stages of the disease or exhibit **uniform, diffuse thickening of the glomerular capillary wall**. By electron microscopy the thickening is seen to be caused by irregular electron dense also deposits containing immune complexes between the basement membrane and the overlying epithelial cells, with effacement of podocyte foot processes. Basement membrane material is laid down between these deposits, appearing as **irregular spikes protruding from the GBM**. Immunofluorescence microscopy demonstrates that the granular deposits contain both immunoglobulins and complement."* - Robbins 9/e p915

Membranous Glomerulonephritis (MGN)

- MGN or *membranous nephropathy* accounts for approximately 30% of cases of nephrotic syndrome in adults
- Peak incidence: 30-50 years; Rare in childhood
- MC cause of nephrotic syndrome in the elderly^Q.
  - Characterized by **diffuse thickening of the glomerular capillary wall** due to the **accumulation of electron-dense, Ig-containing deposits along the subepithelial side** of the **basement membrane**^{Q}

Secondary membranous glomerulonephritis

Infection	Hepatitis B & C, syphilis, malaria, schistosomiasis, leprosy, filariasis
Cancer	**Breast, colon, lung, stomach**, kidney, esophagus, neuroblastoma
Drugs	**Gold^Q, mercury^Q, penicillamine^Q, NSAIDs^Q, probenecid^Q**
Autoimmune diseases	SLE, rheumatoid arthritis, primary biliary cirrhosis, dermatitis herpetiformis, bullous pemphigoid, myasthenia gravis, Sjogren's syndrome, Hashimoto's thyroiditis^Q
Other systemic diseases	**Fanconi's syndrome, sickle cell anemia, diabetes, Crohn's disease, sarcoidosis, Guillain-Barre syndrome**, Weber-Christian disease, angiofollicular lymph node hyperplasia

Pathogenesis:
- Form of **chronic immune complex–mediated disease**^{Q}
- Secondary MGN: **Inciting antigens** can sometimes be identified in the **immune complexes**.

Morphology:

Light microscopy	Electron microscopy	Immunofluorescence microscopy
• **Uniform, diffuse thickening** of the **glomerular capillary wall**^{Q}	• **Granular deposits**^{Q} (Ig + Complement) • **Effacement of podocyte foot processes**^{Q}	• **Granular/Lumpy bumpy electron dense immune complex deposits**^{Q}

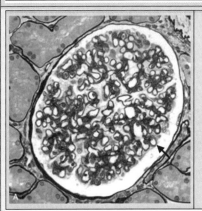 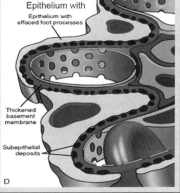 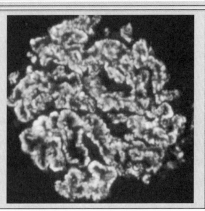

- On silver Methenamine stain: Prominent **"spikes & domes"** of silver staining matrix^Q

Clinical Features:
- **80%** of patients present with **nephrotic syndrome & nonselective proteinuria**^{Q}.
- **Spontaneous remissions** occur in **20-33% of patients**. Persistent proteinuria in 60% patients
- **10% die or progress to renal failure** within 10 years
- **40%** eventually **develop severe CKD or ESRD.**
- **Recurs in 40%** patients who undergo transplantation^Q

Complications:
- MGN has the **highest reported incidences of renal vein thrombosis, pulmonary embolism & DVT** among the causes of nephrotic syndrome^Q.

Prognosis:
- **Male gender, older age, hypertension & persistence of proteinuria** are associated with **worse prognosis**^{Q}
- **Concurrent sclerosis of glomeruli in renal biopsy** at the time of diagnosis is a **predictor of poor prognosis**^{Q}.

43. **Ans. b. Flea bitten kidney of malignant hypertension** *(Ref: Robbins 9/e p940)*
    The image is typically showing a flea bitten kidney that is a granular kidney with multiple petechial spots. Flea bitten kidney is a descriptive term referring to the petechial hemorrhages and micro infarctions on the renal cortical surface, typical of malignant hypertension, which are caused by thrombosis in the arcuate and interlobular arteries.

    "The kidney size varies depending on the duration and severity of the hypertensive disease. Small, pinpoint petechial hemorrhages may appear on the cortical surface from rupture of arterioles or glomerular capillaries, giving the kidney a peculiar "flea-bitten" appearance."- Robbins 9/e p940

"Flea Bitten Kidney" Appearance is seen in	
• Malignant hypertension[Q] • Post-streptococcal glomerulonephritis[Q] • Polyarteritis nodosa[Q] • Subacute bacterial endocarditis[Q] • Wegener's granulomatosis[Q] • Henoch Schonlein purpura[Q] • Systemic lupus erythematosus[Q] • Goodpasture syndrome[Q]	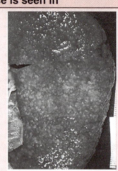

Malignant Hypertension	
Fibrinoid Necrosis of afferent arteriole	**Hyperplastic Arteriolitis (onion-skin lesion)**
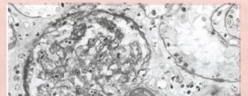	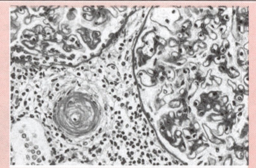

Malignant Nephrosclerosis
• **Renal vascular disorder** associated with **malignant** or **accelerated hypertension**[Q]. • Generally **superimposed on preexisting essential hypertension, secondary forms of hypertension**, or an underlying chronic renal disease, particularly **glomerulonephritis** or **reflux nephropathy**[Q]. • Frequent cause of **renal failure in systemic sclerosis**[Q].
Pathology: • **Fundamental lesion: Vascular injury**[Q]
• **Initiating event injures endothelium** resulting in **increased permeability of small vessels to fibrinogen** & other plasma proteins, **focal death of cells** of vascular wall & **platelet deposition**[Q]. • This can lead to **fibrinoid necrosis of arterioles & small arteries** with **intravascular thrombosis**[Q]. • **Hyperplastic arteriolosclerosis (onion-skinning)** is **typical of malignant hypertension**[Q]
• Associated with **markedly elevated levels of plasma renin**[Q].
• **Small, pinpoint petechial hemorrhages** may appear on the **cortical surface from rupture of arterioles or glomerular capillaries**, giving the kidney a **peculiar "flea-bitten" appearance**[Q].

44. **Ans. c. Rheumatic endocarditis** *(Ref: Robbins 9/e p560)*
    The given image is showing small vegetations in a row along the lines of closure of valves and commissural fusion. This is typically seen in rheumatic endocarditis.

"The rheumatic fever phase of rheumatic heart disease (RHD) is marked by small, warty vegetations along the lines of closure of the valve leaflets. Infective endocarditis (IE) is characterized by large, irregular masses on the valve cusps that can extend onto the chordae. Nonbacterial thrombotic endocarditis (NBTE) typically exhibits small, bland vegetations, usually attached at the line of closure. One or many may be present. Libman-Sacks endocarditis (LSE) has small or medium-sized vegetations on either or both sides of the valve leaflets."- Robbins 9/e p560

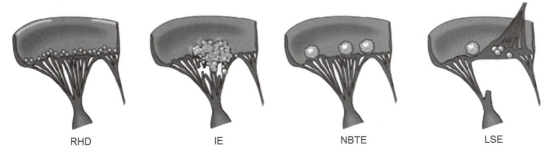

Fig. 22: Comparison of the four major forms of vegetative endocarditis.

Rheumatic Fever (RF) & Rheumatic Heart Disease (RHD)

- **RHD** is characterized principally by **deforming fibrotic valvular disease**, particularly **mitral stenosis**, of which **RHD** is **virtually the only cause**[Q].

Morphology:
- During **acute RF**, focal inflammatory lesions are found in various tissues.
- **Distinctive lesions** occur in **heart**, called **Aschoff bodies**, which **consist of foci of lymphocytes (primarily T cells)**, occasional plasma cells & **plump activated macrophages** called **Anitschkow cells (pathognomonic for RF)**.
  - These **macrophages** have **abundant cytoplasm & central round to ovoid nuclei** in which **chromatin** is **disposed** in a **central, slender, wavy ribbon ("caterpillar cells")** & may become **multinucleated**[Q].
- During acute RF, **diffuse inflammation & Aschoff bodies** may be found in **any of three layers of heart**, causing **pericarditis, myocarditis, or endocarditis (pancarditis)**[Q].
  - Inflammation of endocardium & left-sided valves typically results in **fibrinoid necrosis within the cusps or along tendinous cords**.
  - Overlying these necrotic foci are **small (1-2 mm) vegetations**, called **verrucae, along the lines of closure**[Q].
- **Subendocardial lesions**, perhaps exacerbated by regurgitant jets, may **induce irregular thickenings** called **MacCallum plaques**, usually in the left atrium[Q].
  - Cardinal anatomic changes of mitral valve in chronic RHD are leaflet thickening, commissural fusion & shortening, and **thickening & fusion of tendinous cords**[Q].
  - Fibrous bridging across valvular commissures & calcification create "fish mouth" or "buttonhole" stenoses[Q].

Summary of Salient Features of Vegetations in Different Endocarditis

Rheumatic Fever	Non Bacterial Thrombotic (Marantic) Endocarditis	Libman Sack's Endocarditis	Infective endocarditis
• Small, warty[Q] • Firm[Q] • Friable[Q]	• Small, warty[Q] • Friable[Q]	• Small or medium sized[Q] • Verrucous (warty), irregular[Q]	• Large, bulky[Q] • Irregular[Q] • Most friable[Q]
• Along lines of closure[Q]	• Along lines of closure	• On surface of cusps (both surfaces may be involved but under-surface is more likely affected, less commonly mural endocardium is involved • In pockets of valves[Q]	• Vegetations on the valve cusps[Q] • Less often on mural endocardium extend to chordae[Q]
• Sterile[Q] (no organism)	• Sterile[Q] (no organism)	• Sterile[Q] (no organism)	• Non-sterile[Q] (bacteria)

AIIMS ESSENCE

Summary of Salient Features of Vegetations in Different Endocarditis

• Embolization is uncommon	• Embolization is uncommon	• Embolization is uncommon	• **Embolization very common**[Q] (maximum chances)
• In **rheumatic heart disease**[Q]	• In cancers (**M3-AML**[Q], pancreatic cancer[Q]), **DVT**[Q], Trousseau syndrome[Q]	• In **SLE**[Q]	• In **infective endocarditis**[Q]

MC site for vegetations in rheumatic fever	Mitral valve >Combined mitral & aortic valve[Q]
MC site for vegetations in NBTE	Mitral valve[Q]
MC site for vegetations in Libman Sack's Endocarditis	AV valves, mitral & tricuspid valve[Q]

45. **Ans. d. Predominantly necrotic cells** *(Ref: Robbins 8/e p27 (Not given in 9th edition))*
    A "smeared" pattern of DNA fragmentation is thought to be indicative of necrosis.

    > "A "smeared" pattern of DNA fragmentation is thought to be indicative of necrosis, but this may be a late autolytic phenomenon, and typical DNA ladders are sometimes seen in necrotic cells as well." - *Robbins 8/e p27*

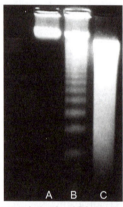

Fig. 23: Agarose gel electrophoresis of DNA extracted from culture cells. Ethidium bromide stain; photographed under ultraviolet illumination.

Lane A	Viable cells in culture[Q]
Lane B	Culture of cells exposed to heat showing extensive apoptosis[Q]
	Note **ladder pattern of DNA fragments**, which **represent multiples of oligonucleosomes**[Q].
Lane C	Culture showing cell necrosis; note **diffuse smearing of DNA**[Q]

DNA and Protein Breakdown

- **Apoptotic cells** exhibit a **characteristic breakdown of DNA** into large **50-to300-kilobase pieces**[Q].
- Subsequently, there is **cleavage of DNA by Ca^{2+}- & Mg^{2+}-dependent endonucleases** into fragments whose **sizes are multiples of 180 to 200 base pairs**, reflecting **cleavage between nucleosomal subunits**[Q].
- The fragments may be **visualized by electrophoresis as DNA "ladders"**[Q].

    > • **Endonuclease activity** also **forms the basis for detecting cell death by cytochemical techniques** that **recognize double-stranded breaks of DNA**[Q].
    > • A "smeared" pattern of DNA fragmentation is thought to be indicative of **necrosis**, but this may be a late autolytic phenomenon, and **typical DNA ladders are sometimes seen in necrotic cells as well**[Q].

46. **Ans. c. Bouin's solution** *(Ref: Surgical Pathology by 'Rosai and Ackerman 9/e p27; Upper Urinary tract Urothelial Carcinoma by Michael Grasso (2015)/p11)*
    Testicular biopsy specimen should be put into Bouin's solution.

    > "Bouin's is a noncoagulate picrate solution which is routinely utilized to fix testicular biopsies because it preserves nuclear detail." -*Upper Urinary tract Urothelial Carcinoma by Michael Grasso (2015)/p11*

Role of Fixative in Histopathology

- An essential part of all histological & cytological techniques is **preservation of cells & tissues as they naturally occur.**
- Tissue blocks, **sections or smears are usually immersed in a fixative fluid**, although in the case of smears, merely drying the preparation acts as a form of preservation.

  - **Fixatives** employed **prevent autolysis by inactivating lysosomal enzymes** & they **stabilize the fine structure, both inside & between cells**, by **making macro-molecules resistant to dissolution by water & other liquids**[Q].
  - **Fixatives** also **inhibit the growth of bacteria** & **molds** that give rise to putrefactive changes[Q].

- Fixatives denature proteins by coagulation, **by forming additive compounds**, or by a **combination of coagulation** and **additive processes**[Q].
- **Fixation changes both chemical** and **antigenic profiles of proteins**[Q].

Tissue-Fixatives

Formalin	• **Formaldehyde** as a **buffered 10% aqueous solution (formalin**[Q]**)** is the **fixative most commonly used** in **histology**[Q] • In routine clinical diagnostics it **offers** the **best possible compromise** between a **simple** and a **reliable method** as well as **extremely good structural preservation**[Q]. • **Strong cross-linking action** of formaldehyde is essential, to protect the tissue from aggressive effect of concentrated solvents in the course of fixation & embedding in paraffin[Q]. • **Fixation of tissue arrests** the **autolysis & putrefaction** and **stabilizes the cellular & tissue contents**[Q]
Glutaraldehyde	• It is an **aldehyde fixative** that **forms cross-links** • Glutaraldehyde causes **deformation of alpha-helix structure**[Q] in proteins so it is **not good for immunoperoxidase staining**[Q] • However, it **fixes quickly**, so it is **good for electron microscopy**[Q].
Alcohols	• **Not used routinely for tissues** because they cause **too much brittleness & hardness**[Q] • However, they are **good for cytologic smears** because they **act quickly** and **give good nuclear detail**[Q].
Mercurials (Mercuric Chloride)	• Mercurials **fix by an unknown mechanism** • These fixatives **penetrate relatively poorly** and cause some tissue hardness but are **fast & give excellent nuclear detail** • **Penetrate rapidly and precipitate all proteins** • **Best application** is **for fixation of hematopoietic** & **reticuloendothelial tissues.**
Picrates (Picric acid, BOUINS solution[Q]**)**	• Composed of **picric acid, acetic acid** & **formaldehyde** in an aqueous solution. • Especially good for **GI tract biopsies** because it allows crisper & better nuclear staining than 10% neutral-buffered formalin. • **Good fixation of tissue for histological evaluation of spermatogenesis**[Q] • It does almost as well as mercurials with **nuclear detail** but does not cause as much hardness. • It **leaves tissue soft** & **penetrates well** precipitating all proteins

Variations of Bouin's solution

Gendre solution	Hollande solution
• It's an **alcoholic version of Bouin solution.** • **An alcoholic solution saturated with picric acids** is used instead of an aqueous solution saturated with picric acid when making this solution. • **Useful when glycogen & other carbohy-drates must be preserved in tissue.**	• It's a **version of Bouin solution** that **contains copper acetate.** • The **copper acetate stabilizes red blood cell membranes** & **granules of eosinophils** and **endocrine cells** so that there is **less lysis of these cell components** than in regular Bouin solution.

AIIMS ESSENCE

Role of Fixative in Histopathology	
Oxidizing Agents (Potassium permagnate, potassium dichromate, osmium tetra oxide)	• They **cross-link proteins**[Q] • **Cause extensive denaturation**[Q] • **Osmium tetra oxide** causes **preservation of fine structures** in **electron microscopy** and is **effective for small specimens**[Q]. • Its **low penetration** limits its application in routine light microscopy. • **Interferes with staining**[Q]

Important Fixatives	
Routine Fixative	• **10% buffered normal formalin**[Q] (Most commonly used)
Electron microscopy	• **Glutaraldehyde**[Q] (Most commonly used) • **Osmium tetraoxide**[Q]
Adrenal medulla	• **Orth's fluid**[Q]
Bone marrow aspirate	• **Helly's fluid**[Q]
Bone marrow biopsy	• **Zenker's fluid**[Q] **& B-5** (Give **excellent nuclear detail, best for fixation of hematopoietic & reticuloendothelial tissues**)
Brain tissue	• **Formalin ammonium bromide**[Q]
Cell blocks	• **Bouin's fluid**[Q]
Cytoplasmic fixatives	• **Champy's fluid**[Q]
Nuclear fixatives	• **Carnoy's fluid**[Q] • **Clarke's fluid**[Q]
Karyotyping fixatives	• **Carnoy's fixative**[Q] (3:1 methanol to glacial acetic acid)
PAP's smear	• **95% ethanol**[Q]
Gastrointestinal biopsies	• **Bouin's fluid**[Q]
Testis & ovary	• **Susa's fixative**[Q]
HOPE Fixative (**H**epes-glutamic acid buffer-mediated **O**rganic solvent **P**rotection **E**ffect)	• Gives formalin-like morphology • **Best for immunohistochemistry, enzyme histochemistry & nucleic acid**

47. **Ans. d. C56789** *(Ref: Robbins 9/e p88-89)*

Complement complex that attacks cell membrane (Membrane attack complex) is C56789.

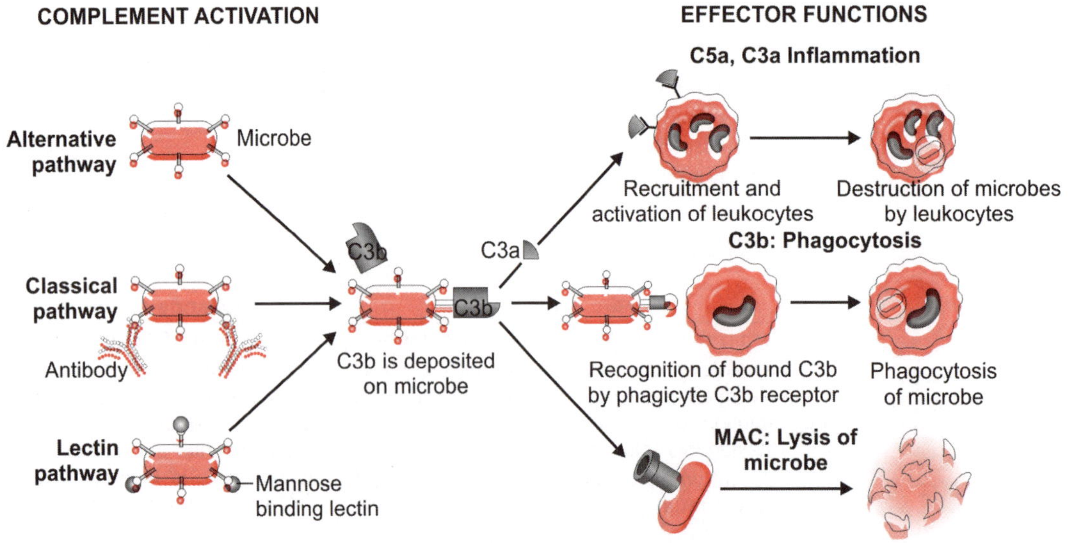

Fig. 24: The activation and functions of the complement system

Complement

- Complement system is a collection of soluble proteins & membrane receptors[Q]
- Synthesized mainly from liver[Q]; Other sites: GIT, macrophages & spleen[Q]
- Function mainly in **host defense against microbes & in pathologic inflammatory reactions**[Q].
- Species non-specific, heat labile & consists of >20 proteins (numbered C1 through C9)[Q]
- Functions in both **innate & adaptive immunity** for defense against microbial pathogens[Q]
- Binds to Fc region of antibody: **IgM**[Q] **(strongly)** >IgG3 > IgG1 > IgG2

Complement Pathways

Classical pathway	Triggered by **fixation of C1 to antibody (IgM or IgG)** that has combined[Q]
Alternative pathway	Triggered by **microbial surface molecules (endotoxin or LPS), complex polysaccharide, cobra venom** & other substances **in the absence of antibody**[Q]
Lectin pathway	Plasma mannose-binding lectin binds to carbohydrates on microbes & directly activates C1[Q]

Stages of Complement Activation

- Initiation of pathway[Q]
- Formation of C3 convertase[Q]
- Formation of C5 convertase[Q]
- Formation of membrane attack complex[Q]

	Classical Pathway	Alternative pathway	Lectin pathway
Activator (Initiator)	Antigen-antibody complex[Q]	Endotoxin[Q] IgA, IgD[Q] Cobra venom[Q] Nephritic factor[Q]	Mannose binding protein[Q]
1st complement activated	C1[Q]	C3b[Q]	C4[Q]
C3 convertase	C4b2a[Q]	C3bBb[Q]	MBL/MASP-C4b2a
C5 convertase (C3 convertase + 3b)	C4b2a3b[Q]	C3bBb3b[Q]	MBL/MASP-C4b2a3b
Complement level in the serum	C1-C9: Low[Q]	C1, C4, C2: Normal[Q] Others: Low[Q]	C1: Normal[Q] Others: Low[Q]
Immunity	Acquired[Q]	Innate[Q]	Innate[Q]

Biological Role of Complement

- **Cell lysis** by the MAC[Q]
- **Vascular phenomena: C3a, C5a** & to a lesser extent, **C4a stimulate histamine release** & **increase vascular permeability**, cause vasodilation (called **anaphylatoxins**)[Q]
- Mediate hypersensitivity reaction type II & III[Q]
- **Leukocyte adhesion, chemotaxis & activation: C5a** is a **powerful chemotactic agent** for neutrophils, monocytes, eosinophils & basophils[Q]
- Opsonisation by C3b & C4b[Q]
- **Removal of immune complex** from blood to spleen **by C3b**[Q]

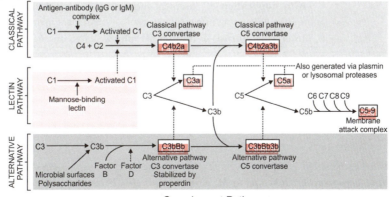

Fig. 25: Complement Pathways

48. Ans. c. C4d *(Ref: Robbins 9/e p234)*

C4d factor is a marker for humoral rejection.

> *"Acute antibody-mediated rejection is manifested mainly by damage to glomeruli and small blood vessels. Typically, the lesions consist of inflammation of glomeruli and peritubular capillaries, associated with deposition of the complement breakdown product C4d, which is produced during activation of the complement system by the antibody- dependent classical pathway. Small vessels may also show focal thrombosis. Cyclosporine, an immunosuppressive drug, is also nephrotoxic, and hence the histologic changes resulting from cyclosporine therapy (e.g., arteriolar hyaline deposits) may be superimposed."- Robbins 9/e p234*

Types of Graft Rejection	
Hyperacute Rejection	• **Immediate** (within minutes to hours) **graft destruction** due to **ABO** or **pre-formed anti-HLA antibodies**[Q]. • Characterized by **intravascular thrombosis**[Q] • **Immunoglobulin & complement** are **deposited in vessel wall** leading to **thrombotic occlusion of capillaries & fibrinoid necrosis** in arterial walls. • **Kidney transplants** are **particularly vulnerable**[Q] to hyperacute graft rejection (kidney rapidly becomes **cyanotic, mottled & flaccid**, and may **excrete few drops of bloody urine**) • **Heart & liver transplants** are **relatively resistant**[Q].

Acute Rejection		
	Acute cellular (T cell-mediated) rejection	**Acute antibody-mediated rejection**
	• Occurs **during first 6 months**[Q] • Most commonly presents **between 5-30**[Q] **days after transplantation** • **T-cell dependent**, characterized by **mononuclear cell infiltration**[Q] • Usually **reversible**[Q] • **Tubulointerstitial pattern (type I)**: Tubulitis associated with presence of both CD4+ & CD8+ T lymphocytes • **Vascular pattern: Endotheliitis (type II)**, sometimes with **necrosis of vascular walls (type III)**[Q].	• Manifested by **damage to glomeruli & small blood vessels**[Q]. • Lesions consist of **inflammation of glomeruli & peritubular capillaries**, with **deposition of** complement breakdown product **C4d**[Q]

Chronic Rejection	Occurs **after the first 6 months**[Q] **MC cause** of **graft failure**[Q] **Non-immune factors** may contribute to pathogenesis Characterized by **myointimal proliferation** in **graft arteries** leading to **ischemia & fibrosis**[Q]

Chronic Rejection in Kidney
• Dominated by **intimal thickening with inflammation, glomerulopathy with duplication** of basement membrane & **peritubular capillaritis** with multilayering of peritubular capillary basement membranes[Q].   • **Interstitial fibrosis & tubular atrophy** with loss of renal parenchyma[Q]

49. Ans. d. Thymocytes *(Ref: Robbins 9/e p625, 788)*

Immature T lymphocytes of thymus are called thymocytes. Thymic epithelial cells are antigen presenting cells (Non-professional) but not thymocytes.

> *"M-cells or microfold cells are a part of GALT (gut associated lymphoid tissue) and an antigen presenting cells in intestine."*

> *"Shigella are resistant to the harsh acidic environment of the stomach, thereby explaining the extremely low infective dose. Once in the intestine, organisms are taken up by M, or microfold cells. These are epithelial cells, which are specialized for sampling and presentation of luminal antigens."- Robbins 9/e p788*

Antigen Presenting Cells (APC)	
Professional APCs	**Nonprofessional APCs**
• **Express MHC class II molecules**[Q] • It includes: • **Dendritic cells**[Q] • **Immature dendritic cells**[Q] • **Macrophages**[Q] • **B-cells**[Q]	• **Do not express MHC class II** for interaction with naïve T cells[Q]. • **Stimulation by cytokines like IFN-γ**[Q]. | **Nonprofessional APCs include**	| |---|---| | • **Fibroblasts**[Q] (skin) • **Thymic epithelial cells**[Q] • **Thyroid epithelial cells**[Q] | • **Glial cells**[Q] (brain) • **Pancreatic beta cells**[Q] • **Endothelial cells**[Q] |

50. Ans. b. 2–6 °C   *(Ref: UK-NHS Guidelines; Harrison 19/e p138e-2)*

RBCs should be stored at a temperature of 2-6 °Celsius.

Characteristics of Selected Blood Components				
Component	**Volume (mL)**	**Storage & duration**	**Content**	**Clinical Response**
Whole Blood	450 ml ± 45[Q]	**2-6°C for 42 days**[Q]	• No elements removed • Contains **RBCs, WBCs, plasma & platelets** (WBCs & platelets may be **non-functional**[Q])	• Not for routine use • Used for **acute massive bleeding, open heart surgery** & neonatal total exchange[Q]
Packed RBCs	180–200[Q]	**2-6°C for 42 days**[Q]	• **RBCs** with variable **leukocyte** content & **small** amount of **plasma**[Q]	• Increase **Hb 1 gm/dL & hematocrit 3%**[Q]
Platelets	50–70[Q]	**22-24°C for 5 days**[Q]	• 5.5 x 10^10/RD unit	• Increase platelet count **5000–10,000/μL**[Q]
FFP	200–250[Q]	**–18°C for 1 year**[Q]	• **Plasma proteins: Coagulation factors**, proteins C & S, antithrombin[Q]	• Increases **coagulation factors** about 2%[Q]
Cryoprecipitate	10–15[Q]	**–18°C for 1 year**[Q]	• Cold-insoluble plasma proteins, fibrinogen, factor VIII, vWF[Q]	• Topical fibrin glue, also **80 IU factor VIII**[Q]

51. Ans. b. With a 18–20 G needle within 4 hours of issue from the blood bank   *(Ref: WHO Clinical Transfusion Guidelines/p22)*

RBCs should be transfused with 18–20 G needle within 4 hours of issue from the blood bank.

Transfusion Protocols

• After collection from donor, blood should be processed for component separation within 6 hours[Q].
• Transfusion should commence within 30 minutes of removing blood bag from refrigerator to decrease the risk of bacterial contamination[Q].
 	
    • **Whole blood or packed RBCs transfusion must be completed within 4 hours**[Q].
    • **Platelet & FFP transfusion must be completed within 20 minutes**[Q].
    • Transfusion set should have **standard filter of 170 micron pore size**[Q] (Standard BT Set).
 	
• Needle size of 18–19 gauge should be used for the transfusion[Q].
• It is not necessary to warm the blood before transfusion[Q].

52. Ans. c. Aplastic anemia   *(Ref: Robbins 9/e p643)*

Direct Coomb's test is negative in aplastic anemia.

Direct Coomb's test	**Indirect Coomb's test**
• Also known as **direct antiglobulin test**[Q] • **Detect antibodies of complement bound to RBC surface antigens** in vivo[Q]. • **It is used for:** • **Immune-mediated hemolytic anemia**[Q] • **Hemolytic disease of the newborn**[Q] • Rh D-hemolytic disease of the newborn[Q] • ABO hemolytic disease of the newborn[Q] • **Drug-induced immune-mediated hemolysis**[Q] • Mismatch transfusion reaction[Q].	• Also known as **indirect antiglobulin test**[Q] • **Detect in vitro antibody-antigen reactions** or **antibodies in serum**[Q]. • **It is used for:** • Detection of very low concentrations of antibodies in a patient's plasma/serum prior to a blood transfusion[Q]. • Used to **screen pregnant women for antibodies** that may cause **hemolytic disease of the new born**[Q]. • **Compatibility testing**[Q] • Antibody identification[Q] • RBC phenotyping[Q] • Titration studies

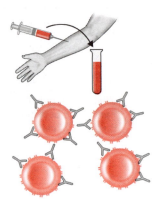
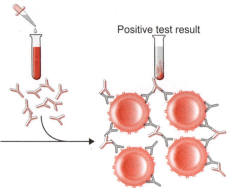

Fig. 26: Direct Coomb's test

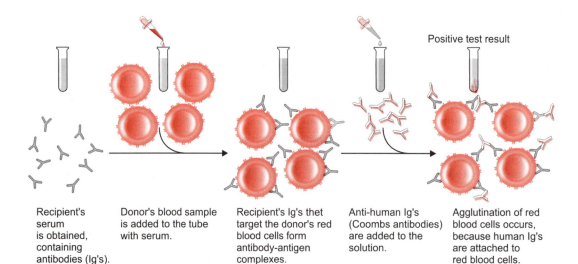

Fig. 27: Indirect Coomb's test

53. Ans. c. Type 3 hypersensitivity reaction *(Ref: Robbins 9/e p207)*
Serum sickness is the prototype of a systemic immune complex disease or type III hypersensitivity reaction.

"Immune Complex–Mediated (Type III) Hypersensitivity: Acute serum sickness is the prototype of a systemic immune complex disease; it was once a frequent sequela to the administration of large amounts of foreign serum (e.g., serum from immunized horses used for protection against diphtheria)." - Robbins 9/e p207

Hypersensitivity Reactions			
Type	Name	Includes	Examples
Type 1	Anaphylactic reaction Mediated by IgE[Q]	Local: Eczema, Hay fever, Asthma (Atopy)[Q] Systemic: Anaphylaxis[Q]	**Theoblad Smith phenomenon:**[Q] This is anaphylaxis in guinea pigs. **PK reaction (Prusnitz Kunster):**[Q] Demonstrate that IgE is homocytotropic i.e. species specific. **Casoni's test:** Immediate type (IgE) Hypersensitivity

Type 2	(IgG & IgM)[Q] Cytotoxic, complement mediated lysis[Q]	• Includes: • **Complement mediated lysis**[Q] • **Antibody dependent cell mediated toxicity** (formerly classified as type I)[Q] • **Changes in cellular function** (former type V)[Q] • **Increased function: Grave's disease**[Q] • **Decreased function: M. gravis**[Q] • Phagocytosis	• Those with **Ag on RBC**: • **Blood transfusion reaction**[Q] • Hemolytic anemia e.g. with I.M. & mycoplasma[Q] • Those with **Ag on neutrophils: Agranulocytosis**[Q] • Those with **Ag on platelets: ITP**[Q] • Those with **Ag on basement membrane: Goodpasture's syndrome**[Q] • **Pemphigus vulgaris**[Q] • ANCA mediated vasculitis[Q] • Acute rheumatic fever[Q] • Insulin resistant diabetes[Q] • Pernicious anemia[Q] • Hemolytic anemia[Q] (quinine, penicillin) • Erythroblastosis fetalis[Q]
Type 3	**Immune complex**[Q] reaction. Antigen antibody complex activates complement[Q]	• Includes: • **Local: Arthus reaction**[Q] • **Systemic: Serum sickness**[Q]	• Shick's test[Q] • Post streptococcal glomerulonephritis[Q] • Detected by RAJI Assay[Q] • Chronic serum sickness-SLE[Q] • Hypersensitivity pneumonitis[Q] • Type 2 Lepra reaction (ENL)[Q]
Type 4	**Delayed hypersensitivity**[Q] **Cell mediated reaction** **T cell mediated**[Q] (initiated by CD4+ T-cells)	• Includes: • **Tuberculin test**[Q] • **Lepromin test**[Q] • **Contact dermatitis**[Q] • **Jones-Mote reaction** (cutaneous basophilic hypersensitivity)[Q] • **Graft rejection (chronic)**[Q]	• Tuberculoid-leprosy[Q] • Graft versus host disease[Q] • Multiple sclerosis. Guillain-Barre syndrome, Hashimoto's thyroiditis[Q]

54. Ans. c. Hydroxyl *(Ref: Robbins 9/e p480)*

Hydroxyl radical (˙OH) is the most potent reactive oxygen species.

"Hydroxyl radical (˙OH): Most reactive oxygen-derived free radical; principal ROS responsible for damaging lipids proteins & DNA"- Robbins 9/e p48

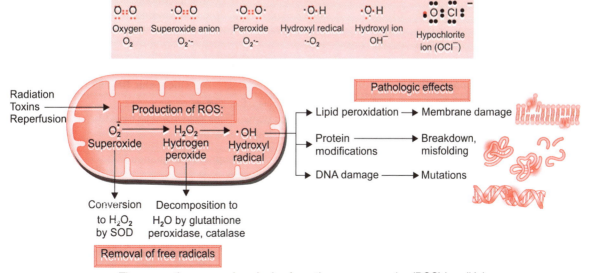

Fig. 28: The generation, removal, and role of reactive oxygen species (ROS) in cell injury.

AIIMS ESSENCE

Properties of the Principal Free Radicals Involved in Cell Injury				
Properties	**$O_{2-\bullet}$ (superoxide anion)**	**H_2O_2 (hydrogen peroxide)**	**OH**	**$ONOO^-$ (Peroxynitrite)**
Mechanisms of production	Incomplete reduction of O_2 during oxidative phosphorylation; by phagocyte oxidase in leukocytes[Q]	Generated by SOD from O_2 & by oxidases in peroxisomes[Q]	Generated from H2O by hydrolysis[Q], e.g., by radiation; from H2O2 by Fenton reaction; from $O_2^{-\bullet}$	Produced by interaction of O2-· & NO generated by NO synthase in many cell types (endothelial cells, leukocytes, neurons)
Mechanisms of inactivation	Conversion to H_2O_2 & O_2 by SOD[Q]	Conversion to H_2O & O_2 by catalase (peroxisomes), glutathione peroxidase (cytosol, mitochondria)[Q]	Conversion to H_2O by glutathione peroxidase[Q]	Conversion to HNO_2 by peroxiredoxins (cytosol, mitochondria)[Q]
Pathologic effects	Stimulates production of degradative enzymes in leukocytes & other cells; may **directly damage lipids, proteins, DNA**; acts close to site of production[Q]	Can be converted to OH & OCl⁻, which destroy microbes & cells; can act distant from site of production	**Most reactive oxygen-derived free radical[Q]; principal ROS responsible for damaging lipids, proteins & DNA[Q]**	Damages lipids, proteins, DNA[Q]

55. Ans. b. Nodular lymphocyte predominant Hodgkin's lymphoma *(Ref: Robbins 9/e p327, 609)*

Among Hodgkin's lymphomas, EBV is not associated with nodular sclerosis & lymphocyte predominant Hodgkin's lymphoma.

*"**Epstein-Barr Virus.** EBV, a **member of the herpes virus family**, has been implicated in the pathogenesis of several human tumors: the **African form of Burkitt lymphoma**; B-cell lymphomas in immunosuppressed individuals (particularly in those with HIV infection or undergoing immunosuppressive therapy after organ or bone marrow transplantation); **a subset of Hodgkin lymphoma**; nasopharyngeal and some gastric carcinomas; and **rare forms of T-cell lymphoma and natural killer (NK) cell lymphoma.**" - Robbins 9/e p327*

Hodgkin's Lymphoma	Immuno-phenotype	Association with EBV	Morphology
Nodular sclerosis	**CD15+, CD30+**[Q]	Usually **EBV–**[Q]	• Frequent lacunar cells (clear space around nucleus) & occasional diagnostic **RS cells**[Q] • Background infiltrate composed of **T lymphocytes, eosinophils, macrophages & plasma cells & fibrous bands**[Q]
Mixed cellularity	**CD15+, CD30+**[Q]	70% EBV+[Q]	• Frequent mononuclear & diagnostic RS cells[Q]
Lymphocyte rich	**CD15+, CD30+**[Q]	40% EBV+[Q]	• Frequent mononuclear & diagnostic RS cell[Q]
Lymphocyte depletion	**CD15+, CD30+**[Q]	Most EBV+[Q]	• Reticular variant: Frequent diagnostic RS cells[Q]
Lymphocyte Predominance	**CD20+, CD15–, C30–**[Q]	EBV–[Q]	• Lymphocytic & Histiocytic (popcorn cell)[Q]

Oncogenic DNA virus	Oncogenic RNA virus
• Human papilloma virus[Q] • Epstein-Barr virus[Q] • Hepatitis B virus[Q]	• Hepatitis C virus[Q] • Human T-cell leukemia virus type-1[Q] • Helicobacter pylori[Q]

Infectious Agent	Lymphoid Malignancy
Epstein-Barr virus	• *Burkitt's lymphoma*[Q] • *Post-organ transplant lymphoma*[Q] • *Primary CNS diffuse large B cell lymphoma*[Q] • *Hodgkin's lymphoma*[Q] *(except nodular sclerosis & lymphocyte predominant Hodgkin's lymphoma)* • *Extranodal NK/T cell lymphoma, nasal type*[Q]
HTLV-I	• *Adult T cell leukemia/lymphoma*[Q]

AIIMS May 2016

Infectious Agent	Lymphoid Malignancy
HIV	• Diffuse large B cell lymphoma[Q] • Burkitt's lymphoma[Q]
Hepatitis C virus	• Lymphoplasmacytic lymphoma[Q]
Helicobacter pylori	• Gastric MALT lymphoma[Q]
Human herpes virus 8	• Primary effusion lymphoma[Q] • Multicentric Castleman's disease[Q]

PHARMACOLOGY

56. Ans. b. Rabeprazole   *(Ref: Goodman Gilman 12/e p1990; Katzung 13/e p1060, 12/e p1089; KDT 7/e p653)*

Rabeprazole is exclusively metabolized by CYP2C19 and does not cause any inhibition of CYP450. Rabeprazole has the highest efficacy, while lansoprazole is the most potent.

*"**Rabeprazole and pantoprazole have no significant drug interactions**. The FDA has issued a warning about a potentially important adverse interaction between clopidogrel and proton pump inhibitors. **Clopidogrel is a prodrug that requires activation by the hepatic P450 CYP2C19 isoenzyme, which also is involved to varying degrees in the metabolism of proton pump inhibitors (especially omeprazole, esomeprazole, lansoprazole, and dexlansoprazole)**. Pending further studies, proton pump inhibitors should be prescribed to patients taking clopidogrel only if they have an increased risk of gastrointestinal bleeding or require them for chronic gastro-esophageal reflux or peptic ulcer disease, in which case agents with minimal CYP2C19 inhibition (pantoprazole or rabeprazole) are preferred."- Katzung 12/e p1089*

*"**Rabeprazole is primarily converted non-enzymatically to rabeprazole-thioether**; some of it is **oxidized to desmethylrabeprazole and rabeprazole sulfone by CYP2C19 and CYP3A4, respectively. CYP2C19 genetic polymorphism has a modest effect on rabeprazole clearance.** Rabeprazole possesses an asymmetric sulfur center; the enantiomers inhibit H^+/K^+-ATPase with equal potency in vitro. ~90% of radiolabeled oral dose is recovered in urine, indicating near-complete gastrointestinal absorption. Incomplete systemic availability is due to instability and first-pass metabolism of rabeprazole."- Goodman Gilman 12/e p1990*

*"**Rabeprazole decreases the concentration of ketoconazole in the plasma (in 33%), increases the concentration of digoxin (in 22%), and does not interact with liquid antacids. Hence, rabeprazole is compatible with any medicine metabolized by CYP450 (theophylline, warfarin, diazepam, phenytoin)."***

PPI	Bioavailability	Protein binding	Metabolism	Biological Half-life	Excretion
Omeprazole	35–76%	95%	Hepatic (**CYP2C19 & CYP3A4[Q] mediated**)	1–1.2 hours	**80% in urine[Q], 20% in feces[Q]**
Lansoprazole	**80% or more[Q]**	97%	Hepatic (**CYP3A4 & CYP2C19[Q] mediated**)	1–1.5 hours	**Renal & fecal[Q]**
Pantoprazole	77%	**98%[Q]**	Hepatic (**CYP3A4[Q]**)	1-2 hours	**Renal[Q]**
Rabeprazole	52%	96%	**Mostly non-enzymatic[Q], partly hepatic (CYP2C19)**	1-1.5 hours	**90% renal[Q]**

57. Ans. c. Epinephrine   *(Ref: Goodman Gilman 12/e p286, 326; Katzung 13/e p161, 12/e p160; The Cornea by Smolin and Thoft's/p504)*

Black deposits on conjunctiva in a patient with glaucoma are seen with use of epinephrine. Latanoprost is associated with iris hyperpigmentation.

*"**Epinephrine is unstable in alkaline solution; when exposed to air or light, it turns pink from oxidation to adrenochrome and then brown from formation of polymers.**"- Goodman Gilman 12/e p286*

*"**Adrenochrome deposits in conjunctiva are common after prolonged use of epinephrine for glaucoma. These are products of oxidation and polymerization of epinephrine. The cornea may also appear black due to deposition of this material over surface.**"- The Cornea by Smolin and Thoft's/p504*

Topical Adrenaline Use

- **Topical use of adrenaline** & related compounds **cause pigmentation of conjunctiva**[Q].
- **Histological appearance** of the lesions: Conjunctival inclusion cysts filled with melanin.
- Deposits **mainly in lower conjunctival fornix**
- **Pigment deposits** may **remain unchanged for long periods of time in spite of stopping adrenaline**.

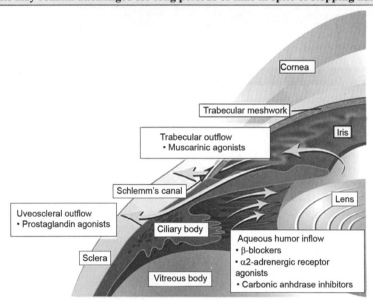

Fig. 29: Mechanism of action of Drugs used for Glaucoma

Drugs for Glaucoma			
Group	**Drugs**	**Mechanism of Action**	**Adverse-effects**
Miotics: • Direct Acting • ACHE inhibitor	**Pilocarpine** **Physostigmine**	↑ Trabecular outflow[Q]	• **Blurred vision**[Q] **(induced myopia)** • Headache, brow pain • **Cataract formation**[Q] • **Retinal detachment**[Q] • **Iris cysts**[Q] & corneal hypoesthesia
Beta-Blockers: • Non-selective (**beta-1 & beta-2**) • Selective (**Beta-1**)	**Timolol,** **Levobunolol,** **Carteolol** **Betaxolol**	↓ Aqueous formation[Q]	• **Allergic blepharoconjunctivitis**[Q] • Transient stinging • **Acquired nasolacrimal duct obstruction**[Q]
• Carbonic Anhydrase Inhibitors	**Dorzolamide** **Brinzolamide**	↓ Aqueous formation[Q]	• Ocular allergy, bitter taste • **Corneal edema**[Q]
• Alpha-2 agonists	**Apraclonidine** **Brimonidine**	↓ Aqueous formation[Q]	• **Lid retraction**[Q] • **Allergic follicular conjunctivitis**[Q] • **Blepharitis**[Q] & **anterior uveitis**[Q] • Dry mouth, drowsiness & apnea in children <6 years with **apraclonidine**[Q]
• Alpha-1 agonists	Dipivefrine Adrenaline	↑ Trabecular & uveoscleral outflow[Q]	• Maculopathy, black adrenochrome deposits with adrenaline[Q] • **Ocular allergy**[Q] • **Conjunctival hyperemia**[Q]
• Prostaglandin F 2-alpha	Latanoprost Bimatoprost Travoprost Unoprostone **Tafluprost**	↑ Uveoscleral outflow[Q]	• **Iris pigmentation**[Q] (Hyperchromia) • **Darkening of periocular skin**[Q] • Conjunctival congestion (Least with latanoprost) • **Growth of eyelashes**[Q] • **Macular edema**[Q] • Mild iridocyclitis[Q]

58. **Ans. c. Paclitaxel** *(Ref: Goodman Gilman 12/e p1708; Katzung 13/e p932, 12/e p963; KDT 7/e p865)*

Paclitaxel is an alkaloid ester derived from the Western yew (Taxus brevifolia) and the European yew (Taxus baccata). Paclitaxel is a taxane, which act by causing disruption of the cell's microtubule function by stabilizing microtubule formation. Paclitaxel acts on the M-phase of cell division.

> *"Paclitaxel: It binds specifically to the β-tubulin subunit of microtubules and antagonizes the disassembly of this key cytoskeletal protein, with the result that bundles of micro-tubules and aberrant structures derived from microtubules appear in the mitotic phase of the cell cycle. Arrest in mitosis follows. Cell killing is dependent on both drug concentration and duration of cell exposure. Drugs that block cell-cycle progression prior to mitosis antagonize the toxic effects of taxanes."* - *Goodman Gilman 12/e p1708*

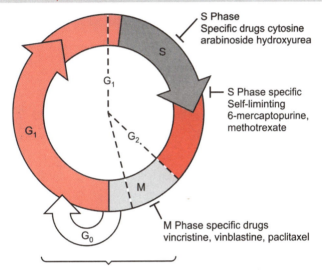

Fig. 30: Cell cycle effects of major classes of anticancer drugs

Cell Cycle Effects of Major Classes of Anticancer Drugs			
Antimetabolites (S phase)		**Alkylating agents**	
• Capecitabine[Q] • Cladribine[Q] • Clofarabine • Cytarabine[Q] • Fludarabine[Q] • 5-Fluorouracil[Q]	• Gemcitabine[Q] • 6-Mercaptopurine[Q] • Methotrexate[Q] • Nelarabine • Pralatrexate • 6-Thioguanine[Q]	• Altretamine • Bendamustine • Busulfan[Q] • Carmustine[Q] • Chlorambucil[Q] • Cyclophosphamide[Q]	• Dacarbazine[Q] • Lomustine[Q] • Mechlorethamine • Melphalan • Temozolomide[Q] • Thiotepa[Q]
Epipodophyllotoxin (topoisomerase II inhibitor) (G$_1$–S phase)		**Antitumor antibiotics**	
Etoposide[Q]		Dactinomycin & Mitomycin[Q]	
Taxanes (M phase)		**Camptothecins (topoisomerase I inhibitors)**	
• Albumin-bound paclitaxel • Cabazitaxel & Paclitaxel[Q]		• Irinotecan[Q] • Topotecan[Q]	
Vinca alkaloids (M phase)		**Platinum analogs**	
• Antimicrotubule inhibitor (M phase)		**Anthracyclines**	
• Ixabepilone[Q]		• Daunorubicin, Doxorubicin, Epirubicin[Q] • Idarubicin • Mitoxantrone	
Antitumor antibiotics (G$_2$–M phase)			
• Bleomycin[Q]			

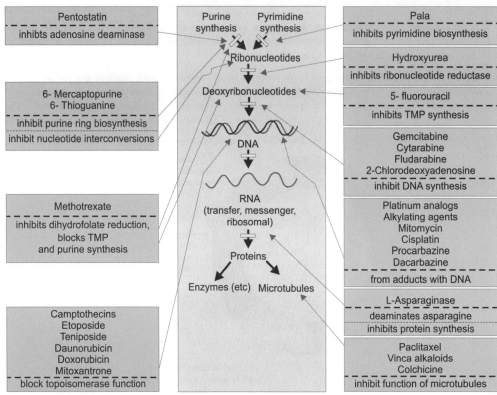

Fig. 31: Chemotherapy of neoplastic diseases

Paclitaxel
• **Paclitaxel** is an alkaloid ester derived from the **Western yew (Taxus brevifolia) & European yew (Taxus baccata)**[Q].
Mechanism of Action: • Drug functions as **a mitotic spindle poison through high-affinity binding to microtubules with enhancement of tubulin polymerization**[Q].   • It **binds to beta-tubulin & enhances its polymerization**[Q] (a mechanism opposite to that of vinca alkaloids)   • **Microtubules are stabilized** & their **depolymerisation is prevented**[Q].   • **Abnormal arrays or 'bundles' of microtubules are produced throughout the cell cycle**[Q].   • **Cytotoxic action of paclitaxel** emphasizes the importance of **tubulin-microtubule dynamic equilibrium**[Q].
Indications: • **Approved indications of paclitaxel**: **Metastatic ovarian & breast carcinoma**[Q] after failure of first line chemotherapy & relapse cases.   • **Paclitaxel** has **significant activity** in a wide variety of solid tumors, including **ovarian, advanced breast, non-small cell & small cell lung, head & neck, esophageal, prostate & bladder cancer** and **AIDS-related Kaposi's sarcoma**[Q].
Side Effects: • Its common side effects are reversible myelosuppression, gastrointestinal mucositis & hair loss, stocking & glove neuropathy[Q].

59. **Ans. b. ALL** *(Ref: Goodman Gilman 12/e p1720; Katzung 13/e p938-939, 12/e p968; KDT 7/e p868)*
    Asparaginase (L-asparagine amidohydrolase) is an enzyme used to treat childhood ALL

    "*Asparaginase (L-asparagine amidohydrolase) is an enzyme used to treat childhood ALL. The drug is isolated and purified from Escherichia coli or Erwinia chrysanthemi for clinical use. It hydrolyzes circulating L-asparagine to aspartic acid and ammonia. Because tumor cells in ALL lack asparagine synthetase, they require an exogenous source of L-asparagine. Thus, depletion of L-asparagine results in effective inhibition of protein synthesis. In contrast, normal cells can synthesize L-asparagine and thus are less susceptible to the cytotoxic action of asparaginase.*"- *Katzung 13/e p938*

L-Asparaginase

- **L-Asparaginase** is **isolated & purified from Escherichia coli**[Q] or **Erwinia chrysanthemi** for clinical use.

Mechanism of Action:
- Most **normal tissues** are **able to synthesize L-asparagine in amounts sufficient for protein synthesis**[Q]
- **Lymphocytic leukemias lack adequate amounts of asparagine synthetase & derive the required amino acid from plasma**[Q].
  - **L-Asparaginase catalyzes the hydrolysis of circulating asparagine to aspartic acid & ammonia**[Q] **deprives these malignant cells of asparagine, leading to cell death**[Q].

Indications:
- **L-Asparaginase** has become a **standard agent for treating ALL**[Q].
- It is used in combination with **methotrexate, doxorubicin, vincristine & prednisone** for the **treatment of ALL & high-grade lymphomas**[Q].

Side-Effects:
- **Main adverse effect: Hypersensitivity reaction**[Q]
- Other side effects: **Increased risk of clotting & bleeding**[Q] (due alterations in various clotting factors), **pancreatitis**[Q], & **neurologic toxicity**[Q].

Miscellaneous anticancer drugs (Clinical activity & toxicities)				
Drug	**Mechanism of Action**	**Clinical Applications**	**Acute Toxicity**	**Delayed Toxicity**
Asparaginase	**Hydrolyzes circulating L-asparagine**, resulting in rapid inhibition of protein synthesis[Q]	**ALL**[Q]	Fever, allergic reactions[Q]	Hepatotoxicity, increased risk of **bleeding & clotting**[Q], **pancreatitis**[Q]
Erlotinib	**Inhibits EGFR tyrosine kinase leading to inhibition of EGFR signaling**[Q]	**Non-small cell lung cancer**[Q], **pancreatic cancer**[Q]	Diarrhea[Q]	Skin rash, diarrhea, anorexia, interstitial lung disease
Gefitinib	Same as erlotinib	**Non-small cell lung cancer**[Q]	**Hypertension & diarrhea**[Q]	Skin rash, diarrhea, interstitial lung disease
Imatinib	**Inhibits Bcr-Abl tyrosine kinase**[Q] **& PDGFR, stem cell factor, & c-kit**[Q]	**CML**[Q], **GIST**[Q], **Philadelphia chromosome-positive ALL**[Q]	Nausea & vomiting	**Fluid retention with ankle & periorbital edema**[Q], diarrhea, myalgias, **CHF**[Q]
Cetuximab	**Binds to EGFR & inhibits down-stream EGFR signaling**[Q]; **enhances response to chemotherapy & radiotherapy**[Q]	**Colorectal cancer**[Q], **head & neck cancer** (used with radiotherapy[Q]), **non-small cell lung cancer**[Q]	**Infusion reaction**[Q]	**Skin rash**[Q], **hypomagnesemia**[Q], fatigue, interstitial lung disease
Panitumumab	Binds to EGFR & inhibits down-stream EGFR signaling; enhances response to chemotherapy & radiotherapy	**Colorectal cancer**[Q]	Infusion reaction (rarely)	**Skin rash**[Q], **hypomagnesemia**[Q], fatigue, interstitial lung disease
Bevacizumab	**Inhibits binding of VEGF to VEGFR leading to inhibition of VEGF signaling**[Q]; **inhibits tumor vascular permeability; enhances tumor blood flow & drug delivery**[Q]	**Colorectal cancer**[Q], **breast cancer**[Q], **non-small cell lung cancer**[Q], **RCC**[Q]	**Hypertension &** infusion reaction	**Arterial thromboembolic events**[Q], **GI perforations**[Q], **wound healing complications, proteinuria**[Q]
Sorafenib	**Inhibits raf kinase, VEGF-R2, VEGF-R3 & PDGFR-beta** leading to **inhibition of angiogenesis, invasion & metastasis**[Q]	**RCC**[Q], **HCC**[Q]	Hypertension	Skin rash, fatigue & asthenia, **bleeding complications, hypophosphatemia**[Q]
Sunitinib	**Inhibits VEGF-R1, VEGF-R2, VEGF-R3, PDGFR-alpha & PDGFR-beta** leading to **inhibition of angiogenesis, invasion & metastasis**[Q]	**RCC**[Q], **GIST**[Q]	Hypertension	Skin rash, fatigue & asthenia, **bleeding complications, cardiac toxicity** leading to CHF in rare cases

60. **Ans. a. Prasugrel** *(Ref: Goodman Gilman 13/e p595, 12/e p870; Katzung 13/e p595, 12/e p612; KDT 7/e p631)*
Prasugrel reduce platelet aggregation by inhibiting the ADP pathway of platelets. It irreversibly blocks the ADP receptor on platelets.

> *"From this list of agents, several targets for platelet inhibitory drugs have been identified: inhibition of prostaglandin synthesis (aspirin), inhibition of ADP- induced platelet aggregation (clopidogrel, prasugrel, ticlopidine), and blockade of glycoprotein IIb/IIIa receptors on platelets (abciximab, tirofiban, and eptifibatide). Dipyridamole and cilostazol are additional antiplatelet drugs."- Katzung 12/e p612*

> *"Ticlopidine, clopidogrel, and prasugrel reduce platelet aggregation by inhibiting the ADP pathway of platelets. These drugs irreversibly block the ADP receptor on platelets. Unlike aspirin, these drugs have no effect on prostaglandin metabolism. Use of ticlopidine, clopidogrel, or prasugrel to prevent thrombosis is now considered standard practice in patients undergoing placement of a coronary stent."- Katzung 13/e p595*

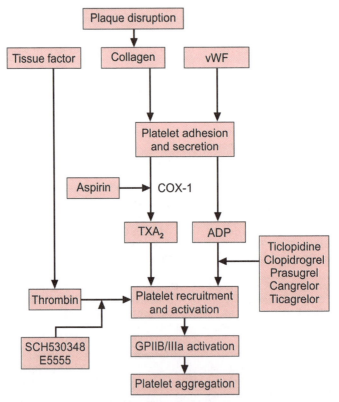

Fig. 32: Site of action of antiplatelet drugs

| Anticoagulants & Antiplatelet Agents ||||
Drug	Mechanisms	Characteristic Features	Adverse Effects
Aspirin	• Acetylates & irreversibly inhibits cyclooxygenase[Q] (both COX-1 & COX2) to prevent conversion of arachidonic acid to thromboxane A_2 → Inhibits platelet aggregation[Q].	• Decreases risk of thrombus in CAD & post-MI & post-operative state. • Antipyretic, analgesic, anti-inflammatory, anti-platelet	• Increased risk of hemorrhagic stroke[Q] • GI ulceration[Q] & bleeding[Q] • Tinnitus[Q] • Reye's syndrome[Q]
Thienopyridines Clopidogrel[Q], Ticlopidine[Q], Prasugrel[Q], Cangrelor[Q], Ticagrelor[Q]	• Block ADP receptors (P2Y12 receptors) to suppress fibrinogen binding & platelet adhesion[Q] to injury sites	• Decreases risk of repeat MI or stroke or PVD[Q] • Decreases thrombus risk in coronary stenting[Q]	• Increased risk of hemorrhage & GI bleeding • Neutropenia (ticlopidine[Q])

Contd...

Contd...

Drug	Mechanisms	Characteristic Features	Adverse Effects
GP IIb/IIIa inhibitors (Abciximab[Q], eptifiba-tide[Q], tirofiban[Q])	• **Inhibit platelet aggregation** by **binding to platelet GP IIb/IIIa**[Q]	• **Decreases risk of thrombus** in **unstable angina** or **following PTCA**[Q]	• Increased risk of **hemorrhage** • **Hypotension** • **Back pain**
Adenosine reuptake inhibitors Dipyridamole[Q]	• **Inhibit activity of adenosine deaminase & phosphodies-terase receptors**[Q]	• **Used in combination with ASA** in patients with **recent stroke** or with **warfarin following artificial heart valve replacement**[Q]	• Dizziness • Headache
Heparin	• **Activates antithrombin III,** which **decreases the activity of thrombin & Xa**[Q] • **Prevents clot formation**[Q]	• **Immediate anticoagulation for MI, DVT, PE, stroke**[Q] • **Post-operative prophylaxis for DVT & PE**[Q] • **Decreases post-MI thrombus risk** • **Safer in pregnancy**[Q] (does not cross placenta)	• Thrombocytopenia[Q] • **Hemorrhage**[Q] • **Osteoporosis**[Q] • **Hypersensitivity**[Q]
Low Molecular Weight Heparin (LMWH) (Enoxparin[Q], dalteparin[Q])	• **Binds to factor Xa to prevent clot formation**[Q]	• Postoperative prophylaxis for DVT & PE • Safest option during pregnancy[Q]	• **Hemorrhage, fever**
Direct thrombin inhibitors **Parenteral: Lepirudin, Argatroban, Bivalirudin** **Oral: Dabigatran**[Q]	• **Highly selective inhibitors of thrombin**[Q] to **suppress activity of factors V, IX & XIII & platelet aggregation**	• Alternative to heparin for anticoagulation in patients with **history of heparin induced thrombocytopenia**	• Hemorrhage & hypotension
Indirect factor Xa inhibitors Fondaparinux[Q]	• **Inhibition of factor Xa**[Q] without activity against thrombin, **require antithrombin as a co-factor & do not inhibit factor Xa bound to prothrombinase complex**[Q]	• **DVT prophylaxis** • Anticoagulation following acute DVT or PE • Given subcutaneously	• Hemorrhage • Fever & anemia • Edema & rash • Constipation
Oral Direct Factor Xa inhibitors (rivaroxaban, apixaban)	• Directly engage the active centre of factor Xa molecule & inhibit both free factor Xa in plasma & factor Xa attached to prothrombinase complex[Q]	• Used for **prevention & treatment of venous thromboembolism & stroke prevention** in **atrial fibrillation**[Q]	
Warfarin	• **Impairs synthesis & carbox-ylation of vitamin K-dependent factors**[Q] **II, VII, IX & X** and **protein C & protein S**[Q] • **Affects extrinsic pathway & PT**[Q]	• Used for **long-term anti-coagulation, post-throm-botic event** or in cases of **increased thrombus risk (post-surgery, atrial fibrillation, artificial valves)**[Q] • Metabolized by **cytochrome P-450 pathway, long half-life**	• Hemorrhage • **Teratogenicity (Conrad's syndrome**[Q]) • **Calciphylaxis**[Q]

61. **Ans. c. Telmisartan**   *(Ref: Yamagishi S, Takeuchi M. Telmisartan is a promising cardiometabolic sartan due to its unique PPAR-gamma-inducing property. Med Hypotheses. 2005;64(3):476-8)*

Angiotensin receptor blocker (ARB) with PPAR-gamma function as well is telmisartan.

"Recently, telmisartan, an ARB, was found to act as a partial agonist of peroxisome proliferator-activated receptor-gamma (PPAR-gamma). In fact lisinopril and valsartan are also PPAR-gamma agonists, though with a lesser potency. PPAR-gamma influences the gene expression involved in carbohydrate metabolism, and pioglitazone and rosiglitazone, ligands for PPAR- gamma, improve insulin resistance in diabetic patients. Furthermore, there is a growing body of

1086 | AIIMS ESSENCE

*evidence that activators of **PPAR-gamma** exert anti-inflammatory, anti-oxidative and anti- proliferative effects on vascular wall cells, thus decreasing the risks for atherosclerosis. Due to its unique PPAR-gamma-modulating activity, telmisartan is a promising 'cardiometabolic sartan', that targets both diabetes and CVD in hypertensive patients. The binding affinity to PPAR-gamma is highest for telmisartan followed by lisinopril and valsartan. Pharmacokinetic differences may explain different potencies of PPAR-gamma stimulation by drugs acting on the renin-angiotensin system in clinical settings."- Yamagishi S, Takeuchi M. Telmisartan is a promising cardiometabolic sartan due to its unique PPAR-gamma-inducing property. Med Hypotheses. 2005;64(3):476-8*

62. **Ans. d. Postsynaptic nicotinic receptors** *(Ref: Goodman Gilman 13/e p108, 12/e p255; Katzung 13/e p108, 12/e p98)*

Ganglionic transmission is mediated by nicotinic receptors present post-synaptically.

> *"The nicotinic acetylcholine (ACh) receptor mediates neurotransmission post-synaptically at the neuromuscular junction and peripheral autonomic ganglia; in the CNS, it largely controls release of neurotransmitters from presynaptic sites. The receptor is called the nicotinic acetylcholine receptor because both the alkaloid nicotine and the neurotransmitter ACh can stimulate the receptor. Distinct subtypes of nicotinic receptors exist at the neuromuscular junction and the ganglia, and several pharmacological agents discriminate between the receptor subtypes."- Goodman Gilman 12/e p255*

63. **Ans. b. Increase in renal perfusion due to agonist action on D1 receptors** *(Ref: Goodman Gilman 13/e p1062, 12/e p355; KDT 7/e p134, 6/e p507)*

Dopamine at low concentrations (2 to 5 mcg/kg per minute) primarily acts on vascular D_1 receptors, especially in the renal, mesenteric, and coronary beds. By activating adenylyl cyclase and raising intracellular concentrations of cyclic AMP, D_1 receptor stimulation leads to vasodilation. Infusion of low doses of dopamine causes an increase in glomerular filtration rate, renal blood flow, and Na^+, K^+-ATPase pump. Increased renal perfusion caused by dopamine due to D1 agonism (at low doses) doesn't improves survival in acute shock.

Dopamine (3,4-dihydroxyphenylethylamine)
• It is **immediate metabolic precursor of norepinephrine & epinephrine**
• **Central neurotransmitter** particularly **important in regulation of movement** & **possesses important intrinsic pharmacological properties**[Q].
• In the periphery, it is **synthesized in epithelial cells of proximal tubule** & is thought to **exert local diuretic & natriuretic effects**[Q].
• **Dopamine** is a **substrate for both MAO & COMT** & is **ineffective when administered orally**[Q].

Pharmacological Properties of Dopamine	
At low concentrations (2–5 mcg/kg per minute)	**At somewhat higher concentrations (5–10 mcg/kg per minute)**

• **Primarily acts on vascular D_1 receptors**, especially in **renal, mesenteric & coronary beds**[Q].
• By **activating adenylyl cyclase** & raising intracellular concentrations of c-AMP, D_1 **receptor stimulation leads to vasodilation**[Q].
 	
  • **Infusion of low doses of dopamine** causes an **increase in GFR, renal blood flow & Na^+, K^+-ATPase pump**[Q].
 	
• **Renal tubular actions of dopamine** that **cause natriuresis** may be **augmented by increase in renal blood flow** & small increase in GFR that follow its administration.
• Resulting **increase in hydrostatic pressure in peritubular capillaries & reduction in oncotic pressure** may contribute to **diminished reabsorption of Na^+** by proximal tubular cells.
 	
  • **Dopamine** has pharmacologically appropriate effects in **management of states of low cardiac output associated with compromised renal function,** such as **severe CHF.**
	• Exerts a **positive inotropic effect on myocardium,** acting on **beta$_1$ adrenergic receptors**[Q].
	• Causes **release of norepinephrine from nerve terminals**, which contributes to its effects on heart.
	• **Dopamine increases SBP & pulse pressure** & either has no effect on diastolic blood pressure or increases it slightly[Q].
	• **Total peripheral resistance usually is unchanged** when low or intermediate doses of dopamine are given, because of **ability of dopamine to reduce regional arterial resistance in some vascular beds,** such as **mesenteric & renal,** while causing only minor increases in others[Q].

64. **Ans. b. D_2 antagonist** *(Ref: Goodman Gilman 12/e p1325; Katzung 13/e p1062, 12/e p1092; KDT 7/e p665)*

Metoclopramide is a dopamine D_2 receptor antagonist, and is also a mixed 5-HT$_3$ receptor antagonist & 5-HT$_4$ receptor agonist. The antiemetic action of metoclopramide is due to its antagonist activity at D_2 receptors in the chemoreceptor trigger zone in the central nervous system-this action prevents nausea & vomiting triggered by most stimuli. At higher doses, 5-HT$_3$ antagonists activity may also contribute to the antiemetic effect.

"Metoclopramide and domperidone also block dopamine D_2 receptors in the chemoreceptor trigger zone of the medulla (area postrema), resulting in potent anti-nausea and antiemetic action."- *Katzung 13/e p1062*

Metoclopramide
• Derivative of para-aminobenzoic acid & structurally related to procainamide. • Prokinetic agent, increases lower esophageal sphincter tone & stimulates antral & small intestinal contractions[Q] (effects are confined largely to the upper digestive tract)

Mechanism of Action:
- Metoclopramide acts through both dopaminergic & serotonergic receptors[Q].

D_2 Antagonism[Q]	5-HT_4 Agonism[Q]	5-HT_3 Antagonism[Q]
• Central antidopaminergic (D_2) action on CTZ is responsible for **antiemetic property**[Q].	• Acts in GIT to **enhance ACh release from myenteric motor neurons**, resulting from 5-HT_4 receptor activation[Q] on primary afferent neurons (PAN) of the enteric nervous system via excitatory interneurons	• At high concentrations it can **block 5-HT_3 receptors present on inhibitory myenteric interneurons & in NTS/CTZ**[Q].

Pharmacokinetics:
- Absorbed rapidly after oral ingestion, undergoes sulfation & glucuronide conjugation by liver[Q]
- Excreted mainly in urine[Q]

Uses:
- Antiemetic: Postoperative, drug-induced, disease associated (especially migraine), radiation sickness but is less effective in motion sickness[Q].
- Gastrokinetic: To accelerate gastric emptying[Q] (emergency general anesthesia, relieve post vagotomy or diabetic gastric stasis)
- Dyspepsia & other functional GI disorders
- Metoclopramide may succeed in stopping persistent hiccups[Q]
- Gastroesophageal reflux disease[Q]

Side-Effects:
- Major side effects include extrapyramidal effects[Q] (dystonias, akathisia, parkinsonian features)
- Extrapyramidal effects more common in children & young adults[Q] (at higher doses).

> • **Elevated prolactin levels (blocking the inhibitory effect of dopamine on prolactin release)** can cause **galactorrhea, gynecomastia, impotence & menstrual disorders**[Q].

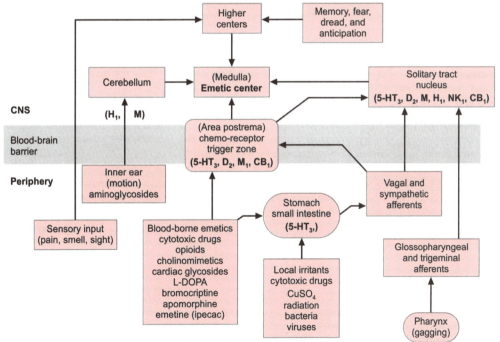

Fig. 33: Pathway of emesis

Types of Antiemetics			
Type	**Mechanism**	**Examples**	**Clinical indications**
Antiemetic agents	H₁ Antihistamines	Promethazine, **cyclizine**[Q] diphenhydramine, dimenhydrinate, **cinnarizine**[Q]	**Motion sickness, inner ear disease**[Q]
	Anticholinergic	**Hyoscine, dicyclomine**[Q]	**Motion sickness, inner ear disease**[Q]
	Antidopaminergic	Prochlorperazine, thiethylperazine	Medication, toxin or metabolic-induced emesis
	5-HT₃ antagonist	**Ondansetron, granisetron**[Q]	**Chemotherapy & radiation-induced emesis**[Q]**, postoperative emesis**[Q]
	Neurokinin (NK-1) antagonist	**Aprepitant**[Q] Fosaprepitant	**Chemotherapy-induced nausea & vomiting**[Q]
	Tricyclic antidepressant	Amitriptyline, nortriptyline	Chronic idiopathic nausea, functional vomiting, cyclic vomiting syndrome
Prokinetic agents	**5-HT₄ agonist & D₂ antagonist** (anti-dopaminergic)	**Metoclopramide**[Q]	Gastroparesis
	Motilin agonist	**Erythromycin**[Q]	Gastroparesis, intestinal pseudo-obstruction
	Peripheral antidopaminergic	**Domperidone**[Q]	Gastroparesis
	5-HT₄ agonist	**Tegaserod**[Q]	Constipation predominant irritable bowel syndrome, gastroparesis
	5-HT₄ agonist with weak 5-HT₃ antagonism	**Cisapride**[Q]	GERD
	Somatostatin analogue	**Octreotide**[Q]	Intestinal pseudo-obstruction
Adjuvant antiemetics	Benzodiazepines	**Lorazepam**[Q]	Anticipatory nausea & vomiting with chemotherapy
	Glucocorticoids	**Methylprednisolone, dexamethasone**[Q]	**Chemotherapy-induced emesis**[Q]
	Cannabinoids	**Tetrahydrocannabinol**[Q]	**Chemotherapy-induced emesis**[Q]

65. **Ans. d. Action on presynaptic alpha-receptors** *(Ref: Goodman Gilman 12/e p209, 302, 308)*

Activation of presynaptic α_2 receptors inhibits the release of NE and other co-transmitters from peripheral sympathetic nerve endings. Activation of α_2 receptors in the pontomedullary region of the CNS inhibits sympathetic nervous system activity and leads to a fall in blood pressure. Action on presynaptic alpha-receptors (α_2 receptors) is not helpful in management of anaphylactic shock.

"Pre-synaptically located α_2 and β_2 receptors fulfill important roles in the regulation of neurotransmitter release from sympathetic nerve endings. Presynaptic α_2 receptors also may mediate inhibition of release of neurotransmitters other than norepinephrine in the central and peripheral nervous systems. Both α_2 and β_2 receptors are located at post-synaptic sites, such as on many types of neurons in the brain. In peripheral tissues, postsynaptic α_2 receptors are found in vascular and other smooth muscle cells (where they mediate contraction), adipocytes, and many types of secretory epithelial cells (intestinal, renal, endocrine). Postsynaptic β_2 receptors can be found in the myocardium (where they mediate contraction) as well as on vascular and other smooth muscle cells (where they mediate relaxation) and skeletal muscle (where they can mediate hypertrophy). Indeed, most normal human cell types express β_2 receptors. Both α_2 and β_2 receptors may be situated at sites that are relatively remote from nerve terminals releasing NE. Such extra-junctional receptors typically are found on vascular smooth muscle cells and blood elements (platelets and leukocytes) and may be activated preferentially by circulating catecholamines, particularly epinephrine."- Goodman Gilman 12/e p209

"The α_2 receptors have an important role in regulation of the activity of the sympathetic nervous system, both peripherally and centrally. As mentioned earlier, activation of presynaptic α_2 receptors inhibits the release of NE and other co-transmitters from peripheral sympathetic nerve endings. Activation of α_2 receptors in the pontomedullary region of the CNS inhibits sympathetic nervous system activity and leads to a fall in blood pressure."- Goodman Gilman 12/e p308

AIIMS May 2016

Treatment of Anaphylaxis (Anaphylactic Shock)

- **Early recognition of an anaphylactic reaction is mandatory,** since **death occurs within minutes to hours** after first symptoms[Q].
- **Mild symptoms** (pruritus & urticaria) can be **controlled by** administration of 0.3 to 0.5 mL of 1:1000 (1 mg/mL) **epinephrine SC or IM,** with repeated doses as required at 5- to 20-min intervals for a severe reaction[Q].
- **If antigenic material was injected into an extremity,** rate of absorption may be reduced by **prompt application of a tourniquet proximal to reaction site,** administration of 0.2 mL of 1:1000 **epinephrine into the site**[Q] & removal without compression of an insect stinger, if present.
  - An **IV infusion** should be initiated to provide a **route for administration of 2.5 mL epinephrine,** diluted 1:10,000, at 5- to 10-min intervals, **volume expanders such as normal saline & vasopressor agents** such as **dopamine if intractable hypotension occurs**[Q].
- Replacement of intravascular volume due to post-capillary venular leakage may require several liters of saline.
  - **Epinephrine provides both alpha & beta-adrenergic effects,** resulting in **vasoconstriction, bronchial smooth-muscle relaxation & attenuation of enhanced venular permeability**[Q].
- When epinephrine fails to control the anaphylactic reaction, hypoxia due to airway obstruction or related to a cardiac arrhythmia, or both, must be considered.
  - **Oxygen alone via a nasal catheter** or **with nebulized albuterol** may be helpful, but either **endotracheal intubation** or a **tracheostomy is mandatory for oxygen delivery if progressive hypoxia develops**[Q].
- Ancillary agents such as **diphenhydramine,** 50-100 mg IM or IV & **aminophylline,** 0.25-0.5 g IV, are appropriate **for urticaria-angioedema & bronchospasm, respectively**[Q].
  - **Intravenous glucocorticoids,** 0.5-1 mg/kg of medrol, are **not effective for acute event** but **may alleviate later recurrence of bronchospasm, hypotension, or urticaria**[Q].

Direct Sympathomimetics

Drug	Selectivity	Indications
Epinephrine	$\alpha_1, \alpha_2, \beta_1, \beta_2, \beta_3$	• **Anaphylactic shock**[Q]**, open angle glaucoma**[Q]**, bronchodilator in acute asthma**[Q]**, hypotension, complete heart block**[Q] • With **local anesthetics to prolong action**[Q]
Norepinephrine	$\alpha_1, \alpha_2 > \beta_1$	• **Hypotension**[Q]
Isoproterenol	$\beta_1 = \beta_2$	• **Bronchodilator in asthma, complete heart block, shock**[Q]
Dopamine	$D_1 = D_2 > \beta > \alpha$	• **Inotropic & chronotropic**[Q]**; used in shock**
Dobutamine	$\beta_1 > \beta_2$	• **Inotropic but not chronotropic**[Q] • **Short term treatment** of **cardiac decompensation** after surgery, or patients with **CHF** or **MI**
Phenylephrine	$\alpha_1 > \alpha_2$	• Used as **pure mydriatic**[Q] when **cycloplegia is not required** (fundus examination), **nasal decongestion, vasoconstriction, antagonizes hypotension of spinal anesthesia**[Q]
Albuterol, terbutaline	$\beta_2 > \beta_1$	• **Albuterol for acute attack of asthma**[Q] • **Terbutaline as tocolytic**[Q]
Ritodrine	β_2	• **To stop premature labour (Tocolytic)**[Q]

66. Ans. c. Decrease in heart rate on adrenaline administration after phentolamine has been given *(Ref: KDT 7/e p131, 140)*

Decrease in heart rate on adrenaline administration after phentolamine has been given depicts vasomotor reversal of Dale.

"Blockade of vasoconstrictor alpha-1 (also alpha-2) receptors reduces peripheral resistance and causes pooling of blood in capacitance vessels →venous return and cardiac output are reduced →fall in BP. Postural reflex is interfered with →marked hypotension occurs on standing →dizziness and syncope. Hypovolemia accentuates the hypotension. The alpha-blocker abolishes the pressor action of adrenaline (injected IV in animals), which then produces only fall in BP due to beta-2 mediated vasodilatation. This was first demonstrated by Sir HH Dale (1913) and is called vasomotor reversal of Dale. Pressor and other actions of selective alpha agonists (phenylephrine) are suppressed."- KDT 7/e p140

67. Ans. d. Phase IV (Ref: Goodman Gilman 12/e p79; Katzung 13/e p17, 12/e p75; KDT 7/e p63-64, 6/e p77)

Surveillance after marketing, i.e. after the drug is out in the market is a part of Phase IV of clinical trials. It includes follow-up of patients taking the drug and adverse drug reaction (ADR) reporting as well as looking for newer treatment indications.

"Once approval to market a drug has been obtained, phase 4 begins. This constitutes monitoring the safety of the new drug under actual conditions of use in large numbers of patients. The importance of careful and complete reporting of toxicity by physicians after marketing begins can be appreciated by noting that many important drug-induced effects have an incidence of 1 in 10,000 or less and that some adverse effects may become apparent only after chronic dosing. The sample size required to disclose drug-induced events or toxicities is very large for such rare events. For example, several hundred thousand patients may have to be exposed before the first case is observed of a toxicity that occurs with an average incidence of 1 in 10,000. Therefore, low-incidence drug effects are not generally detected before phase 4 no matter how carefully the studies are executed. Phase 4 has no fixed duration. As with monitoring of drugs granted accelerated approval, phase 4 monitoring has often been lax."- Katzung 13/e p17

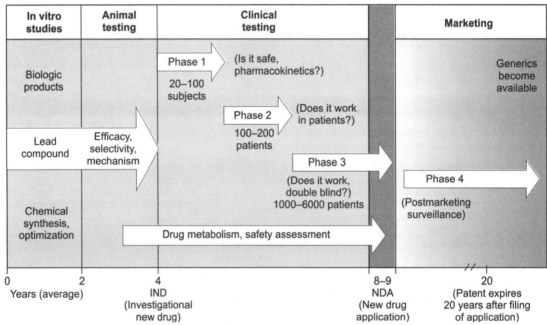

Fig. 34: The development and testing process required to bring a drug to market

Stage of development	Phase 1	Phase 2	Phase 3	Phase 4
End point	Safety	Safety	Safety	Safety
Specific end point	Safety profile[Q]	Cardiac output	Reduction in mortality rate[Q]	Reduction in mortality rate
Types of studies	Different indications: Single or multiple dose	Placebo controlled: Dose Escalation	Placebo controlled: Long term follow up	Comparative new indications

Summary of Clinical Trial				
Phase	Name	Conducted on	Blinding & Control	Purpose
I	Human Pharmacology & safety	**Healthy** volunteers (20-100)	Open Label (No blinding)	To know maximum tolerable dose[Q] Safety & tolerability[Q]
II	Therapeutic exploratory	100-150 **Patients** (**Homogenous** population)	Single blind Controlled	To establish therapeutic efficacy[Q] Dose ranging & ceiling effect[Q]
III	Therapeutic confirmatory	Upto 5000 patients from several centres (**Heterogeneous** population)	Double blind Randomized Controlled	To confirm therapeutic efficacy[Q] To establish the value of drug in relation to existing therapy

Phase	Name	Conducted on	Blinding & Control	Purpose
IV	Post Marketing surveillance	Large no. of patients being treated by practicing physicians	–	To know **rare & long term adverse effects**[Q] Special groups like children, pregnancy can be tested
V	Microdosing studies	**Healthy** volunteers (small number)	–	**Very low dose 1/100th of human dose:** Maximum 100 mg of drug is administered **to know pharmacokinetics**. This could avoid costly phase I studies for candidate drugs with unsuitable pharmacokinetics.

MICROBIOLOGY

68. Ans. c. Gram-negative diplococci, ferments glucose and maltose *(Ref: Ananthanarayan 10/e p230, 8/e p223, 230)*

The clinical-picture given in the question i.e. meningitis with a typical purpuric rash is seen in meningococcemia due to Neisseria meningitidis, which is Gram-negative diplococci and ferments glucose and maltose.

A	Gram-positive cocci catalase negative, bacitracin sensitive	Streptococcus pyogenes
B	Gram-positive diplococci (lanceolate), catalase negative, optochin sensitive	Streptococcus pneumoniae
C	Gram-negative diplococci, ferments glucose and maltose	Neisseria meningitidis
D	Gram-negative diplococci (kidney shaped), oxidase positive	Neisseria gonorrhoea

"Meningococcemia presents as acute fever with chills, malaise and prostration. Typically a petechial rash occurs early in the disease. Meningococci may be isolated from the petechial lesions. Metastatic involvement of the joints, ears, eyes, lungs and adrenals may occur. About 10 percent develop pneumonia."- Ananthanarayan 10/e p230, 8/e p223

Neisseria meningitidis (Meningococci)

- **Gram (-)ve, aerobic, non-motile, lens shaped diplococci**[Q]
- **Oxidase positive**[Q] **(key test for identifying Neisseria)**, catalase positive
- **Ferments glucose & maltose** but not sucrose[Q]
- Can grow both **intracellularly & extracellularly**[Q]
- Categorized as **b-proteobacterium**[Q] on basis of genome sequencing

Classification:
- On the basis of capsular polysaccharide, classified into 13 serogroups
- 5 serogroups are responsible for most meningococcal diseases (**A,B,C,W,Y**)[Q]
- **Group A- epidemic, Group B- both epidemic & outbreak, Group C- Localized outbreak**[Q]

Virulence Factors:
- Capsular polysaccharide
- Outer membrane protein (pilli)
- **Lipooligosaccharide, LOS (endotoxin)**[Q] not the lipopolysaccharide: **Morbidity & mortality** of meningococcal **bacteremia & meningitis** is **directly proportional to** amount of **circulating meningococcal endotoxin**
- IgA proteases & Transferrin binding protein

Pathogenesis:
- **MC source of infection: Human nasopharyngeal carriers**[Q]
- **Mode of transmission: Droplet inhalation**[Q]
  - **Spread of infection: MC route of spread to meninges** from nasopharynx is **hematogenous**[Q] **> direct olfactory nerve spread via cribriform plate**[Q]

Clinical Features:
- **Incubation period: 3-4 days**[Q] (may vary from 2-10 days)
- **Deficiency of** terminal or alternate complement pathway C_5-C_9[Q] **increases the risk of meningococcal infection**
  - **Meningitis** is the result of **blood borne dissemination**[Q] & not the direct invasion
  - **Early symptoms** are **non-specific** & suggest an influenza like illness with **fever, headache & myalgia** accompanied by **vomiting & abdominal pain**[Q].

Neisseria meningitidis (Meningococci)
• **Rash**, if present may appear to be viral early in the course, until petechiae or purpuric lesions develop.
• **Fulminant meningococcemia**, most rapid lethal form of septic shock, with **prominent hemorrhagic skin lesions & characteristic rash**[Q]
• **Fatality** of typically **untreated cases: 80%**[Q]
• With **early diagnosis and treatment, case fatality rates** have declined to **<10%.**
• **Waterhouse-Friedrichsen syndrome:** Severe form of **fulminant meningococcemia with large purpuric rash (purpura fulminans), shock, DIC, bilateral adrenal hemorrhage & multi-organ failure**[Q].
Lab Diagnosis:
• Diagnosis is established by **recovering meningococci from sterile body fluids** such as **blood, CSF** etc
• **Specimen for cases: Blood & CSF; Specimen for carriers: Nasopharyngeal swab**[Q]
• Grow best on **Muller-Hinton**[Q] or chocolate agar at 35⁰C in 5-10% CO_2.
• **Thayer-Martin media** is **selective media**[Q] used **for culturing throat or nasopharyngeal specimen**
Treatment:
• 3rd generation cephalosporin such as **cefotaxime or ceftriaxone**[Q] is **DOC** for initial therapy
• **Prophylaxis: Rifampicin** is **DOC for meningococcal prophylaxis**[Q]
Prevention:
• **Vaccine**: Quadrivalent vaccine Meningococcal polysaccharide vaccine (serogroup **A, C, W, Y**)[Q]
• There is **no vaccine against serogroup B**[Q] as its capsule is non-immunogenic
• Vaccine is **ineffective in Age < 2 years**[Q], so given after 2 years

69. Ans. c. Meningococcus   *(Ref: Ananthanarayan 10/e p230, 10/e p230, 8/e p230)*

History of fever and headache for 3 days with blood pressure 90/60 mm Hg and rash on the legs are suggestive of meningococcemia.

See Q. No. 68 AIIMS May 2016.

70. Ans. c. Streptococcus pneumoniae   *(Ref: Ananthanarayan 10/e p223, 8/e p216)*

Gram stain shows lanceolate Gram-positive cocci in pairs, that is Streptococcus pneumoniae

"Pneumococci are typically small, slightly elongated cocci, with one end broad or rounded and the other pointed, presenting a flame shaped or lanceolate appearance. They occur in pairs (diplococci), with the broad ends in apposition, the long axis of the Coccus parallel to the line joining the two cocci in a pair. They are capsulated, the capsule enclosing each pair. The capsules are best seen in material taken directly from exudates and may be lost on repeated cultivation."- Ananthanarayan 10/e p223

Shape of Bacteria	Appearance
Coccus	
Bacillus	
Vibrio (Comma shaped)	
Spirillum (Spirally coiled, **rigid**)	
Spirochete (Spirally coiled, **flexible**)	

Arrangement of Bacilli	Appearance
Bacilli in cluster	
Bacilli in chains (Bacillus anthrax)	
Diplobacilli (Klebsiella pneumoniae)	

Organism	Shape	Image	Appearance
Streptococci	Gram positive cocci in chains		
Pneumococci	Lanceolate gram positive cocci in pairs		
Gonococci	**Gram negative cocci** arranged in **pairs (kidney shaped)**		
Meningococci	**Gram negative cocci** arranged in **pairs (lens shaped)**		
Moraxella (Neisseria) catarrhalis	**Gram negative cocci** arranged in **pairs (kidney/bean shaped)**		
Gaffkya tetragena	Gram positive cocci in tetrads		
Sarcina	**Gram positive cocci** in octet		
Staphylococci	**Gram positive cocci** found in **grape like clusters**		

Streptococcus Pneumoniae (Pneumococcus)

- **Pneumococcus is flame-shaped or lanceolate gram positive cocci in pairs (diplococci)**[Q]
- **Optochin sensitive**[Q] (differentiates from S. viridans), **catalase & oxidase negative**[Q]
- **Ferments inulin** (differentiates from other streptococci), **bile soluble &** grow best in 5% CO_2[Q]

Culture Characteristics:
- **Alpha hemolytic on blood agar: 'Draughtsman' or 'carom-coin colonies**[Q]
- **Capsule demonstrated with India ink**[Q]
- **Quellung**[Q] **reaction** (Neufeld's capsule swelling reaction) seen

Virulence Factors of Pneumococcus	
Polysaccharide capsule	• **Inhibits phagocytosis**[Q] • Forms basis of **antigenic serotyping & pneumococcal vaccine**[Q] • Diffuses into culture media, tissues & exudates (**specific soluble substance**) • **Type 3 pneumococcus** has **abundant capsular material** & is **more virulent.**
IgA protease	• **Degrades IgA** in mucosal secretions
Pneumolysin (hemolysin)	• Acts as a membrane-damaging cytotoxin • Activates the complement system, causes a release of TNF-alpha & IL-1 • Inhibits neutrophil chemotaxis
Autolysin	• An amidase enzyme, **cleaves peptidoglycan leading to autolysis** of cells • Responsible for **bile solubility & Draughtsman appearance** of colonies[Q]
Cell surface proteins	• Surface protein A, surface adhesin A
Enzymes	• Neuraminidase & hyaluronidase

Pneumococcal Diseases:
- Approximately 50% of normal population will have **pneumococcal colonization in nasopharynx**[Q].
- **Source of infection: Upper respiratory tract of carriers**[Q]
- **Mode of transmission: Inhalation of contaminated droplet nuclei**[Q]

Pneumococcus is MC Cause of	
Community acquired pneumonia[Q] **Acute otitis media & sinusitis**[Q]	**Pyogenic meningitis in all ages**[Q] (except in neonates)

- **Austrian's syndrome or Osler triad: Pneumococcal endocarditis** (usually involves aortic valve) + **Meningitis + Pneumonia**[Q]

- **Laboratory Diagnosis:**

	Pneumococcus	Strep. viridans
Morphology	**Capsulated, lanceolate, flamed-shaped**[Q]	**Round/oval**[Q]
Arrangement	**In pairs**[Q]	**In long chains**[Q]
On blood agar	**Draughtsman or carom coin colony**[Q]	**Dome shaped (convex) colony**[Q]
Liquid medium	**Uniform turbidity**[Q]	**Granular turbidity**[Q]
Bile solubility	**Positive**[Q]	**Negative**[Q]
Inulin fermentation	**Fermenter**[Q]	**Non-fermenter**[Q]
Optochin sensitivity	**Sensitive**[Q]	**Resistant**[Q]
Mice pathogenicity	**Fatal infection**[Q]	**Nonpathogenic**[Q]

Treatment:
- **DOC: Penicillin**[Q] (Penicillin resistance is due to altered penicillin binding protein)
- **DOC for meningitis: Vancomycin + ceftriaxone**[Q]
- **DOC for ASOM: Amoxicillin**[Q]

71. **Ans. a. Amoebiasis** *(Ref: Paniker's 7/e p17; Jawetz 27/e p711; Harrison 19/e p1364)*
History of abdominal pain and bloody diarrhea of one-week duration and the given colonoscopic biopsy, appearance of ulcers on colonoscopy inflammatory infiltrate with Entamoeba histolytica trophozoites is diagnostic of amoebiasis.

AIIMS May 2016

*"The earliest intestinal lesions are microulcerations of the mucosa of the cecum, sigmoid colon, or rectum that release erythrocytes, inflammatory cells, and epithelial cells. Proctoscopy reveals small ulcers with heaped-up margins and normal intervening mucosa. Submucosal extension of ulcerations under viable-appearing surface mucosa causes the classic "flask-shaped" ulcer containing trophozoites at the margins of dead and viable tissues. Although neutrophilic infiltrates may accompany the early lesions in animals, **human intestinal infection is marked by a paucity of inflammatory cells, probably in part because of the killing of neutrophils by trophozoites**. Treated ulcers characteristically heal with little or no scarring. Occasionally, however, full-thickness necrosis and perforation occur." - Harrison 19/e p1364*

Intestinal Amoebiasis

Low Power	High Power

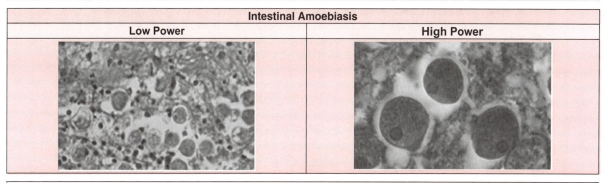

Entamoeba Histolytica

- Entamoeba histolytica causes **intestinal amoebiasis & amebic liver abscess**.
- **Host**: Humans are the only host[Q]
- **Route of infection**: Feco-oral route[Q]; Infective stage: Quadrinucleate cyst[Q]
- **Site of infection**: Large intestine[Q]

Pathogenesis:
- **Virulence factors**: Amebic lectin antigen[Q], cysteine proteinase, amebapore, neuraminidase & metalloproteinase
- Both **trophozoites & cysts** are found **in intestinal lumen**, but **only trophozoites invade tissue**.
- Trophozoites attach to colonic mucus & epithelial cells by **Gal/ GalNAc lectin[Q]**.
- **Earliest intestinal lesions**: Microulcerations[Q] of mucosa of large intestine

  - MC form of invasive disease: Colitis[Q]
  - MC site of amebic colitis: Cecum & ascending colon[Q]
  - In colon: Flask-shaped ulcers[Q] (MC site: Cecum & ascending colon)[Q]
  - **Synchronous hepatic abscess** is found in **one-third** of patients with **active amebic colitis**.

Intestinal amoebiasis:
- **MC type of amebic infection**: Asymptomatic cyst passage[Q]
- Symptomatic amebic colitis develops 2–6 weeks after ingestion of cysts.
- A gradual onset of **lower abdominal pain & mild diarrhea** is followed by **malaise, weight loss & diffuse lower abdominal or back pain[Q]**.
- Cecal involvement may mimic **acute appendicitis[Q]**.
- **Complications**: Toxic megacolon, fulminant amebic colitis

Laboratory diagnosis:
- **Minimum 3 stool samples on consecutive days[Q]** (ameba are **shed intermittently[Q]**)
- **Stool microscopy**: Trophozoite (indicates **active infection[Q]**); Quadrinucleate cyst (indicates **carrier state**)
- Stool culture & stool antigen detection by ELISA

Appearance (Gross & Microscopic):
- Proctoscopy: Small ulcers with heaped-up margins & normal intervening mucosa[Q]

  - **Submucosal extension of ulcerations** under viable-appearing surface mucosa causes classic **"flask-shaped" ulcer** containing **trophozoites at margins of dead & viable tissues[Q]**.
  - **Human intestinal infection** is marked by a **paucity of inflammatory cells**, probably in part because of **killing of neutrophils by trophozoites[Q]**.

Treatment:
- **Metronidazole** is **mainstay of treatment[Q]**.
- **Luminal agents** include **iodoquinol, paromomycin & diloxanide furoate[Q]**.

72. Ans. d. Actinomyces *(Ref: Ananthanarayan 10/e p398, 10/e p398, 8/e p393; Jawetz 27/e p296; Harrison 19/e p1089)*
The given image is Pap smear showing Actinomyces infection. Pelvic actinomycosis is a rare but proven complication of use of intrauterine devices.

> *"Actinomycotic involvement of the pelvis occurs most commonly in association with an IUCD. When an IUCD is in place or has recently been removed, pelvic symptoms should prompt consideration of actinomycosis. The risk, although not quantified, appears small. The disease rarely develops when the IUCD has been in place for <1 year, but the risk increases with time. Actinomycosis can also present months after IUCD removal. Symptoms are typically indolent; fever, weight loss, abdominal pain, and abnormal vaginal bleeding or discharges are the most common. The earliest stage of disease—often endometritis—commonly progresses to pelvic masses or a tuboovarian abscess. Unfortunately, because the diagnosis is often delayed, a "frozen pelvis" mimicking malignancy or endometriosis can develop by the time of recognition. Ca125 levels may be elevated, further contributing to misdiagnosis."* - *Harrison 19/e p1089*

Morphology of Actinomyces

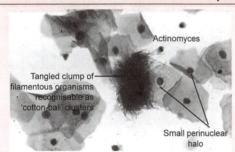

- **Identified cytologically** as **ball-like clusters of bacteria, with radiating filaments**[Q].
- **'Cotton-ball' clusters: Tangled clump of filamentous organisms**, with **acute angle branching**[Q].
- **Radial distribution of filaments** or irregular **'wooly body' appearance**[Q] (also known as **"Gupta bodies"**)
- **Inflammatory perinuclear halo**[Q] may be seen.
- **Masses of leukocytes adherent to micro-colonies** of the organisms **with swollen filaments** or **'clubs'** at the **periphery**[Q].

Actinomycosis

- Actinomycosis is an **indolent, slowly progressive infection** caused by **anaerobic or microaerophilic bacteria**, primarily of the genus **Actinomyces**, that **colonize mouth, colon & vagina**[Q].
- **Mucosal disruption** may **lead to infection at virtually any site in the body**[Q].
- In vivo growth of actinomycetes results in the **formation of characteristic clumps called grains** or **sulfur granules**[Q].

Etiology:
- **Actinomycosis** is most commonly caused by **A. israelii, A. naeslundii, A. odontolyticus, A. viscosus, A. meyeri & A. gerencseriae**[Q].
- **Most** if not all actinomycotic infections **are polymicrobial**[Q].

Clinical Features:
- **Oral, cervical, or facial site**, usually as a **soft tissue swelling, abscess, or mass lesion** that is often mistaken for a neoplasm[Q].
- **Angle of jaw** is **generally involved**[Q].
- **Radiation therapy & bisphosphonate treatment** have been recognized as contributing to an **increasing incidence of actinomycotic infection** of the **mandible & maxilla**[Q].
- **Actinomycotic involvement of the pelvis** occurs **most commonly in association with an IUCD**[Q].

Three "classic" clinical presentations that should prompt consideration of this unique infection
- Combination of **chronicity, progression across tissue boundaries & mass-like features (mimicking malignancy**[Q])
- **Development of a sinus tract**, which may **spontaneously resolve & recur**[Q]
- **A refractory or relapsing infection** after a short course of therapy, since **cure of established actinomycosis requires prolonged treatment**[Q].

Diagnosis:
- Diagnosis is made by **microscopic identification of sulfur granules** (an in **vivo matrix of bacteria, calcium phosphate & host material**) in **pus or tissues**[Q].

Actinomycosis

- Although **sulfur granules are a defining characteristic of actinomycosis**, **granules** also are **found in mycetoma & botryomycosis**[Q].
- **Gram Stain:** **Thin gram-positive filaments** surrounded by a **peripheral zone of swollen radiating club shaped structures**, presenting a **sun-ray appearance**[Q]. The **'clubs'** are believed to be **antigen-antibody complexes**[Q].

Treatment:
- **DOC: Penicillin**[Q]
- Treatment requires **prolonged administration of penicillin (6–12 months)**.
- **Clindamycin or erythromycin** is effective in **penicillin-allergic patients.**
- **Surgical excision & drainage** may be required.

PAP Smear Findings in Sexually Transmitted Infections

Granuloma inguinale	Trichomonas vaginalis	Haemophilus ducreyi
• Caused by **Calymmatobacterium granulomatis**[Q] • **Coccobacilli** seen in **Giemsa-stained specimen**[Q] • **Donovan bodies** are seen **intracellularly in mononuclear cells**[Q].	• In cervical smear, **transparent 'halo' around their superficial cell nucleus**[Q] • **Three-dimensional clusters of neutrophils (polyballs**[Q]**)** may be seen.	• **Moderate small gram-negative rods**[Q] • **School of fish appearance**[Q] is seen with 40–50 WBCs/hpf. • No clue cells observed.

PAP Smear in Bacterial Vaginosis

- Finding of a **watery discharge** & **typical smell**[Q]
- **'Clue cells'** (sloughed epithelial cells coated with Gram-variable pleomorphic coccobacilli): This is **sufficient evidence to diagnose infection with Gardnerella vaginalis**[Q].

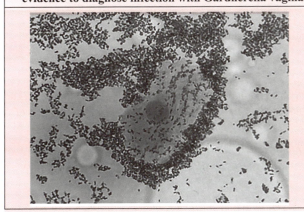 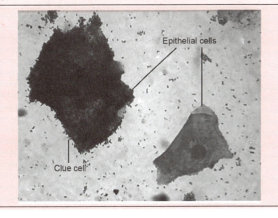

73. **Ans. b. Both adult and larval stages are seen in humans** *(Ref: Paniker's 7/e p135, 6/e p156)*

    The given image is the egg of Hymenolepis nana showing characteristic polar filaments, polar knobs, yolk granules and 6 hooklets (hexacanth) in the oncosphere (embryo). Both adult and larval stages of this species are seen in humans. It causes a transient infection in humans but does not resolve on its own and has to be treated.

"Egg of Hymenolepis nana: Egg is roughly spherical or ovoid, 30-40 mm in size. It has thin colorless outer membrane and inner embryophore enclosing the hexacanth oncosphere. The space between 2 membranes contains yolk granules and 4-8 threads like polar filaments arising from 2 knobs on the embryophore. The eggs float in saturated solution of salt and are non-bile stained. They are immediately infective and unable to survive for more than 10 days in external environment." - Paniker's 7/e p135

Nematodes	Fecal examination
Trichinella spiralis	**Adult worm**[Q]
Trichuris trichiura	**Eggs (barrel shaped)**[Q]
Strongyloides	**Rhabditiform larvae**[Q]
Ancylostoma duodenale & Necator americanus	Egg which may be hatched, so **rhabditiform larvae** can be seen
Enterobius vermicularis	Usually not useful
Ascaris lumbricoides	**Eggs & adult worm**[Q]
Hymenolepis nana	**Eggs: Polar filaments, polar knob, yolk granules & 6 hooklets in oncosphere**[Q]
Filariasis	No role
Dracunculus medinensis	No role

Hymenolepis nana (Dwarf Tapeworm)
• **MC tapeworm infection in humans**: **Hymenolepis nana**[Q].   • **H. nana** is the **only cestode of humans** that **does not require an intermediate host**[Q].   • Both the **larval & adult phases** of life cycle **take place in human**[Q].   • Adult (**smallest tape-worm parasitizing humans**) is ~**2 cm long** & dwells in **proximal ileum**[Q].
Life-Cycle: • **Transmission** is through **ingestion of infected food & water**[Q]   • Both **adult & larval stages** are seen in **human intestine**[Q].   • **Ingestion of egg → Egg develops to cysticercoid larva → Larva develops to adult → Adult under go self-fertilization & produce eggs→ Eggs are released in feces**[Q]   • **Eggs** may **hatch before passing into stool**, causing **internal autoinfection** with increasing numbers of intestinal worms.
Clinical Features: • Usually **asymptomatic**, when **infection is intense, anorexia, abdominal pain & diarrhea** develop.
Diagnosis: • Infection is diagnosed by **finding of eggs in stool**.
Treatment: • **Praziquantel** is **drug of choice**[Q], because it **acts against both adult worms & cysticercoids** in intestinal villi.   • **Nitazoxanide** may be used as an alternative.

74. **Ans. c. Females of these species show parthenogenesis** *(Ref: Paniker's 7/ep178, 6/ep173; Jawetz 27/ep731; Harrison 19/ep1415)*
The given stool mount is showing severe infestation with Strongyloides rhabditiform larvae. The infective stage is filariform larvae only. It is usually transmitted through skin. Females show parthenogenesis in human intestine. Drug of choice is ivermectin.

"Rhabditiform larvae passed in feces can transform into infectious filariform larvae either directly or after a free-living phase of development. Humans acquire strongyloidiasis when filariform larvae in fecally contaminated soil penetrate the skin or mucous membranes." - Harrison 19/e p1415

The minute (2-mm-long) parasitic adult female worms reproduce by parthenogenesis; adult males do not exist. Eggs hatch in the intestinal mucosa, releasing rhabditiform larvae that migrate to the lumen and pass with the feces into soil. Alternatively, rhabditiform larvae in the bowel can develop directly into filariform larvae that penetrate the colonic wall or perianal skin and enter the circulation to repeat the migration that establishes ongoing internal reinfection. This autoinfection cycle allows strongyloidiasis to persist for decades." - Harrison 19/e p1415

"*The ongoing autoinfection cycle of strongyloidiasis is normally constrained by unknown factors of the host's immune system. Abrogation of host immunity, especially with glucocorticoid therapy and much less commonly with other immunosuppressive medications, leads to hyperinfection, with the generation of large numbers of filariform larvae. Disseminated strongyloidiasis, particularly in patients with unsuspected infection who are given glucocorticoids, can be fatal. Strongyloidiasis is a frequent complication of infection with human T cell lymphotropic virus type 1, but disseminated strongyloidiasis is not common among patients infected with HIV-1.*" - Harrison 19/e p1415

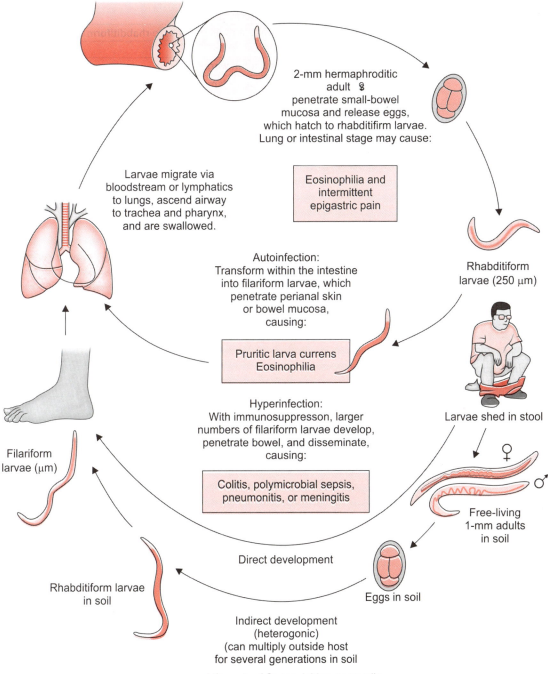

Fig. 35: Life cycle of Strongyloides stercoralis

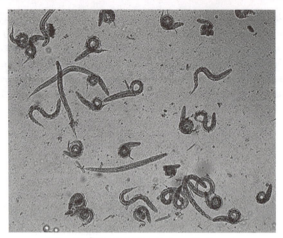

Fig. 36: Strongyloides stercoralis larvae

Strongyloides Stercoralis (Thread worm)
• Adult **females** of **Strongyloides stercoralis do not need to mate with male worms to reproduce**[Q].   • **Minute (2-mm-long) parasitic adult female worms reproduce by parthenogenesis**[Q]
Life-cycle: • **Site of infection: Small intestine**[Q]   • **Mechanism of infection: Larvae in soil penetrate skin** & (rarely) **internal auto-reinfection**[Q]
Clinical Features: • **Disseminated infections**: GIT (severe **diarrhea, abdominal pain, GI bleeding**, nausea, vomiting), lungs (**coughing, wheezing, hemoptysis**) & skin (**rash, pruritus, larva currens**).   • **Larvae migrating from intestine carrying enteric bacteria** can cause **local infections or sepsis**, resulting in death.   • **MC cutaneous manifestation: Recurrent urticaria**[Q] involving buttocks & wrists   • **Migrating larvae** can elicit a **pathognomonic serpiginous eruption, larva currens ("running larva")**[Q].
Diagnosis: • **Stool exam, sputum, bronchial lavage** for ova & parasite (larvae).
Treatment: • **Ivermectin**[Q] **(DOC)** is consistently **more effective than albendazole.**

75. **Ans. d. Ascaris lumbricoides**   *(Ref: Paniker's 7/e p197, 6/e p169)*
Autoinfection is not seen in Ascaris lumbricoides.

Autoinfection
• **Autoinfection**: Infection of a primary host with a parasite, particularly a helminth, in such a way that the **complete life cycle of the parasite happens in a single organism**, without the involvement of another host.   • **Primary host is at the same time the secondary host of parasite.**

Autoinfection is seen in (CHEST)	
• **C**ryptosporidium parvum[Q] • **H**ymenolepis nana[Q] • **E**nterobius vermicularis[Q]	• **S**trongyloides stercoralis[Q] • **T**aenia solium[Q]

76. **Ans. a. Diphyllobothrium latum**   *(Ref: Paniker's 7/e p118, 6/e p142; Jawetz 27/e p731; Harrison 19/e p1434)*
Helminth implicated in causing pernicious anemia is Diphyllobothrium latum.

> "***Diphyllobothrium latum***: Disease caused by tapeworms is chiefly vague abdominal discomfort and loss of appetite, leading to weight loss. **D latum has an unusual capacity to absorb vitamin B$_{12}$**, and among some groups—especially Finns—a vitamin B$_{12}$ deficiency leading to various levels of pernicious anemia may rarely develop." - *Jawetz 27/e p731*

"Diphyllobothrium latum: Because the tapeworm absorbs large quantities of vitamin B_{12} and interferes with ileal B_{12} absorption, vitamin B_{12} deficiency can develop, but this effect has been noted only in Scandinavia, where up to 2% of infected patients, especially the elderly, have megaloblastic anemia resembling pernicious anemia and may exhibit neurologic sequelae of B_{12} deficiency."- Harrison 19/e p1434

Clinical Hints in Parasitology	
Findings	**Organism**
Brain cysts, seizures[Q]	**Taenia solium** (neurocysticercosis)
Hemoptysis[Q]	Paragonimus westermani
Microcytic anemia[Q]	Ancylostoma, Necator
Vitamin B_{12} deficiency (megaloblastic[Q] **& pernicious anemia**[Q]**)**	Diphyllobothrium latum
Hepatic cysts[Q]	Echinococcus granulosus
Biliary tract disease[Q] (cholangiocarcinoma)	Clonorchis sinensis
Portal hypertension[Q]	Schistosoma mansoni
Hematuria, bladder cancer (SCC & TCC)[Q]	Schistosoma hematobium
Perianal pruritus[Q]	Enterobius

Diphyllobothrium Latum (Human Broad/Fish Tapeworm)

- **D. latum** is **longest tapeworm**[Q] **in humans** (up to 25 meters)
- **Attaches to ileal** & **occasionally to jejunal mucosa** by suckers[Q].

Mechanism of Infection:
- Humans acquire the infection by **ingesting infected raw or smoked fish**[Q].
- **Definitive host: Man; Intermediate host: Cyclops**[Q] **(1st), fresh water fish**[Q] **(2nd)**

Clinical Features:
- Generally **mild symptoms** like diarrhea, abdominal pain, vomiting, weight loss, fatigue & constipation.
- **Severe Vitamin B_{12} deficiency: Parasite absorbs 80%** or more of the host's B_{12} **intake** leading to **megaloblastic anemia indistinguishable from pernicious anemia**[Q] (in a small number of cases).
- Anemia can also lead to **subacute combined degeneration of spinal cord**.

Diagnosis:
- Diagnosis is made by **identifying proglottid segments** or **characteristic operculated eggs in feces** (eggs possess a **single shell with an operculum at one end** & a **knob at the other**[Q]).

  - **Contrast medium gastrografin** (interesting potential diagnostic tool & treatment) introduced into the duodenum allows both **visualization of the parasite** & **cause detachment and passing of the whole worm.**

Treatment:
- **Drug of choice: Praziquantel**[Q]
- **Parenteral vitamin B_{12}** should be given if B_{12} deficiency is manifest.

Parasitic Nematodes					
Feature	Ascaris lumbricoides (Roundworm)	Necator Americanus, Ancylostoma duodenale (Hookworm)	Strongyloides stercoralis	Trichuris trichiura (Whipworm)	Enterobius vermicularis (Pinworm)
Infective stage	**Egg**[Q]	**Filariform larva**[Q]	**Filariform larva**[Q]	**Egg**[Q]	**Egg**[Q]

Contd...

Contd...

Parasitic Nematodes					
Route of infection	Oral[Q]	Percutaneous[Q]	Percutaneous or autoinfection[Q]	Oral[Q]	Oral[Q]
Gastro-intestinal location of worms	Jejunal lumen[Q]	Jejunal mucosa[Q]	Small bowel mucosa[Q]	Cecum, colonic mucosa[Q]	Cecum, appendix[Q]
Pulmonary passage of larvae	Yes[Q]	Yes[Q]	Yes[Q]	No[Q]	No[Q]
Principal symptoms	Rarely gastro-intestinal or biliary obstruction	**Iron deficiency anemia** in heavy infection[Q]	Gastrointestinal symptoms; malabsorption or sepsis in hyperinfection	Gastro-intestinal symptoms, **anemia**[Q]	**Perianal pruritus**[Q]
Diagnostic stage	Eggs in stool[Q]	Eggs in fresh stool, larvae in old stool[Q]	Larvae in stool or duodenal aspirate; sputum in hyperinfection	Eggs in stool[Q]	Eggs from perianal skin on cellulose acetate tape[Q]
Treatment	Mebendazole, Albendazole	Mebendazole, Albendazole	**Ivermectin**[Q], Albendazole	Mebendazole, Albendazole	Mebendazole Albendazole

77. Ans. c. It allows Staphylococcus and Candida to grow *(Ref: Ananthanarayan 10/e p39, 10/e p39, 8/e p667)*
Advantage of CLED medium over MacConkey agar is that it allows Staphylococcus and Candida to grow.

CLED (Cystine Lactose Electrolyte Deficient) Agar

- It is a valuable **non-inhibitory, differential culture medium** used in the **isolation & differentiation of urinary organisms**[Q].
- **Advantages over MacConkey agar:** It is **less inhibitory** than MacConkey agar, supports Gram positive bacteria (except beta-hemolytic Streptococcus) & Candida[Q].
- **Advantages over Blood agar:** Being **electrolyte deficient**, it **prevents the swarming of Proteus species**[Q].

Cystine	Promotes formation of **cystine-dependent dwarf colonies**[Q]
Agar	**Solidifying agent**[Q]
Bromothymol blue	**Indicator** used in the agar
	Changes to **yellow** in case of **acid production during fermentation of lactose** or changes to **deep blue in case of alkalinization**[Q].

- Lactose-positive bacteria build **yellow colonies**[Q].
- Bacteria which **decarboxylate L-Cystine** cause an **alkaline reaction** and build **deep blue colonies**[Q]
- **L-Cystine** is added as a **growth supplement for cystine-dependent coliforms**[Q].

> **CLED agar** supports the **growth of all potential urinary pathogens** & a number of contaminants such as **diphtheroids, lactobacilli & micrococci** and **provides distinct colony morphology**[Q].

Benefits of using CLED agar for urine culture

- **Food discrimination of Gram-negative bacteria** on the basis of **lactose fermentation & colony appearance**[Q]
- It is **less inhibitory than MacConkey agar**[Q]
- **Inhibits swarming of Proteus spp**[Q] (Advantage over blood agar)
- Relatively **low cost** (Compared with combined use of blood agar & MacConkey agar for urine culture).

Contd...

Contd...

Typical colony morphology on CLED Agar	
Escherichia coli	• **Opaque yellow** colonies with a slightly deeper yellow center[Q]
Klebsiella spp	• **Yellow to whitish-blue** colonies, **extremely mucoid**[Q]
Proteus spp	• **Translucent blue** colonies[Q]
Pseudomonas aeruginosa	• **Green colonies** with typical **matted surface & rough periphery**[Q]
Enterococci	• **Small yellow** colonies, about 0.5 mm in diameter[Q]
Staphylococcus aureus	• **Deep yellow** colonies, uniform in color[Q]
Coagulase negative Staphylococci	• **Pale yellow** colonies, more opaque than *Enterococcus faecalis*[Q]

Culture media		
Simple (Basal) Media	**Complex Media**	**Special Media**
• **No added ingredients**[Q] • **Nutrient broth**: Simple **liquid** medium, consist of peptone, meat extract, sodium chloride & water. • **Nutrient agar:** Simple **solid** medium prepared by adding 2% agar to nutrient broth; **simplest & MC used medium** in microbiology.	• Contain some **ingredients of unknown chemical composition**[Q] • One common ingredient is **peptone**[Q]	• **Added ingredients** for special purpose or **for bringing out certain characteristics** or **providing special nutrients required for growth** of the bacterium under study[Q].

Media	Features	Example
Enriched	• Nutrients (blood, serum or egg) are added with basal medium	• **Blood agar (blood + nutrient agar):** For growth of **Streptococcus**[Q] • **Chocolate agar (heated blood agar):** For isolation of **Neisseria & H. influenzae**[Q] • **Loeffler's serum slope:** For grouping **C. diphtheria**[Q]
Enrichment media	• Contains **substances in liquid medium** having **stimulating effect on bacteria to be grown** or **inhibits its competitors**	• **Tetrathionate broth:** Allows **typhoid & paratyphoid bacilli** to grow[Q] • **Selenite F broth:** Allows **typhoid & paratyphoid bacilli** to grow[Q] • **Alkaline peptone water:** To grow **Vibrio cholerae**[Q]
Selective media	• Contain **substances that inhibit others** & **facilitate isolation of a particular species**	• **Deoxycholate citrate agar & xylose lysine deoxycholate agar** for enteric bacilli: **Shigella & Salmonella**[Q] • **Thiosulphate citrate bile salt (TCBS) agar:** Vibrio cholera[Q] • **L-J medium:** Mycobacterium tuberculosis[Q] • **Potassium tellurite agar:** C. diphtheria[Q] • **Wilson Blair bismuth sulphite medium:** S. typhi[Q]
Differential media	• Contains **substances** that **help to distinguish differing characteristics** of bacteria	• **MacConkey's medium:** To differentiate **lactose & non-lactose fermenters**[Q] • **CLED (Cystine Lactose Electrolyte Deficient) agar**[Q]
Indicator media	• **Contain an indicator** which **changes colour when a bacterium grows** on them	• **Wilson Blair sulphite medium:** S. typhi[Q] • **MacConkey's agar**[Q]

Organism	Medium
Bacillus anthracis	• **PLET** (Polymyxin Lithium EDTA Thallous acetate) medium[Q]
Bacillus cereus	• **MYPA** (Mannitol Egg Yolk Phenol red Polymyxin agar)[Q]
Bordetella	• **Bordet Gengou medium; Regan Low medium, Lacey's DFP medium**[Q]

Contd...

AIIMS ESSENCE

Contd...

Organism	Medium
Brucella	• **Castaneda method of blood culture**[Q]
Burkholderia	• **Ashdown's medium**[Q]
Campylobacter jejuni	• **Campy Bap, Skirrow's or Butzler's media**[Q]
Chlamydiae	• Tissue culture (**Irradiated McCoy cells, HeLa cells treated with DEAE dextran**)[Q]
Clostridia (anaerobic organisms)	• **Robertson's cooked meat broth, Thioglycollate, Smith Noguchi**[Q]
Corynebacterium diphtheria	• **Potassium Tellurite blood agar**[Q]
Legionella	• **BCYE (Buffered charcoal yeast extract)**[Q]
Listeria	• **PALCAM agar**[Q]
Leptospira	• EMJH medium; Fletcher medium; Korthof medium; Stuart's medium
Mycobacterium tuberculosis	• **Lowenstein Jensen (LJ) medium**[Q] • **Middle Brook's medium, Dorset Egg medium**[Q]
Mycoplasma	• **PPLO medium**[Q]
Neisseria gonorrhoeae	• **Thayer Martin medium & Chacko Nair medium**[Q]
Pseudomonas	• **Cetrimide agar**[Q]
Rickettsiae	• **Yolk sac of developing chick embryo**[Q]
Shigella	• **Deoxycholate citrate agar**[Q]
Spirochaetes	• **Noguchi's medium**[Q]
Staphylococcus	• **Ludlam's medium**[Q]
Trypanosomes	• **Novy-Macneal-Nicolle medium**[Q]

78. **Ans. c. Ehrlichia chaffensis** *(Ref: Ananthanarayan 10/e p416, 8/e p409; Jawetz 27/e p346, 347; Harrison 19/e p1159, 1162)*

Though both Coxiella and Ehrlichia are obligate intracellular pathogens, in 2009 scientists reported a technique allowing the Q-fever pathogen Coxiella burnetii to grow in an axenic culture and suggested the technique may be useful for study of other pathogens. Hence, Ehrlichia is a better answer in this case.

"C. burnetii can be cultivated in cell cultures, but this should only be done in experienced biosafety level 3 laboratories."- Jawetz 27/e p347

"Isolation of C. burnetii from buffy-coat blood samples or tissue specimens by a shell-vial technique is easy but requires a biosafety level 3 laboratory." - Harrison 19/e p1159, 1162

"The Ehrlichia group consists of obligate intracellular bacteria transmitted by tick vectors."- Jawetz 27/e p346

"Ehrlichioses are acute febrile infections caused by members of the family Anaplasmataceae, which is made up of obligately intracellular organisms of five genera: Ehrlichia, Anaplasma, Wolbachia, Candidatus Neoehrlichia, and Neorickettsia. The bacteria reside in vertebrate reservoirs and target vacuoles of hematopoietic cells." - Harrison 19/e p1159

Obligate Intracellular Parasites (CRV CM PTL)		Facultative Intracellular Parasites (MBBS CRY for NHL)	
• **C**hlamydia[Q] • **R**ickettsia[Q] (**Ehrlichia**[Q] **& Anaplasma**) • **V**iruses[Q] • **C**oxiella burnetii[Q] • **C**ryptosporidium parvum[Q]	• **M**ycobacterium leprae[Q] • **P**lasmodium species[Q] • **P**neumocystis jiroveci[Q] • **T**oxoplasma gondii[Q] • **T**rypanosoma cruzi[Q] • **L**eishmania species[Q]	• **M**ycobacterium[Q] • **B**artonella henselae[Q] • **B**rucella[Q] • **S**almonella typhi[Q] • **C**ryptococcus neoformans[Q] • **R**hodococcus equi[Q] • **Y**ersinia[Q]	• **F**rancisella tularensis[Q] • **N**ocardia[Q] • **N**eisseria meningitidis[Q] • **H**istoplasma capsulatum[Q] • **L**isteria monocytogenes[Q] • **L**egionella[Q]

AIIMS May 2016

Ehrlichia chaffeensis
• **Ehrlichia** group consists of **obligate intracellular bacteria transmitted by tick vectors**[Q].
• **Ehrlichia chaffeensis** causes **human monocyte ehrlichiosis**[Q]
• **Ehrlichia infect circulating leukocytes** in which they **multiply within phagocytic vacuoles & form morulae**[Q].

Disease Transmission:
• **Vector: Tick**[Q]
• **Mammalian reservoir: Deer, dogs, humans**[Q]

Clinical Features:
• **Clinical manifestations** are **nonspecific** and include **fever** (96% of cases), **headache** (72%), **myalgia** (68%) & malaise (77%).
• Less frequently observed are nausea, vomiting & diarrhea (25–57%); cough (28%); rash (26% overall, 6% at presentation) & confusion (20%).

Diagnostic test:
• Diagnosis is made by **demonstration of morula within the respective leukocytes** (relatively insensitive) & by **serology or PCR.**

Treatment
• **Doxycycline**[Q] is **drug of choice** for treatment.

79. **Ans. a. Trophozoites**   *(Ref: Paniker's 7/e p77, 6/e p69; Harrison 19/e p1374)*

Transfusion associated malaria has a shorter incubation period because of presence of trophozoites in blood.

"Malaria can be transmitted by blood transfusion, needle-stick injury, sharing of needles by infected injection drug users, or organ transplantation. The incubation period in these settings is often short because there is no pre-erythrocytic stage of development. The clinical features and management of these cases are the same as for naturally acquired infections. Radical chemotherapy with primaquine is unnecessary for transfusion-transmitted P. vivax and P. ovale infections."

"Transfusion Malaria: Blood transfusion can accidentally transmit malaria, if the donor is infected with malaria. The parasites may remain viable in blood bank for 1-2 weeks. As this condition is induced by direct infection of red cells by the merozoites, pre-erythrocytic schizogony and hypnozoits are absent. Relapse does not occur and incubation period is short." - Paniker's 7/e p77

	Mosquito-Borne Malaria	Blood-Transfusion Malaria
Mode of transmission	Mosquito bite[Q]	Blood or blood products transfusion[Q]
Infective stage	**Sporozoite**[Q]	**Trophozoite**[Q]
Incubation period	**Long**[Q]	**Short**[Q]
Pre-erythrocytic schizogony	**Present**[Q]	**Absent**[Q]
Hypnozoites	**May be present**[Q]	**Absent**[Q]
Severity	**Comparatively less**[Q]	**More complications seen**[Q]
Relapse	**May occur**[Q]	**Does not occur**[Q]
Radical treatment	**Required**[Q]	**Not required**[Q]

FORENSIC MEDICINE

80. **Ans. a. Laceration**   *(Ref: Reddy 34/e p180, 34/e p180, 33/e p189; Parikh 6/e p4.10)*

The patient in the question has laceration in the left anterior part of chest.

"Lacerations are splits or tears of skin, mucous membranes, muscle or internal organs produced by application of blunt force to broad area of the body, which crushed or stretched tissues beyond the limit of their elasticity." - Reddy 33/e p189

Lacerations (Tears / Rupture)
• Lacerations are **splits or tears of skin, mucous membranes, muscle or internal organs**[Q]
• Produced by **application of blunt force to broad area of the body,** which **crushed or stretched tissues** beyond the limit of their elasticity[Q].

Contd...

Lacerations (Tears / Rupture)

Characteristic Features:

- When **underlying tissue** is **rigid structure** (skull), lacerations occur easily & **simulate incised wound**, whereas when **underlying tissue is flexible** (cheek & abdomen), lacerations occur less readily & **is jagged & irregular**[Q].
    - **Edges** are **ragged, irregular & bruised**[Q]
    - Margins are commonly abraded & **deeper tissues are unevenly divided & crushed**[Q].
    - **Hair follicles** & blood vessels are crushed; external haemorrhage is **not pronounced**[Q].

- **Hammer-crescentic laceration; blunt pointed metal rod-stellate laceration & stick-linear laceration with a split (Y shaped). Direction of shelving of margins indicates direction of blow**[Q].

Incised like laceration

- **Blunt force on areas where the skin is close to bone & subcutaneous tissues are scanty**, may produce a **wound, which looks like incised wound**[Q].
- **Sites: Scalp, forehead, eye brows, cheek bones, lower jaw, iliac crest, perineum & shin**[Q]

Types of Laceration

Split laceration	• **Incised looking or incised like wound**[Q] due to blunt perpendicular impact causing crushing of skin between two hard objects.
Stretch laceration	• **Due to tangential impact causing over stretching of fixed skin** & producing peeled off flap[Q].
Avulsion	• **Shearing laceration** due to horizontal impact (or shearing & grinding force) at an acute angle resulting in **avulsion** or **degloving of skin**[Q]. e.g. **lorry wheel causing degloving of skin known as flaying**[Q].
Tear	• Due to irregularly directed impact against irregular or semi-sharp object e.g. door handle.
Internal laceration	• Due to impact exceeding tensile strength & elasticity of an internal organ or tissue.
Contused (Bruised) tear	• Laceration producing bleeding into adjacent tissue.
Scraped (abraded) tear	• Has abraded margin

Trait	Incised Wound	Lacerated Wound	Stab Wound
Manner of production	By **sharp objects** or **weapons**[Q]	By **blunt objects** or **weapons**[Q]	By **pointed sharp or blunt weapons**[Q]
Site	**Anywhere**[Q]	Usually over **bony prominences**[Q]	Anywhere; usually **chest & abdomen**[Q]
Margins	**Smooth**, even clean cut & **everted**[Q]	**Irregular & often undermined**[Q]	**Clean-cut, parallel edges**[Q] Lacerated if weapon is blunt pointed
Abrasion on edges	**Absent**[Q]	**Usually present**[Q]	**Absent**[Q]
Bruising	No adjacent bruising of soft tissues	**Bruising of surrounding & underlying tissues**[Q]	Rare
Shape	**Linear or spindle shaped**[Q]	**Usually irregular**[Q]	**Linear or irregular**[Q]
Dimensions	**Usually longer than deep; often gaping**[Q]	**Usually longer than deep**[Q]	**Depth greater than length & breadth**[Q]
Depth of wound	Structures **cleanly cut to the depth of wound**[Q]	Small strands of tissue at the bottom bridge across margins	**Structures cleanly cut**[Q]
Hemorrhage	Usually **profuse & external Spurting** of blood may be seen	**Slight** except scalp & **external**[Q]	Varies; **usually internal**[Q]
Hair bulbs	**Cleanly cut**[Q]	**Crushed or torn**[Q]	**Usually clean cut**[Q]
Bones	May be **cut**	May be **fractured**[Q]	May be **punctured**[Q]
Foreign bodies	**Absent**[Q]	**Present**[Q]	**Absent**[Q]
Clothes	May be **cut**[Q]	May be **torn**[Q]	**May be cut**[Q]

AIIMS May 2016

81. **Ans. b. Intermediate range** *(Ref: Reddy 34/e p204, 34/e p207, 33/e p219; Parikh 6/4.43)*

This is an intermediate range, gunshot entrance wound, in which there is powder "tattooing" seen around the entrance wound site.

> *"Intermediate range shotgun wounds: At a distance of 60–90 cm, **single irregular circular aperture** 4 to 5 cm with **irregular and lacerated edges** is produced. The shots are **scattered after entering the wound** and **cause much damage to the internal tissues**. At a distance of 1.5 meters, the shot mass enters the body in one mass, producing a round defect. The margins are abraded. **At a distance of 2 meters, the shot mass begins to spread**. The **wound of entry is irregular**, with **ragged margins (rat hole)** about 5 cm in a diameter with a **few satellite perforations at the margins of the main defect**."*

Feature	Contact Shot	Close Shot	Near Shot	Distant Shot
Definition, Range and Discharge reaching victim	**In firm (hard or actual) contact**, muzzle end is pushed hard against the skin & all **discharge from muzzle are blown into the track taken by bullet**[Q], producing severe disruption of deeper tissues	When victim is **within the range of flame. Point blank** is used when range is very close to or in near contact with skin & is with in range of all discharge from muzzle.	When victim is **within the range of gun powder** but outside the range of flame.	When victim is **outside the range of all** discharges of muzzle **except bullet.**
Rifled firearm (Revolver, Pistol) range **Shot gun** range (~)	In touch with skin	5-8 cm (2.5-7.5 cm) Short range (1-2 meter)	Up to 50 cm (60cm) Intermediate range (2-4 metres)	>50 cm (or 60cm) Long (distant) range (>4 metres)
Discharge	**Bullet, gun powder, soot,** (smoke, carbon particles), **gases, flame** (fire, burn, heat) with **imprinted barrel marks & tearing in actual contact**[Q]	Bullet, gun powder, soot, gases and burn	Bullet, gun powder, and ± soot	**Only bullet** (± coarse particles of gun powder)
Blast effect	**Muzzle end imprint, eversion of edges, back spatter, soiling** of internal structures & pocket formation, **burst (comminution) fracture of skull and crazy paving fracture of base of skull**[Q] are all seen	**Absent**	**Absent**	**Absent**
Heat Effect on surface & cloths	Absent	**Scorching of skin, singeing of hair & burning melting – ironing of cloths present**	**Absent**	**Absent**
Blackening (smudging)	**Absent outside present inside the track**[Q]	**Present outside**[Q] the wound	Absent (±)	**Absent**
Tattooing	Absent outside present inside	**Present outside**	**Present outside**	Absent (±)
Abrasion / Grease collar	Absent outside present inside	**Present**	**Present**	Present (skin adjacent to hole shows two zones inner grease & outer abrasion collar)
Lead snow storm	**Absent**	**Absent**	**Absent**	Present (on x-ray) in shotgun injury
Carboxy Hb, Cherry red discoloration	Present **in wound track**	**Present in surrounding tissue**	±	±

Contd...

Contd...

Feature	Contact Shot	Close Shot	Near Shot	Distant Shot
Surrounding skin around entrance wound shows	**No** burning, blackening (soot), tattooing, abrasion/ grease collar	**Burning, blackening (soot), tattooing, abrasion / grease collar** present	**Tattooing & abrasion / grease collar** present	**Abrasion** (grease / dirt) **collar & lead storm** present
Entrance Wound Size	Largest	Bullet size	Smaller	**Smallest** due to initial stretching of skin
Shape	**Stellate (star shaped**[q]**), triangular, cruciform (cruciate**[q]**)** or **raged (irregular** with crenated & scalloped **edges)**	Circular (or rat hole[q])	Circular (central big wound with smaller wounds around)	Circular (wide spread[q])
Number	Single	Single	Multiple	Multiple
Edges (Margin)	Scorched, contused, undermined or **everted margins from which tears (lacerations) over skin radiating outwards from entrance hole because of expansion of gases** (between scalp & skull)	**Inverted & well defined**	Inverted	Inverted

82. **Ans. b. <17.5 years** (Ref: Reddy 34/e p73, 33/e p75; Parikh 6/e p2.9)
   In the given X-ray, pisiform has appeared, while the lower ends of radius and ulna have not fused yet. That places the age to be >12 years but <18–19 (Boys) or < 16–18 (Girls). Predicted bone age from the given wrist radiograph <17.5 years.

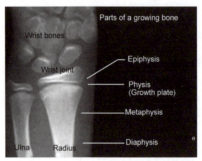

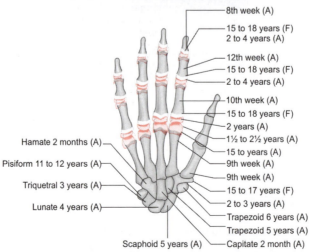

Fig. 37: Appearance and fusion of epiphysis in bones of hand

AIIMS May 2016

Ossification of Carpal Bones			
Bone	Ossification time	Bone	Ossification time
Capitate	1-3 months[Q]	Scaphoid	4-6 years[Q]
Hamate	2-4 months[Q]	Trapezium	4-6 years[Q]
Triquetral	2-3 years[Q]	Trapezoid	4-6 years[Q]
Lunate	2-4 years[Q]	Pisiform	8-12 years[Q]

Ossification of Carpal Bones
- Ossification of carpal bones occurs in a predictable sequence, **starting with capitate & ending with pisiform**.
- **At birth**, there is **no calcification in carpal bones**.

- **Ossification centers of distal radius & ulna (Distal radius: 1 year & Distal ulna: 5-6 years)[Q]**

Appearance of Centres of Ossification & Union of Bones & Epiphysis		
Age	Appearance of Centres of Ossification	Union of Bones & Epiphysis
5th year	Head of radius, trapezoid, scaphoid[Q]	Greater tubercle fuses with head of humerus[Q]
6th year	Lower end of ulna, trapezium[Q]	Rami of pubis & ischium unite[Q]
6th to 7th year	Medial epicondyle of humerus[Q]	–
9th year	Olecranon[Q]	–
9th to 11th year	Trochlea of humerus[Q]	–
10th to 11th year	Pisiform[Q]	–
11th year	Lateral epicondyle of humerus[Q]	–
13th year	Separate centres in triradiate cartilage of acetabulum[Q]	–
12th to 14th year	Lesser trochanter of femur[Q]	–
14th year	Crest of ilium; head & tubercles of ribs[Q]	Medial epicondyle of humerus; lateral epicondyle with trochlea; patella complete[Q]
15th year	Acromian[Q]	Coracoid with scapula; triradiate cartilage of acetabulum[Q]
16th year	Ischial tuberosity[Q]	Lower end of humerus; olecranon to ulna; upper end of radius; metacarpals; proximal phalanges[Q]
17th to 18th year	–	Head of femur; lesser 7 greater trochanter of femur; acromian; lower end of ulna[Q]
18th to 19th year	Inner end of clavicle[Q]	Lower end of femur; upper end of tibia & fibula; head of humerus; lower end of radius[Q]
20th to 21st year	–	Iliac crest; inner head of clavicle; ischial tuberosity, head of ribs[Q]

83. **Ans. a. Pugilistic attitude** *(Ref: Reddy 34/e p300, 33/e p332; Parikh 6/e p4.156)*
The given picture depicts flexion of elbows, knees, hip, and neck, and clenching of hand into a fist known as pugilistic attitude.

Pugilistic Attitude
- **Pugilistic attitude** or **boxing attitude, defense attitude, fencing attitude, heat rigor, heat stiffening** is the characteristic attitude adopted by the body after severe burns[Q].
- A 'defensive' position adopted by pugilists (boxers) found in **severely burned bodies**, characterized by **flexion of elbows, knees, hip & neck** and **clenching of hand into a fist**[Q].

Contd...

Pugilistic Attitude
Causes:
• **Coagulation of proteins of muscles** in burns, falling in hot liquids, high voltage electric shocks[Q]
Mechanism:
• **Pugilistic attitude** is due to **coagulation of muscle proteins, dehydration & contracture of muscles** due to heat[Q].
• **Temperature required >50°C; well established at 75°C**[Q]
• **Myosin coagulates at 50°C & albumin coagulates at 73°C.** If body is subjected to a **temperature >73°C, all these proteins are coagulated**[Q].   • **Contraction of paraspinal muscles** causes a **marked opisthotonos,** an attitude commonly adopted by boxers[Q].
Characteristic Features:
• **Pugilistic attitude rigidity is stronger than** that produced by **rigor mortis**[Q].
Interpretation:
• **Not a sign of ante-mortem burns**[Q]: Occurs irrespective of weather the victim was alive or dead at the time of burning.
• **Pugilistic attitude is never seen in living victims**[Q].

84. **Ans. c. Recent microinjuries** *(Ref: Parikh 6/e p5.36; Forensic Emergency Medicine by Jonathan S. Olshake Pg 100)*

In examination of a victim of sexual assault, toluidine blue dye test is done to identify recent micro injuries.

Examination of a victim of sexual assault	
• Wet mount evaluation for motile sperm[Q]	• Anoscopy[Q]
• Alternative light source[Q]	• Colposcopy[Q]
• Toluidine blue dye test[Q]	

Toluidine Blue Dye (TBD) Test
• Lauber and Souma (1982) were the first to introduce research in this new technique.
• **Most important benefit from TBD** is **ability to identify microtrauma**[Q] caused by **blunt force trauma to genitalia.**
• **Toluidine blue dye**, a nuclear stain, improves the **identification of genital microlacerations**[Q] during the examinations of rape victims.   • It **identifies micro-tears** or **abrasions**[Q], especially in **posterior fourchette**[Q], a common site of trauma from intercourse.
• **Positive results with TBD, does not determine** whether the **injury occurred from consensual or non-consensual intercourse**[Q].
• It can however bear witness that there has been blunt force trauma applied to the area in question.

85. **Ans. c. Little finger** *(Ref: Reddy 34/e p84, 33/e p87; Parikh 6/e p2.15)*

Fingerprint reader (FINDER) is a computerized automatic fingerprint reading system which can record each fingerprint data in half second. Prints of eight fingers are recorded excluding little fingers.

"Computerisation: Fingerprint reader (FINDER) is a computerized automatic fingerprint reading system which can record each fingerprint data in half second. Prints of eight fingers are recorded excluding little fingers. The light reflected from a fingerprint can be measured and converted to digital data which is classified, codified and stored in the computer." - Reddy 34/e p84

86. **Ans. c. Change in partial weight of lungs** *(Ref: Reddy 34/e p411, 33/e p439)*

In assessing infant deaths, Ploucquet's test involves change in partial weight of lungs.

"Ploucquet's test: The blood flow in the lung beds is so increased after breathing that their weight is almost doubled from 1/70 of the body weight before respiration to 1/35 after respiration. This increase in weight is not constant and is not a reliable indication of breathing." - Reddy 33/e p439

Tests for Live Birth		
Stomach Bowel test	**Breslau's Second Life Test (Stomach Bowel test)**	
	Principle: • **It assumes that a live born child would respire and therefore would also swallow some air into stomach & bowel**[Q]. • **Detecting presence of air in stomach & intestine (positive test) proves live birth.** • **Negative test** (absence of air in stomach & bowel) **does not always mean still-birth**.	
	Procedure: • **Stomach & intestine are removed separately after tying double ligature at each end**, place them in water. They **float in water if respiration has taken place**, otherwise they will sink.	
	No medicolegal value: • Because air may be swallowed by child in attempting to free the air passage of fluid obstruction in case of still-birth. • It is **useless in putrefaction.**	
For Lungs	**Static test or Fodere's test**[Q]	• Weight of lung before (30-40 gm) & after respiration (60-66 gm) is measured. • **Increase in weight of lung is due to increased blood flow**[Q].
	Ploucquet's test[Q]	• **Weight of lung is doubled after respiration**[Q] • **Before respiration-1/70 of body weight, after respiration-1/35 of body weight**[Q].
	Hydrostatic test (Raygat's test)[Q]	• It is based on a fact that **on breathing, volume of lungs is increased**[Q], which more than compensates the weight of additional blood, due to which their specific gravity is diminished.
For Middle Ear	**Werdin's test**[Q]: Before birth, middle ear contains gelatinous embryonic connective tissue. **With respiration, sphincter at pharyngeal end of eustachian tube relaxes & air replaces the gelatinous substance in few hours to 5 weeks.** This is **not reliable.**	

87. **Ans. c. 130 cm** *(Ref: Parikh 6/e p2.75, 12.2)*

In general, humerus represents 20%, Tibia 22%, Femur 27% and Spine 34% of the stature. Multiplication factor for humerus is 5.31 for calculation of stature. In the question, length of femur is 24.5 cm. Hence, predicted height = 5.31×24.5 = 130 cm.

Multiplication Factors				
	Bengal, Bihar & Odisha		Uttar Pradesh & Punjab	
Length of	**Male**	**Female**	**Male**	**Female**
Humerus	5.31[Q]	5.31[Q]	5.30	4.97
Radius	6.78	6.70	6.90	6.43
Ulna	6.00	6.00	6.30	5.93
Femur	3.82	3.80	3.70	3.57
Tibia	4.49	4.46	4.48	4.18
Fibula	4.46	4.43	4.48	4.35

88. **Ans. b. Helsinki declaration** *(Ref: Reddy 34/e p600, 33/e p26, 400, 647; Parikh 6/e p1.26)*

Helsinki declaration governs biomedical research in human subjects.

"The declaration of Helsinki is a set of ethical principles regarding human experimentation developed for the medical community by the World Medical Association. It is widely regarded as the cornerstone document on human research ethics."

Declaration of **Geneva (1948)**	• **Modernized version of Hippocratic oath**[Q]
Declaration of **London (1949)**	• International code of **medical ethics**
Declaration of **Helsinki (1964)**	• **Human experimentation & clinical trials**[Q]
Declaration of **Sydney (1968)**	• Definition of **death & recovery of organs**
Declaration of **Oslo (1970)**	• **Therapeutic (legalized) abortion**[Q]
Declaration of **Munich (1973)**	• Discrimination in medicine
Declaration of **Tokyo (1975)**	• **Torture & medicine**[Q]
Declaration of **Lisbon (1981)**	• Rights of patients
Declaration of **Venice (1983)**	• Terminal illness
Declaration of **Malta (1992)**	• Role of doctors in hunger strikes
Declaration of **Istanbul (2008)**	• Organ trafficking & transplant tourism

89. Ans. d. Surgeon doing liver transplant *(Ref: http://mohfw.gov.in/showfile.php?lid=2606; Transplantation of Human Organs and Tissue Rules)*

In the case of brain-stem death of the donor, a certificate has been signed by all the members of the Board of medical experts; Where a neurologist or a neurosurgeon is not available, an anesthetist or intensivist nominated by the Registered Medical Practitioner and who is not member of the transplantation team for the recipient concerned, may certify the brain stem death as a member of the Board. Because of vested interest, surgeon doing liver transplant cannot declare a person brain dead.

"In the case of brain-stem death of the donor, a certificate has been signed by all the members of the Board of medical experts; Where a neurologist or a neurosurgeon is not available, an anesthetist or intensivist nominated by the Registered Medical Practitioner (RMP) and who is not member of the transplantation team for the recipient concerned, may certify the brain stem death as a member of the Board."

"In the case of brain-stem death of a person of less than eighteen years of age, a certificate has been signed by all the members of the Board of medical experts and an authority; has been signed by either of the parents of such person."

Form 10 for Certification of Brainstem Death
• The following are required to announce brain death:
• **RMP: In charge of hospital** in which **brainstem death** has occurred[Q].
• **RMP nominated** from the panel of names sent by the hospitals & approved by the appropriate authority[Q].
• **Neurologist/Neurosurgeon**[Q]
• **RMP treating the aforesaid deceased person (where Neurologist/ Neurosurgeon is not available**, any **surgeon or physician and anesthetist or intensivist**[Q], nominated by medical administrator in charge from the panel of names sent by the hospital and approved by the appropriate authority shall be included)

- • **Minimum interval between 1st & 2nd testing** will be **6 hours in adults**.
- • In case of children **6 to 12 years** of age, **1 to 5 years of age & infants**, the **time interval shall increase** depending on the opinion of the above brainstem death experts.

90. Ans. a. Universal system *(Ref: Reddy 34/e p96-97, 33/e p99-100)*

The given system of depiction of the 32 teeth is in accordance with Universal system.

Most Widely Used Systems for Charting of Permanent Teeth	
Universal system	• **Teeth are numbered 1 to 16 from upper right to upper left, and 17 to 32 from lower left o lower right**[Q]. • This follows the plan advocated by the **American and International Society of Forensic Odontology.**

Right	1	2	3	4	5	6	7	8	9	10	11	12	13	14	15	16	Left
	32	31	30	29	28	27	26	25	24	23	22	21	20	19	18	17	

Contd...

Contd...

Most Widely Used Systems for Charting of Permanent Teeth	
Palmer's notation	• **Numbering of teeth in the quadrant begins at the midline & numbers increase as the teeth become farther from the midline**[Q]. Right 8 7 6 5 4 3 2 1 | 1 2 3 4 5 6 7 8 Left 8 7 6 5 4 3 2 1 | 1 2 3 4 5 6 7 8
Haderup system	• It is similar to **Palmer's notation** except that it uses a **plus sign (+) to designate upper teeth and a minus sign (−) for the lower**[Q].
FDI (Federation Dentaire Internationale) Two digit system	• It bears slight **resemblance to Palmer's system in that both utilize the same numbers**, but the **FDI system substitutes a number for the quadrant side and that number is placed before the tooth number**. • Thus the lower right canine will be number 43 in this system. Right $\dfrac{1}{4}$ $\dfrac{1}{3}$ Left
Diagrammatic or Anatomical Chart	• In this **each tooth is represented by a pictorial symbol** that gives the **same number of teeth surfaces as those on the same teeth in the mouth.** • The **incisors & canines are represented by four surfaces** & premolar & molars by **five** (due to occlusal surface). • The **positions of crowns, caries, fillings, or other abnormalities are marked** on these diagrams. • The diagrams also **includes deciduous teeth**

PREVENTIVE SOCIAL MEDICINE

91. **Ans. d. It is responsible for seasonal epidemics of influenza**   *(Ref: Park 24/e p164, 23/e p154, 22/e p145)*

Antigenic drift is a mechanism for variation in viruses that involves the accumulation of mutations within genes that code for antibody binding sites. This results in a new strain of virus particles, which cannot be inhibited as effectively by the antibodies that were originally targeted against previous strains, making it easier for the virus to spread throughout a partially immune population, responsible for seasonal epidemics of influenza.

"When there is a sudden or major change, it is called a shift, and when the antigenic change is gradual over a period of time, it is called a drift. Antigenic shift appears to result from genetic recombination of human with animal or avian virus, providing a major antigenic change. This can cause a major epidemic or pandemic involving most or all age groups. Antigenic drift involves point mutation in the genes owing to selection pressure by immunity in the host population."- *Park 24/e p164*

Antigenic Shift	Antigenic Drift
• **Major antigenic change**[Q]	• **Minor antigenic change**[Q]
• Occurs as a result of **genome reassortment between difference subtypes**[Q].	• Occurs as a result of **accumulation of point mutations** in the gene[Q]
• An antigenic change which r**esults in drastic or dramatic alteration in HA (hemagglutinin) or NA (neuraminidase) subtypes**[Q]	• An antigenic change can **alter antigenic sites** on the molecule such that a **virion can escape recognition by host's immune system**[Q]
• **Large & sudden mutation**[Q]	• **Random & spontaneous mutation**[Q]
• **Difficult to treat (need new vaccine)**[Q]	• **Easy to treat (antibody & drugs available)**[Q]
• **Occurs only in Influenza virus A**[Q]	• Occurs in **Influenza viruses A, B & C**[Q]
• **Gives rise to pandemics**, which occur **irregularly & unpredictably**[Q]	• Usually **responsible for epidemics** in between pandemics[Q]

Contd...

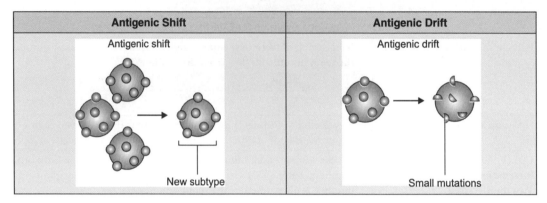

92. **Ans. b. 100 mg of elemental iron and 500 micrograms of folic acid to pregnant women weekly for an entire year**
    (Ref: Park 22/e p596; http://www.nrhmhp.gov.in/sites/default /files/files/Iron%20plus%20 initiative%20for%206%20 months%20-5%20years.pdf)

According to the National Iron Plus Program made to tackle iron-deficiency anemia, 100 mg of elemental iron and 500 micrograms of folic acid should be given to pregnant women weekly for an entire year.

National Iron Plus Program
• Under **National Iron+ Initiative**, the following age groups are covered for **lifelong supplementation of Iron from the age of 6 months onwards:**
• Bi-weekly 20 mg elemental iron & 100 mcg folic acid per ml of liquid formulation & age-appropriate de-worming for **preschool children of 6–59 months**[Q].
• Weekly supplementation of 45 mg elemental iron & 400 mcg folic acid per child per day for children from **1st to 5th grade** in Government & Government aided schools, and at AWC for out of school children **(6 to 10 years)**[Q].
• Weekly dose of 100 mg elemental iron & 500 mcg folic acid with **biannual de-worming in adolescents (10–19 years)** under WIFS 4[Q]
• Weekly supplementation for women in reproductive age, pregnant & lactating women[Q].

IFA supplementation programme and service delivery			
Age group	Intervention/Dose	Regime	Service delivery
6–60 months	1 ml of IFA syrup containing **20 mg** of elemental **iron** & **100 mcg** of **folic acid**[Q]	**Biweekly** throughout the period **6–60 months** of age & **deworming** for **children 12 months & above**[Q]	Inclusion in MCP card Through ASHA/ANM
5–10 years	Tablets of **45 mg** elemental **iron** & **400 mcg** of **folic acid**[Q]	**Weekly** throughout the period **5–10 years** of age & **biannual de-worming**[Q]	In school through teachers & for out of school children through Anganwadi center (AWC)
10–19 years	**100 mg** elemental **iron** & **500 mcg** of **folic acid**[Q]	**Weekly** throughout the period **10–19 years** of age & **biannual de-worming**[Q]	In school through teachers and for those out of school through AWC
Pregnant & lactating women	100 mg elemental **iron** & 500 mcg of **folic acid**[Q]	1 tablet daily for 100 days, starting after 1st trimester, at 14–16 weeks of gestation[Q]. To be repeated for 100 days post-partum[Q]	ANC/ANM/ASHA Inclusion in MCP card
Women in reproductive age group	100 mg elemental **iron** & 500 mcg of **folic acid**[Q]	**Weekly throughout the reproductive period**[Q]	Through FHW during house visit for contraceptive distribution

93. **Ans. c. A and B**   *(Ref: Park 24/e p192, 23/e p182, 22/e p170; http://tbcindia.nic.in/WriteReadData/l892s/9659721466Guideline%20for%20Partnership.pdf)*

AIIMS May 2016

According to RNTCP, sputum samples for testing of TB are packed in two containers labeled as A and B.

"The sputum samples are labeled with a serial number and a suffix a-b with regard to the spot-morning samples respectively. Early morning specimen is always labeled as "b", while the first spot specimen is labeled as "a". It is important to label sputum containers properly. Sputum containers should always be labeled on the side, and never on the lid, as the lid from one container may be placed on another container resulting is specimens being labeled incorrectly."

Guidelines for Sputum Sampling
• The **cup** should be **clean, do not open it until you are ready for sampling.**
• The **early morning (B) sample** should be **as soon as you wake up.**
• The **volume** should be **at least** reach the **5 ml** line in the plastic container provided.
• **The spot sample is labeled as A and the early morning sample as B**[Q].

94. **Ans. c. Administering zero dose of DPT and OPV** *(Ref: Park 24/e p936, 23/e p449, 22/e p414; Ministry of Health and Family Welfare (MoHFW). (2005b). Reading Material for ASHA. Government of India)*

ASHA does'nt receive financial renumeration for administering zero dose of DPT and OPV is not the function of ASHA.

ASHA Payments under Janani Suraksha Yojana (JSY): On 45th Day	Other ASHA Payments
• **6 visits in institutional deliveries**[Q] (Day 3, 7, 14, 21, 28, 42) • **7 visits in home deliveries**[Q] (Day 1, 3, 7, 14, 21, 28, 42) • **Birth weight record**[Q] • **Immunized with BCG, first dose of OPV & DPT**[Q] • **Birth registration**[Q] • Mother & child are safe	• **Institutional deliveries**[Q] • Arrange transport of AN mother • Escort AN mother to facility • **Completed immunization upto 1 & 2 years of age**[Q] • **Pulse polio immunization**[Q] • **Family planning services**[Q] • Sanitary napkins to adolescent girls • Promote use of sanitary toilets • **DOTS provider**[Q] • **Leprosy treatment**[Q] • **Peripheral smear for malaria**[Q] • **Malaria treatment**[Q]

Accredited Social Health Activist (ASHA)
• Launched as part of **National Rural Health Mission (NRHM)** to **strengthen primary health care at village level**
• ASHA will be a **health activist** in the community who will **create awareness on health**
• Expected to act as **interface between community & health care system** and **bridge between ANM & village**
• **Accountable to panchayat**[Q]
• **Resource person for training of ASHA: ANM & anganwadi worker**[Q]
• **General norm of selection: one ASHA for 1000 population**[Q]

Selection of ASHA	
• Must be **resident of the village**[Q] • A **woman (married/widowed/divorced)** in the age group of **25-45 years**[Q]	• Formal **education upto class 8th**[Q] • **Good communication skills & leadership qualities**[Q]

• Under HBNC, ASHA will be paid Rs. 250/- for the care of the mother and the new born. **She will be conducting:**
• **Six visits** in case of **institutional delivery (Days 3, 7, 14, 21, 28 & 42)**
• **Seven visits** in case of **home delivery (Days 1, 3, 7, 14, 21, 28 & 42)**

The payment will be made subject to:
• Ensuring that **birth weight is recorded** in the Maternal & Child Protection card
• Ensuring that the **newborn is immunized** with BCG, first doses of DPT & OPV & entered in MCP card
• **Ensuring birth registration**
• Both **mother & newborn** are safe until the **42nd day** of delivery

Monitoring & Evaluation of ASHA		
Process indicators	**Outcome indicators**	**Impact indicators**
• Number of ASHAs selected by due process • Number of ASHAs trained • Percentage of ASHAs attending review meeting after one year	• **Percentage of newborns who were weighed and families counseled**[Q] • **Percentage of deliveries with skilled assistance**[Q] • **Percentage of institutional deliveries**[Q] • **Percentage of completely immunized children in the 12-23 months age group**[Q] • Percentage of unmet need for spacing contraception among people below poverty line • Percentage of people who received chloroquine within first week in a malaria endemic area	• **Infant mortality rate**[Q] • **Child malnutrition rates**[Q] • **Number of cases of tuberculosis or leprosy reported as compared to the previous year**[Q].

95. Ans. a. PHC   *(Ref: Park 24/e p944, 23/e p906, 22/e p847)*

A psychiatrist is not posted at PHC.

Staff	Essential	
	Type A	**Type B**
Medical officer-MBBS	1	1
Medical officer-AYUSH		–
Accountant cum data entry operator	1	1
Pharmacist	1	1
Pharmacist-AYUSH		
Nurse-midwife (Staff nurse)	3	4
Health workers (Female)	1*	1*
Health assistant (Male)	1	1
Health assistant (Female) /Lady health visitor	1	1
Health educator		
Laboratory technician	1	1
Cold chain & vaccine logistic assistant		–
Multi-skilled group D worker	2	2
Sanitary worker cum watchman	1	1
Total	13	14

*For sub-centre area of PHC
• **Apart from the essential staff, the desirable staff for both type A and type B PHC are:**
• **One of the two medical officers (MBBS) should be lady doctor, if the delivery case load is 30 or more per month**
• **One AYUSH medical officer to provide choice to the people, where as AYUSH facility is not available in the vicinity**
• **One staff nurse/nurse midwife**
• **One health educator at the PHC.**
That makes total staff at type A PHC 18 and at type B PHC 21.

96. Ans. a. Drug inventory   *(Ref: https://www.ncbi.nlm.nih.gov/pmc/articles/PMC3719141/)*

ABC and VED analysis at PHC are done for drug inventory.

"Inventory control is a scientific system which indicates as to what to order, when to order, and how much to order, and how much to stock so that purchasing costs and storing costs are kept as low as possible. It helps to protect against the fluctuation in supply and demand, uncertainty and minimise waiting time. There are various methods involved for inventory control but two are commonly used: Always, better and control (ABC) and vital, essential and desirable (VED)."- https://www.ncbi.nlm.nih.gov/pmc/articles/PMC3719141/

Inventory control
• **Inventory control** is a scientific system which **indicates** as to **what to order, when to order & how much to order**, and **how much to stock** so that **purchasing costs & storing costs** are kept as low as possible. • It helps to **protect against the fluctuation in supply & demand, uncertainty & minimise waiting time.**

Contd...

Contd...

Inventory control	
Methods of Inventory Control	
Always, Better and Control (ABC)	**Vital, Essential and Desirable (VED)**
• **ABC analysis** helps in **identifying the items** that **require greater attention for control**[Q]. • *Group A*: **10%** items consume about **70% of the budget.** • *Group B*: Next **20%** inventory items take away **20% of financial resources**. • *Group C*: Remaining **70%** items account for just **10% of budget**.	• **VED analysis** is **based on critical values** & **shortage cost of item**[Q]. • **Based on their criticality**, the items could be classified into three categories: **Vital, essential & desirable, i.e., VED**[Q].

• A **combination of ABC & VED analysis (ABC-VED matrix)** can be gainfully employed to evolve a meaningful control over the material supplies.

Category I	Category II	Category III
• Category I includes **all V & E items (AV, BV, CV, AE, AD).**	• Category II includes **remaining items of E & B groups (BE, CE, BD)**.	Category III includes **desirable & cheaper** group of **items (CD)**.

97. **Ans. d. The criteria of endemicity is a total goitre rate of >10%** *(Ref: Ghai 8/e p519)*

The term 'endemic goitre' refers to a total goitre rate of >5 percent in a given community. Total goitre rate is an indicator of iodine deficiency, which causes brain damage and mental retardation.

"Endemic goiter is present when the prevalence of goiter in a defined population exceeds 5%. Endemic goiter is graded by the method of WHO. Screening estimates of iodine intake are usually derived from 24-hr urinary excretion values or urinary iodine concentration expressed in relation to creatinine concentration."- Ghai 8/e p519

Estimation of Thyroid Size by Palpation	
Stage 0	• No goiter
Stage 1A	• **Goiter detectable only by palpation** & **not visible** even when the neck is fully extended
Stage 1B	• **Goiter palpable** but **visible** only when the **neck is fully extended** (this stage also includes **nodular glands** even if not goitrous)
Stage 2	• **Goiter visible** when the **neck** is in **normal position**; palpation not needed for diagnosis
Stage 3	• **Very large goiter**, which can be recognized at a considerable distance

98. **Ans. b. Case control study** *(Ref: Park 24/e p76, 23/e p71; 22/e p76)*

Best study design to assess in quick time the strength of association between smoking and lung cancer is case control study.

"Case control studies, often called retrospective studies are a common first approach to test causal hypothesis. In recent years, the case control approach has emerged as a permanent method of epidemiological investigation. The case control method has three distinct features: a. Both exposure and outcome (disease) have occurred before the start of study; b. the study proceeds backwards from effect to cause; c. it uses a control or comparison group to support or refute an inference."- Park 23/e p71

Case control study	Cohort study
• Proceeds from 'effect to cause'[Q]	• Proceeds from 'cause to effect'[Q]
• Starts with the disease[Q]	• Starts with people exposed to risk factor or suspected cause[Q]
• Tests whether the suspected cause occurs more frequently in those with the disease than among those without the disease.[Q]	• Tests whether disease occurs more frequently in those exposed, than in those not similarly exposed[Q].
• Usually the first approach to the testing of a hypothesis[Q], but also useful for exploratory studies.	• Reserved for testing of precisely formulated hypothesis[Q].
• Involves fewer number of subjects[Q].	• Involves larger number of subjects[Q].
• Yields relatively quick results[Q].	• Long follow-up period often needed, involving delayed results[Q].

Contd...

Contd...

Case control study	Cohort study
• Suitable for the study of rare diseases[Q].	• Inappropriate when the **disease or exposure under** investigation is rare.
• Generally **yields only estimate of RR (odds ratio)**[Q].	• **Yields incidence rates, RR as well as AR**[Q].
• Cannot yield information about diseases other than that selected for study[Q].	• **Can yield information about more than one disease outcome**[Q].
• **Relatively inexpensive**[Q]	• **Expensive**[Q]

99. **Ans. c. Blood groups A, B, ABO** *(Ref: High Yield Statistics/p13)*

Blood groups (A, B, ABO) is a discrete variable.

Continuous variable	Discrete Variables
• Have an **infinite number of possible values** between any two observed values[Q]. • **Every interval is divisible into an infinite number of equal parts**[Q] • Measured on nominal or ordinal scale[Q] • **Example: Height, weight, body mass index, mid arm circumference, blood sugar level**[Q]	• **Has separate, indivisible categories**[Q] • **No values exist between two neighboring categories**[Q] • **Measured on a metric scale**[Q] • **Example: ABO blood group, gender, presence of diabetes**[Q]

100. **Ans. c. Stratified random sampling** *(Ref: Park 24/e p886, 23/e p850, 22/e p792; BK Mahajan 6th/100-101)*

Stratified random sampling is used for selecting patients with respect to potential factors that will affect the results.

"Stratified random sample: The sample is deliberately drawn in a systematic way so that each portion of the sample represents a corresponding strata of universe. This method is particularly useful where one is interested in analyzing the data by a certain characteristic of population, viz. Hindus, Christians, Muslims, age-groups etc."- Park 23/e p850

Types of Sampling		
	Random sampling	**Non-random sampling**
Synonyms	• **Probability** sampling[Q] • **Non-purposive** sampling	• **Non-probability** sampling • **Purposive** sampling[Q]
Types	• **Simple** random sampling • **Systematic** random sampling • **Stratified** random sampling • **Multistage** random sampling • **Multiphase** random sampling • **Cluster** random sampling	• **Convenience** sampling • **Quota** sampling • **Snow-ball** sampling • **Clinical trial** sampling

Types of Random Sampling
Simple Random Sampling: • **Every unit of population has equal and known chance of being selected**[Q]   • Is also known as **'unrestricted random sampling'**   • Applicable for **small, homogenous** and **readily available populations**   • Used in clinical trials

Methods of Simple random sampling		
• **Lottery method**[Q]	• **Random number tables**[Q]	• **Computer software**[Q]

Systematic Random Sampling: • **Based on sampling fraction: Every K^{th} unit is chosen in the population list, where K is chosen by sampling interval**[Q]   • **Sampling Interval (K) = Total no. of units in population/ Total no. of units in sample**   • Applicable for **large, non-homogenous populations where complete list of individuals is available**   • For example, if there is a population of 1000 from which sample of 20 is to be chosen, then K = 1000/20 = 50; thus every 50th unit will be included in the sample (i.e. 1st, 51st, 101st, so on…) First unit among first 50 is chosen by simple random sampling.

Types of Random Sampling

Stratified Random Sampling:
- **Non-homogenous population** is **converted to homogenous groups/classes (strata); sample is drawn from each strata at random, in proportion to its size**[Q]
  - **Applicable for large non-homogenous population**[Q]
  - **Gives more representative sample than simple random sampling**[Q]
  - **None of the categories is under or over-represented**[Q]
- For example, In a population of 1000, sample of 100 is to be drawn for Hemoglobin estimation; first convert non-homogenous population is converted to homogenous strata (i.e. 700 males and 300 females), then draw 70 males and 30 females randomly respectively.

Multistage Random Sampling:
- Is **done in successive stages; each successive sampling unit is nested in the previous sampling unit**[Q]
- **Advantage: Introduces flexibility in sampling**[Q]
- For example, in large country surveys, states are chosen, then districts, then villages, then every 10th person in village as final sampling unit

Multiphase Random Sampling:
- Is **done in successive phases; part of information is obtained from whole sample & part from the sub-sample**[Q]
- For example, in a TB survey, Mantoux test done in first phase, then X-ray done in all Mantoux positives, then sputum examined in all those with positive X-ray findings.

Cluster Random Sampling:
- **Applicable when units of population are natural groups or clusters**[Q]
- **Use in India: Evaluation of immunization coverage**[Q]
  - **WHO technique used: 30 × 7 technique (total = 210 children)**[Q]
  - **WHO technique used in CRS: 30 × 7 technique (total = 210 children)**
  - **30 clusters, each containing 7 children,** who are 12-23 months age and are **completely immunized for primary immunization (till Measles vaccine)**[Q]
  - Clusters are heterogeneous within themselves but homogenous with respect to each other
  - **Sampling interval is also calculated in CRS**
- **Accuracy**[Q]**: Low error rate of only ± 5%**
- **Limitation: Clusters cannot be compared with each other**[Q].

Types of Non-Random Sampling

Convenience Sampling:
- **Patients are selected, in part or in whole, at the convenience of the researcher; no/limited attempt to ensure that sample is an accurate representation of population**[Q]
- For example, standing at a shopping mall and selecting shoppers as they walk by to fill out a survey.

Quota Sampling:
- **Population is first segmented into mutually exclusive sub-groups (quotas), just as in stratified sampling;** then **judgment is used to select the units from each group non-randomly**
- Is a **type of convenience sampling.**

- **Snow-ball Sampling:**
- **A technique for developing a research sample where existing study subjects recruit future subjects from among their acquaintances;** thus the **sample group appears to grow like a rolling snowball**
- Is **often used in hidden populations** which are difficult for researchers to access, e.g. **drug users or commercial sex workers**[Q]

- **Clinical Trial Sampling**

---

101. **Ans. b. Weight for age**   (*Ref: Park 24/e p582, 23/e p547, 22/e p506*)
India has adopted the new WHO Child Growth Standards (2006) in February 2009 for monitoring the young child growth and development within the National Rural Health Mission and the ICDS. These are based on weight for age. Weight for age is used at anganwadi centers for growth monitoring in children.

"Growth chart used in India: India has adopted the new WHO Child Growth Standards (2006) in February 2009 for monitoring the young child growth and development within the National Rural Health Mission and the ICDS. These are based on Weight for age. These standards are available for both boys and girls below 5 years of age. With those new standards, the child care workers will know when the nutrition and care needs of the child are being compromised and it will enable them to take timely corrective action at different levels. A joint "Mother and Child Protection Card" has been developed. The chart is easily understood by the health workers and the mother, with a visual record of the health and nutritional status of the child. It is kept by the mother and brought to the health center at each visit. The growth chart shows normal zone of weight for age, under nutrition (below-2 SD) and severely underweight zone (below-3 SD). It is the direction of growth that is more important than the position of dots on the line. Flattening or falling of the child's weight curve signals growth failure, which is the earliest sign of the protein-energy malnutrition and may precede clinical signs by weeks and months. The objective in child care is to keep the child in normal zone."
- Park 24/e p582

Growth Charts

- The **growth or "road to health" chart (first designed by David Morely** and **later modified by WHO)** is a **visible display of the child's physical growth** and **development**[Q].
- **Growth chart is generally plotted between: Weight and Age**[Q]
- It is **designed primarily for longitudinal follow-up (growth monitoring) of a child,** so that changes overtime can be interpreted.
- The **purpose of the chart** is **early identification of growth failure** so that action can be taken to prevent severe malnutrition.
- **Changes in weight** are **most sensitive indicators of growth & nutrition status in young children**[Q].

Growth chart provides information on	
• **Identification & registration**[Q] • **Birth date & birth weight**[Q] • **Chronological age**[Q] • **Weight-for-age**[Q] • Developmental milestones • History of sibling health	• Immunization procedures • Introduction of supplementary foods • Episodes of sickness • Child spacing (Contraceptive/family planning methods used) • Reasons for special care

102. **Ans. b. Type II error** *(Ref: High Yield Biostatistics/p46)*

A study finds no significant association between two variables but truly there exists a difference. This type of error is type II error.

*"Type I error , also known as an **error of the first kind,** occurs **when the null hypothesis (H_0) is true, but is rejected.** It is **asserting something that is absent, a false hit.** A type I error may be compared with a so-called false positive (a result that indicates that a given condition is present when it actually is not present) in tests where a single condition is tested for. **The type I error rate or significance level is the probability of rejecting the null hypothesis, given that it is true. It is denoted by the Greek letter α (alpha) and is also called the alpha level.** Often, the significance level is set to 0.05 (5%), implying that it is acceptable to have a 5% probability of incorrectly rejecting the null hypothesis.*

Type I errors are philosophically a focus of skepticism and Occam's razor. A type I error occurs when we believe in falsehood ("believing in a lie"). In terms of folk tales, an investigator may be "crying wolf" without a wolf in sight (raising a false alarm) (H_0: no wolf)."

*"A type II error, also known as an **error of the second kind,** occurs when the null hypothesis is false, but erroneously fails to be rejected. It is failing to assert what is present, a miss. A type II error may be compared with a so-called false negative (where an actual 'hit' was disregarded by the test and seen as a 'miss') in a test checking for a single condition with a definitive result of true or false. A type II error is committed when we fail to believe a truth. In terms of folk tales, an investigator may fail to see the wolf ("failing to raise an alarm"). Again, H_0: no wolf. The rate of the type II error is denoted by the Greek letter β (beta) and related to the power of a test (which equals $1-\beta$)."*

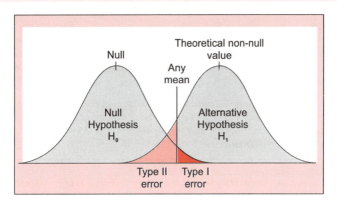

Type I Error	Type II Error
• The **null hypothesis is true but rejected** (False positive)[Q] • Probability of type I error is given by p value[Q] • Significance (alpha) level is the maximum tolerable probability of type I errors[Q] • Keep type I error to be minimum; then results are declared to be statistically significant[Q] • Type I error is more serious than type II error[Q]	• Null hypothesis is not false but is not rejected/accepted (false negative)[Q] • Probability of type II error is given by beta[Q]

103. Ans. c. Odds ratio/Relative risk   *(Ref: Park 24/e p78, 23/e p73, 22/e p75)*
The strength of association between the risk factor and disease is measured by Odds ratio/Relative risk.

"The estimation of disease risk associated with exposure is obtained by an index known as relative risk (RR) or risk ratio, which is defined as the ratio between the incidence of disease among exposed persons and incidence among non-exposed."- Park 23/e p73

"Odds ratio (Cross-product ratio): From a case control study, we can derive what is known as odds ratio (OR) which is a measure of the strength of the association between risk factor and outcome. Odds ratio is closely related to relative risk."- Park 23/e p73

104. Ans. b. 4-16   *(Ref: Park 24/e p887, 23/e p851, 22/e p794)*

Standard Error (SE) of Proportion
$SE = \sqrt{PQ/n}$
P= Prevalence = 10% (10/100)
Q= 1-P = 90% (90/100)
n = Sample size = 100
$SE = \sqrt{PQ/n} = \sqrt{10 \times 90/100} = 3$
Confidence Intervals (CI)
The LL and UL estimates for the Statistic are given as:
Lower Limit: Statistic – C×SE (statistic)
Upper Limit: Statistic + C×SE (statistic)
C = Confidence coefficient
= 1.96 for 95% confidence interval
= 2.58 for 99% confidence interval
= 3.29 for 99.9% confidence interval
For 95% confidence interval
CI = 10–2×3 to 10 + 2×3 = 4–16

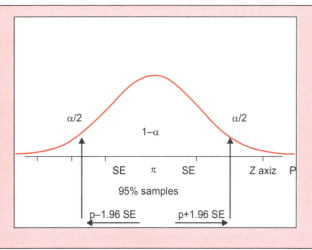

105. Ans. c. Newer and effective treatment modalities decrease the incidence   *(Ref: Park 24/e p67, 23/e p62, 22/e p59)*
Newer and effective treatment modalities do not decrease the incidence. Improvements in treatment may decrease the duration of illness and may decrease prevalence.

AIIMS ESSENCE

"Prevalence is the proportion of a population that has a condition at a specific time, but the prevalence will be influenced by both the rate at which new cases are occurring and the average duration of the disease. Incidence reflects the rate at which new cases of disease are being added to the population (and becoming prevalent cases). Average duration of disease is also important, because the only way you can stop being a prevalent case is to be cured or to move out of the population or die."

"Improvements in treatment may decrease the duration of illness and thereby decrease prevalence of disease. But if the treatment is such that by preventing death, and at the same time not producing recovery, may give rise to the apparently paradoxical effect of an increase in prevalence. Further, if duration is decreased sufficiently, a decrease in prevalence could take place despite an increase in incidence."- Park 24/e p67

Incidence
• **Incidence: Number of new case**[Q] **occurring in a defined population during a specified period of time.**
• It is **expressed as per 1000 per year**[Q].
• **Incidence is a rate**[Q]
• Incidence is **not affected by duration of disease**[Q]
• **Use of in incidence is** generally **restricted to acute conditions**[Q].
• This is a **much more accurate measure of risk than prevalence**[Q].

Prevalence
• Prevalence is the **total current (Old+ new) cases in a given population over a point or period of time**[Q].
• **Types: Point prevalence (at a point of time) & Period prevalence (over a period of time)**[Q]
• **Prevalence = No. of total (old + new) cases of a disease in a year/Total population x 100**[Q]
• **Prevalence = Incidence x Mean duration of disease**[Q]
• **Prevalence is a proportion, not a ratio**[Q]: Numerator is a part of denominator, and is always expressed in percentage.
• **Prevalence can be determined from cross-sectional study**[Q].

Relation between Incidence & Prevalence
• Given the assumption that **population is stable & incidence** and **duration are not changing.**
• **Prevalence = Incidence x Mean duration of disease**[Q]
• **Prevalence describes balance between incidence, mortality & recovery**[Q].
• **Incidence reflects causal factors**[Q].
• **Duration reflects prognostic factors**[Q]

106. Ans. b. Negatively skewed data *(Ref: Park 24/e p886, 23/e p847, 22/e p786; High Yield Statistics/p67)*

Since more number of children has a higher APGAR score, the tail of the distribution curve will be towards the right. Hence, the data will be negatively skewed.

Skewed Data	
Negative skew	**Positive skew**
• **Left tail is longer**[Q] • **Mass of distribution is concentrated on the right of figure**[Q] • **Distribution is said to be left-skewed, left-tailed, or skewed to the left**[Q].	• **Right tail is longer**[Q] • **Mass of distribution is concentrated on the left of figure**[Q]. • **Distribution is said to be right-skewed, right-tailed, or skewed to the right**[Q].
  Negative skew	 Positive skew

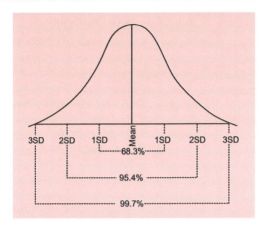

Normal Distribution
• Also known as 'Gaussian distribution' or 'Standard distribution'[Q]
• **Type of distribution**: Distribution of values of a quantitative variable such that they are **symmetric with respect to a middle value with same mean, median and mode & frequencies taper off rapidly & symmetrically on both sides**[Q].
• **Bilaterally symmetrical or bell-shaped**[Q]
• **Mean, Median and Mode coincide (Mean = Median = Mode)**[Q]
• **Mean (μ) = 0 and SD (σ) = 1**[Q]
• SD = √Variance or Variance = $σ^2$
• In normal distribution, SD (σ) = 1, thus Variance = 1[Q]

Actual parameters in a Normal (Gaussian) distribution
• **Mean ± 1SD (μ ± 1σ)** covers 68.27% values[Q]
• **Mean ± 2SD (μ ± 2σ)** covers 95.45% values[Q]
• **Mean ± 3SD (μ ± 3σ)** covers 99.73% values[Q]
• **Mean ± 2.58SD (μ ± 2.58σ)** covers 99% values[Q]

107. Ans. b. 900   *(Ref: Park 23/e p850, 22/e p792)*

$n_0 = Z^2pq/e^2$
n_0 = sample size
Z^2 is the abscissa of the normal curve that cuts off an area α at the tails
(1−α) equals the desired confidence level, e.g. 95%
e is the desired level of precision
p is the estimated proportion of an attribute that is present in the population
q is 1−p
The value for Z is found in statistical tables, which contain the area under the normal curve, e.g. Z = 1.96 for 95% level of confidence
In this question, Alpha = 5%
Z = 1.96
Prevalence, p = 10%
Error, e = 20% of Prevalence (Relative)
e = 2%
Sample size = $(1.96)^2 \times (10) \times (100−10)/(2)^2$ = **900**

MEDICINE

108. Ans. b. Platelet count of less than 40,000 is a contraindication   *(Ref: Dacie Practical Hematology 10/e p163)*
The given image is of Jamshidi bone marrow biopsy needle. Severe thrombocytopenia is not a contraindication to bone marrow aspiration, as long as prolonged pressure is applied to the site to prevent bleeding. Bone marrow aspiration is used in diagnosis of conditions responsible for low platelet counts.

Bone Marrow Biopsy Needles

- Needles most commonly used for obtaining **bone marrow aspirates from sternum** are **Salah, Klima & Jamshidi needles[Q]**.

Salah Needle	Klima Needle	Jamshidi Needle
• **Salah sternal puncture needle is a wide-bore needle** for obtaining samples of **red marrow from sternum.**	• The needle is advanced into the marrow cavity with the stylet locked in place. • The stylet is then removed and a syringe used to aspirate the marrow.	• The stylet is in place for advancement through soft tissue and cortex. • On reaching marrow, the needle is advanced without the stylet to create a core sample. • The probe (hooked) is used to expel the sample into formalin.
5 cms		

Bone Marrow Aspiration

Bone Marrow Aspiration Procedure

- **Clean the skin** with **7% alcohol** (or **0.5% Chlorhexidine**)
- **Infiltrate the skin, subcutaneous tissue & periosteum** overlying the selected site with a 2-5 ml of 2% lignocaine.
- With a **boring movement, pass the bone marrow aspiration needle perpendicularly into the cavity of ilium** at the **centre of oval posterior superior iliac spine** or **2 cm posterior & 2 cm inferior to anterior superior iliac spine[Q]**.
- When the bone has been penetrated, remove the stylet & attach a **1 or 2 ml syringe & suck up marrow contents for making films**.
- **Usual sites for puncture in adults: Posterior > anterior iliac spine[Q]**.
- If serial punctures are being performed, a different site should be selected for each to avoid aspirating marrow that has been diluted by haemorrhage resulting from previous punctures.
- **Posterior iliac spine overlies a large marrow-containing area & relatively large volumes of marrow can be aspirated from this site[Q]**.

Indications for Bone marrow aspiration	Indications for Bone Marrow Trephine Biopsy
• To investigate children with **abnormal peripheral blood findings (atypical cells** or **blasts, pancytopenia, unexplained anemia, leukopenia** or **thrombocytopenia)[Q]** • To diagnose **malignant haematological disorders, hypoplastic anemias,** inherited **bone marrow failure** syndromes & **metastatic spread of tumours[Q]** • To obtain **microbiological cultures** in **pyrexia of unknown origin[Q]** • For investigation of **hypersplenism, lymphadenopathy, mediastinal or abdominal masses[Q]** • For **follow-up after chemotherapy** or **hematopoietic stem cell transplant[Q]**.	• **Inadequate** or **failed marrow aspiration[Q]** • **Suspected bone marrow fibrosis[Q]** • **Investigation & staging of Hodgkin's & non-Hodgkin's lymphoma & small blue round cell tumours of childhood[Q]** (neuroblastoma, rhabdomyosarcoma & Ewing's sarcoma) • Diagnosis of **aplastic anemia, myelodysplastic syndromes & acute megakaryoblastic leukemia[Q]** (AML-M7)

Bone Marrow Aspiration

Contraindications for Bone Marrow Aspiration

- **Hemorrhagic disorders**: Congenital coagulation factor deficiencies (hemophilia), **DIC & concomitant use of anticoagulants**^{Q}.
  - If a **BMA or a BMTB is absolutely indicated** in these patients, then **factor replacement** or **cessation of anticoagulation** should be considered **before the procedure**^{Q}
  - Patient should be **closely monitored for 24 hour post-procedure**^{Q}
  - Severe thrombocytopenia is not a contraindication to BMA, as long as prolonged pressure is applied to the site to prevent bleeding^Q.
  - For **obese patients with severe thrombocytopenia**, in whom a **bone marrow biopsy** is indicated, it is preferable to **perform a platelet transfusion to raise the platelet count >15 × 10⁹/L**^{Q}.
- **Skin infection** or **recent radiation therapy** at the **sampling site.**
- Bone disorders such as **osteomyelitis or osteogenesis imperfecta.**

109. **Ans. a. Electrical cardioversion** *(Ref: Harrison 19/e p1483-1484, 1479 18/e p1888)*

The given ECG shows tachycardia with narrow QRS complex and absent P waves, the diagnosis is Paroxysmal Supraventricular Tachycardia (PSVT). Since the patient is in shock with hypotension, electrical cardioversion is the immediate treatment of choice. Drug of choice for PSVT is Adenosine but it is to be used hemodynamically stable patients.

> *"Acute management of narrow QRS PSVT is guided by the clinical presentation. Continuous ECG monitoring should be implemented and a 12-lead ECG should always be obtained when possible. In the presence of hypotension with unconsciousness or respiratory distress, QRS-synchronous direct current cardioversion is warranted, but this is rarely needed, because intravenous adenosine works promptly in most situations. For stable individuals, initial therapy takes advantage of the fact that most PSVTs are dependent on AV nodal conduction (AV nodal reentry or orthodromic AV reentry) and therefore likely to respond to sympatholytic and vagotonic maneuvers and drugs."* - Harrison 19/e p1483

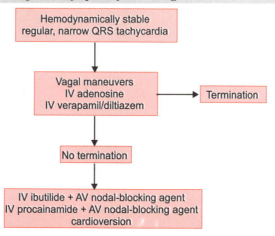

Fig. 38: Treatment Algorithm of PSVT in hemodynamically stable patient

Atrioventricular Nodal Reentry Tachycardia (AVNRT)

- **AVNRT is MC form of PSVT**^{Q}
- Most commonly manifests in **2ⁿᵈ to 4ᵗʰ decades.**

Mechanism:
- **Reentry involving AV node**^{Q}
- **MC form**: A **slowly conducting AV nodal pathway extends from compact AV node** near the bundle of His, **inferiorly along tricuspid annulus,** adjacent to coronary sinus os. **Reentry wave-front propagates up this slow pathway to compact AV node** & then **exits from fast pathway at the top of AV node**^{Q}.

Atrioventricular Nodal Reentry Tachycardia (AVNRT)

Clinical Features:

- It is **often well tolerated**, but **rapid tachycardia**, particularly in the elderly, may **cause angina, pulmonary edema, hypotension, or syncope**[Q].
- Usually not associated with **structural heart disease**[Q].

ECG Findings:

- **Long PR interval, narrow QRS complex tachycardia**[Q]
- **P-wave buried inside QRS complex**[Q] (not visible or distort initial or terminal portion of QRS complex)

Acute Treatment:

- Treatment is directed at **altering conduction within the AV node**[Q].
- **Vagal stimulation** (Valsalva maneuver or carotid sinus massage) can **slow conduction in AV node sufficiently to terminate AVNRT**[Q].
  - If physical maneuvers do not terminate tachyarrhythmia, **1st-line treatment: Adenosine**[Q]
  - **2nd-line treatment:** IV beta blockade or calcium channel therapy[Q]
  - In hemodynamically unstable patients, **R-wave synchronous DC cardioversion using 100–200 J can terminate the tachyarrhythmia**[Q].

Catheter Ablation

- **Catheter ablation** of **slow AV nodal pathway** is recommended for **recurrent or severe episodes** or when **drug therapy is ineffective, not tolerated, or not desired** by the patient[Q].
- **Catheter ablation is curative in over 95% of patients**[Q].
- Major risk: Heart block requiring permanent pacemaker implantation

Adenosine

- **Adenosine** is administered as a **rapid IV bolus for acute termination of re-entrant supraventricular arrhythmias**[Q].
- **Used to produce controlled hypotension**[Q] during some surgical procedures & in diagnosis of coronary artery disease.

Pharmacologic Effects:

- Effects of adenosine are **mediated by interaction with specific G protein-coupled adenosine receptors**[Q].
- **Adenosine activates acetylcholine-sensitive K+ current in the atrium, sinus & AV nodes**, resulting in **shortening of APD, hyperpolarization, & slowing of normal automaticity**[Q].
  - **Adenosine reduces Ca^{2+} currents**, it can be **anti-arrhythmic by increasing AV nodal refractoriness** and by **inhibiting DADs elicited by sympathetic stimulation**[Q].
  - **IV bolus of adenosine** transiently **slows sinus rate & AV nodal conduction velocity & increases AV nodal refractoriness**[Q].

Clinical uses:

- Treatment of **reentrant supraventricular tachycardias**[Q]
- **IV adenosine terminates majority of PSVT by transiently blocking conduction in AV node**[Q].

110. **Ans. d. Low molecular weight heparin**   *(Ref: Harrison 19/e p1597, 18/e p2020)*

EKG in this scenario is showing T-wave inversion (Leads I , aVR , aVL) with a history of retrosternal pain for 6 hours. This is suggestive of Non-ST elevation MI. The primary management of NSTEMI is anti- thrombotic therapy followed by early PCI, if high-risk features are present. In this patient, there are no ST wave changes or any other high-risk feature mentioned. Hence low molecular weight heparin should be the treatment of choice.

"Anticoagulants (For NSTEMI): Four options are available for anticoagulant therapy to be added to antiplatelet agents: (1) unfractionated heparin (UFH), long the mainstay of therapy; (2) the low-molecular-weight heparin (LMWH), enoxaparin, which has been shown to be superior to UFH in reducing recurrent cardiac events, especially in patients managed by a conservative strategy but with some increase in bleeding; (3) bivalirudin, a direct thrombin inhibitor that is similar in efficacy to either UFH or LMWH but causes less bleeding and is used just prior to and/or during PCI; and (4) the indirect factor Xa inhibitor, fondaparinux, which is equivalent in efficacy to enoxaparin but appears to have a lower risk of major bleeding."- Harrison 19/e p1597

Management of NSTEMI (Non ST Segment Elevation MI)

- **Nitrates:** First given **sublingually or by buccal spray**, if patient is **experiencing ischemic pain**. If **pain persists after 3 doses given 5 minutes apart, IV nitroglycerin** is recommended.
- **Beta-Blockers:** Beta-blockers are the other **mainstay of anti-ischemic treatment**.
   - **Heart rate slowing calcium channel blockers** (verapamil or diltiazem), are **recommended for** patients who have **persistent or recurrent symptoms after treatment with full-dose nitrates & beta blockers** and in patients with **contraindications to beta blockade**.
- **Additional medical therapy:** ACE inhibitors & HMG-CoA reductase inhibitors for long-term secondary prevention.
- **Early administration of intensive statin therapy (atorvastatin 80 mg) prior to percutaneous coronary intervention (PCI) has been shown to reduce complications,** suggesting that high-dose statin therapy should be started at the time of admission.
- **Antithrombotic therapy:** This is the other **main component of treatment for NSTEMI**. Initial treatment should begin with **platelet cyclooxygenase inhibitor aspirin.** Typical initial dose is **325 mg/d**, with **lower doses (75–162 mg/d) recommended for long-term therapy**.
- Four options are available for anticoagulant therapy to be added to aspirin and clopidogrel.
   - **Unfractionated heparin (UFH) is mainstay of therapy. LMWH (enoxaparin) has been shown in several studies to be superior to UFH in reducing recurrent cardiac events, especially in conservatively managed patients**.
- **Indirect factor Xa inhibitor, fondaparinux,** is equivalent for **early efficacy** compared with enoxaparin but appears to have a **lower risk of major bleeding**.
- **Bivalirudin,** a **direct thrombin inhibitor**, is **similar in efficacy to either UFH or LMWH** among patients treated with a GP IIb/IIIa inhibitor, but **use of bivalirudin alone causes less bleeding than the combination of heparin and a GP IIb/IIIa inhibitor in patients with NSTEMI undergoing catheterization and/or PCI**.

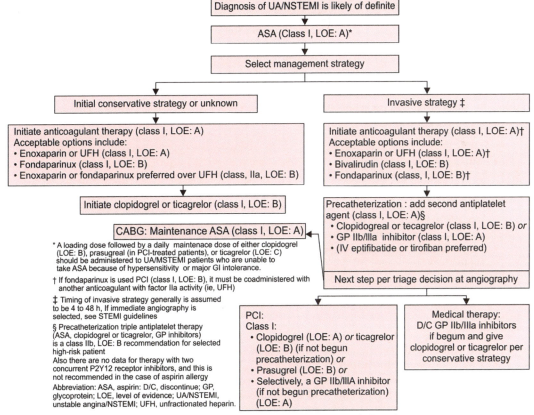

Fig. 39: Initial Management of Unstable Angina/NSTEMI

Class I Recommendations for use of an Early Invasive Strategy (PCI-Percutaneous Intervention)	
• Recurrent angina at rest/low-level activity despite treatment[Q] • Elevated TnT or TnI[Q] • New ST-segment depression[Q] • Recurrent angina/ischemia with CHF symptoms, rales, MR[Q]	• Positive stress test[Q] • EF < 0.40[Q] • Decreased BP[Q] • Sustained VT[Q] • PCI < 6 months, prior CABG[Q] • High-risk score

111. **Ans. c. The guy is performing it in the wrong way**   *(Ref: Ganong 25/e p229)*

This guy is performing the deep tendon reflex in the wrong way. The mistakes in the technique: (1) The feet of the patient should not be touching the bed; (2) The quadriceps muscle in the thigh should be exposed.

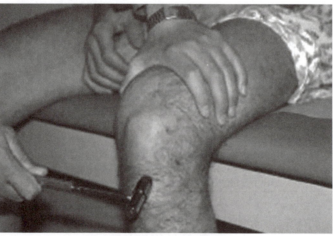

Fig. 40: Knee Jerk Reflex

Knee Jerk Reflex
• **Patellar reflex** or **knee jerk** is a **stretch reflex** which tests the **L2, L3 & L4 segments** of spinal cord[Q]. • Patellar reflex is a **clinical & classical example of monosynaptic reflex arc**[Q]. • **Tapping the patellar tendon elicits** the **knee jerk**, a **stretch reflex of quadriceps femoris** muscle, because the **tap on the tendon stretches the muscle**[Q].

Reflex Arc
• Striking the **patellar ligament with a reflex hammer just below patella stretches the muscle spindle** in quadriceps muscle[Q]. • This produces a signal, which **travels back to spinal cord & synapses** (without interneurons) **at the level of L4 in spinal cord**, completely independent of higher centers[Q]. • From centres there, an **alpha motor neuron conducts an efferent impulse back to quadriceps femoris muscle, triggering contraction**[Q]. • This **contraction, coordinated with relaxation of antagonistic flexor hamstring muscle** causes the **leg to kick**[Q]. • This reflex is a **reflex of proprioception** which **helps maintain posture & balance**[Q].

• **Reflexes may be enhanced** by asking the patient to voluntarily contract other, distant muscle groups (**Jendrassik maneuver**).

> • **After the tap of a hammer, leg is normally extended once** and comes to rest. **Absence or decrease of this reflex is problematic,** and known as **Westphal's sign**.
> • This reflex may be **diminished or absent in lower motor neuron lesions** & during sleep.
> • **Absence of the knee jerk** can signify an **abnormality anywhere within the reflex arc**, including **muscle spindle, Ia afferent nerve fibers,** or **motor neurons to quadriceps muscle**.
> • **MC cause** is a **peripheral neuropathy** from such things as **diabetes, alcoholism & toxins**.

Contd...

Contd...

Knee Jerk Reflex
• Multiple oscillation of leg (**pendular reflex**) following the tap may be a sign of **cerebellar diseases**. • **Exaggerated (brisk) deep tendon reflexes** can be found in **upper motor neuron lesions, hyperthyroidism, anxiety or nervousness**[Q].
Procedure: • **Patient** should be **relaxed** & muscle **positioned midway between full contraction & extension**. • Most easily done with the **patient seated, feet dangling over the edge of exam table**. If they cannot maintain this position, have them lie supine (i.e. on their backs). • **Strike the patellar tendon directly** with reflex hammer[Q]. • **For supine patient, support the back of thigh with your hands such that the knee is flexed and the quadriceps muscles relaxed. Then strike the tendon as described above**[Q]. • **Make sure that the quadriceps is exposed so that you can see muscle contraction.** In the normal reflex, the lower leg will extend at the knee.

112. Ans. a. Pulsus bisferiens   *(Ref: Harrison 19/e p1531, 1536, 18/e p1939)*

Pulsus bisferiens is seen in a patient of aortic stenosis (AS) along with aortic regurgitation (AR) and is rare in isolated AS. The cardiac apex is usually displaced to left because of left ventricular hypertrophy.

"In some patients with AR or with combined AS and AR, the carotid arterial pulse may be bisferiens, i.e., with two systolic waves separated by a trough."- Harrison 19/e p1536

"Aortic Stenosis: The rhythm is generally regular until late in the course; at other times, AF should suggest the possibility of associated mitral valve disease. The systemic arterial pressure is usually within normal limits. In the late stages, however, when stroke volume declines, the systolic pressure may fall and the pulse pressure narrow. The carotid arterial pulse rises slowly to a delayed peak (pulsus parvus et tardus). A thrill or anacrotic "shudder" may be palpable over the carotid arteries, more commonly the left. In the elderly, the stiffening of the arterial wall may mask this important physical sign. In many patients, the a wave in the jugular venous pulse is accentuated. This results from the diminished distensibility of the RV cavity caused by the bulging, hypertrophied interventricular septum."- Harrison 19/e p1531

Types of Pulses	
Pulsus alternans	• **Alternate large & small volume pulse with normal rhythm**[Q] • Difference of **10-40 mm Hg in systolic pressure between beats**[Q] • Due to alternate left ventricular contractile force, i.e., ventricles beats strongly, then weakly, alternating with each other. • Seen in **LV failure, cardiac arrhythmia**[Q]
Pulsus begeminus	• **A pulse wave with normal beat followed by premature beat & compensatory pause, thereby producing irregular rhythm**[Q] • Caused by **coupled ectopic beats (an ectopic beat following each regular beat)**[Q] • Seen in **digitalis toxicity**[Q]
Anacrotic pulse **(Pulsus tardus)**	• **Low amplitude pulse with slow rise & slow fall**[Q] • **Duration of pulse is prolonged**[Q] • Seen in **aortic stenosis**[Q]
Dicrotic pulse **(Pulsus dicrotius)**	• Has **two palpable waves with one peak in systole, one in diastole**[Q] • It is due to a **very low stroke volume with decreased peripheral resistance**[Q] • Seen in **LVF, dilated cardiomyopathy, cardiac tamponade**[Q]
Collapsing or water hammer pulse or Corrigan pulse	• **Large volume pulse with rapid upstroke & rapid downstroke**[Q] • **Rapid upstroke is because of increased stroke volume**[Q] • Rapid downstroke is due to decrease in peripheral resistance & diastolic leak back into left ventricles • **Best felt in radial artery with patient's arm elevated**[Q] • Seen in **aortic regurgitation, patent ductus arteriosus, Hyperdynamic states (anemia, thyrotoxicosis, AV fistula)**[Q]

Contd...

Contd...

Types of Pulses	
Pulsus bisferiens	• **Single pulse wave with two peaks in systole**[Q] • **Due to ejection of rapid jet blood through aortic valve**[Q] • **Best felt in brachial artery & femoral artery**[Q] • Seen in **AR + AS, severe AR, hypertrophic obstructive cardiomyopathy**[Q]
Pulsus parvus	• **Small volume pulse like anacrotic pulse but anacrotic wave is not felt**[Q] • It occurs as a **result of a reduction in left ventricular stroke volume or decrease in systemic arterial pressure**[Q] • Seen in **severe hypotension (shock), severe AS, severe PS**[Q]
Pulsus paradoxus	• **Exaggerated decrease in strength of arterial pulse during inspiration**[Q] • **Radial pulse gets smaller in volume with inspiration & larger in volume with expiration**[Q] • Seen in **cardiac tamponade, SVC obstruction, COPD, acute severe asthma, constrictive pericarditis, pulmonary embolism, hypovolemic shock**[Q]

113. **Ans. b. Dengue virus**   *(Ref: Harrison 19/e p1322)*

Tourniquet test is used in daily follow up of patients with dengue virus

"The tourniquet test (capillary-fragility test) is part of the new WHO case definition for dengue. The test is a marker of capillary fragility and it can be used as a triage tool to differentiate patients with acute gastroenteritis, for example, from those with dengue. It is a clinical diagnostic method to determine a patient's hemorrhagic tendency, fragility of capillary walls and thrombocytopenia."

"Severe dengue is identified by the detection of bleeding tendencies (tourniquet test, petechiae) or overt bleeding in the absence of underlying causes, such as preexisting gastrointestinal lesions. Shock may result from increased vascular permeability. In milder cases of severe dengue, restlessness, lethargy, thrombocytopenia (<100,000/μL), and hemoconcentration are detected 2–5 days after the onset of typical dengue, usually at the time of defervescence. The maculopapular rash that often develops in dengue may also appear in severe dengue. In more severe cases, frank shock is apparent, with low pulse pressure, cyanosis, hepatomegaly, pleural effusions, and ascites; in some patients, severe ecchymoses and gastrointestinal bleeding develop. The period of shock lasts only 1 or 2 days."
- Harrison 19/e p1322

Zika Virus Outbreak
Microbiology: • Zika virus belongs to **family Flaviviridae & genus Flavivirus; Single stranded RNA virus**[Q]
History: • It is named after the **Zika Forest, Uganda** in 1947.   • **Reservoir: Monkeys**[Q]
Transmission: • **Mosquito borne: Mainly spread by the Aedes aegypti**[Q]   • **Mother-to-child transmission through placenta** (common in first trimester),   • **Sexual transmission** is also possible
Current Outbreak: • **Zika virus current outbreak began in April 2015 in Brazil.**   • Subsequently it spread to other countries in South America, Central America, and the Caribbean.   • Imported cases have also been reported from Europe and the United States and Australia.   • In February 2016, WHO declared Zika virus outbreak a public health emergency of international concern.
Situation in India: • **No cases have been reported so far**, but there is evidence of sero-prevalence (i.e. Indian patients have in the past tested positive for Zika virus antibodies).   • As the vector is prevalent, so India may be affected in near future.

Zika Virus Outbreak
Clinical Manifestations:
• **Majority** patients are **asymptomatic**[Q]
• **Zika fever: Minor illness such as fever and a rash**[Q].
• **Congenital transmission** leads to **newborn microcephaly**[Q]
• In very few cases, **Guillain-Barre syndrome** has been reported.
Laboratory Diagnosis:
• **IgM ELISA** is available. But it cross reacts with Dengue antibodies
• **Plaque-reduction neutralization test** may be more specific.
• **RT-PCR** is done in acutely ill patients
Treatment and Vaccine:
• **No effective treatment & vaccine is available so far**.
• **Only symptomatic treatment available** such as fluid replacement & analgesic (acetaminophen).

114. **Ans. d. Hematocrit**   *(Ref: Harrison 19/e p1319, 1322)*

In a patient with dengue hemorrhagic fever (DHF), hematocrit is most important parameter to monitor. Diagnosis of DHF needs the presence of rise in hematocrit of 20% or more i.e. Hemoconcentration. Despite the name, the critical feature that distinguishes DHF from dengue fever is not hemorrhaging, but rather plasma leakage resulting from increased vascular permeability

Expanded WHO definition of Dengue hemorrhagic fever	
• **Fever** lasting from **2-7 days**[Q] • Evidence of **hemorrhagic manifestation** or a **positive tourniquet test**[Q] • **Thrombocytopenia (≤100,000 cells/mm³)**[Q]	• Evidence of **plasma leakage** shown by **hemoconcentration** (an **increase in hematocrit ≥20%** above average for age or **a decrease in hematocrit ≥20% of baseline following fluid replacement therapy**), or **pleural effusion**, or **ascites** or **hypoproteinemia**[Q].

115. **Ans. c. Both early and late inspiratory crackles**   *(Ref: Harrison 19/e p1661-1665, 18/e p2143)*

Post-tuberculous bronchiectasis will usually affect one lung only and produce coarse crackles, which are usually biphasic. Late inspiratory fine crackles are usually heard in COPD or pneumonia. Bibasilar crepitations are typical of fluid overload (due to pulmonary edema). Tubular breathing is heard when there is a consolidation.

"Biphasic crackles occur in both inspiration and expiration. They are combination of coarse and fine crackles. Biphasic crackles are feature of bronchiectasis and are related to a combination of secretions and increased compliance of the walls in larger airways."

"Biphasic crackles occur in both inspiration and expiration. They are combination of coarse and fine crackles. Biphasic crackles are feature of bronchiectasis and are related to a combination of secretions and increased compliance of the walls in larger airways."

Crackles	
• **Crackles** are **brief, discontinuous, popping lung sounds**	
• Classified on the basis of **quality of sound (coarse & fine)** or **phase of respiratory cycle**.	

Fine crackles	Coarse crackles
• Heard during **mid to late inspiration**[Q]	• It occurs in **both phases of respiration**[Q]
• Usually starts in **basal part of lungs**[Q]	• No predilection for any particular area of lung[Q]
• It is **altered by body position change**, but remains **unaltered by coughing**[Q]	• It is **altered by coughing**, but **not by body position** changes[Q]
• It is **not transmitted to mouth**[Q]	• It can be **transmitted to mouth**[Q]
• It is **produced by sudden inspiratory opening of small airways** which were held closed during the previous expiration[Q]	• It is **produced by gas passing through airways which undergo intermittent opening & closing**[Q]

Contd...

Crackles	
Crackles	
Early inspiratory crackles	**Small airway disease (bronchiolitis[Q])**
• Mid-inspiratory crackles	• Pulmonary edema[Q]
• Late inspiratory crackles	• Pulmonary fibrosis (fine)[Q]
	• Pulmonary edema[Q]
	• Bronchial secretions in **COPD**[Q]
	• Pneumonia, lung abscess[Q]
	• Tubercular lung cavities (coarse)[Q]
• **Crackles** throughout **inspiration & expiration**	• **Bronchiectasis (coarse)**[Q]

116. **Ans. d. Albumin** *(Ref: Harrison 19/e p1715-1716)*

The most important diagnostic tests in pleural fluid specimen in a patient with suspected TB are GeneXpert (PCR) and ADA levels. Total protein levels and LDH levels are required to differentiate between transudative and exudative effusion according to Light's Criteria. So doing a pleural fluid albumin level separately will not be very useful. Total protein estimation should be done instead.

Independent Diagnostic Markers for TB Pleuritis
• **Pleural fluid protein > 50 gm/l**[Q]
• **Adenosine deaminase of > 10 U/l**[Q]

Light's Criteria (Satisfying any **one criterion** means it is **exudative**)
• **Pleural total protein/ Serum total protein > 0.5**[Q]
• **Pleural LDH/ Serum LDH > 0.6**[Q]
• **Pleural LDH > 2/3rd of upper limit of normal for serum LDH**[Q]

Pleural Fluid Analysis in TB
• **Protein > 5.0 gm/ dL**[Q]; **Lymphocytes >50%**[Q]; **Mesothelial cells < 3%**[Q]
• HIV infected patients with tuberculosis pleuritis may have **significant number of mesothelial cells** in pleural fluids[Q].
• **Eosinophil >10% excludes the diagnosis of tuberculosis pleuritis**[Q].

Adenosine Deaminase (ADA)
• **ADA:** Enzyme that **catalyzes the conversion of adenosine to inosine**[Q].
• **ADA-1: All cells; ADA-2: Only in monocytes**[Q]
• **Majority of ADA in tuberculosis pleural fluid is ADA-2**[Q]
• **Higher the pleural fluid ADA level, the more likely patient is to have tuberculosis**[Q].
• **High ADA** may be seen in: **Empyema, rheumatoid arthritis (do not have pleural fluid lymphocytosis)**[Q]   • **ADA levels >40-60 U/L** in setting of a **lymphocytic effusion are specific for TB** (Cut off value of ADA <40)[Q]

Polymerase Chain Reaction
• **PCR is certainly not superior to either the pleural fluid ADA or interferon gamma levels**[Q]
• **Sensitivity- 80%, Specificity is not 100%**
• **False positive:** DNA contamination, non-viable organism, latent infection, reactivation due to immunosuppression caused by **primary malignant involvement of pleura.**
• **Xpert MTB/RIF detects DNA sequences specific for** *Mycobacterium tuberculosis* & **rifampicin resistance by PCR**. It is **based on nucleic acid amplification tests (NAAT)**[Q].   • **Xpert® MTB/RIF purifies & concentrates** *Mycobacterium tuberculosis* **bacilliform sputum samples, isolates genomic material from captured bacteria** by sonication & subsequently **amplifies genomic DNA by PCR**[Q].

AIIMS May 2016

117. Ans. b. Sustained BP >185/110 mm Hg despite treatment   *(Ref: Harrison 19/e p759, 1605, 18/e p3273)*

A sustained BP >185/110 mm Hg despite treatment is a contraindication for thrombolytic therapy as it may lead to hemorrhage.

Administration of IV Recombinant Tissue Plasminogen Activator (rtPA) for Acute Ischemic Stroke	
Indication	**Contraindication**
• Clinical diagnosis of stroke[Q] • Onset of symptoms to time of drug administration <3 hours[Q] • CT scan showing no hemorrhage or edema of >1/3 of the MCA territory[Q] • Age ≥ 18 years [Q]	• Sustained BP >185/110 mm Hg despite treatment[Q] • Platelets <100,000; HCT <25%; glucose <50 or >400 mg/dL[Q] • Use of heparin within 48 hours & prolonged PTT, or elevated INR[Q]
Indication	**Contraindication**
• Consent by patient or surrogate	• Rapidly improving symptoms[Q] • Prior stroke or head injury within 3 months[Q] • Prior intracranial hemorrhage[Q] • Major surgery in preceding 14 days[Q] • Minor stroke symptoms[Q] • Gastrointestinal bleeding in preceding 21 days[Q] • Recent myocardial infarction[Q] • Coma or stupor[Q]

Administration of IV Recombinant Tissue Plasminogen Activator (rtPA)
• **IV access with two peripheral IV lines**[Q] (avoid arterial or central line placement) • Review eligibility for rtPA • **Administer 0.9 mg/kg IV** (maximum 90 mg) IV as 10% of total dose by bolus, followed by remainder of total dose over 1 h • **Frequent cuff blood pressure monitoring**[Q] • **No other antithrombotic treatment for 24 hours**[Q] • **For decline in neurologic status or uncontrolled blood pressure, stop infusion, give cryoprecipitate, and reimage brain emergently**[Q] • **Avoid urethral catheterization for >2 hours** [Q]

118. Ans. b. Intravenous tissue plasminogen activator   *(Ref: Harrison 19/e p1634-1636, 18/2170-2177)*

In the given question, patient is a female with underlying hypercoagulable state (history of nephrotic syndrome) and prolonged air travel presenting with hypotension (BP of 90/60 mm Hg) and ventricular dysfunction (dilation of right ventricle with bulging of the interventricular septum to the left) is most probably suffering from massive pulmonary embolism.

"Anticoagulation is the foundation for successful treatment of DVT and PE. Immediately effective anticoagulation is initiated with a parenteral drug: unfractionated heparin (UFH), low-molecular-weight heparin (LMWH), or fondaparinux. One should use a direct thrombin inhibitors (argatroban, lepirudin, or bivalirudin) in patients with proven or suspected heparin-induced thrombocytopenia. Parenteral agents are continued as a transition or "bridge" to stable, long-term anticoagulation with a vitamin K antagonist (exclusively warfarin in the United States). Warfarin requires 5-7 days to achieve a therapeutic effect. During that period, one should overlap the parenteral and oral agents."
- Harrison 19/e p1635

"Successful fibrinolytic therapy rapidly reverses right heart failure and may result in a lower rate of death and recurrent PE by (1) dissolving much of the anatomically obstructing pulmonary arterial thrombus, (2) preventing the continued release of serotonin and other neurohumoral factors that exacerbate pulmonary hypertension, and (3) lysing much of the source of the thrombus in the pelvic or deep leg veins, thereby decreasing the likelihood of recurrent PE. The preferred fibrinolytic regimen is 100 mg of recombinant tissue plasminogen activator (tPA) administered as a continuous peripheral

Contd...

Contd...

*intravenous infusion over 2 hours. Patients appear to respond to fibrinolysis for up to 14 days after the PE has occurred. Contraindications to fibrinolysis include **intracranial disease, recent surgery**, and **trauma**. The only FDA-approved indication for PE fibrinolysis is massive PE."* -Harrison 19/e p1636

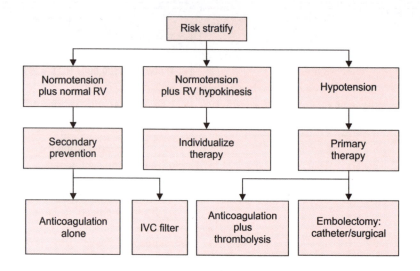

Management of Massive Pulmonary Embolism

- For patients with **massive PE & hypotension**, replete volume with 500 mL of normal saline[Q].
- **Additional fluid should be infused with extreme caution**[Q] because excessive fluid administration exacerbates RV wall stress, causes more profound RV ischemia & worsens LV compliance and filling by causing further interventricular septal shift toward the LV.
- **Dopamine & dobutamine** are first-line inotropic agents for treatment of PE-related shock[Q].

Fibrinolysis in Massive Pulmonary Embolism

- Only FDA approved indication for PE fibrinolysis is massive PE[Q].
- Successful fibrinolytic therapy rapidly reverses right heart failure & may **result in a lower rate of death and recurrent PE** by:
  - **Dissolving** much of **anatomically obstructing pulmonary arterial thrombus**[Q]
  - **Preventing continued release of serotonin** & other neurohumoral factors that exacerbate pulmonary hypertension[Q]
  - Lysing much of the **source of thrombus in pelvic or deep leg veins**, decreasing the likelihood of recurrent PE[Q].
- **Preferred fibrinolytic regimen:** Recombinant tissue plasminogen activator (tPA)[Q]
- **Contraindications:** Intracranial disease, recent surgery & trauma[Q].

Pulmonary Embolism

- Risk factors for pulmonary embolism are the **risk factors for thrombi formation** within **venous circulation**.
- **Calf venous thrombosis:** Low risk for embolism[Q]
- **Thrombosis of larger veins:** High risk for embolism[Q] (due to **loosely attached thrombus** to venous wall)
  - **MC site for DVT: Calf veins**[Q]
  - **MC source for pulmonary emboli: Proximal vein of lower extremity**[Q] (femoro-popliteal & iliac vein)

Contd...

AIIMS May 2016

Contd...

Risk Factors for Pulmonary Thromboembolism		
• Age (Increasing age)^Q • Obesity^Q • Immobility (bed rest >4 days)^Q • Pregnancy^Q & Puerperium^Q • High dose estrogen therapy^Q • Nephrotic syndrome^Q	• Surgery/trauma (especially of pelvis, hip or lower limb)^Q • Malignancy (especially pelvis, abdominal, metastatic) • Heart failure / Recent MI^Q • Inflammatory bowel disease^Q • Polycythemia^Q	• PNH^Q or Lupus anticoagulant • Behcet's syndrome^Q • Homocystinuria^Q • Paralysis of lower limb • Varicose veins, Infection

Clinical features:
- **Symptoms: Dyspnea (MC)^Q, chest pain, hemoptysis & cough**
- **Signs: Tachypnea (MC)^Q, fever, unilateral leg swelling, wheeze, pleural friction rub**

  - Any patient with **high likelihood** of pulmonary embolism on clinical evaluation **straightaway undergoes imaging tests**, while a patient with **low clinical likelihood** should **first undergo D-dimer test^Q**.

Factors for Clinical Assessment of Pulmonary Embolism	
• Clinical **signs** & symptoms of DVT^Q • An alternative diagnosis is less likely than pulmonary embolism • **Heart rate >100/min^Q** • **Hemoptysis^Q**	• **Immobilization** or **previous surgery in 4 weeks^Q** • **Previous DVT/PE^Q** • **Malignancy^Q** (on treatment, treatment in past 6 months)

ECG Changes in Pulmonary Embolism	
(Sinus tachycardia: MC & non-specific finding on ECG^Q)	
Features of Acute Right Heart Strain	**Highly predictive of PE**
• Acute **right axis deviation^Q** • **P pulmonale^Q** • **Right bundle branch block^Q** • **Inverted T waves^Q** • ST segment change	• $S_1Q_3T_3{}^Q$: Seen in **<12%** patients • **S** wave in lead **I** • **Q** wave in lead **III** • Inverted **T** wave in lead **III** • S wave in lead I, II, and III ($S_1S_2S_3$)

Diagnosis:
- **D-dimer: Excellent screening test for the diagnosis of PE^Q.**
- **Best investigation in clinical suspicion of PE: Multidetector CT^Q**
- **Lung scanning** is now a **2nd line** diagnostic test for PE.
- **Pulmonary angiography: Gold standard** for **diagnosis of PE^Q** (but expensive & cumbersome)

Treatment:
- **Anticoagulation is foundation for successful treatment of DVT & PE^Q.**
- **Immediately effective anticoagulation is initiated with a parenteral drug, unfractionated heparin (UFH)^Q.**
- **Only FDA-approved indication for PE fibrinolysis is massive PE^Q.**
- **Pulmonary embolectomy:** Risk of intracranial hemorrhage with fibrinolysis has prompted a renaissance of surgical embolectomy.

119. Ans. c. The cuff should be slowly deflated until the first Korotkoff sound is heard only during expiration *(Ref: Harrison 19/e p1621, 1446 18/e p1825; Ganong 25/e p517)*

The cuff is slowly deflated and the paradoxical pulse is recorded from the point when first Korotkoff sound is heard only during expiration to when it is heard in both expiration and inspiration. Pulsus paradoxus is quantified using a blood pressure cuff and stethoscope (Korotkoff sounds), by measuring the variation of the systolic pressure during expiration and inspiration. Inflate cuff until no sounds (as is normally done when taking a BP) slowly decrease cuff pressure until systolic sounds are first heard during expiration but not during inspiration, (note this reading), slowly continue decreasing the cuff pressure until sounds are heard throughout the respiratory cycle, (inspiration and expiration) (note this second reading). If the pressure difference between the two readings is >10mm Hg, it can be classified as pulsus paradoxus.

"Before the blood pressure measurement is taken, the individual should be seated quietly in a chair (not the exam table) with feet on the floor for 5 min in a private, quiet setting with a comfortable room temperature. At least two measurements should be made. The center of the cuff should be at heart level, and the width of the bladder cuff should equal at least 40% of the arm circumference; the length of the cuff bladder should encircle at least 80% of the arm circumference. It is important to pay attention to cuff placement, stethoscope placement, and the rate of deflation of the cuff (2 mmHg/s). Systolic blood pressure is the first of at least two regular "tapping" Korotkoff sounds, and diastolic blood pressure is the point at which the last regular Korotkoff sound is heard. In current practice, a diagnosis of hypertension generally is based on seated, office measurements."- Harrison 19/e p1621

"Pulsus paradoxus is measured by noting the difference between the systolic pressure at which the Korotkoff sounds are first heard (during expiration) and the systolic pressure at which the Korotkoff sounds are heard with each heartbeat, independent of the respiratory phase. Between these two pressures, the Korotkoff sounds are heard only intermittently and during expiration. The cuff pressure must be decreased slowly to appreciate the finding. It can be difficult to measure pulsus paradoxus in patients with tachycardia, atrial fibrillation, or tachypnea. A pulsus paradoxus may be palpable at the brachial artery or femoral artery level when the pressure difference exceeds 15 mmHg. This inspiratory fall in systolic pressure is an exaggerated consequence of interventricular dependence."- Harrison 19/e p1446

Blood pressure

- Blood pressure is measured by auscultatory method using sphygmomanometer tends to be higher than true intra-arterial pressure measured by arterial cannulation, because some cuff pressure gets dissipated between the cuff & artery[Q], in the soft tissue.
- Systolic pressure is best indicated by 1st korotkoff's sound & diastolic pressure in adults by 5th korotkoff's sound[Q]. Where as diastolic pressure in children, in adults after exercise, hyperthyroidism & aortic insufficiency best correlates with 4th Korotkoff's sound.

- Using relatively small cuff, obesity & persons with thick calcified & sclerotic vessels that are difficult to compress (e.g. in elderly, atherosclerosis, diabetics and Monkenberg's arteriosclerosis)[Q] are the reasons of **spuriously high blood pressure (Pseudohypertension).**

Blood pressure

Technique	Korotkoff's sound	Source of error
• Person should be comfortably seated, with back & arm supported, legs uncrossed & **upper arm at the level of right atrium**[Q]. • **Snugly wrapped cuff** should allow only one finger to be slipped between it & skin. • **The cuff is rapidly inflated to 30 mm Hg above** the point at which radial pulse disappears. **Deflation rate should be 2-3 mm/ second**[Q]. • **Two readings should be at least 1 minute apart**[Q].	• Are produced by turbulent flow in artery. The sound gradually become louder, then dull & muffled. **1.** Faint, clear, tapping sounds It indicates **systolic BP**[Q] **2.** Murmur / swishing sounds **3.** More intense, crisper sounds **4.** Distinct abrupt muffle f sounds Indicates diastolic BP in children, in adults after exercise, hyperthyroidism, & aortic insufficiency. **5.** No sound **Best correlates with diastolic BP in normal adults**[Q]. • It tends to give values for **systolic pressure that are lower than true intra arterial pressure & diastolic values that are higher**[Q].	• **False High values** are found in: • Thick overlying soft tissue causing more dissipation of pressure e.g. obese • **Hard sclerotic vessels with low compressibility** such as • Elderly • Atherosclerosis • Diabetics • **Mokenberg's arteriosclerosis**[Q] • **Relatively small size of cuff (bladder)** e.g. standard arm cuff used in thigh • Too slow inflation rate leading to too high diastolic pressure • **False low** values are found in: • **Large (wide) cuff** e.g. standard arm cuff used in forearm. • **Too fast Deflation rate** leads to too low systolic pressure.

AIIMS May 2016

Blood pressure
Appropriate Cuff size

• Ratio of width of compression cavity of cuff (bladder) to circumference of extremity is of critical importance.
• **According to American Heart Association:**
  – Bladder **width should be 40% of circumference or 1.2 times of diameter of extremity**[Q]
  – Bladder **length** should be **80% of arm circumference**[Q]
  – **Length to width ratio is 2:1**[Q]
• If the person's limb measurement is on the borderline of two different cuff sizes, chance of error is decreased if the larger of two cuff sizes is used.
• So in obese & recording BP in thigh wider cuff size provide more accurate results.

120. **Ans. d. Fulminant hepatitis due to hepatitis E infection**   *(Ref: Harrison 19/e p2018, 18/e p2546)*

In the question, anti-HBc IgG is reactive but HbsAg is negative, the case is a recovered case from hepatitis B. Hepatitis A is rarely chronic, can be ruled out from the given options. Anti-HAV IgG suggests recovered case from HAV infections. Anti-HEV IgM is an indicator of acute hepatitis E infection. History of pregnancy and high serum bilirubin with raised AST and ALT is suggestive of fulminant hepatitis E.

"The most feared complication of viral hepatitis is fulminant hepatitis (massive hepatic necrosis); fortunately, this is a rare event. Fulminant hepatitis is seen primarily in hepatitis B, D, and E, but rare fulminant cases of hepatitis A occur primarily in older adults and in persons with underlying chronic liver disease, including, according to some reports, chronic hepatitis B and C. Hepatitis B accounts for >50% of fulminant cases of viral hepatitis, a sizable proportion of which are associated with HDV infection and another proportion with underlying chronic hepatitis C. Fulminant hepatitis is hardly ever seen in hepatitis C, but hepatitis E, as noted above, can be complicated by fatal fulminant hepatitis in 1–2% of all cases and in up to 20% of cases in pregnant women. Patients usually present with signs and symptoms of encephalopathy that may evolve to deep coma. The liver is usually small and the PT excessively prolonged. The combination of rapidly shrinking liver size, rapidly rising bilirubin level, and marked prolongation of the PT, even as aminotransferase levels fall, together with clinical signs of confusion, disorientation, somnolence, ascites, and edema, indicates that the patient has hepatic failure with encephalopathy. Cerebral edema is common; brainstem compression, gastrointestinal bleeding, sepsis, respiratory failure, cardiovascular collapse, and renal failure are terminal events. The mortality rate is exceedingly high (>80% in patients with deep coma), but patients who survive may have a complete biochemical and histologic recovery. If a donor liver can be located in time, liver transplantation may be life-saving in patients with fulminant hepatitis."- Harrison 19/e p2018

Commonly Encountered Serologic Patterns of Hepatitis B Infection					
HBsAg	Anti-HBs	Anti-HBc	HBeAg	Anti-HBe	Interpretation
+	–	IgM	+	–	• Acute hepatitis B, high infectivity
+	–	IgG	+	–	• **Chronic hepatitis B, high infectivity**[Q]
+	–	IgG	–	+	• **Late acute** or **chronic hepatitis B, low infectivity**[Q] • **HBeAg-negative** ('precore–mutant') hepatitis B (chronic or rarely acute)
+	+	+	+/–	+/–	• HBsAg of one subtype and heterotypic anti-HBs (common) • Process of seroconversion from HBsAg to anti-HBs (rare)
–	–	IgM	+/–	+/–	• **Acute hepatitis B**[Q] • **Anti–HBc 'window'**[Q]
–	–	IgG	–	+/–	• **Low-level hepatitis B carrier**[Q] • **Hepatitis B in remote past**[Q]
–	+	IgG	–	+/–	• **Recovery from hepatitis B**[Q]
–	+	–	–	–	• **Immunization with HBsAg** (after vaccination) • **Hepatitis B in the remote past** (?) • False-positive

121. Ans. c. Intravenous fluids *(Ref: Harrison 19/e p314; 18/e p361)*

Initial therapy of significant hypercalcemia begins with volume expansion because hypercalcemia invariably leads to dehydration; 4–6 L of intravenous saline may be required over the first 24 h, keeping in mind that underlying comorbidities (e.g., congestive heart failure) may require the use of loop diuretics to enhance sodium and calcium excretion.

*"Mild, asymptomatic hypercalcemia does not require immediate therapy, and management should be dictated by the underlying diagnosis. By contrast, **significant, symptomatic hypercalcemia usually requires therapeutic intervention independent of the etiology of hypercalcemia**. Initial therapy of significant hypercalcemia begins with volume expansion because hypercalcemia invariably leads to dehydration; 4–6 L of intravenous saline may be required over the first 24 h, keeping in mind that underlying comorbidities (e.g., congestive heart failure) may require the use of loop diuretics to enhance sodium and calcium excretion. However, loop diuretics should not be initiated until the volume status has been restored to normal. If there is increased calcium mobilization from bone (as in malignancy or severe hyperparathyroidism), drugs that inhibit bone resorption should be considered."*- Harrison 19/e p314

"Zoledronic acid, pamidronate, and ibandronate are bisphosphonates that are commonly used for the treatment of hypercalcemia of malignancy in adults. Onset of action is within 1–3 days, with normalization of serum calcium levels occurring in 60–90% of patients."- Harrison 19/e p314

Hypercalcemia
• **Calcium ion** plays a **critical role in normal cellular function & signaling, regulating neuromuscular signaling, cardiac contractility, hormone secretion & blood coagulation**[Q].
• Hypercalcemia is relatively common & serves as a harbinger of underlying disease.

Causes of Hypercalcemia	
Excessive PTH production	• **Primary hyperparathyroidism**[Q] (adenoma, hyperplasia, rarely carcinoma)
	• **Tertiary hyperparathyroidism**[Q] (long-term stimulation of PTH secretion in renal insufficiency)
	• **Ectopic PTH secretion**[Q] (very rare)
	• **Inactivating mutations in the CaSR or in G proteins (FHH)**[Q]
	• **Alterations in CaSR function (lithium therapy)**[Q]
Hypercalcemia of malignancy	• **Overproduction of PTH-rP (many solid tumors)**[Q]
	• **Lytic skeletal metastases** (breast, myeloma)[Q]
Excessive 1,25(OH)$_2$D production	• **Granulomatous diseases (sarcoidosis, tuberculosis, silicosis)**[Q]
	• **Lymphomas , Vitamin D intoxication**[Q]
Primary increase in bone resorption	• **Hyperthyroidism**[Q]
	• **Immobilization**[Q]
Excessive calcium intake	• **Milk-alkali syndrome & total parenteral nutrition**[Q]
Other causes	• Endocrine disorders (**adrenal insufficiency, pheochromocytoma, VIPoma**)[Q]
	• Medications (**thiazides, vitamin A, antiestrogens**)[Q]

Clinical Features:

Mild hypercalcemia (up to 11–11.5 mg/dL)	Severe hypercalcemia (>12–13 mg/dL)
• Usually asymptomatic, recognized on routine calcium measurements;	• If develops acutely, result in lethargy, stupor, coma
• Neuropsychiatric symptoms, peptic ulcer disease, nephrolithiasis & increased fracture risk in some patients.	• GI symptoms (nausea, anorexia, constipation, pancreatitis)[Q]
	• Polyuria & polydipsia: Hypercalcemia decreases renal concentrating ability)[Q]
	• Bone pain & pathologic fractures in long-standing hyper-parathyroidism[Q]
	• ECG changes: Bradycardia, AV block & short QT interval[Q]

Treatment:

• **Mild, asymptomatic hypercalcemia does not require immediate therapy** & management should be dictated by underlying diagnosis.

• **Significant, symptomatic hypercalcemia requires therapeutic intervention independent of etiology**[Q].

Hypercalcemia

Management of Significant, Symptomatic Hypercalcemia

- **Initial therapy: Volume expansion** (hypercalcemia leads to dehydration) **with 4–6 L of IV saline** over the first 24 h, keeping in mind that underlying comorbidities (e.g., congestive heart failure) may require **use of loop diuretics to enhance Na$^+$ & Ca^{2+} excretion**[Q].
- **Increased calcium mobilization from bone** (in **malignancy** or **severe hyperparathyroidism**): -
  - **Drugs that inhibit bone resorption should be considered**[Q].
    - **Zoledronic acid, pamidronate & ibandronate** are used for **treatment of hypercalcemia of malignancy in adults**[Q].
    - **Onset of action is within 1–3 days**, with **normalization of serum calcium** levels occurring in **60–90%** of patients.

Management of Significant, Symptomatic Hypercalcemia

- **Gallium nitrate:** Alternative to bisphosphonates, effective but **nephrotoxic**[Q]
- **Dialysis** may be necessary inn rare instances

1,25(OH)$_2$ D-mediated Hypercalcemia

- **Preferred therapy: Glucocorticoids (IV hydrocortisone** or **oral prednisone)**[Q]
- **Glucocorticoids decrease 1,25(OH)$_2$D production**[Q].

122. Ans. a. Ventilation with continuous positive airway pressure *(Ref: Harrison 19/e p1731, 18/e p2200)*

The patient here has decreased and increased paO$_2$ as well as paCO$_2$. Hence the patient is in type 2 respiratory failure, which can be seen in bronchial asthma patients. The best management strategy for these patients is assisted ventilation with CPAP (Non-invasive ventilation) rather than controlled mandatory ventilation.

"The mainstays of therapy for type II respiratory failure are directed at reversing the underlying cause(s) of ventilatory failure. Noninvasive positive-pressure ventilation with a tight-fitting facial or nasal mask, with avoidance of endotracheal intubation, often stabilizes these patients. This approach has been shown to be beneficial in treating patients with exacerbations of chronic obstructive pulmonary disease; it has been tested less extensively in other kinds of respiratory failure but may be attempted nonetheless in the absence of contraindications (hemodynamic instability, inability to protect the airway, respiratory arrest)."- Harrison 19/e p1731

Types of Respiratory Failure			
Type I	Type II	Type III	Type IV

• Defined as a **low level of O$_2$ in blood (hypoxemia) without an increased level of CO$_2$ in blood (hypercapnia)**[Q].
• Basic defect is **failure of oxygenation**[Q] characterized by:
• **Low PaO$_2$ (<60 mm Hg)**[Q]
• **Normal** or **low PaCO$_2$ (<50 mm Hg)**[Q]
• **Increased P$_{A-a}$O$_2$**[Q]
• Caused by:
• **Ventilation/perfusion (V/Q) mismatch**[Q] (pulmonary embolism)
• **Low ambient oxygen**[Q] (at high altitude)
• **Alveolar hypoventilation** (acute neuromuscular disease[Q])
• **Diffusion problem**[Q] (pneumonia or ARDS)
	• Represents a **defect in ventilation**[Q] **(hypoventilation)** & is characterized by decreased **PaO$_2$ with increased PaCO$_2$**[Q]
	• Characterized by:
	• **Low PaO$_2$ (<60 mm Hg)**[Q]
	• **Increased PaCO$_2$ (>49 mm Hg)**[Q]
	• **Normal P$_{A-a}$O$_2$**[Q]
	• Caused by:
	  – **Increased airways resistance: COPD, asthma**[Q]
	  – **Reduced CNS drive/breathing effort: Drug overdose, brain stem lesion,** sleep-disordered breathing & **severe hypothyroidism**[Q]
		• Occurs as a result of **lung atelectasis**[Q].
		• Also called **perioperative respiratory failure**[Q] (atelectasis occurs commonly **in perioperative period)**
		• After general anesthesia, **decrease in functional residual capacity** lead to collapse of dependent lung units[Q].
		• Can be **treated by frequent changes in position, chest physiotherapy,** upright positioning & aggressive control of incisional and/or abdominal pain[Q].
			• Results from **hypoperfusion of respiratory muscles** in patients in **shock**[Q].
			• **Intubation & mechanical ventilation** can allow redistribution of cardiac output away from respiratory muscles & back to vital organs while the shock is treated[Q].

AIIMS ESSENCE

Contd...

Type I	Type II	Type III	Type IV
• **Right to left shunts**[Q] • **Alveolar flooding** (pulmonary edema, pneumonia, or alveolar hemorrhage)[Q]	– **Weakness of respiratory muscles: NM disorders (Guillain-Barré syndrome, amyotrophic lateral sclerosis, M. gravis), myopathy**[Q] – **Rib cage deformity; kypho-scoliosis** [Q] – **Rigid chest: Ankylosing spondylitis**[Q]	• **Noninvasive positive-pressure ventilation** may also be used to **reverse regional atelectasis**[Q].	

123. **Ans. d. Amino levulinic acid levels in urine** *(Ref: Harrison 19/e p2689, 427e-2; Harper 30/e p329)*

High levels of lead can affect heme metabolism by combining with SH groups in enzymes such as ferrochelatase and ALA (delta-amino levulinic acid) dehydratase. Elevated levels of protoporphyrin are found in red blood cells, and elevated levels of ALA and of coproporphyrin are found in urine.

*"High levels of lead can affect heme metabolism by combining with SH groups in enzymes such as **ferrochelatase and ALA (delta-amino levulinic acid) dehydratase**. This affects porphyrin metabolism. **Elevated levels of protoporphyrin are found in red blood cells**, and elevated levels of ALA and of coproporphyrin are found in urine."- Harper 30/e p329*

"The most common presentation of lead poisoning is an encephalopathy; however, symptoms and signs of a primarily motor neuropathy can also occur. The neuropathy is characterized by an insidious and progressive onset of weakness usually beginning in the arms, in particular involving the wrist and finger extensors, resembling a radial neuropathy. Sensation is generally preserved; however, the autonomic nervous system can be affected. Laboratory investigation can reveal a microcytic hypochromic anemia with basophilic stippling of erythrocytes, an elevated serum lead level, and an elevated serum coproporphyrin level. A 24-h urine collection demonstrates elevated levels of lead excretion."- Harrison 19/e p2689, 427e-2

"Lead Poisoning: Abdominal pain, irritability, lethargy, anorexia, anemia, Fanconi's syndrome, pyuria, azotemia in children with blood lead level (BPb) >80 μg/ dL; may also see epiphyseal plate "lead lines" on long bone x-rays."- Harrison 19/e p 427e-2

Lead poisoning
• **Metallic lead & all its salts are poisonous**.
• **Principal toxic salts of Lead: Lead acetate**[Q] (Saturn salt or sugar of lead)**, lead carbonate**[Q] (safeda)**, lead chromate**[Q]**, lead tetra oxide (red lead, vermillion, sindur), lead mono oxide** (litharge)**, lead sulphide (Least toxic)**

    • Fatal dose: Lead acetate: 20 gm; Lead carbonate: 40 gm
    • Fatal period: 1-2 days

Metabolism:
- **Absorbed through ingestion or inhalation**; organic lead (e.g., **tetraethyl lead**) **absorbed dermally**[Q].
- In **blood, 95–99% sequestered in RBCs**—thus, must **measure lead in whole blood**[Q] (not serum).
- **Distributed widely in soft tissue**, with **half-life ~30 days**
- **15%** of dose **sequestered in bone** with half-life of >20 years.
- **Excreted mostly in urine**[Q]

    • **Interferes with mitochondrial oxidative phosphorylation, ATPases, calcium-dependent messengers; enhances oxidation & cell apoptosis**[Q].
    • At cellular level **lead interacts with sulfhydryl groups** and **interferes in action of enzymes essential for heme synthesis,** for **hemoglobin & cytochrome production**. It **causes hemolysis**[Q].

Main source:
- Manufacturing of **auto batteries, lead crystal**; demolition or sanding of lead-painted houses, bridges; stained glass–making, plumbing, soldering; exposure to the combustion of leaded fuels[Q].

Lead poisoning

Signs and symptoms of Lead Poisoning

Acute Poisoning	Chronic Lead Poisoning (Plumbism, saturnism)
• Astringent or metallic taste • Dry throat and thirst • **Abdominal pain**[Q], nausea & vomiting, sometimes diarrhea. • **Peripheral circulatory collapse**[Q] • Headache, lethargy & weakness, insomnia, paresthesia, depression, coma & death[Q]. • **Cerebellar ataxia is common in children in acute lead poisoning**[Q]	• **Facial pallor: Earliest & most consistent sign**[Q] • Weakness • **Punctate basophilic or basophilic stippling**[Q] • **Lead line (Burtonian lines in gums)**[Q] • **Colic (Dry belly ache)**[Q] **& constipation is late symptom**[Q] • **Sterility** in males and females. • **Wrist drop & foot drop**[Q] • **Vasoconstriction** leads to **hypertension & arteriolar degeneration**[Q]. • **Lead encephalopathy**[Q]

Diagnosis:
• **Porphyrinuria** (mainly **due to coproporphyrin III inhibition**[Q])

Blood tests	Urine tests
• **>200 punctate basophilia stippling cells /mm³ is diagnostic**[Q] • **Zinc protoporphyrin & free erythrocyte protoporphyrin > 50mg/100ml**[Q] • **Increased lead & aminolaevulinic acid (>25mg/100ml)**[Q]	• Increased **coproporphyrin (CPU) levels.** In nonexposed person it is **<150µg /liter**[Q] • **Aminolaevulinic acid > 5µg** • Presence of **0.25mg lead /liter is diagnostic**[Q]

X-ray Findings in Lead Poisoning

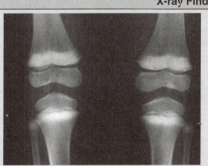

• **Radio-opaque bands /lines at metaphysis of long bones in children**[Q]
• **Radiopaque matter** in GI tract (ingested < 48 hours)
• X-ray in lead poisoning showing dense metaphyseal bands at distal femurs & proximal tibias.

Treatment:
• **Gastric lavage with 1% solution of sodium or magnesium sulphate**[Q]
• **Chelating agent: BAL, DMSA**[Q]

> • Most effective antidote: **Calcium Disodium Versenate**[Q]
> • Intravenous calcium chloride causes deposition of lead in skeleton from blood[Q].

• Peritoneal or hemodialysis.
• Symptomatic treatment

Chronic Lead Poisoning presents with "New-A B C D E F"

New	• **Neuropathy (leading to weakness, wrist drop) & Nephropathy**[Q] **(Late** feature)
A	• **Anemia with punctate basophilia (i.e. basophilic stippling)**[Q] **(Early** feature)
B	• Burtonian or blue stippled lead line on gums[Q]
C	• Colic (abdominal pain) & Constipation[Q]
D	• **Dry belly ache i.e. diarrhea is very rare**[Q] • Dyspepsia, Drop of wrist etc due to **neuropathy**[Q]
E	• **Encephalopathy**[Q], Eosinophilia
F	• **Facial pallor**[Q] (earliest sign)

1142   AIIMS ESSENCE

124. **Ans. a. Before performing the ABG, syringe should be loaded with 0.3 cc of Heparin** *(Ref: Harrison 18/e p364; http://emedicine.medscape.com/article/1902703-overview)*

Care should be taken when measuring blood gases to obtain the arterial blood sample without using excessive heparin. Heparin should be expelled from the syringe after loading as it may lead to false pCO_2 readings.

Arterial Blood for Blood Gas Analysis
• **Blood is most commonly drawn from radial artery**[Q] (easily accessible, can be compressed to control bleeding & less risk for occlusion)
• **Selection of radial artery** to draw is based on the **outcome of an Allen's test**[Q].
• **Brachial artery** (or less often, femoral artery) is also used, especially **during emergency situations** or **with children**[Q].
• **Most syringes come pre-packaged & contain a small amount of heparin, to prevent coagulation**[Q].
• **Other syringes may need to be heparinized, by drawing up a small amount of liquid heparin & squirting it out again to remove air bubbles**[Q].
• **Once the sample is obtained**, care is taken to **eliminate visible gas bubbles**, as **these bubbles can dissolve into the sample & cause inaccurate results**[Q].
• **Patients with poor distal perfusion** (e.g., those in hypovolemic states, with advanced heart failure, or on vasopressor therapy) **may not exhibit a strong arterial pulsation**; the **operator may need to pull back the ABG syringe plunger to get a blood sample**, although this increases the risk of venous blood sampling
• **Puncture of venous structures** can be **identified by lack of pulsatile flow or dark-colored blood**[Q].

Precautions Taken During Taking ABG
• **Incomplete dismissal of heparin solution** from syringe could cause **falsely low values for partial pressure of CO_2**; to avoid this, operator should **expel all heparin solution from syringe** before arterial puncture[Q]
• **Incomplete removal of air bubbles** can cause **falsely elevated values for partial pressure of oxygen**; to avoid this, operator should be sure to **completely remove air bubbles from syringe**[Q]
• **Avoid puncture of brachial artery or femoral artery** in patients with **diminished or absent distal pulse**s; absence of distal pulses may signal **severe peripheral vascular disease**[Q]
• When **femoral or brachial artery puncture** is being considered, use of **ultrasound guidance** during passage of needle aids in providing an accurate roadmap to vessel & helps minimize inadvertent arterial injuries.

125. **Ans. b. Metabolic acidosis** *(Ref: Harrison 19/e p317, 18/e p365)*

In the question, pH is decreased (acidosis) & pCO_2 is decreased (Normal= 40–45 mm Hg). A decreased pCO_2 will try to increase pH, hence it must be secondary compensating mechanism. So, the primary mechanism causing the acid base imbalance must be a decrease in serum bicarbonate concentration i.e. metabolic acidosis.

Acid Base Disorders
pH < 7.35 is acidosis; pH >7.45 is alkalosis
1° change in HCO_3^- is termed as Metabolic (Normal HCO_3^- = 22-30 mEq/l)
• **If change in HCO_3^- is in keeping with the pH** (i.e. if there is acidosis and HCO_3^- is decreased) the problem is **metabolic** one.
• **If change in HCO_3^- is opposite with the pH** (i.e. if there is acidosis and HCO_3^- is increased or normal) the problem is **compensatory metabolic**.
1° change in CO_2 is termed as Respiratory (Normal CO_2 = 35-45 mEq/l)
• **If change in CO_2 is in keeping with the pH** (i.e. if there is acidosis and CO_2 is increased) the problem is **respiratory.**
• **If change in CO_2 is in opposite with the pH** (i.e. if there is acidosis and CO_2 is decreased or normal) the problem is termed as **compensatory respiratory.**

SURGERY

126. **Ans. d. Severe acute pancreatitis** *(Ref: Sabiston 20/e p1528, 19/e p1519-1526; Bailey 27/e p1223-1224, 26/e p1127-1129,; Blumgart 5/e p841-851; Shackelford 7/e p1123-1130)*

The given CT image showing extensive pancreatic necrosis in combination with the acute clinical presentation is typical of severe acute pancreatitis.

Tools for Predicting Severity in Acute Pancreatitis Ready for Clinical Use		
On Admission	**At 24 Hours**	**At 48 Hours**
• **APACHE-II score ≥8**[Q] • **IL-6** • **Urea >60 mmol/L**	• **BISAP score ≥3**[Q] • Polymorphonuclear **elastase** • Urinary **trypsinogen** activation peptide	• **Ranson/Glasgow score ≥3**[Q] • **CRP ≥130**[Q] **mg/mL**

Assessment of severity of Acute Pancreatitis
• **Severe pancreatitis** is diagnosed if ≥ 3[Q] of **Ranson's criteria** are fulfilled (**Main disadvantage: It does not predict the severity of disease at the time of admission because 6 parameters are only assessed after 48 hours of admission.**)   • **APACHE II score** of ≥ 8[Q] defines **severe pancreatitis** (Main advantage: It can be used on admission & repeated at any time)   • **CRP level** ≥ 130 mg/mL[Q] defines **severe pancreatitis**.

BISAP (Bedside Index of Severity in Acute Pancreatitis) Score	
• Incorporates **five clinical & laboratory parameters** obtained **within first 24 h of hospitalization**[Q] • **BISAP score ≥3 indicates severe pancreatitis**[Q]	
BUN[Q]	• **>25** mg/dL (8.9 mmol/L)
Impaired mental status[Q]	• Glasgow coma score **<15**
SIRS[Q]	• ≥2 of 4 present
Age[Q]	• **>60 years**
Pleural effusion[Q]	• On radiography

Ranson's Prognostic Criteria for Non-Gallstone Pancreatitis	
At Admission	**During Initial 48 Hours**
• Age **>55 years**[Q] • WBC **>16,000**[Q] cells/mm • Blood glucose **>200**[Q] mg/dL • Serum LDH **>350**[Q] IU/L • AST **>250**[Q] U/L	• Hematocrit fall **>10**[Q] percentage points • BUN elevation **>5**[Q] mg/ dL • Serum calcium fall to **<8**[Q] mg/ dL • Arterial **PO$_2$ <60**[Q] mm Hg • Base deficit **>4**[Q] mEq/L • Estimated fluid sequestration **>6**[Q] **Litres**

Ranson's Prognostic Criteria for Gallstone Pancreatitis	
At Admission	**During Initial 48 Hours**
• Age **>70** years • WBC **>18,000** cells/mm • Glucose **>220** mg/ dL • Serum LDH **>400** IU/L • AST **>250** U/L	• Hematocrit fall **>10** percentage points • BUN elevation **>2** mg/ dL • Serum calcium fall to **<8** mg/ dL • Base deficit **>5** mEq/L • Arterial PO$_2$ **<60** mm Hg • Estimated fluid sequestration **>4 Litres**

• Patients with **one or two** criteria have a predicted mortality of less than **1%**, with **three** criteria (**10%**) or **four** criteria (**15%**); with more than **seven** criteria **50%.**

Modified Glasgow Criteria	
• This system comprises eight factors. The presence of any **3 or more** within 48 hours of admission defines the patient as having **severe disease.**	
Criteria During initial 48 Hours	
• Age **>55** years • WBC count **>15,000** cell/mm • Blood urea nitrogen **>45** mg/dL • Arterial PO2 **<60** mm Hg	• Blood glucose **>180** mg/dL • Serum LDH **>600** IU/L • Serum calcium **<8** mg/dL • Serum albumin **<3.3** g/dL

Contd...

Contd...

Assessment of severity of Acute Pancreatitis

Acute Physiology And Chronic Health Evaluation (APACHE)-II Scoring System
• **APACHE-II scoring system** incorporates **12[Q]** physiological & laboratory parameters as well as age & comorbid conditions to estimate severity of any disease process. • **Score ≥8** signifies **severe, acute pancreatitis[Q]** • It can be determined on a **daily basis[Q]**.

12 physiologic variables (BT increases HR at CWG SHOP-2)		
• **BP[Q]** (Mean arterial)	• **Creatinine[Q]**	• **Hematocrit[Q]**
• **Temperature[Q]**	• **WBC count[Q]**	• **Oxygenation[Q]**
• **Heart rate[Q]**	• **Glasgow coma scale[Q]**	• Arterial **pH[Q]**
• **Respiratory rate[Q]**	• **Sodium[Q]**	• Serum **potassium[Q]**

Balthazar Grading System for Acute Pancreatitis (CT scan based)	
Grade A	• **Normal** pancreas[Q]
Grade B	• **Focal** or **diffuse** pancreatic **enlargement[Q]**
Grade C	• Intrinsic pancreatic alterations with **peripancreatic fat inflammatory** changes[Q]
Grade D	• **Single fluid collection**/or **phlegmon[Q]**
Grade E	• **Two** or **more** fluid collections or **gas**, in or adjacent to the pancreas[Q]

Computed Tomography Severity Index (CTSI) for Acute Pancreatitis
• **CTSI** (CT severity index scoring system) = Balthazar grade score + necrosis score • **Highest attainable score = 10[Q]**

Pancreatic Inflammation		Pancreatic Necrosis	
Normal pancreas	0	None	0
Focal or **diffuse** pancreatic **enlargement**	1	≤30%	2
Intrinsic pancreatic alterations with **peripancreatic fat inflammatory** changes	2	30%-50%	4
Single fluid collection/or **phlegmon**	3	>50%	6
Two or **more** fluid collections or **gas**, in or adjacent to the pancreas	4		

CTSI score					
0-3		4-6		7-10	
Mortality	Morbidity	Mortality	Morbidity	Mortality	Morbidity
3%	8%	6%	35%	17%	92%

127. Ans. a. IV fluids and antibiotics followed by laparotomy   *(Ref: Sabiston 20/e p1079, 19/e p1100-1102; Bailey 27/e p1051-1052, 26/e p971-974)*

Chest X-ray is showing air under the right dome of diaphragm, which is seen in perforation peritonitis. In cases of perforation peritonitis, laparotomy is the treatment of choice after fluid resuscitation of the patient and IV antibiotics.

Management of Peritonitis
• General care of patient[Q]
• **Correction of fluid & electrolyte imbalance[Q]**
• **Insertion of nasogastric drainage tube & urinary catheter[Q]**
• **Broad-spectrum antibiotic therapy[Q]**
• **Analgesia[Q]**
• **Vital system support** [Q]
• **Operative (laparotomy) treatment** of cause when appropriate[Q]
• **Remove or divert cause[Q]**
• **Peritoneal lavage ± drainage[Q]**

128. **Ans. a. Needle holder, tooth forceps and scissors** *(Ref: Bailey 25/e p234-235)*
Needle holder, tooth forceps and scissors are required for suturing a patient.

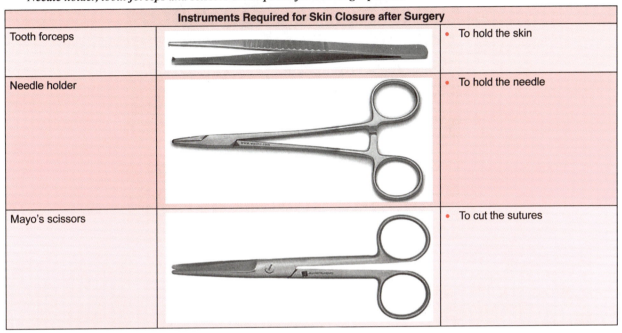

Instruments Required for Skin Closure after Surgery		
Tooth forceps		• To hold the skin
Needle holder		• To hold the needle
Mayo's scissors		• To cut the sutures

129. **Ans. b. Poor prognosis** *(Ref: DeVita's Oncology 10/e p 1243)*

The **IHC profile** depicts a **triple negative breast cancer, as ER, PR and Her-2 are all negative**. Positive staining is seen as brownish dots over the slide. These negative results mean that the growth of the cancer is not supported by the hormones estrogen and progesterone, nor by the presence of too many HER2 receptors. Therefore, **triple-negative breast cancer does not respond to hormonal therapy (such as tamoxifen or aromatase inhibitors) or therapies that target HER2 receptors, such as Herceptin (Trastazumab)**. In general, **survival rates** tend to be **lower with triple-negative breast cancer** compared to other forms of breast cancer:

Immunohistochemistry Interpretation in Breast Cancer			
	ER	PR	Her-2-neu
Positive	ER	ER	
Negative	PR	PR	

ER+/PR+/HER2− ER+/PR+/HER2+ ER−/PR−/HER2+ ER+/PR−/HER2−

	Triple-Negative Breast Cancer (TNBC)
	• **TNBC:** Breast cancer that **does not express** the genes for **ER, PR & Her-2-neu**[Q] • Accounts for **15-25%** of breast cancer cases • More common in **premenopausal women**[Q]
Pathology:	• **Germline mutations of BRCA-1 & BRCA-2** genes are the **causative factor**[Q] • Also known as **basal like (75% of basal-type** breast cancers are **triple negative)**[Q] • Some TNBC **overexpress EGFR & transmembrane glycoprotein NMB (GPNMB)**[Q]

Treatment:	• **Standard treatment: Surgery (Mastectomy/BCS) + Adjuvant chemotherapy + Radiotherapy**[Q]
	
	    • **Didox** (synthetic antioxidant) in addition to chemotherpay **reduces drug resistance**[Q]
	    • **Didox inhibits ribonucleotide reductase M2 (RRM2)**[Q]
	    • **RRM2** contributes to **cell resistance of the chemotherapy resulting in relapse**[Q]
	
	• **TNBC** are **very susceptible to chemotherapy**[Q]
	• **BRCA-1 related TNBC** is particularly **susceptible to platinum-based agents & taxanes**[Q]

Prognosis:	• **High risk of recurrence** after treatment[Q]

130. Ans. a. Monocryl *(Ref: Essentials of Breast Surgery by Michael S. Sabel /p174)*

Monocryl sutures 3-0 or 4-0 (monofilament) are used in closure of MRM wounds by subcuticular suturing. Monofilaments sutures are preferred for subcuticular suturing. Braided or multi-filaments sutures should not be used for subcuticular suturing because of increased risk of infections.

See Q. no. 140 AIIMS November 2016.

Monocryl	• **Trade name of Polyglycaprone** • **Monofilament synthetic absorbable surgical suture** • Copolymer of **glycolite & caprolactone**[Q] • Indicated for use in general **soft tissue approximation and/or ligation**
Vicryl	• **Braided multifilament** • Copolymer of **lactide & glycolide**[Q] in a ratio of 90:10, coated with polyglactin & calcium stearate
Mersilk	• Non-absorbable, braided suture (multifilament)
Chromic catgut	• Tanned with **chromium salts** to **improve handling & resist degradation** in tissue[Q] • **Causes intense reaction, not used commonly**

AIIMS May 2016

131. Ans. d. Immediate needle thoracostomy *(Ref: Sabiston 20/e p428 19/e p1599; Schwartz 9/e p138; Bailey 27/e p367, 919, 26/e p354)*

This case is a classical description of tension pneumothorax of right hemithorax with decreased breath sounds and shock. Since patient is shouting it means her airway is clear. Immediate decompression with large bore needle in mid clavicular line in 2nd intercostal space is the urgent treatment for this patient followed by insertion of IV line and fluid administration.

Features	Cardiac Tamponade	Tension Pneumothorax
Presenting	**Shock**[Q] (**Shortness of breath**[Q] may be seen)	**Respiratory distress**[Q] (Shock may be the presenting feature but less common)
Neck veins	**Distended**[Q]	**Distended**[Q]
Trachea	**Midline**[Q]	**Deviated**[Q]
Breath sounds	**Normal**[Q]	**Decreased or absent on side of injury**[Q]
Percussion Note	**Normal**[Q]	**Hyper-resonant**[Q]
Heart sound	**Muffled**[Q]	**Normal**[Q]

Tension Pneumothorax

- A tension pneumothorax develops when a **'one-way valve' air leak** occurs either **from lung** or **through** the **chest wall**[Q].
- **Air** is **forced into thoracic cavity** without any means of escape, **completely collapsing** the **affected lung**[Q].
  - **Mediastinum** is **displaced to the opposite side, decreasing venous return** and **compressing** the **opposite lung**[Q].

Common Causes of Tension Pneumothorax	
• **Penetrating chest trauma**[Q] • **Blunt chest trauma**[Q] (with **parenchymal injury** & **air leak** that did not spontaneously close)	• **Iatrogenic lung punctures** (e.g. due to **subclavian central venepuncture**) • Mechanical **positive pressure ventilation**[Q]

Clinical Features:
- **Clinical presentation** is **dramatic.**
- Patient is panicky with **tachypnoea, dyspnoea & distended neck veins** (similar to pericardial tamponade)[Q].
- **Clinical examination** can reveal **tracheal deviation** (a **late finding** – not necessary to clinically confirm diagnosis), **hyperresonance & absent breath sounds** over the **affected hemithorax**[Q].

Diagnosis:
- Tension pneumothorax is a **clinical diagnosis** and **treatment should not be delayed**[Q] by waiting for radiological confirmation.

Treatment:
- Treatment consists of **immediate decompression** by **rapid insertion** of a **large-bore needle** into **2nd intercostal space** in the **mid-clavicular line**[Q] of the affected hemithorax.
- This is **immediately followed** by **insertion of a chest tube** through the **5th intercostal space** in **anterior axillary line**[Q].
  - If the **tension in pleural space is not relieved, patient** is likely to **die from inadequate cardiac output** or **marked hypoxemia**[Q].

132. Ans. d. Completely absent *(Ref: Harrison 19/e p280, 18/e p325)*

Absence of urinary urobilinogen is usually suggestive of obstructive jaundice.

*"The **conjugated bilirubin** excreted into bile drains into the duodenum and passes unchanged through the proximal small bowel. Conjugated bilirubin is not taken up by the intestinal mucosa. When the conjugated bilirubin reaches the distal ileum and colon, it is hydrolyzed to unconjugated bilirubin by bacterial β-glucuronidases. The unconjugated bilirubin is reduced by normal gut bacteria to form a group of colorless tetrapyrroles called urobilinogens. About 80–90% of these products are excreted in feces, either unchanged or oxidized to orange derivatives called urobilins. The remaining 10–20% of the urobilinogens are passively absorbed, enter the portal venous blood, and are re-excreted by the liver. A small fraction (usually <3 mg/dL) escapes hepatic uptake, filters across the renal glomerulus, and is excreted in urine."- Harrison 19/e p280*

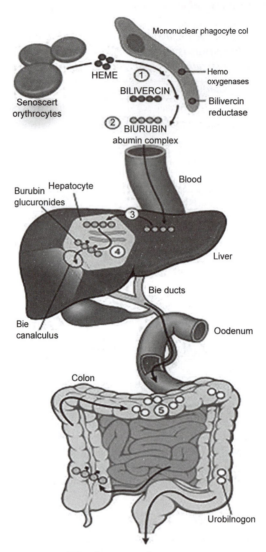

Fig. 41: Bilirubin metabolism and elimination.

Function test	Prehepatic jaundice	Hepatic jaundice	Post-hepatic (Obstructive) jaundice
Total bilirubin	Normal/ increased	Increased[Q]	Increased[Q]
Conjugated bilirubin	Normal	Increased[Q]	Increased[Q]
Unconjugated bilirubin	Normal/ increased	Increased[Q]	Normal
Urobilinogen	Normal/ increased	Decreased[Q]	Decreased/ negative[Q]
Urine color	Normal	Dark (urobilinogen + conjugated bilirubin)[Q]	Dark (conjugated bilirubin)[Q]
Stool color	Normal	Normal/pale[Q]	Pale[Q]
Alkaline phosphatase levels	Normal	Increased[Q]	Increased[Q]
Alanine transferase & aspartate transferase levels	Normal	Increased[Q]	Increased[Q]
Conjugated bilirubin in urine	Absent[Q]	Present[Q]	Present[Q]
Splenomegaly	Present[Q]	Present[Q]	Absent[Q]

Contd...

Bilirubin metabolism and elimination

- Normal bilirubin production from heme (0.2–0.3 gm/day) is derived **primarily from the breakdown of senescent circulating erythrocytes.**
- **Extrahepatic bilirubin** is **bound to serum albumin** and **delivered to the liver.**
- **Hepatocellular uptake**
- **Glucuronidation in the endoplasmic reticulum** generate **bilirubin monoglucuronides & diglucuronides**, which are **water soluble** and **readily excreted into bile.**
- **Gut bacteria deconjugate the bilirubin** and **degrade it to colorless urobilinogens**. The **urobilinogens** and the **residue of intact pigments are excreted in the feces**, with **some reabsorption and excretion into urine.**

133. Ans. a. Basal cell carcinoma   *(Ref: Harrison 19/e p500; Robbins 9/e p1157)*

Lesion on the cheek with raised, pearly borders and with telangiectasia on surface of the lesion is highly suggestive of basal cell carcinoma.

> *"Basal cell carcinomas usually present as pearly papules containing prominent dilated subepidermal blood vessels (telangiectasias). Some tumors contain melanin and superficially resemble melanocytic nevi or melanomas. Advanced lesions may ulcerate, and extensive local invasion of bone or facial sinuses may occur after many years of neglect or in unusually aggressive tumors, explaining the archaic designation rodent ulcers."- Robbins 9/e p1157*

> *"BCC arises from epidermal basal cells. BCC also can present as a small, slowly growing pearly nodule, often with tortuous telangiectatic vessels on its surface, rolled borders, and a central crust (nodular BCC). The occasional presence of melanin in this variant of nodular BCC (pigmented BCC) may lead to confusion with melanoma. Morpheaform (fibrosing), infiltrative, and micronodular BCC, the most invasive and potentially aggressive subtypes, manifest as solitary, flat or slightly depressed, indurated whitish, yellowish, or pink scar-like plaques."- Harrison 19/e p500*

134. Ans. a. 40%   *(Ref: Sabiston 20/e p507, 19/e p523; Schwartz 9/e p199-200; Bailey 26/e p389)*

The best way to measure the area burned accurately is the Lund and Browder chart. Total body surface area affected in burns of a 2 years old child involving face (8.5%), bilateral upper limb (20%), front of chest & abdomen (13%) is 41.5% (approximately 40%).

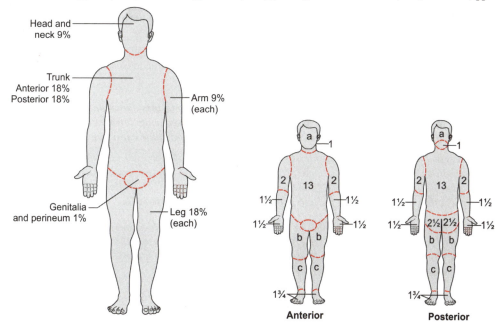

Relative percentage of body surface area (% BSA) affected by growth

Body part	0 yr	1yr	5yr	10yr	15yr
a = 1/2 of head	9 1/2	8 1/2	6 1/2	5 1/2	4 1/2
b = 1/2 of 1 thigh	2 3/4	3 1/4	4	4 1/4	4 1/2
c = 1/2 of 1 lower leg	2 1/2	2 1/2	2 3/4	3	3 1/4

Contd...

Burn Size (% BSA)
• Determination of **burn size estimates** the **extent of injury**.
• **Burn size** is assessed by **Wallace rule of nines** (By **Alfred Russel Wallace**[Q])
• **Children** have a relatively **larger proportion** of body surface area **in their head & neck**, which is compensated for by a relatively smaller surface area in the lower extremities.
• **In infants: Head & neck- 21%**[Q]; **Each leg- 13%**[Q]
• **Berkow formula**[Q] is used to **accurately determine burn size** in **children.**
• **Lund & Browder chart** give a **more accurate accounting of true burn size in children**[Q].
• **For estimating smaller burns: Area of open hand**[Q] (including **palm & extended fingers**) of the **patient** is approximately **1%**[Q] of TBSA.
• This method is helpful in **evaluating splash burns** & burns of **mixed distribution**[Q].

135. Ans. a. Clean and drape from the level of nipple to mid thigh *(Ref: Bailey 27/e p52, 26/e p252)*

For abdominal and pelvic surgeries, patient should be cleaned and draped from the level of nipple to mid thigh.

Area of Cleaning & Draping in Surgeries	
Cranial surgery	• Depends upon surgeon
Thyroid or neck surgery	• **Chin to nipple** with shoulder & axilla[Q]
Eye surgery	• **Cut eyelashes** of affected eye
Nasal surgery	• No shaving unless with mustache
Ear surgery	• **Two & half inches around ear**[Q]
Chest surgery	• **Base of neck to waist**, axilla & inner arm[Q]
Abdominal & pelvic surgery	• **Nipple to symphysis pubis, vulva, perineum & thigh**[Q]
Kidney-anterior	• **Nipple to perineum**, side to side; supra scapular region to buttocks
Vaginal, scrotal, rectal surgery	• **Waist to perineum** plus **anterior & inner aspect of thigh** & 6 inches from groin; posterior- entire buttocks & anus[Q]
Lower extremities	• **Digits 2 inches above knee**, entire extremity and groin[Q]
Upper extremities	• **Distal arm 2 inches above elbow**, elbow up to axilla[Q]

136. Ans. a. Grey *(Ref: Bailey 25/e p291)*

In a patient with massive bleeding, there is always a risk of patient going into shock and widest bore cannula available showed be used for cannulation. The ACLS guidelines recommend securing intravenous access with two large-bore cannulae (14–16G) in a patient needing resuscitation. Color code for 16 Gauge cannulae is grey.

"Primary survey in Trauma: These include blood samples for full blood count (FBC), coagulation studies, plasma chemistry (urea and electrolytes and, sometimes, toxicology or other case-specific indices), transfusion screening (group and cross-match, etc.), 12- electrocardiography (ECG) monitoring and pulse oximetry, if available. ***The blood can be taken at the same time as securing intravenous access with two large-bore cannulae (14–16G)."*** *- Bailey 25/e p291*

"The sizes of needle-based instruments (such as Venflons and needles themselves) ***are measured in 'Gauge'*** *(i.e. how many can be fitted into a tube of a fixed diameter).* ***In Gauge, larger numbers, mean smaller diameter lumens.*** *Catheters use the 'French' system. This is the circumference of the tube in millimeters, e.g. a 30 F catheter has a circumference of 30 mm.* ***In French, larger numbers therefore mean larger diameter lumens."***

Gauge	Color code	External Diameter	Length	Flow Rate
14G	Orange	2.1 mm	45 mm	240 ml/min
16G	Grey	1.8 mm	45 mm	180 ml/min
18G	Green	1.3 mm	32/45 mm	90 ml/min
20G	Pink	1.1 mm	32 mm	60 ml/min
22G	Blue	0.9 mm	25 mm	36 ml/min
24G	Yellow	0.7 mm	19 mm	20 ml/min
26G	Violet	0.6 mm	19 mm	13 ml/min

137. **Ans. d. Use ultrasound guidance to locate and prick the balloon and then remove the catheter** (Ref: http://www.aafp. org/afp/2000/0915/p1397.html)
Best technique in this situation is ultrasound-guided rupture of balloon.

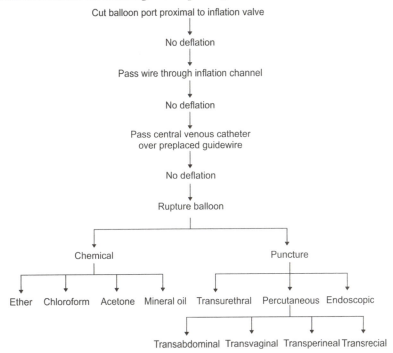

Fig. 42: Management of Non-deflating Urethral Catheter: (Transrectal spelling error)

Management of Non-deflating Urethral Catheter

- **Malfunction of inflation valve** caused by **external clamping, crushing or kinking** of inflation channel is the **primary reason** for non-deflating catheter balloon[Q].
- Valve can also become obstructed by **crystallization** when non-sterile fluid is used to fill the balloon.
  - **First step: Advance the catheter** to ensure that it is actually in bladder. If this does not work, **balloon port should be cut proximal to inflation valve**[Q]. This removes the valve and should allow water to spontaneously drain.
  - If this does not work, **area of obstruction** is likely to be along the **length of catheter** or at **entrance to balloon**. **Next maneuver** is to **pass a lubricated fine-gauge guidewire through the inflation channel**[Q]. Guidewire or stylet should allow fluid to drain along the wire itself. If this does not work, a **22-gauge central venous catheter** can be passed over the guidewire. When the catheter tip is into the balloon, the wire can be removed, and the balloon should drain[Q].
    - If above techniques are unsuccessful, **do not perform hyperinflation** with air or saline. This step may **cause severe pain** & could cause **bladder rupture**[Q].
- It is recommended that **balloon be dissolved chemically** by use of **ether, chloroform, acetone and mineral oil**. **Only mineral oil is recommended** because **other compounds** are potentially **toxic to bladder epithelium**[Q].
- **Final method: Active rupture of Foley balloon** with a sharp instrument percutaneously using transabdominal, transvaginal, transperineal and transrectal approaches[Q].
  - In **women, a transurethral approach can be used** that involves applying continuous, steady pressure on catheter that might cause part of it to show through urethral meatus, followed by piercing the balloon with a lumbar needle. This technique is **not recommended for use in men**[Q].
  - Most people recommend **transrectal approach** in **men,** preferably **with use of transrectal sonography**[Q].

138. **Ans. a. Limiting pCO₂ of the patient** (Ref: Harrison 19/e p1780, 18/e p2257)
Hyperventilation and decreasing pCO₂ is the initial and one of the most important treatment strategies to lower the ICP in a patient of head injury.

"Emergent treatment of elevated ICP is most quickly achieved by intubation and hyperventilation, which causes vasoconstriction and reduces cerebral blood volume. To avoid provoking or worsening cerebral ischemia, hyperventilation, if used at all, is best administered only for short periods of time until a more definitive treatment can be instituted. Furthermore, the effects of hyperventilation on ICP are short-lived, often lasting only for several hours because of the buffering capacity of the cerebral interstitium, and rebound elevations of ICP may accompany abrupt discontinuation of hyperventilation. As the level of consciousness declines to coma, the ability to follow the neurologic status of the patient by examination lessens and measurement of ICP assumes greater importance. If a ventriculostomy device is in place, direct drainage of CSF to reduce ICP is possible. Finally, high-dose barbiturates, decompressive hemicraniectomy, and hypothermia are sometimes used for refractory elevations of ICP, although these have significant side effects and have not been proven to improve outcome." - *Harrison 19/e p1780*

Stepwise Approach to Treatment of Elevated Intracranial Pressure

- Insert **ICP monitor—ventriculostomy**[Q] versus parenchymal device
- **General goals**: maintain **ICP <20 mmHg** and **CPP 60 mmHg**[Q]

For ICP >20–25 mmHg for >5 min

- Drain CSF via **ventriculostomy**[Q] (if in place)
- **Elevate head of** the **bed**[Q]; midline head position
- **Osmotherapy—mannitol**[Q] 25–100 g q4h as needed (maintain serum **osmolality <320**[Q] mosmol) or **hypertonic saline**[Q] (30 mL, 23.4% NaCl bolus)
- **Glucocorticoids**—dexamethasone (4 mg q6h) **for vasogenic edema from tumor, abscess**[Q] (avoid glucocorticoids in head trauma, ischemic and hemorrhagic stroke[Q])
- **Sedation**[Q] (e.g. morphine, propofol, or midazolam); add **neuromuscular paralysis** if necessary (patient will require endotracheal intubation and mechanical ventilation at this point, if not before)
- **Hyperventilation**[Q]—to **PaCO$_2$ 30–35 mmHg**

For ICP >20–25 mmHg for >5 min

- **Pressor therapy**[Q]—**phenylephrine, dopamine, or norepinephrine to maintain adequate MAP** to ensure **CPP 60 mmHg** (maintain euvolemia to minimize deleterious systemic effects of pressors)
- Consider **second-tier therapies for refractory elevated ICP**:
    a. **High-dose barbiturate therapy ("pentobarb coma")**[Q]
    b. **Aggressive hyperventilation to PaCO$_2$ <30 mmHg**[Q]
    c. **Hypothermia**[Q]
    d. **Hemicraniectomy**[Q]

---

139. Ans. d. Subarachnoid hemorrhage *(Ref: Harrison 19/e p1787, 1735; Katzung 13/e p202, 12/e p204)*
Nimodipine is approved for use in subarachnoid hemorrhage.

"Subarachnoid hemorrhage may occur secondary to aneurysm rupture and is often complicated by cerebral vasospasm, re-bleeding, and hydrocephalus. Vasospasm can be detected by either transcranial Doppler assessment or cerebral angiography; it is typically treated with the calcium channel blocker nimodipine, aggressive IV fluid administration, and therapy aimed at increasing blood pressure, typically with vasoactive drugs such as phenylephrine. The IV fluids and vasoactive drugs (hypertensive hypervolemic therapy) are used to overcome the cerebral vasospasm. Early surgical clipping or endovascular coiling of aneurysms is advocated to prevent complications related to re-bleeding. Hydrocephalus, typically heralded by a decreased level of consciousness, may require ventriculostomy drainage." - *Harrison 19/e p1735*

"Vasospasm remains the leading cause of morbidity and mortality following aneurysmal SAH. Treatment with the calcium channel antagonist nimodipine (60 mg PO every 4 h) improves outcome, perhaps by preventing ischemic injury rather than reducing the risk of vasospasm. Nimodipine can cause significant hypotension in some patients, which may worsen cerebral ischemia in patients with vasospasm." - *Harrison 19/e p1787*

"Nimodipine, a member of the dihydropyridine group of calcium channel blockers, has a high affinity for cerebral blood vessels and appears to reduce morbidity after a subarachnoid hemorrhage." - *Katzung 13/e p202*

AIIMS May 2016

OBSTETRICS AND GYNECOLOGY

140. Ans. b. Granulosa cell tumor   *(Ref: Shaw's 16/e p442, 15/e p379; Robbins 9/e p1032)*

In the given PAP smear, predominance of mature cells (orange coloured cells compared to parabasal cells: blue colored), this might be due to estrogen secretion from granulosa cell tumor.

"Granulosa cell tumors are of clinical importance for two reasons: (1) they may elaborate large amounts of estrogen, and (2) they may behave like low-grade malignancies. Functionally active tumors in prepubertal girls (juvenile granulosa cell tumors) may produce precocious sexual development. In adult women they may be associated with proliferative breast disease, endometrial hyperplasia, and endometrial carcinoma, which eventually develops in about 10% to 15% of women with steroid-producing tumors. Occasionally, granulosa cell tumors produce androgens, masculinizing the patient."- Robbins 9/e p1032

Granulosa cell tumor
• Composed of cells that **resemble granulosa cells** of a **developing ovarian follicle**[Q].
• 2/3rd occur in **postmenopausal women**.
• Tumor **secretes estrogens**, which causes **precocious sexual development in girls** or increases the risk for **proliferative breast disease, endometrial hyperplasia and endometrial carcinoma** in adult women[Q]
• Less commonly granulosa cell tumors can secrete **androgens** and **produce masculinization**[Q].

Pathology:
- **Low grade malignancy**[Q]; Almost always unilateral[Q]
- **Encapsulated tumors** and have smooth surface[Q]
- **Microscopy: Coffee bean nucleus** and **Call-Exner bodies**[Q]

> - **MC type of ovarian tumor** that is composed of cells that **stain positively with inhibin**[Q].
> - **Metastasis is peculiar** in case of **granulosa cell tumor**, it first involves opposite ovary followed by metastasis in **lumbar region.**
> - **Mutations of *FOXL2* gene in 97% of adult granulosa cell tumors**[Q].

Clinical Features:
- **MC symptoms: Menometrorrhagia and post-menopausal bleeding**[Q]

Diagnosis:
- **Granulosa cell tumor** secretes **inhibin**[Q] (useful marker)

Treatment:
- **Children and women of reproductive age: Unilateral salpino-oophorectomy**[Q]
- **Post-menopausal: TAH + BSO**[Q]

Body/Figures	Feature	Seen in
Alder-Reiliy bodies[Q]	Deeply **basophilic granules** seen within **neutrophils**[Q]	**Hunter's and Hurler's syndrome**[Q]
Antoni A bodies[Q]	Densely cellular areas with palisaded nuclei, fascicles & **Verocay bodies**[Q]	**Schwannoma**[Q]
Antoni B bodies[Q]	Loose, gelatinous stroma, fewer cells microcystic changes	**Schwannoma**[Q]
Arao-Perkins bodies[Q]	Small fibrous bodies in dermal papilla	Androgenic alopecia[Q]
Aschoff body[Q]	**Small granulomatous lesion composed of macrophages, lymphocytes & giant cells**[Q]	**Rheumatic fever**[Q]
Asteroid body[Q]	Star-like cytoplasmic inclusions in giant cells	**Sarcoidosis**[Q] and other **granulomatous disease** (TB, Botryomycosis, sporotrichosis, actinomycosis, leprosy, Berylliosis)[Q]
Bamboo bodies[Q]	Cylindrical, high density foreign bodies in lung.	**Asbestosis**[Q]
Banana bodies[Q]	**Crescentic shaped bodies within Schwann cells**[Q]	**Disseminated lipogranulomatosis**[Q] Farber disease, Ochronosis[Q]
Birbeck granules[Q]	**Tennis racket structures on EM**[Q]	**Langerhans cells**[Q]

Contd...

Contd...

Body/Figures	Feature	Seen in
Bodies of Arantius[Q]	Small nodules located at cusps of aortic and pulmonary valves[Q]	Aortic valve nodules[Q]
Body of Highmore[Q]	Mass of fibrous tissue continuous with tunica albuginea that project into testis.	Mediastinum testis[Q]
Bollinger bodies[Q]	Intracytoplasmic, eosinophilic inclusions in epithelial cells of birds[Q].	Fowlpox[Q]
Brassy body[Q]	Dark shrunken blood corpuscles[Q]	Malaria[Q]
Bunina bodies[Q]	Small eosinophilic intraneuronal inclusions in lower motor neurons[Q]	Amyotrophic lateral sclerosis[Q]
Call-Exner bodies[Q]	Small eosinophilic, fluid-filled spaces found in ovary between granulosa cells[Q]	Granulosa cell tumor[Q]
Caterpillar bodies[Q]	Elongated epidermal eosinophilic bodies[Q]	Porphyria cutanea tarda[Q]
Chromatid bodies[Q]	Cytoplasmic elongated cigar-shaped bars with bluntly rounded ends[Q]	Entamoeba histolytica precyst[Q]
Cigar bodies[Q]	Elongated, cigar like[Q]	Sporotrichosis[Q]
Citron bodies[Q]	Boat or leaf shaped pleomorphic bacteria[Q]	Clostridium septicum[Q]
Civatte bodies (colloid bodies)[Q]	Spherical, eosinophilic hyaline bodies seen in or below the epidermis[Q]	Lichen planus[Q]
Councilman bodies[Q]	Cytoplasmic inclusion[Q]	Viral hepatitis[Q] yellow fever[Q]
Cowdry type A bodies[Q]	Lipschutz inclusions, intranuclear eosinophilic inclusions surrounded by clear halo[Q]	Herpes simples, Varicella Zoster lesions[Q]
Cowdry type B bodies[Q]	Droplet like masses of acidophilic material surrounded by clear halo within nuclei	Polio & adenovirus[Q]
Coccoid X bodies[Q]	Minute bodies (elementary & reticulate) found in the blood[Q]	Psittacosis[Q]
Comma shaped bodies[Q]	Two electron dense membranes within histiocytes[Q]	Juvenile Xanthogranuloma, histiocytosis[Q]
Creola bodies[Q]	Clumps of benign respiratory epithelium in sputum indicative of asthma[Q]	Asthma[Q]
Cystoid bodies[Q]	Heterogeneous round, oval, or polygonal deposit, usually in dermis	Collective form for colloid bodies, Russell bodies amyloid, elastic globes[Q]
Davidson bodies[Q]	Nuclear chromatin buds[Q]	Female's neutrophils[Q]
Donovan bodies[Q]	Single or clustered rod safety pin like bacteria in macrophages	Granuloma inguinale[Q]
Dutcher bodies[Q]	Intranuclear, eosinophilic globules found in plasma cells.	B-cell lymphoma, multiple myeloma, Farber disease[Q]
Farber bodies[Q]	Comma-shaped tubular structures in cytoplasm of fibroblasts	Farber disease[Q]
Ferruginous bodies (Asbestos bodies)[Q]	Thin, curved or drumstick appearance; stain positively with Perl's Prussian blue[Q].	Asbestosis, silicosis[Q]
Flame Figures[Q]	Poorly circumscribed, small areas of amorphous eosinophilic material adherent to dermal collagen	Eosinophilic cellulitis + flame figures was syndrome > arthropod bites, parasites, BP, of eosinophilic panniculi
Floret cells[Q]	Multinucleated giant cells with marginally placed nuclei	Pleomorphic (spindle cell) lipoma[Q]
Flower cells[Q]	Atypical CD4+ T cells, prominent nuclear lobation	HTLV-1, ATL[Q]
Gamma Gandy bodies[Q]	Nodules secondary to accumulation of hemosiderin	CML, sickle cell anemia, cirrhosis of liver[Q]
Guarnieri bodies (Paschen bodies)[Q]	Cytoplasmic, eosinophilic inclusion in keratinocytes	Smallpox, Vaccinia[Q]

Contd...

Body/Figures	Feature	Seen in
Heinz bodies (Ehrlich or Heinz-Ehrlich bodies)[Q]	Small rounded distensions that deform RBCs. Ehrlich or Heinz-Ehrlich bodies	G-6-PD deficiency[Q]
Henderson-Patterson bodies[Q]	Large, cytoplasmic eosinophilic inclusions in keratinocytes	Molluscum contagiosum[Q]
Herring bodies[Q]	Large eosinophilic masses of neurosecretory granules located in posterior lobe of pituitary at dilatations along the axons and their endings.	Neurohypophysis[Q]
Hirano bodies[Q]	Intracellular, eosinophilic rod-shaped structures in nerve cells.	Alzheimer's disease, Creutzfeldt-Jacob disease[Q]
Homer-Wright rosettes	Central nerve fibrils, peripheral small tumor cells	Cutaneous neuroblastoma[Q]
Kamino bodies[Q]	Eosinophilic globoid bodies, probably apoptotic lesional cells.	Spindle cell naevi[Q]
Lafora bodies[Q]	Concentric amyloid deposits (**polyglucosan bodies**)[Q]	Lafora disease[Q]
Levinthal-Coles-Lillie bodies[Q]	Cytoplasmic inclusion bodies in macrophages of lung	Psittacosis[Q]
Lewy bodies[Q]	**Round eosinophilic structures found in cytoplasm of neurons**[Q].	Parkinsonism, Alzheimer's disease[Q]
Lipofuscin-like granules	Yellow-brown granules in dermal macrophages	Amiodarone hyperpigmentation[Q]
Marquee sign[Q]	Organisms at the periphery of macrophages	Leishmania[Q]
Medlar (sclerotic) bodies[Q]	Muriform cells, "copper pennies, "round thick-walled brown fungi	Chromoblastomycosis[Q]
Michaelis-Gutmann bodies[Q]	Calcified, degraded bacteria in macrophages, lamellated	Malakoplakia[Q]
Mikulicz cells[Q]	**Large macrophages containing Klebsiella rhinoscleromatis**[Q]	Rhinoscleroma[Q]
Morulae[Q]	**Leukocyte intracytoplasmic inclusions, Ehrlichia multiplying in cell vacuoles**[Q]	Ehrlichiosis[Q]
Mooser bodies[Q]	Large mononuclear cells filled with Rickettsia typhi in patients with endemic typhus fever	Endemic typhus[Q]
Mott bodies (Mott cells)[Q]	Plasma cells with spherical inclusions (Russell bodies) packed in their cytoplasm.	Multiple myeloma[Q]
Negri bodies[Q]	Eosinophilic, cytoplasmic inclusions in neutrons	Rabies[Q]
Odland bodies[Q]	Small, granular, membrane-bound vacuoles found in cytoplasm of skin keratinocytes	Derived from the Golgi apparatus Shows synthesis of epidermal lipids
Psammoma bodies[Q]	Concentrically laminated, round calcified bodies	Papillary carcinoma thyroid, Serous cystadenoma of ovary, Meningioma, Malignant Mesothelioma[Q]
Pustule-ovoid bodies of Milian[Q]	Large eosinophilic granules with clear halo	Granular cell tumor[Q]
Reilly bodies[Q]	**Granular inclusions found in WBCs in Alder-Reilly anomaly**[Q]	Hurler's syndrome[Q]
Rokitansky bodies[Q]	Yellowish appearance of adipose tissue on CT	Benign cystic teratomas[Q]
Ross's bodies[Q]	**Spherical copper-coloured bodies**[Q]	Syphilis[Q]
Rushton bodies[Q]	Intraepithelial, curvilinear and eosinophilic lamellar structures	Odontogenic cyst[Q]
Russell bodies[Q]	Immunoglobulin deposits in plasma cells	Rhinoscleroma, plasmacytosis[Q]

Contd...

Contd...

Body/Figures	Feature	Seen in
Sandstorm bodies[Q]	Synonymous with parathyroid glands	Parathyroid glands[Q]
Schaumann bodies[Q]	Shell-like, lamellated, basophilic, calcified protein complexes in giant cells[Q]	Sarcoidosis[Q]
Schiller-Duval bodies[Q]	Perivascular structures consisting of tumor cells arranged around a blood vessel[Q].	Yolk sac tumor[Q]
Sclerotic bodies[Q]	Rounded cells surrounded by thick walls often known as **Medlar bodies or copper pennies**[Q].	Chromoblastomycosis[Q]
Spiderweb cells[Q]	Globular, striated, vacuolated cells	Adult rhabdomyoma[Q]
Verocay bodies[Q]	Palisading nuclei in rows around eosinophilic cytoplasm[Q]	Schwannoma[Q]
Winkler bodies[Q]	Spherical structures in lesions in syphilis	Syphilis[Q]
Weibel-Palade bodies[Q]	Dense rod or oval organelles on EM[Q]	Endothelial cells[Q]
Zebra bodies[Q]	Vacuoles with transverse membrane with endothelial cells[Q]	Metachromatic leukodystrophy[Q]

141. **Ans. d. Hydatidiform mole** *(Ref: Williams 24/e p399)*

The given ultrasonography is showing snowstorm appearance, which is typically seen in a hydatidiform mole.

> "Although sonographic imaging is the mainstay of trophoblastic disease diagnosis, not all cases are confirmed initially. Sonographically, a complete mole appears as an echogenic uterine mass with numerous anechoic cystic spaces but without a fetus or amnionic sac. The appearance is often described as a "snowstorm". A partial mole has features that include a thickened, multicystic placenta along with a fetus or at least fetal tissue. In early pregnancy, however, these sonographic characteristics are seen in fewer than half of hydatidiform moles. The most common misdiagnosis is incomplete or missed abortion. Occasionally, molar pregnancy may be confused for a multifetal pregnancy or a uterine leiomyoma with cystic degeneration."-*Williams 24/e p399*

Sonograms of hydatidiform moles	
Complete hydatidiform mole	**Partial hydatidiform mole**
• **"Snowstorm"** appearance is due to an **echogenic uterine mass** having **numerous anechoic cystic spaces**[Q]. • Fetus and amnionic sac are absent[Q].	• Fetus is seen above a multicystic placenta[Q]

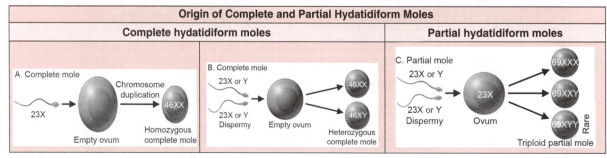

Origin of Complete and Partial Hydatidiform Moles

Feature	Complete mole	Partial mole
Karyotype	46 XX, 46 XY[Q]	Triploid, 69, XXY or 69, XYY[Q]
Villous edema	All villi[Q]	Some villi[Q]
Trophoblast proliferation	Diffuse, circumferential[Q]	Focal, slight[Q]
Atypia	Often present[Q]	Absent[Q]
Serum hCG	Elevated[Q]	Less elevated[Q]
hCG in tissue	++++[Q]	+[Q]
Behavior	2% choriocarcinoma[Q]	Rare choriocarcinoma[Q]
Fetal parts	Rarely seen[Q]	More common[Q]

Hydatidiform Mole

- A **benign neoplasm of trophoblastic cells** that **carries a risk of malignant transformation**[Q].
- **Complete mole**: 46, XX; 2 sperm + empty egg; completely paternal in origin[Q].
- **Partial mole**: 69, XXY[Q]; 2 sperm + 1 egg; made up of 3 or more parts (triploid or tetraploid[Q]); may contain fetal parts.

Risk factors:
- **Low socioeconomic status, age > 40 years, Asian heritage, tobacco use**[Q].

Pathology:
- **Classic appearance**: Delicate, friable mass of thin-walled, translucent, cystic, grapelike structures consisting of swollen edematous (hydropic) villi[Q].
- **Complete mole**: Microscopic abnormalities involve **all or most of the villous tissue**[Q].
- **Partial moles**: Only a fraction of the villi are **enlarged and edematous**[Q].

	Clinical Features of Hydatidiform Mole

Symptoms	- **Vaginal Bleeding**: MC presentation[Q], may be preceded by a brownish or watery discharge. **Blood may be mixed with fluid from ruptured cysts** giving the appearance of discharge "white currant in red currant juice"[Q]
	- **Varying degree of lower abdominal pain**[Q]
	- **Constitutional symptoms:**
	  – Patient may become **sick**[Q] without any apparent reason
	  – **Excessive vomiting of pregnancy**[Q]
	  – **Breathlessness**[Q] due to pulmonary embolization of trophoblastic cells
	- **Thyrotoxic features** of **tremors** or **tachycardia** are present on occasion (2%), due to **increased chorionic thyrotropin**[Q]. Thyrotoxicosis resulting in supraventricular tachycardia, dyspnoea & increased T_4, T_3 is seen in 3% of cases & is due to fact that **subunits of both TSH & hCG share a similar structure**[Q].
	- **Expulsion of grape like vesicles per vaginum: Diagnostic of vesicular mole**[Q]

Signs	- Features are suggestive of early months of pregnancy are evident - **Patient looks more ill**[Q] than can be accounted for. - **Pallor**[Q] is unusually **prominent** - Features of **pre-eclampsia**[Q] (hypertesnsion, edema and/or proteinuria) are present **in about 50%.**

Diagnosis:
- Suspect in patients with **1st trimester uterine bleeding** and **excess nausea & vomiting**[Q].
- Also suspect if **preeclampsia occurs in first half (<24 weeks) of pregnancy**[Q].
- Other signs—**Uterine size > gestational age (MC with complete mole**[Q]); hyperthyroidism; expulsion of "grape-like" vesicles from the vagina, no detectable fetal heartbeat[Q].
- **Beta-hCG ↑↑ for gestational age**[Q] (usually > 100,000 mIU/dL)
- **USG: "Snowstorm" appearance** with **no gestational sac in complete mole**[Q]

  - **Complete mole** appears as an **echogenic uterine mass** with **numerous anechoic cystic spaces without a fetus or amnionic sac ("Snowstorm" appearance**[Q])
  - **Partial mole**: Thickened, multicystic placenta along **with a fetus** or **at least fetal tissue**[Q].

Hydatidiform Mole

Principles of Management of Hydatidiform Mole
• Supportive therapy to **restore blood loss** & to **prevent infection**[Q] • To **evacuate the uterus as soon as the diagnosis is made**[Q] • **Regular follow-up** for early detection of **persistent trophoblastic disease**[Q]

Patients are grouped into:
- **Mole is in process of expulsion: Suction evacuation is best**[Q]
- **Uterus remain inert**:
  - **Vaginal evacuation (suction evacuation)**[Q]
  - **Hysterotomy**, rarely in cases of **profuse vaginal bleeding**[Q] & unfavorable cervix for immediate vaginal evacuation
  - **Hysterectomy** in patients **>35 years**[Q] & patients **completed the family**[Q] irrespective of age.

Complications of Vaginal Evacuation
• Acute pulmonary insufficiency due to **pulmonary embolization**[Q] of trophoblastic cells • **Thyroid storm**[Q] in presence of hyperthyroid state

- Remember: **Following hysterectomy, persistent GTN is observed in 3-5% cases. As such it does not eliminate the necessary of follow up**[Q].

Indications of Prophylactic Chemotherapy
• If the **hCG levels fails to become normal** by the stipulated time (**4-6 weeks**) or there is **re-elevation (>20,000 mIU/ml) at 4-6 weeks**[Q] • **Evidence of metastasis irrespective on the level of hCG**[Q] • In cases, where the **malignant sequelae is higher** as judged by **risk factors** & where proper **follow up facilities are not available**[Q]

Chemotherapy Regimes
• **Methotrexate 5 mg TDS × 5 days**[Q], a total of 3 courses at intervals of 2 weeks. • Alternatively, **IV Actinomycin D 12 mg/kg body weight daily for 5 days**[Q] may be given. It is less toxic than methotrexate.

Follow-up:
- **Routine follow-up** is mandatory for all cases **for at least 6 months**[Q].

Contraceptive advice:
- If the patient desires, she may be pregnant **after 6 months**[Q], following the **negative hCG titre**.
- **IUD is contraindicated**[Q], because of its frequent association of irregular bleeding—a feature often co-exists with choriocarcinoma.
- **hCG levels should be checked 3 weeks** after the end of any pregnancy, **subsequent to molar one**[Q].

142. **Ans. d. Anencephaly** *(Ref: Williams 24/e p201)*

The ultrasound appearance (absence of cranial vault and varying amount of brain) is classically seen in anencephaly of fetus, though usually detectable in a first trimester sonogram at 11–14 weeks.

> *"Anencephaly is characterized by absence of the cranium and telencephalic structures, with the skullbase and orbits covered only by angiomatous stroma. Acrania is absence of the cranium, with protrusion of disorganized brain tissue. Both are generally grouped together, and anencephaly is considered to be the final stage of acrania. These lethal anomalies can be diagnosed in the late first trimester, and with adequate visualization, virtually all cases may be diagnosed in the second trimester. An inability to view the biparietal diameter should raise suspicion. Hydramnios from impaired fetal swallowing is common in the third trimester."-Williams 24/e p201*

Anencephaly

Acrania	Anencephaly
• **Absence of cranium**, with **protrusion of a disorganized mass of brain tissue** that resembles a **"shower cap" (arrows)**[Q] • Characteristic **triangular facial appearance**[Q].	• **Absence of forebrain & cranium** above skull base & orbit. • **Long white arrow** points to **fetal orbit** & short white arrow indicates **nose**[Q].

Anencephaly

- **Absence of a major portion of brain, skull & scalp** that occurs during embryonic development.
    - It is **a cephalic disorder** that **results from a neural tube defect** that occurs when **rostral (head) end of neural tube fails to close**, usually between 23rd & 26th day following conception.
- **Largest part of brain consisting mainly of cerebral hemispheres**, including neocortex, which is responsible for cognition[Q].
- The **remaining structure is usually covered only by a thin layer of membrane**—skin, bone, meninges, etc. are all lacking[Q].

Encephalocele	Cystic Hygroma	Omphalocele
• Image depicts a **large defect in occipital region of cranium** (arrows) through which **meninges & brain tissue have herniated.**	• **Massive multiseptated hygromas** (arrowheads) in the setting of hydrops fetalis at 15 weeks.	• Omphalocele as a **large abdominal wall defect** with **exteriorized liver covered by a thin membrane.**

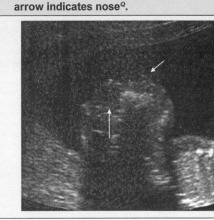

Head Malformations	
Anencephaly	• Due to failure of closure of the rostral neuropore[Q]
Holoprosencephaly	• **Incomplete separation**[Q] of the cerebral hemispheres • Seen in **Patau's syndrome**[Q]
Porencephaly	• **Cysts or cavities**[Q] **in the brain** may result from developmental defect or acquired lesions including infarction of tissue
Lissencephaly	• Bat like brain with **no cerebral convolutions**[Q] & a poorly formed sylvian fissure (agyria)

Contd...

Contd...

Head Malformations	
Schizencephaly	• Unilateral or bilateral **cleft in cerebral hemispheres,** microgyria[Q]
Encephalocele	• **Malformed diverticulum of CNS tissue** extending through a defect in cranium[Q]
Arnold-Chiari deformity	• **Elongation of cerebellar tonsils** & drawing of cerebellum into 4th ventricle[Q] • Associated with myelomeningocele.
Dandy-Walker malformation	• Enlarged posterior fossa, **absent cerebellar vermis** & a large midline cyst[Q].
Shapiro's syndrome	• Agenesis of **corpus callosum**[Q]

143. Ans. c. Dilatation and curettage *(Ref: Shaw's 16/e p316, 15/e p246)*

The given instrument is a plastic, flexible Karman's cannula, used for dilatation and curettage. For dye instillation in hysterosalpingography, Rubin's cannula is used.

Karman Cannula
• It is a long tubular structure made of plastic or metal.
Types: • Rigid or flexible (A **plastic cannula** is preferred because it is **less traumatic, transparent & disposable**)
Sizes: • 4-12 mm (number of cannula corresponds to diameter of cannula in millimeters)
Parts: • **Distal end:** Double whistle at the terminal end; **Proximal end:** Fixes into syringe. • Superior overhanging edge acts as a curette.
Used for: • Endometrial aspiration; Dilatation & curettage • To **remove retained products of conception in missed abortion**

144. Ans. b. Amniotic sac and yolk sac *(Ref: Williams 24/e p170)*

A double bleb sign is a sonographic feature where there is visualization of a gestational sac containing a yolk sac and amniotic sac giving an appearance of two small bubbles. The embryonic disc is located between the two bubbles. It is an important feature of an intrauterine pregnancy and thus distinguishes a pregnancy form a pseudogestational sac or decidual cast cyst.

Ultrasound Findings in Early Pregnancy
• **Gestational sac:** Mean sac diameter
• **Yolk sac**
• **Fetal pole**: Crown rump length
• **Confirming intrauterine gestation:** Double decidual sac sign, intra-decidual sign & double bleb sign[Q]

Sonographic Recognition of Pregnancy

• **Transvaginal sonography** is commonly used to **accurately establish gestational age & confirm pregnancy location**[Q].
• A gestational sac (a **small anechoic fluid collection within endometrial cavity**) is **first sonographic evidence of pregnancy**. It may be seen with transvaginal sonography by **4 to 5 weeks gestation**[Q].
    • **Pseudo-gestational sac** (pseudosac): A **fluid collection** can also be seen **within endometrial cavity** with an **ectopic pregnancy**[Q]
    • A **normal gestational sac** implants eccentrically in endometrium[Q]
    • **Pseudosac** is seen in the **midline of endometrial cavity**[Q].
• Other **potential indicators of early intrauterine pregnancy**:
• **Intradecidual sign**: Anechoic center surrounded by a **single echogenic rim**[Q]
• **Double decidual sign**: Two concentric echogenic rings surrounding the gestational sac[Q]
• **Visualization of yolk sac** (a **brightly echogenic ring with an anechoic center**) **confirms** with certainty an **intrauterine location for pregnancy** & can normally be seen by **middle of 5th week**[Q].
• Up to **12 week's gestation, crown-rump length** is predictive of **gestational age within 4 days**[Q].

Double bleb sign	Double decidual sac sign	Intradecidual sac sign
• Visualization of a **gestational sac** containing a **yolk sac & amniotic sac** giving an **appearance of two small bubbles**[Q] • Feature of an **intrauterine pregnancy**[Q] • **Distinguishes a pregnancy form a pseudo-gestational sac** or **decidual cast cyst**[Q].	• **Two concentric echogenic rings surrounding the gestational sac** • Helps in **distinguishing between an early intrauterine pregnancy & a pseudo-gestational sac**[Q].	• **Site of implantation** is seen as an **early gestational sac** or **an intrauterine fluid collection** or an **echogenic area in markedly thickened decidua** on one side of uterine cavity[Q] • Useful feature for **identifying an early intrauterine pregnancy**[Q]

Decidual reaction surrounding the gestational sac — Endometrial cavity — Geastational sac

Ultrasound Signs of Pregnancy	
Twin peak sign	• Presence of a **dichorionic-diamniotic**[Q] twin gestation (multiple gestation) • Also called **lambda sign**[Q] • Most useful in **assessing the chorionicity of pregnancies after 10 weeks**[Q].
T sign	• Denotes a **monochorionic pregnancy** (it is really the **absence of a twin-peak sign**[Q])
Intradecidual sac sign	• **Anechoic center** surrounded by a **single echogenic rim**[Q] • Useful feature for **identifying an early intrauterine pregnancy**[Q]
Double decidual sac sign	• **Two concentric echogenic rings surrounding the gestational sac**[Q] • Helps in **distinguishing between an early intrauterine pregnancy & a pseudo-gestational sac**[Q].
Double bleb sign	• Visualization of a **gestational sac** containing a **yolk sac & amniotic sac** giving an **appearance of two small bubbles**[Q] • **Distinguishes a pregnancy from a pseudo-gestational sac** or **decidual cast cyst**[Q].
Interstitial line sign	• Finding in **interstitial ectopic pregnancy**[Q]
Tubal ring sign	• Sign of a **tubal ectopic pregnancy**[Q] • Comprises of an **echogenic ring** surrounding an **unruptured ectopic pregnancy**[Q]
Empty amnion sign	• Visualization of an **amnionic sac without concomitant visualization of an embryo**[Q]. • **Indicator of pregnancy failure** regardless of mean sac diameter[Q].

145. Ans. d. Cardiac output *(Ref: Dutta 8/e p60-61, 7/e p51-53; Williams 24/e p59)*

All the four options given in the question increases during pregnancy. Even cardiac output at term is more as compared to a non-pregnant female, but it is lesser than first and second trimester, mainly due to IVC compression. Hence, cardiac output it is the best answer.

"Cardiac output increases from the fifth week of pregnancy and reaches its maximum levels at approximately 32 weeks, after which there is only a slight increase until labor, delivery, and the postpartum period."-Miller Anesthesia 7/chapter 69

Hemodynamic Changes during Pregnancy			
	Non-Pregnant	**Pregnancy near Term**	**Change**
Cardiac output (litre/min)	4.5	6.26	+40%
Stroke volume (ml)	65	75	+27%
Heart rate (per minute)	70	85	+17%

Blood pressure	Unaffected or mid-pregnancy drop of diastolic pressure by 5-10 mm Hg		
Venous pressure	8-10 cm (femoral)	20 cm water	+100% water
Colloid oncotic pressure	20	18	-14%
Systemic vascular resistance			-21%
Pulmonary vascular resistance			-34%

Physiological Changes in Cardiovascular System During Pregnancy

- **Peripheral vasodilation** leading to a decrease in systemic vascular resistance is thought to be the **first cardiovascular change associated with pregnancy (induced by progesterone^Q)**.

    - **Cardiac output increases in response to this, by 20% at 8 weeks gestation** & by up to **40-50% at 20-28 weeks gestation^Q**.
    - This is achieved **predominantly via an increase in stroke volume** (due to an increase in ventricular end-diastolic volume, wall muscle mass & contractility) but **also by an increase in heart rate^Q**.

    - **Labour** leads to **further increases in cardiac output by 15% in first stage & 50% in second stage** due to combination of **auto-transfusion** of 300-500 ml of blood back into the circulation with each uterine contraction & **sympathetic stimulation** caused **by pain & anxiety^Q**.

- **Cardiac output increases again immediately after delivery** due to **auto-transfusion of blood** via uterine contraction and **relief of aortocaval compression.** This may increase cardiac output by as much as 60-80%, followed by a **rapid decline to pre-labour values within 1 hour^Q**.

Physiological Changes in Blood Volume During Pregnancy

- **Hypervolemia associated with normal pregnancy** averages **40-45% above** the non-pregnant blood volume after 32 to 34 weeks^Q.
- It **meets the metabolic demands of enlarged uterus** & greatly **hypertrophied vascular system**.
- **Provides abundant nutrients & elements** to support the **rapidly growing placenta & fetus^Q**.

    - **Increased intravascular volume protects the mother & fetus**, against the deleterious effects of impaired venous return in supine & erect positions^Q.
    - It **safeguards the mother** against the adverse effects of **parturition- associated blood loss^Q**.

- Maternal blood volume **begins to increase during 1st trimester,** expands **most rapidly during 2nd trimester.** It then rises at a **much slower rate** during **3rd trimester to plateau during last several weeks** of pregnancy^Q.

    - Blood volume expansion results from an **increase in both plasma & erythrocytes^Q**.
    - **More plasma than erythrocytes** is **added to the maternal circulation** (hence **fall in hematocrit)^Q**.

Physiological Changes in Respiratory System During Pregnancy

- **FRC decreases** by approximately **20-30%** or **400-700 mL during pregnancy^Q**.
- This capacity is composed of expiratory reserve volume—which decreases 15-20% or 200-300 mL—and residual volume— which decreases 20-125% or 200-400 mL.

    - **FRC & residual volume decline due to diaphragm elevation^Q**.
    - **Inspiratory capacity increases by 5-10% or 200-250 mL during pregnancy^Q**.
    - **Total lung capacity** is unchanged or decreases by **<5% at term^Q**.

- **Respiratory rate** is essentially **unchanged, but tidal volume and resting minute ventilation increase significantly as pregnancy advances^Q**.
- **Peak expiratory flow rates increase progressively as gestation advances^Q**.
- **Lung compliance is unaffected by pregnancy^Q**.

    - **Airway conductance** is **increased & total pulmonary resistance reduced**, as a result of progesterone^Q.
    - **Maximum breathing capacity** & forced or timed vital capacity are **not altered** appreciably^Q.

Physiological Changes in Kidney During Pregnancy

- **Kidney size increases** approximately 1.5 cm.
- **GFR & renal plasma flow increase early in pregnancy**[Q].
- **GFR increases** as much as **25% by 2nd week after conception & 50% by** beginning of **2nd trimester.**
- **Hyperfiltration result from:**
  - **Hypervolemia-induced hemodilution lowers protein concentration & oncotic pressure** of plasma entering the glomerular microcirculation[Q].
  - **Renal plasma flow increases** by 80% before the end of 1st trimester.
    - **Elevated GFR persists until term,** even though **renal plasma flow decreases during late pregnancy**[Q].
    - Primarily as a consequence of **elevated GFR**, approximately **60% of women** report **urinary frequency** during pregnancy[Q].
- During the **puerperium**, a **marked GFR persists during 1st postpartum day** principally **from reduced glomerular capillary oncotic pressure**[Q].
- **Relaxin increases endothelin & nitric oxide production in renal circulation**, leading to **renal vasodilation & decreased renal afferent & efferent arteriolar resistance**, with a resultant increase in renal blood flow & GFR[Q].

146. Ans. a. Mullerian agenesis   *(Ref: Williams 24/e p149; Shaw's 16/e p128, 15/e p145)*

Findings of amenorrhea with normally developed breast, pubic hairs and blind vagina with absent uterus is highly suggestive of Mullerian agenesis. Presence of pubic hair and well-developed breasts confirms that ovaries are functioning and rules out Turner's syndrome or Gonadal dysgenesis.

Feature	Mullerian Agenesis	Turner's syndrome (Gonadal Dysgenesis)	Androgen Insensitivity Syndrome
Presentation	Amenorrhea[Q]	Amenorrhea[Q]	Amenorrhea[Q]
Breasts	Normally developed	Poorly developed[Q]	Enhanced (Tanner Stage 5)[Q]
Pubic/Axillary Hair	Present	Present	Absent[Q]
Stature	Normal	Short[Q]	Normal
Uterus	Absent[Q]	Present	Absent[Q]
Vagina	Blind[Q]	Present/Ambiguous[Q]	Absent proximal (upper) vagina[Q]
Ovaries	Present	Streak gonads[Q]	Abdominal testis present[Q]

Rokitansky-Kuster-Hauser syndrome

- **Mullerian agenesis** is the cause of **primary amenorrhea,** which is characterized by **absence of uterus /vagina**, also known as **Rokitansky-Kuster- Hauser syndrome**[Q].
- **Rare** disorder; Prevalence: 1:4000-5000 female births
- Patients have a **46,XX karyotype & normal secondary sex characteristics**[Q].

Characteristic Features of Rokitansky-Kuster-Hauser Syndrome

- **External genitalia appear normal**, but only a **shallow vaginal pouch** is present[Q].
- **Ovarian function is normal**[Q].
- **Absence of both the vagina & uterus**[Q].
- **Only symmetric uterine remnants** (the muscular buds), **normal fallopian tubes**, and **normal ovaries are present**[Q].

147. Ans. d. Hypomenorrhea   *(Ref: Shaw's 16/e p250; Novak's 13/e p351)*

Hypomenorrhea is seen in Asherman syndrome

"Asherman's syndrome, which is more common with secondary amenorrhea or hypomenorrhea, may occur in patients with risk factors for endometrial or cervical scarring, such as a history of uterine or cervical surgery, infections related to use of an intrauterine device, and severe pelvic inflammatory disease. It is found in 39% of patients undergoing hysterosalpingography who have previously undergone postpartum curettage. Infections such as tuberculosis and schistosomiasis may cause Asherman's syndrome but are rare in the United States."- Novak's 13/e p351

Asherman Syndrome
• **Asherman's syndrome** or **Fritsch syndrome** is a condition characterized by **adhesions and/or fibrosis of the endometrium most often associated** with *dilation & curettage* of intrauterine cavity[Q]. • **MC type of adhesions: Bands of scar tissue** that **span from one wall of uterus to another**[Q].
Etiology: • Related to **procedures involving the uterus after pregnancy**, such as a **D&C**[Q]. • **Curettage for postpartum complications** such as postpartum haemorrhage or retained placenta[Q] • **Dilation & evacuation** (D&E) or **dilation & curettage (D&C)** for a miscarriage, abortion, or retained products of conception[Q]. • **Pelvic infection** after a delivery, miscarriage or abortion[Q] • **Pelvic tuberculosis** is a **common cause of intrauterine adhesions** in the **developing world**[Q].
Clinical Features: • Can be asymptomatic • **Infertility (43%) >Amenorrhea (37%) > Hypomenorrhea (32%)**[Q] • **Recurrent pregnancy loss, cyclic pelvic pain**[Q] <blockquote>• **Menstrual anomalies are often but not always correlated with severity: adhesions restricted to only the cervix or lower uterus may block menstruation**[Q].</blockquote>
Diagnosis: • **Hysterosalpingogram (HSG)**[Q] • **Gold standard investigation: Hysteroscopy**[Q] (directly visualize uterine cavity & define extent & nature of any adhesions) • **Transvaginal ultrasound**: To evaluate & measure the endometrial stripe (thickness of endometrial lining). • **Endometrial biopsy:** To sample the lining to the uterus as a way of determining if any abnormal endometrium is present.
Treatment: • **Hysteroscopic lysis of adhesions & removal of scar tissue**[Q] • Preventing reformation of the scar tissue after the initial lysis of adhesions

148. **Ans. a. Observation and follow-up for cyst after 2–3 months** *(Ref: Shaw's 15/e p369)*

The patient is premenopausal, 3 weeks after LMP (likely to have ovulated) with a 5 cm cyst. The scenario presented here likely represents the patient having a corpus luteum cyst. These cysts need not be approached aggressively unless causing significant symptoms.

Corpus Luteum Cyst
• **Type of functional cyst**, occurs after an **egg has been released from a follicle.** • Follicle becomes a **secretory gland** known as **corpus luteum**. • Ruptured follicle begins **producing large quantities of estrogen & progesterone** in preparation for conception[Q].
Pathophysiology: • If a pregnancy doesn't occur, **corpus luteum breaks down & disappears**[Q]. • It **may fill with fluid or blood, causing corpus luteum to expand into a cyst** & stay in the ovary[Q].
Clinical Features: • In women of reproductive age, **cysts <5 cm are common**, clinically **inconsequential & physiological condition** • It can grow to **almost 10 cm** in diameter. • If it **fills with blood, cyst may rupture**, causing **internal bleeding & sharp pain**[Q]. • Rarely, it may cause **ovarian torsion** & causes **pain**.
Diagnosis: • Cysts that **persist beyond 2 or 3 menstrual cycles**, or occur **in post-menopausal women** should be investigated through **ultrasonography & laparoscopy**, especially with **family history of ovarian cancer**[Q]. • Such cysts may require **surgical biopsy**. • **CA-125:** Increased levels in ovarian cancer

Corpus Luteum Cyst	
Management:	
• **Functional cysts & hemorrhagic ovarian cysts** usually **resolve spontaneously[Q].**	
• **Treatment** may be required if **cysts persist over several months, grow** or **cause increasing pain[Q].**	

Indications for Surgery	
• Persistent complex ovarian cysts[Q] • Persistent symptomatic cysts[Q] • Complex ovarian cysts >5 cm[Q]	• Simple ovarian cysts >10 cm or >5 cm in postmenopausal patients[Q] • Menopausal or perimenopausal patients[Q]

149. **Ans. a. Less chance of extension**   *(Ref: Williams 24/e p551)*

A mediolateral episiotomy is preferred because it has a much lesser chance of extension through the perineum till anal sphincter, though there is increased risk of blood loss and it is difficult to repair.

Type of Episiotomy		
Characteristic	**Midline**	**Mediolateral**
Surgical repair	Easy[Q]	More difficult[Q]
Faulty healing	Rare[Q]	More common[Q]
Postoperative pain	Minimal[Q]	Common[Q]
Anatomical results	Excellent[Q]	Occasionally faulty[Q]
Blood loss	Less[Q]	More[Q]
Dyspareunia	Rare[Q]	Occasional[Q]
Extensions	Common[Q]	Uncommon[Q]

Episiotomy
• Episiotomy is **incision of pudendum**—the **external genital organs**.   • Incision may be **made in midline**, creating a **median or midline episiotomy**.   • It may also **begin off the midline & directed laterally & downward** away from rectum, termed a **mediolateral episiotomy.**
Indications & Consequences: • **Restricted use of episiotomy** is preferred to routine use.   • Applied selectively for **shoulder dystocia, breech delivery, macrosomic fetuses, operative vaginal deliveries, persistent occiput posterior positions &** instances in which **failure to perform an episiotomy will result in significant perineal rupture[Q].**
Episiotomy Timing: • Before episiotomy, **analgesia** may be provided by existing labor epidural analgesia, by **bilateral pudendal nerve blockade**, or by **infiltration of 1% lidocaine**.   • Typically, **episiotomy is completed when the head is visible during a contraction to a diameter of approximately 4 cm**, that is, **crowning[Q].**   • When used **in conjunction with forceps delivery**, most perform an **episiotomy after application of blades[Q].**
Technique: • For **midline episiotomy, fingers** are **insinuated between crowning head & perineum**. Scissors are positioned at 6 o'clock on the vaginal opening & directed posteriorly. **Incision length** varies from **2 to 3 cm** depending on perineal length & degree of tissue thinning. **Incision** should **stop well before reaching the external anal sphincter[Q].**   • With **mediolateral episiotomy**, scissors are **positioned at 7 o'clock or at 5 o'clock** & incision is **extended 3 to 4 cm toward the ipsilateral ischial tuberosity[Q].**

150. **Ans. d. Placenta succenturiata**   *(Ref: Williams 24/e p117)*

A succenturiate lobe is a variation in placental morphology and refers to a smaller accessory placental lobe that is separate to the main disc of the placenta. There can be more than one succenturiate lobes. In this case, typically an accessory lobe seems to have been left inside, which caused postpartum hemorrhage. One or more small accessory lobes (succenturiate lobes) may develop in the membranes at a distance from the main placenta. These lobes have vessels that course through the membranes. If these vessels overlie the cervix to create a vasa previa, they can cause dangerous fetal hemorrhage if torn. An accessory lobe may also be retained in the uterus after delivery and cause postpartum uterine atony and hemorrhage.

1166 AIIMS ESSENCE

> *"A placenta containing three or more equally sized lobes is rare and termed multilobate. However, more frequently, one or more small accessory lobes—succenturiate lobes—may develop in the membranes at a distance from the main placenta. These lobes have vessels that course through the membranes. If these vessels overlie the cervix to create a vasa previa, they can cause dangerous fetal hemorrhage if torn. An accessory lobe may also be retained in the uterus after delivery and cause postpartum uterine atony and hemorrhage."*-Williams 24/e p117

151. Ans. d. Remove intrauterine contraceptive device   *(Ref: Novaks 14/e p263; Dutta 8/e p618-619, 6/e p540)*

Women who become pregnant with an IUCD in situ should be informed of the increased risks of second-trimester miscarriage, preterm delivery and infection if the intrauterine method is left in situ. Removal would reduce adverse outcomes but is associated with a small risk of miscarriage.

Women with IUCD in-situ with Amenorrhea
• A woman with an **IUCD in place**, **with amenorrhea** should have **a pregnancy test & pelvic examination**.
• **An intrauterine pregnancy can occur** & continue successfully to term with an IUCD in place.

Intrauterine pregnancy with visible IUCD strings	IUCD should be removed as soon as possible in order to prevent septic abortion, premature rupture of membranes & premature birth

Intrauterine pregnancy with non-visible IUCD strings[Q]	• **USG** should be performed **to localize IUCD & determine whether expulsion has occurred.**
	• **If IUCD is present, three options for management:**
	  – **Therapeutic abortion**[Q]
	  – **If IUCD is not fundal in location: USG guided intrauterine removal of IUCD**[Q].
	  – **If IUCD is present in fundus of uterus:** It should be **left in place** & pregnancy continued with the device left in place[Q].

- If **pregnancy continues with the device in place**, the patient should be warned of the **symptoms of intrauterine infection** like fever or flu-like symptoms, **abdominal cramping or bleeding**[Q].
- At the **earliest sign of infection**, **high dose IV antibiotics therapy** should be given & **pregnancy evacuated promptly**[Q].

152. Ans. c. 5   *(Ref: Williams 24/e p525-526; Dutta 8/e p600, 7/e p722)*

Cervical Station: -1 = 2; Cervical Dilatation: 1 cm = 1; Effacement: 30% = 0 ; Cervix Position: Posterior = 0; Consistency: Soft = 2. Hence, Bishop Score = 5.

Bishop Scoring System Used for Assessment of Inducibility					
Score	Cervical Factor				
	Dilatation (cm)	Effacement (%)	Station (-3 to +2)	Consistency	Position
0	Closed	0-30	−3	Firm	Posterior
1	1-2	40-50	−2	Medium	Midposition
2	3-4	60-70	−1	Soft	Anterior
3	≥ 5	≥ 80	+1, +2	–	–

Bishop Score
• **Quantifiable method** used to **predict labor induction outcomes**.
• **As favorability or Bishop score decreases, rate of induction to effect vaginal delivery** also **declines**.
• A **Bishop score of 9** conveys a high likelihood for a successful induction.
• Woman whose **cervix is 2-cm dilated, 80% effaced, soft & mid-position and with fetal occiput at −1 station** would have a **successful labor induction**.
• For research purposes, a **Bishop score of 4 or less** identifies an **unfavorable cervix** & may be an **indication for cervical ripening**.

Modified Bishop Score
• According to **Modified Bishop's pre-induction cervical scoring system**, effacement has been replaced by **cervical length in cm**, with scores as follows: **0 for >3 cm, 1 for >2 cm, 2 for >1 cm, 3 for >0 cm**.
• **Another modification** for the Bishop's score is the **modifiers**.

Contd...

Contd...

Points are added or subtracted according to special circumstances	
One point is added for	**One point is subtracted for**
• **Existence of pre-eclampsia**[Q] • **Every previous vaginal delivery**[Q]	• **Postdated pregnancy**[Q] • **Nulliparity**[Q] • **PPROM**[Q] (preterm premature rupture of membranes)

153. Ans. d. Adenomyosis   *(Ref: Shaw's 16/e p413-415, 15/e p475; Novak's 13/e p184; Robbins 9/e p1012)*

Clinical features like abdominal pain and menorrhagia with normal endometrial biopsy and on ultrasound diffuse, symmetrical enlargement of uterus, in a perimenopausal women without any focal lesion is highly suggestive of Adenomyosis.

"A related disorder, adenomyosis, is defined as the presence of endometrial tissue within the uterine wall (myometrium). Adenomyosis remains in continuity with the endometrium, presumably signifying down growth of endometrial tissue into and between the smooth muscle fascicles of the myometrium. Adenomyosis occurs in up to 20% of uteri. On microscopic examination, irregular nests of endometrial stroma, with or without glands, are arranged within the myometrium, separated from the basalis by at least 2 to 3 mm. Like endometriosis, the clinical symptoms of adenomyosis include menometrorrhagia (irregular and heavy menses), colicky dysmenorrhea, dyspareunia, and pelvic pain, particularly during the premenstrual period. It can coexist with endometriosis."- Robbins 9/e p1012

"Adenomyosis often is asymptomatic. Symptoms typically associated with adenomyosis include excessively heavy or prolonged menstrual bleeding and dysmenorrhea, often beginning up to a week before the onset of a menstrual flow."- Novak's 13/e p184

"The uterus is diffusely enlarged, although usually less than 14 cm in size, and is often soft and tender, particularly at the time of menses. Mobility of the uterus is not restricted, and there is no associated adnexal pathology."- Novak's 13/e p184

Adenomyosis

- **Adenomyosis** is characterized by **presence of ectopic glandular tissue in the muscular wall of uterus (myometrium)**[Q].
- Typically found in women **35 to 50 years**
- **Extension of endometrium into myometrium.**[Q]
- It is due to **dysfunction of junctional zone**[Q]

Pathology:
- **Irregular nests of endometrial stroma, with or without glands,** are arranged within myometrium[Q]

Clinical Features:
- Adenomyosis often is **asymptomatic**[Q].
- **Clinical symptoms include menometrorrhagia (irregular & heavy menses), colicky dysmenorrhea, dyspareunia & pelvic pain, particularly during the premenstrual period**[Q].
  - **Uterus is diffusely enlarged, boggy, soft & tender**, particularly at the time of menses **without associated adnexal pathology. Mobility of uterus is not restricted**[Q].

Diagnosis:
- Adenomyosis is a **clinical diagnosis & imaging studies**, although helpful, are **not definitive**.
- Uterus may be imaged using **transvaginal ultrasound (TVS) or MRI** (better diagnostic capability due to increased soft tissue differentiation).

Diagnostic Features of Adenomyosis on TVS	
• **Globular enlarged uterus**[Q] • Sign of **endometrial invasion to myometrium**[Q] • Heterogenous echogenicity • Ill-defined endometrial echo	• Hypoechoic myometrium with **multiple small cysts in myometrium (honeycomb appearance, Swiss cheese pattern**[Q]**)** • Increased vascularity within myometrium

Management:
- **Hysterectomy: Most effective treatment** for adenomyosis[Q]
- **Levonorgestrel-releasing IUCD, GnRH analogues (**Danazol), uterine embolization & endometrial ablation.

1168   AIIMS ESSENCE

154. Ans. a. Ventricular septal defect   *(Ref: Nelson 20/e p898)*

Most common congenital abnormality in a baby of diabetic women is ventricular septal defect.

"The incidence of congenital anomalies is increased threefold in infants of diabetic mothers; cardiac malformations (ventricular or atrial septal defect, transposition of the great vessels, truncus arteriosus, double-outlet right ventricle, tricuspid atresia, coarctation of the aorta) and lumbosacral agenesis are most common. Additional anomalies include neural tube defects, hydronephrosis, renal agenesis and dysplasia, duodenal or anorectal atresia, situs inversus, double ureter, and holoprosencephaly. These infants may also demonstrate abdominal distention caused by a transient delay in development of the left side of the colon, the small left colon syndrome."- Nelson 20/e p898

<table>
<tr><th colspan="2">Effects of Diabetes Mellitus on Pregnancy</th></tr>
<tr><th>Maternal Complications</th><th>Fetal Complications</th></tr>
<tr>
<td>

During pregnancy:
- **Recurrent abortions in uncontrolled diabetes[Q]**
- **Preterm labour because of infection, polyhydramnios[Q]**
- **Infection specially UTI[Q]**
- **Increased incidence of pre-eclampsia (25%)[Q]**
- **Polyhydramnios[Q]**

During labour: increased incidence of
- **Prolongation of labour** due to big baby[Q]
- **Shoulder dystocia** due to disproportionate growth with increased shoulder / head ratio[Q]
- Perineal injuries, postpartum hemorrhage

Puerperium:
- Puerperal sepsis, lactational failure

</td>
<td>

- Fetal macrosomia (30-40%) due to maternal hyperglycemia & elevation of maternal free fatty acids
- Congenital malformations (6-10%) is related to the severity of diabetes affecting organogenesis, in the first trimester.

Major Birth Defects in Infants of Diabetic Mothers	
CNS & skeletal	• **NTD** • **Anencephaly[Q] (MC)** • **Microcephaly** • **Sacral agenesis**
Cardiac	• **VSD[Q], ASD** • Coarctation of aorta • **Transposition of great vessels[Q]** • Cardiomegaly
Renal	• Renal agenesis • Hydronephrosis, ureteral duplication
GIT	• Duodenal atresia, anorectal atresia
Others	• Single umbilical artery

</td>
</tr>
</table>

Neonatal complications	
• Hypoglycemia[Q] • Respiratory distress syndrome[Q] • Hyperbilirubinemia[Q] • Polycythemia[Q]	• Hypocalcemia[Q] • Hypomagnesemia[Q] • Cardiomyopathy[Q]

MC fetal association with maternal diabetes	• **Fetal macrosomia[Q]**
MC congenital fetal malformation with maternal diabetes	• **Congenital heart disease[Q]**
MC congenital heart disease with maternal diabetes	• **VSD[Q]**
Most specific congenital heart disease with maternal diabetes	• **TGA[Q]**
Most specific congenital malformation with maternal diabetes	• **Sacral agenesis[Q] (Caudal regression syndrome[Q])**

PEDIATRICS

155. Ans. a. Decrease mechanical ventilation   *(Ref: Ghai 8/e p393)*

In the given chest X-ray, there is hyperinflated left lung with increased cardiac shadow and bilateral diffuse haziness. In a patient of pneumonia on mechanical ventilation with the above clinical picture, it is indicative of the child developing acute respiratory distress syndrome as a result of volutrauma. Hence, decreasing mechanical ventilator settings is the management of choice.

"There are many pulmonary and systemic complications of mechanical ventilation. Lung injury may result from positive pressure (barotrauma), oxygen toxicity, or excessive volume changes in the lung-volutrauma. Volutrauma may be manifested acutely as pulmonary air leak, such as pneumothorax, pneumomediastinum, pulmonary interstitial emphysema, and bronchopleural fistula. Volutrauma may also be a cause of chronic repetitive lung injury, exacerbating the primary disease. Evidence of decline in lung function as measured by pulmonary function testing can occur as quickly as 24 hours of continuous exposure to 100% oxygen, with evidence of diffuse alveolar damage and the onset of acute respiratory distress syndrome usually occurring after 48 hours on 100% oxygen."

156. **Ans. b. Facioscapulohumeral dystrophy** *(Ref: Harrison 19/e p462e-11)*

The picture is showing winging of the left scapula. It can be seen in Facioscapulohumeral dystrophy or long thoracic nerve palsy. Long thoracic nerve palsy is usually due to sports trauma or breast surgeries, and hence unlikely in a child. So FSHD is a better answer. It is one of the muscular dystrophies, which can present asymmetrically and unilaterally.

"Facioscapulohumeral Dystrophy: The condition typically has an onset in childhood or young adulthood. In most cases, facial weakness is the initial manifestation, appearing as an inability to smile, whistle, or fully close the eyes. Weakness of the shoulder girdles, rather than the facial muscles, usually brings the patient to medical attention. Loss of scapular stabilizer muscles makes arm elevation difficult. Scapular winging becomes apparent with attempts at abduction and forward movement of the arms. Biceps and triceps muscles may be severely affected, with relative sparing of the deltoid muscles. Weakness is invariably worse for wrist extension than for wrist flexion, and weakness of the anterior compartment muscles of the legs may lead to footdrop."
-Harrison 19/e p462e-11

Facioscapulohumeral Dystrophy (FSHD)
<ul><li>Also known as **Landouzy-Dejerine disease**[Q]; **Autosomal dominant**[Q]</li><li>Shows the **earliest & most severe weakness in facial & shoulder girdle muscles**[Q].</li><li>Most patients have **FSHD type 1 (95%)**, whereas approximately **5% have FSHD2**.</li></ul>
Clinical Features: <ul><li>Typically onset in **childhood or young adulthood**.</li><li>In **most cases, facial weakness is the initial manifestation**[Q] (inability to smile, whistle, or fully close the eyes)</li><li>**Weakness of shoulder girdles** usually brings the **patient to medical attention**[Q].</li><li>**Loss of scapular stabilizer** with **winging of scapula**[Q]</li></ul> <ul><li>**Scapular winging** is prominent, often **even in infants**[Q].</li><li>**Flattening** or **even concavity of deltoid contour is seen**[Q]</li><li>**Biceps & triceps brachii muscles are wasted & weak**[Q].</li></ul> <ul><li>**Weakness** is invariably **worse for wrist extension** than for wrist flexion & **footdrop**[Q].</li></ul>
Laboratory Features: <ul><li>**Serum CK level**: Normal or mildly elevated</li><li>**EMG**: **Indicates a myopathic pattern**.</li><li>**Muscle biopsy**: Nonspecific features of a **myopathy**</li></ul>
Treatment: <ul><li>**No specific treatment** is available; **ankle-foot orthoses** are helpful for footdrop.</li><li>**Scapular stabilization procedures improve scapular winging** but may not improve function.</li></ul>

157. **Ans. a. Pneumothorax is present** *(Ref: Nelson 20/e p2131)*

The chest X-ray above is showing bilateral intercostal chest drainage tubes in place with the mediastinum shadow slightly shifted to the right. As the patient is having intercostal chest tube in place, it is unlikely that he will develop a pneumothorax. There is pleural effusion on the left side which is likely contributing to mediastinal shift to the right.

158. **Ans. b. Absence of murmur** *(Ref: Nelson 20/e p2212; Ghai 8/e p422)*

During cyanotic spell, temporary disappearance or a decrease in intensity of the systolic murmur is usual as flow across the right ventricular outflow tract diminishes.

"Paroxysmal hypercyanotic attacks (hypoxic, "blue," or "tet" spells) are a particular problem during the 1st 2 years of life. The infant becomes hyperpneic and restless, cyanosis increases, gasping respirations ensue, and syncope may follow. The spells occur most frequently in the morning on initially awakening or after episodes of vigorous crying. Temporary disappearance or a decrease in intensity of the systolic murmur is usual as flow across the right ventricular outflow tract diminishes. The spells may last from a few minutes to a few hours. Short episodes are followed by generalized weakness and sleep. Severe spells may progress to unconsciousness and, occasionally, to convulsions or hemiparesis. The onset is usually spontaneous and unpredictable."- Nelson 20/e p2212

Tetralogy of fallot

Four abnormalites that results in insufficently oxygenated blood pumped to the body

1. Narrowing of the pulmonary valve
2. Thickening of wall of right ventricle
3. Displacement of aorta over ventricular septal defect
4. Ventricular septal defect-opening between the left and right ventricles

Tetralogy of Fallot

- **Components:** Pulmonary stenosis[Q] + Ventricular septal defect[Q] + Right ventricular hypertrophy[Q] + **Overriding** or **dextroposed aorta**[Q]
- **MC congenital cyanotic congenital heart disease**[Q] in children >2 years constituting almost **75% of all blue patients.**

Hemodynamics:

- **Pulmonary stenosis** causes **concentric right ventricular hypertrophy without cardiac enlargement**[Q] & an increase in right ventricular pressure.
- **Severity of cyanosis** is **directly proportional** to **severity of pulmonic stenosis**, but **intensity of systolic murmur** is **inversely proportional** to **severity of pulmonic stenosis**[Q].
- Since the right ventricle is effectively decompressed by VSD, **congestive failure never occurs in TOF**[Q].
- **Late & soft P$_2$** is generally **inaudible in TOF; S$_2$** is **single** & **audible sound is A$_2$.**
- On auscultation, **diastolic interval** is **completely clear in TOF,** as there is no third or fourth sound or diastolic murmur.

Clinical Features:

- **MC symptoms** are **dyspnea on exertion** & **exercise intolerance**[Q].

Infancy	Childhood
• **Infant: Progressively deeper cyanosis** occurs[Q] • **Cyanotic spells**[Q] (Hypoxemic spells or Tet spells): Characterized by **sudden onset of cyanosis** or **deepening of cyanosis**[Q], dyspnea with **alteration of consciousness** & decrease or **disappearance of systolic murmur**[Q] (as right ventricular outflow tract becomes completely **obstructed**[Q]).	• **Squatting after exertion to overcome dyspnea**[Q] • **Squatting** is **not specific for TOF**[Q] • **TOF** is **MC congenital lesion** in which squatting is noted[Q]

- **Signs: Central cyanosis**[Q], **clubbing**[Q], **right ventricular heave**[Q], single S$_2$ with ejection systolic murmur at left 3rd interspace[Q]

Investigations:

- **ECG: Right axis deviation, inverted T wave & P pulmonale**[Q]

Characteristic Radiological Features of TOF

- **Normal sized heart** with **upturned apex**[Q] (suggestive of RVH)
- **Absence of main pulmonary artery segment** gives it the shape described as **"Cor-en Sabot"** (Boot shaped heart)[Q]
- **Pulmonary fields** are **oligemic**[Q]
- **Aortic-mitral valve continuity** is **maintained**[Q]
- **Right aortic arch**[Q] (in **25%** patients)

| AIIMS May 2016 | 1171 |

- **Complications:**
- Anemia, infective endocarditis, venous thrombosis
- **Paradoxical embolism**, hemiplegia, **brain abscess**[Q]

Treatment:
- Medical management for anemia & management of complications.

Management of Anoxic Spells in Tetralogy of Fallot
• Knee chest position; humidified oxygen; **Morphine**[Q] 0.1 to 0.2 mg/kg SC
• **Obtain venous pH; sodium bicarbonate**[Q] 1-3 ml/kg (diluted) IV
• **Propranolol 0.1 mg/kg/IV (during spell)**[Q]; 0.5-1 mg/kg/6 hourly orally (alternatives: metoprolol, esmolol)
• **Vasopressors: Methoxamine** IM or IV drip (*Phenylephrine* is a *vasopressor*)[Q]
• Correct anemia & consider surgery

Palliative operations in TOF
• **Blalock-Taussig shunt: Subclavian artery-pulmonary artery anastomosis**[Q]
• **Potts shunt: Descending aorta is anastomosed to pulmonary artery**[Q]
• **Waterston's shunt: Ascending aorta-right pulmonary artery anastomosis**[Q]

- **Definitive operations: Closing the VSD & resecting the infundibular obstruction**[Q].

Fallot's		
Trilogy	**Tetralogy**	**Pentalogy**
• **Pulmonary stenosis**[Q] • **Atrial septal defect**[Q] • **Right ventricular hypertrophy**[Q]	• **Pulmonary stenosis**[Q] • **Ventricular septal defect**[Q] • **Right ventricular hypertrophy**[Q] • **Overriding or dextroposed aorta**[Q]	• **Tetralogy of Fallot + ASD**[Q] or **patent foramen ovale**[Q]

159. Ans. a. Allergy due to the food content *(Ref: Nelson 20/e p1139; Ghai 8/e p90)*

Babies should receive only breast milk or infant formula for the first 6 months of life. Most important reason for this is allergy due to the food content. Gastrointestinal infection may be there but is not that common.

"Exclusive breastfeeding for the first 4-6 months of life may reduce allergic disorders in the first few years of life. Potentially allergenic foods (eggs, milk, wheat, soy, peanut and fish) should be introduced after this period of exclusive breastfeeding to decrease chances of food allergy."- Nelson 20/e p1139

160. Ans. d. Debranching enzyme *(Ref: Nelson 20/e p717-720; Harrison 19/e p433 e-2, 18/e p3200, 3201)*

In this child, a combination of liver and muscle involvement with ketoacidosis and raised liver enzymes points towards Type III glycogen storage disease, i.e. Cori's disease caused by deficiency of debranching enzyme.

In contrast to type I glycogen storage disease, the administration of glucagon 2 hours after a carbohydrate meal provokes a normal increase in blood glucose, but after an overnight fast, glucagon may provoke no change in blood glucose level.

"Type IIIa Glycogen Storage Disease or Cori's Disease or Forbes Disease: Type III GSD is caused by a deficiency of glycogen debranching enzyme activity. Debranching enzyme, together with phosphorylase, is responsible for complete degradation of glycogen. When debranching enzyme is defective, glycogen breakdown is incomplete and an abnormal glycogen with short outer branch chains and resembling limit dextrin accumulates. Deficiency of glycogen debranching enzyme causes hepatomegaly, hypoglycemia, short stature, variable skeletal myopathy, and variable cardiomyopathy."- Nelson 20/e p719

"Hypoglycemia and hyperlipidemia are common. In contrast to type I GSD, elevation of liver transaminase levels and fasting ketosis are prominent, but blood lactate and uric acid concentrations are usually normal. Serum creatine kinase levels can be useful to identify not rule out muscle enzyme deficiency. The administration of glucagon 2 hr after a carbohydrate meal provokes a normal increase in blood glucose; after an overnight fast, glucagon may provoke no change in blood glucose level."-Nelson 20/e p719

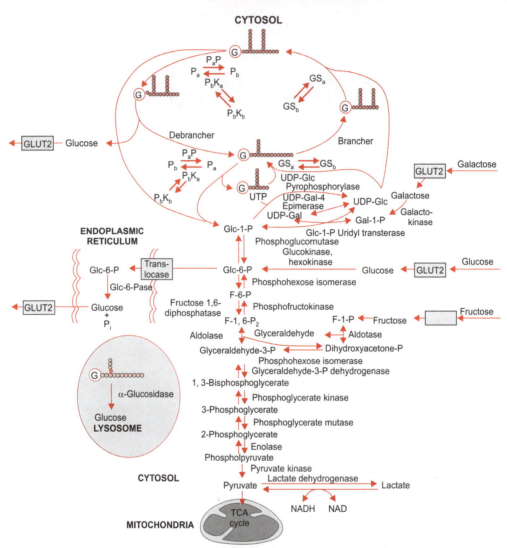

Fig.43: Metabolic pathways related to glycogen storage diseases and galactose and fructose disorders (GS_a, active glycogen synthase; GS_b, inactive glycogen synthase; P_a, active phosphorylase; P_b, inactive phosphorylase; P_aP, phosphorylase *a* phosphatase; P_bK_a, active phosphorylase *b* kinase; P_bK_b, inactive phosphorylase *b* kinase; G, glycogenin, the primer protein for glycogen synthesis)

Type IIIa Glycogen Storage Disease or Cori's Disease or Forbes Disease
• Caused by a **deficiency of glycogen debranching enzyme**[Q]. • **Debranching** & phosphorylase enzyme are responsible for complete degradation of glycogen. • When the **debranching enzyme is defective, glycogen breakdown is incomplete**[Q]. • **Abnormal glycogen accumulates** with short outer chains & **resembles dextrin**[Q].
Clinical & Laboratory Findings: • Deficiency of glycogen debranching enzyme causes **hepatomegaly, hypoglycemia, short stature, variable skeletal myopathy & cardiomyopathy.** Disorder usually **involves both liver & muscle** and is termed **type IIIa glycogen storage disease**[Q]. • **Hypoglycemia, hyperlipidemia & elevated liver transaminases** occur in children[Q].
• Administration of glucagon 2 hour after a carbohydrate meal provokes a normal increase in blood glucose; after an overnight fast, glucagon may provoke no change in blood glucose level[Q].

Contd...

Type IIIa Glycogen Storage Disease or Cori's Disease or Forbes Disease
Diagnosis:
• **Deficient debranching enzyme activity** can be demonstrated in **liver, skeletal muscle & heart**^{Q}
• **DNA-based analyses** now provide a noninvasive way of subtyping these disorders in most patients.
Treatment:
• **Frequent high-carbohydrate meals** with **cornstarch supplements** or nocturnal gastric drip feedings are usually **effective in treating hypoglycemia**^{Q}.
• A **high-protein diet** is recommended as **gluconeogenesis is intact**, providing a source for glucose.

161. **Ans. d. 20 mL/kg of 0.9% normal saline**   *(Ref: Ghai 8/e p718)*

In hypovolemic or septicemic shock, replacement of intravascular volume by isotonic fluids is the main stay of treatment. Hence, normal saline resuscitation with 20 ml/kg boluses is the best answer here.

Management of Septicemic Shock in Children
• **Two large-bore peripheral IV catheters**^{Q} should be placed & **prompt administration of crystalloid** begun.
• **Isotonic solutions** such as **normal saline & Ringer lactate** solution should be **given rapidly** in aliquots of **20 mL/kg**^{Q} **until perfusion, tachycardia & hypotension resolve**^{Q}.
• **Successful outcomes depend on rapidity of infusion**^{Q} & may require drawing fluid into syringes & manually administering the fluid.
• If the administration of **60 mL/kg of crystalloid results in no improvement, myocardial dysfunction should be considered. Inotropic agents (dopamine or epinephrine) improve contractility** by stimulating dopaminergic & β-adrenergic receptors, respectively^Q. • **Pressor agents (norepinephrine) restore SVR through α-adrenergic receptors**^{Q}.
• **Phosphodiesterase inhibitors (milrinone, amrinone) improve contractility**, **facilitate diastolic relaxation & decrease SVR**^{Q}. Milrinone has been shown to improve the cardiac index by 20% in pediatric patients with septic shock.
• Endogenous **vasopressin levels decrease during vasodilatory septic shock** & administration of **low-dose vasopressin** (0.02-0.04 unit/min) restores SVR^Q.
• **Correction of metabolic deficiencies** can also **improve myocardial function**^{Q}.
• **Metabolic acidosis & elevated lactate levels** occur **secondary to tissue hypoperfusion**^{Q}; administration of sodium bicarbonate has not been shown to decrease morbidity or mortality. • Rather, the **base deficit & serum lactate** are **used to monitor the adequacy of resuscitation**.
• **Calcium & potassium** ions are **integral to conduction & contractility of myocardium** & their levels must be **monitored & supplemented** as needed.

162. **Ans. a. Reassure the parents and follow up after 6 months**   *(Ref: Nelson 20/e p2585; Ghai 8/e p504)*

Bed-wetting is normal till 5 years of age. In a child with only night-time bed wetting, when urinalysis (to rule out infections) and urine osmolality (to rule out diabetes) are normal, only regular follow up is required. An anatomic abnormality requiring USG-KUB is unlikely. The decision on whether to start treatment should be guided by degree of concern and motivation on part of the child rather than the parents. General advice can be given, but active treatment need not be started before 6 years. In this case, only a behavioral and motivational therapy is required. A referral to psychiatrist should be done only if behavioral therapy fails or it is causing significant distress to the child. If the option says Referral to a psychologist instead of a psychiatrist, you may consider that option as well with regard to behavioral therapy.

*"**The best approach to treatment is to reassure the child and parents that the condition is self-limited and to avoid punitive measures that can affect the child's psychologic development adversely.** Fluid intake should be restricted to 2 oz after 6 or 7 pm. The parents should be certain that the child voids at bedtime. Avoiding extraneous sugar and caffeine after 4 pm also is beneficial. If the child snores and the adenoids are enlarged, referral to an otolaryngologist should be considered, because adenoidectomy can cure the enuresis." -Nelson 20/e p2585*

"Active treatment should be avoided in children <6 years of age, because enuresis is extremely common in younger children. Treatment is more likely to be successful in children approaching puberty compared with younger children."- *Nelson 20/e p2585*

Nocturnal Enuresis
• **Nocturnal enuresis** refers to **occurrence of involuntary voiding at night after 5 years**[Q].
• By 5 years of age, 90-95% of children are nearly completely continent during the day & 80-85% are continent at night.
• **Primary (75-90%):** Children with enuresis; **nocturnal urinary control never achieved**
• **Secondary (10-25%):** **Child was dry at night** for at least a few months & then enuresis developed

Epidemiology

• More common in **boys**.

• **Family history is positive** in 50% of cases.

Clinical Manifestations:

• A careful history with respect to **fluid intake at night** & **pattern of nocturnal enuresis**.

• **History of snoring** loudly at night.

• Examined carefully for **neurologic & spinal abnormalities**.

Diagnosis:

• **Urine examination:** Increased incidence of bacteriuria in enuretic girls

• Absence of glycosuria should be confirmed.

• If there are **no daytime symptoms, physical examination & urinalysis are normal & urine culture is negative, further evaluation** for urinary tract pathology generally is **not warranted**.

• **Renal USG** is in an **older child** with enuresis or in **children who do not respond to therapy**.

Treatment

• **Best approach: Reassure the child & parents** that the **condition is self-limited** & to **avoid punitive measures** that can affect the child's psychologic development adversely[Q].

• **Fluid intake should be restricted to 2 oz after 6 or 7 pm; child should void at bedtime**[Q].

• Avoiding **extraneous sugar & caffeine after 4 pm** is beneficial[Q].

• **Snoring & enlarged adenoids**: Referral to an otolaryngologist because **adenoidectomy** can cure enuresis[Q].

• **Active treatment should be avoided in children <6 years of age**, because **enuresis is extremely common in younger children**[Q].

• Treatment is more likely to be **successful in children approaching puberty compared with younger children**.

• **Simplest initial measure: Motivational therapy** & includes a star chart for dry nights[Q].

Conditioning therapy	• Use of a loud auditory or vibratory alarm attached to a moisture sensor in the underwear. **Most effective in older children**[Q].
Psychologic therapy	• **Primary role** of psychologic therapy is **to help the child deal with enuresis psychologically** & help **motivate the child to void at night** if he or she awakens with a full bladder[Q].
Pharmacologic therapy	• **Pharmacologic therapy** is regarded as **second-line** and is **not curative**. • **Desmopressin acetate**[Q] is effective in 40% of children. • **Anticholinergic therapy (Oxybutynin or tolterodine**[Q]**):** For therapy-resistant enuresis or children with symptoms of an overactive bladder • **Imipramine**[Q] (Tricyclic antidepressant)

ORTHOPAEDICS

163. **Ans. b. Monteggia fracture** *(Ref: Apley's 9/e p770-771)*

In the given X-ray, head of radius is dislocated forwards with fracture of upper third of ulna with forward bowing[Q].

> *"**Monteggia Fracture:** With isolated fractures of the ulna, it is essential to obtain a true anteroposterior and true lateral view of the elbow. **In the usual case, the head of the radius (which normally points directly to the capitulum) is dislocated forwards, and there is a fracture of the upper third of the ulna with forward bowing. Backward or lateral bowing of the ulna (which is much less common) is likely to be associated with, respectively, posterior or lateral displacement of the radial head.** Trans-olecranon fractures, also, are often associated with radial head dislocation."-Apley's 9/e p770*

Monteggia Fracture

- **Fracture of shaft of ulna associated with dislocation of proximal radio-ulnar joint**[Q]
- **Radio- capitellar joint is inevitably dislocated or subluxated as well**[Q].

Mechanism of injury:
- **Fall on the hand**; if at the moment of impact the body is twisting, its momentum may forcibly pronate the forearm.
- **Radial head usually dislocates forwards & upper third of ulna fractures & bows forwards**[Q].
- Sometimes the causal force is **hyperextension**[Q].

Clinical features:
- **Ulnar deformity** is **usually obvious** but **dislocated head of radius is masked by swelling**[Q].
- **Pain & tenderness on lateral side of the elbow**[Q]

X-ray:
- **Head of radius is dislocated forwards** with **fracture of upper third of ulna with forward bowing**[Q].

Treatment:
- **Key to successful treatment: Restore the length of fractured ulna**; only then can the dislocated joint be fully reduced & remain stable.
- **Very unstable fracture, always treated by open reduction & external fixation (OREF)**
- **Adults: Operation through a posterior approach**

Complications:
- **Nerve injury** caused by over- enthusiastic manipulation of radial dislocation or during surgical exposure.
- **Malunion & Non-union**

Galeazzi's Fracture

- It is a **fracture of lower one-third of radius with dislocation of distal radioulnar joint**[Q].

Mechanism of injury:
- **Fall on the hand; probably with a superimposed rotation force**[Q].
- **Radius fractures in its lower third & inferior radio-ulnar joint subluxates or dislocates**[Q].

Clinical features:
- **More common** than Monteggia
- **Striking feature: Prominence or tenderness over the lower end of ulna**[Q]

  - It may be possible to demonstrate the **instability of radio-ulnar joint by 'ballotting' the distal end of the ulna ('piano-key sign') or by rotating the wrist**[Q].

X-ray:
- **A transverse or short oblique fracture** is seen in lower third of radius, **with angulation or overlap**. The **distal radio-ulnar joint is subluxated or dislocated**[Q].

Treatment:
- **Perfect reduction is essential for complete restoration of all functions**; called **fracture of necessity** because **surgery is absolutely necessary**
- Restore the length of the fractured bone.
- **Children: Closed reduction is often successful**;
- **Adults**: **Reduction by open operation & compression plating of radius.**

Colles' fracture	• Fracture of distal radius in forearm with **dorsal (posterior) & radial displacement of wrist & hand.** • Occurs as a result of **falling onto wrists in extension.** • Referred to as a **'dinner fork' or 'bayonet' deformity** due to shape of resultant forearm.
Smith's fracture (reverse Colles' fracture)	• **Fracture of distal radius** caused by a direct blow to dorsal forearm or falling onto flexed wrists • **Distal fracture fragment is displaced ventrally,** as opposed to a Colles' fracture in which the fragment is displaced dorsally

164. Ans. a. Radial nerve *(Ref: Apley's 9/e p749, 760)*

The given X-ray is showing Holstein-Lewis fracture of the lower shaft of humerus. The most commonly involved nerve is radial nerve, which passes in its groove on the posterior aspect of humerus bone.

"Radial nerve palsy (wrist drop and paralysis of the metacarpophalangeal extensors) may occur with shaft fractures, particularly oblique fractures at the junction of the middle and distal thirds of the bone (Holstein–Lewis fracture)."
– Apley's 9/e p749

Injury	Common nerve involved
Surgical neck of humerus	• **Axillary nerve**[Q]
Shaft of humerus	• **Radial nerve**[Q]
Medial condyle of humerus	• **Ulnar nerve**[Q]
Monteggia fracture dislocation	• **Posterior interosseus nerve**[Q]
Volkmann's ischemic contracture	• **Anterior interosseous nerve**[Q]
Lunate dislocation	• **Median nerve**[Q]
Hip dislocation	• **Sciatic nerve**[Q]

165. Ans. d. Gaenslen's *(Ref: Apley's 9/e p499)*

The given X-ray is showing features of Developmental dysplasia of Hip. All the tests mentioned in the options maybe seen except the Gaenslen's test.

"Gaenslen's test is used to detect musculoskeletal abnormalities and primary-chronic inflammation of the lumbar vertebrae and sacroiliac joint. This test is often used to test for spondyloarthritis, sciatica, or other forms of rheumatism."

"DDH is usually suspected in the early neonatal period due to the widespread adoption of clinical examination (including Ortolani's test, Barlow maneuvers, Galeazzi's sign). The diagnosis is then usually confirmed with ultrasound, although the role of ultrasound in screening is controversial."

Developmental Dysplasia of Hip (DDH)
• DDH comprises a spectrum of disorders including **acetabular dysplasia without displacement, subluxation & dislocation**[Q]. • More common in **girls & in left hip**[Q]
Etiology & Pathogenesis: • **Genetic factors**[Q] • **Hormonal factors** (e.g. high levels of maternal estrogen, progesterone & relaxin in the last few weeks of pregnancy) may **aggravate ligamentous laxity in the infant**[Q]. • **Intrauterine malposition** (especially a **breech position with extended legs**[Q]) favors dislocation • **Plagiocephaly, congenital torticollis & postural foot deformities** are associated with a higher than usual incidence of DDH.

Contd...

AIIMS May 2016

Contd...

Developmental Dysplasia of Hip (DDH)

Clinical Features:

Testing for Instability in Developmental Dysplasia of Hip	
Ortolani's test[Q]	• Baby's thighs are held with the thumbs medially & fingers resting on the greater trochanters; hips are flexed to 90° & gently abducted. Normally there is smooth abduction to almost 90°. • In congenital dislocation, movement is usually impeded, but if pressure is applied to greater trochanter there is a soft 'clunk' as the dislocation reduces & then the hip abducts fully (**'jerk of entry'**). • If **abduction stops halfway and there is no jerk of entry**, there may be an **irreducible dislocation**.
Barlow's test[Q]	• Examiner's thumb is placed in the groin & by grasping the upper thigh, an attempt is made to lever the femoral head in and out of the acetabulum during abduction and adduction. • If femoral head is normally in reduced position, but can be made to slip out of the socket & back in again, **hip is classed as 'dislocatable' (i.e. unstable).**
Galeazzi's sign[Q]	• **With unilateral dislocation, skin creases look asymmetrical & leg is slightly short & externally rotated**[Q]
Vascular Sign of Narath[Q]	• **Tests for presence of head of femur. Palpate femoral artery pulse bilaterally to evaluate volume, intensity & position.** • **If very readily palpated:** Possible **unreduced anterior hip dislocation.** • **If palpated with great difficulty or not felt at all,** it implies **femoral head displaced from the hip joint due to hip dislocation,** most commonly **posterior hip dislocation**[Q].

• **Late features:** An observant mother may spot **asymmetry, a clicking hip, or difficulty in applying the napkin** (diaper) because of **limited abduction.**

Imaging:
• **Ultrasonography:** Ultrasound scanning has replaced radiography for imaging hips in the newborn. Radiographically 'invisible' acetabulum & femoral head can be displayed with static & dynamic ultrasound.
• **Plain x-rays:** X-rays of infants are **difficult to interpret, more useful after first 6 months**

166. **Ans. c. Congenital pseudoarthrosis of tibia**   *(Ref: Apley's 9/e p185)*

The image is showing anterolateral bowing of tibia, which is commonly seen in congenital pseudoarthrosis of tibia.

*"**Congenital Pseudarthrosis of Tibia**: This rare condition is usually diagnosed in early infancy. **The child may be born with a fractured tibia, or the bone may be attenuated and then fracture some months later. In either case, the fracture fails to unite, or heals very poorly only to fracture again shortly afterwards. By the age of two years the leg is noticeably short and bowed anterolaterally.** By then it has become obvious that this is an intractable condition which will not yield to ordinary forms of fracture treatment."-Apley's 9/e p185*

Congenital Pseudarthrosis of Tibia

• Characterized by **anterolateral bowing of tibia** that **can lead to a fracture that fails to reunite**[Q]
• Diagnosed in **early infancy**.
• Linked to **type I neurofibromatosis**[Q]

Clinical Features:
• Child may be born with a **fractured tibia,** or the bone may be **attenuated** & then **fracture some months later**. In either case, **fracture fails to unite**, or **heals very poorly only to fracture again shortly afterwards**[Q].
• **By 2 years of age, leg is noticeably short & bowed anterolaterally**[Q].

Contd...

Contd...

Congenital Pseudarthrosis of Tibia
Diagnosis: • **X-ray: Gap, or marked thinning of tibial shaft.** Sometimes the fibula also is affected. • **Biopsy: Histological features of neurofibromatosis**[Q]
Treatment: • **Excise the affected segment of bone, correcting the deformity & closing the gap** gradually by bone transport in a circular external fixator (**Ilizarov technique**). • **Excision of abnormal segment & replacement by a vascularized fibular graft.** • Limb can be 'stabilized' & held in reasonable alignment with a clamshell orthosis & an intramedullary device until the child is old enough to undergo limb reconstruction.

167. Ans. a. Ankylosing spondylitis *(Ref: Harrison 19/e p2170, 18/e p2775; Apley's 9/e p68)*

Given X-rays showing irregular subchondral erosions, sclerosis of articulating surfaces and widening of sacro-iliac joint space with squaring of vertebra and loss of lumbar lordosis is seen in ankylosing spondylitis.

"Ankylosing Spondylitis: The cardinal sign – and often the earliest – is erosion and fuzziness of the sacroiliac joints. Later there may be peri-articular sclerosis, especially on the iliac side of the joint and finally bony ankylosis.

The earliest vertebral change is flattening of the normal anterior concavity of the vertebral body ('squaring'). Later, ossification of the ligaments around the intervertebral discs produces delicate bridges (syndesmophytes) between adjacent vertebrae. Bridging at several levels gives the appearance of a 'bamboo spine'."- Apley's 9/e p68

Ankylosing Spondylitis/Marie-Strumpell or Bechterew's Disease
• **Generalized chronic inflammatory disease** in which effects are seen **mainly in spine & sacroiliac joints**. • Characterized by **pain & stiffness of back**, with variable involvement of **hips & shoulders** (rarely the peripheral joints)
Etiology & Pathogenesis: • **More than 90% patients of AS are HLA B27 positive**[Q]. • The **enthesis**, the **site of ligament attachment to bone** is **primary site of pathology in AS**[Q]. • **Sacroilitis** is the **earliest manifestation** with features of both **enthesitis & synovitis**[Q].

Clinical Presentation:
• More common in **males**
• **Age of onset** is **15-25 years (late adolescence & early adulthood)**[Q].
• The **initial symptom** is usually **dull pain**, insidious in onset, accompanied by **low back morning stiffness of up to few hours duration that improves with activity and returns following period of inactivity**[Q].
• Arthritis in hips & shoulders (root joints) occur in **25-35%**[Q].
 	
    • **Peripheral joints (usually shoulder, hips & knees) are involved in one third of patients**[Q].
    • **Most serious complication of spinal disease** is **spinal fracture** with even minor trauma.
    • **MC extra-articular manifestation is acute anterior uveitis (iridocyclitis)**[Q].

Diagnosis:

Radiological Examination	
(The following changes may be seen on an X-ray of the pelvis)	
• **Earliest change: Haziness** of **sacro-iliac joints**[Q] (Sacroileitis) • **Irregular subchondral erosions** in **SI joints**[Q] • **Sclerosis of articulating surfaces** of **SI joints**[Q] • **Widening** of **sacro-iliac joint space**[Q] • **Bony ankylosis** of the **sacro-iliac joints**[Q] • **Dagger sign:** Single radiodense line related to supraspinous & interspinous ligaments	• **Calcification** of **sacro-iliac ligaments & sacro-tuberous ligaments** • **Evidence of enthesopathy: Calcification** at the attachment of muscles, tendons & ligaments, **particularly around pelvis & heel**[Q]. • **Andersson lesion: Discovertebral fracture** in AS • **Trolley/Tram Track sign:** Three vertical linear increased density lines

Contd...

Contd...

Ankylosing Spondylitis/Marie-Strumpell or Bechterew's Disease
X-ray of Lumbar spine in Ankylosing Spondylitis
<ul><li>**Squaring of vertebra**[Q]: Normal anterior concavity of vertebral body is lost due to calcification of anterior longitudinal ligament</li><li>**Loss of lumbar lordosis**[Q]</li><li>**Shiny corner sign (Romanus lesion)**</li></ul> <ul><li>**Bridging osteophytes (syndesmophytes)**[Q]</li><li>**Bamboo spine appearance**[Q] due to syndesmophytes & paravertebral ossification</li></ul>
Treatment: <ul><li>**Phenylbutazone** is **most effective drug**[Q] (causes aplastic anemia).</li><li>**Indomethacin** is **most commonly used NSAID**[Q].</li></ul>

168. **Ans. a. Giant cell tumor**   *(Ref: Apley 9/e p202, 215)*
A 30 years old male patient presents with pain in hip for last 6 months and X-ray of hip joint shows lytic lesion on the right femur near hip joint. In the given X-ray, epiphyseal lytic lesion in femur with a 'soap bubble' appearance is characteristic of giant cell tumor (osteoclastoma). The tumour always abuts against the joint margin in osteoclastoma.

"**X-ray (Giant cell tumor): Radiolucent area situated eccentrically at the end of a long bone & bounded by subchondral bone plate**. The **centre** sometimes has a **soap-bubble appearance** due to ridging of the surrounding bone. Appearance of a 'cystic' lesion in mature bone, extending right up to the subchondral plate, is so characteristic that the diagnosis is seldom in doubt."- *Apley 9/e p202*

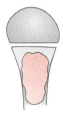
Solitary bone cyst upper limb metaphyseal? Fracture

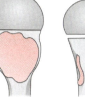
Aneurysmal bone cyst metaphyseal expanding eccentric

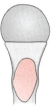
Fibrous cortical defect lower limb cortical lesion

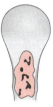
Fibrous cortical defect lower limb cortical lesion

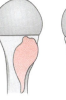
Chondroma calcification

Chondromyxoid fibroma eccentric dense endosteal margin

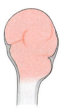
Chondro-blastoma epiphysis

Giant cell tumour mature bone always extends to subarticular margin

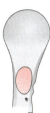
Brown tumour think of it! Look for signs of HPT

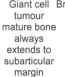

Fig. 44: Cysts and cyst-like lesions of bone
(Thumb-nail sketches of lesions which appear as 'cysts' on X-ray examination)

Simple Bone Cyst	Adamantinoma	Multiple Myeloma
<ul><li>**Fills the medullary cavity but does not expand the bone**[Q]</li><li>**X-rays:** Well-defined radiolucent cyst, often trabeculated & eccentrically placed[Q].</li><li>In a growing tubular bone it is **always situated in the metaphysis**[Q].</li></ul>	<ul><li>**X-ray** shows a typical **bubble-like defect in the anterior tibial cortex**; sometimes there is thickening of the surrounding bone[Q].</li></ul>	<ul><li>X-rays: The 'classical' lesions are multiple punched-out defects with 'soft' margins (lack of new bone) in the skull, pelvis and proximal femur, a crushed vertebra, or a solitary lytic tumour in a large-bone metaphysis[Q].</li></ul>

169. Ans. c. Osteoclast giant cells constitute the proliferative component of the tumor *(Ref: Robbins 9/e p1204; Apley's 9/e p202)*

In giant cell tumors, osteoclast giant cells are the malignant cells, which induce the proliferation of mononuclear macrophage lineage cells, hence the dividing cell population is the mononuclear cells which form the matrix. Osteoclast giant cells do not constitute the proliferative component of the tumor.

See Q. no. 168 AIIMS May 2016.

"Histologically, the tumor consists of sheets of uniform oval mononuclear cells and numerous osteoclast-type giant cells with 100 or more nuclei. The nuclei of the mononuclear cells and the osteoclasts are similar, ovoid with prominent nucleoli. Thus, the neoplastic population of osteoblast precursors is difficult to identify on routine histology. Necrosis and mitotic activity may be prominent. Although reactive bone, especially at the periphery of a lesion, may be present, the tumor cells do not synthesize bone or cartilage."-Robbins 9/e p1204

"Giant cell tumors are typically treated with curettage, but 40% to 60% recur locally. Up to 4% of tumors metastasize to the lungs, but these sometimes spontaneously regress and they are seldom fatal."-Robbins 9/e p1204

OPHTHALMOLOGY

170. Ans. a. Nocardia asteroides *(Ref: Yanoff & Duker 4/e p219; Smolin and Thoft's The Cornea 4/e p248)*

Keratitis caused by Nocardia asteroides, which is a filamentous bacteria, closely resembles the morphology of corneal ulcers caused by fungi.

"Corneal infections with Nocardia, Actinomyces, and Streptomyces typically follow an indolent clinical course, which may simulate mycotic keratitis with hyphal edges, satellite lesions, and elevated epithelial lesions."- Smolin and Thoft's The Cornea 4/e p248

"Nocardia infections tend to follow trauma, especially if there is soil contamination. The ulcer is characteristically superficial, with a wreath-shaped gray-white infiltrate and an undermined necrotic edge. The base might assume a cracked windshield appearance. Nocardia keratitis often resembles fungal infection, with a filamentous appearing border and satellite lesions. Infection appears to be indolent; the anterior chamber reaction is often minimal. However, rarely, more severe anterior chamber reaction and hypopyon can be seen."

Nocardia
• **Gram-positive, branching pleomorphic rods** with **intermittent or beaded staining patterns[Q]**, especially when invading tissues.
• **Nocardiae** are **gram-positive weakly acid-fast branching rod- shaped bacteria** and can be **visualized by a modified Ziehl-Neelsen stain** like **Fite-Faraco method[Q]**.
• **Nocardia asteroides** is **most frequently found species infecting humans[Q]**
• Most cases occur as an **opportunistic infection in immunocompromised patients.**
Staining & Culture Characteristics:
• Because it is **acid-fast to some degree**, it **stains only weakly Gram-positive[Q]**.
• Visualized by a **modified Ziehl-Neelsen stain** like **Fite-Faraco method[Q]**.
• **Stain black** with the **methenamine-silver stain.**
• In culture, **Nocardia are not fastidious** but do tend to **grow slowly.**
• Colonies will **grow on most bacterial, fungal, or mycobacterial media that lack antibiotics.**
• *Blood & Sabouraud's agars* are good substrates for pathogenic organisms that usually grow satisfactorily at temperatures between *35-37°C[Q]*.
• *Growth of N. asteroides* is facilitated by *10% carbon dioxide[Q]*.
Clinical Features:
• **MC form of human nocardial disease** is a **slowly progressive pneumonia[Q]**, the common symptoms of which include **cough, dyspnea & fever**.
• Nocardia species are deeply involved in the process of **endocarditis** as one of its main pathogenic effects.
• Nocardia infection takes the form of **encephalitis** and/or **brain abscess formation** (In 25–33%)
• **Cutaneous infections:** Actinomycetoma (especially **N. brasiliensis**), **lymphocutaneous disease, cellulitis, & subcutaneous abscesses[Q]**.

Contd...

AIIMS May 2016

Contd...

Nocardia
Nocardia keratitis
• **Nocardia infections tend to follow trauma,** especially if there is **soil contamination**[Q].
• **Ulcer is characteristically superficial,** with a **wreath-shaped gray-white infiltrate** & an **undermined necrotic edge. Base** might assume a **cracked windshield appearance**[Q].
• **Nocardia keratitis** resembles **fungal infection**[Q], with a **filamentous appearing border & satellite lesions**.

Diagnosis:

- **First step in diagnosis: Examination of sputum or pus for crooked, branching, beaded, gram-positive filaments *1 mm wide and up to 50 mm long*[Q].**

- **Most Nocardiae are acid-fast in direct smears if a weak acid is used for decolorization** (e.g., in the **modified Kinyoun, Ziehl-Neelsen, and Fite-Faraco methods)**[Q].

- **Recovery from specimens** containing a mixed flora **can be improved with selective media (colistin-nalidixic acid agar, modified Thayer-Martin agar,** or **buffered charcoal-yeast extract agar)**[Q].

  - **Nocardiae grow relatively slowly;** colonies may take up to 2 weeks to appear and may not develop their **characteristic appearance, white, yellow, or orange, with aerial mycelia and delicate, dichotomously branched substrate mycelia,** for up to 4 weeks[Q].

- **Nocardia isolation from biological specimens** can be performed using **buffered charcoal-yeast extract agar (BCYE),** the same **used for Legionella species**[Q].

171. **Ans. a. Aspergillosis**   *(Ref: Yanoff & Duker 4/e p225; Parson 22/e p203, 21/e p199)*

Pain and watering in the eye for 36 hours with presence of corneal ulcer having elevated margins, feathery hyphae, finger like projections and minimal hypopyon is highly suggestive of fungal corneal ulcer. In the question, Aspergillus is the only fungus.

"Mycotic or fungal keratitis is frequently seen in tropical countries, rural areas and in immunocompromised individuals. It is commonly due to Aspergillus, Fusarium or Candida albicans. Fungal ulcers are typically seen after injury with vegetable matter such as a thorn or wooden stick and are characterized by a relatively indolent course. Symptoms are much milder than the clinical signs would suggest. The slough in these ulcers is dry in appearance with feathery borders, surrounded by a yellow line of demarcation, which gradually deepens into a gutter and there may also be a hypopyon. An immune ring (Wessely) may be visible due to deposition of immune complexes and inflammatory cells around the ulcer. Satellite lesions may also be seen. There is marked ciliary and conjunctival congestion, but symptoms of pain, watering and photophobia are disproportionately less as compared to those in cases of bacterial corneal ulcers. The hypopyon, if present, is thick and immobile, and is due to direct invasion into the anterior chamber of fungal hyphae enmeshed in thick exudates."-Parson 22/e p203

172. **Ans. a. Volume of tears is measured as it changes color on contact with tears**   *(Ref: Yanoff & Duker 4/e p277)*

Phenol red dye test measures the production of tears without topical anesthesia, as the dye changes its color to red on contact with tears. It doesn't require pH meter for reading the result.

*"Hamano et al. developed the **phenol red thread test to obviate the disadvantages of Schirmer's test by eliminating the need for anesthesia.** Three millimeters of a fine dye-impregnated 75 mm cotton thread is placed under the lateral one-fifth of the inferior palpebral lid margin for 15 seconds; alkalinity changes its color to bright orange from tear contact."*

"The Schirmer's test is used to test aqueous tear production. Traditionally, instilling a topical anesthetic and then placing a thin strip of filter paper in the inferior cul-de-sac perform the basic secretion test. The corners of a soft tissue paper may be used to wick all liquid from the inferior fornix by capillary attraction without any wiping or direct irritation before the paper is placed. The patients' eyes are then closed for 5 minutes, and the amount of wetting in the paper strip is measured. Less than 5 mm of wetting is abnormal; 5–10 mm is equivocal."

Phenol Red Thread Test
• **Phenol red** is a **pH indicator used in cell biopsy** as it **changes colour from yellow to red** on pH range from **6.8 to 8.2**[Q].
• **Used to measure residual tears in inferior conjunctival sac,** especially in **dry eye patients**[Q].

Contd...

Contd...

Phenol Red Thread Test
Procedure: • Phenol red impregnated thread is taken, which is yellow. • 3 mm folded edge is placed in conjunctival sac **without anesthesia**^{Q} • After 15 seconds, amount of wetting of thread, which now shows red colour in contact with tears is measured. • **Wetting of <10 mm: Dry eye**^{Q}; **Wetting of 20 mm: Normal tear volume**^{Q}
Advantages: • **Better than Schirmer's test**^{Q} • **Time taken is very short**^{Q} (15 seconds) as compared to 5 minutes in Schirmer's test • **Less reflex tear stimulation** as compared to Schirmer's test^Q

173. **Ans. a.** Unchanged   *(Ref: Yanoff & Duker 4/e p589)*

Photodynamic therapy (PDT) is used in the treatment of wet ARMD. Verteporfin dye and diode laser is used. Immediately after PDT, there is no colour change but after sometime (1 day after PDT) hypopigmentation or whitening of treated area occurs.

Verteporfin Photodynamic Therapy (PDT)

• **PDT** is a technology that **uses low-energy light to activate an intravenously injected photosensitizing agent & induce closure of a neovascular complex**^{Q}.
• **Goal of PDT** is to **specifically target neovascular tissue** while sparing surrounding & overlying retinal structures.
• **No immediate, permanent laser-induced scotoma** is produced & there is no corresponding RPE defect.
   • At day 1 after PDT, a circular region of hypopigmented retina, with a well-demarcated border corresponding to the site of photodynamic activation, is **clearly visible**^{Q}.
   • **Discoloration & whitening decrease gradually**^{Q}, but the border of lesion remains visible.
• *Dynamic changes in distribution, visible color & amount of macular pigment occur.*
• *After initial bleaching (days 1–3), gradual recovery with irregularly shaped distribution is noticeable until 1 month (day 28). After that, the appearance is stable.*
   • **Whitening of the deep retinal layers** & mild graying of treatment area plus **early hypo fluorescence** of the spot up to 4 weeks occurs^Q.

174. **Ans. c.** 50 minutes   *(Ref: Yanoff & Duker 4/e p42; Parson 22/e p98, 21/e p98-100)*

The angular spacing between the bars of the C or E in Snellen's chart is 1 minute for the 6/6 letter (smallest letter). The largest letter on the Snellen's chart is the 6/60 letter. When viewed from a distance of 6 meter, this letter subtends an angle of 50 minutes in the eye and the bars of the letter subtend an angle of 10 minutes

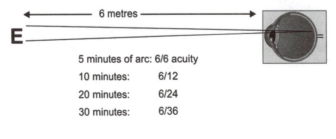

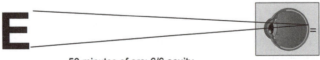

The human eye is just able to discern separate objects if the angle between them is 30 seconds of arc.

"Snellen defined "standard vision" as the ability to recognize one of his optotypes when it subtended 5 minutes of arc. Thus the optotype can only be recognized if the person viewing it can discriminate a spatial pattern separated by a visual angle of 1 minute of arc. 6/60 vision means that the patient can see at 6 m what Snellen's assistant could see at 60 m. The essence of correct identification of the letters on the Snellen's chart is to see the clear spaces between the black elements of the letter. At exactly 6 meters distance from the patient, the letters on the 6/6 line shall subtend 5 minutes of arc (such that the individual limbs of the letters subtend 1 minute of arc), which means that the chart should be sized such that these letters are 8.86 mm tall and the topmost (6/60) "E" should be 88.6 mm tall. Putting it another way, the eye should be at a distance 68.75 times the height of the top (6/60) letter. Another calculation for United States clinics using 20 foot chart distances (slightly closer vice 6 m), and using a 17 mm model eye for calculations, and a letter which subtends 5 minutes of arc, gives a vertical height of the 20/20 letter to be 8.75 mm."

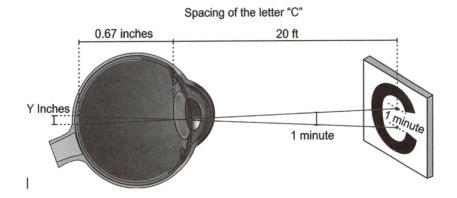

ENT

175. **Ans. c. Allergic fungal sinusitis**   *(Ref: Scott-Brown's 7/e p2734; Byron J. Bailey, Jonas T. Johnson Head & Neck Surgery 4/e p434)*

Complaints of nasal congestion, stuffiness, discharge and anosmia with CT scan of showing peripheral rim of low density, edematous mucosa and there is complete opacification of the central cavity by homogenous high-attenuation material is highly suggestive of allergic fungal sinusitis.

"Allergic fungal sinusitis, a hypersensitivity reaction to fungal antigens, typically occurs among patients with atopy and nasal polyposis. Allergic fungal sinusitis can involve one or many sinus cavities. On CT scans, the involved sinus has a peripheral rim of low density, edematous mucosa and there is complete opacification of the central cavity by homogenous high-attenuation material corresponding to fungus and thick allergic mucin. There are often scattered flecks of calcific material. The sinus wall can be surprisingly expanded and destroyed." -Byron J. Bailey, Jonas T. Johnson Head & Neck Surgery 4/e p434

Allergic Fungal Sinusitis
• **Allergic fungal sinusitis, a hypersensitivity reaction to fungal antigens,** typically occurs among patients with **atopy & nasal polyposis**[Q].   • **Can involve one or many sinus cavities**[Q].
Etiopathogenesis:
• Most patients have a **history of allergic rhinitis**[Q]   • **Thick fungal debris & mucin**[Q] are developed in sinus cavities & must be surgically removed so that the inciting allergen is no longer present.
Clinical Features:
• Signs & symptoms of **nasal airway obstruction, allergic rhinitis, or chronic sinusitis** that includes **nasal congestion, purulent rhinorrhea, postnasal drainage, or headaches**[Q].

Contd...

Allergic Fungal Sinusitis

Diagnosis of Allergic Fungal Sinusitis

CT scan	MRI
• Majority of sinuses show **near complete opacification**[Q]. • **Unenhanced CT**: Sinuses are typically **opacified by centrally (often serpiginous) hyperdense material** with a **peripheral rim of hypodense mucosa**[Q]. • **Heterogeneous areas of signal intensity** within paranasal sinuses filled with **allergic fungal mucin**[Q]. • **Expansion, remodeling, or thinning of involved sinus walls**[Q] caused by expansile nature of the accumulating mucin. • **Areas of high attenuation**[Q] within expanded paranasal sinuses.	• **MC finding: Hypointensity on T1WI & T2WI** • **T1**: Hypointense inflamed mucosal thickness[Q] • **T2**: Hyperintense peripheral inflamed mucosal thickness; **Low T2 signal or signal void**[Q] is due to high concentration of various metals such as iron, magnesium & manganese concentrated by fungal organisms and high protein & low free water content in allergic mucin • **T1 C+ (Gd)**: Inflamed mucosal lining has contrast enhancement[Q]; **No enhancement in the center** or **majority of sinus contents** (c.f. neoplasms)[Q]

Treatment:
- **Treated by local excision & steroid therapy**
- **Antifungal therapy** in some cases

Prognosis:
- **Recurrence after surgery is not uncommon**; inclusion of **steroid therapy significantly reduces relapse**.

176. **Ans. b. Sinus tympani** *(Ref: Scott-Brown's 7/e p1570)*
Encircled structure of middle ear in the given image is sinus tympani.

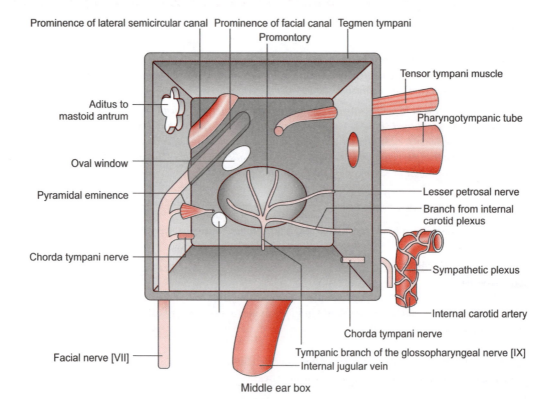

Sinus Tympani

• **Sinus tympani**: **MC & constant depression** present in **retrotympanic area**[Q].
• Located at **junction of lateral & posterior walls** of tympanic cavity.
• Lies between ponticulus superiorly & subiculum inferiorly[Q].
• Bounded by **pyramidal ridge externally & promontory internally**[Q].
• Extend posteriorly up to the round window niche.
      • **Visualization** of this area during middle ear surgery proves **to be a challenge**.
      • It is the most inaccessible site in the middle ear & mastoid.
      • **Cholesteatoma**, which has **extended up to sinus tympani**, is very **difficult to eradicate**[Q].

Subiculum	• Posterior extension of promontory separating oval & round windows[Q].
Ponticulus	• Ponticulus is **a spicule of bone**, which **arises from promontory above subiculum & runs to the pyramid on posterior wall** of middle ear cavity[Q].

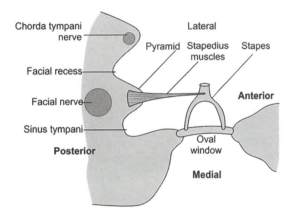

Posterior Wall of Middle Ear

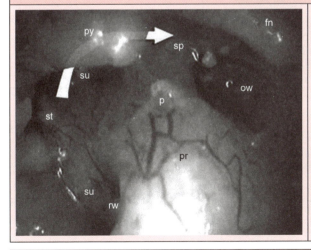 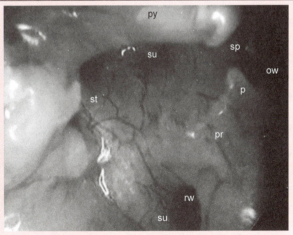

Posterior Wall of Middle Ear
• *It lies close to the mastoid air cells. It has the following main features:* • **Aditus:** An opening through which **attic communicates with mastoid antrum**[Q]. • **Pyramid**: Bony projection from which **originates stapedius muscle**[Q]. • **Facial nerve** runs in **posterior wall just behind the pyramid**[Q].

Contd...

Posterior Wall of Middle Ear
• **Facial recess:** Also called **suprapyramidal recess;** a **depression in posterior wall lateral to pyramid**[Q]; bounded medially by external genu of facial nerve, laterally by chorda tympani nerve, superiorly by fossa incudis & anterolaterally by tympanic membrane. • **Fossa Incudis: Depression on the posterior wall & contains short process of incus**[Q]. • **Sinus tympani:** Lies medial to pyramid; bounded by subiculum below & ponticulus above. • **Round window opening** is **separated from oval window opening by a bony ridge** called the **subiculum**[Q]. • **Ponticulus:** Bony ridge below oval window.

177. **Ans. a. Respiratory papillomatosis** *(Ref: Dhingra 7/e p345-346, 6/e p305)*

Abnormality marked on the fiberoptic laryngoscopy is respiratory papillomatosis. Respiratory papillomatosis is a recurrent condition, common in children and presents with respiratory polyps, which can lead to voice change and stridor.

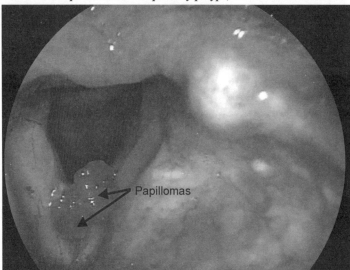

Fig. 45: Respiratory papillomatosis

Juvenile Papilloma (Recurrent Laryngeal Papillomatosis or Recurrent Respiratory Papillomatosis)
• Disease of **viral origin**[Q] characterized by presence of **multiple recurrent papillomas in the larynx**[Q] • Common in **anterior part of glottis**[Q], especially **anterior commissure**[Q] **(MC site: Vocal fold**[Q]) • **More common in children <5 years of age**[Q], equally common in males & females • **First born vaginally delivered child** of a teenage mother is most prone (**Vertical transmission**[Q])
Etiology: • Associated with **HPV infection (HPV-6 & HPV-11)**[Q] • **HPV-11: More aggressive disease** & more prone to malignant change.
Pathology: • **Multiple sessile or pedunculated papilloma, friable & bleed on touch**[Q]
Transmission: • The exact mode is not known. • **Recognized association** between **maternal genital warts** (condylomata acuminata) & **recurrent laryngeal papillomatosis** both conditions being caused by HPV-6 & HPV-11.
Clinical Features: • **Presenting features: Hoarseness & abnormal cry**[Q] • **Dyspnea, stridor**[Q] & eventually complete airway obstruction may occur.
Treatment: • **Surgery:** Primary modality of treatment[Q] • **Endoscopic surgical removal** is the **preferred treatment**[Q] • **CO_2 laser:** MC used modality[Q]

Contd...

Contd...

Juvenile Papilloma (Recurrent Laryngeal Papillomatosis or Recurrent Respiratory Papillomatosis)
• **Recurrence is common** and **multiple procedures are often required**[Q]
Other Treatments Options
• Systemic interferon   • Interferon alpha-2a
• Photodynamic therapy   • 13-cis-retinoic acid
• Intralesional injection of antiviral drug (cidofovir)[Q]
Prognosis:
• **More severe in juvenile onset disease** as compared to adult onset
• **Remission** of recurrent papillomatosis may take place **at any time; more likely to undergo remission in larynx (48%)** than in tracheobronchial tree
• **Malignant transformation is rare** but may be seen (**squamous cell carcinoma**).

178. **Ans. b. Conductive hearing loss of right ear**   (Ref: Scott-Brown's 7/e p1156)

This patient is showing improved hearing in left hear with constant difference in air and bone conduction, i.e. decreased air conduction with normal bone conduction. This is seen typically in conductive hearing loss.

Symbols Used in Audiogram
• **Blue line for left ear**[Q]
• **Red line for right ear**[Q] (Remember **R-R**)
• **Continuous line** for **air conduction**[Q]
• **Broken line for bone conduction**[Q] (Remember **B-B**)

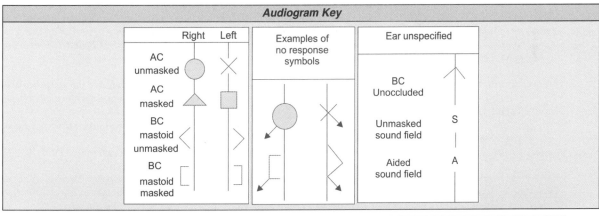

Audiogram		
Normal hearing	**Conductive hearing loss**	**Sensorineural hearing loss**
• This is the **PTA graph seen in normal persons.** • In normal persons, **hearing threshold values with both air & bone remain between 0 and 10 dB**	• Sound cannot properly conduct through outer and/or middle ear to reach the normal-hearing cochlea • **AC thresholds** will be **abnormal in presence of normal BC thresholds** in **disorders of outer and/or middle ear only** • Air-bone gap ≥15 dB difference between AC & BC • In the graph, **bone-air gap is seen** which means a **patient can hear by bone under 10-20 dB**, while with **air hearing is much below**, depending on severity, indicating **conductive hearing loss.**	• **SNHL: Disorder of inner ear and/or auditory nerve** • **AC thresholds will be equal to BC thresholds (no air-bone gap) & both will be abnormal** • Both **bone & air conduction** value are **decreased** and may **even overlap each other.** • In this graph air-bone is not seen. Thus in **SNHL, air bone gap is <15-20 dB.**

Contd...

Contd...

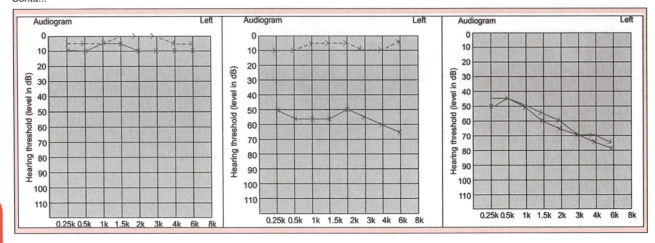

179. Ans. c. Microdebrider   *(Ref: Scott-Brown's 7/e p3576; Cummings Pediatric Otolaryngology By Marci M. Lesperance, Paul W. Flint/p51; Dhingra 6/e p430)*

All these four instruments are used in different techniques of tonsillectomy. Microdebrider is less commonly used than others as it leaves behind a small amount of tissue covering the constrictor muscle. So, preferred answer would be microdebrider.

"The classic technique of tonsillectomy was the so-called cold dissection, in which the tonsil was grasped, the anterior tonsillar pillar was incised, and the capsule was dissected off the pharyngeal constrictors using blunt and sharp dissection. Hemostasis was obtained by suture ligature or electrocautery. Monopolar electrocautery has become the most popular technique of tonsil dissection in the past two to three decades, because it affords greater hemostasis during the dissection. It may be associated with increased postoperative pain and longer healing times."- Cummings Pediatric Otolaryngology By Marci M. Lesperance, Paul W. Flint/p51

"Newer techniques include bipolar cautery, plasma excision (coblation), Harmonic Scalpel, and powered Intracapsular tonsillectomy (PITA). Bipolar cautery allows precise coagulation with less tissue injury and may be performed using a small, bipolar bayonet forceps with the operating room microscope or bipolar electrosurgical scissors. Coblation uses current conducted through normal saline fluid or gel. The Harmonic Scalpel uses ultrasonic vibrations to transfer mechanical energy sufficient to break hydrogen bonds. Its vibrating titanium blades cut at a frequency of 55.5 kHz and generate minimal heat and tissue damage."- Cummings Pediatric Otolaryngology By Marci M. Lesperance, Paul W. Flint/p51

"The most common extracapsular techniques use a "cold" knife (sharp dissection), monopolar electrocautery, bipolar cautery (or bipolar scissors), or harmonic scalpel. Intracapsular techniques may use the micro-debrider, bipolar radiofrequency ablation (which can also be used to remove the entire tonsil), and carbon dioxide laser.
Bipolar radiofrequency ablation can be used to perform an extracapsular or intracapsular tonsillectomy; however, it is most commonly used to perform a partial tonsillectomy."

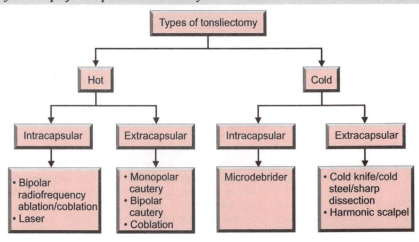

| AIIMS May 2016 | 1189 |

Tonsillectomy
• **Position** of patient during tonsillectomy: **Rose position**[Q]
• **Boyle-Davis mouth gag** is used & held in position with **Draffin's bipods**[Q].
• **Method of performing tonsillectomy: Dissection & snaring method**[Q]

Indications of Tonsillectomy		
Tonsillar indications		**Non-tonsillar indications**
Absolute	**Relative**	
• **Huge hypertrophic tonsil** causing **oro-pharyngeal obstruc-tion**[Q] • **Suspected malignancy** of tonsil[Q]	• **2nd attack of peritonsillar abscess** in children • **Chronic tonsillitis**[Q] • Tonsillitis causing **febrile seizures**[Q] • Tonsillitis in **cardiac valvular disease** patient • Long term management of **IgA nephropathy**[Q] • Severe infectious mononucleosis with upper airway obstruction • **Obstructive sleep apnea & dysphagia due to hypertrophied tonsil**[Q]	• As an approach for elongat-ed styloid process (**Styal-gia or eagle syndrome**)[Q] • **Glossopharyngeal neuralgia**[Q] • As a part of **uvulopalato-pharyngoplasty in ob-structive sleep apnea**[Q]

Contraindications of Tonsillectomy	
Absolute	**Others**
• **Polio epidemic**[Q] • **Submucous cleft palate**[Q]	• **Acute tonsillar infection**[Q] • **Children <3 years of age**[Q] • **Recent acute URTI**[Q]

Types of Tonsillectomy	
Extracapsular (Total or **subcapsular) tonsillectomy**	**Intracapsular (Partial** or **subtotal) tonsillectomy**
• Involves **dissecting lateral to tonsil** in the plane **between tonsillar capsule & pharyngeal musculature** & tonsil is generally removed as a single unit[Q]. • MC extracapsular techniques use a **"cold" knife (sharp dissection)**, **monopolar electrocautery**, **bipolar cautery** (or bipolar scissors), or **harmonic scalpel**[Q]. • **Only extracapsular techniques** should be used for patients undergoing **tonsillectomy as a result of tonsillitis or peritonsillar abscess**[Q].	• Also known as **tonsillotomy**[Q] • Involves **removal of most of tonsil**, while **preserving a rim of lymphoid tissue & tonsillar capsule**[Q]. • **Preservation of this margin of tissue**, this "**biologic dressing**," may **promote an easier recovery**, with **lower haemorrhage rates** and **better recovery of diet & activity**[Q]. • Intracapsular techniques may use the **microdebrider, bipolar radiofrequency ablation** (which can also be used to remove the entire tonsil) & **CO_2 laser**[Q].

Complications of Tonsillectomy
• **MC complication** of tonsillectomy: **Hemorrhage**[Q]   • **Average blood loss** during tonsillectomy: **50-80 ml**[Q]   • **MC cause of bleeding** during tonsillectomy: **Paratonsillar vein**[Q] (**Denis Browne vein**[Q])   • **MC arterial cause of bleeding** during tonsillectomy: **Tonsillar branch of facial artery**[Q] (known as artery of tonsillar hemorrhage[Q])

SKIN

180. **Ans. c. Molluscum contagiosum**   *(Ref: Robbins 9/e p1176; Fitzpatrick 6/e p2347)*

Lesions on the face in a young patient of 5 years with findings of cuplike verrucous epidermal hyperplasia and large, ellipsoid, homogeneous, cytoplasmic inclusion in cells of the stratum granulosum and the stratum corneum on microscopic examination is highly suggestive of Molluscum contagiosum, which is caused by the poxvirus.

"Molluscum contagiosum: On microscopic examination, lesions show cuplike verrucous epidermal hyperplasia. The diagnostically specific structure is the molluscum body, which occurs as a large (up to 35 μm), ellipsoid, homogeneous, cytoplasmic inclusion in cells of the stratum granulosum and the stratum corneum. In the hematoxylin and eosin stain, these inclusions are eosinophilic in the blue-purple stratum granulosum and acquire a pale blue hue in the red stratum corneum. Numerous virions are present within molluscum bodies." -Robbins 9/e p1176

Molluscum contagiosum

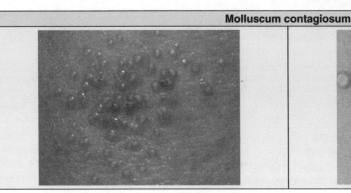
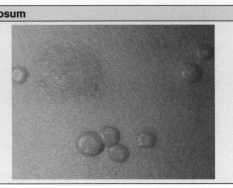

"The histologic appearance of the hypertrophied and hyperplastic epidermis is characteristic. Above the normal-appearing basal layer are lobules of enlarged epidermal cells that contain multiple Feulgen-positive intracytoplasmic inclusion bodies (molluscum bodies or Henderson-Paterson bodies). These inclusion bodies, which contain the viral particles, increase in size as the infected cell moves toward the surface. In the horny layer, the molluscum bodies are enmeshed in a fibrous network that dissolves in the center of the lesions, forming the central core, which is composed primarily of molluscum bodies."- Fitzpatrick 6/e p2347

181. Ans. b. Alopecia areata *(Ref: Rooks 8/e p66.13, Fitzpatrick 6/e p732)*

Discoid patch of alopecia with no scarring, no scaling, papules, inflammation or atrophy and exclamation mark hair (broken-off hair, about 4 mm from the scalp due to constriction in shaft) are highly suggestive of alopecia areata.

"The scalp appears normal in alopecia areata. In affected areas, anagen is abruptly terminated prematurely and affected hairs move prematurely into telogen, with resultant often precipitous hair shedding. The near pathognomonic 'exclamation point' hairs may be present, particularly at the periphery of areas of hair loss. These short broken hairs, whose distal ends are broader than the proximal ends, illustrate their inherent sequence of events: follicular damage in anagen and then a rapid transformation to telogen. White or graying hairs are frequently spared and probably account, in cases of fulminant alopecia areata, for the mysterious phenomenon of 'going gray overnight.' - Fitzpatrick 6/e p732

Alopecia Areata
• **Recurrent, non-scarring alopecia** which can **affect any hair-bearing area**[Q]
• Also known as **spot baldness** or **'Davey Kirts syndrome'**[Q]
• **Associated with other autoimmune diseases**[Q] e.g., myxedema, pernicious anemia etc.
Genetic Factors:
• 10-20% patients give a **family history** & **inheritance is polygenic**[Q]
• Strong association between **alopecia areata** & **MHC class II antigens HLA DR4, DR II (DR 5) & DQ3**[Q]
• **DR4, DR5, DQ3** are associated with **severe alopecia**[Q]
• **DQ3 & DR11** (allele DRB1* 1104) is associated with **alopecia totalis & universalis.**
Pathology:
• It's a **chronic organ specific autoimmune disease**, mediated by **CD8+ T-cells affecting hair follicles**[Q] (**Peribulbar lymphocytic infiltrate** known as **"swarm of bees"**)[Q] & sometimes nail.
• AR autoimmune polyglandular syndrome type 1 (APS-1, autoimmune polyendocrinopathy-candidiasis -ectodermal dystrophy syndrome) & **Down's syndrome** have **high incidence of alopecia areata**[Q].
Clinical Features:
• **Peak incidence** between **2nd and 4th decade (M=F)**
• Characteristic **initial lesion** is a **circumscribed, totally bald, smooth patch**[Q]
• **Short easily extractable broken hairs** known as **exclamation mark hairs**[Q] are seen at margins of bald patch.
• **Scalp is the first affected site in most cases**[Q]

Alopecia totalis	• **Total** or **almost total loss of scalp hair**[Q]
Alopecia universalis	• **Loss of all body hair**[Q]
Ophiasis	• **Alopecia along scalp margin** (Hair loss on sides & the **lower back of scalp**[Q])
Sisaipho pattern	• **Hair loss spares** the **sides & back of head**[Q]
	• Also known as **Ophiasis spelled backward**[Q]

Contd...

Contd...

Alopecia Areata
• **Classical feature** is **sparing of gray/white hairs**[Q] & preferentially affecting pigmented (black) hair. • This results in a **dramatic change in hair colour, if alopecia progress rapidly** & known as "**going white overnight phenomenon**"[Q] • **Nail Involvement: MC finding is pitting** (**fine stippled pitting**[Q]), trachyonychia (roughening of nail plate), onychomadesis, modesis, mottled lunula.
Treatment: • **Intralesional & topical glucocorticoids**[Q] • **Topical antralin or tazarotene**[Q]; **topical contact sensitizers**[Q] (diphencyprone, squaric acid dibutylester)

182. **Ans. a. Methotrexate**   *(Ref: Fitzpatrick 6/e p2676)*

Methotrexate or oral retinoids (Acitretin) are the drug of choice for management of erythrodermic psoriasis.

"Current use of methotrexate to treat psoriasis is most common in patients with severe or refractory plaque-type disease that requires systemic treatment. It is also very useful for erythrodermic and pustular psoriasis, as well as psoriatic arthritis."- Fitzpatrick 6/e p2676

Treatment of Psoriasis vulgaris		
	Treatment of choice	**Alternatives in resistant cases**
Localized (<10% BSA)	• **Topical coal tar + salicylic acid**[Q] • **Topical dithranol**[Q] (short constant)	• Topical steroids + salicylic acid
Moderately extensive (10-30% BSA)	• **Narrow band UVB therapy**[Q] • **PUVA/PUVA sol**[Q]	• Methotrexate
Extensive (> 30% BSA)	• Topical **low-mid potency steroids**[Q]	
Palmoplantar psoriasis	• Topical **high potency steroid** combined with **salicylic acid** even under occlusion[Q]	• Methotrexate (small dose) in debilitating cases

Treatment of Choice in Various Types of Psoriasis		
Type	**Treatment of choice**	**Alternatives in resistant cases**
Erythrodermic psoriasis	• **Methotrexate**[Q] • **Acitretin + Emollients**[Q]	• **Cyclosporine**[Q]
Guttate psoriasis	• **Antibiotics + Emollients** [Q] • **PUVA/PUVA sol**[Q]	• *Coal tar* • *Tacrolimus* • *Mild topical steroids*
Flexural psoriasis	• **Topical low-medium potency steroids** + antifungal agents[Q]	–
Localized pustular psoriasis (Hands & feet)	• **Topical high-potency steroids + Salicylic acid**[Q] • **Topical PUVA/PUVA sol**[Q]	• Methotrexate (small dose)
Generalized pustular psoriasis	• **Retinoids (oral acitretin)**[Q]	• **Methotrexate + Emollients (2nd choice)**[Q]; Cyclosporine • **Oral steroids used only in pregnant women**[Q]

Psoriasis
• **Genetically determined T-cell mediated chronic relapsing disease of skin** with **unknown etiology**[Q] • **Skin lesions** are **erythrosquamous**, which indicates that **both vasculature (erythema) & epidermis (increased scale formation) are involved**[Q]. • Affects **1-2%** of **population; worsens in winter**[Q]
Etiopathogenesis: • **Associated with HLA CW6**[Q] • **Positive family history**[Q] in **>50%** of patients with psoriasis • **Pathology: MC abnormality is increased epidermal proliferation rate**[Q] (**Normal skin: 27 days**[Q]; **Psoriatic skin: 4 days**[Q])

Contd...

Psoriasis

Histological Features of Psoriasis

- **Epidermal mass** is **increased 3-5 times**[Q]
- **Granular layer is constantly absent** over tips of dermal papillae with **parakeratosis**
- **Thick granular layer** between rete ridges[Q]
- **Mitotic figures** above basal layer[Q]
- **Exaggeration of rete pattern**[Q]
- **Prominent elongated papillae** containing dilated, tortuous capillaries[Q]
- **Munro microabscesses**[Q]: Aggregates of neutrophils within the **stratum corneum**
- **Spongiform pustules of Kogoi**[Q]: Aggregates of neutrophils in **stratum spinosum**
- **Squirting papillae**[Q]: Migration of neutrophils out of dilated papillary capillaries.
- **Suprapapillary thinning**[Q] with edematous dermal papillae

Aggravating Factors

- **Sepsis**[Q]
- **Stress**[Q] (emotional)
- **Shivering**[Q] (cold injury)
- **Trauma**[Q]
- **Drugs: Beta-blockers**[Q], **lithium**[Q], **antimalarials**[Q], **ibuprofen, stoppage of steroids**[Q]

Clinical Features:

- **Chronic inflammatory skin disorder** characterized by **erythematous, sharply demarcated papules & round plaques covered by silvery mica like scales**[Q].
- **Scales** of psoriasis are **typically absent in groin & flexures**[Q].
- **MC age of onset: 2nd & 3rd decade;** More common in **males**[Q]
- **Common sites: Extensor aspect of elbows & knees, trunk (back & lumbosacral area**[Q]), **scalp & hands**
- **Skin lesions** are **variably pruritic** (mild or no itching[Q])

Signs in Psoriasis

Auspitz sign[Q]	• When scales are forcefully removed, **pinpoint bleeding from dilated superficial capillaries** occurs **through Bulkeley's membrane**[Q].
Bulkeley's membrane[Q]	• Removal of scales reveals a **glistening red membrane of Bulkeley**[Q].
Candle-grease sign[Q] **(Tache de bouge)**	• When a lesion is scratched with the point of a dissecting forceps, a **candle-grease-like scale**[Q] can be repeatedly produced even from non-scaling lesions.
Grattage test[Q]	• On scratching the lesion, **mica like scales appear**
Koebner/isomorphic phenomenon[Q]	• **Traumatized areas** (scratching, wounds, hat band pressure, sunburn) **develop lesions of psoriasis**[Q]
Woronoff's ring[Q]	• **Whitish halo** around the lesion[Q]

Nail Involvement	• **MC nail finding: Thimble pitting**[Q] • **Onycholysis:** Separation of nail from nail bed[Q] • **Salmon patches** of nail bed[Q] • **Subungal hyperkeratosis:** Keratinous material under nail plate[Q] • **'Oil drop' sign:** Staining of nail bed[Q] • **Thickening & tunneling** of nail plate[Q]
Joint Involvement	• **Skin changes precedes joint disease**[Q] • **Psoriatic arthritis in 30% patients**[Q] • **Nail changes** occur in **90% of psoriatic arthritis**[Q] • **Features of psoriatic arthritis: Distal interphalangeal joint predominant; dactylitis**[Q] **(sausage digits); Arthritis mutilans: Severe destructive arthritis**[Q] • **DOC for psoriatic arthritis: Methotrexate**[Q]

Psoriasis	
X-ray Signs of Psoriatic Arthritis	
Opera glass hand[Q]	• Telescoping of one bone into its neighbor with shortening of digits
Pencil in cup appearance[Q]	• Tapering of proximal phalanx & bony proliferation of distal terminal phalanx
Whiskering[Q]	• Marginal erosions with adjacent bony proliferation

Stable plaque psoriasis | Rupioid psoriasis | Guttate psoriasis | Inverse or seborrhoeic psoriasis

Pustular psoriasis | Erythrodermic psoriasis | General pustular or von Zumbusch psoriasis | Impetigo herpetiformis

Types of Psoriasis	
Stable Plaque psoriasis	• **MC type of psoriasis**[Q] • Commonly involves **elbows, knees, lower back, scalp, nails & napkin area** • In infants, can present as **"nappy rash"**[Q].
Rupioid psoriasis	• **Limpet-like cone-shaped hyperkeratotic lesions** of psoriasis[Q]
Guttate (Eruptive) or raindrop psoriasis	• More common in **children & adolescents** • Frequently preceded by **tonsillitis or pharyngitis by beta-hemolytic streptococci**[Q]
Inverse or seborrhoeic psoriasis	• **Classical lesions on scalp** associated with **less typical moist lesions in body folds**[Q] (groins, **axillae, submammary region, navel**); **No visible scales**[Q] • Can be very **resistant to therapy**.
Pustular psoriasis	• Rare but **serious type** of psoriasis; May be **precipitated by steroid use**[Q] • **Sudden onset with small sterile pustules**[Q] on an erythematous base • **Palms & soles** maybe involved[Q] (**Acrodermatitis pustulosa**[Q]: More common in **smokers**); **Treated with retinoids**[Q]
Erythrodermic psoriasis	• **Precipitated by irritants like tar, dithranol or withdrawal of steroids**[Q] • **Skin** becomes **universally red & scaly**[Q] • **Treatment of choice: Methotrexate**[Q]
General pustular or Von Zumbusch psoriasis	• Combination of **erythroderma & sterile pustular psoriasis**. • **Skin** first becomes **erythrodermic** & then develops **sheets of sterile pustules over trunk & limbs**[Q]. • **Treatment of choice: Retinoids (oral acitretin)**[Q]
Impetigo herpetiformis	• **Generalized pustular eruption of pregnancy**[Q] • Associated with **hypoparathyroidism & hypocalcemia**[Q] • **Treatment of choice: Corticosteroids**[Q] >Cyclosporine • **Methotrexate & retinoids** are **contraindicated in pregnancy**[Q]

AIIMS ESSENCE

183. Ans. a. Patch test *(Ref: Rooks 8/e p26.93, Fitzpatrick 6/e p1451, 1309)*

The clinical picture mentioned above is suggestive of air-borne contact dermatitis, which is a type of allergic contact dermatitis. Most common source is Parthenium exposure and it leads to dermatitis involving the exposed parts, i.e. Face, upper neck, cubital and popliteal fossa. The only useful and reliable method for the diagnosis of allergic contact dermatitis remains the patch test.

> "The only useful and reliable method for the diagnosis of allergic contact dermatitis remains the patch test."- *Fitzpatrick 6/e p1309*

Patch Test	• Detect allergens responsible for type IV hypersensitivity • Finds the cause of allergic contact dermatitis but not of irritant dermatitis.
Prick Test	• Detects type I hypersensitivity, helpful in diagnosing atopic dermatitis.
IgE levels	• May be used to detect atopic states.
Skin Biopsy	• Shows non-specific changes in all dermatitis

Patch Test

- **Patch Test:** Gold-standard method for diagnosis of allergic contact dermatitis resulting from type IV delayed hypersensitivity (allergic contact dermatitis & airborne contact dermatitis)[Q].
- **Patch test** should be **avoided in active flaring dermatitis involving >25% body surface & excited skin (angry back) syndrome,** a major cause of false positive patch test[Q]

Closed patch test	Open patch test
• Battery of suspected allergen is applied to patients back under occlusive dressing[Q] • Allowed to **remain in contact with skin**[Q] • Adhesive bandage is removed after 48 hours (2 days) for initial interpretation[Q] • **Second reading** is taken at **96 hours (4 days) or at 3-7 days**[Q] • **Second reading** is important **for elderly**[Q], who mount an allergic reaction more slowly than young patients & in **neomycin allergy**[Q]	• **Allergen is applied on outer arm skin & left uncovered**[Q].

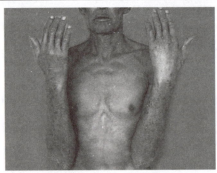

Fig. 46: Airborne contact dermatitis (ABCD)

Airborne Contact Dermatitis (ABCD)

- **ABCD** encompasses all **acute or chronic dermatoses** predominantly of **exposed parts of body,** which are **caused by substances** which when **released into air, settle on the exposed skin**[Q].
- Involvement of exposed areas of face, "V" of neck, hands & forearms, "Wilkinson's triangle," both eyelids, nasolabial folds & under the chin[Q].
- Involvement of both light-exposed & protected areas helps to differentiate ABCD from a photo-related dermatitis[Q].
- **Photopatch tests** can be **useful for excluding light as a factor** in the pathogenesis of lesions[Q].
- During patch testing, **volatile allergens** sometimes also cause **irritant dermatitis**; therefore, **high dilutions should be used**[Q].

> • **Patch Test: Gold-standard method for diagnosis of allergic contact dermatitis** resulting from type IV delayed hypersensitivity (allergic contact dermatitis & airborne contact dermatitis)[Q]

184. **Ans. a. Tinea cruris** *(Ref: Fitzpatrick 6/e p2217)*

Itchy annular scaly plaques in groin with peripheral extension is highly suggestive of Tinea cruris, also known as Jack itch, which is a dermatophytosis of the groin region caused by usually Trichophyton rubrum.

> "Tinea cruris usually appears as multiple erythematous papulovesicles with a well-marginated, raised border. Pruritus is common, as is pain with maceration or secondary infection." - *Fitzpatrick 6/e p2217*

Type	Affected body part	Causative agent
Tinea carporis (glabrosa)	Skin of body or limbs[Q] (usually non-hairy)	T. verrucosum[Q]
Tinea cruris (Dhobi/jack itch)	Groin, perineum, thighs, scrotum[Q] (least & late involvement)	Trichophyton rubrum[Q] E. floccosum
Tinea capitis[Q]	Scalp[Q]	Microsporum canis (MC)[Q] T. schoenleini, T. tonsurans
Tinea pedis (Athlete foot)	Feet, MC 4th web space[Q]	T. rubrum[Q] T. mentagrophyte, E. floccosum
Tinea manuum	Palms	T. rubrum[Q]
Tinea unguum (Onychomycosis)	Nail plate >nail bed[Q]	T. rubrum[Q] T. mentagrophyte, E. floccosum

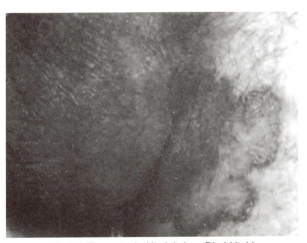

Fig. 47: Tinea cruris (Jack itch or Dhobi itch)

Tinea Cruris (Jack Itch or Dhobi Itch)
• It is the 2nd MC dermatophytosis worldwide involving groin, pubic, perineal skin & genitalia[Q]. • More common in males & adults[Q]
Etiology: • Most cases of Tinea cruris are caused by Trichophyton rubrum[Q] • Other agents: **Epidermophyton floccosum**
Predisposing Factors: • Summers & rainy season, use of synthetic clothes (Warm & moist environment)[Q]
Clinical Features: • Seen on **inner aspect of aspect of thighs** as arcuate sharply demarcated plaques with peripheral scaling, papulo-vesiculation & pustulation[Q]. • **Chronic lesions** may show **hyperpigmentation, nodulation & lichenification in center**[Q] • Lesions expand centrifugally and center clears • Involvement of scrotum & genitalia is unusual.
Treatment: • **DOC: Griseofulvin** (Active against most dermatophytes[Q])

185. Ans. c. Borderline lepromatous leprosy *(Ref: Rooks 7/e p29.1-29.19, Fitzpatrick 6/e p2181)*

The patient here has multiple hypoaesthetic patches (seen in borderline leprosy) and bilateral symmetrical nerve thickening (suggestive of lepromatous leprosy). Now in lepromatous leprosy, there is normal anesthesia. Hence, the patient fits in the category of borderline lepromatous leprosy.

"Borderline Lepromatous Leprosy: Skin lesions are often hypoaesthetic or anesthetic, but not necessarily so. Nerve trunk palsies have their highest prevalence in BL disease, but are variable in number, ranging from none to serious neurologic deficits, both motor and sensory, in all four extremities. Involvement of both median and ulnar nerves, not infrequently bilateral, is characteristic." - Fitzpatrick 6/e p2181

Feature	TT	BT	BB	BL	LL
Skin Lesions					
Number	**Single/few**	Few	Several	Numerous	Innumerable
Size	**Variable**	May be large	Variable	**Small[Q]**	**Small[Q]**
Sensations	**Anesthetic[Q]**	Hypoesthetic	Hypoesthetic	**Hypoesthetic**	**Normoesthetic**
Symmetry	**Asymmetrical[Q]**	Asymmetrical	Bilateral, Asymmetrical	**Nearly Symmetrical**	**Symmetrical[Q]**
Morphology	Well defined macule/ plaque	Well defined plaques with satellite lesions	Plaques with sloping edge (inverted saucer appearance)	Macule, nodules, Ill defined plaques	Macule, nodules, Ill defined plaques
Nerves	**Single trunk[Q]**	Asymmetrical involvement of few nerves with thickening	Several nerves involved asymmetrically with thickening	**Glove & stocking anesthesia[Q]**	**Symmetrical nerve thickening[Q]**
Reactions	**Stable[Q]**	**Type I[Q]**	**Type I[Q]**	Type I/II	**Type II[Q]**
Lepromin Test	+	+/–	–	–	–
Histology					
Granuloma	**Well defined epitheloid cell granulomas[Q]**	**Epitheloid cell granuloma[Q]**	–	**Ill-defined** macrophage granulomas with many lymphocytes	**Ill-defined foamy macrophage granulomas[Q]**
Grenz Zone	–	+	++[Q]	++[Q]	++[Q]
AFB	–	–	+/–	+	++[Q]

Type of Leprosy	Characteristic Features

Polar Tuberculoid (TT)	• **Increased CMI[Q]** & low bacillary load; **Lepromin test positive**
	• Skin lesions are often **solitary, non-infectious**
	• **Typical lesion:** Firmly indurated, elevated, erythematous, scaly, dry, hairless, hypopigmented, characteristically **hypoaesthetic** & anhidrotic plaque, often assuming an **annular configuration[Q]**
	    • **Histology: Small tubercles** with **large lymphocytic mantles** along with **abundant Langerhans giant cells** & exocytosis into epidermis[Q].
	• Only type in which **granuloma invades papillary zone & may even erode epidermis** but **AFB are not seen; Not infections & not associated lepra reactions[Q].**
	    • **MC type in India[Q]** & Africa but (virtually absent in south east Asia)
	• **Strong immunity** manifested by **spontaneous cure & absence of downgrading**; but **antibiotic therapy is recommended[Q]**

Borderline Tuberculoid (BT)	• **Immunological resistance is strong enough** to restrain the infection, but **host response is insufficient to self-cure (does not heal spontaneously).** • It is **unstable**; primary skin lesions are **plaques & papules** or **annular lesions** with **sharply marginated satellite papules[Q].**

Contd...

Type of Leprosy	Characteristic Features
	• **Little or no scaling, less erythema, less induration & less elevation,** but **lesions may become much larger (>10 cm)** • **Nerve trunk enlargement** or palsies, usually **asymmetrical & affecting no >2 nerves** are common; **Nerve abscesses** are more common in **males.** • **MC type in South-East Asia; Associated with type I lepra reaction**[Q]**.** • **Histology: Epitheloid cell granuloma** is more diffuse than in TT with a **free but narrow papillary zone** with **foreign body giant cells**

Borderline Leprosy (BB)	• **Characteristic skin lesions:**
	  – Classical **annular lesions** with **well defined centers**
	  – **Plaques with punched out appearance**
	  – **Swiss cheese appearance** or **classic dimorphic lesion.**
	• Because of **instability**, it is the **rarest type.**
	• **Histology: Diffuse epitheloid cell granuloma; papillary zone is clear,** nerves are slightly swollen by cellular infiltrate

Indeterminate leprosy	Pure neuritic leprosy
• **Early & transitory stage** of leprosy • **Histology: Scattered nonspecific histiocytic & lymphocytic infiltration** • **Clinically: Hypopigmented macule or patch with or without sensory deficit & AFB**[Q]**,** if found, are present in **very small numbers**	• **Asymmetrical involvement of peripheral nerve trunks** • **No visible skin lesions** • **Non-infectious, slit smear negative** • Seen **most frequently**, but not exclusively, in **India & Nepal**

Type of Leprosy	Characteristic Features

Borderline Lepromatous (BL)	• Classic **borderline** or **dimorphic lesion** is most characteristic which is an **indurated & elevated annular plaque;** Inverted saucer-shaped annular lesions are characteristic.
	  • **Poorly or sharply marinated plaques** with **punched out or Swiss cheese sharply marginated areas of normal skin** in the interior of plaque are also **characteristic.**
	  • **Symmetrical involvement** of bilateral ulnar & median nerve is characteristic[Q]**.**
	• **Histology:** Classic response is **dense lymphocytic infiltrate** confined to **space occupied by macrophages, lamination of perineurium** with a **lymphocytic infiltrate**
	• **Formation of small granulomas is characteristic**

Lepromatous Leprosy (LL)	• **Lack of CMI**[Q] & increased bacillary replication (**Lepromin test negative**) & **widely disseminated multiorgan disease.**
	• **Bacilli are plentiful in circulating blood & in all organ systems except lungs & CNS**[Q]**.**
	• **MC lesions: Symmetrically distributed,** poorly defined nodules (anywhere apart form hairy **scalp, axillae, groins & perineum**)
	  • **Diffuse dermal infiltration** is always **present subclinically** & is manifested by **enlargement of ear lobes, widening of nasal root & fusiform selling of fingers.**
	  • **Late manifestations: Leonine facies, madarosis, saddle nose,** hoarseness of voice, upper incisor teeth loosen or fall out, pendulous & dry scaling skin particularly on feet.
	• **Acral, distal, symmetric peripheral neuropathy & nerve trunk enlargement.**
	  • **Testicular involvement: Elevated FSH & LH levels, impotence, infertility, loss of libido & testicular sensation, atrophy & gynaecomastia**[Q]**.**

	• **Upper respiratory tract involvement** (from tip of nose to vocal cord): Present as **rhinitis, septal perforation, nasal collapse &** hoarseness from **vocal cord nodules.**

Histology
• **Thinning of epidermis** with **clear (free) subepidermal grenz zone**[Q]**.** • **Foamy macrophages** laden with **acid-fast bacilli (Virchow's or lepra cells)** • **Dermis contains enormous number of AFB**, singly or in clumps (globi)[Q]**.** • **Onion-skin perineural lamination** but not infiltration[Q]**.**

• **Mucous membrane involvement & ulceration; Regurgitation due to perforation of palate.**

186. Ans. d. Cholinergic urticaria *(Ref: Roxburgh 17 /e p71-75; Rooks 7/e p47.1-47.29, Fitzpatrick 6/e p1265)*
Complaints of rash on exposure to sun, after exercise, after getting angry or on eating spicy food are highly suggestive of cholinergic urticaria.

> *"Cholinergic urticaria develops after an increase in core body temperature, such as during a warm bath or shower, exercise, or episodes of fever. The highest prevalence is observed in individuals aged 23 to 28 years. The eruption appears as distinctive, pruritic, small, 1- to 2-mm wheals that are surrounded by large areas of erythema; occasionally, the lesions may become confluent, or angioedema may develop. Systemic features include dizziness, headache, syncope, flushing, wheezing, shortness of breath, nausea, vomiting, and diarrhea."- Fitzpatrick 6/e p1265*

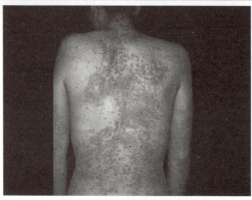

Fig. 48: Cholinergic Urticaria

Cholinergic Urticaria

- Urticaria develops due to acetylcholine liberated from post ganglionic cholinergic enervated sweat glands **under the influence of any stimuli** which **induces sweating** by **increasing core body temperature**[Q].
- Characteristic feature is **small size pruritic wheals surrounded by large erythema**[Q].

Precipitating Factors	
• Exercise or physical exertion[Q]	• Exposure to sun/heat[Q]
• Emotion upset[Q]	• Hot bath/food[Q]

Clinical Features:
- Mostly seen in **adolescents; Worse in winters.**
- Cholinergic urticaria **appears rapidly**[Q], usually within a few minutes after the onset of sweating & lasts from a half hour to an hour or more.

> • **Morphology:** Eruption appears as distinctive, pruritic, small, 1-2 mm wheals that are surrounded by large areas of erythema[Q]

- **Systemic features:** Dizziness, headache, syncope, flushing, wheezing, shortness of breath, nausea, vomiting, & diarrhea.

Diagnosis:
- **Pilocarpine stimulation test**[Q]

Treatment:
- In cholinergic urticaria, **hydroxyzine & cetirizine** are the **initial agents of choice**[Q].

ANESTHESIA

187. Ans. a. Atracurium *(Ref: Goodman Gilman 12/e p263; Morgan 4/e p221; Lee 13/e p191-192)*
Atracurium has unique metabolism, Hoffmann elimination, independent of hepatic & renal functions.

> *"Atracurium is converted to less active metabolites by plasma esterases and spontaneous Hofmann elimination. Cisatracurium is also subject to this spontaneous degradation. Because of these alternative routes of metabolism, atracurium and cisatracurium do not exhibit an increased $t_{1/2}$ in patients with impaired renal function and therefore are good choices in this setting."-Goodman Gilman 12/e p263*

Atracurium

- Available as **atracurium besylate**[Q]
- To be stored at **4°C**[Q]

Pharmacokinetics:

- **Acidic compound, can precipitate if given in IV line containing alkaline solution** like **thiopentone**[Q].
- **Dose: 0.5 mg/kg**[Q]
- **Onset of action: 2-3 minutes; Duration of action: 10-15 minutes**[Q]

Metabolism of Atracurium
• It has **unique method of degradation**[Q].
• It's **metabolism is independent of hepatic & renal functions**[Q].
• It undergoes **spontaneous degradation** in plasma called as **Hoffman degradation**[Q].

Systemic Effects:

- **Histamine release** is much **less than d-tubocurare.**
- **CVS**: Can cause **bronchospasm** because of release of histamine.
- **CNS: At higher doses** its metabolic product **laudanosine can cross blood brain barrier & produce convulsions**[Q].
- **Allergic reactions** ranging from **pruritic rash to angioneurotic edema** can occur.

Atracurium is relaxant of choice in	
(Because of **unique metabolism independent of hepatic & renal functions** and **ensured degradation**)	
• **Hepatic failure**[Q]	• **Myasthenia gravis**[Q]
• **Renal failure**[Q]	• **Newborn**[Q]
• **If reversal agent is contraindicated**[Q]	• **Old age**[Q]

Cis-Atracurium
• It is an **isomer of atracurium, 4 times more potent**

Chief advantage of Cis-Atracurium over atracurium
• It **does not release histamine**[Q]
• **Laudanosine production is 5 times lesser than atracurium**[Q].
• Whenever available it is **always preferred over atracurium**[Q].

Drug	Duration	Metabolism	Elimination by kidney (%)	Elimination by liver (%)
Succinylcholine	**Ultra-short**[Q]	**Butyrylcholinesterase (98–99%)**[Q]	<2%	None
Mivacurium	**Short**[Q]	**Butyrylcholinesterase (95–99%)**[Q]	<5%	None
Atracurium	Intermediate	**Hofmann elimination & nonspecific ester hydrolysis**[Q] **(60–90%)**	10–40%	None
Cisatracurium	Intermediate	**Hofmann elimination**[Q]	**77%**[Q]	16%
Vecuronium	Intermediate	Liver (30–40%)	40–50%	**60%**[Q]
Rocuronium	Intermediate	**None**[Q]	10–25%	**>70%**[Q]
Pancuronium	**Long**[Q]	Liver (10–20%)	**85%**[Q]	15%
d-Tubocurarine	**Long**[Q]	**None**[Q]	**80%**[Q]	20%

Important Muscle Relaxants	
Shortest & fastest acting neuromuscular blocker	• Succinylcholine[Q]
Shortest acting competitive (non-depolarizing) neuromuscular blocker	• Mivacurium[Q]
Fastest acting non-depolarizing neuromuscular blocker	• Rocuronium[Q]
Longest acting & most potent non-depolarizing neuromuscular blocker	• Doxacurium
Maximum ganglion blockade	• d-TC

188. Ans. c. Dantrolene (Ref: Goodman Gilman 12/e p266; 13/e p467, Katzung 12/e p479; Miller 8/e p1291)

Dantrolene sodium is a postsynaptic muscle relaxant that lessens excitation-contraction coupling in muscle cells. It achieves this by inhibiting Ca^{2+} ions release from sarcoplasmic reticulum stores by antagonizing ryanodine receptors. Hence, it is direct acting on muscle cells rather than the neuromuscular junction.

> "Dantrolene is a hydantoin derivative related to phenytoin that has a unique mechanism of spasmolytic activity. In contrast to the centrally acting drugs, dantrolene reduces skeletal muscle strength by interfering with excitation-contraction coupling in the muscle fibers. The normal contractile response involves release of calcium from its stores in the sarcoplasmic reticulum. This activator calcium brings about the tension-generating interaction of actin with myosin. Calcium is released from the sarcoplasmic reticulum via a calcium channel, called the **ryanodine receptor (RyR) channel** because the plant alkaloid ryanodine combines with a receptor on the channel protein. **In the case of the skeletal muscle RyR1 channel, ryanodine facilitates the open configuration. Dantrolene interferes with the release of activator calcium through this sarcoplasmic reticulum calcium channel by binding to the RyR1 and blocking the opening of the channel. Motor units that contract rapidly are more sensitive to the drug's effects than are slower-responding units.** Cardiac muscle and smooth muscle are minimally depressed because the release of calcium from their sarcoplasmic reticulum involves a different RyR channel (RyR2)."-Katzung 13/e p467

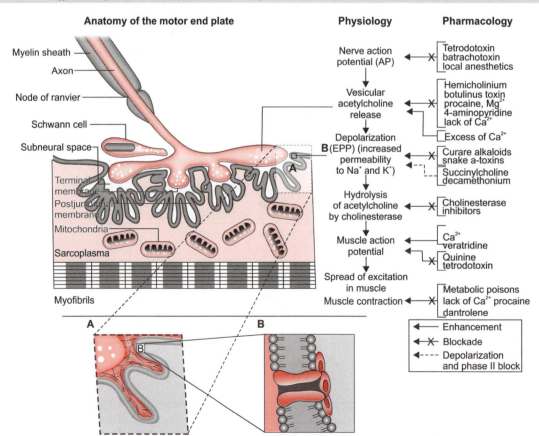

Fig. 49: Sites of action of agents at NM junction & adjacent structures

Classification of Muscle Relaxants

Neuromuscular blocking agents			Directly acting
Depolarizing	Non-depolarizing		
	Steroidal	Benzylisoquinoline	
• Succinylcholine[Q] • Decamethonium[Q]	• Pancuronium • Pipecuronium • Vecuronium • Rocuronium • Rapacuronium	• d-Tubocurare • Metocurine • Atracurium • Cis-atracurium • Mivacurium • Doxacurium	• Dantrolene[Q] • Quinine[Q]

Dantrolene

- **Dantrolene reduces skeletal muscle strength** by **interfering with excitation-contraction coupling** in the muscle fibers[Q]
- Dantrolene **interferes with the release of activator calcium through sarcoplasmic reticulum calcium channel** by **binding to the RyR1[Q] & blocking the opening of channel[Q]**.

Mechanism of Action:
- **Blocks RyR1 Ca^{2+}-release channels in the sarcoplasmic reticulum of skeletal muscle[Q]**

Effects:
- **Reduces actin-myosin interaction & weakens skeletal muscle contraction[Q]**

Clinical Applications:
- **IV: Malignant hyperthermia[Q]**
- **Oral: Spasm due to cerebral palsy[Q], spinal cord injury[Q], multiple sclerosis[Q]**

Adverse-Effects:
- **Muscular weakness** is the **dose limiting side effect[Q]**.
- Sedation, malaise, light headedness; Troublesome diarrhea is another problem.
- Long term use causes **dose dependent serious liver toxicity** in 0.1–0.5% patients.

---

189. **Ans. a. Level of needle insertion should be L1-L2 vertebral junction** *(Ref: Harrison 19/e p443-e2)*

The spinal cord ends at L3 vertebrae in children and L1 in adults. With a safe margin, A lumbar puncture should be performed at L3-L4 or L4-L5 interspace.

"The spinal cord terminates at approximately the L1 vertebral level in 94% of individuals. In the remaining 6%, the conus extends to the L2–L3 interspace. LP is therefore performed at or below the L3–L4 interspace. A useful anatomic guide is a line drawn between the posterior superior iliac crests, which corresponds closely to the level of the L3–L4 interspace. The interspace is chosen following gentle palpation to identify the spinous processes at each lumbar level."
- Harrison 19/e p443-e2

"The LP needle (typically 20- to 22-gauge) is inserted in the midline, midway between two spinous processes, and slowly advanced. The bevel of the needle should be maintained in a horizontal position, parallel to the direction of the dural fibers and with the flat portion of the bevel pointed upward; this minimizes injury to the fibers as the dura is penetrated."
- Harrison 19/e p443-e2

Lumbar Puncture

- **Normal extent of spinal cord: From foramen magnum to lower border of L1 vertebra in adults[Q] & to upper border of L3 vertebra in infants[Q]**
- **LP** is therefore performed **at or below the L3–L4 interspace[Q]**
- Patients with an **altered level of consciousness**, a **focal neurologic deficit**, **new-onset seizure**, **papilledema**, or an **immunocompromised state** are at **increased risk for potentially fatal cerebellar or tentorial herniation** following LP. **Neuroimaging** should be **obtained in these patients prior to LP to exclude a focal mass lesion** or diffuse **swelling[Q]**.
- **A low platelet count of <20,000/µL** is considered to be a **contraindication to LP[Q]**.

Contd...

Contd...

Lumbar Puncture

During lumbar puncture, the needle passes through the following anatomic structures before it enters the subarachnoid space:	
1. Skin[Q]	5. Ligamentum flavum[Q]
2. Subcutaneous tissue[Q]	6. Dura mater[Q]
3. Supraspinous ligament[Q]	7. Arachnoid mater[Q]
4. Interspinous ligament[Q]	

Positioning:
- Performed on a **firm surface**
- If performed **at bedside**, patient should be positioned **at the edge of bed[Q]** (not in middle).
- Patient is asked to **lie on his or her side, facing away from examiner** & to **"roll up into a ball"[Q]**.
- **Neck is gently anteflexed** & thighs pulled up toward abdomen[Q]
- **Shoulders & pelvis** should be **vertically aligned without forward or backward tilt[Q]**.

- Performed at or below the **L3–L4 interspace[Q]**
- **Useful anatomic guide:** Line drawn between posterior superior iliac crest, which **correspond closely to level of L3–L4 interspace[Q].**

- **Interspace** is chosen following **gentle palpation to identify spinous processes** at each lumbar level.
- An **alternative to lateral recumbent position** is the **seated position**.
- Patient **sits at the side of bed**, with **feet supported on a chair**.
- Patient is **instructed to curl forward**, trying to **touch the nose to umbilicus**.
- LP is sometimes **more easily performed in obese patients if they are sitting**.
- **Disadvantage of seated position:** Measurement of opening pressure is **not accurate[Q]**.

Technique:
- **Proper local disinfection** reduces the risk of introducing skin bacteria into subarachnoid space (SAS).
- Local anesthetic (**1% lidocaine**), **3–5 mL total**, is injected into subcutaneous tissue.
- **LP** should be **delayed for 10–15 min** following the injection of anesthetic to decrease pain from the procedure.

- **LP needle** (typically **20-22 gauge[Q]**) is **inserted in midline, midway between two spinous processes[Q]** & slowly advanced.
- **Bevel of needle** should be **maintained in a horizontal position, parallel to direction of dural fibers** & with **flat portion of bevel pointed upward[Q]**; this **minimizes injury to fibers as dura is penetrated.**

- When **LP** is performed **in sitting position**, bevel should be **maintained in vertical position**.
- In most adults, **needle is advanced 4–5 cm** before the SAS is reached; examiner recognizes **entry as a sudden release of resistance, a "pop"[Q]**.
- If **no fluid appears despite apparently correct needle placement**, then the **needle may be rotated 90°–180°**. If there is **still no fluid, stylet is reinserted & needle is advanced slightly[Q]**.
- If the **needle cannot be advanced** because it hits bone, if the patient **experiences sharp radiating pain down one leg**, or **if no fluid appears ("dry tap")**, needle is partially withdrawn & reinserted at a different angle.
- Once the **SAS is reached**, a manometer is attached to needle & opening pressure measured.
- **Upper limit of normal opening pressure** with the **patient supine** is **180 mm H$_2$O** in adults but may be **as high as 200–250 mm H$_2$O in obese adults[Q]**.
- **CSF is allowed to drip into collection tubes**; it **should not be withdrawn with a syringe[Q]**.

CSF Obtained for	
1. **Cell count with differential[Q]**	7. **PCR amplification** of DNA or RNA of microorganisms (e.g., herpes simplex virus, enteroviruses)[Q]
2. **Protein & glucose concentrations[Q]**	
3. **Culture[Q]** (bacterial, fungal, mycobacterial, viral)	8. **Immunoelectrophoresis** for determination of γ-globulin level & **oligoclonal banding[Q]**
4. **Smears** (e.g., Gram's & acid-fast stained smears)	
5. **Antigen tests[Q]** (e.g., latex agglutination)	9. **Cytology[Q]**
6. **Antibody levels** against microorganisms[Q]	

Contd...

AIIMS May 2016

1203

Contd...

Lumbar Puncture

• Although **15 mL of CSF** is **sufficient to obtain all of the listed studies**[Q], yield of fungal & mycobacterial cultures & cytology increases when larger volumes are sampled (20–30 mL may be safely removed from adults).
 	
    • A **bloody tap** due to penetration of a meningeal vessel (a **"traumatic tap"**) may result in confusion with subarachnoid hemorrhage (SAH).
    • **Specimen of CSF should be centrifuged immediately** after it is obtained[Q]
    • **Clear supernatant following CSF centrifugation supports the diagnosis of a bloody tap**, whereas **xanthochromic supernatant suggests SAH**[Q].
    • **Bloody CSF due to penetration of a meningeal vessel clears in successive tubes**, whereas **blood due to SAH does not**[Q].
    • **Xanthochromic CSF** may also be present **in patients with liver disease** & when **CSF protein concentration is markedly elevated (>1.5–2 g/L)**[Q].
 	
• Prior to removing LP needle, stylet is reinserted to avoid the possibility of entrapment of a nerve root in the dura as the needle is being withdrawn; **entrapment could result in a dural CSF leak, causing headache**[Q].

190. Ans. d. Vapor pressure *(Ref: Miller 7/e p683)*

In a closed container, molecules from a volatile liquid escape the liquid phase and become vapor. These gaseous molecules strike the wall of the container, exerting what's known as vapor pressure. Vapor pressure is directly proportional to temperature. Increasing temperature will increase the ratio of gas:liquid molecules, thereby increasing vapor pressure.

> *"Contemporary inhaled volatile anesthetics exist in the liquid state at temperatures below 20°C. **When a volatile liquid is in a closed container, molecules escape from the liquid phase to the vapor phase until the number of molecules in the vapor phase is constant. These molecules in the vapor phase bombard the wall of the container and create a pressure known as the saturated vapor pressure. As the temperature increases, more molecules enter the vapor phase, and the vapor pressure increases.** Vapor pressure is independent of atmospheric pressure and is contingent only on the temperature and physical characteristics of the liquid."-Miller 7/e p683*

Vaporizers
• **Vaporizer** is a device that **changes liquid anesthetic into vapor & adds a clinical useful amount of** this **vapor to** the **fresh gas flow** or **anesthetic system**[Q]. • **Vaporizer** materials are made of **copper** due to **high specific heat & thermal conductivity**[Q]. • Boyles anesthetic apparatus contains **two vaporizers:** one for **ether** & one for **trichloroethylene**[Q].

Old vaporizers	Newer vaporizers
• **Boyles vaporizer, Goldman vaporizer** • **Out** is highly **affected by temperature change** • **Don't deliver accurate concentrations**	• **TEC 4, TEC 5, TEC 7** used for delivery of **halothane, isoflurane, enflurane, sevoflurane** • **TEC 6** is specially designed for desflurane. • **Aladin Cassette:** Latest vaporizer, used for delivery of **halothane, isoflurane, enflurane, sevoflurane & desflurane.**

Sequence of Vaporizers:
• Multiple vaporizers are present in the anesthetic machine.

Order of Placement of Vaporizers
• **More volatile agents (highest SVP)** are placed **downstream** • **Potent agents** are placed **downstream** (overdose is unlikely during subsequent use, even if contaminations occurs) • **Agents with toxic byproducts** should be placed **downstream** (to prevent contamination of other vaporizers)

AIIMS ESSENCE

Contd...

Vaporizers		
Agent	**Boiling point (°C)**	**Standard vapor pressure (SVP) at 20°C (mm Hg)**
Trichloroethylene	**87.2**	**60[Q]**
Chloroform	**61.2**	**160**
Sevoflurane	**58.5**	**170**
Enflurane	56.5	172
Isoflurane	48.5	184
Halothane	50.2	243
Diethyl ether	34.6	425
Desflurane	**22.8**	**669[Q]**

- Isoflurane is placed before halothane & sevoflurane.

Safety Features in Vaporizers	
• **Clear color coding indicator** on the **vaporizer** & **agent bottle** • Agent specific filling systems with sealed bottles • **Agent level indicators**	• **Mounting system** with interlock to prevent simultaneous use of two vaporizers • Filling port is low to avoid overfilling

191. Ans. d. Induction should be done with thiopentone sodium and succinylcholine for muscle relaxation *(Ref: Miller 7/e p34, 887)*

Thiopentone induction is contraindicated in cardiac patients because of direct negative inotropic effects on the heart and depressant effects on systemic BP. Etomidate is the preferred induction agent in such a patient.

Rapid Sequence Intubation (RSI)

• **Rapid sequence intubation** is an **advanced airway management procedure,** used to **achieve tracheal intubation under GA** in patients who are at **high risk of pulmonary aspiration[Q]**.
 • **Objective: To secure airway rapidly & prevent aspiration of gastric contents[Q]**.
 • **RSI involves pre-filling the patient's lungs with a high concentration of oxygen gas,** followed by administering **rapid-onset hypnotic & NM-blocking drugs** that **induce prompt unconsciousness & paralysis,** allowing **insertion** of an endotracheal tube **with minimal delay[Q]**.
 • **No artificial ventilation from the time of drug administration till intubation to minimize insufflation of air into stomach to avoid regurgitation[Q]**.
      • **Sellick's maneuver (cricoid Pressure): To prevent aspiration[Q]**
      • **Intubate with cuffed endotracheal tube & establish lung ventilation[Q]**.
      • **Manual mask ventilation before intubation is avoided[Q]**.

192. Ans. b. Infants > Neonates > Adults *(Ref: Miller 8/e p2764, 7/e p517, 1243; Wylie 7/e p966, 967, 988)*

MAC, the minimum alveolar concentration at 1 atmosphere that prevents movement in 50% of patients exposed to a surgical incision, decreases with age after 1 year. It is lesser in neonates followed by increase up to 1 year of age and then gradual decline to values lesser then those in neonates.

"The lower MAC of halothane in neonates compared with infants may be related to immaturity of the central nervous system and attenuation of the pain response due to high levels of plasma peptides (beta-endorphin and beta-lipoprotein). The higher MAC in infants compared with older children and adults may be due to an increase in the brain water content." - Wylie 7/e p966

"Beginning in young adulthood, MAC, the ED_{50} equivalent for inhalational anesthesia, declines linearly with increasing age." - Wylie 7/e p988

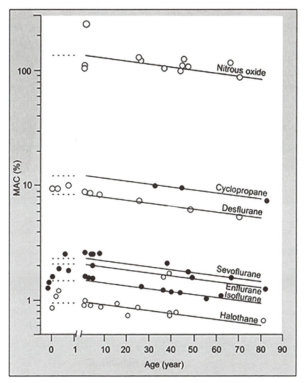

Fig. 50: Age related changes in MAC

Properties of Volatile Anesthetic Agents			
	Halothane	Isoflurane	Sevoflurane	Desflurane
Odor	Sweet, non-pungent	Markedly pungent, ethereal	Minimally pungent	Markedly pungent, ethereal
Blood–gas partition coefficient				
Neonates	2.1	1.2	0.7	–
Adults	2.3	1.4	0.7	0.4
MAC (%)				
Neonates	0.9	1.6	3.3	9.2
Infants	1.2	1.9	2.5	9.9
Adults	0.8	1.2	2.0	6.0
Rate of metabolism (%)	20.0	0.2	2.0	0.02
Myocardial depression	++	+	?+	+
Peripheral vasodilation	+	++	?++	++
Respiratory depression	+	++	++	++

193. **Ans. d. Neuromuscular blockers** (Ref: Miller 7/e p884)
  Most common cause of perioperative anaphylaxis is muscle relaxants and antibiotics followed by opioids and intravenous anesthesia.

AIIMS ESSENCE

"The frequency of life-threatening anaphylactic (immune-mediated) or anaphylactoid reactions occurring during anesthesia has been estimated to be between 1 in 1,000 and 1 in 25,000 anesthetizations, with about a 5% mortality rate. In France, the most common causes of anaphylaxis in patients who experienced allergic reactions were reported to be neuromuscular blocking drugs (58.2%), latex (16.7%), and antibiotics (15.1%). Anaphylactic reactions are mediated through immune responses involving immunoglobulin E antibodies fixed to mast cells. Anaphylactoid reactions are not immune mediated and represent exaggerated pharmacologic responses in very rare and very sensitive individuals."- Miller 7/e p884

Most Common Drugs Involved in Perioperative Anaphylaxis		
Substance	**Incidence (%)**	**Most commonly associated**
Muscle relaxants	69.2[Q]	**Succinylcholine, rocuronium, atracurium**[Q]
Natural rubber latex	12.1[Q]	**Latex gloves, tourniquets, Foley catheters**
Antibiotics	8[Q]	**Penicillin & other beta-lactams**[Q]
Hypnotics	3.7[Q]	**Propofol, thiopental**[Q]
Colloids	2.7	**Dextran, gelatin**[Q]
Opioids	1.4	**Morphine, meperidine**[Q]
Other substances	2.9	Paracetamol, aprotinin, chymopapain, protamine, bupivacaine

Muscle Relaxants
• **Muscle relaxants** are **MC cause of anaphylaxis during anesthesia**[Q].
• **IgE antibodies to the two quaternary** or **tertiary ammonium ions mediate anaphylaxis**[Q].

Muscle Relaxants
• **Succinylcholine** contains **flexible molecule** that can **crosslink two mast cell IgE receptors** & **induce mast cell degranulation**[Q].   • **Succinylcholine** is **more likely to cause anaphylaxis than nondepolarizing muscle relaxants** with a rigid backbone between their **two ammonium ions**[Q] (e.g., pancuronium or vecuronium).

- **Incidence of anaphylaxis** is also **more frequent with benzylisoquinolinium compounds than with aminosteroid compounds**[Q].
- Many over-the-counter **drugs, cosmetics & food products contain quaternary or tertiary ammonium ions** that could **sensitize people**. Therefore, **anaphylaxis may develop on the first exposure to a muscle relaxant** in a **sensitized patient**[Q].
- **Neostigmine & morphine** also contain **ammonium ions** that may **cross-react with muscle relaxants**.

194. Ans. a. Bezold-Jarisch reflex   *(Ref: 8/e p1970, Miller 7/e p409)*

The Bezold-Jarisch reflex involves a variety of cardiovascular and neurological processes which cause hypopnea (excessively shallow breathing or an abnormally low respiratory rate) and bradycardia (abnormally low resting heart rate). The Bezold-Jarisch reflex has been suggested as a possible cause of profound bradycardia and circulatory collapse after spinal anesthesia.

"The Bezold-Jarisch reflex responds to noxious ventricular stimuli sensed by chemoreceptors and mechanoreceptors within the LV wall by inducing the triad of hypotension, bradycardia, and coronary artery dilatation. The activated receptors communicate along unmyelinated vagal afferent type C fibers. These fibers reflexively increase parasympathetic tone. Because it invokes bradycardia, the Bezold-Jarisch reflex is thought of as a cardioprotective reflex. This reflex has been implicated in the physiologic response to a range of cardiovascular conditions such as myocardial ischemia or infarction, thrombolysis, or revascularization and syncope. Natriuretic peptide receptors stimulated by endogenous ANP or BNP may modulate the Bezold-Jarisch reflex. Thus, the Bezold-Jarisch reflex may be less pronounced in patients with cardiac hypertrophy or atrial fibrillation."-Miller 7/e p409

"The Bainbridge reflex is elicited by stretch receptors located in the right atrial wall and the cavoatrial junction. An increase in right-sided filling pressure sends vagal afferent signals to the cardiovascular center in the medulla. These afferent signals inhibit parasympathetic activity, thereby increasing the heart rate. Acceleration of the heart rate also results from a direct effect on the SA node by stretching the atrium. The changes in heart rate are dependent on the underlying heart rate before stimulation." -Miller 7/e p409

"A reverse Bainbridge reflex has been proposed to explain the decreases in heart rate observed under conditions in which venous return is reduced, such as during spinal and epidural anesthesia, controlled hypotension, and severe hemorrhage."

Major Cardiovascular Reflexes

Reflex	Receptors and location	Afferent limb	Efferent limb and response
Arterial baroreceptor reflex	Stretch receptors in vessel wall of carotid sinus & aortic arch, which respond to changes in arterial blood pressure[Q]	Fibers in glossopharyngeal & vagus nerves to medulla[Q]	Homeostatic control of arterial blood pressure via changes in cardiac output & systemic vascular resistance mediated by autonomic nervous system[Q]
Bezold-Jarisch reflex (coronary chemoreflex)	Mechanical & chemosensitive receptors in ventricular walls[Q]	Non-myelinated vagal C-fibers to medulla[Q]	Inhibition of sympathetic outflow resulting in bradycardia, peripheral vasodilation & hypotension[Q]
Bainbridge reflex	Stretch receptors at junction of vena cava & right atrium & at junction of pulmonary vein & left atrium, which respond to changes in volume in central thoracic compartment[Q]	Fibers in vagus nerve to medulla[Q]	Inhibition of vagal outflow & enhancement of sympathetic outflow to sinoatrial node causing tachycardia[Q]

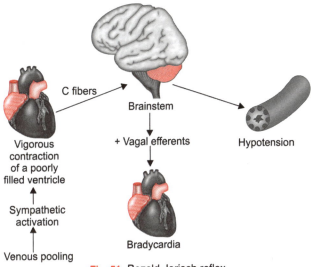

Fig. 51: Bezold-Jarisch reflex

RADIOLOGY

195. Ans. a. Ovary *(Ref: Perez and Brady's Principles of Radiation Oncology 6/e p65)*

Among the given options, most radiosensitive organ is ovary >rectum >bladder >vagina (Radiation tolerance dose: Ovary = 2-3 Gy ; Rectum = 60 Gy; Bladder = 65 Gy; Vagina = 90 Gy).

Radiotherapy

- **MC radiations used** to treat cancers: **X-rays & gamma rays**[Q]
- **X-rays** are **generated by linear accelerators**[Q]
- **Gamma rays** are generated **from decay of atomic nuclei** in radioisotopes like **cobalt**[Q].
- **Radiation energy** is absorbed by tissue causing **ionization** or **excitation**[Q], which are responsible for various biological effects.
- **Susceptibility of various phases of cell cycle to radiation: G_2M[Q] $>G_2 >M >G_1 >$Early S $>$Late S Phase**[Q].

Phase of cell cycle	Comment
$G_2M >G_2$	• **Most sensitive**[Q] to radiation
End of S phase	• **Most resistant**[Q] to radiation
G_1	• Radiation exposure leads to **chromosomal aberration**[Q]
G_2	• Radiation exposure leads to **chromatid aberration**[Q]

Radiosensitiser	Radiation protectors
• **Oxygen**[Q] (most effective radiosensitiser) • **Metronidazole**[Q], misonidazole, tinidazole • **5-FU**[Q] (non-hypoxic cell sensitizer) • **Hydroxyurea**[Q] (non-hypoxic cell sensitizer) • **BUDR & IUDR**[Q] (non-hypoxic cell sensitizer) • **Cisplatin**[Q], paclitaxel, gemcitabine • **Mitomycin**[Q], topotecan, vinorelbine • **Dactinomycin (Actinomycin D)**[Q]	• **Amifostine**[Q] • **IL-1**[Q] • **GM-CSF**[Q]

	Most radiosensitive	Least radiosensitive
Tissue	**Bone marrow**[Q]	**Nervous tissue**[Q]
Blood cell	**Lymphocyte**[Q]	**Platelet**[Q]
Stage of cell cycle	**G2-M interphase**[Q] (mitosis or M phase)	**S phase**[Q]
Cell type	**Rapidly dividing**[Q] (Vegetative intermitotic cells)	**Quiescent**[Q] (Fixed postmoitotic cells)
Ocular structure	**Lens**[Q]	**Sclera**[Q]
Layer of retina	**Rods**[Q] (more than cones)	**Ganglion cell layer**[Q]

- **Most radiosensitive tissue of body: Bone marrow**[Q]
- **Least** radiosensitive tissue of body: **Nervous tissue/Brain**[Q]
- **Most radiosensitive blood cell: Lymphocyte**[Q] (lymphocytic predominant Hodgkins lymphoma has best prognosis)
- **Least radiosensitive blood cell: Platelet**[Q]
- **MC organ** to be affected by radiation: **Skin**[Q] (Erythema earliest change, MC affected layer: Stratum basalis[Q])
- **Sebaceous gland function doesn't recover after radiotherapy**[Q].
- **Pinna & axillae** are **common sites of radionecrosis** i.e. for skin doses[Q].

- **Most radiosensitive abdominal organ: Kidney**[Q]
- Most **radio resistant** organ: **Vagina**[Q]
- **MC mucosa** affected by radiation: **Intestinal mucosa**[Q] (Earliest symptom is diarrhea[Q])

Effect of Radiation on Testes & Ovaries
• **Type B spermatogonia** are **exquisitely sensitive** to the effects of **radiation**[Q].
• **Sertoli cells & Leydig cells** are **less radiosensitive** than spermatogonia[Q].
• The **single dose** required for **permanent sterilization** on **human males** is **6-10 Gray (Gy)**[Q].
• The radiation dose necessary to induce ovarian failure is age dependent.
• A **single dose of 3-4 Gray (300-400 rads)** can induce **amenorrhea in** almost all **women >40 years of age**[Q].
• In young women, **oogenesis** is much **less sensitive to radiation than is spermatogenesis** in men.

Most radiosensitive ovarian tumor	• **Dysgerminoma**[Q]
Most radiosensitive **brain** tumor	• **Medulloblastoma**[Q]
Most radiosensitive **testicular** tumor	• **Seminoma**[Q]
Most radiosensitive **lung** tumor	• **Small cell CA**[Q]
Most radiosensitive **kidney** tumor	• **Wilm's tumor**[Q]
Most radiosensitive **bone** tumor	• **Ewing's sarcoma**[Q] & **multiple myeloma**[Q]

PSYCHIATRY

196. Ans. c. ECG *(Ref: Kaplan & Sadock 11/e p376; Niraj Ahuja 7/e p90)*

A complains of ghabrahat, palpitations, profuse sweating and sense of impending doom is suggestive of panic attack. Most close differential of this condition is myocardial infarction, which can be differentiated by ECG in emergency.

"Panic disorder must be differentiated from a number of medical conditions that produce similar symptomatology. Panic attacks are associated with a variety of endocrinological disorders, including both hypo- and hyperthyroid states, hyperparathyroidism, and pheochromocytomas. Episodic hypoglycemia associated with insulinomas can also produce panic-like states, as can primary neuropathological processes. These include seizure disorders, vestibular dysfunction, neoplasms, or the effects of both prescribed and illicit substances on the CNS. Finally, disorders of the cardiac and pulmonary systems, including arrhythmias, chronic obstructive pulmonary disease, and asthma, can produce autonomic symptoms and accompanying crescendo anxiety that can be difficult to distinguish from panic disorder."-Kaplan & Sadock 11/e p376

197. Ans. a. Food preference *(Ref: Kaplan & Sadock 11/e p189-190; Niraj Ahuja 7/e p9-10)*

Though food preference is an important part of personal history elsewhere, it is not as important as the other options in diagnosing psychiatric conditions or planning their management.

"Components of Personal and Social History: Perinatal history; Childhood history; Educational history; Puberty history; Menstrual and obstetric history; Occupational history; Sexual and Marital history."

Parts of Initial Psychiatric Interview	
• Identifying data	• Developmental & social history
• Source & reliability	• Review of systems
• Chief complaint	• Mental status examination
• Present illness	• Physical examination
• **Past psychiatric history**	• Formulation
• **Substance use/abuse**	• DSM-V diagnoses
• **Past medical history**	• Treatment plan
• **Family history**	

198. Ans. d. Disorder of content of thought *(Ref: Fish's Clinical Psychopathology/p22-24; Niraj Ahuja 7/e p95; Kaplan Synopsis 10/e p234; CDTP 2/e p106, 274, 749)*

Strictly speaking, obsessions are disorders of "possession" of thought and not "content" of thought.

"Obsessions as defined by (1), (2), (3), and (4): (1) Recurrent and persistent thoughts, impulses, or images that are experienced, at some time during the disturbance, as intrusive and inappropriate and that cause marked anxiety or distress. (2) The thoughts, impulses, or images are not simply excessive worries about real-life problems. (3) The person attempts to ignore or suppress such thoughts, impulses, or images, or to neutralize them with some other thought or action. (4) The person recognizes that the obsessional thoughts, impulses, or images are a product of his or her own mind (not imposed from without as in thought insertion) [Ego-Dystonic]."

Thought Disorders			
Disorders of Form (Form is structure of thought)	**Disorders of Stream** (Flow of thought)	**Disorders of Possession** (Control of thought)	**Disorders of Content** (Themes)
• **Loosening of association** • **Derailment** • **Tangentiality** • **Substitution** • **Omission** • **Transitory thinking** • **Driveling** • **Desultory thinking** • **Neologism**, poverty of speech • **Poverty of content of speech**, word salad	• **Flight of ideas** • **Thought block** • Circumstantiality • Prolixity • Thought retardation • **Preservation**	• **Obsessions & compulsion**[Q] • **Thought insertion** • **Thought withdrawal** • **Thought broadcast**	• **Delusion of reference** • Persecution, misinterpretation • **Grandiosity** • **Guilt** • **Nihilism** • **Depressive cognitions** • **Overvalued ideas**

199. **Ans. b. Cognition**   *(Ref: Kaplan & Sadock 11/e p201, 225; Niraj Ahuja 7/e p13)*

The mini-mental state examination (MMSE) or Folstein test is a 30-point questionnaire that is used extensively in clinical and research settings to measure cognitive impairment. It is a screening tool for dementia. It assesses cognitive functions. The total score in MMSE is 30. A score <24 is suggestive of dementia.

"Mini-Mental State Examination (MMSE). The MMSE is a 30-point cognitive test developed in the mid-1970s to provide a bedside assessment of a broad array of cognitive function, including orientation, attention, memory, construction, and language."- Kaplan & Sadock 11/e p201

Mini-Mental State Examination (MMSE)	
Orientation[Q] • Name: Season/date/day/month/year • Name: Hospital/floor/town/state/country	 5 (1 for each name) 5 (1 for each name)
Registration[Q] • Identify three objects by name and ask patient to repeat	 3 (1 for each object)
Attention and calculation[Q] • Serial 7s: subtract from 100 (e.g. 93-86-79- 72-65)	 5 (1 for each subtraction)
Recall[Q] Recall the three objects presented earlier	 3 (1 for each object)
Language[Q] • Name pencil and watch • Repeat "No ifs, ands, or buts" • Follow a 3-step command ("Take this paper, fold it in half & place it on table") • Write "close your eyes" and ask patient to obey written command • Ask Patient to write a sentence • Ask patient to copy a design (e.g. intersecting pentagons)	 2 (1 for each object) 1 3 (1 for each command) 1 1 1
Total	**30**

200. **Ans. c. Events**   *(Ref: Kaplan & Sadock 11/e p116-117; Niraj Ahuja 7/e p14)*

Semantic memory is one of the two types of declarative or explicit memory. Semantic memory refers to general word knowledge that we have accumulated throughout our lives. This general knowledge (facts, ideas, meaning and concepts) is intertwined in experience and dependent on culture. Semantic memory is distinct from episodic memory, which is our memory of experiences and specific events that occur during our lives, from which we can recreate at any given point.

AIIMS May 2016

"Declarative memory depends on medial temporal and midline diencephalic structures along with large portions of the neocortex. This system provides for the rapid learning of facts (semantic memory) and events (episodic memory). Nondeclarative memory depends on several different brain systems. Habits depend on the neocortex and the neostriatum, and the cerebellum is important for the conditioning of skeletal musculature, the amygdala for emotional learning, and the neocortex for priming."- Kaplan & Sadock 11/e p116

"Declarative memory is phylogenetically more recent than nondeclarative memory. In addition, declarative memories are available to conscious recollection. The flexibility of declarative memory permits the retrieved information to be available to multiple response systems."- Kaplan & Sadock 11/e p116

"Nondeclarative memory is inaccessible to awareness and is expressed only by engaging specific processing systems. Nondeclarative memories are stored as changes within these processing systems—changes that are encapsulated such that the stored information has limited accessibility to other processing systems."- Kaplan & Sadock 11/e p116

"Semantic memory, which concerns general knowledge of the world, has often been categorized as a separate form of memory. Facts that are committed to memory typically become independent of the original episodes in which the facts were learned. Amnesic patients can sometimes acquire information that would ordinarily be learned as facts, but the patients learn it by relying on a different brain system than the system that supports declarative memory."- Kaplan & Sadock 11/e p116

Types of Memory	
Declarative memory	**Nondeclarative memory**
• Facts[Q] • Events[Q]	• Skill & habbits[Q] • Priming[Q] • Simple classical conditioning[Q] • Non-associative learning[Q]

Note

Note

Note

AIIMS NOVEMBER 2015

Multiple Choice Questions

ANATOMY

1. Identify the nerve in the given diagram whose palsy causes lateral gaze palsy.

   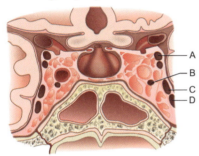

   a. A
   b. B
   c. C
   d. D

2. The nerve supplying the superior oblique muscle exits the brainstem at which of the following sites:

   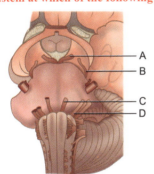

   a. A
   b. B
   c. C
   d. D

3. Which of the muscles marked in the given diagram helps in the protrusion of jaw?

   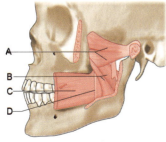

   a. A
   b. B
   c. C
   d. D

4. Identify the vagus nerve in this given cross-sectional diagram of the neck:

   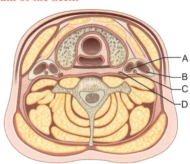

   a. A
   b. B
   c. C
   d. D

5. A 37-year-old patient presented to you with hyperextension of 4th and 5th metacarpophalangeal joint with flexion at proximal interphalangeal joint. This deformity is due to injury to:
   a. Deep branch of ulnar nerve
   b. Median nerve
   c. Radial nerve
   d. Superficial branch of median nerve

6. Which of the following nerves supplies the ear lobule?
   a. Greater auricular nerve
   b. Lesser occipital nerve
   c. Facial nerve
   d. Auriculotemporal nerve

7. Which of the following structures are not involved in development of diaphragm?
   a. Somatic body wall
   b. Septum transversum
   c. Pleuroperitoneal membrane
   d. Pleuropericardial membrane

8. Which of these is an immune-privileged site?
   a. Area postrema
   b. Loop of Henle
   c. Optic nerve
   d. Seminiferous tubules

9. Craniovertebral joint does not include:
   a. Occipital condyle
   b. Axis
   c. Atlas
   d. Wings of sphenoid

10. In pronator teres syndrome, the nerve involved is:
    a. Radial nerve
    b. Anterior interosseous nerve
    c. Ulnar nerve
    d. Median nerve

11. Maxillary bone does not articulate with:
    a. Ethmoid
    b. Sphenoid
    c. Frontal
    d. Lacrimal

12. **True statements about osteoblasts are all except:**
    a. Derived from osteoprogenitor cells
    b. Regulated by BMP
    c. Have a plasma membrane showing multiple folds
    d. Have neuropeptide receptors

13. **Which of the following vessels does not supply the anal canal?**
    a. Superior rectal artery   b. Middle rectal artery
    c. Inferior rectal artery   d. Median sacral artery

14. **Buccinator is pierced by all of the following except:**
    (AIIMS November 2015, November 2008)
    a. Labial branch of facial nerve
    b. Buccal branch of mandibular nerve
    c. Parotid duct
    d. Molar mucous glands

15. **All of the following are true about location of otic ganglia except:**
    a. Inferior to foramen ovale
    b. Lateral to tensor veli palatini
    c. Lateral to mandibular nerve
    d. Anterior to middle meningeal artery

PHYSIOLOGY

16. **All of the following are true about basal electrical rhythm of intestines except:**

    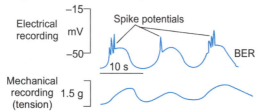

    a. Tone of contraction is related to amplitude of the stimulus
    b. Tone of contraction is related to frequency of stimulation
    c. Frequency of contraction is 6 per minute
    d. Threshold of contraction is –50 mV

17. **The given graph likely depicts which of the following disease?**

    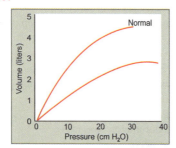

    a. Bronchial asthma   b. Emphysema
    c. Interstitial lung disease   d. Normal study

18. **Calculate the ejection fraction from the given volume pressure curve:**

    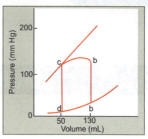

    a. 40%   b. 50%
    c. 55%   d. 60%

19. **Sodium iodine symporter is not present in:**
    a. Pituitary gland   b. Placenta
    c. Parotid   d. Thyroid

20. **Interstitial fluid volume can be determined by:**
    a. Radioactive iodine and radiolabelled water
    b. Radioactive water and radiolabelled albumin
    c. Radioactive sodium and radioactive water
    d. Radioactive sodium and radioactive labelled albumin

21. **Considering the latent period of a muscle twitch to be 10 ms, contraction time 40 ms and relaxation time 50 ms, what will be the tetanizing frequency for this muscle?**
    a. 25 Hz   b. 50 Hz
    c. 100 Hz   d. 75 Hz

22. **All of these are actions of Atrial Natriuretic Peptide except:**
    a. Afferent arteriole dilation
    b. Mesangial constriction
    c. Decreased sodium absorption in PCT
    d. Inhibition of sodium reabsorption in medullary collecting duct

23. **The extracellular potassium concentration is 100 mEq/mmol and intracellular potassium concentration is 10 mEq/mmol. What will be the equilibrium potential for potassium according to Nernst equation?**
    (AIIMS May 2016, November 2015)
    a. 0 V   b. –60 V
    c. –90 V   d. +30 V

24. **In the formula for urea clearance, $C = U \times V/P$, what does U stands for:** *(AIIMS May 2016, November 2015)*
    a. Urinary concentration in g/24 hour
    b. Urinary concentration in mg/ml
    c. Urine osmolarity
    d. Urine volume per minute

25. **Which of the following methods is used for calculation of anatomical dead space?**
    a. Xenon dilution technique   b. Bohler's method
    c. Spirometry
    d. Single breath nitrogen test

BIOCHEMISTRY

26. **Which of these is not a cofactor for glycogen phosphorylase, an important enzyme of the glycogenolysis pathway?**
    a. Calmodulin   b. c-AMP
    c. Protein Kinase A   d. Glycogenin

27. After a point mutation, glutamic acid is replaced by valine, which leads to formation of sickle cell hemoglobin. The mobility of HbS as compared with normal hemoglobin on gel electrophoresis will be:
    a. Decreased
    b. Increased
    c. Dependent on HbS concentration
    d. Unchanged

28. Thiamine is a cofactor for all of the following enzymes except:
    a. Alpha ketoglutarate dehydrogenase
    b. Branched-chain keto-acid dehydrogenase
    c. Succinate dehydrogenase
    d. Pyruvate dehydrogenase

29. The cofactor vitamin B12 is required for the following conversion:
    a. Dopamine to Norepinephrine
    b. Propionyl CoA to methyl malonyl CoA
    c. Methyl malonyl CoA to succinyl CoA
    d. Cysteine to homocysteine

30. Glycogen synthesis and breakdown takes place in the same cell, having enzymes necessary for both the pathways. Why the glucose-6-phosphate, freshly synthesized during glycogenesis in cytoplasm of hepatocytes, is not immediately degraded by the enzyme glucose-6-phosphatase?
    a. The thermodynamics does not favor such a reaction to occur
    b. Glucose-6-phosphatase is present in the endoplasmic reticulum and cannot act on glycogen formed in the cytoplasm
    c. Glycogenesis and glycogenolysis are tightly regulated such that enzymes of only one of those is present at a time.
    d. Steric hindrance due to albumin

31. In lead poisoning, there is an inhibition of some of the enzymes of the heme biosynthetic pathway. This is reflected by the accumulation of what substance in blood?
    a. Uroporphyrinogen III
    b. Ferrochelatase
    c. Porphobilinogen
    d. Delta amino levulinic acid

32. Sites of heme synthesis are all of these except:
    a. RBC
    b. Hepatocytes
    c. Osteocytes
    d. Bone marrow

33. What is the codon for selenocysteine?
    a. UAG
    b. UGA
    c. UAA
    d. GUA

34. All of these substrates are glucogenic except:
    (AIIMS May 2016, November 2015)
    a. Acetyl CoA
    b. Pyruvate
    c. Glycerol
    d. Lactate

35. Which of the following conversions does not require Biotin as a cofactor?
    a. Gamma carboxylation of glutamate
    b. Acetyl Co-A to Malonyl Co-A
    c. Propionyl Co-A to methyl malonyl Co-A
    d. Pyruvate to oxaloacetate

36. Which of the following is not a technique for protein precipitation?
    a. Trichloroacetic acid
    b. Heat precipitation
    c. Isoelectric point method
    d. Titration with reducing sugar

PATHOLOGY

37. The following microscopic appearance is that of schwannoma—a nerve sheath tumor most commonly involving the cerebellopontine angle. What does the area marked with arrow represent?

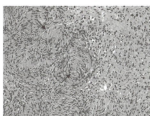

    a. Myxoid tissue
    b. Antony A pattern
    c. Antony B pattern—Verocay body
    d. Antony C pattern—Verocay body

38. A 12-year-old boy presents with enlargement of bilateral cervical lymph nodes for 2 years. A biopsy from the lymph node reveals the following picture. Which of the following is the correct set of diagnosis, etiology and the cell described?

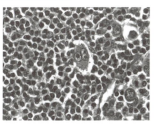

    a. Hodgkin's lymphoma; Epstein Barr Virus and Reed Sternberg cells
    b. Hodgkin's lymphoma; Epstein Barr Virus and Embryo cell
    c. Non-Hodgkin's lymphoma; HIV and Giant B cell
    d. Tuberculosis, Mycobacterium and Tiny granuloma

39. A liver biopsy reveals following findings. What is true about this condition?

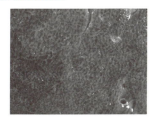

a. Nutmeg liver with dark areas of perivenular dead hepatocytes and gray areas of periportal viable hepatocytes
b. Nodular regenerative hyperplasia of liver induced due to OCPs
c. Nutmeg liver with pale areas of necrosis and dark congested areas of perivenular viable hepatocytes
d. Cirrhotic liver with fibrotic nodules.

40. A 30-years-old male patient presents with a history of heartburn. An upper GI endoscopy was done and a biopsy from a suspicious lesion showed the following picture. What does this show? Which special stains will you do for confirmation and what will you look for?

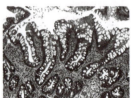

a. H. pylori infection, Silver stain, Gram-negative coccobacilli
b. Adenocarcinoma esophagus, mucin stain, mitotic figures
c. Squamous cell carcinoma, keratin stain
d. Barrett's esophagus, mucin stain, dysplasia

41. Cell growth can be stopped at some specific checkpoints in the cell cycle as depicted. Which stage of cell cycle demonstrates the primary point in regulation of cell growth?

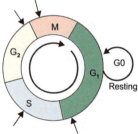

a. End of M
b. End of G_1
c. End of S
d. End of G_2

42. For what procedure is the instrument depicted in the diagram used?

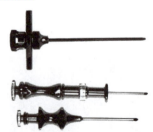

a. Bone marrow biopsy
b. Pleural biopsy
c. Kidney biopsy
d. Liver biopsy

43. Most important but nonspecific regulator of iron metabolism is:
a. Hepcidin
b. DMT1
c. Ferroportin
d. Ferritin

44. Which of these is the most important prognostic factor in ALL?
a. Hyperploidy
b. Total leucocyte count greater than 50,000
c. Age
d. Response to steroids

45. In genomic imprinting, DNA is modified by:
a. Acetylation
b. Methylation
c. Phosphorylation
d. Deamination

46. About intraoperative histopathological analysis, all are true except:
a. Gives an immediate definitive diagnosis of tumor
b. Used for detecting positive margins after resection
c. Used to confirm suspected metastasis
d. Sentinel lymph node biopsy in breast carcinoma is an example

PHARMACOLOGY

47. Some gram-negative bacteria produce an enzyme that blocks the action of beta lactam antibiotics in periplasmic space. Which arrow in the structural diagram of Penicillin G denotes the site of action of this enzyme?

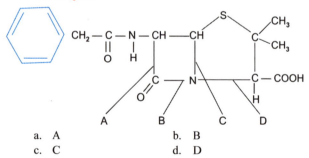

a. A
b. B
c. C
d. D

48. A guinea pig is dissected and a portion of its intestine is fixed in the modified Dales chamber to study the effects of some drugs on intestinal contractility. A substance X was infused in the broth following which the graph comes out as depicted. Substance X most closely resembles which of these substances?

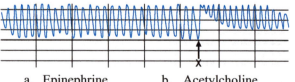

a. Epinephrine
b. Acetylcholine
c. KCl
d. $BaCl_2$

49. Drugs prescribed by registered medical practitioners mostly fall under which class of drugs?
a. Schedule X
b. Schedule S
c. Schedule H
d. Schedule P

50. Which of these drugs is a calcineurin inhibitor?
a. Cyclosporine
b. Methotrexate
c. Azathioprine
d. Mycophenolate mofetil

51. Which of the following is an antifibrinolytic agent?
    a. Dabigatran
    b. Protamine
    c. Alteplase
    d. Epsilon aminocaproic acid

52. At low infusion rates of 3–5 mcg/kg/min, what action is produced by dopamine?
    a. Vasoconstriction
    b. Increased renal blood flow
    c. Increased cardiac contractility
    d. Decreased blood pressure

53. Platelet aggregation is blocked by aspirin due to its action on:
    a. Prostacyclin
    b. PGF 2 alpha
    c. Thromboxane A2
    d. Phospholipase C

54. Phase 1 clinical trial is done for:
    a. Drug safety
    b. Pharmacodynamics
    c. Efficacy
    d. Dosing

55. Which of the following drugs acting on dilator pupillae has an action analogous to that of pilocarpine on sphincter papillae?
    a. Timolol
    b. Epinephrine
    c. Neostigmine
    d. Tropicamide

56. Which of the following drugs does not affect DNA synthesis?
    a. Rifampicin
    b. Linezolid
    c. Nitrofurantoin
    d. Metronidazole

57. What does low volume of distribution of a drug mean?
    a. Low bioavailability
    b. Does not accumulates in tissues
    c. Low absorption
    d. Not metabolized in the body

58. Which of the following drugs is not used in treatment of bird flu?
    a. Oseltamivir
    b. Ribavirin
    c. Zanamivir
    d. Peramivir

59. What are the appropriate instructions to be given while prescribing bisphosphonates to a patient:
    a. To be given empty stomach with a glass of water
    b. Taken along with food
    c. Stop if features of gastritis develop
    d. Stop if bone pains occur

60. Absorption of which of the following drugs is increased after a fatty meal?
    a. Amphotericin B
    b. Griseofulvin
    c. Ampicillin
    d. Aspirin

61. Steroids do not have a role in management of which of these tumors?
    a. Kaposi sarcoma
    b. Chronic lymphoid leukemia
    c. Hodgkin's lymphoma
    d. Multiple myeloma

62. Which of these anticonvulsants causes contraction of visual field?
    a. Levetiracetam
    b. Phenytoin
    c. Vigabatrin
    d. Ethosuximide

63. Which one of the following is a gender specific side-effect of valproate?
    a. Polycystic ovarian syndrome
    b. Alopecia
    c. Weight loss
    d. Tremor

64. Etanercept is a disease-modifying drug used in management of rheumatoid arthritis. What is its mechanism of action?
    a. Inhibition of TNF alpha
    b. COX-2 inhibition
    c. IL-6 inhibition
    d. Stabilization of mast cells

65. Which of the following drugs is not used in detoxification of chronic alcoholics?
    a. Flumazenil
    b. Disulfiram
    c. Acamprosate
    d. Naltrexone

MICROBIOLOGY

66. Stool examination in a patient reveals the following finding. What is the likely route of infection of this parasite?

    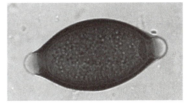

    a. Ingestion of food contaminated with the egg of larva
    b. Insect bite
    c. Improperly cooked beef
    d. Swimming in dirty water pool

67. A 35-year-old male farmer presents with multiple discharging cervical sinuses. Which of these stains will be useful for the diagnosis? Where does this organism normally colonise in the body?

    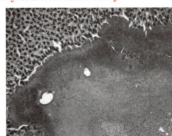

    a. Gram-stain, oropharynx
    b. PAS, intestine
    c. AFB, mouth
    d. Grocott Methenamine silver, skin

68. The following picture was seen in nasal biopsy from a patient with brain abscess. Identify the organism seen and the stain used?

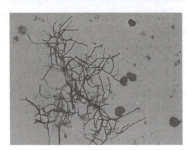

a. Staphylococcus, Gram-stain
b. Streptococcus, Gram-stain
c. Cryptococcus, India ink   d.   Nocardia, Gram-stain

69. **A smear was prepared from the genital ulcer. Identify the organism responsible:**

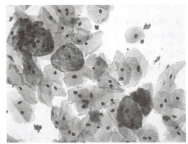

a. Chlamydia   b. Treponema pallidum
c. Trichomonas vaginalis d. Neisseria gonorrhoea

70. **A 24-year-old female presented with an ulcer in the genital area. A Giemsa stained cervical smear was taken which showed the following image. Identify the causative agent:**

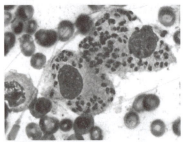

a. Chlamydia   b. Gardnerella vaginalis
c. Hemophilus ducreyi
d. Calymmatobacterium donovani

71. **A patient presented with headache and projectile vomiting along with alteration in sensorium. The following parasite demonstrated on India ink staining. What is the likely diagnosis?**

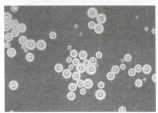

a. Coccidioides   b. Histoplasma
c. Blastomyces   d. Cryptococcus

72. **This is a schematic diagram depicting body structure of which of these helminths?**

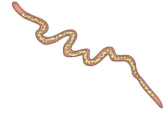

a. Onchocerca volvulus   b. Brugia malayi
c. Loa loa   d. Wuchereria bancrofti

73. **A patient presents with progressive dyspnoea. Chest X-ray revealed a cavitary lesion in lower lobe of right lung. The following histopathological appearance was seen of resection of the cavity. What is the most likely cause of this disease and the number of layers that can be seen in the wall of the parasite?**

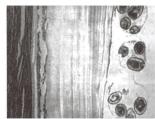

a. Cysticercosis with 3 layers
b. Strongyloides with 2 layers
c. Echinococcus with 2 layers
d. Paragonimus with 2 layers

74. **The following diagram depicts blood smear of which species?**

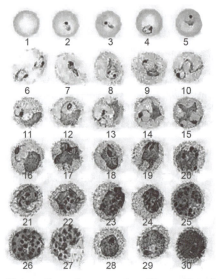

a. Plasmodium vivax   b. Plasmodium falciparum
c. Plasmodium ovale   d. Plasmodium malariae

75. A patient comes to your clinic with a complaint of multiple episodes of loose watery stool for 3 days. On probing, you discover that these episodes start after he had ingested shellfish at a local restaurant 3 days back and other people who had food from that restaurant had similar symptoms. What is the most common cause of viral diarrhoea in adults?
    a. Calicivirus
    b. Rotavirus
    c. Adenovirus
    d. Norovirus

76. Antibody-dependent enhancement is implicated in the immunopathogenesis of which disease?
    a. Influenza
    b. Staphylococcal toxic shock syndrome
    c. Waterhouse-Friderichsen syndrome
    d. Dengue hemorrhagic fever

77. Phage mediated change in C. diphtheria is due to which of the following?
    a. Conjugation
    b. Transformation
    c. Transduction
    d. None of the above

FORENSIC MEDICINE

78. Shoe polish like smell is seen in:
    a. Mercaptans
    b. Lacquer
    c. Paraldehyde
    d. Nitrobenzene

79. Which acid does not show coagulation necrosis on contact?
    a. HCl
    b. H_2SO_4
    c. HF
    d. HNO_3

80. Ashley rule is for determination of what:
    a. Age
    b. Sex
    c. Height
    d. Ethnicity

81. A man throws sulphuric acid on the face of his wife after a fight following which she comes to the emergency for supportive management. All of these statements are true about chemical burns except:
    a. Blisters are present
    b. Ulcerated patches are present
    c. Absence of singeing of hairs
    d. Coagulation necrosis occurs at the site of burn

82. A doctor who performed the autopsy on a 26-year-old married woman, committing suicide found the cause of death to be aluminium phosphide poisoning. She was summoned in a court of law where he willingly hides this information. This is punishable under which section?
    a. IPC 193
    b. CrPC 175
    c. CrPC 69
    d. IPC 189

83. Ewing's postulates concerns with which of the following:
    a. Growth at the site following trauma
    b. Growth after a neurological injury
    c. Age related changes in the teeth
    d. Old seminal stains

84. Boiled lobster syndrome is seen in poisoning of:
    a. Boric acid
    b. HNO_3
    c. H_2SO_4
    d. Phenol

85. An autopsy was performed on a case of accidental death. It showed two linear fractures on petrous part of temporal bone. Which of the following rules gives the sequence of fractures?
    a. McNaughton's rule
    b. Puppe's rule
    c. Young's rule
    d. Dunlop's rule

86. Which of these findings is not specific of blast injury?
    a. Abrasion
    b. Bruise
    c. Puncture laceration
    d. Fracture

87. According to National Crime Bureau, most common mode of suicide in India is:
    a. Drowning
    b. Poisoning
    c. Fall from height
    d. Hanging

88. Which of the following statement is false statement about snake-bites?
    a. Anti-venom is not effective in humpnosed pit viper bite
    b. Cobra venom is neurotoxic
    c. Atropine premedication should be used before administering Neostigmine
    d. Neostigmine has a role in krait bite

PSM

89. What is the name of disease transmitted by this vector?

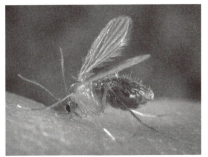

    a. Filaria
    b. Leishmaniasis
    c. Yellow fever
    d. Malaria

90. Identify the disease in which the following treatment is used?

MB adult blister pack

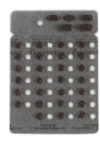

    a. Influenza
    b. Kala-Azar
    c. Tuberculosis
    d. Leprosy

91. The following life cycle most closely resembles that of which of the following viruses?

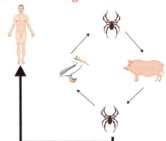

   a. Influenza A b. Dengue
   c. Japanese encephalitis virus
   d. Kyasanur forest disease virus

92. The following box plot shows the distribution of three sets of data around the mean. What is the correct sequence of inference from this box plot?

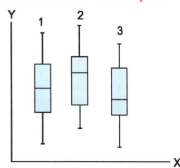

   a. 1-Normal distribution, 2-Positive skewed, 3-Negative skewed
   b. 1-Normal distribution, 2-Negative skewed, 3-Positive skewed
   c. 1-Negative skewed, 2-Positive skewed, 3-Normal distribution
   d. 1-Positive skewed, 2-Normal distribution, 3-Negative skewed

93. The following scatter plot of 4 different samples shows the correlation between weight and height in the samples. All 4 samples have the same coefficient of correlation of 0.6 taken together, what will be the net correlation coefficient?

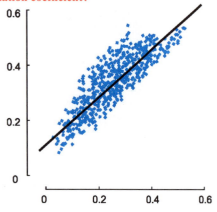

   a. More then 0.6 b. Less then 0.6
   c. 0.6 d. Cannot be calculated

94. What is following type of data description called?

5	3				
6	8	9	5		
7	9	2	0	2	
8	4	7	9	5	3
9	0	4			

   a. Stem and leaf diagram b. Box whisker plot
   c. Forrest plot d. Funnel plot

95. A latex agglutination test for detection of meningitis was approved. Calculate the sensitivity and specificity of the test based on the data given below:

	Test Positive	Test Negative
Diseased	27	3
Non-diseased	5	95

   a. Sensitivity 90%, Specificity 95%
   b. Sensitivity 95%, Specificity 90%
   c. Sensitivity 80%, Specificity 90%
   d. Sensitivity 75%, Specificity 95%

96. A patient of diabetes and hypertension comes to your clinic. As a doctor, you explain to him the risks of various complications. Which of these is the best tool to demonstrate the complications?
   a. Pie chart b. Histogram
   c. Scatter plot d. Venn diagram

97. Which of these is the best study to evaluate effect and outcome?
   a. Clinical trial b. Cohort
   c. Case control study d. Cross sectional study

98. A researcher selected all possible samples from a population and plotted their means on a line graph. This distribution is called as:
   a. Sample distribution
   b. Sampling distribution
   c. Population distribution
   d. Parametric distribution

99. Some medicine comes with a label of 'store at a cool place only'. At what temperature should these medicines be kept?
   a. 8–15 °C b. 2–8 °C
   c. 0 °C d. 25–28 °C

100. The mean systolic blood pressure was measured in a sample population of elderly females and came out to be 125 mm Hg with a standard deviation of 10. 95 percent of people would have blood pressure above:
   a. 105 mm Hg b. 110 mm Hg
   c. 115 mm Hg d. 140 mm Hg

AIIMS November 2015

101. A drug, which does not cure a disease but decreases its symptoms and increases survival, leads to?
    a. Increased prevalence
    b. Increased incidence
    c. Decreased prevalence
    d. Decreased incidence

102. Which of these is not true about randomization in a clinical trial?
    a. Reduces confounding
    b. Decreases selection bias
    c. Ensures comparability of two groups
    d. Increases external validity of the trial

103. Which of these statements is true about Rashtriya Swasthya Bima Yojana?
    a. Cashless benefit on presenting smartcard and fingerprints
    b. Valid for up to 4 family members
    c. Can be used only in 1 district
    d. Treatment only in government hospitals

104. A recently delivered woman with a 15 days old child suffering from cough, sneezing and fever needs help. She has no money for transportation to nearby hospital. Which of the national programme can help this woman?
    a. JSSK
    b. Indira Gandhi Yojana
    c. F-IMNCI
    d. Home-based Care

105. According to the new WHO 2013 malaria treatment guidelines, which of the following statements is true?
    a. No ACT in falciparum malaria
    b. Presumptive treatment with chloroquine should be given
    c. Primaquine is contraindicated in infants and pregnant women
    d. Primaquine is to be given for 7 days in falciparum malaria

106. The trivalent influenza vaccine contains all of the following strains except:
    a. H1N1
    b. H3N2
    c. H2N1
    d. Influenza B

107. Most cost-effective method of infection control is:
    a. Repeated disinfectant use
    b. Alcohol based rubbing
    c. Prophylactic antibiotic therapy
    d. Hand washing

MEDICINE

108. A 29-year-old male athlete suddenly collapsed and died during a football game. At autopsy the following finding was seen on gross examination. He had a history of two similar deaths in the family previously. What is the most likely cause of death?

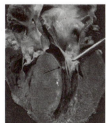

    a. Hypertrophic cardiomyopathy
    b. RHD
    c. Coronary heart disease
    d. Dilated cardiomyopathy

109. A 65-year-old patient presents to your clinic with a history of chest pain for last 24 hours associated with sweating and diaphoresis. The following ECG findings are seen. BP is 150/90 mm Hg. Which of the following is not given in management of this patient?

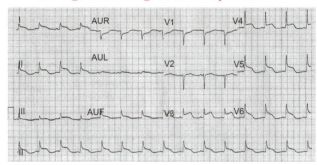

    a. Thrombolysis
    b. Aspirin
    c. Statin
    d. Morphine

110. A following ECG was recorded from a patient presenting to the emergency. What is the likely diagnosis?

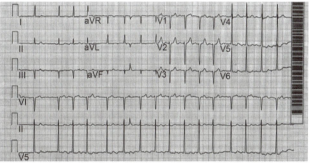

    a. Sinus arrhythmia
    b. Atrial Fibrillation
    c. PSVT
    d. Heart block

111. Which of the following drugs is not indicated in the management of the condition seen in the following ECG?

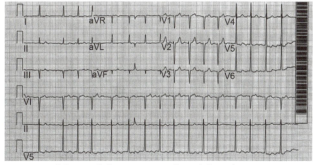

    a. Metoprolol
    b. Adenosine
    c. Amiodarone
    d. Diltiazem

112. All of these are true about microalbuminuria except:
    a. Urine protein levels range from 20 mg/d to 200 mg/d
    b. It is an independent risk factor for cardiovascular morbidity in diabetic patients
    c. It is the earliest marker of diabetic nephropathy
    d. It is not detected by routine dipstick method
113. Which of the following is a new drug available to treat multi drug resistant tuberculosis?
    a. Bedaquiline   b. Rifampicin
    c. Linezolid   d. Cefepime
114. According to WHO guidelines, latent TB should be ruled out in all the following situations except:
    a. Before treatment with TNF-alpha inhibitors
    b. Chronic alcoholics
    c. Silicosis   d. Hemodialysis
115. A 65-year-old male adult presents with chronic sinusitis, nasopharyngeal ulcers, cavitatory lung nodules and renal failure. What will be the appropriate next diagnostic step?
    a. Lung biopsy
    b. Sputum AFB and PCR for TB
    c. ANCA and evaluation for vasculitis
    d. ESR
116. Serology profile done for a patient is mentioned below. What is the likely cause of the abnormal findings:
    HbsAg-Non-reactive
    HBV DNA-Undetectable
    HbeAg-Non-reactive
    IgG Anti-HbC-Reactive
    a. Chronic hepatitis inactive state
    b. Chronic hepatitis recovery state
    c. Pre-core mutant infection
    d. Window period
117. A 23-year-old male patient presented with a history of back pain, which is more in the morning and relieved by bathing in warm water. What is the likely additional finding present in this patient?
    a. Marrow fibrosis
    b. Distal phalangeal joint involvement
    c. Pleural nodules
    d. Decreased chest wall expansion
118. Which of these is a new oral drug used in treatment of chronic Hepatitis C?
    a. Interferon alpha   b. Ledipasvir
    c. Oseltamivir   d. Lamivudine
119. In a patient of jaundice, absence of urobilinogen in urine indicates?
    a. Obstructive jaundice   b. Hemolysis
    c. Liver failure   d. Hepatitis
120. Most specific sign of metabolic encephalopathy is:
    a. Asterixis   b. Abulia
    c. Akinetic mutism   d. Apraxia
121. A patient presented with a steering wheel injury to the right side of chest with breathlessness and shock. How will you differentiate tension pneumothorax and cardiac tamponade?
    a. Pulse pressure   b. JVP
    c. Breath sound   d. Heart sounds
122. All of the following are features of glucocorticoid deficiency except:
    a. Fever   b. Hyperkalemia
    c. Postural hypotension   d. Weight loss
123. Naming and fluency is impaired in:
    a. Broca's aphasia
    b. Wernicke's aphasia
    c. Anomic aphasia
    d. Transcortical sensory aphasia
124. A 9-year-old boy presented with difficulty in climbing stairs and combing. On examination, bilateral calves are swollen and the child uses his feet to stand up on his legs. What is the next diagnostic step?
    a. Creatine kinase levels
    b. EMG
    c. Nerve conduction velocity
    d. RA factor
125. All are features of benign intracranial hypertension except:
    a. Proptosis   b. Normal size ventricles
    c. Headache   d. Papilledema

SURGERY

126. Identify this crystal found in urine analysis:

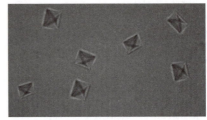

    a. Calcium carbonate stone
    b. Ammonium phosphate stone
    c. Uric acid
    d. Calcium oxalate stone
127. A 17-year-old patient develops intussusception for which he was operated and a segment of intestine showing multiple polyps was resected. Microscopy showed the following pathology. What is the likely diagnosis?

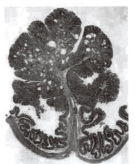

    a. Tubulovillous polyps   b. Hamartomatous polyps
    c. Inflammatory polyps   d. Adenocarcinoma

128. **Peau d'orange in carcinoma breast is due to:**
   (AIIMS November 2015, DNB 2012, PGI June 95, December 95)
   a. Obstruction of sub-dermal lymphatics
   b. Infiltration of Coopers ligament
   c. Hematogenous dissemination
   d. Nipple involvement

129. **A patient underwent thyroidectomy for Hyperthyroidism. Two days later he presented with features of thyroid storm. What is the most likely cause?**
   (AIIMS November 2015, COMED K 2007)
   a. Poor antibiotic coverage
   b. Rough handling during surgery
   c. Removal of parathyroid
   d. Inadequate preoperative preparation

130. **A 60-year-old chronic smoker presented with progressive jaundice, pruritus and clay colored stools for 2 months. History of waxing and waning of jaundice was present. A CT scan revealed dilated main pancreatic duct and common bile duct. What is the likely diagnosis?**
   a. Carcinoma head of pancreas
   b. Periampullary carcinoma
   c. Chronic pancreatitis
   d. Hilar cholangiocarcinoma

131. **What is false about Meckel's diverticulitis?**
   a. Present in 3% of the population
   b. Presents with periumbilical pain
   c. Remnant of proximal part of vitellointestinal duct
   d. Lies on the anti-mesenteric border

132. **A child presented with a swelling in the right groin region. When the swelling was reduced, a gurgling sound was heard. Which of the following is an incorrect statement?**
   a. The sac contains omentum only
   b. The hernia lies above and medial to pubic tubercle
   c. Patent processus vaginalis
   d. This type of hernia is most common in children

133. **During laparoscopic inguinal hernia repair a tacker was accidently placed below and lateral to the iliopubic tract. Postoperatively the patient complained of pain and soreness in the thigh. This is due to the involvement of:** *(AIIMS November 2015, May 2015)*
   a. Lateral cutaneous nerve of thigh
   b. Ilioinguinal nerve
   c. Genital branch of genitofemoral nerve
   d. Obturator nerve

134. **Which of these is the most reliable method for monitoring fluid resuscitation?**
   (AIIMS November 2015, PGI December 97, All India 94)
   a. Urine output
   b. CVP
   c. Pulse rate
   d. Blood pressure

135. **What are the minimum and maximum possible values of Glasgow Coma Score?**
   a. Minimum = 3, Maximum = 15
   b. Minimum = 0, Maximum = 13
   c. Minimum = 0, Maximum = 15
   d. Minimum = 3, Maximum = 18

136. **A patient had a massive bleeding during surgery. Which sized cannula should be used?**
   (AIIMS May 2016, November 2015)
   a. 16 Gauge
   b. 20 Gauge
   c. 22 Gauge
   d. 24 Gauge

OBSTETRICS & GYNAECOLOGY

137. **A 28-year-old female patient presented with lower abdominal pain along with dysmenorrhea. The following finding was seen on laparoscopic examination. What is the likely diagnosis?**

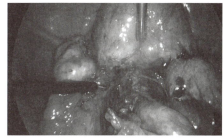

   a. Krukenberg tumor
   b. Polycystic ovaries
   c. Endometriosis
   d. Cystadenoma of ovary

138. **Following fetal tocographic finding was seen in a 30-year-old female patient in labor. What does it suggest?**

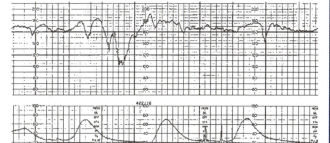

   a. Early cord compression
   b. Fetal distress
   c. Head compression
   d. Fetal anemia

139. **HSG image below shows:**

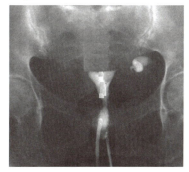

   a. Endometrial polyp
   b. Genital TB
   c. Fibroid uterus
   d. Asherman syndrome

140. Which of the following statements is true about Swyer syndrome?
    a. Can be fertile with surrogacy
    b. Can be fertile with ovum donation
    c. Presents with primary fertility
    d. Gonadectomy is indicated for all patients

141. Which of these is seen in Asherman syndrome?
    (AIIMS May 2016, November 2015)
    a. Oligomenorrhea   b. Hypomenorrhea
    c. Metromenorrhagia   d. Polymenorrhea

142. What is the most likely cause for beaded appearance of fallopian tubes with clubbed ends of fimbriae on HSG?
    a. Genital tuberculosis   b. Chlamydia
    c. Neisseria gonorrhoea   d. Endometriosis

143. Which of these is diagnostic of menopause?
    a. Serum FSH > 40   b. Serum LH > 20
    c. Serum FSH < 40   d. Serum estradiol < 30

144. What is the first sign of puberty in a girl?
    a. Thelarche   b. Menarche
    c. Adrenarche   d. Pubarche

145. A 23-year-old lady taking antiepileptics for a seizure disorder gets married. When should folic acid supplementation advised to the patient?
    a. Any time as soon as she presents to the clinic irrespective of pregnancy
    b. Three months before becoming pregnant
    c. 1st trimester
    d. As soon as pregnancy is confirmed

146. In the pelvic inlet, which is the shortest anteroposterior diameter?
    a. True conjugate   b. Obstetric conjugate
    c. Anatomical conjugate d. Bispinous diameter

147. Estrogen and progesterone in the first 2 months of pregnancy are produced by:
    a. Fetal ovaries   b. Fetal adrenal
    c. Placenta   d. Corpus luteum

148. Drug of choice for pregnancy-induced hypertension is: *(AIIMS November 2015, May 2015)*
    a. Atenolol   b. Nitroprusside
    c. Enalapril   d. Alpha-methyldopa

149. A G3P2, pregnant comes to your clinic at 18 weeks of gestation for genetic counselling. She has a history of two kids born with thalassemia major. Which test would you recommend now?
    a. Amniocentesis
    b. Chorionic villus sampling
    c. Cordocentesis
    d. Non-invasive prenatal testing

150. Modified BPP consists of:
    a. NST with AFI
    b. NST with fetal breathing
    c. NST with fetal movement
    d. NST with fetal tone

151. Which of these is not a non-contraceptive use of levonorgestrel?
    a. Endometriosis
    b. Premenstrual tension
    c. Complex endometrial hyperplasia
    d. Emergency contraception

152. All of these can be used for post-coital contraception except:
    a. Desogestrel   b. Copper-T
    c. Levonorgestrel   d. OCP

153. Ulipristal acetate is a/an:
    a. GnRH agonist
    b. Androgen antagonist
    c. Selective estrogen receptor modulator
    d. Selective progesterone receptor modulator

154. What is the approved dose of misoprostol in emergent management of postpartum hemorrhage?
    a. 200 mcg   b. 400 mcg
    c. 600 mcg   d. 1000 mcg

155. What is the best time to give anti-D to a pregnant patient?
    a. 12 weeks   b. 28 weeks
    c. 36 weeks   d. After delivery

PEDIATRICS

156. Identify the following congenital defect:

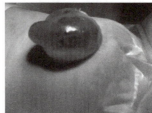

    a. Spina bifida occulta b. Dermoid cyst
    c. Meningocele   d. Cystic hygroma

157. A 2-year-old child with fever and barking cough for last 2 days presented to the pediatric emergency at 2.30 am. On examination, respiratory rate is 36/min, temperature of 39 °C and stridor heard only on crying. No other abnormality is found. What is the next best step in management?
    (AIIMS November 2015, May 2013)
    a. High-dose dexamethasone
    b. Racemic epinephrine nebulization
    c. Reassurance
    d. Intravenous antibiotics

158. A 1-year old infant presents with 10–12 episodes of watery stools per day for the last 9 days. Along with zinc supplementation, what else should be prescribed to the child?
    a. ORS with antibiotics
    b. ORS only
    c. ORS with low-lactose diet
    d. ORS with low-lactose diet and probiotics

159. **Milk is deficient in:**
    a. Iron and vitamin C
    b. Iron and vitamin A
    c. Phosphorus and vitamin A
    d. Saturated fats

160. **All of these are criteria for severe acute malnutrition in a 6-month-old child except:**
    a. Mid-upper arm circumference
    b. Symmetrical edema
    c. Weight for height
    d. Height for age

161. **How is under-nutrition defined?**
    a. Weight for age < –2 SD
    b. Weight for height < –2 SD
    c. Weight for age < –3 SD
    d. Weight for height < –3 SD

162. **A 3.5 kg male infant born at term after an uncomplicated pregnancy and delivery develops respiratory distress shortly after birth and requires mechanical ventilation. The chest radiograph reveals a normal cardiothymic silhouette but a diffuse ground glass appearance to the lung fields. Surfactant replacement fails to improve gas exchange. Over the first week life, the hypoxemia worsens. Results of routing culture and echocardiographic findings are negative. A term female sibling died at 1 month of age with respiratory distress. Which of the following is the most likely diagnosis?**
    (AIIMS November 2015, May 2011)
    a. Neonatal pulmonary alveolar proteinosis
    b. Meconium aspiration
    c. Total anomalous pulmonary venous return
    d. Disseminated herpes simplex infection

ORTHOPEDICS

163. **Identify the deformity seen in the given picture:**

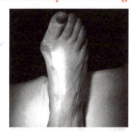

    a. Hallux valgus
    b. Hallux varus
    c. Cubitus valgus
    d. Rheumatoid nodule

164. **Which of the following test is being demonstrated by the given image?**

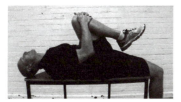

    a. Straight leg raising test
    b. Thomas test
    c. Narath sign
    d. Trendelenburg test

165. **A 9-year-old child presents to your clinic with the following deformity. Which is the most likely fracture leading to such a defect?**

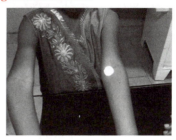

    a. Colle's fracture
    b. Lateral epicondyle fracture
    c. Medial epicondyle fracture
    d. Supracondylar fracture

166. **A child presented with pain in the forearm following a trauma. An AP and lateral X-ray of the forearm reveal the findings as shown. What is the most likely diagnosis?**

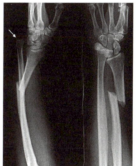

    a. Colle's fracture   b. Smith fracture
    c. Monteggia fracture   d. Galeazzi's fracture

167. **Meralgia paresthetica is due to involvement of:**
    a. Lateral cutaneous nerve of thigh
    b. Genitofemoral nerve
    c. Ilioinguinal nerve
    d. Saphenous nerve

168. **All the following can lead to damage of the axillary nerve except:**
    a. Fracture of surgical neck of humerus
    b. Intramuscular injection
    c. Improper use of crutches
    d. Shoulder dislocation

OPHTHALMOLOGY

169. **Keyhole-shaped visual field defect is seen in lesion involving which of the following regions?**
    a. Optic disk
    b. Optic chiasma
    c. Lateral geniculate body
    d. Occipital lobe

170. Which of the following is the most common fungal infection of the eye seen in an HIV positive patient?
    a. Aspergillus   b. Candida
    c. Toxoplasma   d. Rhinosporidium

ENT

171. Which is the most common type of congenital ossicular dysfunction?
    a. Isolated stapes defect
    b. Stapes defect with fixation of footplate and lenticular process involvement.
    c. Defective lenticular process of incus
    d. None of the above

172. Auditory neurotherapy is an effective modality of treatment for which of the following abnormalities of hearing?
    a. CSOM
    b. Meniere's disease
    c. Malignant otitis externa
    d. Otosclerosis

173. Which of the following tests is recommended for neonatal screening of hearing?
    a. Automated auditory brainstem response
    b. Spontaneous OAE
    c. Evoked OAE
    d. Distorted product OAE

174. A patient presents to your clinic for evaluation of defective hearing. Rinne's test shows air conduction greater than the bone conduction on both sides with Weber test lateralized to right ear. What is the next logical step?
    a. Normal test
    b. Schwabach's test
    c. Repeat Rinne's test on right side
    d. Wax removal

SKIN

175. A lady presents with history burning sensation on eating spicy food. On examination bilateral white lacy streaks are present in buccal mucosa. There is no history tobacco abuse but amalgamated third molar is present. What is the diagnosis?

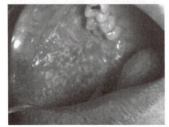

    a. Leukoplakia   b. Lichen planus
    c. Candidiasis   d. Aphthous stomatitis

176. A young male presents with the following itchy lesion for one month. All of the following genera can cause this kind of lesion except:

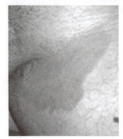

    a. Aspergillus   b. Trichophyton
    c. Microsporum   d. Epidermophyton

177. An 18-year-old female presents to you with a hypopigmented patch on the medial aspect foot with feathery margin. The rest of the physical examination is normal. Which of the following drug should not be used in the treatment of this patient?

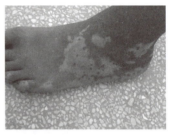

    a. Topical tacrolimus   b. Clobetasol
    c. Isotretinoin   d. PUVA

178. A young boy with oily skin presents with acne as shown. What is the appropriate treatment?

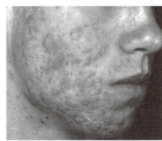

    a. Oral isotretinoin   b. Oral steroid
    c. Topical retinoic acid   d. Benzoyl peroxide

179. A 28-year-old lady has asymptomatic dome shaped small lesions on forehead for last 2 months. She has a 2-year-old daughter with similar lesions. What is the causative agent of the lesion?

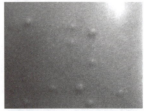

    a. Papillomavirus   b. Poxvirus
    c. Herpes virus   d. Coxsackie virus

180. A young male presented with anesthetic patch on right forearm. A thickened nerve was palpable on examination. Skin biopsy shows the following picture. What is the diagnosis?

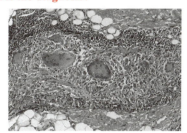

   a. TT
   b. LL
   c. Histiocytosis
   d. Lymphoma

181. A 28-year-old patient of neurocysticercosis develops generalized peeling of skin all over except palms and soles starting one month after taking anti-epileptics. What is the most probable diagnosis?
   a. Fixed drug eruption
   b. Pemphigus
   c. Steven Johnson syndrome
   d. TEN

182. Which type of oral candidiasis does not presents with white patch?
   a. Chronic atrophic candidiasis
   b. Chronic hyperplastic candidiasis
   c. Chronic mucocutaneous candidiasis
   d. Pseudomembranous candidiasis

ANESTHESIA

183. The given instrument is used for?

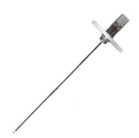

   a. Pleural biopsy
   b. Lumbar puncture
   c. Liver biopsy
   d. Bone marrow biopsy

184. Identify the use of the following instrument:

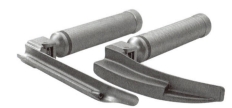

   a. Laryngoscopy
   b. Bone marrow aspiration
   c. Intraoperative retraction
   d. None of these

185. The diagram of a correctly positioned proseal-type Laryngeal Mask Airway is provided below. Above what site is the arrow marked area of the airway positioned?

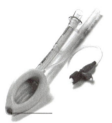

   a. Carina
   b. Upper end of trachea
   c. Vocal cords
   d. Above esophagus

186. A patient was in surgery when suddenly a resident noticed the following plot on the capnograph monitor. What should be the immediate next step in management of the patient?

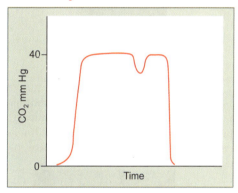

   a. Increase muscle relaxant
   b. Increase the depth of anesthesia
   c. Check tubes for any blockage
   d. Change soda-lime

187. What is color of medical oxygen cylinder?
   a. Black body with grey shoulder
   b. Grey body with black and white shoulder
   c. Black body with white shoulder
   d. Grey body with black shoulder

188. What is the most reliable site to measure core temperature during general anesthesia?
   a. Pulmonary artery
   b. Distal esophagus
   c. Rectum
   d. Tympanic membrane

189. While performing a lumbar puncture, a snap is felt just before entering into the epidural space. This is due to piercing of which structure?
   a. Ligamentum flavum
   b. Supraspinous ligament
   c. Duramater
   d. Posterior longitudinal ligament

190. A pregnant woman with placenta previa started to bleed as she went into labor. Her blood pressure was 80/50 mm Hg. A lower segment caesarean section was planned in view of acute shock. What type of anesthesia will you plan for this patient?

a. General anesthesia with IV induction by ketamine
b. Spinal anesthesia up to L4 level
c. General anesthesia with IV induction by propofol followed by maintenance with fluranes
d. Sedation and epidural analgesia

191. Which of these is most commonly used as pre-anesthetic medication?
    a. Atropine
    b. Promethazine
    c. Scopolamine
    d. Glycopyrrolate

RADIOLOGY

192. A 20-year old male patient presents with pain on movement. X-ray of knee joint shows lytic lesion on the upper end of tibia. What is the likely diagnosis?

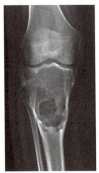

    a. Simple bone cyst
    b. Adamantinoma
    c. Multiple myeloma
    d. Osteoclastoma

193. The following chest X-ray was recorded from a patient presenting to emergency with breathlessness. What is the most likely diagnosis?

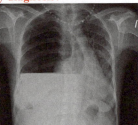

    a. Emphysema
    b. Hydropneumothorax
    c. Pneumothorax
    d. Cardiac tamponade

194. A patient presented with neck pain and rigidity, which gets relieved after bathing in hot water and also after exercise. Cervical X-ray is shown below. What is the likely diagnosis?

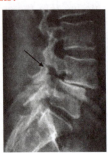

    a. Spondylolisthesis
    b. Spondylosis
    c. Compression fracture
    d. Osteoporosis

PSYCHIATRY

195. A 30-year old pregnant woman comes to your clinic with decreased sleep, increased appetite and hyperactivity for 2 weeks. A diagnosis of mania is made. Further probing reveals four episodes of major depression in the past two years. What drug will you prescribe to this patient?
    a. Haloperidol
    b. Lithium
    c. Promethazine
    d. Clonazepam

196. Which of the following is not a component of cognitive triad of Beck?
    a. Hopelessness
    b. Worthlessness
    c. Helplessness
    d. Guilt

197. A young female on antidepressants presents to the emergency with altered sensorium and hypotension. ECG reveals wide QRS complexes and right axis deviation. Next best step for the management of this patient:
    a. Sodium bicarbonate
    b. Hemodialysis
    c. Fomepizole
    d. Flumazenil

198. A 23-year old young boy with schizophrenia is well maintained on risperidone for the last 2 months. He has no family history of the disease. For how long medication should be continued in this patient?
    a. 5 years
    b. 6 months
    c. 2 years
    d. 12 months

199. A child with pervasive developmental disorder will have all of the following except:
    a. Stereotype behaviour
    b. Reduced social interaction
    c. Poor language skills
    d. Impaired cognition

200. A male patient of bipolar disorder with history of 5 episodes of mania and 1 episode of depression in last 8 years, under control by mood stabilizer, and manic symptoms appear as he tapered down the drugs. Which of the following intervention should be carried out to improve drug compliance?
    a. Psychoeducation
    b. CBT
    c. Supportive psychotherapy
    d. Insight-oriented psychotherapy

Explanations

ANATOMY

1. **Ans. b. B** *(Ref: Gray's 41e p437, 664, 670; 40/e p430; Snells 9/e p544)*

   Lateral gaze palsy is due to paralysis of lateral rectus, which is supplied by the abducens nerve.

	Structures Marked in the Diagram
A	• Oculomotor nerve
B	• Abducens nerve
C	• Ophthalmic nerve
D	• Maxillary nerve

   *"**The abducens nerve** is the **sixth cranial nerve** and **innervates lateral rectus exclusively**. It emerges from the brain stem between the pons and the medulla oblongata and usually **runs through** the inferior venous compartment of the **petroclival venous confluence in a bow-shaped canal, Dorello's canal**. It then bends sharply across the upper border of the petrous part of the temporal bone to enter the cavernous sinus, where **it lies lateral to the internal carotid artery** (unlike the oculomotor, trochlear, ophthalmic and maxillary nerves, which merely invaginate the lateral dural wall of the sinus). The abducens nerve **enters the orbit through the superior orbital fissure**, within the common tendinous ring, at first below, and then between, the two divisions of the oculomotor nerve and lateral to the nasociliary nerve. It **passes forwards to enter the medial (ocular) surface of lateral rectus**."- Gray's 40/e p430*

   Fig. 1: The nerves of the left orbit and the ciliary ganglion

   ### Cavernous Sinus

   - It is a **large venous space** situated **in middle cranial fossa** on either side of **body of the sphenoid**.

   #### Contents of the Cavernous Sinus

   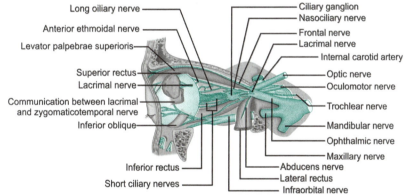

Structures in the lateral wall of sinus from above downwards	Structures passing through centre of the sinus (content)
• Oculomotor (IIIrd) nerve[Q] • Trochlear nerve (IVth)[Q] • Ophthalmic (V₁) nerve[Q] • Maxillary (V₂) nerve[Q] • Trigeminal ganglion[Q]	• *Abducent (VIth) nerve*[Q] • *Internal carotid artery*[Q]

AIIMS ESSENCE

Tributaries of cavernous sinus		
From the orbit	**From the brain**	**From the meninges**
• **Superior ophthalmic vein**[Q] • A branch of the **inferior ophthalmic vein**[Q] • **Central vein of retina**[Q]	• **Superficial middle cerebral vein**[Q] • **Inferior cerebral veins**[Q]	• **Sphenoparietal sinus**[Q] • Frontal trunk of the middle meningeal vein

Draining channels of cavernous sinus	
• Into the **transverse sinus** through **superior petrosal sinus**[Q] • Into the **internal jugular vein** through **inferior petrosal sinus**[Q]	• Into the **pterygoid plexus of veins** through **emissary veins**[Q] • Into the **facial vein** through **superior ophthalmic vein**[Q]

Cranial Nerve	Characteristic Features
Olfactory (I) Nerve	• Only cranial nerve to enter cerebrum directly[Q] • Only sensory afferent pathway that reaches cerebral cortex with out synapsing in one of the thalamic nuclei[Q]
Trochlear (IV) Nerve	• **Smallest cranial nerve**[Q] • **Most slender cranial nerve**[Q] • **Only nerve to emerge from dorsal (posterior) surface of brain stem**[Q] (mid brain) • Passes anteriorly around the brain stem, running the **longest intracranial (subarachnoid) course**[Q] • Nerve crosses the midline within the midbrain, emerges from its dorsal aspect and immediately **decussates with the nerve of opposite side**[Q] • **Sole supply is superior oblique**[Q] the only extra ocular muscle that uses pulley/ trochlea to redirect its line of action
Trigeminal (V) Nerve	• **Largest cranial nerve**[Q] (if atypical optic nerve is excluded) • Large sensory root is composed of central processes of **pseudounipolar neurons**[Q], whose cell bodies make up the crescent shaped trigeminal /semilunar ganglion, which is housed with in a dural recess the **trigeminal** or **Meckel's cave** lateral to the cavernous sinus.
Abducent (VI) Nerve	• **Longest intradural course**[Q] **with in the cranial** cavity (from clivus to superior orbital fissure) • **Involved most commonly in raised intracranial tension**[Q] (due to long course of the sharp bend it makes over the petrous temporal bone) • **Only the cranial nerve passing through cavernous sinus**[Q]
Facial (VII) Nerve	• **Longest intraosseous course**[Q] • Most commonly paralyzed of all cranial nerves

2. **Ans. b. B** *(Ref: Gray's 41e p664, 670, 40/e p276)*
   Superior oblique muscle is supplied by the fourth cranial nerve (Trochlear nerve). It is the only nerve that exits the brainstem from its posterior aspect.

Structures Marked in the Diagram	
A	• **Oculomotor nerve**
B	• **Trochlear nerve**
C	• **Abducens nerve**
D	• **Facial nerve**

*"The trochlear nerve is the **fourth cranial nerve** and **innervates superior oblique exclusively**. It is the only cranial nerve to emerge from the dorsal surface of the brain stem, passing from the midbrain onto the lateral surface of the crus of the cerebral peduncle. It runs through the lateral dural wall of the cavernous sinus and then crosses the oculomotor nerve to enter the orbit through the superior orbital fissure, above the common tendinous ring and levator palpebrae superioris, and medial to the frontal and lacrimal nerves. The trochlear nerve travels but a short distance to enter the superior (orbital) surface of superior oblique."* - Gray's 40/e p276

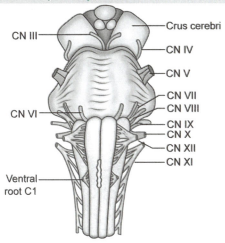

Fig. 2: Location of cranial nerves

Trochlear (IVth) Nerve

- It is **crossed cranial nerve** or the **only cranial nerve whose fibers originate completely from the contralateral nucleus**. Therefore, the **trochlear nerve nucleus**[Q] supplies the **contralateral superior oblique muscle**[Q].
- **Trochlear nerve** is the only cranial nerve to **emerge dorsally from the brain stem**[Q] & has **longest intra cranial course**[Q] and **most slender (thinnest/smallest) cranial nerve** (in terms of axons it contains).

  - Longest intracranial course makes it highly susceptible to raised intracranial tension[Q]
  - **Trochlear nucleus** is situated in **ventromedial central gray matter** of **midbrain** at the level of **inferior colliculus**[Q].
  - The nerve fibers **cross the midline & decussate** with the **opposite nerve fibers to emerge on opposite side of posterior (dorsal), surface of midbrain**[Q].

- It then winds around the superior cerebellar & cerebral peduncle between posterior cerebral & superior cerebellar arteries → to undersurface of free edge of tentorium cerebelli → through middle cranial fossa in lateral wall of cavernous sinus → and **enters the orbit through lateral part of superior orbital fissure (i.e. lateral to annulus of zinn)**[Q]
- Its pure motor nerve supplying superior oblique muscle (SO_4)[Q]

Cranial Nerves Location	
Cribriform plate (CN I)	• Olfactory nerve[Q]
Middle cranial fossa (CN II–VI) through sphenoid bone	• Optic canal (optic nerve, ophthalmic artery, central retinal vein) • Superior orbital fissure [oculomotor, trochlear, Ophthalmic (V_1) nerve[Q], abducens, ophthalmic vein, sympathetic fibers] • Foramen rotundum [Maxillary (V_2) nerve[Q]] • Foramen ovale [Mandibular (V_3) nerve[Q]] • Foramen spinosum (middle meningeal artery)
Posterior cranial fossa (CN VII–XII) through temporal or occipital bone	• Internal auditory meatus (Facial & Vestibulocochlear nerve)[Q] • Jugular foramen (Glossopharyngeal, vagus, spinal accessory nerve, internal jugular vein)[Q] • Hypoglossal canal (Hypoglossal nerve)[Q] • Foramen magnum (Spinal roots of spinal accessory nerve, brainstem & vertebral arteries)[Q]

AIIMS ESSENCE

Functions of Extraocular Muscles

Muscle	Nerve Supply	Action
Superior rectus	Oculomotor (Superior division)[Q]	Elevation, Adduction, Intortion[Q]
Inferior rectus	Oculomotor (Inferior division)[Q]	Depression, Adduction, Extortion[Q]
Medial rectus	Oculomotor (Inferior division)[Q]	Abduction[Q]
Lateral rectus	Abducens[Q]	Adduction[Q]
Superior oblique	Trochlear[Q]	Depression, Abduction, Intortion[Q]
Inferior oblique	Oculomotor (Inferior division)[Q]	Elevation, Abduction, Extortion[Q]

3. **Ans. a. A** *(Ref: Gray's 41/e p547, 40/e p539)*

Protrusion of jaw is carried out by the bilateral action of lateral pterygoid muscle which is represented by 'A' in the diagram, originating by two heads from sphenoid bone and getting inserted at anterior surface of mandibular condyle.

Muscles Marked in the Diagram

A	• Lateral Pterygoid
B	• Medial Pterygoid
C	• Buccinator
D	• Pterygomandibular Raphe

*"Lateral pterygoid is a **short, thick muscle** consisting of **two parts**. The **upper head arises from** the **infratemporal surface** and **infratemporal crest** of the **greater wing of the sphenoid bone**. The **lower head arises from** the **lateral surface of the lateral pterygoid plate**. From the two origins, the fibres converge, and pass backwards and laterally, to be **inserted into a depression on the front of the neck of the mandible (the pterygoid fovea)**." - Gray's 40/e p539*

*"**Actions of Lateral Pterygoid:** When **left and right muscles contract together** the **condyle is pulled forward** and **slightly downward**. If only one **lateral pterygoid contracts**, the **jaw rotates about a vertical axis** passing roughly through the opposite condyle and is **pulled medially toward the opposite side**. This contraction **together with that of the adjacent medial pterygoid** (both attached to the lateral pterygoid plate) provides most of the strong medially directed component of the force used when **grinding food** between teeth of the same side. It is arguably the **most important function of the inferior head of lateral pterygoid**." - Gray's 40/e p539*

4. **Ans. c. C** *(Ref: Gray's 41/e p982, 40/e p438)*

In the given diagram, the vagus descends vertically in the neck in the carotid sheath, between the internal jugular vein and the internal carotid artery, to the upper border of thyroid cartilage, and then passes between the internal jugular vein and the internal carotid artery to the root of the neck.

Structures Marked in the Diagram

A	• Carotid artery
B	• Internal jugular vein
C	• Vagus nerve
D	• Sympathetic trunk

*"**The vagus exits the skull through the jugular foramen accompanied by the accessory nerve**, with which it shares an arachnoid and a dural sheath. Both nerves lie anterior to a fibrous septum that separates them from the glossopharyngeal nerve. The **vagus descends vertically in the neck in the carotid sheath, between the internal jugular vein and the internal carotid artery**, to the upper border of the thyroid cartilage, and then passes between the vein and the **common carotid artery to the root of the neck**."- Gray's 40/e p438*

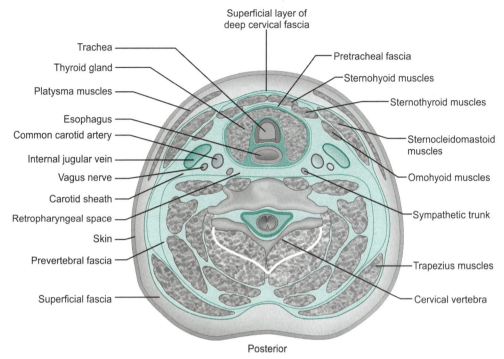

Fig. 3: Transverse section through the neck

Vagus Nerve
• **Large mixed nerve**, has a **more extensive course & distribution** than any other cranial nerve
• Runs through the **neck, thorax & abdomen**
Course:
• Vagus exits the skull through jugular foramen accompanied by accessory nerve[Q], with which it shares an arachnoid and a dural sheath. Both nerves lie anterior to a fibrous septum that separates them from the glossopharyngeal nerve.
• **Vagus descends vertically in neck in carotid sheath**, between **internal jugular vein & internal carotid artery**, to the **upper border of the thyroid cartilage**, and then passes between vein & CCA to root of the neck[Q].

Right Vagus	Left Vagus
• Right vagus **descends posterior to IJV to cross the first part of subclavian artery** and enter thorax[Q].	• Left vagus **enters thorax between left CCA & subclavian arteries** and behind **left brachiocephalic vein**[Q].

• After emerging from the jugular foramen, **vagus bears two marked enlargements, a small, round, superior ganglion & a larger inferior ganglion.**

Superior (jugular) Ganglion	Inferior (nodose) Ganglion
• It is **connected to cranial root of accessory nerve, inferior glossopharyngeal ganglion & sympathetic trunk**[Q], latter by a filament from superior cervical ganglion.	• It is **connected with hypoglossal nerve**, loop between **1st & 2nd cervical spinal nerves** & with **superior cervical sympathetic ganglion**[Q].

Branches of Vagus in the Neck	
Meningeal branches	• **Start from superior vagal ganglion & pass through jugular foramen** to be distributed to dura mater in **posterior cranial fossa**[Q].
Auricular branch	• **Arises from superior vagal ganglion**[Q] & joined by a branch from inferior ganglion of the glossopharyngeal nerve.
Pharyngeal branch	• It **emerges from upper part of inferior vagal ganglion** and consists chiefly of filaments from the cranial accessory nerve.
	• **Join rami of sympathetic trunk & glossopharyngeal nerve** to form a **pharyngeal plexus**[Q].
	• Supply muscles of pharynx & soft palate except **stylopharyngeus & tensor veli palatini**[Q].

Contd...

Contd...

Branches to the carotid body	• Form a plexus with glossopharyngeal rami & branches of cervical sympathetic trunk[Q].
Superior laryngeal nerve	• Divides into internal & external laryngeal nerves.

Internal Laryngeal Nerve	External Laryngeal Nerve
• **Sensory to laryngeal mucosa down to** level of **vocal folds**[Q]. • It **descends to the thyrohyoid membrane, pierces it above the superior laryngeal artery** and divides into an **upper & lower branch**[Q]. • **Upper branch** supplies **mucosa of pharynx, epiglottis, vallecula & laryngeal vestibule.** • **Lower branch** supplies **aryepiglottic fold, mucosa on back of arytenoid cartilage & transverse arytenoid**[Q].	• External laryngeal nerve **descends behind sternohyoid with superior thyroid artery**[Q]. • It gives **branches to pharyngeal plexus & inferior constrictor**[Q].

Recurrent laryngeal nerve	• The recurrent laryngeal nerve differs, in origin and course, on the two sides.

Right RLN	Left RLN
• **On the right** it **arises from the vagus anterior to the first part of the subclavian artery,** and curves backwards below and then behind it to **ascend obliquely to side of trachea behind CCA**[Q]. • It is **closely related to the inferior thyroid artery,** and crosses either in front of, behind, or between, its branches.	• **On the left,** the **nerve arises from vagus on left of aortic arch, curves below it immediately behind attachment of ligamentum arteriosum** to the concavity of the aortic arch and **ascends to side of the trachea**[Q]. • It gives **cardiac filaments to deep cardiac plexus**[Q].

	• **RLN supplies all laryngeal muscles, except the cricothyroid**[Q] • **RLN communicates with the internal laryngeal nerve,** supplying **sensory filaments** to laryngeal mucosa **below vocal folds**[Q].
Anterior vagal trunk	• Anterior vagal trunk to **anterior stomach & liver**[Q]
Posterior vagal trunk	• Posterior vagal trunk to **posterior stomach** and then **via celiac plexus to liver, kidney, small intestine & large intestine up to right 2/3rd of transverse colon**[Q].

5. **Ans. a. Deep branch of ulnar nerve** *(Ref: Gray's 41/e p784, 866, 40/e p888)*

A 37-year-old patient presented with hyperextension of 4th and 5th metacarpophalangeal joint with flexion at proximal interphalangeal joint is having claw hand. This deformity is due to injury of deep branch of ulnar nerve.

See Q. No. 11 AIIMS May 2016

6. **Ans. a. Greater auricular nerve** *(Ref: Gray's 41/e p627, 40/e p620)*

Greater auricular nerve supplies the ear lobule.

"The sensory nerves involved are the great auricular nerve, which supplies most of the cranial surface and the posterior part of the lateral surface (helix, antihelix, lobule); the lesser occipital nerve, which supplies the upper part of the cranial surface; the auricular branch of the vagus, which supplies the concavity of the concha and posterior part of the eminentia; the auriculotemporal nerve, which supplies the tragus, crus of the helix and the adjacent part of the helix; and the facial nerve, which together with the auricular branch of the vagus probably supplies small areas on both aspects of the auricle, in the depression of the concha, and over its eminence."- Gray's 40/e p620

Nerve supply of Ear

External Ear

Auricle/Pinna	External Acoustic Meatus	Tympanic Membrane
A. Lateral or Outer (Front) Surface: – **Auriculotemporal nerve (branch of V3)** supplies skin anterior to external acoustic meatus (helix, & adjacent part of helix)[Q] – **Greater auricular nerve (C_2, C_3)** supplies **posterior part (helix, antihelix & lobule) of lateral surface**[Q] **B. Medial or Cranial (Back) Surface:** – **Lesser occipital nerve (C_2)** supplies **upper part**[Q] – **Greater auricular nerve (C_2, C_3)** supplies **most of cranial surface**[Q] – **Auricular branch of vagus nerve (Arnold's nerve)** supplies root of auricle (concavity of concha)[Q], posterior part of eminentia. It also supplies posterior wall & floor of external auditory canal/meatus and adjoining tympanic membrane. – **Facial nerve with auricular branch of vagus** supplies **small areas on both aspects of auricle,** in **depression of concha & over its eminence (concha & retroauricular groove)**[Q]. – **Auricular muscles** are supplied by **facial nerve**[Q].	• Anterior half by auriculotemporal nerve[Q] • Posterior half by auricular branch of vagus nerve. Through this posterior wall also receives sensory fibers from facial nerve[Q].	**A. Outer or Lateral Surface:** – **Auriculotemporal nerve** supply anterior half[Q] – **Auricular branch of vagus nerve (Arnold's nerve)** supply posterior half[Q] **B. Inner or Medial Surface:** – **Tympanic branch of glosso-pharyngeal nerve (Jacobson's nerve)**[Q] through tympanic plexus

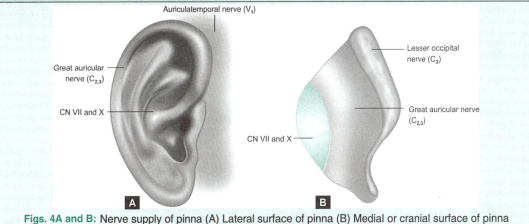

Figs. 4A and B: Nerve supply of pinna (A) Lateral surface of pinna (B) Medial or cranial surface of pinna

Middle Ear

Cavity (Mucosa mastoid, antrum, air cells, auditory tube)	Muscles
• Tympanic plexus formed by: • **Tympanic branch of glossopharyngeal nerve**[Q] • **Superior & inferior carotympanic nerves**[Q] (Sympathetic plexus around internal carotid artery)	• **Tensor tympani by mandibular division of trigeminal nerve**[Q] • **Stapedius by Facial nerve**[Q]

7. **Ans. d. Pleuroperitoneal membrane** *(Ref: Gray's 40/e p1015; Langman 11/e p161; IB Singh 10/e p187)*

Pleuropericardial membrane is a supradiaphragmatic structure and not involved in formation of diaphragm.

Development of Diaphragm
• **Septum transversum** →**Central tendon**[Q] • **Pleuroperitoneal membranes** →Small **intermediate muscular portion**[Q] • **Mesentery** of **esophagus** →**Crura**[Q] • **Body wall** →**Peripheral muscular diaphragm**[Q] • **Cervical myotomes** (muscular input)[Q]

	Diaphragm		
	• Diaphragm is a **musculo tendinous, dome-shaped partition** between the thoracic & abdominal cavities • **Develops from 4 major structures:** Septum transversum, pleuroperitoneal membranes, dorsal esophageal mesentery & body wall
Septum Transversum	**Pleuroperitoneal Membranes**	**Dorsal Esophageal Mesentery**	**Body Wall**
• **Septum transversum (most important component)** forms the **central tendon**[Q] • First seen as a **thick mesodermal plate cranial to pericardial cavity**[Q] between base of thoracic cavity & stalk of yolk sac. • Septum **does not separate thoracic & abdominal cavities entirely**, but after the head fold forms (**week 4**), it becomes a **thick incomplete partition between the cavities**[Q] with an opening on each side of the gut, the pleural canals. • **Septum fuses dorsally with primitive mediastinal mesenchyme** below esophagus & **later with pleuroperitoneal membranes**[Q].	• **Pleuroperitoneal membranes fuse with dorsal mesentery of esophagus** & with **dorsal part of septum transversum to complete the partition between thoracic & abdominopelvic cavities** to form **primitive diaphragm**[Q]. • They represent only a **small portion of final adult structure**[Q].	• **Dorsal esophageal mesentery (meso-esophagus)** fuses with both & this mesentery **forms median portion of diaphragm**[Q]. • **Crura of diaphragm develop from muscle fibers**[Q], which grow into esophageal mesentery.	• **The body wall:** During **weeks 9-12**, the pleural cavities enlarge & invade lateral body walls. **Body wall tissue, at this time, splits off medially to form the peripheral parts of diaphragm**[Q] outside that formed by membranes. • **Extensions of pleural cavities into body walls** form **costo-diaphragmatic recesses**[Q].

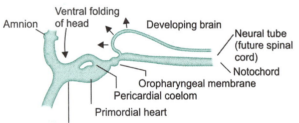

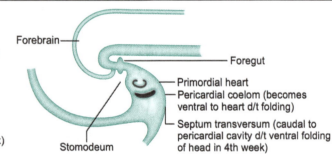

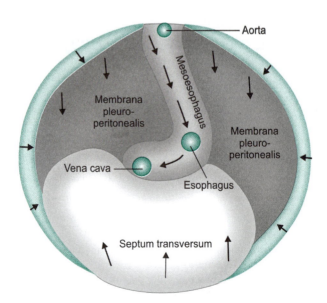

Small Openings in the Diaphragm		
Opening	Location	Passing structure
Medial lumbocostal Arch	Behind medial arcuate ligament	Sympathetic chain[Q]
Lateral lumbocostal arch	Behind arcuate ligament	Subcostal nerve & vessels[Q]
Larry's space / Foramen of Morgagni	Between xiphoid & costal origin of diaphragm	Superior epigastric vessels[Q] some lymphatics

Opening	Vertebral level	Part of diaphragm	Passing structure
Vena Caval	$T_8{}^Q$	*Central tendon[Q]*	• *Inferior vena cava[Q]* • *Right phrenic nerve[Q]*
Esophageal	$T_{10}{}^Q$	*Muscular portion derived from right crus[Q]*	• *Esophagus[Q]* • Esophageal branch of left gastric artery • *Gastric or vagus nerve[Q]*
Aortic	$T_{12}{}^Q$	*Osseoaponeurotic between right & lateral crus.[Q]*	• Aorta • *Thoracic duct[Q]* • *Azygous vein[Q]*

8. **Ans. d. Seminiferous tubules**   *(Ref: Gray's 40/e p52; Robbins 9/e p214; Ganong 25/e p418, 24/e p420)*

Seminiferous tubule of testis is an immune-privileged site.

*"**Some antigens are hidden (sequestered) from the immune system**, because the **tissues in which these antigens are located do not communicate with the blood and lymph**. As a result, **self-antigens in these tissues fail to elicit immune responses** and are **essentially ignored by the immune system**. This is believed to be the case for the **testis, eye,** and **brain**, all of which are called **immune- privileged sites** because it is **difficult to induce immune responses to antigens introduced into these sites**. If the antigens of these tissues are released, for example, as a consequence of trauma or infection, the result may be an immune response that leads to prolonged tissue inflammation and injury. This is the postulated mechanism for post-traumatic orchitis and uveitis."*- Robbins 9/e p214

*"**The fluid in the lumen of the seminiferous tubules is quite different from plasma**; it contains very little protein and glucose but is rich in androgens, estrogens, K^+, inositol, and glutamic and aspartic acids. **Maintenance of its composition depends on the blood-testis barrier**. The **barrier also protects the germ cells from blood borne noxious agents, prevents antigenic products of germ cell division** and **maturation from entering the circulation** and **generating an autoimmune response**, and may help establish an osmotic gradient that facilitates movement of fluid into the tubular lumen."*- Ganong 24/e p420

*"**Endogenous** derangements of the immune system may also contribute to the loss of immunologic tolerance to self-antigens and the development of autoimmunity. Some autoantigens reside in **immunologically privileged sites**, such as the **brain** or **the anterior chamber of the eye**. These sites are characterized by the **inability of engrafted tissue to elicit immune responses**. **Immunologic privilege results from** a number of events, including the **limited entry of proteins from those sites into lymphatics**, the **local production of immunosuppressive cytokines** such as transforming growth factor β, and the **local expression of molecules (including Fas ligand)** that can induce apoptosis of activated T cells. **Lymphoid cells remain in a state of immunologic ignorance** (neither activated nor anergized) **with regard to proteins expressed uniquely in immunologically privileged sites**."*- Harrison 19/e p377e-2

Immune- Privileged Sites
• **Some antigens are hidden (sequestered) from the immune system**, because **tissues in which these antigens are located do not communicate with blood & lymph**.
• As a result, **self-antigens in these tissues fail to elicit immune responses** and are **essentially ignored by the immune system**.

Immune- Privileged Sites	
• **Testis[Q]**	• **Placenta & fetus[Q]**
• **Eye (Anterior camber)[Q]**	• **Brain[Q]**

Circumventricular Organs

- These organs have **fenestrated capillaries** & because of their permeability they are said to be **outside the blood brain barrier**.
- Some of them function as **neurohemal organ** (areas in which polypeptides secreted by neurons enter the circulation).

Circumventricular Organs includes (SAMPO)	
• **S**ubfornical organ[Q]	• **P**osterior pituitary (neurohypophysis)[Q]
• **A**rea postrema[Q]	• **O**rganum vasculosum of lamina terminalis[Q]
• **M**edian eminence of hypothalamus[Q]	

9. **Ans. d. Wings of sphenoid** *(Ref: Gray's 40/e p733)*

   Craniovertebral joint consists of the occipital condyles, atlas & axis.

   "Craniovertebral Joint: The articulation between the cranium and vertebral column is specialized to provide a wider range of movement than those which occur in the rest of the axial skeleton. It consists of the occipital condyles, the atlas and the axis, and functions like a universal joint that permits horizontal and vertical scanning movements of the head, and is adapted for eye-head co-ordination." - Gray's 40/e p733

Craniovertebral Joint

- The articulation between **cranium & vertebral column** is specialized to provide a wider range of movement than those, which occur in the rest of the axial skeleton.
- It **consists of occipital condyles, atlas & axis**[Q].
- CV joint **functions like a universal joint that permits horizontal** and **vertical scanning movements of the head,** and is **adapted for eye-head co-ordination**[Q].

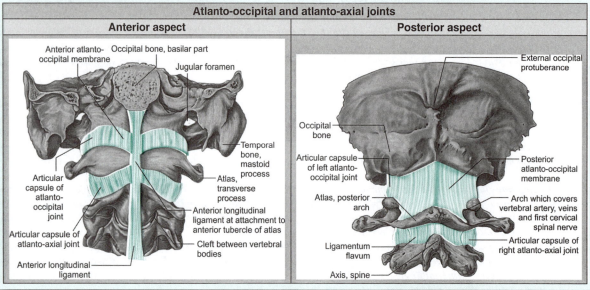

Atlanto-occipital and atlanto-axial joints

10. **Ans. d. Median nerve** *(Ref: Gray's 41/e p784-786, 40/e p845)*

    In pronator teres syndrome, the nerve involved is median nerve.

    *"Pronator syndrome: This is an uncommon **entrapment neuropathy of the median nerve** occurring **in the elbow region**. Entrapment can occur typically at four sites. The **first** occurs at the site of the **ligament of Struthers**. This ligament represents an anatomical variant and when present connects a small supracondylar spur of bone to an accessory origin of pronator teres. The median nerve can be compressed as it passes under this ligament. The nerve may also be **trapped as it passes deep to the bicipital aponeurosis; the aponeurotic edge of the deep head of pronator teres muscle; or the tendinous aponeurotic arch forming the proximal free edge of the radial attachment of flexor digitorum superficialis." - Gray's 40/e p845*

Pronator Teres Syndrome

- This is an uncommon **entrapment neuropathy of the median nerve** occurring **in the elbow region**.

Sites of Entrapment of Median Nerve

1. **Site of ligament of Struthers**[Q]
2. **Deep to bicipital aponeurosis**[Q]
3. Aponeurotic edge of **deep head of pronator teres muscle**[Q]
4. **Tendinous aponeurotic arch** forming the **proximal free edge of radial attachment of flexor digitorum superficialis**[Q].

Clinical Features:

- **Pain on the volar aspect** of the **distal arm & proximal forearm**[Q].
- Symptoms may be **aggravated by flexing the elbow against resistance, pronating the forearm against resistance, or flexion of superficialis to the middle finger against resistance**, depending on the precise cause of the entrapment.
  - If the **anterior interosseous nerve** is also **compressed** there is **weakness of all the muscles innervated by the median nerve**, including **abductor pollicis brevis & long finger flexors**, and **sensory impairment on the palm** of hand[Q].

Treatment:

- Treatment involves **exploration of the nerve & surgical decompression**.

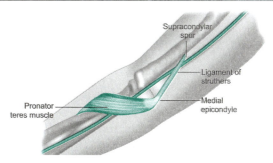

Fig. 5: Pronator teres syndrome

11. **Ans. b. Sphenoid** *(Ref: Gray's 41/e p484, 40/e p473-476)*

    Maxillary bone does not articulate with sphenoid.

Maxilla

- Maxillae are largest of facial bones, other than mandible & jointly form whole of upper jaw.
- Each bone **forms the greater part of floor & lateral wall of nasal cavity & of floor of the orbit, contributes to the infratemporal & pterygopalatine fossae, and bounds inferior orbital & pterygomaxillary fissures**[Q].

Parts of Maxilla

- **Body**
- **Four processes:**
  1. Zygomatic process[Q]
  2. Frontal process of maxilla[Q]
  3. Alveolar process[Q]
  4. Palatine process[Q]
- **Infraorbital foramen**
- **The maxillary sinus**

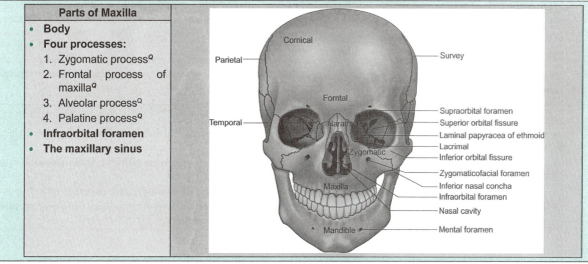

Maxilla

Articulations of Maxilla

• **Each maxilla articulates with nine bones:**
  – **Two of the cranium: Frontal & ethmoid**[Q]
  – **Seven of the face: Nasal, zygomatic, lacrimal, inferior nasal concha, palatine, vomer** & adjacent fused **maxilla**[Q]
• Sometimes it articulates with orbital surface & sometimes with the lateral pterygoid plate of the sphenoid.

12. **Ans. c. Have a plasma membrane showing multiple folds** *(Ref: Gray's 40/e p87, 88, 91)*

Plasma membrane showing multiple folds, i.e. ruffled borders are characteristic of osteoclasts which are involved in resorption of osteocytes.

*"**Osteoclasts** are large (40 μm or more) polymorphic cells containing up to 20 oval, closely packed nuclei. They lie in close contact with the bone surface in resorption bays (Howship's lacunae). The cytoplasm also **contains numerous coated transport vesicles** and **microtubule arrays involved in the transport of the vesicles between the Golgi stacks** and **the ruffled membrane**, which is the **highly infolded cell surface of active osteoclasts at sites of local bone resorption."** - Gray's 40/e p88*

*"**Osteoblasts are derived from osteoprogenitor (stem) cells of mesenchymal origin**, which are present in the bone marrow and other connective tissues. They **proliferate and differentiate, stimulated by bone morphogenetic proteins (BMPs), into osteoblasts prior to bone formation."** - Gray's 40/e p87*

*"**Bone** has a complex autonomic and sensory innervation; osteoblasts possess receptors for several neuropeptides that are found in the nerves which supply bone, e.g. neuropeptide Y, calcitonin gene-related peptide, vasoactive intestinal peptide and substance P."- Gray's 40/e p91*

Osteoblasts
• Osteoblasts are **derived from osteoprogenitor (stem) cells of mesenchymal origin**, which are present in the bone marrow and other connective tissues. • They **proliferate and differentiate, stimulated by bone morphogenetic proteins (BMPs), into osteoblasts prior to bone formation**[Q]. • Found on the **forming surfaces of growing or remodelling bone**, where they **constitute a covering layer**[Q]. • In relatively **quiescent adult bones** they appear to be **present mostly on endosteal** rather than periosteal **surfaces**, but they also occur deep within compact bone where osteons are being remodelled.

Contd...

Contd..

Osteoblasts
• **Responsible for the synthesis, deposition & mineralization of the bone matrix**, which they secrete. • Their **plasma membranes display many extensions**, some of which **contact neighbouring osteoblasts** and embedded osteocytes at intercellular gap junctions[Q].

- **Osteoblasts synthesize & secrete organic matrix**, i.e. **type I collagen, small amounts of type V collagen**, and numerous other macromolecules involved in bone formation and resorption[Q].
    - **Osteoblasts possess receptors for several neuropeptides** that are **found in nerves** which **supply bone**, e.g. **neuropeptide Y** [Q], calcitonin gene-related peptide, vasoactive intestinal peptide & **substance P**[Q].

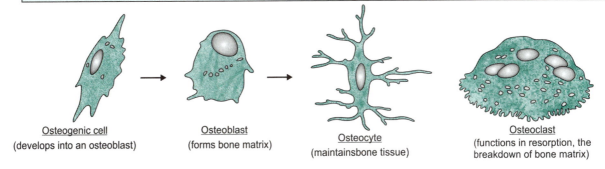

Osteogenic cell (develops into an osteoblast) → Osteoblast (forms bone matrix) → Osteocyte (maintains bone tissue) | Osteoclast (functions in resorption, the breakdown of bone matrix)

13. **Ans. is d.** Median sacral artery   *(Ref: Gray's 41/e p1058, 40/e p1155-1159; Manual of Total Mesorectal Excision by Moran, Richard John Heald (2013)/p40)*
Anal canal is supplied by superior rectal, middle rectal, inferior rectal arteries and occasionally by median sacral artery.

> *"The **arterial supply to the anal canal** is derived from **terminal branches of the superior rectal artery, the inferior rectal branch of the pudendal artery** and **branches of the median sacral artery**."- Gray's 40/e p1159*

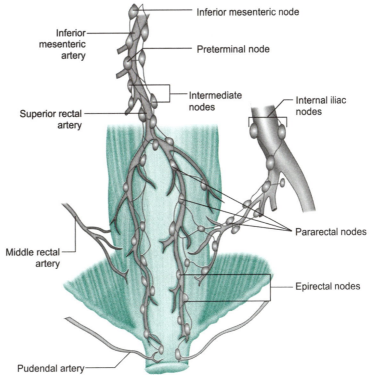

Fig. 6: Lymph nodes of the rectum and anal canal

Contd...

> *"As the rectum is derived from the hindgut, the rectum including the upper anal canal is supplied by the inferior mesenteric artery via the superior rectal artery. The middle and inferior rectal arteries originate from the internal iliac vessels and contribute to the blood supply of the lower anal canal and minor parts of the rectum via intramural anastomoses. Occasionally, the posterior part of the anal canal and internal anal sphincter are additionally supplied by median sacral artery."-Manual of Total Mesorectal Excision by Moran, Richard John Heald (2013)/p40*

Anal Canal

- Anal canal **begins at anorectal junction** and **ends at anal verge.**
- **Length: 4 cm** (2.5-5 cm) long in adults

Anal canal		
Upper (Mucous) zone	**Middle (Transitional) zone**	**Lower (cutaneous) zone**
• Length: **15 mm**[Q] • Lined by **simple columnar mucous membrane** showing **anal columns** of **Morgagni, anal valves, anal sinus, anal papilla**[Q]. • **Pain insensitive**[Q]	• Length: **15 mm**[Q] • Lined by **non-keratinized stratified squamous epithelium** without sweat & sebaceous gland[Q] • **Pain sensitive**[Q]	• Length: **8 mm**[Q] • Lined by non-keratinized stratified squamous epithelium **with sweat** & **sebaceous gland**[Q] • **Pain sensitive**[Q]

- **Dentate/ Pectinate line** lies **between upper & middle part**[Q]
- **White line of Hilton** lies **at lower limit of middle**[Q] (transitional) part
- **Anal glands open at the dentate line**[Q]

Arterial supply	Venous drainage	Lymphatics
• Terminal branches of **superior rectal artery**[Q] • **Middle rectal artery** • **Inferior rectal branch of pudendal artery**[Q] • **Occasionally,** branches of the **median sacral artery**[Q] (which supplies **posterior part of the anal)** *canal*	• **Upper anal canal mucosa, internal anal sphincter & conjoint longitudinal coat:** Passes via the **terminal branches of the superior rectal veins into the inferior mesenteric vein**[Q]. • **Lower anal canal & external sphincter** drain via the **inferior rectal branch of pudendal vein** into **internal iliac vein**[Q].	• **Upper anal mucosa, internal anal sphincter & conjoint longitudinal coat** drain **upwards into submucosal & intramural lymphatics of rectum**[Q] • **Lower anal canal** epithelium & **external anal sphincter** lymphatics **drain downwards via perianal plexuses into vessels** that drain into **external inguinal lymph nodes**[Q]. • **Lymphatics of puborectalis** drain into **internal iliac lymph nodes**[Q].

Anal Sphincter	
External Anal Sphincter	**Internal Anal Sphincter**
• **Voluntary**[Q] • Sphincter complex of **striated muscles,** composed mainly of **type 1 (slow twitch) skeletal muscle fibers**[Q] suited for prolonged contraction • Contributed by fibers from **Puborectalis part of levator ani muscle**[Q] (in upper most part); **superficial transverse perineal muscles anteriorly**[Q] and **anococcygeal raphe posteriorly** (in **upper third);** and **anococcygeal ligament**[Q] (in **middle third).** • It is **innervated by inferior rectal branch of pudendal nerve** (**anterior divisions** of **S2, S3, S4**[Q] sacral spinal nerves) **mainly** and by **perineal branch of S4**. • It also receives **nerve to levator ani (Puborectalis),** with which it contracts in unison to maintain continence when internal sphincter is relaxed (except during defecation).	• **Involuntary**[Q] • Formed by **thickening of inner circular smooth muscle layer**[Q] of upper end of anal canal. • This sphincter remains in **state of tonic contraction most of the time to maintain resting tone or pressure**[Q] (90 cm H_2O) and to prevent leakage of fluid and flatus. • Its **contraction is maintained by sympathetic fibers** from **superior rectal** (periarterial) and **hypogastric plexuses**; and inhibited (relaxed) by parasympathetic pelvic splanchnic nerves

Contd...

Contd...

Anal Canal
Anal Canal Physiology
• **Resting pressure** or **tone**: Due to **Internal sphincter** (90 cm H_2O)[Q] • **Squeeze pressure**: Contraction of the **external anal sphincter** & **puborectalis muscle**[Q] • **Principal mechanism that provides continence**: Pressure differential between the **rectum** (6 cm H_2O) & **anal canal** (90 cm H_2O)[Q]. • **Anorectal angle** is produced by the **anterior pull of** the **puborectalis muscle** as it encircles the rectum at the anorectal ring and contributes to fecal continence. **This angle** may act as a **flap valve** or have a **sphincter-like function**[Q].

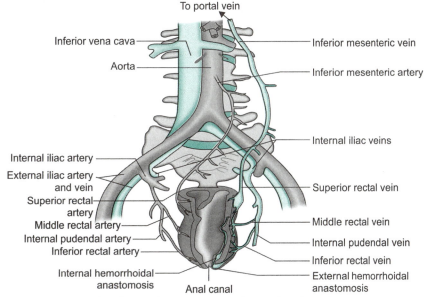

Fig. 7: Arterial supply and venous drainage of anal canal

14. **Ans. b. Buccal branch of facial nerve** *(Ref: Gray's 41/e 495, 40/e p487; Snells 9/e p582)*

   The buccal branch of facial run crosses the buccinator muscle and innervates it, without piercing it.

   "*Anteriorly, the superficial surface of buccinator is related to zygomaticus major, risorius, levator and depressor anguli oris, and the parotid duct. It is crossed by the facial artery, facial vein and branches of the facial and buccal nerves. The parotid duct pierces buccinator opposite the third upper molar tooth, and lies on the deep surface of the muscle before opening into the mouth opposite the maxillary second molar tooth.*"- *Gray's 41/e p495*

Buccinator
Origin:
• From the **outer surface of alveolar margins of maxilla** & **mandible** opposite the **molar teeth** and from the **pterygomandibular ligament**[Q]
Insertion:
• **Buccinator is pierced by parotid duct**[Q]. • At angle of mouth central fibers decussate, those from below entering the upper lip and those from above entering the lower lip; **highest** & **lowest fibers continue into the upper** & **lower lips, respectively**[Q], without intersecting. • Buccinator muscle **blends** & **forms part of orbicularis oris muscle**[Q].
Nerve supply:
• **Buccal branch of facial nerve**[Q]
Action:
• **Compresses** the **cheeks** & **lips** against the **teeth**[Q]

Structures Piercing the Buccinator		
• **Parotid duct (Stenson's duct)**[Q]	• **Molar glands of cheeks**[Q]	• **Buccal branch of mandibular nerve**[Q]

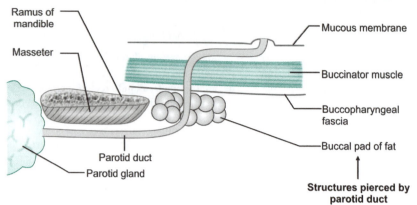

Fig. 8: Structures pierced by parotid duct

15. **Ans. c. Lateral to mandibular nerve** *(Ref: Gray's 41/e p552, 40/e p543)*

The mandibular nerve lies lateral to the otic ganglion. Otic ganglion is medial to mandibular nerve.

*"Otic ganglion: This is a **small, oval, flat reddish-grey ganglion situated just below the foramen ovale**. It is a **peripheral parasympathetic ganglion related topographically to the mandibular nerve**, but **connected functionally with the glossopharyngeal nerve**. Near its junction with the trigeminal motor root, the **mandibular nerve lies lateral to the ganglion**; tensor veli palatini lies medially, separating the ganglion from the cartilaginous part of the pharyngotympanic tube, and the **middle meningeal artery is posterior to the ganglion**. The otic ganglion usually surrounds the origin of the nerve to medial pterygoid."- Gray's 41/e p552*

Otic Ganglion
• Otic ganglion lies **medial to the mandibular nerve**[Q]
• Otic ganglion is a small parasympathetic ganglion **located in the infratemporal fossa**[Q].
• It is functionally **associated with glossopharyngeal nerve & innervates parotid gland for salivation**[Q].
• It is **connected to the chorda tympani nerve** & to **nerve of pterygoid canal**. These pathways **provide an alternate pathway of taste** from **anterior two-thirds of tongue**[Q].

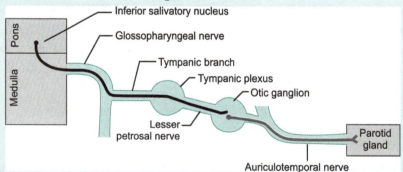

- The **preganglionic parasympathetic fibers originate** in the **inferior salivatory nucleus** of the **glossopharyngeal nerve**[Q].
- They **leave the glossopharyngeal nerve by its tympanic branch** and then **pass via the tympanic plexus and the lesser petrosal nerve to the otic ganglion**[Q].
- Here the **fibers synapse**, and the **postganglionic fibers pass by communicating branches to the auriculotemporal nerve**, which **conveys them to the parotid gland**[Q].
- They produce **vasodilator & secretomotor effects**[Q].

Relations of Otic Ganglion	
• **Just below foramen ovale**[Q]	• **Middle meningeal artery lies posterior to the ganglion**[Q]
• **Medial to mandibular nerve**[Q]	• Surrounds the origin of nerve to medial pterygoid
• **Lateral to tensor veli palatini**[Q]	

Contd...

Contd...

Otic Ganglion		
Connections of Otic Ganglion		
Sympathetic root	**Sensory root**	**Motor Root**
• Derived from the **plexus on middle meningeal artery**[Q]. • **Contains postganglionic fibers** arising in superior cervical ganglion. • Fibers **pass through the ganglion without relay & reach parotid gland via auriculotemporal nerve**[Q]. • **Vasomotor** in function	• Sensory root comes from auriculotemporal nerve[Q] • Sensory to parotid gland[Q]	• **Motor fibers supplying medial pterygoid & tensor palate, tensor tympani** pass through the ganglion without relay[Q].

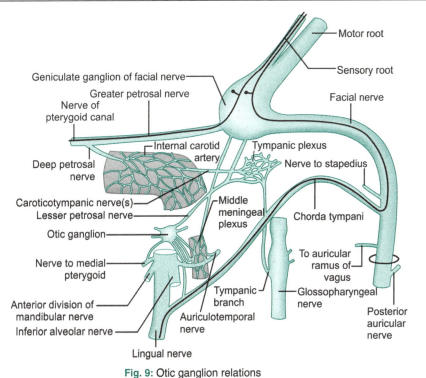

Fig. 9: Otic ganglion relations

PHYSIOLOGY

16. **Ans. a. Tone of contraction is related to amplitude of the stimulus** (Ref: Ganong 25/e p496-497, 24/e p498-499)
    The tone of contraction depends on the frequency of the stimulus rather than the amplitude.

    The threshold for action potential can be seen clearly to be 50 mV, i.e. the potential required to trigger an action potential and contraction. One contraction in 10 seconds implies frequency is 6 contractions/minute.

Basic Electrical Activity and Regulation of Motility

• **Except in esophagus & proximal portion of stomach**, the **smooth muscle of GI tract** has **spontaneous rhythmic fluctuations in membrane potential** between about **−65 & −45 mV**[Q].
   • This **basic electrical rhythm (BER)** is initiated by the **interstitial cells of Cajal**[Q], stellate mesenchymal **pacemaker cells with smooth muscle-like features** that send long multiply branched processes into the intestinal smooth muscle.
   • In the **stomach & small intestine**, these cells are **located in outer circular muscle layer near the myenteric plexus**; in **colon**, they are at **submucosal border of circular muscle layer**[Q].

Contd...

Contd...

Basic Electrical Activity and Regulation of Motility

- In the stomach and small intestine, there is a descending gradient in pacemaker frequency, and as in the heart, the pacemaker with the highest frequency usually dominates.
- The **BER itself rarely causes muscle contraction**, but **spike potentials superimposed on the most depolarizing portions of the BER waves do increase muscle tension**[Q].
- The **depolarizing portion of each spike** is due to Ca^{2+} **influx**, and the **repolarizing portion** is **due to K^+ efflux**[Q].
- Many polypeptides and neurotransmitters affect the BER. For example, **acetylcholine increases number of spikes & tension of smooth muscle**, whereas **epinephrine decreases number of spikes & tension**[Q].

  - Rate of BER: 4/min in stomach; 12/min in duodenum; 8/min in distal ileum[Q].
  - In the colon: BER rate 2/min at cecum; 6/min at sigmoid[Q].

- **Function of the BER: Coordinate peristaltic & other motor activity**, such as **setting the rhythm of segmentation**; contractions can occur only during the depolarizing part of the waves.
- **After vagotomy or transection of the stomach wall, peristalsis in stomach becomes irregular & chaotic.**

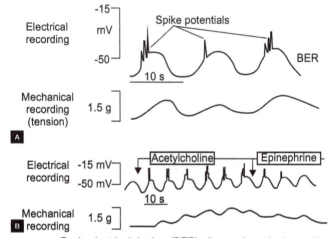

Figs. 10A and B: Basic electrical rhythm (BER) of gastrointestinal smooth muscle

(A) Morphology, and relation to muscle contraction.

(B) Stimulatory effect of acetylcholine and inhibitory effect of epinephrine.

Migrating Motor Complex

- **During fasting between periods of digestion**, the **pattern of electrical and motor activity in gastrointestinal smooth muscle becomes modified** so that **cycles of motor activity migrate from the stomach to the distal ileum**[Q].

  - Each cycle, or **migrating motor complex (MMC),** starts with a **quiescent period (phase I)**, continues with a period of **irregular electrical and mechanical activity (phase II),** and ends with a burst of **regular activity (phase III)**[Q].

- **MMCs are initiated by motilin**[Q]. The circulating level of this hormone increases at intervals of approximately 100 min in the interdigestive state, coordinated with the contractile phases of the MMC.
- **Contractions migrate aborally** at a rate of about **5 cm/ min**, and also occur at **intervals of approximately 100 min**[Q].
- **Gastric secretion, bile flow & pancreatic secretion increase during each MMC**[Q]. They likely serve to clear the stomach and small intestine of luminal contents in preparation for the next meal.
- Conversely, when a **meal is ingested, secretion of motilin is suppressed** (ingestion of food suppresses motilin release via mechanisms that have not yet been elucidated), and the **MMC is abolished, until digestion & absorption are complete**. Instead, there is a return to peristalsis and the other forms of BER and spike potentials during this time.

Contd...

Contd...

Migrating Motor Complex
• **Erythromycin binds to motilin receptors**, and derivatives of this compound **may be of value in treating patients in whom gastrointestinal motility is decreased**[Q].

17. **Ans. c. Interstitial lung disease**   *(Ref: Ganong 24/e p631)*

The pressure-volume loop shown above is the compliance curve, which is showing decreased slope, implying decreased compliance (ΔV/ΔP). This is typically seen in restrictive lung diseases, and interstitial lung disease is a typical example. Emphysema is an obstructive lung conditions and shows increased compliance.

Static Expiratory Pressure-Volume Curves of Lungs		
Shift	**Condition**	**Compliance**
Downward & to right	• **Pulmonary edema**[Q] • **Interstitial pulmonary fibrosis**[Q]	**Compliance is decreased**[Q]
Upward & to left	• **Emphysema**[Q]	**Compliance is increased**[Q]

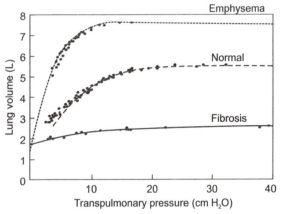

Fig. 11: Static expiratory pressure-volume curves of lungs in normal subjects and subjects with severe emphysema and pulmonary fibrosis

Compliance of the Lungs & Chest Wall

• **Compliance** is developed due to the **tendency for tissue to resume its original position** after an applied force has been removed.
• After an inspiration during quiet breathing, the lungs have a tendency to collapse and the chest wall has a tendency to expand.
    • **Compliance of the lung & chest wall** is measured as the **slope of the transpulmonary pressure & volume curve**, or, as a **change in lung volume per unit change in airway pressure (ΔV/ΔP)**.
• It is normally measured in the pressure range where the relaxation pressure curve is steepest, and **normal values** are **~0.2 L/cm H$_2$O** in a healthy adult male.
• However, **compliance depends on lung volume** and thus can vary. In an extreme example, an individual with **only one lung** has approximately **half the ΔV for a given ΔP**.
• **Compliance** is also **slightly greater when measured during deflation** than when measured during inflation. Consequently, it is more informative to examine the whole pressure-volume curve.
    • The **curve is shifted downward & to right (compliance is decreased)** by pulmonary edema & interstitial pulmonary fibrosis. Pulmonary fibrosis is a **progressive restrictive airway disease** in which there is **stiffening & scarring** of the lung[Q].
    • The **curve is shifted upward & to left (compliance is increased)** in emphysema[Q].

18. **Ans. d. 60%** *(Ref: Ganong 25/e p540, 24/e p542)*

Ejection fraction calculated from the given volume pressure curve is 60%.

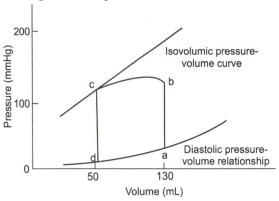

Fig. 12: Normal pressure-volume loop of the left ventricle

During diastole, the ventricle fills and pressure increases from d to a. Pressure then rises sharply from a to b during isovolumetric contraction and from b to c during ventricular ejection. At c, the aortic valves close and pressure falls during isovolumetric relaxation from c back to d.

Pressure Volume Loop
• ab: Isovolumetric contraction
• bc: Ventricular contraction during systole
• cd: Isovolumetric relaxation

- End-Diastolic Volume (EDV) (Point a) = **130 mL**
- End Systolic Volume (ESV) (Point d) = **50 mL**
- Stroke Volume (SV) = EDV–ESV = **80 mL**
- Ejection Fraction = SV/EDV = 80/130 = 0.6 i.e. **% EF = 60%**

19. **Ans. a. Pituitary gland** *(Ref: Ganong 25/e p339, 24/e p341)*

Sodium iodine symporter is not present in pituitary gland.

"The salivary glands, the gastric mucosa, the placenta, the ciliary body of the eye, the choroid plexus, the mammary glands, and certain cancers derived from these tissues also express NIS and can transport iodide against a concentration gradient, but the transporter in these tissues is not affected by TSH. The physiologic significance of all these extrathyroidal iodide-concentrating mechanisms is obscure, but they may provide pathways for radioablation of NIS-expressing cancer cells using iodide radioisotopes. This approach is also useful for the ablation of thyroid cancers." – Ganong 25/e p339

Sodium-Iodide Symporter (NIS) is present in	
• Thyroid[Q]	• Ciliary body of the eye[Q]
• Salivary glands[Q]	• Choroid plexus[Q]
• Gastric mucosa[Q]	• Mammary glands[Q]
• Placenta[Q]	• Certain cancers derived from these tissues

Iodide Transport Across Thyrocytes
• The **basolateral membranes of thyrocytes** facing the capillaries **contain a symporter** that **transports two Na⁺ ions and one I⁻ ion into the cell with each cycle**, against the electrochemical gradient for I⁻.
• This **Na⁺/ I⁻ symporter (NIS)** is capable of producing intracellular I⁻ concentrations that are 20–40 times as great as the concentration in plasma. The process involved is **secondary active transport**, with the energy provided by active transport of Na⁺ out of thyroid cells by Na, K ATPase.
• NIS is regulated both by transcriptional means and by active trafficking into and out of the thyrocyte basolateral membrane; in particular, **TSH induces both NIS expression and the retention of NIS in the basolateral membrane**, where it can **mediate sustained iodide uptake**.

Contd...

Contd...

Iodide Transport Across Thyrocytes

- Iodide must also exit the thyrocyte across the apical membrane to access the colloid, where the initial steps of thyroid hormone synthesis occur.
    - This transport step is believed to be mediated, at least in part, by a **Cl⁻/ I⁻ exchanger** known as **pendrin**.
    - This protein was first identified as the **product of the gene responsible for the Pendred syndrome**, whose patients suffer from **thyroid dysfunction & deafness**[Q].
    - **Pendrin** (SLC26A4) is one member of the larger **family of SLC26 anion exchangers**[Q].
- Iodide is essential for normal thyroid function, but **iodide deficiency & iodide excess both inhibit thyroid function.**
    - **Salivary glands, gastric mucosa, placenta, ciliary body of the eye, choroid plexus, mammary glands & certain cancers derived from these tissues also express NIS** and **can transport iodide against a concentration gradient**, but the **transporter in these tissues is not affected by TSH**[Q].
    - The physiologic significance of all these extrathyroidal iodide-concentrating mechanisms is obscure, but they **may provide pathways for radioablation of NIS-expressing cancer cells using iodide radioisotopes**. This approach is also **useful for the ablation of thyroid cancers**[Q].

20. **Ans. d. Radioactive sodium and radioactive labeled albumin**   *(Ref: Ganong 25/e p3, 24/e p2; Guyton 13/e p309, 310)*

    Interstitial fluid volume cannot be directly calculated and is calculated using extracellular fluid volume and plasma volume, which are measure respectively by radioactive sodium and radiolabelled albumin.

    "Measurement of Extracellular Fluid Volume: The volume of extracellular fluid can be estimated using any of several substances that disperse in the plasma and interstitial fluid but do not readily permeate the cell membrane. They include radioactive sodium, radioactive chloride, radioactive iothalamate, thiosulfate ion, and inulin. When any one of these substances is injected into the blood, it usually disperses almost completely throughout the extracellular fluid within 30 to 60 minutes. Some of these substances, however, such as radioactive sodium, may diffuse into the cells in small amounts. Therefore, one frequently speaks of the sodium space or the inulin space, instead of calling the measurement the true extracellular fluid volume."- Guyton 13/e p309

    "Measurement of Plasma Volume: To measure plasma volume, a substance must be used that does not readily penetrate capillary membranes but remains in the vascular system after injection. One of the most commonly used substances for measuring plasma volume is serum albumin labeled with radioactive iodine (¹²⁵I albumin). Also, dyes that avidly bind to the plasma proteins, such as Evans blue dye (also called T-1824), can be used to measure plasma volume."– Guyton 13/e p310

    "Calculation of Interstitial Fluid Volume: Interstitial fluid volume cannot be measured directly, but it can be calculated as: Interstitial fluid volume = Extracellular fluid volume − Plasma volume."- Guyton 13/e p310

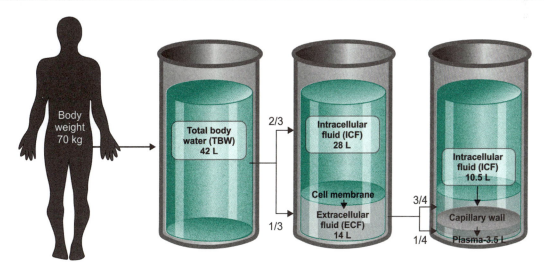

Body Fluids

- **Water** constitutes approximately **60% of total body weight**[Q].
- Of this 60%, **40%** is present in cells in the form of **intracellular fluid (ICF)** and **20%** is present outside the cells in the form of **extracellular fluid (ECF)**[Q].
- 20% of body weight water in ECF is divided into **interstitial fluid (15% of body weight)** and plasma (**5% of body weight)**[Q].

Total Body Water (60% of body weight)[Q]		
Intracellular fluid (ICF)	**Extracellular fluid (ECF)**	
2/3rd of TBW[Q] **(40% of body weight)**	**1/3rd of TBW (20% of body weight)**[Q]	
	ECF	
	Plasma	**Interstitial fluid**
	• 25% or 1/4th of ECF • **5% of body weight**[Q]	• 75% or 3/4th of ECF • **15% of body weight**[Q]

- **Most of the fluids are calculated directly from dilution methods, except for ICF & interstitial fluids. Both of these are calculated indirectly by calculating other body fluids.**

> • **ICF= Total body water volume – ECF volume**
> • **Interstitial fluid = ECF volume – Plasma volume**

Fluid volume	Indicator used
Total body water volume	• **Deuterium oxide: D$_2$O (MC used)**[Q] • **Tritium oxide**[Q]**, Aminopyrine**[Q]**, Antipyrine**[Q]
Extracellular fluid volume	• **Inulin (most accurate)**[Q] • **^{22}Na, ^{125}I-iothalamate, thiosulfate**[Q]
Plasma volume	• **Evans blue**[Q] • **Serum albumin labeled with radioactive iodine**[Q] **(I-125)**
Intracellular fluid	• (Calculated as **total body water − extracellular fluid volume**)
Blood volume	• ^{51}**Cr-labeled RBCs**[Q], or calculated as **blood volume = plasma volume/ (1 − hematocrit)**
Interstitial fluid	• (Calculated as **extracellular fluid volume − plasma volume**)

21. **Ans. a. 25 Hz** *(Ref: Ganong 25/e p107, 24/e p104, 105)*

> *"The stimulation frequency at which summation of contractions occurs is determined by the twitch duration of the particular muscle being studied. For example, if the twitch duration is 10 ms, frequencies less than 1/10 ms (100/s) cause discrete responses interrupted by complete relaxation, and frequencies greater than 100/s cause summation."– Ganong 25/e p107*

- **Tetany** is the **continuous contraction of muscle fibers, without latent period & relaxation time.**
- Hence, the tetanizing frequency depends only on the contraction time, i.e. the twitch duration.
- **Twitch duration = 40 milliseconds = 0.04 sec**
- **Tetanizing frequency = 1/0.04 = 25 Hz**

Summation of Contractions

- The electrical response of a muscle fiber to repeated stimulation is like that of nerve.
- The **fiber is electrically refractory only during rising phase & part of the falling phase of the spike potential.** At this time, the contraction initiated by the first stimulus is just beginning.

  - However, because the **contractile mechanism does not have a refractory period, repeated stimulation before relaxation has occurred produces additional activation of the contractile elements** and **a response that is added to the contraction already present.** This phenomenon is known as **summation of contractions**[Q].

Contd...

Contd...

Summation of Contractions
• **Tension developed during summation** is **considerably greater than that during the single muscle twitch**[Q].
• **With rapidly repeated stimulation, activation of contractile mechanism occurs repeatedly before any relaxation has occurred & individual responses fuse into one continuous contraction**. Such a response is called a **tetanus (tetanic contraction)**[Q].

Complete tetanus	Incomplete tetanus
• When **no relaxation occurs between stimuli** • **Tension developed** is about **4 times** that developed by the **individual twitch contractions**.	• When **periods of incomplete relaxation take place between the summated stimuli**.

- **The stimulation frequency at which summation of contractions occurs is determined by the twitch duration of the particular muscle being studied**[Q].
- For example, if the **twitch duration is 10 ms, frequencies less than 1/10 ms (100/s) cause discrete responses interrupted by complete relaxation, and frequencies greater than 100/s cause summation**[Q].

22. **Ans. b. Mesangial constriction** *(Ref: Ganong 25/e p705, 24/e p707)*

ANP causes mesangial relaxation leading to sodium excretion, not the mesangial constriction.

*"**ANP and BNP** in the circulation act on the kidneys to **increase Na^+ excretion** and injected CNP has a similar effect. They appear to **produce this effect by dilating afferent arterioles and relaxing mesangial cells**. Both of these actions increase glomerular filtration. In addition, they **act on the renal tubules to inhibit Na^+ reabsorption**. Other actions include an **increase in capillary permeability, leading to extravasation of fluid** and a decline in blood pressure. In addition, they **relax vascular smooth muscle in arterioles and venules**. CNP has a greater dilator effect on veins than ANP and BNP. These peptides also **inhibit renin secretion** and **counteract the pressor effects of catecholamines and angiotensin II**."* – *Ganong 25/e p705*

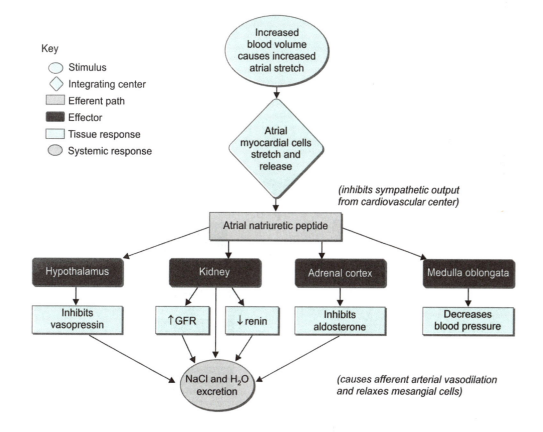

Natriuretic Hormones

- Two **natriuretic hormones** are **secreted by the heart**. The **muscle cells in atria** and, to a much lesser extent in the **ventricles**, contain secretory granules.
- **Granules increase in number** when **NaCl intake is increased** and **ECF expanded**, and extracts of atrial tissue cause natriuresis.

Atrial Natriuretic Peptide (ANP)	• Isolated from **atria & brain**[Q]
Brain natriuretic peptide (BNP; B-type natriuretic peptide)	• Present in **ventricles (mainly) & brain** in humans[Q]
C-type natriuretic peptide (CNP)	• Present in **brain, pituitary, kidneys & vascular endothelial cells**[Q]

Actions of Natriuretic Hormones

- **ANP & BNP** in the circulation **act on kidneys to increase Na⁺ excretion** and injected CNP has a similar effect. They appear to **produce this effect by dilating afferent arterioles** and **relaxing mesangial cells**. Both of these actions increase glomerular filtration[Q].
- In addition, they **act on renal tubules to inhibit Na⁺ reabsorption**[Q].
- **Other actions** include an **increase in capillary permeability, leading to extravasation of fluid** and a **decline in blood pressure**. In addition, they relax vascular smooth muscle in arterioles and venules[Q].
- **CNP** has a **greater dilator effect on veins** than ANP and BNP. These peptides also **inhibit renin secretion** and **counteract the pressor effects of catecholamines & angiotensin II**[Q].

- In the brain, **ANP is present in neurons**, and an ANP-containing neural pathway projects from anteromedial part of hypothalamus to areas in lower brain stem that are concerned with **neural regulation of cardiovascular system**[Q].

  - In general, the **effects of ANP in the brain are opposite to** those of **angiotensin II**, and **ANP-containing neural circuits** appear to be **involved in lowering BP** and **promoting natriuresis**[Q].

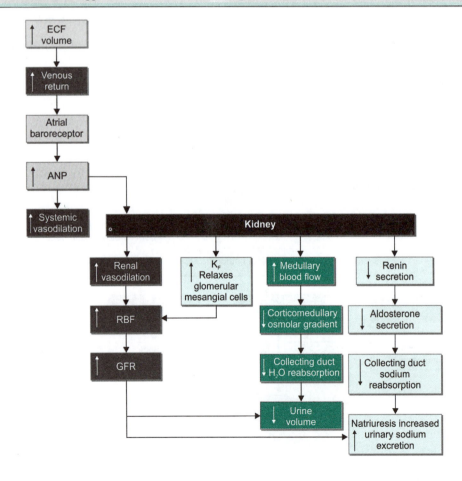

AIIMS November 2015

23. Ans. b. –60 V *(Ref: Ganong 25/e p9-10, 24/e p9-10)*

Equilibrium Potential
• **Equilibrium potential** is the **membrane potential at which equilibrium exists between influx & efflux of ions.**
• The **Nernst equation** has a physiological application when **used to calculate the potential of an ion of charge z across a membrane.** This potential is **determined using the concentration of the ion both inside and outside the cell:**

$$E = \frac{RT}{zF} \ln \frac{[\text{ion outside the cell}]}{[\text{ion inside the cell}]} = 2.3026 - \frac{RT}{zF} \log_{10} \frac{[\text{ion outside the cell}]}{[\text{ion inside the cell}]}$$

When the membrane is in thermodynamic equilibrium (i.e. no net flux of ions), the membrane potential must be equal to the Nernst potential.

E_m = The membrane potential

P_{ion} = The permeability for that ion (in meters per second)

$[\text{ion}]_{out}$ = The extracellular concentration of that ion

$[\text{ion}]_{in}$ = The intracellular concentration of that ion

R = The ideal gas constant

T = The temperature in kelvin

F = Faraday's constant (coulombs per mole)

z is the number of moles of electrons transferred in the cell reaction (Valence of K^+).

Hence, $E_k = 61.5 \log K_o/K_i$

$K_o = 100; K_i = 10$

$E_k = -61.5 = -60$ mV

Concentration (mmol/L of H_2O) of some ions inside and outside mammalian motor neurons			
Ion	Inside cell	Outside cell	Equilibrium potential (mv)
Na^+	15.0	150.0	+60
K^+	150.0	5.5	–90
Cl^-	9.0	125.0	–70
Resting membrane potential = –70 mV[Q]			

24. Ans. b. Urinary concentration in mg/ml *(Ref: Ganong 25/e p676, 24/e p678)*

In the Given Formula:
- C = Clearance of the substance
- U = Urinary concentration of the substance in mg/ml
- P = Plasma concentration of the substance in mg/ml
- V = Volume of urine

Measuring Glomerular filtration rate (GFR)
• **GFR** is the **amount of plasma ultrafiltrate formed each minute** and can be measured in intact experimental animals and humans by measuring the plasma level of a substance and the amount of that substance that is excreted.
• A substance to be used to measure GFR must be freely filtered through the glomeruli and must be neither secreted nor reabsorbed by the tubules; should be nontoxic & not metabolized by the body[Q].
• Inulin, a polymer of fructose with a molecular weight of 5200, meets these criteria in humans & most animals and can be used to measure GFR[Q].
• **Renal plasma clearance** is the **volume of plasma from which a substance is completely removed by the kidney in a given amount of time** (usually minutes)[Q].
• The amount of that substance that appears in the urine per unit of time is the result of the renal filtering of a certain number of milliliters of plasma that contained this amount.

Contd...

Contd...

Measuring Glomerular filtration rate (GFR)

- **GFR & clearance are measured in mL/min.**

  - Therefore, if the substance is designated by the letter X, the **GFR is equal to the concentration of X in urine (U_X) times the urine flow per unit of time (V) divided by the arterial plasma level of X (P_X), or $U_X V/P_X$**
  - This value is called the **clearance of X (C_X).**

- In practice, a loading dose of inulin is administered intravenously, followed by a sustaining infusion to keep the arterial plasma level constant. After the inulin has equilibrated with body fluids, an accurately timed urine specimen is collected and a plasma sample obtained halfway through the collection.
- Plasma and urinary inulin concentrations are determined and the clearance is calculated:

  - U_{IN} = 35 mg/mL
  - V = 0.9 mL/min
  - P_{IN} = 0.25 mg/mL
  - $C_{IN} = U_{IN} V/P_{IN}$ = 35 x 0.9/0.25 = **126 mL/min**

- **Clearance of creatinine** can also be **used to determine GFR,** however **some creatinine is secreted by the tubules thus the clearance of creatinine will be slightly higher than inulin[Q].**

25. **Ans. d. Single breath nitrogen test**   *(Ref: Ganong 25/e p633, 634, 24/e p633, 634)*

   Anatomical dead space is calculated by the Bohr's equation, which uses single breath nitrogen inhalation technique.

   Xenon/Helium dilution technique is used to measure functional residual capacity of lung. Spirometry cannot measure the residual or the dead space volumes.

   "Anatomic dead space can be measured by analysis of the single-breath N_2 curves. From mid-inspiration, the subject takes as deep a breath as possible of pure O_2, then exhales steadily while the N_2 content of the expired gas is continuously measured. The initial gas exhaled (phase I) is the gas that filled the dead space and that consequently contains no N_2. This is followed by a mixture of dead space and alveolar gas (phase II) and then by alveolar gas (phase III). The volume of the dead space is the volume of the gas expired from peak inspiration to the mid portion of phase II. Phase III of the single-breath N_2 curve terminates at the closing volume (CV) and is followed by phase IV, during which the N_2 content of the expired gas is increased."- Ganong 25/e p633

Dead Space & Uneven Ventilation

- Because **gaseous exchange in respiratory system occurs only in terminal portions of airways,** gas that occupies rest of respiratory system is not available for gas exchange with pulmonary capillary blood.
- Normally, the volume (in mL) of this **anatomic dead space** is approximately **equal to body weight in pounds.** As an example, in a man who weighs **150 lb (68 kg), only the first 350 mL of the 500 mL inspired with each breath at rest mixes with air in the alveoli.**
- Conversely, **with each expiration, first 150 mL expired is gas that occupied dead space,** and **only last 350 mL is gas from alveoli.**
- Consequently, **alveolar ventilation,** i.e., **amount of air reaching alveoli per minute,** is less than RMV. Note that because of the dead space, rapid shallow breathing produces much less alveolar ventilation than slow deep breathing at the same RMV.

  - It is important to distinguish between **anatomic dead space (respiratory system volume exclusive of alveoli)** & **total (physiologic) dead space (volume of gas not equilibrating with blood; i.e., wasted ventilation)[Q].**
  - **In healthy individuals, two dead spaces are identical** and **can be estimated by body weight[Q].**
  - However, **in disease states, no exchange may take place between gas in some of alveoli & blood,** and **some of alveoli may be over ventilated[Q].**

- Volume of gas in non-perfused alveoli & any volume of air in alveoli in excess of that necessary to arterialize blood in alveolar capillaries is part of the dead space (non-equilibrating) gas volume.

Contd...

Contd...

Dead Space & Uneven Ventilation

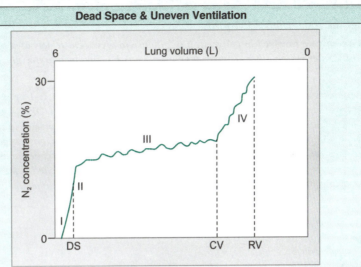

Single-breath N_2 curve

From mid-inspiration, subject takes a deep breath of pure O_2 then exhales steadily. Changes in the N_2 concentration of expired gas during expiration are shown, with the various phases of the curve indicated by roman numerals.

Notably, **region I is representative of dead space (DS); from I–II is a mixture of DS and alveolar gas; transition form III–IV is closing volume (CV) & end of IV is residual volume (RV).**

- **Anatomic dead space** can be **measured by analysis of single-breath N_2 curves.**
- From mid-inspiration, subject takes as deep a breath as possible of pure O_2, then exhales steadily while the N_2 content of expired gas is continuously measured.

  - **Initial gas exhaled (phase I)** is the **gas that filled the dead space** and that **consequently contains no N_2.** This is **followed by a mixture of dead space and alveolar gas (phase II)** and then **by alveolar gas (phase III)**^{Q}.
  - **Volume of dead space** is the **volume of the gas expired from peak inspiration to the mid portion of phase II**^{Q}.
  - **Phase III of single-breath N_2 curve terminates at closing volume (CV) & is followed by phase IV**, during which N_2 **content of expired gas is increased**^{Q}.

- **Total dead space** can be calculated from **PCO_2 of expired air, PCO_2 of arterial blood & TV.**
- Tidal volume (V_T) times the PCO_2 of the expired gas ($PeCO_2$) equals the arterial PCO_2 ($PaCO_2$) times the difference between the TV and the dead space (V_D) plus the PCO_2 of inspired air ($PiCO_2$) times V_D **(Bohr's equation):**

$$PeCO_2 \times V_T = PaCO_2 \times (V_T - V_D) + PiCO_2 \times V_D$$

- Term $PiCO_2 \times V_D$ is so small that it can be ignored and the equation solved for V_D, where $V_D = V_T - (PeCO_2 \times V_T) / (PaCO_2)$
- If, for example: **$PeCO_2$ = 28 mm Hg; $PaCO_2$ = 40 mm Hg and V_T = 500 mL, then V_D = 150 mL**
- **The equation can also be used to measure the anatomic dead space if one replaces $PaCO_2$ with alveolar PCO_2 ($PACO_2$),** which is the PCO_2 of the last 10 mL of expired gas.
- PCO_2 is an average of gas from different alveoli in proportion to their ventilation regardless of whether they are perfused.
- This is in contrast to $PACO_2$, which is gas equilibrated only with perfused alveoli, and consequently, in individuals with under-perfused alveoli, is greater than PCO_2.

Contd...

BIOCHEMISTRY

26. Ans. d. Glycogenin *(Ref: Harper 30/e p181)*

Glycogenin is an enzyme involved in conversion of glucose to glycogen. It acts as a primer, by polymerizing the first few glucose molecules, after which other enzymes take over. Thus it is involved in the glycogen synthesis pathway rather than glycogenolysis.

> *"Glycogen synthase catalyzes the formation of a glycoside bond between C-1 of the glucose of UDPGlc and C-4 of a terminal glucose residue of glycogen, liberating uridine diphosphate (UDP). A preexisting glycogen molecule, or "glycogen primer," must be present to initiate this reaction. The glycogen primer in turn is formed on a protein primer known as glycogenin. Glycogenin is a 37 kDa protein that is glucosylated on a specific tyrosine residue by UDPGlc. Further glucose residues are attached in the 1→4 position (catalyzed by glycogenin itself) to form a short chain that is a substrate for glycogen synthase. In skeletal muscle, glycogenin remains attached in the center of the glycogen molecule; in liver the number of glycogen molecules is greater than the number of glycogenin molecules."* – Harper 30/e p181

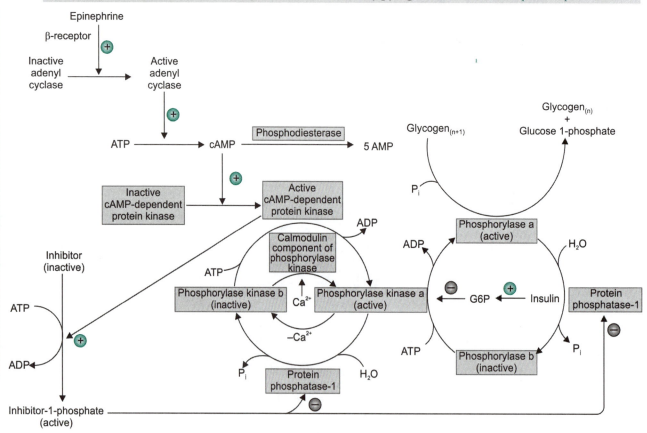

Fig. 13: Control of phosphorylase in muscle

Glycogenolysis

Glycogen phosphorylase

- **Glycogen phosphorylase** catalyzes the **rate-limiting step in glycogenolysis**, the **phosphorolytic cleavage of the 1→ 4 linkages of glycogen to yield glucose 1-phosphate**[Q].
- There are **different isoenzymes of glycogen phosphorylase in liver, muscle & brain,** encoded by different genes[Q].
- **Glycogen phosphorylase** requires **pyridoxal phosphate as its coenzyme**[Q].

Contd...

Contd...

Glycogenolysis
Cyclic-AMP Integrates the regulation of Glycogenolysis & Glycogenesis
• **Principal enzymes controlling glycogen metabolism—glycogen phosphorylase & glycogen synthase—are regulated by allosteric mechanisms & covalent modification by reversible phosphorylation & dephosphorylation** of enzyme protein in response to hormone action[Q].   • **Phosphorylation is increased in response to cAMP** formed from ATP by **adenylyl cyclase** at inner surface of cell membranes in response to hormones such as **epinephrine, norepinephrine & glucagon**[Q].   • **cAMP is hydrolyzed by phosphodiesterase,** so terminating hormone action; **in liver insulin increases the activity of phosphodiesterase**[Q].
c-AMP Activates Phosphorylase
• **Phosphorylase kinase is activated in response to cAMP**[Q].   • Increasing concentration of cAMP activates **cAMP-dependent protein kinase,** which catalyzes phosphorylation by ATP of inactive **phosphorylase kinase b** to active **phosphorylase kinase a,** which in turn, phosphorylates phosphorylase b to phosphorylase a[Q].   • In **liver, cAMP is formed in response to glucagon**, which is secreted in response to falling blood glucose[Q].   • **Muscle is insensitive to glucagon**[Q]; in muscle, signal for increased cAMP formation is action of norepinephrine, which is secreted in response to fear or fright, when there is a need for increased glycogenolysis to permit rapid muscle activity.
Ca²⁺ Synchronizes the Activation of Phosphorylase with Muscle Contraction
• **Glycogenolysis in muscle increases several hundred-fold at the onset of contraction**; the same signal (**increased cytosolic Ca²⁺ ion concentration**) is **responsible for initiation of both contraction & glycogenolysis**[Q].   • Muscle phosphorylase kinase, which activates glycogen phosphorylase, is a tetramer of four different subunits, α, β, γ, and δ. The α and β subunits contain serine residues that are phosphorylated by cAMP- dependent protein kinase.   • **The δ subunit is identical to the Ca²⁺binding protein calmodulin**[Q], and binds four Ca²⁺.   • The binding of Ca²⁺ activates the catalytic site of the γ subunit even while the enzyme is in the dephosphorylated b state; the phosphorylated a form is only fully activated in the presence of high concentrations of Ca²⁺.
Protein Phosphatase-1 Inactivates Phosphorylase
• Both phosphorylase a & phosphorylase kinase a are dephosphorylated and inactivated by **protein phosphatase- 1.**   • **Protein phosphatase-1 is inhibited by a protein, inhibitor-1**[Q], which is active only after it has been phosphorylated by cAMP-dependent protein kinase.   • Thus, cAMP controls both the activation and inactivation of phosphorylase. **Insulin reinforces this effect by inhibiting the activation of phosphorylase b**[Q]. It does this indirectly by increasing uptake of glucose, leading to increased formation of glucose 6-phosphate, which is an inhibitor of phosphorylase kinase.

27. **Ans. a. Decreased**   *(Ref: Harper 30/e p460, 28/e p49, 357, 397-398; Lippincott 5/e p475-477; Lehninger 5/e p168-169)*

The mobility of HbS as compared with normal hemoglobin on gel electrophoresis will be decreased. A molecule of Hb S contains two normal α-globin chains and two mutant β-globin chains (β), in which glutamate at position six has been replaced with valine. Therefore, during electrophoresis at alkaline pH, Hb S migrates more slowly toward the anode (positive electrode) than does HbA. This altered mobility of Hb S is a result of the absence of the negatively charged glutamate residues in the two β chains, thus rendering Hb S less negative than Hb A.

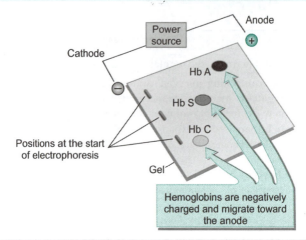

*"Sickle-cell disease, which is **caused by mutation of a single base (T-to-A DNA substitution)**, which in turn results in an **A-to-U change in the mRNA corresponding to the sixth codon of the β-globin gene**. The altered codon specifies a different amino acid (**valine rather than glutamic acid**), and this causes a **structural abnormality of the β-globin molecule leading to hemoglobin aggregation and red blood cell 'sickling'**. A molecule of Hb S contains two normal α-globin chains and two mutant β-globin chains (β), in which glutamate at position six has been replaced with valine. Therefore, during **electrophoresis at alkaline pH, Hb S migrates more slowly toward the anode (positive electrode) than does HbA**. This altered mobility of Hb S is a result of the absence of the negatively charged glutamate residues in the two β chains, thus rendering Hb S less negative than Hb A."*

*"**Electrophoresis of hemoglobin obtained from lysed red blood cells** is routinely used in the diagnosis of sickle cell trait and sickle cell disease. **Sequence of Movement: HbA2 < HbC < HbS < HbF < HbA**."*

Sickle Cell Hemoglobin (HbS)

- A **point mutation** involving **T- to – A** DNA substitution (which in turn results in an '**A – to- U**' change in the m-RNA) corresponding to the 6th codon of β globin gene result in sickle cell disease
- The corresponding single nucleotide change within the codon would be **GAA or GAG of glutamic acid to GUA or GUG of valine**. This is a **partially accepted missense mutation**; partially accepted because HbS does bind & release O_2, albeit abnormally; missense because it hinders normal function & result in sickle cell anemia.

  - **Restriction fragment length polymorphism (RFLP)** is an inherited difference in the pattern of restriction (endonuclease) enzyme digestion due to presence or absence of an extra restriction site.
  - This single base change in sickle cell disease result in RFLP[Q].

- The mutation results in **single amino acid substitution (GLu ⁶(β) – Val)**: i.e. **a surface localized charged (polar, hydrophilic) aminoacid glutamate is replaced by hydrophobic (non polar) amino acid valine (without any charge)** [Q] **at position 6 in two β-chains**. The R group of valine has no electric charge, whereas glutamate has a negative charge at pH 7.4. So HbS has 2 fewer negative charges than HbA (1 for each β-chain).

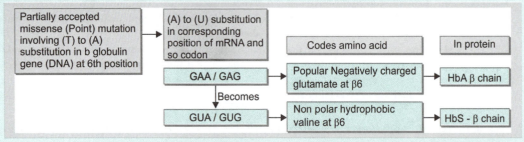

- This replacement creates a **'Sticky hydrophobic patch'** (contact point) on the outer surface at position 6 of β-chain of both oxy HbS and deoxy HbS (but not in Hb A).
  - **Complementary sticky patch** is found in both **HbA and HbS**, but is exposed only in their **deoxygenated (T) state**.

Contd...

Contd...

Sickle Cell Hemoglobin (HbS)

- HbA remains a true solute at rather higher concentrations because of polar exterior surface that is compatible and non reactive with nearby Hb molecules. In contrast **HbS when deoxygenated is less soluble[Q]**.
- Thus at low PO_2, deoxy HbS can polymerize to form long, insoluble fibers. These twisted helical fibers **distort the erythrocyte into characteristic sickle shape[Q]**.
- Binding of **deoxy Hb A** terminates fiber polymerization, since HbA lacks the second sticky patch necessary to bind another Hb molecule.

  - In **heterozygous (Hb A/ HbS, sickle cell trait)** individuals, **sickling decreases by at least a factor of 1000**, thereby **accounting for the asymptomatic nature except during extreme physical exertion**.
  - For reasons that remain to be elucidated, **heterozygosity is associated with an increased resistance to malaria[Q]**, specially for lethal forms like plasmodium falciparum.
  - HbS trait causes parasites to grow poorly or die at low O_2 concentration because of low K^+ levels caused by potassium efflux from RBC on hemoglobin sickling[Q].

28. Ans. c. Succinate dehydrogenase   *(Ref: Harper 30/e p555, 28/e p321, 473)*

Thiamin is the coenzyme for these multienzyme complexes that catalyze oxidative decarboxylation reactions, while succinate dehydrogenase is involved in a redox reaction, which is catalyzed by FMN and FAD.

> "**Pyruvate, formed in the cytosol, is transported into the mitochondrion by a proton symporter.** Inside the mitochondrion, it is **oxidatively decarboxylated to acetyl-CoA by a multienzyme complex** that is associated with the inner mitochondrial membrane. This **pyruvate dehydrogenase complex** is analogous to the **alpha-ketoglutarate dehydrogenase complex of the citric acid cycle**. Pyruvate is decarboxylated by the pyruvate dehydrogenase component of the enzyme complex to a **hydroxyethyl derivative of the thiazole ring of enzyme-bound thiamin diphosphate**, which in turn reacts with oxidized lipoamide, the prosthetic group of dihydrolipoyl transacetylase, to form acetyl lipoamide. **Thiamin is vitamin B1 and in deficiency, glucose metabolism is impaired**, and there is **significant (and potentially life-threatening) lactic and pyruvic acidosis**." *- Harper 30/e p555*

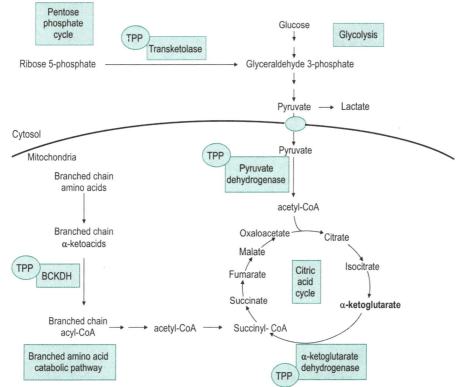

BCKDH, branched chain α-ketoacid dehydrogenase complex; CoA, coenzyme, A; TPP, thiamin pyrophosphate

AIIMS ESSENCE

Thiamin (Vitamin B1)	
• **Thiamin diphosphate (TDP)**[Q] also known as **Thiamin pyrophosphate (TPP)**[Q] is **biologically active & storage form of vitamin B1,** formed by **transfer of pyrophosphate group from ATP.**	

Physiological Role:

- **Thiamin** has a **central role in energy yielding metabolism** and especially of **carbohydrates.**
- **Thiamin requirements increase in excess intake of carbohydrates** and its **deficiency leads to decreased energy production.**

Thiamin diphosphate	• Thiamin diphosphate is the coenzyme for: • **3 multi-enzyme complexes that catalyze oxidative decarboxylation reactions:** • **Branched-chain ketoacid dehydrogenase**[Q] involved in the metabolism of **leucine, isoleucine & valine** • **Alpha-ketoglutarate dehydrogenase**[Q] in the **citric acid cycle** • **Pyruvate dehydrogenase**[Q] in carbohydrate metabolism • **Transketolase**[Q] reaction in the **pentose phosphate pathway**
Thiamin triphosphate	• **Thiamin triphosphate** has a **role in nerve conduction**; it phosphorylates, and so **activates a chloride channel**[Q] in the nerve membrane

Thiamine Deficiency Diseases:

- Chronic peripheral Neuritis, Beriberi & Wernicke Encephalopathy with Korsakoff's Psychosis

Beriberi	Wernicke Encephalopathy with Korsakoff's Psychosis
• **Wet beriberi:** Patients present with an **enlarged heart, tachycardia, high-output congestive heart failure**, peripheral edema & peripheral neuritis[Q]. • **Dry beriberi: Symmetric peripheral neuropathy** of the motor and sensory systems, with diminished reflexes. **Neuropathy affects the legs most markedly**[Q] • **Infantile beriberi:** Occurs in infants born to thiamin deficiency mothers and show tachycardia, vomiting, convulsions & death.	• Alcoholic patients with **chronic thiamin deficiency** also may have **CNS manifestations** known as *Wernicke's encephalopathy*[Q]. • *Wernicke's encephalopathy*: Consists of **horizontal nystagmus, ophthalmoplegia** (due to weakness of one or more extraocular muscles), **cerebellar ataxia, & mental impairment**[Q]. • When there is an **additional loss of memory** and a **confabulatory psychosis**, the syndrome is known as *Wernicke-Korsakoff syndrome*[Q].

29. **Ans. c. Methylmalonyl CoA to succinyl CoA**   *(Ref: Harper 30/e p550, 558, 28/e p346)*

Methylmalonyl CoA mutase, leucine aminomutase, and methionine synthase are vitamin B_{12} –dependent enzymes. Methylmalonyl CoA is formed as an intermediate in the catabolism of valine and by the carboxylation of propionyl CoA arising in the catabolism of isoleucine, cholesterol, and, rarely, fatty acids with an odd number of carbon atoms or directly from propionate, a major product of microbial fermentation in the rumen. It undergoes a vitamin B_{12} –dependent rearrangement to succinyl CoA, catalyzed by methylmalonyl CoA mutase.

*"Methylmalonyl CoA mutase, leucine aminomutase, and methionine synthase are vitamin B_{12} –dependent enzymes. Methylmalonyl CoA is formed as an **intermediate in the catabolism of valine** and by the **carboxylation of propionyl CoA** arising in the catabolism of isoleucine, cholesterol, and, rarely, fatty acids with an odd number of carbon atoms or directly from propionate, a major product of microbial fermentation in the rumen. It undergoes a **vitamin B_{12} –dependent rearrangement to succinyl CoA**, catalyzed by methylmalonyl CoA mutase. The activity of this enzyme is greatly reduced in vitamin B_{12} deficiency, leading to an **accumulation of methylmalonyl CoA** and **urinary excretion of methylmalonic acid**, which provides a means of assessing vitamin B_{12} nutritional status."-Harper 30/e p558*

*"Cobalamin (vitamin B_{12}) exists in a number of different chemical forms. All have a cobalt atom at the center of a corrin ring. In nature, the vitamin is mainly in the 2-deoxyadenosyl (ado) form, which is located in mitochondria. It is the **cofactor for the enzyme methylmalonyl coenzyme A (CoA) mutase**. The other major natural cobalamin is methylcobalamin, the form in human plasma and in cell cytoplasm. It is the **cofactor for methionine synthase**."- Harrison 19/e p640*

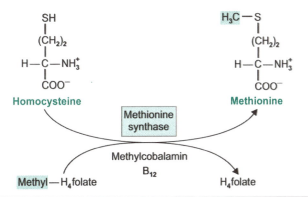

Fig. 14: Metabolism of propionate

*"Propionate is a major precursor of glucose in ruminants; it enters gluconeogenesis via the citric acid cycle. After esterification with CoA, propionyl-CoA is carboxylated to D-methylmalonyl-CoA, catalyzed by **propionyl-CoA carboxylase**, a biotin-dependent enzyme. **Methylmalonyl-CoA racemase** catalyzes the conversion of D-methylmalonyl-CoA to L-methylmalonyl-CoA, which then **undergoes isomerization to succinyl-CoA catalyzed by methylmalonyl-CoA mutase**. Methylmalonyl-CoA mutase is a vitamin B_{12}-dependent enzyme, and in deficiency methylmalonic acid is excreted in the urine (methylmalonic aciduria)."* - Harper 30/e p558

Vitamin B_{12}

- Vitamin B_{12} or cobalamin is **cobalt containing compound possessing corrin ring**.
- Central portion of B_{12} consists of **4 pyrrole rings surrounding a single cobalt atom**.
- **Methylmalonyl CoA mutase, leucine aminomutase, and methionine synthase** are vitamin B_{12} –dependent enzymes[Q].

Vitamin B_{12} is Cofactor for		
Methylmalonyl CoA mutase	**Methionine synthase**	**Homocysteine methyl transferase**
• It converts **methylmalonyl CoA rearrangement to succinyl CoA**[Q]. • The activity of this enzyme is greatly reduced in vitamin B_{12} deficiency, leading to an **accumulation of methylmalonyl CoA** and **urinary excretion of methylmalonic acid**, which provides a **means of assessing vitamin B_{12} nutritional status**[Q].	• When acting as a methyl donor, **S-adenosyl methionine forms homocysteine**, which may be remethylated by methyl tetrahydrofolate catalyzed by **methionine synthase**[Q]. • **Impairment of methionine synthase** in **vitamin B_{12} deficiency** results in the accumulation of methyl tetrahydrofolate that cannot be used — the **'folate trap'**[Q] (functional deficiency of folate, secondary to vitamin B_{12} deficiency)	Transfers CH_3 groups as methylcobalamin[Q]

Contd...

Contd...

Vitamin B$_{12}$
Source & Absorption: • Synthesized **exclusively by microorganisms found only in foods of animal origin** • It is **absorbed from distal third of ileum.**
Metabolic roles of Vitamin B$_{12}$
• Isomerization of methylmalonyl co-A to succinyl co-A by methylmalonyl co-A mutase[Q] • Methylation of homocysteine to methionine by homocysteine methyl transferase[Q] • Methylation of pyrimidine ring to form thymine[Q] • Metabolism of diols[Q] • In bacteria for interconversion of glutamate & beta-methyl aspartate[Q]
Deficiency of Vitamin B$_{12}$ leads to
• **Methylmalonic aciduria:** Methylmalonyl-CoA mutase is a vitamin B$_{12}$-dependent enzyme, and in deficiency methylmalonic acid is excreted in the urine[Q] • Folate trap & pernicious anemia[Q] • Subacute combined degeneration & demyelination of spinal cord[Q]

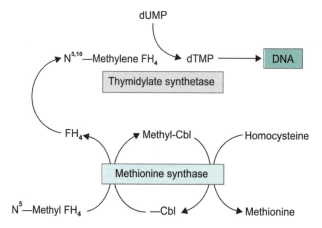

30. **Ans. b. Glucose-6-phosphatase is present in the endoplasmic reticulum and cannot act on glycogen formed in the cytoplasm**   *(Ref: Harper 30/e p178)*

Glucose-6-phosphate is formed in the cytoplasm of hepatocytes while glucose-6-phosphatase is present in the endoplasmic reticulum of cell. Hence, the reaction does not take place until gluconeogenesis is favored.

> "Glucose-6-phosphate is formed in the cytoplasm of hepatocytes while glucose-6-phosphatase is present in the endoplasmic reticulum of cell. Hence, the reaction does not take place until gluconeogenesis is favored. In liver, but not muscle, glucose-6-phosphatase catalyzes hydrolysis of glucose-6-phosphate, yielding glucose that is exported, leading to an increase in the blood glucose concentration. Glucose-6-phosphatase is in the lumen of the smooth endoplasmic reticulum, and genetic defects of the glucose-6-phosphate transporter can cause a variant of type I glycogen storage disease."

See Q. No. 31 AIIMS May 2016

31. **Ans. d. Delta amino levulinic acid**   *(Ref: Harper 30/e p329)*

High levels of lead can affect heme metabolism by combining with SH groups in enzymes such as ferrochelatase and ALA (delta-amino levulinic acid) dehydratase. Elevated levels of protoporphyrin are found in red blood cells, and elevated levels of ALA and of coproporphyrin are found in urine.

"High levels of lead can affect heme metabolism by combining with SH groups in enzymes such as ferrochelatase and ALA (delta-amino levulinic acid) dehydratase. This affects porphyrin metabolism. Elevated levels of protoporphyrin are found in red blood cells, and elevated levels of ALA and of coproporphyrin are found in urine."- Harper 30/e p329

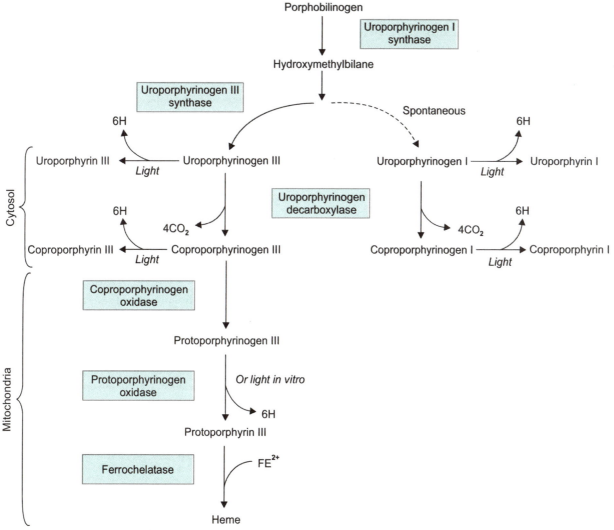

Fig. 15: Steps in the biosynthesis of the porphyrin derivatives from porphobilinogen.

32. **Ans. a. RBC** *(Ref: Harper 30/e p325)*

Heme biosynthesis occurs in most mammalian cells except mature erythrocytes, which lack mitochondria.

*"Heme biosynthesis occurs in most mammalian cells with the exception of mature erythrocytes, which do not contain mitochondria. However, approximately 85% of heme synthesis occurs in erythroid precursor cells in the bone marrow and the **majority of the remainder in hepatocytes**."*– Harper 30/e p325

Heme biosynthesis
• **Heme biosynthesis** occurs in **most mammalian cells** with the **exception of mature erythrocytes**, which do not contain mitochondria[Q].
• **Sites:** 85% of heme synthesis occurs in erythroid precursor cells in the **bone marrow**, and the **majority of the remainder in hepatocytes**[Q].

Contd...

Contd...

Heme biosynthesis
• The enzymatic process that produces heme is properly called **porphyrin synthesis**. In humans, this pathway serves almost exclusively to form heme. • The pathway is **initiated by the synthesis of D-Aminolevulinic acid (dALA or δALA)** from **amino acid glycine & succinyl- CoA from the citric acid cycle** (Krebs cycle)[Q]. • **Rate-limiting enzyme** responsible for this reaction, **ALA synthase**, is **negatively regulated by glucose & heme concentration**[Q]. • It **involves both cytoplasm & mitochondria**[Q].   • Hemes are **most commonly recognized as components of hemoglobin**, but are **also found in** a number of other **biologically important hemoproteins** such as **myoglobin, cytochrome, catalase & endothelial nitric oxide synthase**[Q].

33. Ans. b. UGA   *(Ref: Harper 30/e p18, 286)*

Selenocysteine is commonly termed the "21st amino acid" which unlike other amino acids present in biological proteins, is not coded for directly in the genetic code. Instead, it is encoded by a UGA codon, which is normally a stop codon. Such a mechanism is called translational recoding.

"The ability of the protein synthetic apparatus to identify a selenocysteine-specific UGA codon involves the selenocysteine insertion element, a stem-loop structure in the untranslated region of the mRNA."– Harper 30/e p286

Selenocysteine (the 21st Amino Acid)

• While its occurrence in proteins is uncommon, **selenocysteine** is **present at the active site of several human enzymes** that **catalyze redox reactions**[Q]. **Examples: thioredoxin reductase, glutathione peroxidase, & deiodinase** (that converts thyroxine to triiodothyronine)
• Significantly, **replacement of selenocysteine by cysteine** can significantly **decrease catalytic activity**[Q].
    • Impairments in human selenoproteins have been implicated in tumorigenesis & atherosclerosis, and are associated with **selenium deficiency cardiomyopathy (Keshan disease**[Q]**)**.
• **Biosynthesis of selenocysteine requires cysteine, selenate, ATP, a specific tRNA**, and several enzymes.
• **Serine provides the carbon skeleton of selenocysteine**. Selenophosphate, formed from ATP and selenate, serves as the selenium donor. Unlike hydroxyproline or hydroxylysine, selenocysteine arises co-translationally during its incorporation into peptides.
    • **UGA anticodon of the unusual tRNA designated tRNA**[Sec] **normally signals STOP**[Q].
    • The ability of the protein synthetic apparatus to identify a **selenocysteine-specific UGA codon** involves the **selenocysteine insertion element, a stem-loop structure in the untranslated region of the mRNA**[Q].
• **Selenocysteine- tRNA**[Sec] **is first charged with serine** by the ligase that charges tRNA[Ser]. Subsequent replacement of the serine oxygen by selenium involves selenophosphate formed by selenophosphate synthase.
• Successive enzyme-catalyzed reactions convert cysteyl- tRNA[Sec] to aminoacryl- tRNA[Sec] and then to selenocysteyl- tRNA[Sec].
• In the presence of a specific elongation factor that recognizes selenocysteyl- tRNA[Sec], selenocysteine can then be incorporated into proteins.

34. Ans. a. Acetyl CoA   *(Ref: Harper 30/e p185, 29/e p187)*

Acetyl CoA is not a substrate for gluconeogenesis and cannot be converted back to glucose.

"Acetyl CoA is not a substrate for gluconeogenesis and cannot be converted back to glucose[Q]. This is because acetyl CoA cannot be converted back to pyruvate[Q] since its carbon backbone is lost in citric acid cycle as CO_2."

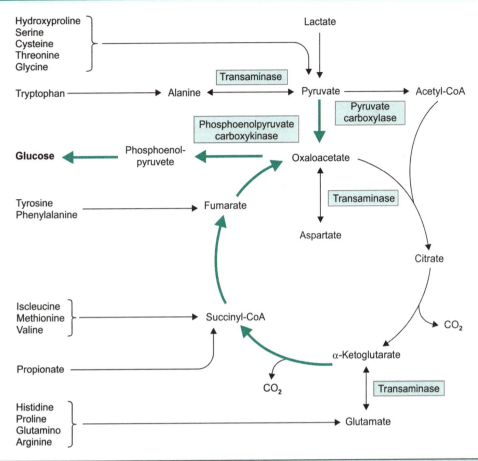

Gluconeogenesis

- **The carbon skeletons** for gluconeogenesis are **derived primarily from glucogenic amino acids & lactate from muscle & glycerol** from adipose tissues[Q].
- Although the **lactate produced in muscle, is used by liver for gluconeogenesis**[Q].

  - Liver & kidneys are the **major gluconeogenic tissues**[Q].
  - **Glucogenic key enzymes** are **expressed in small intestine** but their role in fasting state is unclear.

- Gluconeogenesis prevent hypoglycemia during short & long term fasting.
- Gluconeogenesis is stimulated by excess of acetyl Co-A & decrease in fructose 2, 6 biphosphate concentration[Q].

Substrates for Gluconeogenesis	
• Glucogenic amino acids (all except Leucine & lysine which are purely ketogenic): Most important is alanine[Q] • Lactate[Q]	• Pyruvate[Q] • Propionate[Q] • Glycerol[Q] • Fumarate[Q]

35. **Ans. a. Gamma carboxylation of glutamate** *(Ref: Harrison 19/e p96e-5; Harper 30/e p550, 561)*

   Gamma carboxylation of glutamate is carried out by Gamma-glutamyl carboxylase. It is a Vitamin-K dependent enzyme that catalyzes the post-translational modification of vitamin K-dependent proteins. Biotin functions to transfer carbon dioxide in a small number of reactions: acetyl-CoA carboxylase, pyruvate carboxylase, propionyl-CoA carboxylase, and methylcrotonyl-CoA carboxylase.

   "Biotin functions to transfer carbon dioxide in a small number of reactions: acetyl-CoA carboxylase, pyruvate carboxylase, propionyl-CoA carboxylase, and methylcrotonyl-CoA carboxylase."–Harper 30/e p561

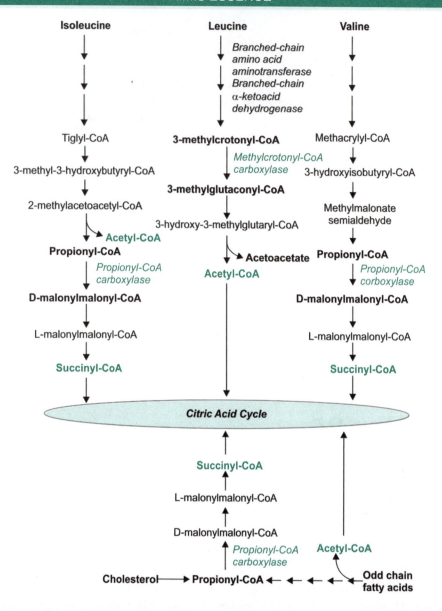

Biotin
• **Biotin** functions to **transfer carbon dioxide** in a small number of reactions: **acetyl-CoA carboxylase, pyruvate carboxylase, propionyl-CoA carboxylase,** and **methylcrotonyl-CoA carboxylase**[Q].
• Other functions: **Catabolism of specific amino acids (leucine)** & gene regulation by histone biotinylation.

Biotin functions to transfer carbon dioxide in reactions	
Pyruvate carboxylase	• Pyruvate (3C) to oxaloacetate (4C) in **gluconeogenesis**[Q]
Acetyl-CoA carboxylase	• Acetyl-CoA (2C) to malonyl-CoA (3C) in **lipid synthesis**[Q]
Propionyl-CoA carboxylase	• Propionyl-CoA (3C) to methylmalonyl-CoA (4C) in **gluconeogenesis**[Q]
Methylmalonyl CoA carboxyl transferase	• Propionic acid synthesis in bacteria[Q]
Methylcrotonyl-CoA carboxylase	• Leucine catabolism[Q]

Contd...

Contd...

Biotin
Source:
• Organ meat such as **liver or kidney, soy & beans, yeast** & egg yolks
• **Egg white contains protein avidin,** which **strongly binds** the vitamin & reduces its bioavailability[Q].
Deficiency:
• Biotin deficiency due to low dietary intake is **rare (deficiency is due to inborn errors of metabolism)**
• **Mental changes** (depression, hallucinations), paresthesia, anorexia & nausea.
• A **scaling, seborrheic, erythematous rash** around eyes, nose, mouth & extremities.
Diagnosis:
• **Laboratory diagnosis: Decreased** concentration of **urinary biotin** (or its major metabolites), **increased** urinary excretion of **3-hydroxyisovaleric acid** after a leucine challenge, or **decreased activity of biotin-dependent enzymes in lymphocytes (propionyl-CoA carboxylase).**
Treatment:
• Treatment requires pharmacologic doses of biotin–i.e., up to **10 mg/d.**

Vitamin	Name	Functions	Deficiency disease
		Lipid-soluble	
A	**Retinal, β-carotene**	**Visual pigments** in retina[Q]; regulation of gene expression & cell differentiation (β**-carotene is an antioxidant**)	**Night blindness, xerophthalmia; keratinization of skin**[Q]
D	**Calciferol**	Maintenance of calcium balance, **enhances intestinal absorption of Ca^{2+} & mobilizes bone mineral**[Q]; regulation of gene expression & cell differentiation	**Rickets**[Q] (poor mineralization of bone); **osteomalacia**[Q] (bone demineralization)
E	**Tocopherols tocotrienols**	**Antioxidant,** especially in **cell membranes;** roles in cell signaling	Extremely rare- serious neurologic dysfunction
K	**Phylloquinone: menaquinones**	Coenzyme in formation of γ**-carboxyglutamate in enzymes of blood clotting & bone matrix**[Q]	**Impaired blood clotting, hemorrhagic disease**[Q]
		Water-soluble	
B1	**Thiamin**	Coenzyme in **pyruvate and α-ketoglutarate dehydrogenases & transketolase**[Q]; regulates Cl$^-$ channel in nerve conduction	Peripheral nerve damage (**beriberi**[Q]) or central nervous system lesions (**Wernicke-Korsakoff syndrome**[Q])
B2	**Riboflavin**	Coenzyme in oxidation & reduction reactions (**FAD & FMN); prosthetic group of flavoproteins**[Q]	Lesions of **corner of mouth, lips, & tongue, seborrheic dermatitis**
Niacin	**Nicotinic acid, nicotinamide**	Coenzyme in **oxidation & reduction reactions,** functional part of **NAD & NADP**[Q]; role in intracellular calcium regulation & cell signaling	**Pellagra**[Q]-photosensitive dermatitis, depressive psychosis
B6	**Pyridoxine, pyridoxal, pyridoxamine**	Coenzyme in **transamination & decarboxylation** of **amino acids & glycogen phosphorylase**[Q]; modulation of steroid hormone action	Disorders of amino acid metabolism, convulsions
	Folic acid	Coenzyme in **transfer of one-carbon fragments**	Megaloblastic anemia
B12	**Cobalamin**	Coenzyme in **transfer of one-carbon fragments & metabolism of folic acid**[Q]	**Pernicious anemia, megaloblastic anemia with degeneration of spinal cord**[Q]
	Pantothenic acid	**Functional part of CoA & acyl carrier protein:** fatty acid synthesis and metabolism[Q]	**Peripheral nerve damage (nutritional melalgia**[Q] or **burning foot syndrome**[Q])
H	**Biotin**	Coenzyme in **carboxylation reactions** in **gluconeogenesis & fatty acid synthesis**[Q]; role in regulation of cell cycle	Impaired fat and carbohydrate metabolism, dermatitis
C	**Ascorbic Acid**	Coenzyme in **hydroxylation of proline & lysine** in **collagen synthesis**[Q]; antioxidant; **enhances absorption of iron**[Q]	**Scurvy-impaired wound healing,** loss of dental cement, subcutaneous hemorrhage[Q]

| 1270 | AIIMS ESSENCE |

36. Ans. d. Titration with reducing sugar *(Ref: Harper 30/e p26)*

Protein precipitation is widely used to concentrate proteins and purify them from various contaminants. Titration with reducing sugar is not used for protein precipitation.

"Highly purified protein is essential for the detailed examination of its physical and functional properties. Cells contain thousands of different proteins, each in widely varying amounts. The isolation of a specific protein in quantities sufficient for analysis thus presents a formidable challenge that may require multiple successive purification techniques. Classic approaches exploit differences in relative solubility of individual proteins as a function of pH (isoelectric precipitation), polarity (precipitation with ethanol or acetone), or salt concentration (salting out with ammonium sulfate). Chromatographic separations partition molecules between two phases, one mobile and the other stationary. For separation of amino acids or sugars, the stationary phase, or matrix, may be a sheet of filter paper (paper chromatography) or a thin layer of cellulose, silica, or alumina (thin-layer chromatography [TLC])."– Harper 30/e p26

See Q. NO. 36 AIIMS May 2016

PATHOLOGY

37. Ans. c. Antony B pattern—Verocay body *(Ref: Robbins 9/e p257, 854, 8/e p1340)*

Area marked with arrow represents the pattern of growth, in which the tumor is less densely cellular and consists of a loose meshwork of cells, microcysts and myxoid stroma, Antoni B pattern of growth.

"Schwannoma: In the Antoni A^Q pattern of growth, elongated cells with cytoplasmic processes are arranged in fascicles in areas of moderate to high cellularity and scant stromal matrix; the "nuclear-free zones" of processes that lie between the regions of nuclear palisading are termed Verocay bodies^Q. In the Antoni B^Q pattern of growth, the tumor is less densely cellular and consists of a loose meshwork of cells, microcysts and myxoid stroma."- Robbins 9/e p854

38. Ans. a. Hodgkin's lymphoma, Epstein Barr Virus and Reed Sternberg cells *(Ref: Robbins 9/e p608, 8/e p617)*

The given slide of histopathology demonstrates Reed-Sternberg cells typical of Hodgkin's Lymphoma. EBV infection is a risk factor for Hodgkin's Lymphoma.

"Identification of Reed-Sternberg cells and their variants is essential for the diagnosis. Diagnostic Reed-Sternberg cells are large cells (45 μm in diameter) with multiple nuclei or a single nucleus with multiple nuclear lobes, each with a large inclusion-like nucleolus about the size of a small lymphocyte (5 to 7 μm in diameter)."- Robbins 9/e p608

Diagnostic Reed-Sternberg cell (Two nuclear lobes, large inclusion-like nucleoli, abundant cytoplasm)	Reed-Sternberg cell, mononuclear variant	Reed-Sternberg cell, lacunar variant (folded or multilobated nucleus, lies within open space)	Reed-Sternberg cell, lymphohistiocytic variant.

Hodgkin's Lymphoma (HL)

- **Arises in a single LN** or **chain (MC-cervical region^Q)**, follow **orderly spread to anatomically contiguous lymphoid tissues.**
- Presence of **distinctive neoplastic giant cells called Reed-Sternberg Cells**, derived from **germinal centre** or **post germinal centre of B-cells^Q.**

Contd...

Contd...

Hodgkin's Lymphoma (HL)

Pathology:
- **Activation of NF-κB is a common event in classical Hodgkin's Lymphoma**[Q]
- **Latent membrane protein-1 (LMP-1) of EBV up regulate NF-κB**[Q].
- **Reed-Sternberg cells** secrete **cytokines (IL-5, IL-10, M-CSF), chemokines (eotaxin)** & other factors **(Immunomodulatory factor galactin-1).**

Reed-Sternberg Cells

- **Reed-Sternberg cells alone are not diagnostic**, since they are **also seen in infectious mononucleosis, immunoblastic NHL, carcinoma & sarcoma**[Q].
- **Histological diagnosis** is established by **presence of Reed-Sternberg cells** along with **background of mixed inflammation** consisting of **neutrophils, plasma cells, eosinophils & histiocytes**[Q].

- *Reed–Sternberg cells are large and are either multinucleated or have a bilobed nucleus (thus resembling an "owl's eye" appearance*[Q]*) with prominent eosinophilic inclusion-like nucleoli*[Q].
- *Reed–Sternberg cells are CD30 & CD15 positive, usually negative for CD20 & CD45*[Q].
- *The presence of these cells is necessary in the diagnosis of Hodgkin's lymphoma – the absence of Reed–Sternberg cells has very high negative predictive value.*

Clinical Features:
- **MC presentation: Painless cervical lymphadenopathy**[Q]
- **Pel-Ebstein fever (Internittent fever every alternate week**[Q])
- **Paraneoplastic syndromes: Affected LN become painful with alcohol ingestion** & secondary amyloidosis **(AA type**[Q])

WHO Classification of Hodgkin's Lymphoma	
Classical Variety (CD15+, CD30+)	**Non-Classical Variety (CD20+, CD15–, C30–)**
• Nodular sclerosis • Mixed cellularity • Lymphocyte rich • Lymphocyte depletion	• Lymphocyte Predominance

- **Prognosis: Lymphocytic predominant**[Q] **> Nodular sclerosis > Mixed cellularity > Lymphocyte depletion**
- **Nodular sclerosis** is **MC type all over the world**[Q] whereas **mixed cellularity** is **MC in India**[Q]
- **Nodular sclerosis** is **MC in females** and **mediastinal involvement**[Q] is particularly common

Hodgkin's Lymphoma	
Subtype	**Characteristic Features**
Nodular sclerosis	• **MC subtype**; usually **stage I or II** disease; frequent **mediastinal involvement**[Q] • **More common in females, most patients young adults**[Q]
Mixed cellularity	• **MC subtype in India**[Q]; >50% present as stage **III or IV** disease; **M > F**; • **Biphasic incidence**, peaking in young adults & again in >55 years • **Good prognosis**
Lymphocyte rich	• **Uncommon; M > F**; seen in **older adults; Good prognosis**[Q]
Lymphocyte depletion	• Uncommon; more common in **older males, HIV-infected individuals** & in **developing countries**; often presents with advanced disease • **Worst prognosis**[Q]
Lymphocyte predominance	• Uncommon; **young males** with **cervical or axillary lymphadenopathy** • **Best prognosis**[Q]

Contd...

Contd...

Hodgkin's Lymphoma (HL)

Hodgkin's Lymphoma	Immuno-phenotype	Association with EBV	Morphology
Nodular sclerosis	CD15+, CD30+	Usually EBV–	Frequent lacunar cells (clear space around nucleus) & occasional diagnostic RS cells Background infiltrate composed of T lymphocytes, eosinophils, macrophages & plasma cells & fibrous bands
Mixed cellularity	CD15+, CD30+	70% EBV+	Frequent mononuclear & diagnostic RS cells
Lymphocyte rich	CD15+, CD30+	40% EBV+	Frequent mononuclear & diagnostic RS cell
Lymphocyte depletion	CD15+, CD30+	Most EBV+	Reticular variant: Frequent diagnostic RS cells
Lymphocyte Predominance	CD20+, CD15–, C30–	EBV–	Lymphocytic & Histiocytic (popcorn cell)

Adverse Prognostic Factors of Hodgkin's Lymphoma

- Age >45 years[Q]
- Male gender[Q]
- Hb <10.5 gm/dL[Q]
- Leucocyte count >15,000/mm³[Q]

- Lymphocytopenia (Absolute lymphocyte count <600/µL; Lymphocytes <8% of leucocyte)[Q]
- S. albumin <4 gm/dl[Q]
- Stage IV[Q]

Hodgkin's Lymphoma	Non-Hodgkin's Lymphoma
• Localized to single axial group of LNs[Q] (MC-cervical) • Orderly spread to anatomically contiguous lymphoid tissues[Q]. • Mesenteric & Waldeyer's rings are rarely involved[Q] • Extranodal presentation is rare	• Involve multiple peripheral LNs[Q] • Non-contiguous spread • Mesenteric & Waldeyer's rings are commonly involved[Q] • Extranodal presentation is common[Q]

39. **Ans. a. Nutmeg liver with dark areas of perivenular dead hepatocytes and gray areas of periportal viable hepatocytes** *(Ref: Robbins 9/e p864, 8/e p872)*

This is a classical picture of nutmeg liver seen in chronic passive venous congestion on liver. The dark congested areas consist of necrotic hepatocytes while the surrounding paler and brownish appearing regions are viable hepatocytes.

"The combination of hypoperfusion and retrograde congestion acts synergistically to cause centrilobular hemorrhagic necrosis. The liver takes on a variegated mottled appearance, reflecting hemorrhage and necrosis in the centrilobular regions. This finding is known as nutmeg liver due to its resemblance to the cut surface of a nutmeg." - Robbins 9/e p864

Passive Congestion and Centrilobular Necrosis

- **Hepatic manifestations of systemic circulatory compromise-passive congestion & centrilobular necrosis** can be seen in **both left & right-sided heart failure[Q].**

Pathology:

- **Right-sided cardiac decompensation** leads to **passive congestion of the liver.** The **liver** is slightly **enlarged, tense, and cyanotic,** with rounded edges. Microscopically there is **congestion of centrilobular sinusoids.** With time, centrilobular hepatocytes become atrophic, resulting in **markedly attenuated liver cell plates[Q].**
- **Left-sided cardiac failure or shock** may lead to **hepatic hypoperfusion & hypoxia,** causing **ischemic coagulative necrosis of hepatocytes in the central region** of the lobule (**centrilobular necrosis[Q]**).

    - **Combination of hypoperfusion & retrograde congestion acts synergistically to cause centrilobular hemorrhagic necrosis.** The liver takes on a **variegated mottled appearance,** reflecting **hemorrhage & necrosis in the centrilobular regions.** This finding is known as **nutmeg liver** due to its **resemblance to the cut surface of a nutmeg[Q].**

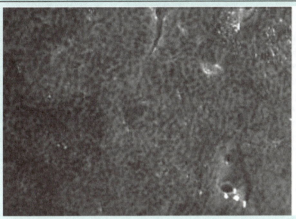
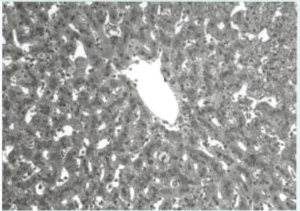

| Central areas are red & slightly depressed compared with the surrounding tan viable parenchyma, forming a "nutmeg liver" pattern | Centrilobular necrosis with degenerating hepatocytes and hemorrhage |

Liver with chronic passive congestion and hemorrhagic necrosis

40. **Ans. d. Barrett's esophagus, mucin stain, dysplasia** *(Ref: Robbins 9/e p757, 758, 8/e p771)*

The histopathological image of esophagus is showing intestinal type epithelium with goblet cells, typical of Barrett's esophagus. Extent of dysplasia is better delineated with mucin stain to rule out malignant transformation.

"Esophageal adenocarcinoma usually occurs in the distal third of the esophagus and may invade the adjacent gastric cardia. Initially appearing as flat or raised patches in otherwise intact mucosa, large masses of 5 cm or more in diameter may develop. Alternatively, tumors may infiltrate diffusely or ulcerate and invade deeply. Microscopically, Barrett esophagus is frequently present adjacent to the tumor. Tumors most commonly produce mucin and form glands, often with intestinal-type morphology; less frequently tumors are composed of diffusely infiltrative signet-ring cells (similar to those seen in diffuse gastric cancers) or, in rare cases, small poorly differentiated cells (similar to small-cell carcinoma of the lung)."
– Robbins 9/e p758

"Goblet cells contain acid mucin, usually sialomucin (Alcian blue+ at pH 2.5, although stain generally not needed or recommended), columnar cells contain neutral mucins (PAS+); intestinal metaplastic cells are often CK7+/CK20- (or CK20+ only superficially, although varies by fixative); also CDX2+ (but non-goblet columnar cells are also CDX2+)."
– http://www.pathologyoutlines.com/topic/esophagusBarrettsgeneral.html

41. **Ans. b. End of G_1** *(Ref: Robbins 9/e p289, 8/e p286)*

G_1-S, i.e. end of G_1 phase is the primary and most important cell cycle checkpoint where both the cell cycle regulators p53 & RB gene act.

"There are two main cell cycle checkpoints, one at the G_1/S transition and the other at G_2/M. The S phase is the point of no return in the cell cycle. Before a cell makes the final commitment to replicate, the G_1/S checkpoint checks for DNA damage; if damage is present, the DNA-repair machinery and mechanisms that arrest the cell cycle are put in motion. The delay in cell cycle progression provides the time needed for DNA repair; if the damage is not repairable, apoptotic pathways are activated to kill the cell. Thus, the G_1/S checkpoint prevents the replication of cells that have defects in DNA, which would be perpetuated as mutations or chromosomal breaks in the progeny of the cell. DNA damaged after its replication can still be repaired as long as the chromatids have not separated."- Robbins 9/e p289, 8/e p286

"The G_2/M checkpoint monitors the completion of DNA replication and checks whether the cell can safely initiate mitosis and separate sister chromatids. This checkpoint is particularly important in cells exposed to ionizing radiation. Cells damaged by ionizing radiation activate the G_2/M checkpoint and arrest in G_2; defects in this checkpoint give rise to chromosomal abnormalities."- Robbins 9/e p289, 8/e p286

Tumor Suppressor Genes	
RB (Retinoblastoma) gene	p53 gene
• Located on **chromosome no 13q14**[Q] • **Tumor suppressive pocket protein** that **binds E2F transcription factors in hypophophorylated state**[Q] • **Key negative regulator** of G_1/S cell cycle transition[Q] • **Tumors associated: Retinoblastoma, osteosarcoma, Glioblastoma, small cell carcinoma of lung, CA breast & CA bladder**[Q]	• Located on **chromosome no 17q13.1**[Q] • p53 is universally expressed in all cells & encodes a 53 kDa protein[Q] • **Regulates cell cycle progression, DNA repair, cellular senescence & apoptosis**[Q] • p53 activates CDK inhibitor (p21) → Inhibits cyclin-CDK complexes → Inhibits phosphorylation of RB → arrests cell cycle at G_1S phase[Q] • p53 gene is the **tumor suppressor gene altered in >50% of human cancers**[Q] • **p53 mutation causes: Brain tumors, CA breast, Leukemia, adrenal carcinoma & sarcoma**[Q]

42. **Ans. a. Bone marrow biopsy** *(Ref: Dacie Practical Hematology 10/e p163)*
    The given diagram shows various types of bone marrow biopsy needles.
    See Q. No. 108 AIIMS May 2016

43. **Ans. a. Hepcidin** *(Ref: Robbins 9/e p650, 848, 8/e p660)*
    The main regulator of iron absorption is the protein hepcidin, encoded by the HAMP gene and secreted by the liver.

    "Iron absorption is regulated by hepcidin, a small circulating peptide that is synthesized and released from the liver in response to increases in intrahepatic iron levels." – Robbins 9/e p650

    *"The main regulator of iron absorption is the **protein hepcidin**, encoded by the **HAMP gene** and **secreted by the liver**. Hepcidin is named for its originally elucidated properties as a hepatocellular protein with bac- bactericidal activities. Transcription of hepcidin is increased by inflammatory cytokines and iron, and decreased by iron deficiency, hypoxia, and ineffective erythropoiesis. Hepcidin binds to the cellular iron efflux channel ferroportin, causing its internalization and proteolysis, thereby **inhibiting the release of iron from intestinal cells** and **macrophages**. Therefore, hepcidin lowers plasma iron levels. Conversely, a deficiency in hepcidin causes iron overload." – Robbins 9/e p848*

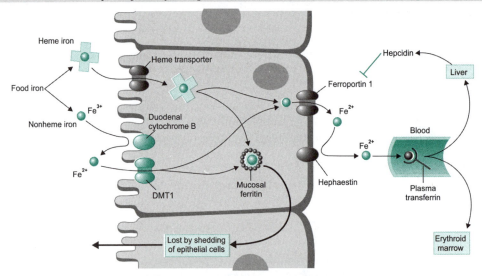

Fig. 16: Regulation of iron absorption

Iron Metabolism

• **Normal daily Western diet** contains about **10-20 mg of iron**[Q], most in the form of **heme contained in animal products**.
 • **20% of heme iron** (in contrast to **1-2% of nonheme iron**) is absorbable[Q].
     • **Total body iron content: 2.5 gm in women & 6 gm in men**[Q]
     • About **80% of functional iron** is found in **hemoglobin; myoglobin & iron-containing enzymes** such as **catalase** and the **cytochromes** contain the rest[Q].

Contd...

Contd...

Iron Metabolism
• **Storage pool** represented by **hemosiderin & ferritin** contains about **15-20% of total body iron**[Q].   • **Major sites of iron storage**: Liver & mononuclear phagocytes[Q].

Iron Transportation & absorption:
 • **Iron is transported** in plasma **by transferrin**[Q], which is synthesized in the liver.
 • **Major function of plasma transferrin** is **to deliver iron to cells**, including **erythroid precursors**[Q], which require iron to synthesize hemoglobin.
 • **Storage iron is sequestered by** binding of iron in the storage pool to either **ferritin or hemosiderin**.
 • **Ferritin** is found at **highest levels in liver, spleen, bone marrow & skeletal muscles**[Q].
 • In the **liver, most ferritin is stored within parenchymal cells**; in **spleen & bone marrow**, it is found mainly **in macrophages**[Q].
      • **Hepatocyte iron** is **derived from plasma transferrin**, whereas **storage iron in macrophages** is derived from **breakdown of red cells**[Q].
      • **Iron in hemosiderin** is **chemically reactive** and **turns blue-black when exposed to potassium ferrocyanide**, which is the basis for the **Prussian blue stain**[Q].
 • **Luminal nonheme iron** is mostly in the Fe^{3+} (ferric) state and **must first be reduced to Fe^{2+} (ferrous) iron by ferrireductases**, such as b-cytochromes & STEAP3[Q].
 • Fe^{2+} iron is then **transported across the apical membrane by divalent metal transporter 1 (DMT1)**[Q].
 • **Iron that enters duodenal cells** can follow one of two pathways: **transport to the blood or storage as mucosal iron**.
      • **Newly absorbed Fe^{3+} iron binds rapidly to transferrin**[Q].
      • Both **DMT1 & ferroportin** are widely distributed in the body and are **involved in iron transport** in other tissues as well[Q].

Regulation of iron absorption:
 • **Iron absorption is regulated by hepcidin,** a small circulating peptide that is **synthesized & released from liver** in response to **increases in intrahepatic iron levels**[Q].
 • **Hepcidin inhibits iron transfer from enterocyte to plasma** by binding to ferroportin and causing it to be endocytosed and degraded[Q].
      • As a result, as **hepcidin levels rise, iron becomes trapped within duodenal cells** in the form of **mucosal ferritin** and is **lost as these cells are sloughed**. Thus, when the body is replete with iron, **high hepcidin levels inhibit its absorption into the blood**[Q].
      • Conversely, **with low body stores of iron, hepcidin synthesis falls** and this in turn **facilitates iron absorption**[Q].
 • **By inhibiting ferroportin, hepcidin not only reduces iron uptake from enterocytes** but also **suppresses iron release from macrophages**, which are an important source of the iron that is used by erythroid precursors to make hemoglobin[Q].

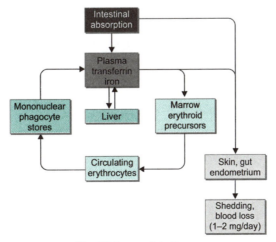

Fig. 17: Iron metabolism

AIIMS ESSENCE

44. Ans. d. Response to steroids *(Ref: Wintrobes Clinical Hematology 12/e p1892; Robbins 9/e p590-593, 8/e p627, 628)*

Three of the most important predictive factors are the age of the patient at the time of diagnosis, the initial leukocyte count, and the speed of response to treatment (i.e. how rapidly the blast cells can be cleared from the marrow or peripheral blood). Among these, response to the treatment with steroids is the most consistent prognostic marker.

*"Prognosis. Pediatric ALL is one of the great success stories of oncology. With aggressive chemotherapy **about 95% of children with ALL obtain a complete remission, and 75% to 85% are cured**. Despite these achievements, however, **ALL remains the leading cause of cancer deaths in children**, and only 35% to 40% of adults are cured. **Several factors are associated with a worse prognosis: (1) age younger than 2 years, largely because of the strong association of infantile ALL with translocations involving the MLL gene; (2) presentation in adolescence or adulthood; and (3) peripheral blood blast counts greater than 100,000**, which probably reflects a high tumor burden. Favorable prognostic markers include (1) age between 2 and 10 years, (2) a low white cell count, (3) hyperdiploidy, (4) trisomy of chromosomes 4, 7, and 10, and (5) the presence of a t(12;21). Notably, the molecular detection of residual disease after therapy is predictive of a worse outcome in both B- and T-ALL and is being used to guide new clinical trials."- Robbins 9/e p592*

Acute Lymphoblastic Leukemia (ALL)

- **ALL is neoplasms of immature B (pre-B) or T (pre-T) cells,** which are referred to as **lymphoblasts**
- **B-ALLs (85%)** typically manifest as **childhood acute "Leukemias"[Q]**
- **T-ALLs** tend to present in **adolescent males as thymic "lymphomas"[Q]**

Epidemiology:

- **ALL: MC cancer of children[Q]; Peak Incidence: 3rd year[Q]; Whites**> blacks; **Boys**>girls
- **Highest incidence in Hispanics**

  - **Mature B-cell ALL is an uncommon type ALL[Q]** (1-2% of ALL cases) **in children.**

Pathology:

- **T-ALLs** have **gain of function mutations in NOTCH-1[Q]**
- **B-ALLs** have **loss of function mutations PAX5[Q], E2A[Q] & EBF[Q], or t(12;21)[Q]** involving genes ETV6 & RUNX1, 2 genes that are needed in very early hematopoietic precursor.

  - **Mature B-cell ALL is associated with t(8;14) & over expression of the c-myc oncogene**
  - **T-ALL are aggressive lymphomas[Q]**
  - In **T-ALL, cells are positive for markers of blasts like-Tdt,[Q] CD34 & T cell markers CD1, CD2, CD5, CD7[Q]**

Classification of ALL			
Immunologic Subtype	**% of Cases**	**FAB Subtype**	**Cytogenetic Abnormalities**
Pre-B ALL	75	L1, L2[Q]	t(9;22), t(4;11), t(1;19)
T-cell ALL	20	L1, L2[Q]	14q11 or 7q34
B-cell ALL	5	L3[Q]	t(8;14), t(8;22), t(2;8)

Clinical Features:

- **Abrupt stormy onset;** Symptoms related to **depression of marrow function[Q]**
- **Fatigue due to anemia; Fever due to neutropenia & Bleeding due to thrombocytopenia[Q]**

  - **Marrow expansion & infiltration of sub-periosteum: Sternal tenderness[Q]**
  - Generalized **lymphadenopathy, hepatosplenomegaly & testicular enlargement** due to **neoplastic infiltration[Q]**

- **CNS features: headache, vomiting & nerve palsies** due to meningeal spread

  - **T-ALL commonly presents with Mediastinal mass (Superior mediastinal syndrome)[Q]**

Diagnosis:

- **Hypercellular bone marrow with >20% lymphoblasts[Q]**
- Compared with myeloblasts, **lymphoblasts have more condensed chromatin, less conspicuous nucleoli & scanty agranular cytoplasm[Q]**
- **Cytochemistry: Myeloperoxidase (MPO)–ve, Sudan Black B (SBB)–ve[Q]**

Contd...

Contd...

Acute Lymphoblastic Leukemia (ALL)			
FAB (French American British) Classification			
ALL-subtype	L1	L2	L3 (Mature B-cells)
Morphology	• Small homogenous blasts[Q] • Little cytoplasm[Q] • Regular nucleus • Small indistinct nucleoli	• Large heterogeneous blasts • One or more nucleoli	• Large homogenous blasts • Abundant basophilic cytoplasm • Prominent cytoplasmic vacuolation • Resemble Burkitt lymphoma[Q]
Age group	Children	Adults	Adults
Prognosis	Good[Q]	Intermediate[Q]	Poor[Q]
Cytochemistry	PAS+	PAS+	PAS-, SBB+[Q]

• **Both B-cell ALL & Burkitt lymphoma** are characterized by **FAB L3[Q] morphology**

Prognostic Factors in ALL		
Determinants	Favorable	Unfavorable
WBC counts	$<10 \times 10^9$/L (Low)[Q]	$>200 \times 10^9$/L (High)[Q]
Age	3-7 years[Q]	<1 year, >10 years
Gender	Female[Q]	Male[Q]
Ethnicity	White[Q]	Black[Q]
Node, liver, spleen enlargement	Absent	Massive[Q]
Testicular enlargement	Absent	Present[Q]
Central nervous system	Absent	Overt (blasts + pleocytosis)
FAB morphologic features L1	L1[Q]	L2[Q]
Ploidy	Hyperdiploidy[Q]	Hypodiploidy <45
Cytogenetic markers	Trisomies 4, 10 and/or 17 t(12;21) (TEL-AML1)	t(9;22) (BCR-ABL) t(4;11) (MLL-AF4)
Time to remission	<14 days[Q]	> 28 days[Q]
DNA index	> 0.16[Q]	< 0.16[Q]
Immunophenotype	Early Pre-B cell	T cell

45. **Ans. b. Methylation**   *(Ref: Robbins 9/e p180, 8/e p172)*

In genomic imprinting, DNA is modified by methylation.

"Gene expression frequently correlates with the level of methylation of DNA, usually of cytosines specifically in CG dinucleotide-rich promoter regions known as CpG islands. As discussed earlier in the section on genomic imprinting, increased methylation of these loci is associated with decreased gene expression and is accompanied by concomitant specific patterns of histone methylation and acetylation. An ever increasing number of disease states warrant analysis of promoter methylation—for example, in the diagnosis of fragile X syndrome, in which hypermethylation results in FMR1 silencing. Methylation analysis is also essential in the diagnosis of Prader-Willi and Angelman syndromes."- Robbins 9/e p180

Genomic Imprinting
• Genomic imprinting is an **epigenetic process** resulting in **differential inactivation of either maternal or paternal alleles of certain genes**[Q] • **Maternal imprinting** refers to **transcriptional silencing of maternal allele**[Q] • **Paternal imprinting** refers to **transcriptional silencing of paternal allele**[Q] • **Imprinting** occurs in the **ovum or sperm before fertilization** and then is **stably transmitted to all somatic cells through mitosis**[Q]

Contd...

Contd...

Genomic Imprinting
Mechanism: <ul><li>DNA methylation at CG nucleotide[Q]</li><li>Histone H4 deacetylation[Q]</li><li>Methylation[Q]</li></ul> **Examples:** <ul><li>Prader-Willi syndrome & Angelman syndrome</li></ul>

Mechanism in Prader-Willi syndrome & Angelman syndrome		
Deletions (70% cases)	**Uniparental Disomy (20-25% cases)**	**Defective Imprinting (1-4%)**
<ul><li>(P for P, M for M)</li><li>Deletion of **P**aternal genes after maternal gene silencing: **P**rader-Willi syndrome[Q]</li><li>Deletion of **M**aternal genes after paternal gene silencing: Angel**M**an syndrome[Q]</li></ul>	<ul><li>Inheritance of both chromosomes of a pair from one parent</li><li>Uniparental disomy of **paternal chromosome 15**: Angelman syndrome[Q]</li><li>Uniparental disomy of **Maternal chromosome 15**: Prader-Willi syndrome[Q]</li></ul>	<ul><li>Paternal chromosomes carries the **maternal imprint** in **Prader-Willi syndrome**[Q]</li><li>Maternal chromosomes carries the **paternal imprint** in **Angelman syndrome**[Q]</li></ul>

Prader-Willi syndrome	Angelman syndrome
Characterized by: <ul><li>Mental retardation, short stature, hypotonia[Q]</li><li>Profound hyperphagia, obesity, small hands & feet[Q]</li><li>Hypogonadism[Q]</li></ul>	**Characterized by:** <ul><li>Mental retardation, ataxic gait, seizure[Q]</li><li>Inappropriate laughter (happy puppets)[Q]</li></ul>

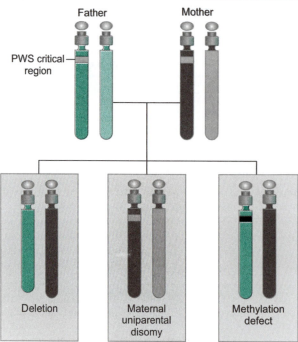

Fig. 18: Mechanism in Prader-Willi syndrome

46. **Ans. a. Gives an immediate definitive diagnosis of tumor**   *(Ref: http://www.ncbi.nlm.nih.gov/pmc/articles/PMC3347896)*
    In frozen section presumptive diagnosis can be rendered in many cases but fixed tissue processing is required for more accurate diagnosis.

AIIMS November 2015

"The intraoperative consultation is the name given to the *whole intervention by the pathologist,* which includes not only *frozen section* but also *gross evaluation of the specimen, examination of cytology preparations taken on the specimen* (e.g. touch imprints), and *aliquoting of the specimen for special studies* (e.g. molecular pathology techniques, flow cytometry). The report given by the pathologist is usually *limited to a 'benign' or 'malignant' diagnosis,* and communicated to the surgeon operating via intercom. When operating on a previously confirmed malignancy, the *main purpose of the pathologist is to inform the surgeon if the surgical margin is clear of residual cancer, or if residual cancer is present at the surgical margin."*

Intraoperative Histopathological Analysis

- The **frozen section procedure/cryosection** is **rapid microscopic analysis of a specimen**[Q].
- It is **used most often in oncological surgery**.
- The **quality of the slides produced by frozen section is lower than formalin-fixed paraffin-embedded tissue processing**[Q].
  - While presumptive diagnosis can be rendered in many cases, **fixed tissue processing is required for more accurate diagnosis**[Q].

- The **intraoperative consultation** is the name given to the **whole intervention by the pathologist**, which includes not only **frozen section** but also **gross evaluation of the specimen, examination of cytology preparations taken on the specimen** (e.g. touch imprints), and **aliquoting of the specimen for special studies** (e.g. molecular pathology techniques, flow cytometry). The report given by the pathologist is usually **limited to a 'benign' or 'malignant' diagnosis**, and communicated to the surgeon operating via intercom. When operating on a previously confirmed malignancy, the **main purpose of the pathologist is to inform the surgeon if the surgical margin is clear of residual cancer, or if residual cancer is present at the surgical margin.**

Intraoperative Histopathological Analysis: Examples

- In the performance of **Moh's micrographic surgery**—a simple method for real-time **margin control of a surgical specimen.**
- If a tumor appears to have **metastasized**, a sample of the **suspected metastasis is sent for cryosection to confirm its identity.**
- If a **tumor has been resected** but it is unclear whether the **surgical margin** is **free of tumor.**
- In a **sentinel node procedure**, a sentinel node containing tumor tissue prompts a further lymph node dissection, while a benign node will avoid such a procedure.

  - If **surgery is explorative, rapid examination of a lesion** might help identify the possible cause of a patient's symptoms. It is important to note, however, that the **pathologist is very limited by the poor technical quality of the frozen sections**. A **final diagnosis is rarely offered intra-operatively**[Q].

PHARMACOLOGY

47. Ans. b. B *(Ref: Goodman Gilman 12/e p1478; Katzung 13/e p770, 12/e p791; KDT 7/e p716, 6/e p694)*

Beta-lactam is an amide bond found in structure of Penicillin G, as represented by 'B' above.

Beta-lactamases

- **Beta-lactamases** are **enzymes produced by some bacteria** that **provide resistance to** *β-lactam antibiotics* like **penicillins, cephamycins, and carbapenems** by breaking the antibiotic's structure.
- These antibiotics all have a **common element in their molecular structure: a four-atom ring known as a** *β-lactam*. Through hydrolysis, the **lactamase enzyme breaks the β-lactam ring open, deactivating the molecule's antibacterial properties.**
- The term 'penam' is used to describe the **common core skeleton of a member of the penicillins.** This core has the molecular formula **R-C$_9$H$_{11}$N$_2$O$_4$S**, where R is the variable side chain that differentiates the penicillins from one another.

  - The **key structural feature of the penicillins** is the **four-membered β-lactam ring**; this structural moiety is **essential for penicillin's antibacterial activity**[Q].

- The **β-lactam ring is itself fused to a five-membered thiazolidine ring.** The fusion of these two rings causes the β-lactam ring to be more reactive than monocyclic β-lactams because the **two fused rings distort the β-lactam amide bond** and therefore **remove the resonance stabilization normally found in these chemical bonds.**

Gram-positive bacteria	Gram-negative bacteria
<ul><li>**Gram-positive bacteria produce & secrete a large amount of beta-lactamase**[Q].</li><li>Most of these enzymes are **penicillinases**[Q].</li><li>**Information for staphylococcal penicillinase is encoded in a plasmid** & this may be **transferred by bacteriophage** to other bacteria[Q].</li></ul>	<ul><li>In **gram-negative bacteria, beta-lactamase** are **found in relatively small amounts** but are **located in the periplasmic space** between inner & outer cell membranes[Q].</li><li>**Beta-lactamases** are **strategically located for maximal protection of the microbe**, encoded either in **chromosomes or in plasmids**[Q].</li><li>**Plasmids** can be **transferred between bacteria by conjugation**[Q].</li></ul>

Molecular classification of Beta Lactamases

- Molecular classification of beta-lactamases is **based on the amino acid sequence**
- Class **A, C & D enzymes** which, **utilize serine for β-lactam hydrolysis** & class B metalloenzymes require **divalent zinc ions for substrate hydrolysis**[Q]

Group 1 (class C)	Group 2 (classes A & D)	Group 3
• Cephalosporinases[Q]	• Broad-spectrum, inhibitor-resistant & extended-spectrum β-lactamases & serine carbapenemases[Q]	• Metallo-β-lactamases[Q]

Beta-Lactamases are grouped into four classes			
Class A	**Class B**	**Class C**	**Class D**
• **Include** extended-spectrum beta-lactamases **(ESBLs) & degrade penicillins**, and some **cephalosporins & carbapenems**[Q]	• **Zn^{2+}-dependent enzymes that destroy all beta-lactams except aztreonam**[Q]	• Beta-lactamases, which are **active against cephalosporins**[Q]	• **Includes Cloxacillin degrading enzymes**[Q]

- **Only Class A & D are inhibited by β-lactamase inhibitors like Clavulanic acid & sulbactam**[Q].

Fig. 19: Structure of penicillins and products of enzymatic hydrolysis

48. **Ans. a. Epinephrine** *(Ref: Goodman Gilman 12/e p188, 285; Katzung 13/e p89, 12/e p90; KDT 7/e p132, 6/e p120)*

This graph is showing decreased contractility after infusion of substance X. Intestinal muscles show increase in contractility on action of acetylcholine on M3 receptors while epinephrine inhibits contraction. Hence, the substance X is likely to be a sympathomimetic drug, i.e. Epinephrine.

> "The effects of epinephrine on the smooth muscles of different organs and systems depend on the type of adrenergic receptor in the muscle. The effects on vascular smooth muscle noted above are of major physiological importance, whereas those on smooth muscle of the GI tract are relatively minor. GI smooth muscle is, in general, relaxed by epinephrine. This effect is due to activation of both α and β receptors. Intestinal tone and the frequency and amplitude of spontaneous contractions are reduced. The stomach usually is relaxed and the pyloric and ileocecal sphincters are contracted, but these effects depend on the pre-existing tone of the muscle. If tone already is high, epinephrine causes relaxation; if low, contraction."–Goodman Gilman 12/e p285

> "Application of ACh to isolated intestinal muscle causes a decrease in the resting potential (i.e., the membrane potential becomes less negative) and an increase in the frequency of spike production, accompanied by a rise in tension. A primary action of ACh in initiating these effects through muscarinic receptors is probably partial depolarization of the cell membrane brought about by an increase in Na^+ and, in some instances, Ca^{2+} conductance. ACh also can produce contraction of some smooth muscles when the membrane has been depolarized completely by high concentrations of K^+, provided that Ca^{2+} is present. Hence, ACh stimulates ion fluxes across membranes and/or mobilizes intracellular Ca^{2+} to cause contraction."
> – Goodman Gilman 12/e p188

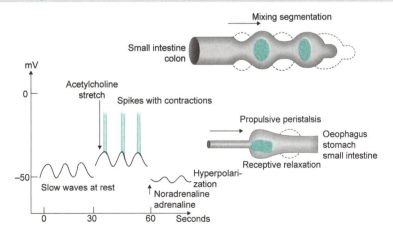

AIIMS ESSENCE

Effects of Epinephrine on the Smooth Muscles
• **Effects of epinephrine on smooth muscles** of different organs and systems **depend on type of adrenergic receptor in muscle.**
• **GI smooth muscle is relaxed by epinephrine due to activation of both alpha & beta receptors**[Q].
• **Intestinal tone, frequency & amplitude of spontaneous contractions are reduced**[Q].
• **Stomach is relaxed & pyloric and ileocecal sphincters are contracted**, but these effects depend on the pre-existing tone of the muscle. **If tone already is high, epinephrine causes relaxation; if low, contraction**[Q].
• During the **last month of pregnancy & at parturition, epinephrine inhibits uterine tone & contractions.**
• **Epinephrine relaxes detrusor muscle of bladder** as a **result of activation of beta-receptors** & contracts trigone & sphincter muscles owing to its alpha-agonist activity. This can result in **hesitancy in urination** and may **contribute to retention of urine in bladder**[Q].
• **Activation of smooth muscle contraction in prostate promotes urinary retention**[Q].

49. **Ans. c. Schedule H**   *(Ref: Drugs and Cosmetics Rules, 1945)*

Schedule H is a class of prescription drugs in India appearing as an appendix to the Drugs and Cosmetics Rules, 1945 introduced in 1945. These are drugs, which cannot be purchased over the counter without the prescription of a qualified doctor.

The Drugs and Cosmetics Rules, 1945
• The **Drugs and Cosmetics Rules, 1945** contains **provisions for classification of drugs under given schedules** and there are **guidelines for the storage, sale, display and prescription of each schedule.**
• The **Rule 67** details the **conditions of licenses**. The **Rule 97** contains the **labeling regulations.**

Important Schedules of Drugs and Cosmetics Rules, 1945	
Schedule	**Deals with**
Schedule C & C1	• **Biological & special products**. Examples: Serums, Adrenaline, etc.
Schedule E	• Various poisons
Schedule F & F1	• **Bacterial vaccines**[Q]
Schedule G	• Drugs to be labeled with the word **"Caution"-it is dangerous to take this prescription except under medical supervision**[Q]
Schedule H	• Drugs that must be sold by retail only when a prescription by registered medical practitioner is produced • **'Schedule H drug Warning: To be sold by retail on the prescription of a Registered Medical Practitioner only.'**[Q]
Schedule J	• List of various **diseases & conditions that cannot be treated under any drug currently in market.** • **No drug may legally claim to treat these diseases**[Q]
Schedule M	• **Good manufacturing practices**
Schedule P	• **Expiry period of drug formulation**
Schedule T	• Regulations & requirements for manufacture of **Ayurvedic, Siddha & Unani products**
Schedule W	• Drugs that shall be **marketed under generic names only**
Schedule X	• **Psychotropic drugs requiring special license for manufacture & sale**
Schedule Y	• Requirement & guidelines for **clinical trials, import & manufacture of new drugs**

50. **Ans. a. Cyclosporine**   *(Ref: Goodman Gilman 12/e p1008; Katzung 13/e p626-627, 12/e p986; KDT 7/e p880, 6/e p837-839)*

Cyclosporine is a calcineurin inhibitor, which targets intracellular signaling pathways induced as a consequence of T cell–receptor activation.

*"**Perhaps** the **most effective immunosuppressive drugs** in routine use are the **calcineurin inhibitors, cyclosporine** and **tacrolimus**, which **target intracellular signaling pathways induced as a consequence of T cell-receptor activation**. Although they are structurally unrelated and **bind to distinct (albeit related) molecular targets**, they **inhibit normal T-cell signal transduction** essentially by the same mechanism. Cyclosporine and tacrolimus do not act per se as immunosuppressive agents. Instead, these drugs **bind to an immunophilin (cyclophilin for cyclosporine** or **FKBP-12 for tacrolimus)**, resulting in **subsequent interaction with calcineurin to block its phosphatase activity." – Goodman Gilman 12/e p1008*

Cyclosporine
• Cyclosporine is produced by fungus ***Beauveria nivea***[Q].   • **Cyclosporine suppresses some humoral immunity** but is **more effective against T cell dependent immune mechanisms** such as those **underlying transplant rejection** and **some forms of autoimmunity**[Q].
Mechanism of Action:

• It preferentially **inhibits antigen-triggered signal transduction in T lymphocytes**, blunting expression of many lymphokines, including IL-2 & expression of anti-apoptotic proteins.
     • Cyclosporine **forms a complex with cyclophilin**, a cytoplasmic-receptor protein present in target cells. **This complex binds to calcineurin, inhibiting Ca^{2+}-stimulated dephosphorylation of the cytosolic component of NFAT**[Q].
     • **Calcineurin phosphatase activity is inhibited after physical interaction with the cyclosporine/cyclophilin complex**[Q].
 • **Cyclosporine increases expression of TGF-β**, a **potent inhibitor of IL-2–stimulated T-cell proliferation** and **generation of cytotoxic T lymphocytes (CTLs)**[Q].

Therapeutic Uses:
• **Clinical indications for cyclosporine** are **kidney, liver, heart & other organ transplantation; rheumatoid arthritis; and psoriasis**[Q].   • Approved by the FDA to **prevent & treat graft-versus-host disease** in bone-marrow transplantation[Q]
Side-effects:
• **Renal dysfunction, hypertension; tremor, hirsutism, hyperlipidemia & gum hyperplasia**[Q]   • **Hypertension** occurs in ~50% of renal **transplant** and **almost all cardiac transplant patients**[Q].   • **Hyperuricemia may lead to worsening of gout, increased P-glycoprotein activity**, and **hypercholesterolemia**[Q].   • **Nephrotoxicity** occurs in the **majority of patients** and is the major reason for cessation or modification of therapy[Q].   • It is **nephrotoxic, neurotoxic, causes hypertension** (due to **renal vasoconstriction & increased sodium reabsorption**), and **increases the risk of squamous cell carcinoma & infections**[Q].

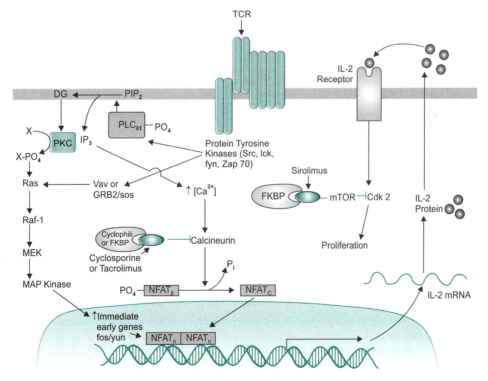

Fig. 20: Mechanism of action of cyclosporine

51. Ans. d. Epsilon aminocaproic acid (Ref: Goodman Gilman 12/e p867; Katzung 13/e p599-600, 12/e p616; KDT 7/e p628, 6/e p608)

Epsilon-aminocaproic acid is a synthetic inhibitor of the plasmin-plasminogen system. It is the only potent antifibrinolytic agent, which is commercially available.

"Aminocaproic acid is a lysine analog that competes for lysine binding sites on plasminogen and plasmin, blocking the interaction of plasmin with fibrin. Aminocaproic acid is thereby a potent inhibitor of fibrinolysis and can reverse states that are associated with excessive fibrinolysis."– *Goodman Gilman 12/e p867*

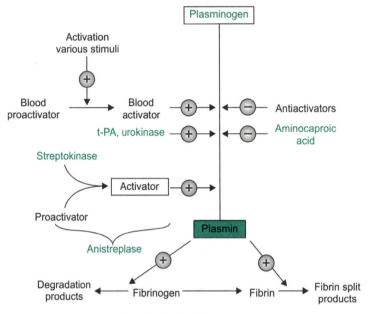

Fig. 21: Fibrinolytic system

Aminocaproic Acid
• EACA is a **synthetic inhibitor of the plasmin-plasminogen system**[Q].   • It is the **only potent antifibrinolytic agent, which is commercially available**[Q].
Mechanism of Action: • **Aminocaproic acid** is a **lysine analog that competes for lysine binding sites on plasminogen & plasmin, blocking the interaction of plasmin with fibrin**[Q].   • **Aminocaproic acid** is a **potent inhibitor of fibrinolysis & can reverse states that are associated with excessive fibrinolysis**[Q].
Therapeutic Uses: • Used to **reduce bleeding after prostatic surgery** or **after tooth extractions in hemophiliacs**[Q].   • Used to **treat the overdose and/ or toxic effects of the thrombolytics** like **tissue plasminogen activator & streptokinase**[Q].
Side-effects: • **Hypotension, cardiac arrhythmias, rhabdomyolysis & generation of thrombi**[Q].

52. Ans. b. Increased renal blood flow (Ref: Goodman Gilman 12/e p355; KDT 7/e p134, 6/e p507)

Dopamine at low concentrations (2 to 5 mcg/kg per minute) primarily acts on vascular D_1 receptors, especially in the renal, mesenteric, and coronary beds. By activating adenylyl cyclase and raising intracellular concentrations of cyclic AMP, D_1 receptor stimulation leads to vasodilation. Infusion of low doses of dopamine causes an increase in glomerular filtration rate, renal blood flow, and Na^+, K^+-ATPase pump.

See Q. No. 63 AIIMS May 2016

53. **Ans. c. Thromboxane A2** *(Ref: Goodman Gilman 12/e p868; Katzung 13/e p621, 12/e p638; KDT 7/e p195, 6/e p186, 609)*

Aspirin causes several different effects in the body, mainly the reduction of inflammation, analgesia, the prevention of clotting, and the reduction of fever. Much of this is believed to be due to decreased production of prostaglandins and TXA2.

"*In platelets, the major cyclooxygenase product is TxA$_2$ (thromboxane A$_2$), a labile inducer of platelet aggregation and a potent vasoconstrictor. Aspirin blocks production of TxA$_2$ by acetylating a serine residue near the active site of platelet cyclooxygenase-1 (COX-1), the enzyme that produces the cyclic endoperoxide precursor of TxA$_2$. Because platelets do not synthesize new proteins, the action of aspirin on platelet COX-1 is permanent, lasting for the life of the platelet (7-10 days). Thus, repeated doses of aspirin produce a cumulative effect on platelet function.*" – *Goodman Gilman 12/e p868*

Drugs affecting Thromboxane A$_2$
• COX inhibitors like **aspirin** decreases the synthesis of TXA$_2$[Q]
• **Daltroban & Sultroban** are TXA$_2$ receptor antagonists[Q]
• **Dazoxiben** inhibits the enzyme thromboxane synthetase[Q]

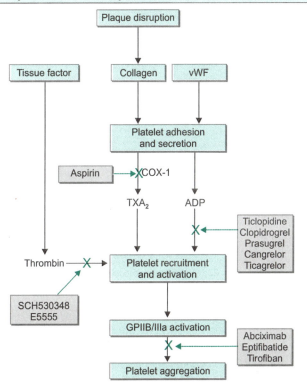

Fig. 22: Site of Action of antiplatelet drugs

Aspirin
• **Aspirin** is now **rarely used as an anti-inflammatory medication** and **used for its anti-platelet effects**[Q] (doses of 81–325 mg once daily).
Mechanisms of Action:
• In **platelets**, the **major cyclooxygenase product** is **TxA$_2$**, a labile inducer of platelet aggregation & a potent vasoconstrictor[Q].
• Aspirin blocks production of TxA$_2$ by acetylating a serine residue near active site of platelet cyclooxygenase-1 (COX-1), enzyme that produces cyclic endoperoxide precursor of TxA$_2$[Q].
• Because **platelets do not synthesize new proteins**, the action of aspirin on platelet COX-1 is **permanent, lasting for the life of the platelet (7-10 days)**[Q].

Contd...

Contd...

Aspirin
Clinical Uses
• Aspirin decreases the incidence of **transient ischemic attacks, unstable angina, coronary artery thrombosis with myocardial infarction** & thrombosis after coronary artery bypass grafting[Q].
• Epidemiologic studies suggest that **long-term use of aspirin at low dosage is associated with a lower incidence of colon cancer**, possibly related to **its COX-inhibiting effects**[Q].
Adverse Effects
• Gastric upset (intolerance) and **gastric & duodenal ulcers**[Q].
• **Hepatotoxicity, asthma, rashes, GI bleeding & renal toxicity rarely** if ever occur at antithrombotic doses.
• **Antiplatelet action of aspirin contraindicates its use by patients with hemophilia**[Q].

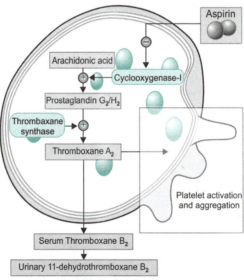

Fig. 23: Mechanism of action of aspirin

54. **Ans. a. Drug safety** (Ref: Goodman Gilman 12/e p79; Katzung 13/e p12, 12/e p75; KDT 7/e p63-64, 6/e p77)

Safety, pharmacodynamics and dosing are all tested in Phase 1 clinical trial, but drug safety is the most important primary end point.

> "In phase 1, the effects of the drug as a function of dosage are established in a small number (20–100) of healthy volunteers. Although a goal is to find the maximum tolerated dose, the study is designed to prevent severe toxicity. If the drug is expected to have significant toxicity, as may be the case in cancer and AIDS therapy, **volunteer patients with the disease are used in phase 1 rather than normal volunteers**. Phase 1 trials are done to determine the probable limits of the safe clinical dosage range. These trials may be nonblind or "open"; that is, both the investigators and the subjects know what is being given. Alternatively, they may be "blinded" and placebo controlled. The choice of design depends on the drug, disease, goals of investigators, and ethical considerations. **Many predictable toxicities are detected in this phase. Pharmacokinetic measurements of absorption, half-life, and metabolism are often done**. Phase 1 studies are usually performed in research centers by specially trained clinical pharmacologists."– Katzung 12/e p75

See Q. No. 67 AIIMS May 2016

55. **Ans. b. Epinephrine** (Ref: Goodman Gilman 12/e p326; Katzung 13/e p162, 12/e p160; KDT 7th/e p153, 6th/e p123)
Epinephrine acts on dilator pupillae, causing the dilatation of pupil analogous to that of pilocarpine on sphincter pupillae.

> "There are two types of muscle that control the size of the iris: the iris sphincter, composed of circularly arranged muscle fibers, and the **iris dilator, composed of radially arranged muscle fibers**. The sphincter is innervated by the parasympathetic nervous system; the **dilator by the sympathetic nervous system (alpha-1)**. Sympathetic stimulation of the adrenergic receptors causes the contraction of the radial muscle and subsequent dilation of the pupil. Conversely, parasympathetic stimulation causes contraction of the circular muscle and constriction of the pupil.

Muscles Controlling Iris	
Iris Sphincter	**Iris Dilator**
• Made up of circular arranged muscle fibers • Innervated by parasympathetic nervous system (M1 receptors) • Parasympathetic stimulation of the muscle →Contraction of the circular muscle of iris sphincter→Constriction of pupil • Pilocarpine is a parasympathomimetic drug → Contraction of the circular muscle of iris sphincter→Miosis	• Made up of radially arranged muscle fibers • Innervated by sympathetic nervous system (alpha-1 receptor) • Stimulation of adrenergic receptors→ Contraction of the radial muscle→ dilatation of pupil • Epinephrine is a sympathetic drug (produces analogous action to pilocarpine, on dilator pupillae) → Contraction of dilator pupillae→ Mydriasis

Eyes	Parasympathetic Nervous System	Sympathetic Nervous System	
		Receptor Type	**Response**
Radial muscle of iris	—	$\alpha_1{}^Q$	Contraction (mydriasis)^Q
Sphincter muscle of iris	Contraction (miosis)^Q	—	—
Ciliary muscle	Contraction for near vision^Q	—	—

Miotics	Mydriatics (with or without cycloplegia)
Cholinergics (parasympathomimetic): Pilocarpine, Physostigmine, Methacholine^Q Sympatholytics: Timolol, Propranolol^Q	Sympathomimetics: Phenylephrine, adrenaline, cocaine ^{Q} Anticholinergics (parasympatholytic): Tropicamide, cyclopentolate, atropine, hyoscyamine & scopolamine^Q

See Q. No. 57 AIIMS May 2016

56. Ans. b. Linezolid *(Ref: Goodman Gilman 13/e p796, 12/e p1537; Katzung 12/e p817; KDT 7/e p758, 817, 6/e p669)*

Linezolid inhibits protein synthesis by binding to the P site of the 50S ribosomal subunit and preventing formation of the larger ribosomal-fMet-tRNA complex that initiates protein synthesis.

> *"Linezolid inhibits protein synthesis by binding to the P site of the 50S ribosomal subunit and preventing formation of the larger ribosomal-fMet-tRNA complex that initiates protein synthesis. Because of its unique mechanism of action, linezolid is active against strains that are resistant to multiple other agents, including penicillin-resistant strains of S. pneumoniae; methicillin-resistant, vancomycin-intermediate, and vancomycin-resist- ant strains of staphylococci; and vancomycin-resistant strains of enterococci. Resistance in enterococci and staphylococci is due to point mutations of the 23S rRNA. Because multiple copies of 23S rRNA genes are present in bacteria, resistance generally requires mutations in two or more copies."– Goodman Gilman 12/e p1537*

Drug	Mechanism of Action
Nitrofurantoin	• Works by **damaging bacterial DNA^Q**
Metronidazole	• Forms toxic free radical metabolites in the bacterial cell that **damage DNA^Q**
Rifampicin	• **Inhibit DNA-dependent RNA polymerase^Q**

Linezolid
• Synthetic antimicrobial agent of the **oxazolidinone class**
• **Well absorbed after oral administration^Q** (oral bioavailability approaching **100%**)
Antimicrobial Activity:
• Linezolid is **active against gram-positive organisms (staphylococci, streptococci, enterococci, gram- positive anaerobic cocci) & gram-positive rods (Corynebacterium** spp. **& Listeria monocytogenes)^Q**
Mechanism of Action:
• **Linezolid inhibits protein synthesis** by **binding to the P site of the 50S ribosomal subunit & preventing formation of larger ribosomal-fMet-tRNA complex** that **initiates protein synthesis^Q.**

Linezolid is FDA approved for treatment of infections caused by	
• **Vancomycin-resistant E. faecium^Q** • **Community-acquired pneumonia** caused by **penicillin-susceptible** strains of **S. pneumoniae^Q**	• **Nosocomial pneumonia** caused by **methicillin-susceptible & resistant** strains of **S. aureus^Q**

Contd...

Contd...

Linezolid
• **Linezolid** is **bacteriostatic for staphylococci & enterococci**; it **should not be first-line therapy for treatment of suspected endocarditis**[Q].
Toxicity:
• **Bone marrow suppression** (especially **thrombocyto penia**[Q]), **peripheral neuropathy**[Q], **serotonin syndrome**[Q].
Mechanism of resistance:
• **Point mutation of ribosomal RNA**[Q]

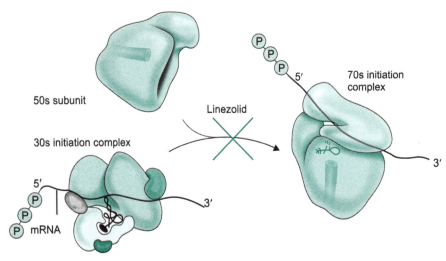

Fig. 24: Mechanism of Action of Linezolid

Classification of antibiotics according to the type of action	
Bacteriostatic	**Bactericidal**
Protein synthesis inhibitors: • Tetracyclines[Q] • Tigecycline[Q] • Chloramphenicol[Q] • Macrolides[Q] • Lincosamide[Q] • Linezolid[Q]	**Protein synthesis inhibitors:** • Aminoglycosides[QQ] • Streptogramins
Drugs affecting DNA: • Nitrofurantoin[Q] • Novobiocin[Q]	**Drugs affecting DNA:** • Quinolones[Q] • Metronidazole[Q]
Drugs affecting metabolism: • Sulfonamides[Q] • Dapsone[Q] • PAS • Trimethoprim[Q] • Ethambutol[Q]	**Cell wall synthesis inhibitors:** • Fosfomycin • Cycloserine[Q] • Bacitracin[Q] • Vancomycin[Q] • Penicillins[Q] • Cephalosporins[Q]

57. **Ans. b. Does not accumulates in tissues** *(Ref: Goodman Gilman 12/e p30; Katzung 13/e p42, 12/e p38; KDT 7/e p17, 18, 6/e p18)*

Low volume of distribution implies that the drug remains confined to the plasma compartment without getting distributed in the body tissues.

"Volume of distribution can vastly exceed any physical volume in the body because it is the volume apparently necessary to contain the amount of drug homogeneously at the concentration found in the blood, plasma, or water. Drugs with very high volumes of distribution, have much higher concentrations in extravascular tissue than in the vascular compartment, i.e., they are not homogeneously distributed. Drugs that are completely retained within the vascular compartment, on the other hand, have a minimum possible volume of distribution equal to the blood component in which they are distributed, for a drug that is restricted to the plasma compartment." –Katzung 13/e p42

"A drug's volume of distribution therefore reflects the extent to which it is present in extravascular tissues and not in the plasma." – Goodman Gilman 12/e p30

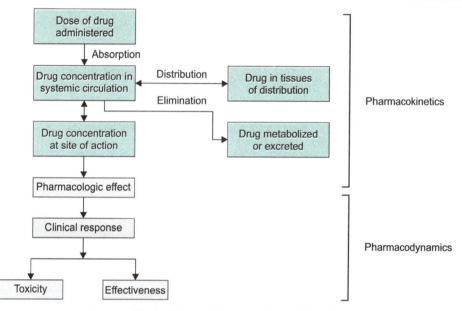

Fig. 25: Effect of tissue binding on volume of distribution

Volume of distribution (V_D)

- Volume of distribution (V_D) is the theoretical **volume** that would be **necessary to contain the total amount of an administered drug at the same concentration**, which is **observed in the blood plasma**.
- The V_D of a drug represents the **degree to which a drug is distributed in body tissue rather than the plasma**.
    - V_D is directly correlated with the amount of drug distributed into tissue; a higher V_D indicates a greater amount of tissue distribution[Q].
    - A V_D greater than the total volume of body water (approximately 42 liters in humans) is possible, and would **indicate that the drug is highly distributed into tissue**[Q].
- In rough terms, **drugs with a high lipid solubility** (non-polar drugs), **low rates of ionization, or low plasma binding capabilities** have **higher volumes of distribution than drugs** which are **more polar, more highly ionized or exhibit high plasma binding in the body's environment**.
    - **Volume of distribution** may be **increased by renal failure** (due to fluid retention) and **liver failure** (due to altered body fluid and plasma protein binding). Conversely it may be **decreased in dehydration**[Q].
- The **initial volume of distribution describes blood concentrations prior to attaining the apparent volume of distribution** and uses the same formula.

$$V_D = \text{Total amount of drug in the body/Drug blood plasma concentration}$$

Drug	V_D	Comments
Warfarin	8 L	• Reflects a **high degree of plasma protein binding**
Theophylline, Ethanol	30 L	• Represents **distribution in total body water**
Chloroquine	15000 L	• Shows **highly lipophilic molecules**, which **sequester into total body fat**.
NXY-059	8 L	• **Highly charged hydrophilic molecule**

58. Ans. b. Ribavirin *(Ref: Harrison 19/e p1214; Goodman Gilman 12/e p1609, 1615; Katzung 13/e p861, 12/e p886, 887; KDT 7/e p798, 804, 6/e p777)*

Oral ribavirin is used for chronic HCV infection, not the bird flu.

"Oral ribavirin in combination with injected pegIFN alfa-2A or -2B has become standard treatment for chronic HCV infection."– Goodman Gilman 12/e p1615

"Ribavirin is a nucleoside analogue with activity against influenza A and B viruses in vitro. Its efficacy against influenza when administered as an aerosol is reportedly variable, and it is ineffective when administered orally. Its efficacy in the treatment of influenza A or B has not been established."– Harrison 19/e p1214

"Ribavirin is used primarily to treat hepatitis C, viral hemorrhagic fevers and RSV."

"The neuraminidase inhibitor peramivir, a cyclopentane analog, has activity against both influenza A and B viruses. Peramivir received temporary emergency use authorization by FDA for intravenous administration in November 2009 due to the H1N1 pandemic."– Katzung 13/e p861, 12/e p887

Specific Antiviral Therapy for influenza
• Neuraminidase inhibitors zanamivir, oseltamivir & peramivir are used for both **influenza A & B**[Q]
• **Amantadine & rimantadine** are used for **influenza A**[Q]

Oseltamivir	• **DOC for bird flu (H5N1)**[Q] • Treatment of **uncomplicated influenza A or B** in healthy adults.
Zanamivir	• **Administered by inhalational route**[Q] • Treatment of **uncomplicated influenza A or B** in healthy adults[Q].
Peramivir	• **Administered IV**[Q] • Activity against both **influenza A & B viruses**[Q]
Laninamivir	• **Long acting neuraminidase inhibitor**[Q] • Effective against **oseltamivir resistant virus**[Q]
Amantadine	• Active against **influenza A** only[Q]
Rimantadine	• **Longer acting than Amantadine**, active against **influenza A** only[Q]

Drug of Choice in Viral Diseases	
Disease	**Drug of Choice**
• **Viral hemorrhagic fever (Lass virus, Rift valley fever, Congo Crimean hemorrhagic fever, Hanta virus)** • **Respiratory syncytial virus** (in high risk patients) • **Measles**	**Ribavirin**[Q]
• **Seasonal influenza** • **Avian influenza (bird flu)**	**Oseltamivir**[Q]
• **Oseltamivir resistant influenza**	**Zanamivir**[Q]
• **Prion disease**	**Flupirtine**[Q]
• **Herpes simplex** • **Varicella**	**Acyclovir**[Q]
• **Acute herpes zoster**	**Valacyclovir**[Q]
• **Cytomegalovirus retinitis**	**Gancicyclovir**[Q]

59. Ans. a. To be given empty stomach with a glass of water *(Ref: Goodman Gilman 12/e p1296; Katzung 13/e p754, 12/e p776; KDT 7/e p344, 6/e p334; Harrison 19/e p2499)*

Esophageal irritation can be minimized by taking the drug with a full glass of water and remaining upright for 30 minutes or by using the intravenous forms of these compounds.

"Oral bisphosphonates, including alendronate, ibandronate, and risedronate, can cause heartburn, esophageal irritation, or esophagitis. Other GI side effects include abdominal pain and diarrhea. Symptoms often abate when patients take the medication after an overnight fast, with tap or filtered water (not mineral water), and remain upright."– Goodman Gilman 12/e p1296

AIIMS November 2015

"A major adverse effect of oral forms of the bisphosphonates (risedronate, alendronate, ibandronate) is esophageal and gastric irritation, which limits the use of this route by patients with upper gastrointestinal disorders. This complication can be circumvented with infusions of pamidronate, zoledronate, and ibandronate."– Katzung 13/e p754

"Esophageal irritation can be minimized by taking the drug with a full glass of water and remaining upright for 30 minutes or by using the intra-venous forms of these compounds."– Katzung 13/e p754

Bisphosphonates
• **Analogs of pyrophosphate** in which the P-O-P bond has been replaced with a nonhydrolyzable P-C-P bond.   • Currently available bisphosphonates include **etidronate**, **pamidronate**, **alendronate**, **risedronate**, **tiludronate**, **ibandronate**, and **zoledronate**.
Mechanism of Action:
• Pyrophosphate analogs; **bind hydroxyapatite in bone, inhibiting osteoclast activity**[Q].
Clinical Uses:
• **Osteoporosis, hypercalcemia associated with malignancy, Paget disease of bone**[Q].
Side-effects:
• **Corrosive esophagitis, osteonecrosis of jaw**[Q].
• **Esophageal irritation can be minimized by taking the drug with a full glass of water and remaining upright for 30 minutes or by using the intravenous forms of these compounds**[Q].

60. Ans. b. Griseofulvin *(Ref: Goodman Gilman 12/e p1585; Katzung 13/e p832, 12/e p855; KDT 7/e p790, 6/e p760)*

Absorption of griseofulvin is increased after a fatty meal.

"The oral administration of a 0.5 g dose of griseofulvin produces peak plasma concentrations of ~1 μg/mL in ~4 hours. Blood levels are quite variable, however. Some studies have shown improved absorption when the drug is taken with a fatty meal."– Goodman Gilman 12/e p1585

"Griseofulvin is a very insoluble fungistatic drug derived from a species of penicillium. Its only use is in the systemic treatment of dermatophytosis. It is administered in a microcrystalline form at a dosage of 1 g/d. Absorption is improved when it is given with fatty foods."– Katzung 13/e p832

Drug Absorption Reduced/Delayed by Food		Drug Absorption increased by food	
• **Ampicillin**[Q]	• **Isoniazid**[Q]	• **Atovaquone**[Q]	• Lovastatin
• **Aspirin**[Q]	• Loratidine	• **Carbamazepine**[Q]	• Methylphenidate
• **Atenolol**[Q]	• Naficillin	• **Chlorthiazide**[Q]	• **Metoprolol**[Q]
• **Azithromycin**[Q]	• **Penicillin G or V**[Q]	• **Cefuroxime**[Q]	• Nelfinavir
• **Captopril**[Q]	• **Phenobarbital**[Q]	• **Clofazimine**[Q]	• Nitrofurantoin
• Cefaclor	• **Phenytoin**[Q]	• **Diazepam**[Q]	• **Propranolol**[Q]
• Cephalexin	• **Rifampin**[Q]	• **Erythromycin estolate**[Q]	• Propoxyphene
• Ciprofloxacin	• **Sucralfate**[Q]	• **Ganciclovir**[Q]	• **Ritonavir**[Q]
• Didanosine	• **Tetracycline**[Q]	• **Hydrochlorothiazide**[Q]	• **Saquinavir**[Q]
• **Indinavir**[Q]	• **Doxycycline**[Q]	• **Itraconazole**[Q]	• **Spironolactone**[Q]
		• **Lithium**[Q]	• **Hydralazine**[Q]

Griseofulvin
• **Griseofulvin inhibits microtubule function** and thereby **disrupts assembly of the mitotic spindle**[Q].   • Prominent morphological manifestation of the action of griseofulvin is the **production of multinucleate cells** as the **drug inhibits fungal mitosis**[Q].   • In addition to its **binding to tubulin, griseofulvin interacts with microtubule-associated protein**[Q].
Pharmacokinetics:
• **Improved absorption when the drug is taken with a fatty meal**[Q].   • Primary metabolite is **6-methylgriseofulvin**.

Contd...

Contd...

Griseofulvin
• **Barbiturates decrease griseofulvin absorption** from the GI tract[Q].
• **Griseofulvin is deposited in keratin precursor cells**; when these cells differentiate, the drug is tightly bound to, and **persists in, keratin, providing prolonged resistance to fungal invasion**[Q].   • For this reason, the **new growth of hair or nails** is the **first to become free of disease**[Q].
Antifungal Activity:
• **Fungistatic for** various species of the dermatophytes **Microsporum, Epidermophyton, & Trichophyton**[Q]. • **No effect on bacteria or on other fungi**[Q].
Therapeutic Uses:
• **Mycotic disease of the skin, hair, and nails** due to *Microsporum, Trichophyton,* or *Epidermophyton* **responds to griseofulvin therapy**[Q]. • **For tinea capitis in children, griseofulvin remains the drug of choice**[Q]. • Griseofulvin also is **highly effective in tinea pedis**[Q].
Side-Effects:
• Headache, peripheral neuritis, lethargy, mental confusion • Hematological effects (leukopenia, neutropenia, punctate basophilia & monocytosis)
• **Griseofulvin induces hepatic CYPs**, thereby **increasing the rate of metabolism of warfarin**. The drug **may reduce the efficacy of low-estrogen OCPs**[Q].

61. Ans. a. Kaposi sarcoma *(Ref: Harrison 19/e p1270, 716; Goodman Gilman 12/e p1755; Katzung 13/e p954-955, 12/e p706; KDT 7/e p284-285, 6/e p285)*

Glucocorticoids are not used in the treatment of Kaposi sarcoma.

*"Glucocorticoids act through their **binding to a specific physiological receptor** that **translocates to the nucleus & induces anti-proliferative and apoptotic responses in sensitive cells**. Because of **lympholytic effects & ability to suppress mitosis in lymphocytes**, glucocorticoids are **used as cytotoxic agents in the treatment of acute leukemia** in children & **malignant lymphoma** in children & adults. Glucocorticoids are a valuable component of **curative regimens for other lymphoid malignancies**, including Hodgkin's disease, non-Hodgkin's lymphoma, multiple myeloma, and chronic lymphocytic leukemia (CLL). Glucocorticoids are **extremely helpful in controlling autoimmune hemolytic anemia** and thrombocytopenia associated with CLL."– Goodman Gilman 12/e p1755*

Glucocorticoids in Cancer Chemotherapy
• **Glucocorticoids** act through their **binding to a specific physiological receptor** that **translocates to the nucleus & induces anti-proliferative and apoptotic responses in sensitive cells**[Q]. • Because of **lympholytic effects & ability to suppress mitosis in lymphocytes**, glucocorticoids are **used as cytotoxic agents in treatment of acute leukemia** in children & **malignant lymphoma** in children & adults[Q].
Antitumor Effect:
• Antitumor effects are mediated by their **binding to the glucocorticoid receptor**, which **activates a program of gene expression that leads to apoptosis**[Q].
Therapeutic Uses in Cancer:
• **Used as cytotoxic agents in treatment of acute leukemia** in children & **malignant lymphoma** in children & adults[Q].
• Component of **curative regimens for Hodgkin's & non-Hodgkin's lymphoma, multiple myeloma & CLL**[Q].   • **Glucocorticoids** are **extremely helpful in controlling autoimmune hemolytic anemia** and **thrombocytopenia associated with CLL**[Q].
• **Dexamethasone** is used in **conjunction with radiotherapy to reduce edema related to tumors in critical areas** such as **superior mediastinum, brain & spinal cord**[Q].

AIIMS November 2015

Management of AIDS associated Kaposi Sarcoma		
• Observation and optimization of **antiretroviral therapy**[Q]		
	Single or limited number of lesions	**Extensive disease**
	• Radiation • Intralesional **vinblastine**[Q] • Cryotherapy	• **Initial therapy:** Interferon α (if CD4+ T cells >150/μL), Liposomal **daunorubicin**[Q] • **Subsequent therapy:** Liposomal **doxorubicin, Paclitaxel**[Q]
• **Combination chemotherapy** with **low-dose doxorubicin, bleomycin, and vinblastine (ABV)**		
• Targeted radiation		

62. **Ans. c. Vigabatrin** *(Ref: Goodman Gilman 12/e p1792; Katzung 13/e p411, 12/e p417; KDT 7/e p421, 6/e p410; Nelson 20/e p2846)*

Vigabatrin causes irreversible diffuse atrophy of the retinal nerve fiber layer. This has the most effect on the outer area (as opposed to the macular, or central area) of the retina, leading to contraction of visual field. These changes may be demonstrable in up to 50% of Vigabatrin users. The retinal toxicity of vigabatrin can be attributed to a taurine depletion.

*"**Vigabatrin: Typical toxicities** include **drowsiness, dizziness, and weight gain**. Less common but more troublesome adverse reactions are **agitation, confusion, and psychosis; preexisting mental illness is a relative contraindication**. The drug was delayed in its worldwide introduction by the appearance in rats and dogs of a **reversible intramyelinic edema**. This phenomenon has now been detected in infants taking the drug; the clinical significance is unknown. In addition, long-term therapy with vigabatrin has been associated with development of peripheral visual field defects in 30–50% of patients. The lesions are located in the retina, increase with drug exposure, and are usually not reversible. Newer techniques such as optical coherence tomography may better define the defect, which has proved difficult to quantify."* – Katzung 13/e p411

*"The anti-seizure drug **vigabatrin causes progressive and permanent bilateral concentric visual field constriction in a high percentage of patients**. The mechanism is not known, but **vigabatrin is more effectively transported into the retina than into the brain, and consequently, elevations of retinal GABA concentrations may contribute to the vision loss."* – Goodman Gilman 12/e p1792

Vigabatrin
• Vigabatrin is approved by the FDA as **adjunctive therapy of refractory partial complex seizures** in adults. • Due to **progressive & permanent bilateral vision loss**, vigabatrin must be **reserved for patients who have failed several alternative therapies**[Q].
Mechanism of Action:
• Vigabatrin is a **structural analog of GABA** that **irreversibly inhibits the major degradative enzyme for GABA, GABA-transaminase**, leading to **increased concentrations of GABA in the brain**[Q]. • Its mechanism of action is thought to involve **enhancement of GABA-mediated inhibition**[Q].
Therapeutic Use:
• Vigabatrin is usually **reserved for use in patients with infantile spasms** or with **complex partial seizures refractory to other treatments**[Q].
Side-effects:
• Typical toxicities include **drowsiness, dizziness & weight gain**[Q]. • Others: **Agitation, confusion & psychosis (preexisting mental illness is a relative contraindication)**[Q]
• **Long-term therapy with vigabatrin** has been associated with **development of peripheral visual field defects in 30–50% of patients**[Q]. • **Lesions are located in retina, increase with drug exposure & are usually not reversible**[Q].

63. **Ans. a. Polycystic ovarian syndrome** *(Ref: Goodman Gilman 12/e p597; Katzung 13/e p412-413, 12/e p418; KDT 7/e p405-409, 6/e p407)*

Contd...

There is evidence that shows valproic acid may increase the chance of polycystic ovary syndrome (PCOS) in women with epilepsy or bipolar disorder.

"There is evidence that shows valproic acid may increase the chance of polycystic ovary syndrome (PCOS) in women with epilepsy or bipolar disorder. However, studies have shown this risk of PCOS is higher in women with epilepsy compared to those with bipolar disorder."

Valproic Acid
• Valproic acid is **effective in absence, partial & generalized tonic-clonic seizures**[Q].
Mechanism of Action:
• Action is **similar to phenytoin & carbamazepine**[Q]
• Mediated by a **prolonged recovery of voltage-activated Na$^+$ channels from inactivation**[Q].
• Valproate can **stimulate the activity of GABA synthetic enzyme, glutamic acid decarboxylase & inhibit GABA degradative enzymes, GABA transaminase & succinic semialdehyde dehydrogenase**[Q].
Therapeutic Uses:
• **Valproate** is a **broad-spectrum anti- seizure drug effective in the treatment of absence, myoclonic, partial, and tonic-clonic seizures**[Q].

Side-effects of Valproic Acid	
• **MC side effects** are **transient GI symptoms**[Q] (anorexia, nausea & vomiting)	• **Elevation of hepatic transaminases, microvesicular steatosis**[Q]
• **Effects on the CNS: Sedation, ataxia & tremor**[Q]	• **Acute pancreatitis**[Q]
• **Rash, alopecia**	• **Hyperammonemia**[Q]
• **Stimulation of appetite & weight gain**[Q]	• **Neural tube defects**[Q]

• There is evidence that shows that **valproic acid** may **increase** the **chance of polycystic ovary syndrome (PCOS) in women** with **epilepsy** or **bipolar disorder**[Q].

Drug of Choice for Various Types of Seizures	
Type of Seizures	**Drug of Choice**
• **Absence seizures** • **GTCS (Grand mal)** • **Tonic seizures** • **Clonic seizures** • **Myoclonic seizures** • **Atonic (Akinetic) seizures**	**Valproate**[Q]
• **Partial seizures**	**Carbamazepine**[Q]
• **Infantile spasm**	**ACTH**[Q]
• **Infantile spasm with tuberous sclerosis**	**Vigabatrin**[Q]
• **Febrile seizures**	**Diazepam**[Q] **(per rectal)**
• **Status epilepticus**	**Lorazepam**[Q] **(IV)**
• **Seizures in eclampsia**	**Magnesium sulphate**[Q]

64. Ans. a. Inhibition of TNF alpha *(Ref: Goodman Gilman 12/e p1826; Katzung 13/e p630, 12/e p648; KDT7/e p883, 6/e p205; Harrison 19/e p348)*

Etanercept is a fusion protein produced by recombinant DNA. It fuses the TNF receptor to the constant end of the IgG1 antibody. It reduces the effect of naturally present TNF, and hence is a TNF inhibitor, functioning as a decoy receptor that binds to TNF.

"Etanercept is a soluble, recombinant, fully human TNF receptor fusion protein consisting of two molecules of the ligand-binding portion of the TNF receptor fused to the Fc portion of IgG$_1$. Etanercept binds soluble and membrane-bound TNF, thereby inhibiting the action of TNF."– Goodman Gilman 12/e p1826

Etanercept
• Etanercept is a **fusion protein produced by recombinant DNA**[Q].
• It **fuses TNF receptor to the constant end of IgG1 antibody**[Q].
• **It reduces the effect of naturally present TNF,** and hence is a **TNF inhibitor, functioning as a decoy receptor that binds to TNF**[Q].

Mechanism of Action:
• Etanercept is a **recombinant fusion protein** consisting of **two soluble TNF p75 receptor moieties linked to the F$_c$ portion of human IgG$_1$**; it binds TNF-α molecules & inhibits lymphotoxin-α[Q].

Clinical use:
• **US-FDA approved for rheumatoid arthritis, juvenile rheumatoid arthritis & psoriatic arthritis, plaque psoriasis & ankylosing spondylitis**[Q].

Side-effects:
• **Serious infections & sepsis**, reactivation of latent tuberculosis & hepatitis B infections[Q].
• Report of **Strongyloides hyperinfection** after use of Etanercept[Q].

65. **Ans. a. Flumazenil** *(Ref: Goodman Gilman 12/e p468; Katzung 13/e p377, 394, 12/e p381, 399; KDT 6/e p385; Harrison 19/e p2727, 18/e p2727)*

Flumazenil is a GABA$_A$ receptor antagonist primarily used intravenously to treat benzodiazepine overdoses and to help reverse anesthesia. It is not used in alcohol detoxification, while rest of the given drugs have a role.

Drugs Used in Acute Ethanol Withdrawal		
Drug	**Mechanism of Action**	**Clinical Applications**
Benzodiazepines (chlordiazepoxide, diazepam, lorazepam)	**BDZ receptor agonists** that facilitate **GABA-mediated activation of GABA$_A$ receptors**[Q]	• **Prevention & treatment of acute ethanol withdrawal syndrome**[Q]
Thiamine (vitamin B$_1$)	Essential vitamin required for synthesis of the **coenzyme thiamine pyrophosphate**[Q]	• Administered to patients suspected of having alcoholism (those exhibiting **acute alcohol intoxication** or **alcohol withdrawal syndrome**) to prevent **Wernicke-Korsakoff syndrome**[Q]

Drugs Used in Chronic Alcoholism		
Drug	**Mechanism of Action**	**Clinical Applications**
Naltrexone	**Nonselective competitive antagonist of opioid receptors**[Q]	**Reduced risk of relapse** in individuals with alcoholism[Q]
Acamprosate	Poorly understood **NMDA receptor antagonist & GABA$_A$ agonist effects**[Q]	**Reduced risk of relapse** in individuals with alcoholism[Q]
Disulfiram	**Inhibits aldehyde dehydrogenase**, resulting in **aldehyde accumulation** during ethanol ingestion[Q]	**Deterrent to drinking** in individuals with alcohol dependence[Q]

Flumazenil
• Flumazenil is an **imidazobenzodiazepine** that behaves as a **specific benzodiazepine receptor antagonist**[Q].

Mechanism of Action:
• Flumazenil **binds with high affinity to specific sites on the GABA$_A$ receptor**, where it **competitively antagonizes** the **binding & allosteric effects of benzodiazepines** and other ligands[Q].
• Flumazenil **antagonizes both electrophysiological & behavioral effects of agonist & inverse-agonist benzodiazepines & beta-carbolines**[Q].

Therapeutic Uses:
• **Primary indication: Management of suspected benzodiazepine overdose & reversal of sedative effects produced by benzodiazepines administered** during various procedures[Q].
• A total of **1 mg flumazenil given over 1-3 minutes usually is sufficient to abolish the effects of therapeutic doses of benzodiazepines**[Q].
• Flumazenil is **not effective in single-drug overdoses with either barbiturates or tricyclic antidepressants.**

MICROBIOLOGY

66. **Ans. a. Ingestion of food contaminated with egg of larva** *(Ref: Paniker's Parasitology 7/e p172, 6/e p166; Jawetz 27/e p724; Harrison 19/e p1416)*

Elongated, barrel-shaped eggs with a polar 'plug' at each end shown here are characteristic of Trichuris egg, which causes trichuriasis via feco-oral transmission.

Nematodes	Fecal examination
Trichinella spiralis	**Adult worm**[Q]
Trichuris trichiura	**Eggs (barrel shaped)**[Q]
Strongyloides	**Rhabditiform larvae**[Q]
Ancylostoma duodenale & Necator americanus	Egg which may be hatched, so **rhabditiform larvae** can be seen
Enterobius vermicularis	Usually not useful
Ascaris lumbricoides	**Eggs & adult worm**[Q]
Filariasis	No role
Dracunculus medinensis	No role

See Q. No. 74 AIIMS November 2016

67. **Ans. c. AFB, mouth** *(Ref: Ananthanarayan 10/e p398, 8/e p391-392; Harrison 19/e p1088)*

In this farmer, who presented with multiple discharging cervical sinuses, the most likely diagnosis is actinomycosis. The Actinomyces is not acid-fast organism.

"Actinomycosis occurs most commonly at an oral, cervical, or facial site, usually as a soft tissue swelling, abscess, or mass lesion that is often mistaken for a neoplasm. The angle of the jaw is generally involved, but a diagnosis of actinomycosis should be considered with any mass lesion or relapsing infection in the head and neck." – Harrison 19/e p1088.

"The diagnosis is most commonly made by microscopic identification of sulfur granules (an in vivo matrix of bacteria, calcium phosphate, and host material) in pus or tissues. Occasionally, these granules are identified grossly from draining sinus tracts or pus. Although sulfur granules are a defining characteristic of actinomycosis, granules also are found in mycetoma and botryomycosis (a chronic suppurative bacterial infection of soft tissue or, in rare cases, visceral tissue that produces clumps of bacteria resembling granules). These entities can easily be differentiated from actinomycosis with appropriate histopathologic and microbiologic studies."– Harrison 19/e p1090.

Actinomyces	Nocardia
• **Facultative anaerobes**[Q]	• Obligate aerobes
• Growth at **35–37°C**[Q]	• Variable temperatures
• **Endogenous infection**: Commensals in mouth, colon, vagina[Q]	• **Exogenous: Saprophytes**[Q]
• **Nonacid fast**[Q]	• **Acid fast**[Q]
• **DOC: Penicillin**[Q]	• **DOC: Sulfonamides**[Q]

See Q. No. 72 AIIMS May 2016

Acid fast Stain
• Acid fastness is a **physical property of certain organisms** by which they **resist decolorization by acids during staining procedures.**
• **Appearance:** Acid fast organisms stain **red with Ziehl-Neelsen Stain**[Q]

Acid fast Stains	
Ziehl-Neelsen stain[Q]	**Kinyoun stain**[Q]
Background stains **blue**[Q]	**Background** will stain **green**[Q]

Contd...

Contd...

Acid fast Stain			
Acid fast organisms	**Acid fast Oocysts**	**Acid fast parasites**	**Other acid fast structures**
• All Mycobacteria (M. tuberculosis, M. leprae, M. smegmatis) & atypical Mycobacterium[Q] • Actinomycetes (except Actinomyces & Streptomyces, which are non-acid fast genera of Actinomycetes) including Nocardia & Rhodococcus • Legionella micdadei[Q] • Bacterial spores [Q]	• Cryptosporidium parvum[Q] • Isospora belli[Q] • Cyclospora cayetanensis[Q]	• Sarcocystis[Q] • Taenia saginata eggs stain well[Q] but Taenia solium eggs do not (Can be used to distinguish) • Hydatid cysts[Q], especially their 'hooklets' stain irregularly with ZN stain but emanate bright red fluorescence under green light[Q]	• Head of sperm[Q]

68. Ans. d. Nocardia, Gram stain *(Ref: Ananthanarayan 10/e p400, 8/e p393; Harrison 19/e p1085, 1086)*

The given picture shows branching pleomorphic rods of Nocardia species. They are also acid fast and can be stained by Modified Ziehl-Nieelsen technique.

Nocardia
• **Gram-positive, branching pleomorphic rods** with **intermittent or beaded staining patterns[Q]**, especially when invading tissues. • **Nocardiae** are **gram-positive weakly acid-fast branching rod- shaped bacteria** and can be **visualized by a modified Ziehl-Neelsen stain** like **Fite-Faraco method[Q]**. • **Nocardia asteroides** is **most frequently found species infecting humans[Q]** • Most cases occur as an **opportunistic infection in immunocompromised patients.**

Staining & Culture Characteristics:
• Because it is **acid-fast to some degree**, it **stains only weakly Gram-positive[Q]**.
• Visualized by a **modified Ziehl- Neelsen stain** like **Fite-Faraco method[Q]**.
• **Stain black** with the **methenamine-silver stain.**
• In culture, **Nocardia are not fastidious** but do tend to **grow slowly.**
• Colonies will **grow on most bacterial, fungal, or mycobacterial media that lack antibiotics.**
    • **Blood & Sabouraud's agars** are good substrates for pathogenic organisms that usually **grow satisfactorily at temperatures between 35-37°C[Q]**.
    • **Growth of N. asteroides** is facilitated by **10% carbon dioxide.**

Clinical Features: • **MC form of human nocardial disease** is a **slowly progressive pneumonia[Q]**, the common symptoms of which include **cough, dyspnea & fever**. • Nocardia species are deeply involved in the process of **endocarditis** as one of its main pathogenic effects. • Nocardia infection takes the form of **encephalitis** and/or **brain abscess formation** (In 25–33%) • **Cutaneous infections: Actinomycetoma** (especially **N. brasiliensis**), **lymphocutaneous disease, cellulitis, & subcutaneous abscesses[Q]**.
Diagnosis: • **First step in diagnosis: Examination of sputum or pus for crooked, branching, beaded, gram-positive filaments** 1 μm wide and up to 50 μm long[Q]. • **Most Nocardiae are acid-fast in direct smears if a weak acid is used for decolorization** (e.g. in the **modified Kinyoun, Ziehl-Neelsen, and Fite-Faraco methods**)[Q]. • **Recovery from specimens** containing a mixed flora **can be improved with selective media (colistin-nalidixic acid agar, modified Thayer-Martin agar, or buffered charcoal-yeast extract agar)[Q]**.

Contd...

Contd...

Nocardia
• Nocardiae grow relatively slowly; colonies may take up to 2 weeks to appear and may not develop their **characteristic appearance, white, yellow, or orange, with aerial mycelia and delicate, dichotomously branched substrate mycelia**, for up to 4 weeks[Q]. • **Nocardia isolation from biological specimens** can be performed using **buffered charcoal-yeast extract agar (BCYE)**, the same **used for Legionella species**[Q].

69. **Ans. c. Trichomonas vaginalis**   *(Ref: Paniker's Parasitology 7/e p34, 6/e p41; Jawetz 27/e p713)*
The given smear shows the infestation of Trichomonas vaginalis.

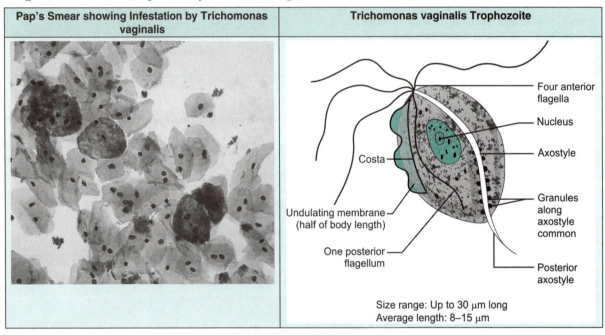

Trichomonas vaginalis
• *Trichomonas vaginalis* is an **anaerobic, flagellated protozoa, exists only as a trophozoite (no cyst stage**[Q]) • It has **four free flagella** that arise from a single stalk and a **fifth flagellum**, which forms an **undulating membrane**[Q]. • MC pathogenic protozoan infection of humans **in industrialized countries**.   • **'Frothy', greenish vaginal discharge with a 'musty' malodorous smell is characteristic**[Q].
Life Cycle and Epidemiology:
• T. vaginalis is a **pear-shaped, actively motile organism**, replicates by **binary fission**, and **inhabits the lower genital tract of females & urethra & prostate of males**. • **Sexual transmission** accounts for virtually all cases of trichomoniasis. • **Prevalence is greatest** among persons with **multiple sexual partners**.
Clinical Manifestations:
• Many **men** infected with **T. vaginalis** are **asymptomatic**, although some **develop urethritis, epididymitis or prostatitis**. • **Women:** Usually symptomatic & manifests with **malodorous vaginal discharge (often yellow), vulvar erythema &** itching, dysuria or urinary frequency & **dyspareunia**[Q]. • **'Frothy', greenish vaginal discharge** with **a 'musty' malodorous smell** is **characteristic**[Q].   • **Vaginal walls are tender** with **multiple small punctuate strawberry sport on the vaginal vault &** **portio vaginalis of cervix** known as **strawberry vagina**[Q].

Contd...

Contd...

Trichomonas vaginalis

Diagnosis:

- Detection of **motile** flagellated **trichomonads by microscopic examination of wet mounts of vaginal or prostatic secretions** has been the **conventional means of diagnosis**.
- Culture done on **Feinberg- Whittington media**[Q]
  - **Classically, with a cervical smear**, infected women have a **transparent 'halo' around their superficial cell nucleus**[Q].
  - **T. vaginalis** was traditionally diagnosed via a **wet mount, in which 'corkscrew' motility was observed**[Q].
- **Direct immunofluorescent antibody staining** is **more sensitive (70–90%) than wet-mount examinations**.
- A new **NAAT, APTIMA**, is **FDA approved and is highly sensitive & specific for urine** and for endocervical & vaginal swabs from women.

Treatment:

- **DOC: Metronidazole**[Q] **(tinidazole** is also effective)
- **All sexual partners must be treated concurrently to prevent reinfection**, especially from asymptomatic males.

70. **Ans. d. Calymmatobacterium donovani** *(Ref: Ananthanarayan 10/e p404, 8/e p396; Jawetz 27/e p761; Harrison 19/e p198e-1)*

Coccobacilli seen in the Giemsa-stained specimen suggest a diagnosis of granuloma inguinale. Donovan bodies are seen intracellularly in mononuclear cells. Granuloma inguinale, or donovanosis, is a chronic inflammatory disease caused by Calymmatobacterium donovani, a minute, encapsulated, coccobacilli that is closely related to the Klebsiella genus. The organism is sexually transmitted.

Organism	Microscopic Examination	Characteristic Features
Chlamydia	 • *Chlamydia trachomatis* grown in McCoy cells and **stained with iodine.** The McCoy cells stain a faint yellow in the background. • **The glycogen- rich intracytoplasmic inclusions of C trachomatis stain a dark brown**[Q].	• **Elementary bodies** stain **purple with Giemsa stain**[Q]. • **Larger, non-infective reticulate body** (RB) **stain blue with Giemsa stain**[Q]. • **Gram reaction of chlamydiae** is **negative or variable** and is **not useful in identification**[Q]. • **Chlamydial particles & inclusions stain brightly by immunofluorescence, with group—specific, species-specific**, or **serovar-specific antibodies**[Q].
Gardnerella vaginalis		• Diagnosis of **bacterial vaginosis** is made by finding of a **watery discharge & typical smell**[Q] • **Wet mounts** may show **trichomonas**, but if negative, a Gram stain should be done to rule out Gardnerella. • **'Clue cells'** (sloughed epithelial cells coated with Gram-variable pleomorphic coccobacilli): This is **sufficient evidence to diagnose infection with Gardnerella vaginalis**[Q]. • Culture is not necessary.
Hemophilus ducreyi		• **School of fish appearance**[Q] • No clue cells observed. • **Moderate small gram-negative rods**, suggestive of *Hemophilus ducreyi*.

Granuloma Inguinale

- **Granuloma inguinale or donovanosis**, is a chronic inflammatory disease **caused by *Calymmatobacterium donovani*,** a minute, encapsulated, coccobacillus that is **closely related to the *Klebsiella* genus**[Q].
- Donovanosis is a **chronic, progressive bacterial infection**, involves **genital region**.
- **Sexually transmitted infection** of **low infectivity**.

Etiology:

- Characteristic **Donovan bodies** in **macrophages & stratum malpighii**[Q].
- Donovanosis is **associated with poor hygiene, more common in lower socioeconomic groups**.

Clinical Features:

- A lesion starts as a **papule or subcutaneous nodule** that later **ulcerates after trauma**[Q].
- **Genitals** are affected in **90%** & **inguinal region** in **10%**.

Four types of lesions have been described:	
- **Classic ulcerogranulomatous lesion**, a **beefy red ulcer** that **bleeds readily when touched**[Q]	- A **necrotic, offensive-smelling ulcer** causing **tissue destruction**[Q]
- A **hypertrophic or verrucous ulcer** with a raised irregular edge[Q]	- A **sclerotic or cicatricial lesion** with fibrous & scar tissue[Q].

- **Most common sites of infection**: **Prepuce, coronal sulcus, frenulum & glans** in men; labia minora & fourchette in women.
- **Cervical lesions** may **mimic cervical carcinoma**.

Diagnosis:

- **Diagnosis is confirmed by microscopic identification of Donovan bodies** in tissue smears[Q].
- **Donovan bodies** can be seen in large, **mononuclear (Pund) cells** as **gram-negative intracytoplasmic cysts filled with deeply staining bodies** that may have a **safety-pin appearance**[Q].
- **PCR analysis with a colorimetric detection system** can now be used in routine diagnostic laboratories.

> - **Microscopic examination of active lesions** reveals marked epithelial hyperplasia at the borders of the ulcer, sometimes mimicking carcinoma (**pseudoepitheliomatous hyperplasia**[Q]).
> - **A mixture of neutrophils & mononuclear inflammatory cells is present at the base of the ulcer and beneath the surrounding epithelium**[Q].
> - **Organisms** are demonstrable in **Giemsa-stained** smears of the **exudate** as **minute, encapsulated coccobacilli (Donovan bodies) in macrophages.**[Q]

Treatment:

- **Drug of choice: Azithromycin**[Q]
- **Alternatives; Cotrimoxazole, erythromycin & tetracycline.**

71. **Ans. d. Cryptococcus** *(Ref: Ananthanarayan 10/e p616, 8/e p611; Harrison 19/e p1340; Jawetz 27/e p687-688)*

The diagram above shows capsule of Cryptococcus stained with India ink. Alternate staining methods are nigrosin and mucicarmine

"A diagnosis of cryptococcosis requires the demonstration of yeast cells in normally sterile tissues. Visualization of the capsule of fungal cells in cerebrospinal fluid (CSF) mixed with India ink is a useful rapid diagnostic technique. Cryptococcal cells in India ink have a distinctive appearance because their capsules exclude ink particles."– Harrison 19/e p1340.

See Q. No. 49 AIIMS November 2016

72. **Ans. b. Brugia malayi** *(Ref: Paniker's Parasitology 7/e p214, 6/e p203)*

The microfilariae given in the question has morphology typical of Brugia malayi. In Brugia malayi, head space is twice as long as it is broad, nuclei in body appears crowded & tail tapers around to two nuclei that appears to be connected by a fine thread.

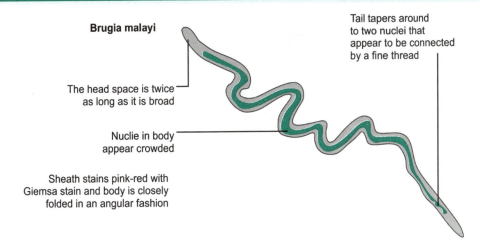

Brugia malayi
- The head space is twice as long as it is broad
- Nuclie in body appear crowded
- Sheath stains pink-red with Giemsa stain and body is closely folded in an angular fashion
- Tail tapers around to two nuclei that appear to be connected by a fine thread

Brugia malayi
• Brugia malayi is one of the **tissue roundworm** responsible for **filariasis in Asia & Indian** subcontinent.
Life-cycle host:
• **Definitive host: Human**^{Q}
• **Intermediate host: Mosquito (Mansonia, Anopheles)**^{Q}
• Characteristic Features:
• **Periodicity: Nocturnal**^{Q}
• **Location of adult: Lymphatic tissue**^{Q}; **Location of microfilariae: Blood**^{Q}
<ul><li>**Morphology of Brugia malayi Microfilariae**</li><li>**Head-space** is twice as long as it is broad^Q</li><li>**Nuclei in body** appears **crowded**^{Q}</li><li>**Sheath** stains **pink-red with Giemsa stain** & body is **closely folded in angular fashion**</li><li>**Tail tapers** around **to two nuclei** that appears to be **connected by a fine thread**^{Q}.</li></ul>
Diagnosis:
• **Microscopic examination** of differential morphological **features of microfilariae in stained blood films** can aid in diagnosis^Q.
• **Giemsa staining** will uniquely **stain Brugia malayi sheath pink**^{Q}.
Treatment:
• **DOC: Diethylcarbamazine (DEC)**^{Q}.

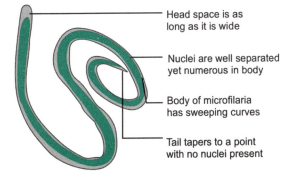

- Head space is as long as it is wide
- Nuclei are well separated yet numerous in body
- Body of microfilaria has sweeping curves
- Tail tapers to a point with no nuclei present

Wuchereria bancrofti microfilariae are found in the blood and are sheathed. The sheath typically stains pale pink with Giemsa.

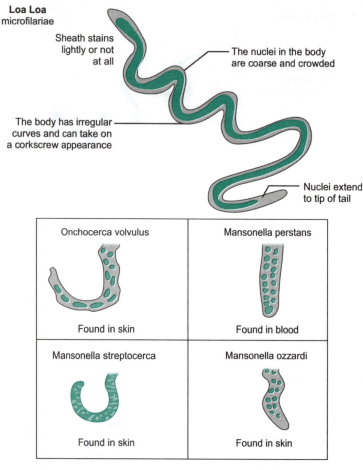

73. **Ans. c. Echinococcus with 2 layers** *(Ref: Paniker's Parasitology 7/e p127, 6/e p153; Jawetz 27/e p736; Sabiston 20/e p1452, 19/e p1447-1449; Blumgart 5/e p1035-1048; Shackelford 7/e p1459-1462)*

The histopathology image given is typical of hydatid cyst, caused by Echinococcus granulosus. Cysts of Echinococcus is enclosed by inner, nucleated, germinative layer & outer, opaque, non-nucleated layer.

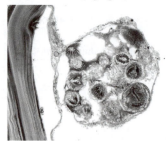

Fig. 29: Histologic section of a hydatid cyst showing several protoscolices (arrows) within a brood capsule.

Hydatid Disease
• Hydatid disease is a **zoonosis**, occurs primarily in **sheep-grazing areas**[Q] of the world
• Endemic in **Mediterranean countries**, Middle East, Far East, South America, Australia, New Zealand, and **East Africa**.
• **Humans** contract the **disease from dogs**, and there is **no human-to-human transmission**[Q].
• Hydatid cyst is caused by **Echinococcus granulosus**[Q].
• Other species affecting human beings: E. **multilocularis**, E. **vogeli**, E. **oligarthus**[Q].

Contd...

Contd...

Hydatid Disease

Life-cycle:

- **Dogs** are the **definitive host**[Q] of E. granulosus
- Eggs are passed (up to thousands of ova daily) and deposited with the dog's feces.
  - **Sheep**: Usual **intermediate host**[Q]
  - **Human: Accidental dead end intermediate host**[Q] without human to human transmission

- In the **human duodenum**, parasitic embryo releases an **oncosphere** that **penetrate mucosa**, allowing access to **bloodstream**[Q].
- In the blood, **oncosphere** reaches **liver (MC)**[Q] or **lungs**, develops its **larval stage**, **hydatid cyst**.
- Organs most commonly involved are: **Liver >Lungs >Spleen >Kidney >Brain >Bone**[Q].

Hydatid Cyst

- Three weeks after infection, a visible hydatid cyst develops
- **The cyst wall has two layers:**
  1. **Ectocyst**: Outer **gelatinous** membrane[Q]
  2. **Endocyst**: Inner **germinal** membrane[Q]
- **Pericyst**: Fibrous capsule **derived from host tissues**, develops around the hydatid cyst.

- **Scoleces develop** into an **adult tapeworm in definitive host**[Q]
- Scoleces **differentiate into** a **new hydatid cyst in intermediate host**[Q]
- **Hydatid sand: Freed brood capsules** and **scoleces** in the hydatid fluid

Clinical Features:

- **Equally common** in males and females, age of **45 years**.
- **Most** (75%) are **singular,** located in **right liver** (VII & VIII)[Q].
- **Mostly asymptomatic**[Q] until complications occur
  - **MC presenting symptoms**: Abdominal pain, dyspepsia & vomiting.
  - **MC sign: Hepatomegaly**[Q]

- **Complications**: Rupture of the cyst into the **biliary tree (MC)**[Q] or **bronchial tree**, or free rupture into **peritoneal, pleural**, or **pericardial cavities**.
- **Intrabiliary rupture** is **MC complication** of **hydatid liver cysts**[Q]
- Free ruptures can result in disseminated echinococcosis and a potentially fatal anaphylactic reaction.

Diagnosis:

- **USG & CT** are the **main diagnostic modalities**[Q]
- **Daughter cyst** within the **large cyst (rosette appearance)** & **calcification** of the **wall** are **highly suggestive** of **hydatid cyst**[Q].
  - **Diagnosis is confirmed** by **serological tests**[Q] (**ELISA, Immunoblot, Arc-5, IHA**) for antibodies.
- In cases of **suspected biliary involvement (Jaundice)**, **ERCP (gold standard)**[Q] or PTC is necessary.

Characteristic Signs of Pulmonary Hydatidosis	
- Meniscus sign[Q]	- Water lily sign[Q]
- Double arc sign[Q]	- Crescent sign[Q]
- Moon sign[Q]	

Treatment:

- **Most cysts** are **treated surgically**[Q]
- **Conservative management** is appropriate in **elderly** patients with **small, asymptomatic, densely calcified cysts**[Q].
- **Treatment options**: PAIR, pericystectomy, marsupialization, leaving the cyst open, drainage of the cyst, omentoplasty, or partial hepatectomy to encompass the cyst.

Surgery remains the **treatment of choice** for cysts where

- **PAIR is not possible** or **cysts are refractory to PAIR**[Q]
- For **complicated cysts** (communicating with biliary tract)[Q]

- **Radical (resection)** and **conservative (drainage & evacuation)** surgical approaches appear to be **equally effective** at controlling disease.

Contd...

Contd...

Hydatid Disease

- **Pericystectomy** is the **preferred surgical approach**[Q] (complete cyst with surrounding fibrous tissue are removed)
- If surgical **cystectomy** is **not** technically **feasible**, then formal **liver resection** can be done.

Chemotherapy in Hydatid Disease

- Chemotherapy with **albendazole** or **mebendazole** is effective at **shrinking** the **cysts**
- **Cyst disappearance** occurs in **fewer than 50%** of patients[Q].
- **Preoperative treatment** may **decrease the risk for spillage**[Q] and is a reasonable and safe practice.
- **Chemotherapy without definitive resection** or drainage is only considered **for:**
  – Widely disseminated disease[Q]
  – Patients with **poor surgical risk**[Q]

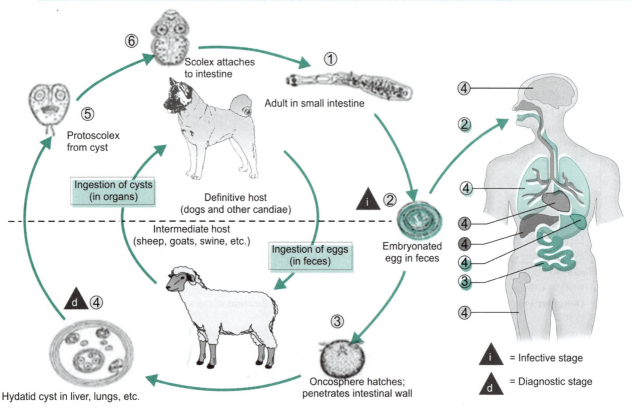

Fig. 26: Life cycle of Echinococcus granulosus (Hydatid cyst)

74. **Ans. a. P. vivax** *(Ref: Paniker's Parasitology 6/e p79; Jawetz 27/e p)*
    In the given image, irregularly shaped large rings and trophozoites are seen with enlarged erythrocytes, which are the characteristic features of Plasmodium vivax.
    See Q. No. 73 AIIMS November 2016

75. **Ans. d. Norovirus** *(Ref: Harrison 19/e p1285, 1286; Jawetz 27/e p537)*
    History of multiple episodes of loose watery stool for 3 days & history of ingestion shellfish with similar symptoms in other patients who consumed the shellfish is suggestive of acute viral gastroenteritis. Most likely organism responsible for this clinical scenario is Norovirus.

> "**Noroviruses may be the most common infectious agents of mild gastroenteritis in the community and affect all age groups**, whereas **sapoviruses primarily cause gastroenteritis in children**." *– Harrison 19/e p1285*

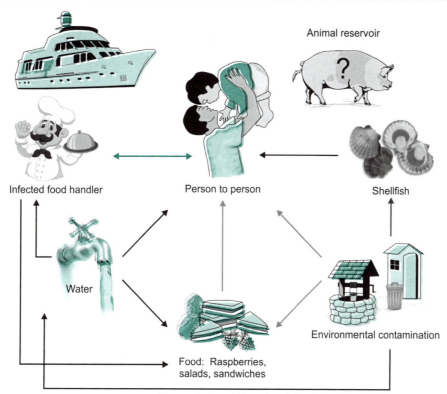

Fig. 27: Transmission of Norovirus Infection

"Gastroenteritis caused by Norwalk and related human caliciviruses has a sudden onset following an average incubation period of 24 h (range, 12–72 h). The illness generally lasts 12–60 h and is characterized by one or more of the following symptoms: nausea, vomiting, abdominal cramps, and diarrhea." – Harrison 19/e p1286

"Shellfish and salad ingredients are the foods most often implicated in norovirus outbreaks. Ingestion of shellfish that have not been sufficiently heated poses a high risk for norovirus infection. Foods other than shellfish may be contaminated by infected food handlers."

"Norovirus is a leading cause of food-borne illness and outbreaks. Seafood harvested from sewage-contaminated waters has caused outbreaks of norovirus gastroenteritis. Large outbreaks have been associated with consumption of raw or inadequately cooked shellfish, such as a series of oyster-and clam-associated outbreaks in which northeastern coastal waters were implicated. Shellfish can accumulate large numbers of viruses. Additionally, insufficient cooking, such as steaming clams only until they open rather than to higher temperatures that kill noroviruses, has contributed to illness and outbreaks."

Norovirus
• **Norovirus (small RNA virus)** is **MC cause of viral gastroenteritis in humans**[Q].
• **Family: Caliciviridae**[Q]
• **Genus: Norovirus** is derived from **Norwalk virus, the only species of the genus.**
• The species causes **90% of epidemic nonbacterial outbreaks of gastroenteritis around the world**[Q].
Epidemiology:
• **Transmitted by fecally contaminated food or water**, by **person-to-person contact** & via **aerosolization of the virus** & subsequent **contamination of surfaces**[Q].
• Most outbreaks are reported from **child-care centers, cruise ships, long-term care facilities** and other **closed populations**[Q].
• **Shellfish & salad ingredients** are the **foods most often implicated in norovirus outbreaks**[Q].
• **Ingestion of shellfish** that have **not been sufficiently heated** poses a high risk for norovirus infection[Q].
• **Foods** other than shellfish may be **contaminated by infected food handlers**[Q].

Contd...

Contd...

Norovirus
Clinical Features:
• It affects **people of all ages**.
• Norovirus infection is characterized by **nausea, vomiting, watery diarrhea, abdominal pain**, and in some cases, loss of taste.
• General lethargy, weakness, muscle aches, headache, and low-grade fever may occur.
Diagnosis:
• The virus may be identified by **electron microscopy or reverse transcriptase PCR of stool samples** and by **enzyme immunoassay for detection of viral antigen in serum samples**[Q].

76. **Ans. d. Dengue hemorrhagic fever** *(Ref: Harrison 19/e p1322)*

Antibody-dependent enhancement is implicated in the immunopathogenesis of Dengue hemorrhagic fever.

"Antibody-dependent enhancement (ADE) occurs when non-neutralizing antiviral proteins facilitate virus entry into host cells, leading to increased infectivity in the cells. Some cells do not have the usual receptors on their surfaces that viruses use to gain entry. The antiviral proteins (i.e. the antibodies) bind to antibody Fc receptors that some of these cells have in the plasma membrane. The viruses bind to the antigen-binding site at the other end of the antibody. The most widely known example of ADE occurs in the setting of infection with the dengue virus (DENV). The phenomenon of ADE may be observed when a person who has previously been infected with one serotype of DENV becomes infected many months or years later with a different serotype. In such cases, the clinical course of the disease is more severe, and these people have higher viremia compared with those in whom ADE has not occurred. This explains the observation that while primary (first) infections cause mostly minor disease (DF) in children, secondary infection (reinfection at a later date) is more likely to be associated with severe disease (DHF and/or DSS) in both children and adults."

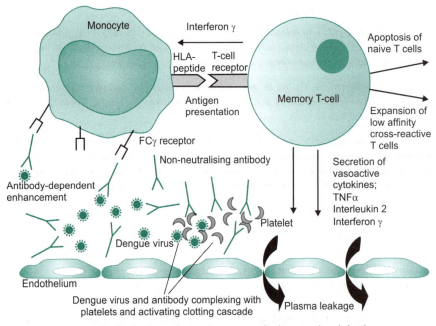

Fig. 28: Antibody dependent enhancement in dengue virus infection

Antibody Dependent Enhancement (ADE)
• **Antibody-dependent enhancement (ADE)** occurs when **non-neutralizing antiviral proteins facilitate virus entry into host cells, leading to increased infectivity in the cells.** Some cells do not have the usual receptors on their surfaces that viruses use to gain entry.

Contd...

AIIMS November 2015

Contd...

Antibody Dependent Enhancement (ADE)
• **The antiviral proteins (i.e. the antibodies) bind to antibody Fc receptors that some of these cells have in the plasma membrane.** The viruses bind to the antigen-binding site at the other end of the antibody.
• **Most widely known example of ADE** occurs in setting of infection with **dengue virus (DENV).**
• **Phenomenon of ADE** may be observed **when a person who has previously been infected with one serotype of DENV becomes infected many months or years later with a different serotype[Q].**
• In such cases, **clinical course of disease is more severe** & these people have higher viremia compared with those in whom ADE has not occurred.
• This explains the observation that **while primary (first) infections cause mostly minor disease (DF) in children, secondary infection** (reinfection at a later date) is **more likely to be associated with severe disease (DHF and/or DSS)** in both children & adults.
• **Four antigenically different serotypes of DENV: DENV-1 to DENV-4**
• **Infection with DENV induces the production of neutralizing homotypic immunoglobulin G (IgG) antibodies,** which provide **lifelong immunity against the infecting serotype.**
• **Infection with DENV** also produces some degree of **cross-protective immunity against the other three serotypes.**
• **Neutralizing heterotypic** (cross-reactive) **IgG antibodies are responsible for this cross-protective immunity**, which typically persists for a period of several months to a few years.
• Heterotypic antibody titers decrease over long time periods (4-20 years).
• While heterotypic IgG antibody titers decrease, **homotypic IgG antibody titers increase over long time periods.** This could be due to the **preferential survival of long-lived memory B cells producing homotypic antibodies.**
• Infection with **DENV can induce heterotypic antibodies, which neutralize the virus only partially or not at all**.
• **Production of such cross-reactive but non-neutralizing antibodies** could be the **reason for more severe secondary infections[Q].**
• It is thought that by binding but not neutralizing the virus, these antibodies cause it to behave as a 'trojan horse', where it is delivered into the wrong compartment of dendritic cells that have ingested the virus for destruction.
• **Once inside the white blood cell, virus replicates undetected,** eventually **generating very high virus titers,** which cause **severe disease.**
• **ADE of infection** has also been reported **in HIV.** Like DENV, **non-neutralizing level of antibodies** have been found to **enhance viral infection through interactions of complement system & receptors[Q].**

77. **Ans. c. Transduction**   *(Ref: Ananthanarayan 10/e p59, 8/e p65-67; Jawetz 27/e p112)*

Phage mediated change in C. diphtheria is due to Transduction.

"In transduction, donor DNA is carried by a phage coat and is transferred into the recipient by the mechanism used for phage infection." – *Jawetz 27/e p537*

Mechanism of Genetic Exchange		
Conjugation	**Transduction**	**Transformation**
• During conjugation, a **gram-negative bacterium transfers plasmids containing resistant genes to an adjacent bacterium** often **via** an elongated proteinaceous structure termed as **"pilus"**, which joins two organisms[Q]. • This process involves **direct cell to cell contact of two bacterias[Q]**	• During transduction, **resistant genes are transferred from one bacterium to another via bacteriophages[Q].** • When a bacteriophage destroys its current host and invades a new one, it may carry pieces of chromosomal DNA or plasmids from previous host.	• **Bacteria acquire and incorporate DNA segments from other bacteria** that have **released their DNA into the environment after cell lysis[Q].** • During transformation, bacterial cell take up DNA from the surrounding environment, such as after cell lysis.

(a) Conjugation:

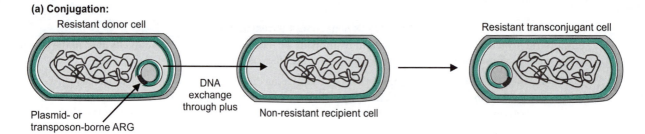

(b) Transduction:

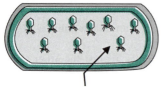 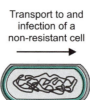 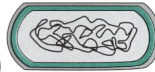

(c) Natural transformation:

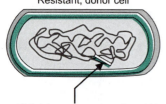 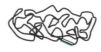 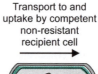 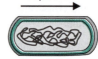 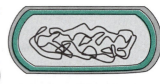

Methods of transfer	Mechanism	Nature of DNA transferred
Conjugation	**Transfer of DNA** form one bacterium to another **through the sex pilus**[Q]	**Chromosomal or plasmid DNA**[Q]
Transduction	**Transfer of DNA** form one bacterium to another **by bacteriophage**[Q]	**Any gene in generalized transduction**, only selected genes in specialized transduction[Q]
Transformation	**Transfer of DNA** from one bacterium to another[Q]	**Any gene**[Q]

FORENSIC MEDICINE

78. **Ans. d. Nitrobenzene** *(Ref: Reddy 34/e p468, 33/e p507; Industrial Hygiene and Toxicology, General Principles/p174)*
    Shoe polish like smell is seen in Nitrobenzene.

    "Nitrobenzene is an oily yellow to yellow-brown liquid that smells like bitter almonds or shoe polish. Nitrobenzene dissolves only slightly in water and easily in other chemicals. It is man-made. The most common exposure is at workplaces that use nitrobenzene to produce dyes, drugs, pesticides or some types of rubber."

    See Q. No. 89 AI IMS November 2016

79. **Ans. c. HF** *(Ref: Reddy 34/e p493, 33/e p530; Principles of Clinical Toxicology 3/e p220; Forensic Pathology 3/e p241, 110)*
    HF does not show coagulation necrosis on contact. Hydrofluoric acid causes liquefaction necrosis.

AIIMS November 2015

"Acids cause greatest damage to the stomach and pylorus. The oropharynx and esophagus usually have minimal involvement. The hydrogen ions from the acid are neutralized fairly quickly and deep penetrating tissue destruction does not occur. Hydrofluoric acid causes liquefaction necrosis."– Reddy 34/e p493

"Acids are hydrogen containing substances that on dissociation in water produce hydronium ions. They are potent desiccants with the ability to produce coagulation necrosis of tissues on contact. Hydrofluoric acid is a prominent exception, since it produces liquefactive necrosis."

Corrosive	MC Site of Injury	Type of injury
Acid	Stomach	Coagulative necrosis
Alkali	Esophagus	Liquefactive necrosis

Acid injury

- Acids are **hydrogen containing substances** that on dissociation in water **produce hydronium ions.**
  - They are **potent desiccants** with the ability to **produce coagulation necrosis** of tissues on contact.
  - **Hydrofluoric acid is a prominent exception**, since it produces liquefactive necrosis.
- There is **eschar (slough) formation** which has a **self-limiting effect, minimising the extent of further damage.**
- When a strong acid is dissolved in a solvent, an exothermic reaction ensues resulting in **emanation of heat** (heat of solution). This should be differentiated from heat of neutralisation which occurs when an acid is neutralised by any alkali. This **thermochemical reaction** is the cause for **eschar formation.**

  - **Lower the pH of an acid, higher is its corrosive effect.**
  - Other **important determinants** include **molarity, concentration & complexing affinity for hydroxyl ions.**
  - **Ingestion of acid causes more damage to stomach than oesophagus** because **squamous epithelium of latter is more resistant to acids**, while it is **just opposite in case of alkali ingestion** where **columnar epithelium of stomach is more resistant.**

- Acid burns of the stomach most commonly involve antrum & pylorus

80. **Ans. b. Sex** *(Ref: Modern Medical Toxicology/p4)*

Ashley's rule is used to know the sex of sternum; It is also known as '149 rule'

Differences between Male & Female sternum		
Features	**Male sternum**	**Female sternum**
Body	**Bigger, longer** & **more than twice** the length of manubrium	**Shorter & less than twice** the length of manubrium
Ashley's rule	Total length **>149 mm**	Total length **<149 mm**
Level of upper border	At the level of **lower part of body of 2nd** thoracic vertebrae	At the level of **lower part of 3rd** thoracic vertebrae
Manubrium	Smaller	Bigger
Sternal index	46.2	54.3
Sternal index = Length of manubrium x 100/length of body of sternum		

Differences between Male & Female pelvis		
Features	**Male pelvis**	**Female pelvis**
General framework	**Deep, funnel shaped** **Massive & rough**	**Shallow, bowl shaped** **Less massive & smooth**
True pelvis	**Narrow deep & funnel shaped**	**Wide & shallow**
Pelvic brim	**Heart shaped**	**Circular**
Ilium	**Smaller**	**Larger**

Contd...

Contd...

Differences between Male & Female pelvis		
Iliac crest	Curve is more prominent, more sloped with less rounded margins	Curve is less prominent, less sloped with more rounded margins
Anterior superior iliac spine	**More prominent**	**Less prominent**
Preauricular sulcus	**Not widely separated**	**Widely separated**
Acetabulum	**Wide & deep**, diameter about 52 mm	Prominent, **broad & deep**
Symphysis pubis	Higher & bigger in depth & narrow in width. **Margins of pubic arch** are **everted** & no parturition pits on the dorsal border	Small & narrow, diameter 46 mm **Lower, wider & rounded** Margins of pubic arch are **not everted** & **parturition pits** are present on dorsal border
Subpubic angle	**70°–75° (acute)** subpubic arch is **V shaped**	**90°** subpubic arch is **U shaped**
Greater sciatic notch	Smaller, deeper & narrower & less than right angle	Wider, larger & shallower & forming a right angle
Sciatic notch index = Width of sciatic notch x 100 Depth of sciatic notch	**4–5**	**5–6**
Obturator foramen	Large, oval shaped with base upwards	Small, triangular with the apex directed forwards
Ischial tuberosity	**More or less inverted**	**Everted**
Pubis (body)	**Narrow & triangular**	**Broad & square**
Pubis (ramus)	Is continuation of body	**Narrow appearance**
Pelvic index = AP diameter of pelvis/Transverse diameter x 100	**More**	**Less**
Kell index = Surface area of acetabulum/Surface area of illium x 100	**More**	**Less**

81. **Ans. a. Blisters are present** *(Ref: Parikh 6/e p4.168)*
    Vesicles & blisters are usually absent in chemical burns.

> **"A chemical burn** *occurs when living tissue is exposed to a corrosive substance such as a strong acid or base. Chemical burns follow standard burn classification and may cause extensive tissue damage. The main types of irritant and/or corrosive products are: acids, bases, oxidizers/reducing agents, solvents, and alkylants. Additionally, chemical burns can be caused by some types of chemical weapons, e.g. vesicants such as mustard gas and lewisite, or urticants such as phosgene oxime."*

Chemical burns may:	
• **Need no source of heat** • **Occur immediately** on contact • Not be immediately evident or noticeable	• Be **extremely painful** • **Diffuse into tissue & damage structures** under skin without immediately apparent damage to skin surface.

	Burns (dry Heat)	Scalds (Moist heat)	Chemicals
Cause	Flame, heated solid substance or radiant heat	Steam or any liquid at or near boiling point	Corrosive acids & alkalis
Site	At & above the site of flame	At & below the site of contract	At & below the site of contact
Clothing	Burnt & may be adherent to the body	Usually wet but not burnt	Characteristic stains
Skin	**Dry, shriveled, charred**	**Sodden & bleached**	**Stained, corroded**

Contd...

Contd...

	Burns (dry Heat)	Scalds (Moist heat)	Chemicals
Vesicles	At circumference of burnt area	Most marked over burnt area	Rarely found
Red line	Present	Present	Absent
Singeing	Present	Absent	In case of mineral acids
Charring (Soot)	Present	Absent	In case of mineral acids
Trickle marks	Absent	Present	Present
Discoloration	Skin roasted & charred	Skin bleached	From action of chemical on skin
Ulceration	Absent	Absent	Present
Scar	Thick & causes disfigurement	Thin & causes less disfigurement	Keloid scar & much disfigurement

82. **Ans. a. IPC 193** *(Ref: Parikh 6/e p1.10; Reddy 34/e p13, 33/e p392; Textbook on the Indian Penal Code by Krishna Deo Gaur 4/e p594; the-indian-penal-code-pdf-d74214920)*

Section 193 in the Indian Penal Code deals with punishment for giving false evidence.

Section 193 Indian Penal Code
• Whoever intentionally gives false evidence in any stage of a judicial proceeding, or fabricates false evidence for the purpose of being used in any stage of a judicial proceeding, shall be punished with imprisonment of either description for a term which may extend to seven years, and shall also be liable to fine, and whoever intentionally gives or fabricates false evidence in any other case, shall be punished with imprisonment of either description for a term which may extend to three years, and shall also be liable to fine.

See Q. No. 83 AIIMS November 2016

83. **Ans. a. Growth at the site following trauma** *(Ref: Parikh 6/e p4.89)*

Ewing's postulates concerns with growth at the site following trauma

Ewing's Postulates
• Certain criteria, known as 'Ewing's postulates', must be satisfied before a relationship between trauma and new growth is accepted: 1. The tumor must arise exactly at the site injured 2. Definite and substantial trauma must be proved 3. The tumor must be confirmed pathologically 4. The tissue at the site must have been healthy before the trauma 5. A reasonable interval-neither too long or too short—must elapse between the time of the trauma and the appearance of the tumor 6. Though not one of the Ewing's original postulates, there should be some good scientific reason for ascribing the tumor formation to the injury and this is rarely possible.

84. **Ans. a. Boric acid** *(Ref: Principles of Clinical Toxicology 3/e p221)*

Boiled lobster syndrome is seen in poisoning of Boric acid.

"In boric acid poisoning, the major symptom is erythema, desquamation and exfoliation. The skin of the patient looks like a 'boiled lobster'."

Boric acid
• Boric acid is used as antiseptics & fungistatic agent in baby talcum powder & as a pesticide against ants & cockroaches. • Although chronic toxicity seldom occurs now, acute ingestion by children at home is common.
Mechanism of toxicity:
• Boric acid is irritating to mucous membranes. • It acts as a general cellular poison. • Most commonly affects skin, GIT, brain, liver, kidneys.

Contd...

Contd...

Boric acid
Toxic dose: • **Acute:** 1-3 gm in newborns, 5 gm in infants & 20 gm in adults. • **Chronic serious toxicity & death in infants:** 5-15 gm; serum borate levels were 400-1600 mg/L.

Clinical presentation:
• **Earliest symptoms** are gastrointestinal, with **vomiting & diarrhea**.
  • **Emesis & diarrhea** may have a **blue-green color**[Q].
• **Significant dehydration & renal failure** can occur, with **death caused by profound shock**.
• Neurologic symptoms of hyperactivity, agitation & seizures may occur early.
  • **An erythrodermic rash (boiled-lobster appearance) is followed by exfoliation after 2-5 days**[Q].

Diagnosis: • Based on a history of exposure, presence of gastroenteritis (possibly with **blue-green emesis**), **erythematous rash, acute renal failure** & **elevated serum borate levels**.
Treatment: • **Emergency and supportive measures**: Maintain an open airway and assist ventilation if necessary; Treat coma, seizures, hypotension & renal failure if they occur. • **Spcific antidote: Not available** • **Decontamination**: Activated charcoal is not very effective. • Consider **gastric lavage for very large ingestions**. • **Enhanced elimination: Hemodialysis is effective**, **indicated after massive ingestions** & for supportive care of renal failure.

85. **Ans. b. Puppe's rule** *(Ref: Reddy 34/e p213, 33/e p225; Forensic Pathology 3/e p241, 110)*

Puppe's rule is used to determine that which fracture line has occurred before the second one.

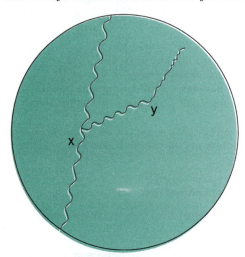

> "*Puppe's Rule: It can determine the sequence of shots, when several bullets have struck the cranium. This rule is applicable to any blunt force, causing skull fractures.* This rule has been developed by Madea in relation to bullet injuries. *The test depends on the observation of the fracture lines either when they intersect each other or when they intersect a cratered lesion, so that one can determine which crack or defect must have been formed first."*– Reddy 34/e p213

> "*Puppe's rule: When 2 or more separate fractures occur from successive impacts and meet each other the later fracture (Y) will terminate at, that is not cross, the earlier fracture line (X) which naturally interrupts the cranial distortion which proceeds fracturing."*

McNaughten's Rule (Legal test or right or Wrong Test)

- Deals with **responsibilities of mentally ill persons in criminal cases.**
- An **accused person is not legally responsible, if it is clearly proved, that at the time of committing the crime**, he was suffering from such a defect of reason from abnormality of mid, that he did not know the nature and quality of the act he was doing, or that what he was doing was wrong.
  - **Section 84 IPC** states that: **Nothing is an offence** which is **done by a person, who at the time of doing it, by reason of unsoundness of mind, is incapable of knowing the nature of the act, or that he is doing what is either wrong or contrary to the law."**

It must be clearly proved that:
1. The **offence is directly related to the insanity**
2. The **offence could not have occurred if there was no mental abnormality**
3. **Insanity subsequent to the act is not a defence.**

---

86. **Ans. d. Fracture** *(Ref: Reddy 34/e p225-227, 33/e p239-240; Parikh 6/e p4.183; Sabiston 19/e p612-613; Bailey 26/e p430, 25/e p422-423)*

Fracture is not specific of blast injury.

"Marshall's triad is diagnostic of explosive injury. Marshall's triad includes bruises, abrasions & puncture lacerations."

Blast Injuries

- **Primary blast injuries** result from the rapid overpressure or shock waves produced by an explosion
- These injuries result from the **dramatic changes in barometric pressure** projected from the point of detonation
- Primary blast injuries predominantly cause **damage to air filled hollow organs** of the body **from rapid pressure change (barotraumas).**
  - Damage to air filled organs includes **middle ear, lungs & GIT.[Q]**
- **Most sensitive & most frequently injured hollow organ: Tympanic membrane[Q] >Lungs**
- **Blast damage to the lungs** is the **MC cause of life threatening injury[Q]** following an explosion.

Most Severely Affected Organs	Most Commonly Affected Organs
• **Air Blast: Lungs[Q]** • **Underwater: GIT[Q]**	• **Air: Tympanic membrane[Q]** • **Underwater (Fully submerged): TM[Q]** • **Underwater (Head is out): GIT[Q]**

Types of Blast Injuries

Type	Mechanism of Injury	Health Impact
Primary	Rapid, crushing over pressure	• **Damage to hollow organs[Q]** (ears, eyes, lungs, GIT)
Secondary	**Flying debris**	• **Marshall's triad of bruises, abrasions & puncture lacerations are diagnostic[Q]** • Penetrating & blunt trauma injuries
Tertiary	**Blast wind**	• Victim is **thrown in air[Q]** & strikes other objects leading to fracture & blunt trauma
Quaternary	**Any complicating factor not in other three categories**	• Burns, crush injuries, histotoxic anoxia, respiratory problem

---

87. **Ans. d. Hanging** *(Ref: http://ncrb.gov.in/ADSI2014/adsi-2014%20full%20report.pdf)*

According to National Crime Bureau, most common mode of suicide in India is hanging.

National Crime Record Bureau Records

- **Accidental deaths and suicides in India 2014 :** The means adopted for committing suicide varied from the easily available means such as consumption of poison, jumping into the well, etc. to more painful means such as self inflicted injuries, hanging, shooting, etc.

Prominent means of committing suicides	
• **Hanging (41.8%)**	• **Self-Immolation (6.9%)**
• **Consuming Poison (26.0%)**	• **Drowning (5.6%).**

AIIMS ESSENCE

88. **Ans. d.** Neostigmine has a role in krait bite   *(Ref: Parikh 6/e p9.47; Harrison 19/e p2736; Snake Bite: Indian Guidelines and Protocol p 425)*

*Neostigmine is an anticholinesterase, which is **particularly effective in postsynaptic neurotoxins such as those of cobra** and is **not useful against presynaptic neurotoxin, i.e. common krait and the Russell's viper**. Polyvalent Anti-snake venom is ineffective against humpnosed pit viper (Hypnale).*

> *"Role of neostigmine in snake-bite: Neostigmine is an anticholinesterase, which is **particularly effective in postsynaptic neurotoxins such as those of cobra** and is **not useful against presynaptic neurotoxin, i.e. common krait and the Russell's viper.**"*

Feature	Elapids (Cobra, Coral, Krait)	Vipers	Sea Snakes
Type of venom	**Neurotoxic**[Q]	**Vasculotoxic**[Q]	**Myotoxic**[Q]
Site of action	**Motor nerve cells**[Q] & resembles curare	**Endothelial cells & RBC leads to hemolysis**[Q]	**Muscles**[Q]
Local symptoms at site of bite	Minimal	**Severe**[Q] (severe swelling, oozing of blood & cellulites)	Minimal
Clinical presentation	Muscle weakness of legs & face **Cobra** venom produces **convulsions**[Q] **Krait** venom produces only **paralysis**[Q]	Venom causes enzymatic destruction of cell walls & **Coagulation disorder**[Q]	**Generalized muscle pain**, weakness, polymyositis, myoglobinuria[Q]

Management of Snake-bite

- The **three types of venomous snakes** that cause the majority of major clinical problems are **vipers, kraits, and cobras.**
- **Snake identification:** While identifying the species is desirable in certain regions, risking further bites or delaying proper medical treatment by attempting to capture or kill the snake is not recommended.
- **First aid:** Protect the person and others from further bites.
- **Keep the person calm**: Acute stress reaction increases blood flow and endangers the person.
- **Call for help to arrange for transport** to the nearest hospital emergency room, where antivenom for snakes common to the area will often be available.

  > - Make sure to keep the **bitten limb in a functional position and below the person's heart level** so as to minimize blood returning to the heart and other organs of the body.
  > - **Do not give the person anything to eat or drink.** This is especially important with consumable alcohol, a known vasodilator, which will speed up the absorption of venom.

- Do not administer stimulants or pain medications, unless specifically directed to do so by a physician.
- Remove any items or clothing which may constrict the bitten limb if it swells (rings, bracelets, watches, footwear, etc.)
- **Keep the person as still as possible.**
- **Do not incise/suture the bitten site.**
- Pain can be relieved with oral paracetamol or tramadol. **Aspirin or NSAIDs should not be administered.**
- **Handling tourniquets though not recommended**, current practices being followed would see many snakebite victims reaching the emergency with tight tourniquets.

  > - Care must be taken while removing these as sudden removal can lead to a massive surge of venom, leading to paralysis, hypotension, etc.

- Before removal of the tourniquet, check for the presence of pulse distal to it. If it is absent, ensure doctors presence before removal, who should be able to handle complications such as sudden respiratory distress or hypotension. If the tourniquet has occluded the distal pulse, then blood pressure cuff should be applied and pressure should be slowly reduced.
- Clinical evidence for pressure immobilization via the use of elastic bandage is limited.
- **Anti-Snake Venom (ASV) is the mainstay of treatment.**

In India, polyvalent ASV (effective against all the four common species)	
Russell's viper	**Common krait**
Common cobra	**Saw-scaled viper**

| AIIMS November 2015 | | 1315 |

Contd...

Management of Snake-bite
• **No monovalent ASVs are available.**
• **Polyvalent ASV is ineffective against humpnosed pit viper (Hypnale)**
• Although some people may develop serious adverse reactions to antivenom, such as anaphylaxis, in emergency situations this is usually treatable and hence the benefit outweighs the potential consequences of not using antivenom.
• Giving **adrenaline to prevent adverse effect to antivenom before they occur** might be reasonable where they occur commonly.
• **Antihistamines do not appear to provide any benefit** in preventing adverse reactions.

PSM

89. **Ans. b. Leishmaniasis**   *(Ref: Park 24/e p812, 23/e p775, 304, 22/e p716-721)*

The given image is of sand fly (hairy body and erect wing). Sandfly is the primary vector of leishmaniasis and pappataci fever.

	Mosquito	Sandfly
Size	4–5 mm	2.5 mm
Color	Black	Yellowish brown
Eggs laid	100–250	40–60
Flight range	2–3 km	200 yards
Life span	2–3 weeks	2 weeks

Sandfly (Phlebotomus)
• **Sandfly** is the **primary vectors of leishmaniasis & pappataci fever[Q]**.
• Viruses carried by sandflies: **Chandipura virus** (cousin of rabies virus)

Species	Acts as vector for
Phlebotamus **argentipes**	• **Kala-Azar[Q]**
Phlebotamus **papatasii**	• **Sandfly fever[Q]**
Phlebotamus **sergenti**	• **Oriental Sore[Q]**

Description of Sandfly	
Adults	• **Adults** are about **1.5–3.0 mm long** and **yellowish in color**, with conspicuous **black eyes, hairy bodies**, wings, & legs[Q].
	• The **oval lanceolate wings** are carried erect on the humped thorax.
	• **Males possess** long prominent genital terminalia known as **claspers. Females** have a pair of **anal recti**.
Distribution	• Found in the **warm countries**
Bites	• **Only female sandfly can bite** in the dwelling at night.
	• It takes shelter during day in holes & crevices in wall, in dark room & store room, etc.
Breeding	• Mostly species are **nocturnal in habit.**
Feeding	• Mostly species are **nocturnal in habit.**
Dispersal	• **Range of flight** is **200 yard** from their breeding places.
Life Span	• Average life of sandfly is about **2 weeks**.

Body of sandfly consists of three parts		
Head	**Thorax**	**Abdomen**
• Head bear a **pair of long & hairy antenna.**	• Thorax bears a **pair of wings & three pair of legs.**	• Abdomen has **ten segments & is covered with hairs**.
• Palpi & proboscis & one pair of **prominent black eyes** are present.	• **Wings are upright** in shape & hairy.	• In the **female, tip of abdomen** is **rounded** while in **male claspers** are **attached to last abdominal segment.**
	• **Second longitudinal vein is branched twice.**	
	• **Legs are long & slender** and **out of proportion** to size of body.	

Contd...

Contd...

Sandfly (Phlebotomus)			
Lifecycle of sandfly			
Egg	**Larva**	**Pupa**	**Adult**
• Female lays eggs in the **damp dark places** in the **cattle sheds & poultry**. • **Number: 40–60** • **Colour: brownish** • **Length: 0.4 mm** • Eggs hatch in **1–2** weeks.	• **Larva is maggot like structure**, having large head, thorax, abdomen & **two long bristle on last abdominal segment**. • Larva feed on decaying organic matter & **become a pupa in about 2 weeks**.	• **Pupa** is found **in cracks & cervices** in the wall. • Pupa stage lasts for about **1 week**.	• **Average life span** of a sandfly is **2 weeks**.

Control Measures:

• Sandflies are **easily controlled** because they **do not move long distance from their breeding places**.
• **Insecticide: Lindane** has been proved effective.
• **Sanitation:** Removal of shrubs & vegetation, filling of cracks & crevices in the wall & floor and distance of cattle sheds & poultry from human habitations.

Visceral Leishmaniasis (VL)

• It is a **systemic protozoan disease** that is **transmitted by phlebotomine sandflies^Q**.
• **Vector: Female phelebotomine sandflies^Q**
• **Incubation period: 2-6 months**

Leishmaniasis	
Types	**Causative agent**
Visceral	• Leishmania **donovani**^{Q}
Cutaneous	• Leishmania **tropica**^{Q}
Mucocutaneous	• Leishmania **braziliensis**^{Q}

Epidemiology:

• **Poor & neglected populations in East Africa & Indian subcontinent** are particularly affected.

Lifecycle:

• **Promastigote of form of L.donovani is transmitted into the skin by female phlebotomine sandfies^Q**.
• Once transmitted, the **parasites are internalized by dendritic cells & macrophages** in the dermis where they **lose their flagella, transforming into the amastigote from^Q**.
• **Amastigotes multiply**, destroy the host cell & **infect other phagocytic cells**.
• **Amastigotes disseminate through lymphatic & vascular systems**, eventually **infiltrating bone marrow, liver & spleen^Q**.

Clinical features:

• **Symptoms & signs of persistent systemic infection**: Fever, fatigue, weakness, anorexia & weight loss

> • **Parasitic invasion of blood & reticuloendothelial system: Enlarged lymph nodes & hepatosplenomegaly^Q**
> • **Fever (intermittent)** is usually associated with **rigor & chills^Q**

• **Fatigue & weakness** are worsened by **anaemia**, which is by the **persistent inflammatory state, hypersplenism** (the peripheral destruction of erythrocytes in the enlarged spleen) and sometimes by bleeding.

> • **Hyperpigmentation**, which probably led to the **name kala-azar** (black fever in hindi), has only been described in VL patients from the Indian subcontinent, but today **this symptom is uncommon^Q**.

Contd...

Contd...

Visceral Leishmaniasis (VL)
Diagnosis: • **Gold standard for diagnosis**: **Demonstration of amastigotes in smears of tissue aspirates** is the gold standard for the diagnosis of VL[Q].   • **Sensitivity of splenic smears is >95%,** whereas smears of **bone marrow (60–85%)** and **lymph node aspirates (50%)** are less sensitive.
• A rapid immunochromatographic test based on detection of antibodies to a recombinant antigen (**rK39**) consisting of 39 amino acids conserved in kinesin region of L. infantum is used worldwide.   • Test **requires only a drop of fingerprick blood or serum** & result can be **read within 15 min.**   • Except in East Africa (where both its sensitivity and its specificity are lower), **sensitivity of the rK39 rapid diagnostic test (RdT) in immunocompetent individuals is ~98%** and its **specificity is 90%**[Q].   • **In Sudan**, an RdT based on a new synthetic polyprotein, **rK28**, was **more sensitive (96.8%) & specific (96.2%) than rK39-based RdTs**[Q].
Treatment: • **First-line treatment for VL: Pentavalent antimonials sodium stibogluconate & meglumine antimoniate**[Q]   • **Antimonials are toxic drugs** with frequent adverse side effects, including **cardiac arrhythmia & acute pancreatitis**[Q].   • **Miltefosine**, which was initially developed as **an anticancer drug** is the **first effective oral drug for VL**[Q].

90. **Ans. d. Leprosy** *(Ref: Park 24/e p339, 23/e p322, 22/e p297; Neena Khanna 4/e p267)*
The given image is of multibacillary adult blister pack, which is used in multibacillary leprosy.

"WHO has designed blister pack medication kits for both paucibacillary leprosy and for multibacillary leprosy. Each easy to use kit contains medication for 28 days. The blister pack medication kit for single lesion paucibacillary leprosy contains the necessary medication for the one time administration of the 3 medications."

"Any patient with a positive skin smear must be treated with the MDT regimen for multibacillary leprosy. The regimen for paucibacillary leprosy should never be given to a patient with multibacillary leprosy. Therefore, if the diagnosis in a particular patient is uncertain, treat that patient with the MDT regimen for multibacillary leprosy."

91. **Ans. c. Japanese encephalitis virus** *(Ref: Park 24/e p302, 23/e p284, 22/e p260; Ananthanarayan 10/e p527, 8/e p513-514)*
It is clear from the given diagram below that the lifecycle given in the question is that of Japanese Encephalitis Virus. Humans are dead end and incidental hosts in the lifecycle of these viruses.

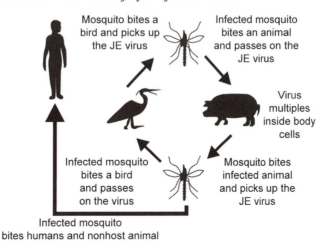

Fig. 29: Cycle of Japanese Encephalitis

Japanese Encephalitis

- It is a **zoonotic disease**[Q].
- **Causative agent: Group B Arbovirus (Flavivirus)**[Q]
- **Incubation period: 5-15 days (in man);** 9-12 days (in mosquito)
- **Case fatality rate:** 20-40%.

Epidemiology: Cycle **(Pig → mosquito → Pig)**[Q], (Pond heron →Mosquito → Pond heron)[Q]
- **Man** is **incidental dead end host** without human to human transmission[Q]
- **Pig is the amplifier**[Q] **host.**

- **Only animal which show encephalitis sign/symptom is horse**[Q].
- **Vector: Culex tritaeniorhynchus (most important)**[Q], **C. Vishnui**[Q], C. Gelidus
- **Gorakhpur** district of UP contributes to **largest no of cases**[Q].

- **85%** cases of JE are reported in **age <15 years (JE is infrequent in infancy**[Q])
- **Endemicity of JE in India: 1-2 cases per village**[Q]

Japanese Encephalitis Vaccine

Routine Japanese Encephalitis vaccination:

- Recommended only for **individuals living in endemic areas**
- The vaccine should be offered to the **children residing in rural areas only** and those **planning to visit endemic areas** (depending upon the duration of stay).

Types of Japanese Encephalitis Vaccine

Live attenuated, Cell Culture Derived Vaccine	Inactivated Cell Culture Derived	Mouse Brain Derived Inactivated Vaccine
- **Strain: SA-14-14-2 strain**[Q] - Minimum age: **8 months**[Q] - **Two dose schedule**, first dose at 9 months along with measles vaccine and second at 16 to 18 months along with DPT booster	- **Strain: Beijing P3 strain**[Q] - **Minimum age: 1 year** (US-FDA: **2 months**)[Q] - Primary immunization schedule: **2 doses** of 0.25ml each administered IM on days 0 and 28 for children **aged ≥ 1 to ≤ 3 years**[Q] - **2 doses of 0.5 ml for children >3 years** and adults aged **≥ 18 years**[Q]	- **Strain: Nakayama strain, Beijing strain**[Q] - **2 primary doses** 4 weeks apart, **booster after 1 year** and **3 years** until the age of 10-15 years - **Dose: 0.5 ml for children <3 years (1 ml for >3 years)**[Q] - **Route: Subcutaneous**[Q] - Vaccine is **most useful in interepidemic period**[Q] - **Pre-exposure prophylaxis: 3 primary doses** on day 0, 7, 28 (or 2 primary doses 4 weeks apart) - **Booster after 1 year** and **then repeated every 3 years**[Q]

Catch-up Vaccination

- **All susceptible children up to 15 years**[Q] **should** be administered **during disease outbreak/ ahead of anticipated outbreak in campaigns.**

---

92. **Ans. b. 1-Normal distribution, 2- Negative skewed, 3- Positive skewed** *(Ref: http://www.physics.csbsju.edu/stats/box2.html)*

Positive or negative skewed data is defined by the direction of the tail, i.e. direction of the least frequency values. Similarly in this box plot we can see that the data is equally distributed on either sides of the mean box in Plot (1). In Plot (2), the median is towards the higher side and most values are distributed towards the higher side hence it is negatively skewed. And similarly vice versa for Plot (3).

Distribution		
Symmetric	**Skewed right (positive)**	**Skewed left (negative)**
- **Mean = Median**[Q] - **Tail** of the distribution **is in centre**[Q].	- **Mean > Median**[Q] - **Tail** of the distribution on **right hand (positive) side** is **longer than on left hand side**[Q]. - **Median is closer to first quartile** than third quartile[Q].	- **Mean < Median**[Q] - **Tail** of the distribution is **longer on left hand side** than on right hand side[Q]. - **Median is closer to third quartile** than to first [Q]uartile[Q].

Contd...

Distribution

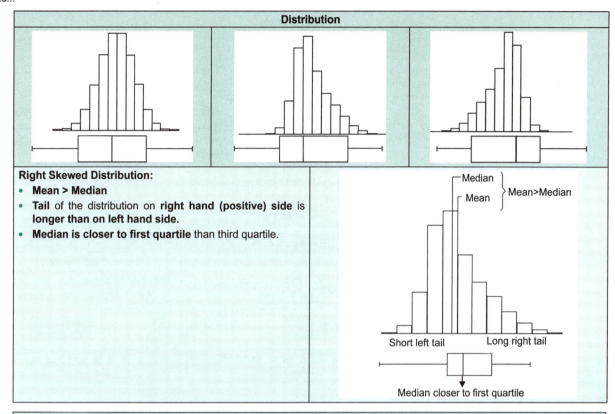

Right Skewed Distribution:
- **Mean > Median**
- **Tail** of the distribution on **right hand (positive) side** is **longer than on left hand side**.
- **Median is closer to first quartile** than third quartile.

Boxplot

- **A boxplot splits the data set into quartiles.**
- The **body of the boxplot consists of a 'box'** (hence, the name), which goes from the **first quartile (Q1) to the third quartile (Q3).**
- Within the box, a **vertical line is drawn at the Q2, the median of the data set**.
- **Two horizontal lines**, called **whiskers**, extend from the front & back of box.

Front whisker	Back whisker
• Front whisker goes **from Q1 to smallest non-outlier** in the data set	• Back whisker goes **from Q3 to largest non-outlier**

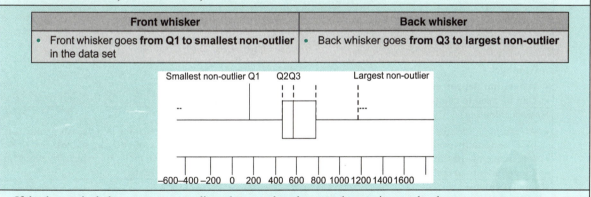

- If the data set includes one or more outliers, they are plotted separately as points on the chart.
- In the boxplot above, two outliers precede the first whisker; and three outliers follow the second whisker.
- Median is indicated by the vertical line that runs down the center of the box. In the boxplot above, the median is about 400.
- Additionally, **boxplots display two common measures of the variability** or **spread in a data set**.

Contd...

Contd...

Boxplot	
Range	**Interquartile range (IQR)**
• If you are interested in the spread of all the data, it is represented on a boxplot by the horizontal distance between the smallest value and the largest value, including any outliers. • In the boxplot above, data values range from about -700 (the smallest outlier) to 1700 (the largest outlier), so the range is 2400. • If you ignore outliers, the **range is illustrated by the distance between the opposite ends of the whiskers** — about 1000 in the boxplot above.	• The middle half of a data set falls within the interquartile range. • In a boxplot, the **interquartile range is represented by the width of the box (Q3 minus Q1)**. • In the chart above, the interquartile range is equal to 600 minus 300 or about 300.

• **Boxplots provide information about the shape of a data set**.

Examples of Boxplot		
Symmetric	**Skewed right (positive)**	**Skewed left (negative)**
• Observations evenly split at the median	• Most of observations are concentrated on lower end of scale	• Most of observations are concentrated on higher end of scale
2 4 6 8 10 12 14 16 Symmetric	2 4 6 8 10 12 14 16 Skewed right	2 4 6 8 10 12 14 16 Skewed left

93. Ans. c. 0.6 *(Ref: Park 24/e p889, 23/e p852)*
Coefficient of correlation is given by the slope of the graph, since the slope of all four populations are same i.e. 0.6, overall correlation coefficient will remain as 0.6.

Correlation Coefficient (*r*)
• The quantity **r**, called the **linear correlation coefficient, measures the strength and the direction of a linear relationship between two variables**. • The **linear correlation coefficient** is sometimes referred to as the **Pearson product moment correlation coefficient** in honor of its developer Karl Pearson.
Formula of Correlation Coefficient (*r*) 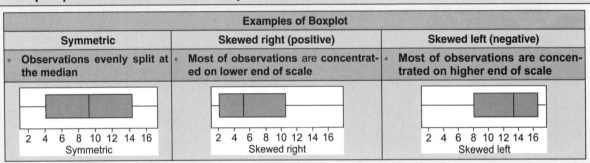

Advantage:
• **It does not depend on the units of X & Y** • **Can be used to compare any two variables regardless of their units.**
How to calculate?
• An essential first step in calculating a correlation coefficient is **to plot the observations in a "scattergram" or "scatter plot"** to visually evaluate the data for a potential relationship or the presence of outlying values. • It is frequently possible to visualize a smooth curve through the data and thereby identify the type of relationship present. • **Independent variable is plotted on X-axis, dependent variable is plotted on Y-axis.**
Range of values:
• **Pearson's Correlation Coefficient (r) has a value of between –1 and +1.**

Interpretation	
–1	**+1**
• **Strong negative correlation**	• **Strong positive correlation**

Contd...

Contd...

Positive correlation	No correlation	Negative correlation
• If **x & y have a strong positive linear correlation**, r is close to + 1[Q]. • **An r value of exactly +1 indicates a perfect positive fit**[Q]. • Positive values indicate a relationship between x and y variables such that as values for x increases, values for y also increase.	• If there is **no linear correlation** or a **weak linear correlation**, r is close to 0[Q]. • A value near zero means that there is a random, nonlinear relationship between the two variables.	• If **x & y have a strong negative linear correlation**, r is close to –1[Q]. • **An r value of exactly –1 indicates a perfect negative fit**[Q]. • Negative values indicate a relationship between x and y such that as values for x increase, values for y decrease.
r = 0.4 Positive Correlation	r = 0 No Correlation	r = –0.4 Negative

94. Ans. a. Stem and leaf diagram   *(Ref: https://en.wikipedia.org/wiki/Stem-and-leaf_display)*

The type of data description given is Stem and Leaf Plot.

Stem and Leaf Plot

- **Stem and Leaf Plot** is a special table where **each data value is split into a 'stem'** (**the first digit or digits**) and a **'leaf'** (**usually the last digit**).
- A **stem-and-leaf display** is a **device for presenting quantitative data in a graphical format, similar to a histogram, to assist in visualizing the shape of a distribution**.
- A basic stem-and-leaf display contains two columns separated by a vertical line.
- The left column contains the stems and the right column contains the leaves.

Advantages	Disadvantages
• **Stem-and-leaf displays** are **useful for displaying the relative density** and **shape of the data**, giving the reader a **quick overview of distribution**. • They **retain (most of) the raw numerical data, often with perfect integrity**. • They are also **useful for highlighting outliers and finding the mode**.	• **Only useful for moderately sized data sets** (around 15–150 data points). • With **very small data** sets a **stem- and-leaf displays can be of little use**. A dot plot may be better suited for such data. • With **very large data sets**, a stem-and-leaf display will **become very cluttered**. A box plot or histogram may become more appropriate as the data size increases.

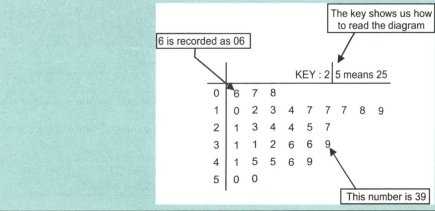

Box Plot

- A **box plot** is a convenient way of **graphically depicting groups of numerical data through their quartiles.**
- Box plots may also have lines extending vertically from the boxes (whiskers) indicating variability outside the upper and lower quartiles, hence the terms **box-and-whisker plot** and **box-and-whisker diagram**. Outliers may be plotted as individual points.

  - **Box plots are non-parametric:** they **display variation in samples of a statistical population without making any assumptions of the underlying statistical distribution.**
  - The **spacing between the different parts of the box indicate the degree of dispersion** (spread) and **skewness in the data**, and **show outliers.**

- In addition to the points themselves, they a**llow one to visually estimate various L-estimators, notably the interquartile range, mid-hinge, range, mid-range, and tri-mean.**
- Boxplots can be drawn either horizontally or vertically.

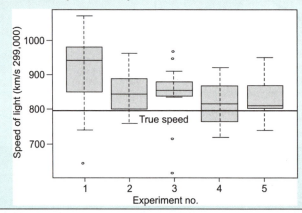

Funnel plot

- A **funnel plot** is a **graph designed to check for the existence of publication bias**.
- Funnel plots are **commonly used in systematic reviews** and **meta-analyses**.
- In the absence of publication bias, it assumes that the **largest studies will be plotted near the average**, and **smaller studies will be spread evenly on both sides of the average,** creating a **roughly funnel-shaped distribution.**
- **Deviation from this shape can indicate publication bias**.

An example funnel plot showing no publication bias.
Each dot represents a study (measuring the effect of a certain drug)
y-axis: Size of the study (number of experimental subjects)
x-axis: Show the study's (drug's measured average effect)

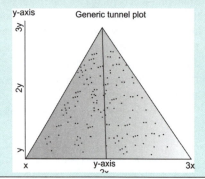

Forest plot

- A **forest plot**, also known as a **blobbogram**, is a **graphical display of estimated results from a number of scientific studies addressing the same question, along with the overall results.**
- It was developed for **use in medical research** as a means of **graphically representing a meta-analysis of the results of randomized controlled trials.**
- In the last twenty years, similar meta-analytical techniques have been applied in observational studies (e.g. environmental epidemiology) and forest plots are often used in presenting the results of such studies also.
- Although forest plots can take several forms, they are **commonly presented with two columns**.

Contd...

Contd...

Forest plot

- The **left-hand column lists the names of the studies** (frequently randomized controlled trials or epidemiological studies), **commonly in chronological order from the top downwards.**
- The **right-hand column** is a **plot of the measure of effect** (e.g. an odds ratio) **for each of these studies** (often represented by a square) **incorporating confidence intervals represented by horizontal lines.**
- The graph may be plotted on a natural logarithmic scale when using odds ratios or other ratio-based effect measures, so that the confidence intervals are symmetrical about the means from each study and to ensure undue emphasis is not given to odds ratios greater than 1 when compared to those less than 1.
- The **area of each square is proportional to the study's weight in the meta-analysis.**
- The overall meta-analyzed measure of effect is often represented on the plot as a dashed vertical line. This meta-analyzed measure of effect is commonly plotted as a diamond, the lateral points of which indicate confidence intervals for this estimate.
- A vertical line representing no effect is also plotted. If the confidence intervals for individual studies overlap with this line, it demonstrates that at the given level of confidence their effect sizes do not differ from no effect for the individual study.
- The **same applies for the meta-analyzed measure of effect: if the points of the diamond overlap the line of no effect the overall meta-analyzed result cannot be said to differ from no effect at the given level of confidence.**

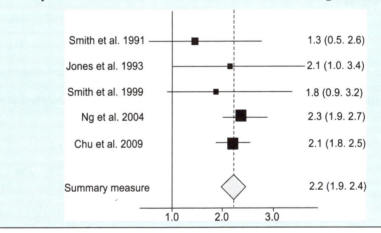

95. Ans. a. Sensitivity 90%, Specificity 95%   *(Ref: Park's 24/e p149, 23/e p125, 22/e p131)*

*"The term **sensitivity** was introduced as a **statistical index of diagnostic accuracy**. It has been defined as the **ability of a test to identify correctly all those who have the disease, that is 'true positive'.**"*

*"**Specificity** measures the proportion of negatives that are correctly identified as such, e.g., the **percentage of healthy people who are correctly identified as not having the condition, that is true negative.**"*

Assessment & Value of A Diagnostic Test		Condition Present	Condition Absent
	Positive Test	a (True positive)	b (False positive)
	Negative Test	c (False negative)	d (True negative)

Sensitivity	Proportion of persons with the condition who test positive: a/(a + c)[Q]
Specificity	Proportion of persons without the condition who test negative: d/(b + d)[Q]
Positive predictive value (PPV)	Proportion of persons with a positive test who have the condition: a/(a + b)[Q]
Negative predictive value (NPV)	Proportion of persons with a negative test who do not have the condition: d/(c + d)[Q]

Contd...

Contd...

Assessment & Value of A Diagnostic Test
Predictive Value
• **Prevalence, sensitivity, and specificity determine predictive value**[Q]   • **PPV** = Prevalence × Sensitivity/(Prevalence × Sensitivity) + (1 − Prevalence)(1 − Specificity)[Q]   • **NPV** = (1 − Prevalence)(Specificity)/(1 − Prevalence) (Specificity) + (1 − Sensitivity) (Prevalence)[Q]
In this 2 × 2 distribution, from the table

	Test Positive	Test Negative
Diseases	a (True positive): 27	b (False positive): 3
Non-diseased	c (False negative): 5	d (True negative): 95

- Sensitivity = **Proportion of persons with the condition who test positive: a /(a + c)**[Q] = 27/30 = **90%**
- Specificity = **Proportion of persons without the condition who test negative: d /(b + d)**[Q] = 95/100 = **95%**

96. Ans. d. Venn diagram *(Ref: https://en.wikipedia.org/wiki/Venn_diagram)*

A Venn diagram is an easy tool to make people understand overlapping risk factors, complications and comorbidities to a patient in a simple language.

Venn Diagram
• **Venn diagram** (also known as a **set diagram** or **logic diagram**) is a diagram that shows **all possible logical relations between finite collections of different sets.**   • They are **used to teach elementary set theory**, as well as **illustrate simple set relationships in probability, logic, statistics, linguistics & computer science.**   • **Complex connections are represented with the help of this diagram, so use it when learning gets more difficult**   • **An Example**:

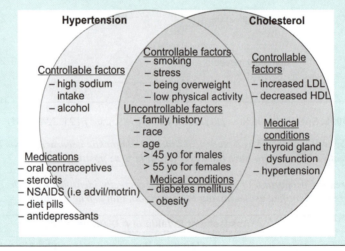

97. Ans. a. Clinical trial *(Ref: Park 24/e p80, 24/e p86; 23/e p75)*

Among the given options, clinical trial is the best study to evaluate effect and outcome.

"Randomized control trial (Experimental study or Intervention study): The randomized control trial is considered as the ideal design to evaluate the effectiveness and the side-effects of new forms of intervention."

"Cohort Study: A study design where one or more samples (called cohorts) are followed prospectively and subsequent status evaluations with respect to a disease or outcome are conducted to determine which initial participants exposure characteristics (risk factors) are associated with it. As the study is conducted, outcome from participants in each cohort is measured and relationships with specific characteristics determined."

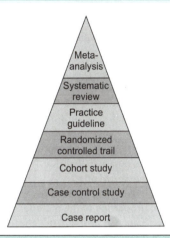

Evidence-Pyramid in Research (From top to bottom)[Q]
• Meta-analysis (Highest clinical relevance: Gold standard[Q])
• Systematic review[Q]
• Cohort study[Q]
• Case control study[Q]
• Case series[Q]
• Case report[Q]
• Ideas, Editorials, Opinions[Q]
• Animal research
• In-vitro (test-tube) research (Lowest clinical relevance[Q])

Types of Epidemiological Studies	
Observational studies[Q]	**Experimental studies (Hypothesis confirmation)[Q]**
• Descriptive studies (Hypothesis formulation[Q]) • Analytical studies (Hypothesis testing[Q])	

Analytical studies	
Type	**Unit**
Cohort study	Individual
Case control study	Individual
Cross sectional study	Individual
Ecological study	Population[Q]

Experimental studies	
Type	**Unit**
Randomized controlled trial	Patients[Q]
Field trial	Healthy people
Community trial	Community
Clinical trial	Patients

See Q. No. AIIMS November 2016

98. **Ans. b. Sampling distribution** *(Ref: Research Methods For Communication Science James H. Watt; http://ciosmail.cios.org:3375/readbook/rmcs/ch09.pdf; Kothari Research methodology p155)*

When a researcher selected all possible samples from a population and plotted their means on a line graph. This distribution is called as sampling distribution.

"In statistics, a sampling distribution or finite-sample distribution is the probability distribution of a given statistic based on a random sample. They allow analytical considerations to be based on the sampling distribution of a statistic, rather than on the joint probability distribution of all the individual sample values."

Types of Distribution		
Sample Distribution	**Population Distribution**	**Sampling Distribution**
• A sample distribution is an **observed distribution of the values** that **a variable is observed to have** for a sample of individuals.	• A population distribution is a **theoretical distribution of the values** that **a variable can take on** in a population of individuals. • Example: Normal & binomial	• A sampling distribution is a **theoretical distribution of the values** that a **specified statistic of a sample takes on in all of the possible samples of a specific size** that can be made from a given population.

AIIMS ESSENCE

99. Ans. a. 8–15 °C *(Ref: Park 22/e p100)*

Some medicines come with label of 'store at a cool place only'. These medicines should be kept at 8–15 °C.

Definitions of Storage Conditions of Drugs as per Ip 6 (Indian Pharmacopoeia 1996)	
Cold	• Any temperature not exceeding **8°C** and usually between **2–8°C**. A **refrigerator** is a cold place in which the temperature is maintained thermostatically between **2–8°C**.
Cool	• Any temperature between **8–25°C**.
	• An article, for which storage in a cool place is directed may alternately, be stored in a refrigerator unless otherwise specified in the individual monograph.
Room Temperature	• The temperature prevailing in a **working area**.
Warm	• Any temperature between **30-40°C**.
Excessive heat	• Any temperature **above 40°C**.
Light resistant containers	• A light-resistant container **protect the content from the effect of actinic light by virtue of the specific properties of the material** of which it is made.
Well closed container	• A well-closed container **protects the contents from contamination by extraneous liquid & from loss of the article** under normal condition of handling, shipment, storage & distribution.
Tightly closed containers	• A tightly closed container **protects the contents from contamination by extraneous liquid & solids or vapor, from loss or deterioration of the article from effervescence**, deliquescent or evaporation under normal condition of handling, shipment, storage & distribution.

"Humidity: When product labels say 'protect from moisture', store the product in a space with no more than 60% relative humidity."

"Store frozen: Some products, such as certain vaccines, need to be transported within a cold chain and stored at –20 °C (4 °F). Frozen storage is normally for longer-term storage at higher-level facilities."

100. Ans. b. 110 mm Hg *(Ref: Park 24/e p886)*

Confidence Intervals
C = Confidence coefficient
= **1 for 68%** confidence interval
= **1.96 for 95%** confidence interval
= **2.58 for 99%** confidence interval
= **3.29 for 99.9%** confidence interval

- This implies that **95% of population** is covered between **Mean –2 SD to Mean + 2 SD**.
- About 2.5% population will have a value less than Mean –2 SD (i.e. half of 5% on either sides.)
- In this question, **Mean = 125**
- **SD = 10**
- **Mean–2SD = 105 mm Hg**
- **Mean–1SD = 115 mm Hg**
- Hence, **97.5% population** will have a **BP of more than 105 mm Hg** and about **84%** will have a **BP above 115** mm Hg. Extrapolating, **95% of the population** will have a **BP above around 110 mm Hg**.

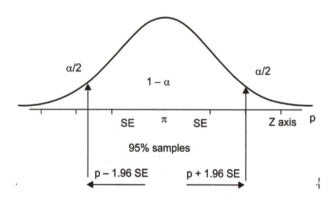

AIIMS November 2015

101. Ans. a. Increased prevalence *(Ref: Park 24/e p66, 23/e p61, 22/e p59)*

A drug, which does not cure a disease but decreases its symptoms and increases survival, means its leads to increased duration of disease and increased prevalence.

Prevalence = No. of total (old + new) cases of a disease in a year/Total population × 100
Prevalence = Incidence × Mean duration of disease

"Prevalence is the proportion of a population that has a condition at a specific time, but the prevalence will be influenced by both the rate at which new cases are occurring and the average duration of the disease. Incidence reflects the rate at which new cases of disease are being added to the population (and becoming prevalent cases). Average duration of disease is also important, because the only way you can stop being a prevalent case is to be cured or to move out of the population or die."

Prevalence
• Prevalence is the total current (Old+ new) cases in a given population over a point or period of time[Q].
• Types: Point prevalence (at a point of time) & Period prevalence (over a period of time)[Q]
Prevalence = No. of total (old + new) cases of a disease in a year/Total population x 100[Q]
• Prevalence is a proportion, not a ratio: Numerator is a part of denominator, and is always expressed in percentage.
• Prevalence can be determined from cross-sectional study[Q].

Relation between Incidence & Prevalence
• Given the assumption that **population is stable & incidence and duration are not changing.**
• **Prevalence = Incidence × Mean duration of disease**[Q]
• **Prevalence describes balance between incidence, mortality and recovery**[Q].
• **Incidence reflects causal factors**[Q].
• **Duration reflects prognostic factors**[Q]

102. Ans. d. Increases external validity of the trial *(Ref: Park 24/e p87, 23/e p82, 22/e p79)*

External validity is the validity of generalized (causal) inferences in scientific research, usually based on experiments as experimental validity. In other words, it is the extent to which the results of a study can be generalized to other situations and to other people. This cannot be ensured by randomization.

Randomization
• **Randomization** is a **statistical procedure by which participants are allocated into two groups, experimental & reference group**[Q].
• Randomization is **best done by random number tables**[Q].

Essential Purposes of Randomization in RCT
• Participants have **equal & known chance of falling into either experimental group** or **reference group**[Q]
• To **eliminate selection bias**[Q]
• To **ensure comparability among groups**[Q]
• To have **similar prognostic factors among two groups**[Q]

• Randomization is known as '**heart of a trial**'[Q].
• **Randomization removes both confounding & bias**[Q].
• **Randomization is superior to matching: Randomization ensures both known and unknown confounding factors are distributed equally among the two groups**, thereby **nullifying their effect on result**, whereas matching is useful for only known confounding factors[Q].

Validity and Reliability
• **Validity** refers to **what degree the research reflects the given research problem.**
• **Reliability** refers to **how consistent a set of measurements are.**
• **Validity** is also known as **accuracy and is measured in terms of sensitivity and specificity of a test.**

Contd...

Contd...

Validity and Reliability

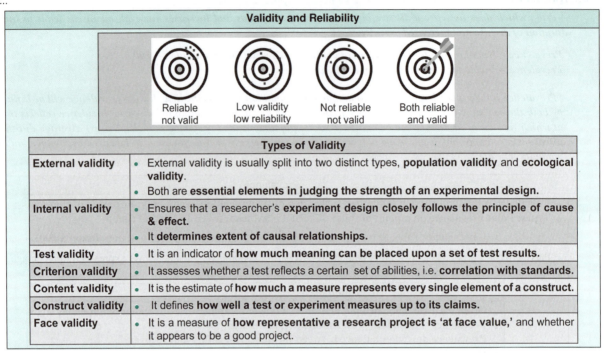

Types of Validity	
External validity	• External validity is usually split into two distinct types, **population validity** and **ecological validity**. • Both are **essential elements in judging the strength of an experimental design.**
Internal validity	• Ensures that a researcher's **experiment design closely follows the principle of cause & effect.** • It **determines extent of causal relationships.**
Test validity	• It is an indicator of **how much meaning can be placed upon a set of test results.**
Criterion validity	• It assesses whether a test reflects a certain set of abilities, i.e. **correlation with standards.**
Content validity	• It is the estimate of **how much a measure represents every single element of a construct.**
Construct validity	• It defines **how well a test or experiment measures up to its claims.**
Face validity	• It is a measure of **how representative a research project is 'at face value,'** and whether it appears to be a good project.

103. **Ans. a. Cashless benefit on presenting smartcard and fingerprints** *(Ref: http://www.rsby.gov.in/about_rsby.aspx)*

Rashtriya Swasthya Bima Yojana (RSBY) is a government- run health insurance scheme for the Indian poor. It provides for cashless insurance for hospitalization in public as well as private hospitals.

"Rashtriya Swasthya Bima Yojana provide health insurance coverage for Below Poverty Line (BPL) families. Objective is to provide protection to BPL households from financial liabilities arising out of health shocks that involve hospitalization."

Rashtriya Swasthya Bima Yojana

• Also known as **National Health Insurance Scheme (NHIS)**
• **Rashtriya Swasthya Bima Yojana** or RSBY started rolling from **1st April 2008.**
• Government sponsored scheme **for the BPL population of India**^{Q}
    – **Rs. 600 (75%) by Central government**^{Q}
    – **Rs. 200 (25%) by State government**^{Q}
• Government of India contribution is 90% in case of North-eastern states & Jammu and Kashmir
• **Launched by Ministry of Labour and Employment**, Government of India.
    • Provide health insurance coverage for **Below Poverty Line (BPL) families**^{Q}.

Objective: • To **provide protection to BPL households from financial liabilities** arising out of **health shocks** that involves **hospitalization**^{Q}.
Beneficiaries: • Beneficiaries under RSBY are entitled to **hospitalization coverage up to Rs. 30,000 per family per year** for hospitalization in public and private hospitals • Cover in case of **death of a family member: Rs. 25,000/-**^{Q} • **Pre-existing conditions** are **covered from day one** and there is **no age limit.** • **Coverage extends to five members of the family,** which includes the **head** of household, **spouse** and **up to three dependents**^{Q}.   • **Beneficiaries need to pay** only **Rs. 30/-** as **registration fee** while **Central** and **State Government pays** the **premium** to the insurer selected by the State Government on the basis of a competitive bidding.

AIIMS November 2015

104. Ans. a. JSSK *(Ref: Park 24/e p476, 23/e p456, 22/e p420; http://nrhm.gov.in/janani-shishu-suraksha-karyakram.html)*

A recently delivered woman with a 15 days old child suffering from cough, sneezing and fever needs help. She has no money for transportation to nearby hospital. Janani Shishu Suraksha Karyakaram (JSSK), the national programme can help this woman.

Janani-Shishu Suraksha Karyakram (JSSK):

- The initiative entitles all pregnant women delivering in public health institutions to **absolutely free and no expense to delivery,** including cesarean section.
- The entitlements include **free drugs and consumables, free diet up to 3 days during normal delivery and up to 7 days for cesarean section, free diagnostics, and free blood** wherever required.
- This initiative also provides for **free transport from home to institution,** between facilities in case of referral and drop back home.
- Similar entitlements have been put in place for **all sick newborns accessing public health institutions for treatment till 30 days after birth.**
- This has been **expanded to cover sick infants**
- The scheme aims to **eliminate out of pocket expenses incurred by the pregnant women and sick new borns** while accessing services at Government health facilities.

Janani-Shishu Suraksha Karyakram (JSSK)	
Pregnant women components	**Child health components**
• **Free deliveries**^{Q} (including caesarean section) in public health institutions • **Free drugs and consumables**^{Q} • **Free diet**^{Q} (Normal delivery: 3 days; Caesarean section: 7 days) • **Free diagnostics**^{Q} • **Free blood transfusion**^{Q} (whenever required) • **Free transport**^{Q} from home to institution	• Nutritional rehabilitation centres (NRCs): **Inpatient treatment of severely malnourished children and counselling of mothers on proper feeding** • Integrated management of neonatal and childhood illnesses (IMNCI): **Management of common childhood illnesses** • Pre-service IMNCI: **Included in medical curriculum to generate trained IMNCI manpower** • Facility based IMNCI (F-IMNCI): **Focus on inpatient management of major causes of neonatal and childhood mortality, viz. asphyxia, sepsis, low birth weight, pneumonia, diarrhoea, malaria, meningitis and severe** malnutrition^Q

Facility based newborn care		
Health facility	**All new-borns at birth**	**Sick newborns**
MCH level I: PHC, Subcentre	Newborn care corner **(NBCC)** in labour room	**Prompt referral**
MCH level II: CHC, First referral unit (FRU)	**NBCC in labour room & operation theatre**	**Newborn stabilization unit** (NBSU)
MCH level III: District hospital	**NBCC in labour room & operation theatre**	**Special newborn care unit** (SNCU)

- **Newborn care corner (NBCC): Space within delivery room for immediate care to newborns mandatory for all health facilities**
- **Newborn stabilization unit (NBSU): Facility within or near maternity ward where sick and low birth weight newborns can be cared for short periods**
  - Location: CHCs, FRUs
  - Space required: 4 bedded unit and 2 beds for post-natal ward for rooming-in
- **Special newborn care unit (SNCU): Neonatal unit near labour room to provide special care for sick newborns (EXCEPT assisted ventilation, major surgery)**
  - Location: District hospitals, Sub-district hospitals having >3000 deliveries per year
  - Space required: 12 bedded unit and 4 additional beds for adult step-down

Contd...

Contd...

Janani-Shishu Suraksha Karyakram (JSSK)		
Triage of Sick Newborns		
Emergency signs	**Priority signs**	**Non-urgent signs**
• **Hypothermia** (<36ºC) • **Apnoea, gasping** • **Severe respiratory distress** • **Central cyanosis** • **Shock** • **Coma, convulsions** • Encephalopathy	• Cold stress • Respiratory distress • Irritable/ restless/ jittery • Abdominal distension • Severe jaundice • Severe pallor • Bleeding from other sites • Major congenital malformation • Weight <1.8 or >4.0 kg	• Transitional stools • Posseting • Minor birth trauma • Superficial infections • Minor malformations • Jaundice • All other cases
Initiate emergency treatment	**Assess & act rapidly**	**Assess & counsel**

- **Home-based newborn care (HBNC):**
  - **Main person involved: ASHA**
  - Other health personnel involved: ANM, Anganwadi worker, Medical officer
  - **ASHA 6 visits in Institutional deliveries:** Day 3, 7, 14, 21, 28, 42
  - **ASHA 7 visits in Homebased deliveries:** Day 1, 3, 7, 14, 21, 28, 42
  - **Other functions of ASHA (Paid Rs. 250/-):**
    - Record birth weight
    - BCG, OPV, DPT to newborn
    - Birth registration
    - Mother/newborn safety till 42nd day

105. **Ans. c. Primaquine is contraindicated in infants and pregnant women** *(Ref: Harrison 19/e p1383; http://nvbdcp.gov.in/ Doc/Diagnosis-Treatment-Malaria-2013.pdf)*

Primaquine is contraindicated during pregnancy and in lactation unless the infant being breast-fed has a documented normal G6PD level.

"Primaquine is contraindicated in persons with G6PD deficiency. It is also contraindicated during pregnancy and in lactation unless the infant being breast-fed has a documented normal G6PD level." – Harrison 19/e p1383.

"Primaquine is used to prevent relapse but is contraindicated in pregnant women, infants and individuals with G6PD deficiency." - http://nvbdcp.gov.in/Doc/Diagnosis-Treatment-Malaria-2013.pdf.

"P. falciparum cases should be treated with ACT (Artesunate 3 days + Sulfadoxine Pyrimethamine 1 day). This is to be accompanied by single dose primaquine preferably on day 2." – http://nvbdcp.gov.in/Doc/Diagnosis-Treatment-Malaria-2013.pdf

"In cases where parasitological diagnosis is not possible due to non-availability of either timely microscopy or RdT, suspected malaria cases will be treated with full course of chloroquine, till the results of microscopy are received. Once the parasitological diagnosis is available, appropriate treatment as per the species, is to be administered. Presumptive treatment with chloroquine is no more recommended." – http://nvbdcp.gov.in/Doc/Diagnosis-Treatment-Malaria-2013. pdf

Treatment of Uncomplicated Malaria

- It is stressed that **all fever cases should be suspected of malaria after ruling out other common causes** and **should be investigated for confirmation of malaria by Microscopy or Rapid Diagnostic Kit (RdK)** so as to ensure treatment with full therapeutic dose with appropriate drug to all confirmed cases.
- The malaria case management is very important for preventive serious cases and death due to malaria. So, the private healthcare providers should also follow the common **National Guidelines for treatment of malaria as per the Drug Policy 2013.**

Contd...

Contd...

Treatment of Uncomplicated Malaria

- *P. vivax* cases should be **treated with chloroquine for 3 days** & **Primaquine for 14 days**[Q].
  - Primaquine is used to prevent relapse but is **contraindicated in pregnant women, infants and individuals with G6PD deficiency**[Q].
  - Note: Patients should be instructed to **report back in case of hematuria or high colored urine/cyanosis or blue coloration of lips** and **Primaquine should be stopped in such cases**. Care should be taken in patients with anemia[Q].

- *P. falciparum* cases should be treated with **ACT** (Artesunate 3 days + Sulfadoxine Pyrimethamine 1 day). This is to be **accompanied by single dose primaquine preferably on day 2**[Q].

- However, considering the reports of resistance to partner drug SP in North-eastern States, the Technical Advisory Committee has recommended to use the Co-formulated tablet of Artemether (20 mg)—Lumefantrine (120 mg ACT- AL) as per the age-specific dose schedule for the treatment of Pf cases in North Eastern States (not recommended during the first trimester of pregnancy and for children weighing < 5 kg).

- **Production and sale of Artemisinin monotherapy** has been **banned in India**[Q].
  - Pregnant women with uncomplicated *P. falciparum* should be treated as follows:
    - 1st Trimester: Quinine
    - 2nd & 3rd Trimester: ACT
  - Note: Primaquine is contraindicated in pregnant woman[Q].

- In cases where parasitological diagnosis is not possible due to non-availability of either timely microscopy or RdT, **suspected malaria cases will be treated with full course of chloroquine**, **till the results of microscopy are received**. Once the parasitological diagnosis is available, appropriate treatment as per the species, is to be administered.
  - **Presumptive treatment with chloroquine is no more recommended**[Q].

- Resistance should be suspected if in spite of full treatment with no history of vomiting, diarrhea, patient does not respond within 72 hours, clinically and parasitologically.

- Such **cases not responding to ACT**, **should be treated with oral quinine with Tetracycline/Doxycycline**. These instances should be reported to concerned District Malaria/State Malaria Officer/ROHFW for initiation of therapeutic efficacy studies.

Treatment of Severe Malaria

- **Severe malaria** is an **emergency** and **treatment should be given as per severity & associated complications**, which can be best decided by the treating physicians.

- Before admitting or referring patients, the attending doctor or health worker, whoever is able to do it, should do **RdT** and take **blood smear**; give a **parenteral dose of artemisinin derivative** or **quinine in suspected cerebral malaria cases** and send case sheet, details of treatment history and blood slide with patient.

- **Parenteral artemisinin derivatives** or **quinine should be used irrespective of chloroquine resistance status** of the area with one of the following options:
  - **Chemotherapy of severe and complicated malaria**.
  - Initial parenteral treatment for at least 48 hours with one of following four options:
    - **Quinine:** 20 mg quinine salt/kg body weight on admission (IV infusion or divided IM injection) followed by maintenance dose of 10 mg/kg 8 hourly; infusion rate should not exceed 5 mg/ kg per hour. Loading dose of 20 mg/kg should not be given, if the patient has already received quinine.
    - **Artesunate:** 2.4 mg/kg IV or IM given on admission (time = 0), then at 12 h and 24 h, then once a day or
    - **Artemether:** 3.2 mg/kg IM given on admission then 1.6 mg/kg per day or
    - **Arteether:** 150 mg daily IM for 3 days in adults only (not recommended for children).

Contd...

<table>
<tr><th colspan="2">Treatment of Severe Malaria</th></tr>
<tr><td colspan="2">Follow-up treatment, when patient can take oral medication following parenteral treatment.</td></tr>
</table>

- **Quinine** 10 mg/kg three times a day **with doxycycline** 100 mg once a day or **clindamycin in pregnant women and children under 8 years of age** to complete the 7 days of treatment.
- After parenteral artemisinin therapy, patients will receive a **full course of area-specific oral ACT for 3 days.**
- Those patients who received parenteral quinine therapy should receive oral quinine 10 mg/kg body weight three times a day for 7 days (including the days when parenteral quinine was administered) plus doxycycline 3 mg/kg body weight once a day or clindamycin 10 mg/kg body weight 12-hourly for 7 days (**Doxycycline is contraindicated in pregnant women and children under 8 years of age**) or area-specific ACT as described.
- **Note: Pregnant women with severe malaria in any trimester** can be **treated with artemisinin derivatives**, which, in contrast to quinine, **do not risk aggravating hypoglycemia**. The parenteral treatment should be given for minimum of 48 hours. Once the patient can take oral therapy, give: Quinine 10 mg/kg three times a day with doxycycline 100 mg once a day or clindamycin in pregnant women and children under 8 years of age, to complete 7 days of treatment, in patients started on parenteral quinine. Full course of ACT to patients started on artemisinin derivatives.
- **Use of mefloquine should be avoided in cerebral malaria due to neuropsychiatric complications associated with it.**

106. Ans. c. H2N1 *(Ref: http://www.who.int/influenza/vaccines/en/)*

Each seasonal influenza vaccine contains antigens representing three (trivalent vaccine) or four (quadrivalent vaccine) influenza virus strains: one influenza type A subtype H1N1 virus strain, one influenza type A subtype H3N2 virus strain, and either one or two influenza type B virus strains.

Currently circulating influenza viruses in world	
H_1N_1 *(Type A):* Cause of **Swine flu**[Q]	H_5N_1 *(Type A):* Cause of **Avian influenza (Bird flu)**[Q]
H_2N_2 *(Type A)*	H_7N_9
H_3N_2	*Type B*

<table>
<tr><th>Influenza vaccines</th></tr>
</table>

- Each seasonal **influenza vaccine contains antigens** representing **three (trivalent vaccine) or four (quadrivalent vaccine) influenza virus strains:**
  - One influenza **type A subtype H1N1** virus strain
  - One influenza **type A subtype H3N2** virus strain
  - Either one or two **influenza type B** virus strains.
- **Influenza vaccines** may be administered as an **injection or as a nasal spray.**
- The **US Centers for Disease Control and Prevention recommend** that **everyone over the ages of 6 months should receive the seasonal influenza vaccine.**
- **Vaccination campaigns** usually focus on **people who are at high-risk of serious complications** if they catch the flu, **such as the elderly and people living with chronic illness** or **those with weakened immune systems**, as well as health care workers.
- **Most flu vaccines provide modest protection against contracting influenza**, with the effect seasonably variable depending on antigenic drift.

WHO recommends that influenza vaccines for use in the 2016 southern hemisphere influenza season contain the following viruses:

- An **A/California/7/2009 (H1N1) pdm09-like virus**[Q]
- An **A/Hong Kong/4801/2014 (H3N2)-like virus**[Q]
- A **B/Brisbane/60/2008-like virus**[Q]

  - It is recommended that **quadrivalent vaccines containing two influenza B viruses contain the above three viruses** and a **B/ Phuket/3073/2013-like virus**[Q].

WHO recommends seasonal influenza vaccination for:	
Highest priority	**Priority (in no particular order)**
Pregnant women[Q]	**Children aged 6–59 months**[Q]
	Elderly[Q]
	Individuals with **specific chronic medical conditions**[Q]
	Health care workers[Q]

AIIMS November 2015

107. Ans. d. Handwashing   *(Ref: Park 24/e p378, 22/e p333)*

In developing countries, handwashing with soap is recognized as a cost-effective, essential tool for achieving good health, and even good nutrition.

Handwashing
• **Handwashing** is like a **'do-it-yourself' vaccine**—it involves five simple and effective steps (**Wet, Lather, Scrub, Rinse, Dry**) you can take **to reduce the spread of diarrheal and respiratory illness** so you can stay healthy.
• **Medical handwashing** is for a **minimum of 15 seconds**, using generous amounts of soap and water or gel to lather and rub each part of the hands.
• Hands should be rubbed together with digits interlocking.
• Since germs may remain in the water on the hands, it is important to rinse well and wipe dry with a clean towel.
• After drying, the paper towel should be used to turn off the water (and open any exit door if necessary). This avoids re-contaminating the hands from those surfaces.
• The **purpose of handwashing in the health care setting** is **to remove pathogenic microorganisms ('germs') & avoid transmitting them.**

The World Health Organization has 'Five Moments' for washing hands:	
• Before patient care	• Before an aseptic task
• After environmental contact	• After patient care
• After exposure to blood/body fluids	

• The **addition of antiseptic chemicals to soap confers killing action to a hand washing agent**. Such killing action may be desired prior to performing surgery or in settings in which antibiotic-resistant organisms are highly prevalent.
• **To 'scrub' one's hands for a surgical operation, it is necessary to have a tap that can be turned on and off without touching it with the hands**, some chlorhexidine or iodine wash, sterile towels for drying the hands after washing, and a sterile brush for scrubbing and another sterile instrument for cleaning under the fingernails.
• All jewelry should be removed. This procedure requires washing the hands and forearms up to the elbow, **usually 2–6 minutes.** Long scrub-times (10 minutes) are not necessary.
• When rinsing, water on the forearms must be prevented from running back to the hands.

• Washing with plain soap results in more than triple the rate of bacterial infectious disease transmitted to food as compared to **washing with antibacterial soap.**
• Comparing hand-rubbing with alcohol-based solution with hand washing with antibacterial soap for a median time of 30 seconds each showed that the **alcohol hand-rubbing reduced bacterial contamination 26% more than the antibacterial soap.**
• But soap and water is more effective than alcohol-based hand rubs for reducing H1N1 influenza A virus & Clostridium difficile spores from hands.

Effectiveness:
• Interventions that promote **handwashing** can **reduce diarrhea episodes by about a third,** and this is **comparable to providing clean water in low-income areas.**

MEDICINE

108. Ans. a. Hypertrophic cardiomyopathy   *(Ref: Harrison 19/e p1568, 18/e p1967; Robbins 9/e p, 8/e p576)v*

History of sudden death during exertion and on autopsy hypertrophy of ventricular wall is highly suggestive of Hypertrophic cardiomyopathy.

*"**Hypertrophic cardiomyopathy**: Macroscopically, **hypertrophy** is typically manifest as **nonuniform ventricular thickening**. The **interventricular septum is the typical location of maximal hypertrophy**, although other patterns of hypertrophic remodeling include concentric and midventricular." - Harrison 19/e p1568*

Hypertrophic Obstructive Cardiomyopathy (HOCM)
• **HOCM** is defined as **left ventricular hypertrophy** that **develops in the absence of causative hemodynamic factors**, such as hypertension, aortic valve disease, or systemic infiltrative or storage diseases.

Contd...

AIIMS ESSENCE

Pathophysiology:

- Macroscopically, **hypertrophy** is typically manifest as **nonuniform ventricular thickening**. The **interventricular septum is the typical location of maximal hypertrophy**[Q].

  - **Septal hypertrophy:** Asymmetrical septal hypertrophy is characteristic[Q], **thickness of ventricular septum is disproportionately increased** when compared with the free wall[Q]

- **Left ventricular outflow tract obstruction** represents **MC focus of diagnosis & intervention**[Q].

Clinical Features:

- **Many patients are asymptomatic**[Q]
- **Sudden death**[Q] may be **first clinical manifestation of disease** (commonly seen in **young adults after competitive sports**).

Clinical Features of HOCM	
Symptoms	**Signs**
- **MC symptom: Dyspnea**[Q] - **Angina pectoris/chest pain**[Q] - **Fatigue**[Q] - **Syncope**[Q]	- **Double or triple precordial impulse**[Q] - **Brisk carotid upstroke**[Q] (Rapidly rising carotid pulse) - **Fourth heart sound**[Q] - **Systolic murmur (Hallmark of disease): Harsh**[Q], **diamond shaped** (crescendo decrescendo), best heard at lower left sternal border as well as at apex[Q]

Condition increasing obstruction & intensity of murmur	Conditions decreasing obstruction & intensity of murmur
- **Factors that increase myocardial contractility:** Sympathomimetic amines[Q], Digitalis glycosides[Q] - **Factors which decrease Ventricular volume:** Valsalva maneuver[Q], sudden standing[Q], nitroglycerine[Q], amyl nitrite[Q], tachycardia[Q] - **Decreased aortic impedance & afterload**[Q]	- **Factors that decrease myocardial contractility:** Beta blockers, Calcium channel blockers[Q] - **Factors which increase Ventricular volume:** Augmentation of venous return by passive leg raising[Q], expansion of blood volume[Q], supine position[Q] - **Increased aortic impedance & afterload:** Elevation of arterial pressure by phenylephrine, sustained hand grip[Q], squatting

Diagnosis:

- **Cardiac imaging** is **central to diagnosis due to the insensitivity of examination and ECG & need to exclude other causes for hypertrophy**[Q].

Management of HOCM:

- **Avoidance of strenuous physical activity**[Q]

  - **Beta-blockers should be the initial drug in symptomatic individuals**[Q]. They reduce heart rate, BP, stiffness of left ventricle, fatal arrhythmias[Q]
  - **Calcium channel blockers**[Q] (verapamil & diltiazem) are alternative drugs. They **reduce-stiffness of ventricle & elevated diastolic pressures**[Q].

- **Amiodarone** may be **used to reduce arrhythmias**[Q].
- **Surgical myomectomy**[Q]

Features	Dilated	Restrictive	Hypertrophic
Ejection fraction (Normal 55%)	**<30%**[Q]	**> 30-50%**[Q]	**>60**[Q]
Left ventricular diastolic dimension (Normal <55 mm)	**≥60 mm**[Q]	**<60 mm**[Q]	**Often decreased**[Q]
Left ventricular wall thickness	**Decreased**[Q]	**Normal or increased**[Q]	**Markedly increased**[Q]
Atrial size	**Increased**[Q]	**Increased**[Q]	**Increased**[Q]

Contd...

Contd...

Features	Dilated	Restrictive	Hypertrophic
Valvular regurgitation	Related to annular dilation; Mitral appears earlier, during decompensating; Tricuspid regurgitation in late stages	Related to endocardial involvement; Frequent mitral and tricuspid regurgitation, rarely severe	Related to valve-septum interaction; Mitral regurgitation
Common first symptoms	**Exertional intolerance**[Q]	**Exertional intolerance, Early fluid retention**[Q]	**Exertional intolerance; May have chest pain**[Q]
Congestive symptoms	Left before right, except right prominent in young adults	Right often dominates	Left-sided congestion may develop late
Arrhythmia	**Ventricular tachyarrhythmia; Conduction blocks** in **Chagas' disease**, atrial fibrillation.	Ventricular tachyarrhythmia **uncommon except in sarcoidosis** **Conduction block in sarcoidosis** & atrial fibrillation.	**Ventricular tachyarrhythmia's; Atrial fibrillation**

109. Ans. a. Thrombolysis   *(Ref: Harrison 19/e p1603-1605, 18/e p2027-2029)*

Symptoms and ECG findings are suggestive of ST-elevation MI. Since the patient has come to the hospital 24 hours after onset of symptoms, there will be no benefit from thrombolysis.

*"Management of Patients with ST-segment Elevation Myocardial Infarction: In the absence of contraindications, it is reasonable to **administer fibrinolytic therapy to patients with symptoms of STEMI beginning within the prior 12 to 24 hours who have continuing ischemic symptoms and electrocardiographic evidence of STEMI**. Fibrinolytic therapy should not be administered to asymptomatic patients whose initial symptoms of STEMI began more than 24 hours earlier nor to patients whose 12-lead ECG shows only ST-segment depression, except if a true posterior myocardial infarction (MI) is suspected."*

"Aspirin is essential in the management of patients with suspected STEMI and is effective across the entire spectrum of acute coronary syndromes. Rapid inhibition of cyclooxygenase-1 in platelets followed by a reduction of thromboxane A levels is achieved by buccal absorption of a chewed 160–325-mg tablet in the Emergency Department. This measure should be followed by daily oral administration of aspirin in a dose of 75–162 mg." – *Harrison 19/e p1603*

*"Morphine is a very effective analgesic for the pain associated with STEMI. However, it may reduce sympathetically mediated arteriolar and venous constriction, and the **resulting venous pooling may reduce cardiac output and arterial pressure**. These hemodynamic disturbances usually respond promptly to elevation of the legs, but in some patients, **volume expansion with intravenous saline is required**. The patient may experience diaphoresis and nausea, but these events usually pass and are replaced by a feeling of well-being associated with the relief of pain. Morphine also has a vagotonic effect and **may cause bradycardia or advanced degrees of heart block, particularly in patients with inferior infarction**. These side effects usually respond to atropine (0.5 mg intravenously). Morphine is routinely administered by repetitive (every 5 min) intravenous injection of small doses (2–4 mg),* rather than by the subcutaneous administration of a larger quantity, because absorption may be unpredictable by the latter route."* – *Harrison 19/e p1603*

Management of Patients with ST-segment Elevation Myocardial Infarction
• **Prehospital, emergency medical service providers should administer aspirin** (162 to 325 mg) **to all patients not already taking aspirin, obtain a 12-lead electrocardiogram (ECG) in patients suspected of having STEMI**[Q], review a reperfusion checklist, and relay this information to a medical facility.
• Patients with **STEMI** who have **cardiogenic shock**, those with **contraindications to lytics**, and those at **high-risk of dying because of heart failure** should be **channeled immediately to a facility capable of cardiac catheterization**[Q].
Initial Recognition and Evaluation in the Emergency Department
• Initial evaluation in the emergency department focuses on **identification of STEMI**, **early therapy**, and **reperfusion strategy**.
• Selection of reperfusion strategy depends on hospital and patient characteristics.
• **Time to reperfusion therapy strongly influences outcomes in STEMI.**

Contd...

Contd...

Management of Patients with ST-segment Elevation Myocardial Infarction
• **Patients presenting to a hospital** with percutaneous coronary intervention **(PCI) capability** should undergo **PCI within 90 minutes of first medical contact** as a systems goal^Q.
• Patients with **STEMI presenting to a non-PCI-capable hospital** should be considered for **transfer to a PCI-capable hospital** based on patient characteristics time from symptom onset, and time to available PCI therapy.
• STEMI patients presenting to a hospital **without PCI capability** and **who cannot be transferred to a PCI center** and **undergo PCI within 90 minutes of first medical contact** should **receive fibrinolytic therapy within 30 minutes of hospital presentation** as a systems goal in the absence of contraindications.
• If pharmacologic reperfusion is selected, **fibrinolytic therapy should be administered to STEMI** patients with symptom **onset within** the prior **12 hours**^{Q}.
• **In the absence of contraindications**, it is reasonable to **administer fibrinolytic therapy** to patients with symptoms of STEMI beginning within the prior **12 to 24 hours** who have **continuing ischemic symptoms & electrocardiographic evidence of STEMI**^{Q}.
• Fibrinolytic therapy should **not be administered to asymptomatic patients** whose **initial symptoms of STEMI** began **more than 24 hours earlier** nor to patients whose 12-lead ECG shows **only ST-segment depression**, except if a true posterior myocardial infarction (MI) is suspected^Q.
• Patients should be evaluated for **contraindications to fibrinolytic therapy** such as a **history of intracranial hemorrhage (ICH)**, significant closed head or facial trauma within the past 3 months, uncontrolled hypertension, or ischemic stroke within the past 3 months.
• **STEMI patients at substantial (4%) risk of ICH should be treated with PCI rather than with fibrinolytic therapy**^{Q}.

110. **Ans. b. Atrial fibrillation** *(Ref: Harrisons 19/e p2080)*

The ECG shows absent P waves with baseline variation. This is seen in atrial fibrillation.

"The ECG in AF is characterized by the lack of organized atrial activity and the irregularly irregular ventricular response. Occasionally, one needs to record from multiple ECG leads simultaneously to identify the chaotic continuous atrial activation. Lead V_1 frequently shows the appearance of organized atrial activity that mimics AFL. This occurs because the crista terminalis serves as an effective anatomic barrier to electrical conduction, and the activation of the lateral right atrium may be represented by a more uniform activation wavefront that originates over the roof of the right atrium. ECG assessment of the PP interval (< 200 ms) and the chaotic P-wave morphology in the remaining ECG leads will confirm the presence of AF."

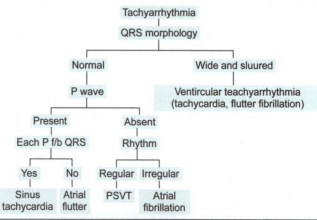

Atrial fibrillation (AF)
• It is characterized by **disorganized, rapid & irregular atrial activation** with loss of atrial contraction & with an **irregular ventricular rate** that is determined by AV nodal conduction^Q.
• **Ventricular rate in AF:** In an untreated patient, **120–160 beats/min, may exceed 200 beats/min**; Patients with high vagal tone or AV nodal conduction disease may have slow rates^Q.

Atrial fibrillation (AF)		

Epidemiology:

- It is the **MC sustained arrhythmia**
- **Prevalence increases with age**, and >**95% of AF** patients are >**60 years** of age.
- AF is slightly **more common in men & whites**

Risk factors for developing AF	
• **Age**[Q] • **Hypertension**[Q] • **Diabetes mellitus**[Q] • **Hyperthyroidism**[Q] • **Pulmonary embolism**[Q]	• **Cardiac disease: RHD (MS & MR), cardiomyopathy, CHD, myocarditis, pericarditis**[Q] • Post cardiac surgery

- **Other precipitating factors for AF**: Heart failure, stroke & dementia.

Pathophysiology:

- It is **often initiated by small re-entrant** or **rapidly firing foci in sleeves of atrial muscle**[Q]
- Episodes may be **initiated by rapidly firing foci**, but **persistence of the arrhythmia is likely due to single** or **multiple areas of reentry facilitated by structural & electrophysiologic atrial abnormalities**[Q].

Clinical features:

- Presentations vary with the ventricular rate and underlying heart disease and comorbidities.
- **Many patients** are **asymptomatic.**
- Rapid rates may cause **hemodynamic collapse or heart failure exacerbations,** particularly in patients with impaired cardiac function, hypertrophic cardiomyopathy & heart failure with preserved systolic function.
- **Exercise intolerance & easy fatigability** are common.
- Occasionally **dizziness or syncope** occurs due to pauses when AF terminates to sinus rhythm

  - In **long standing persistent AF (>1 year), significant structural changes** occur in the atrium that support **reentry & automaticity**[Q].

Clinical types:

- **Paroxysmal AF:** Episodes of AF that **start & stop spontaneously**.
- **Persistent AF lasts >7 days**, & may continue unless cardioversion is performed.

Treatment:

- **Cardioversion within 48 h of the onset of AF is common practice** in patients **who have not been anticoagulated**, provided that they are **not at high risk for stroke** due to a prior history of embolic events, rheumatic mitral stenosis, or hypertrophic cardiomyopathy with marked left atrial enlargement.
- **Acute rate control**: Beta-blockers and/or the calcium channel blockers verapamil & diltiazem[Q].
- **Patients who remain in AF chronically**: β-Adrenergic blockers, calcium channel blockers & digoxin[Q]
- **Prevention: Amiodarone**[Q].

111. **Ans. b. Adenosine** *(Ref: Harrison 19/e p1480, 18/e p1882)*

The given ECG is showing atrial fibrillation. Adenosine is used in the treatment of PSVT, not in atrial fibrillation.

Commonly Used Antiarrhythmic Agents		
Drug	**Primary indication**	**Class**
Acebutolol	AF rate control/SVT; Long QT/RVOT VT	II
Amiodarone	AF/VT prevention[Q]	III
Atenolol	AF rate control/SVT; Long QT/RVOT VT[Q]	II
Digoxin	AF rate control[Q]	—
Diltiazem	AF rate control/SVT[Q]	IV
Disopyramide	AF/SVT prevention	Ia
Dofetilide	AF prevention[Q]	III
Dronedarone	AF prevention	IIIb
Flecainide	AF/SVT/VT prevention[Q]	Ic
Metoprolol	AF rate control/SVT; Long QT/RVOT VT[Q]	II

Contd...

Contd...

Commonly Used Antiarrhythmic Agents		
Mexiletine	**VT prevention**[Q]	**Ib**
Nadolol	**AF rate control/SVT; Long QT/RVOT VT**[Q]	**II**
Propafenone	AF/SVT/VT prevention	Ic
Drug	**Primary indication**	**Class**
Quinidine	**AF/SVT/VT**[Q]	**Ia**
Sotalol	AF/VT prevention	III
Verapamil	**AF rate control/RVOT VT; Idiopathic LV VT**[Q]	**IV**

Classification of antiarrhythmic drugs	
Class **I**	• Agents that primarily **block inward sodium current**
Class **II**	• **Antisympathetic** agents
Class **III**	• Agents that primarily **prolong action potential duration**
Class **IV**	• **Calcium channel-blocking agents**

- **Amiodarone & dronedarone** both are grouped in **class III**, but both **also have class I, II & IV properties.**
- *Abbreviations:* AF, atrial fibrillation; LV, left ventricular; RVOT, right ventricular outflow tract; SVT, supraventricular tachycardia; VT, ventricular tachycardia.

Adenosine

- **Adenosine** is administered as a **rapid IV bolus for the acute termination of re-entrant supraventricular arrhythmias**[Q].
- **Used to produce controlled hypotension**[Q] during some surgical procedures & in the diagnosis of coronary artery disease.

Pharmacologic Effects:

- **Effects of adenosine are mediated by its interaction with specific G protein-coupled adenosine receptors**[Q].
- **Adenosine activates acetylcholine-sensitive K$^+$ current in the atrium, sinus & AV nodes**, resulting in **shortening of APD, hyperpolarization, & slowing of normal automaticity**[Q].

  - **Adenosine reduces Ca^{2+} currents**, it can be **anti-arrhythmic by increasing AV nodal refractoriness** and by **inhibiting DADs elicited by sympathetic stimulation**[Q].
  - **IV bolus of adenosine** transiently **slows sinus rate & AV nodal conduction velocity & increases AV nodal refractoriness**[Q].

Clinical uses:

- Treatment of **reentrant supraventricular tachycardias**[Q]
- **IV adenosine terminates majority of PSVT by transiently blocking conduction in AV node**[Q].

---

112. **Ans. a. Urine protein levels range from 20 mg/d to 200 mg/d** *(Ref: Harrison 19/e p2425, 1582, 1813 18/e p2982, 2985)*

Microalbuminuria is defined as 30–299 mg/d in a 24-h collection or 30–299 mcg/mg creatinine in a spot collection.

"The American Diabetes Association (ADA) recently suggested that the terms previously used to refer to increased urinary protein (microalbuminuria as defined as 30–299 mg/d in a 24-h collection or 30–299 µg/mg creatinine in a spot collection or macroalbuminuria as defined as >300 mg/24 h) be replaced by the phrases "persistent albuminuria (30–299 mg/24 h)" and "persistent albuminuria (≥300 mg/24 h)" to better reflect the continuous nature of albumin excretion in the urine as risk factor for nephropathy and cardiovascular disease (CVD)."– Harrison 19/e p2425

"Microalbuminuria is also a risk factor for CVD. Once macroalbuminuria is present, there is a steady decline in GFR, and ~50% of individuals reach ESRd in 7–10 years. Once macroalbuminuria develops, blood pressure rises slightly and the pathologic changes are likely irreversible."– Harrison 19/e p2425

"The urine should be examined for evidence of diabetes mellitus and renal disease (including microalbuminuria) since these conditions accelerate atherosclerosis."– Harrison 19/e p1582

"Microalbuminuria refers to the excretion of amounts of albumin too small to detect by urinary dipstick or conventional measures of urine protein. It is a good screening test for early detection of renal disease, and may be a marker for the presence of microvascular disease in general. If a patient has a large amount of excreted albumin, there is no reason to test for microalbuminuria."– Harrison 19/e p1813

> *"Albuminuria in the range of 30–300 mg/24 h is called microalbuminuria. Microalbuminuria appears 5–10 years after the onset of diabetes. It is currently recommended to test patients with type 1 disease for microalbuminuria 5 years after diagnosis of diabetes and yearly thereafter and, because the time of onset of type 2 diabetes is often unknown, to test type 2 patients at the time of diagnosis of diabetes and yearly thereafter. Microalbuminuria is a potent risk factor for cardiovascular events and death in patients with type 2 diabetes."– Harrison 19/e p1844*

Microalbuminuria
• **Microalbuminuria** is defined **as 30–299 mg/d in a 24-h collection or 30–299 mcg/mg creatinine in a spot collection (preferred method)**[Q].
• **Microalbuminuria is a risk factor for cardiovascular disease**[Q].
• **Once macroalbuminuria is present**, there is a **steady decline in GFR & 50% of individuals reach ESRd in 7–10 years**[Q].
• **Once macroalbuminuria develops, blood pressure rises slightly & pathologic changes are likely irreversible**[Q].

Nephropathy that develops in type 2 DM differs from that of type 1 DM in the following respects:
• **Microalbuminuria or macroalbuminuria may be present** when type 2 DM is diagnosed, reflecting its long asymptomatic period
• **Hypertension more commonly accompanies microalbuminuria or macroalbuminuria in type 2 DM**
• **Microalbuminuria may be less predictive of diabetic nephropathy** and progression to macroalbuminuria in type 2 DM.

• It should be noted that **albuminuria in type 2 DM may be secondary to factors unrelated to DM**, such as **hypertension, CHF, prostate disease, or infection**[Q].

Interventions effective in slowing progression from microalbuminuria to macroalbuminuria include:	
• **Normalization of glycemia**[Q]	• **Administration of ACE inhibitors or ARBs**[Q]
• **Strict blood pressure control**[Q]	• **Dyslipidemia should also be treated**[Q]

• **Increase in cardiovascular morbidity & mortality** rates appears to relate to the **synergism of hyperglycemia** with other **cardiovascular risk factors**[Q].

113. Ans. a. Bedaquiline   *(Ref: Harrison 19/e p1115, 205e-7)*

Two novel drugs belonging to two new antibiotic classes—the diarylquinoline bedaquiline and the nitroimidazole delamanid—have recently been approved for use in severe cases of MDR-TB by stringent regulatory authorities.

> *"Two novel drugs belonging to two new antibiotic classes—the diarylquinoline bedaquiline and the nitroimidazole delamanid—have recently been approved for use in severe cases of MDR-TB by stringent regulatory authorities (the U.S. Food and Drug Administration [FDA] and the European Medicine Agency [EMA] in the case of bedaquiline; the EMA and the Pharmaceuticals and Medical Devices Agency of Japan in the case of delamanid)."– Harrison 19/e p1115*

Bedaquiline
• **Bedaquiline** is a **new diarylquinoline** with a novel mechanism of action: **inhibition of the mycobacterial ATP synthetase proton pump**[Q].
• It is **bactericidal for drug-susceptible and MDR strains of M. tuberculosis**[Q].
Mechanism of action:
• **Inhibition of the mycobacterial ATP synthetase proton pump.**
Therapeutic Uses:
• **Provisional recommendation** for the use of bedaquiline for 24 weeks in **adults with laboratory-confirmed pulmonary MDR-TB** when no other effective treatment regimen can be provided.
Side-Effects:
• **Arrhythmias** (induce **long QT syndrome** by blocking the hERG channel)
Resistance:
• **Resistance** has been reported and is **due to point mutations in the atpE gene encoding for subunit c of ATP synthetase.**

Anti-Tubercular Drugs		
First line (WHO Group 1)	**Second line**	**Third line**
• **Ethambutol**^{Q} (EMB or E) • **Isoniazid**^{Q} (INH or H) • **Pyrazinamide**^{Q} (PZA or Z) • **Rifampicin**^{Q} (RMP or R) • **Streptomycin**^{Q} (SM or S)	• **Second line drugs** (WHO groups 2, 3 & 4) are **only used to treat disease** that is **resistant to first line therapy**, i.e., **for extensively drug-resistant tuberculosis (XDR-TB)** or **multidrug-resistant tuberculosis (MDR-TB)**. • **Aminoglycosides** (WHO group 2): **Amikacin, kanamycin**^{Q} • **Polypeptides** (WHO group 2): **Capreomycin, viomycin, enviomycin**^{Q} • **Fluoroquinolones** (WHO group 3): **Ciprofloxacin, levofloxacin, moxifloxacin**^{Q} • **Thioamides** (WHO group 4): **Ethionamide, prothionamide**^{Q} • **Cycloserine**^{Q} (WHO group 4) • **Terizidone**^{Q} (WHO group 5)	• **Third-line drugs (WHO group 5)** include drugs that may be **useful**, but have **doubtful or unproven efficacy.** • **Rifabutin**^{Q} • **Clarithromycin**^{Q} • **Linezolid**^{Q} • **Thioacetazone**^{Q} • **Thioridazine**^{Q} • Arginine • Vitamin D • **Bedaquiline**^{Q} • **Delamanid**^{Q}

114. Ans. b. Chronic alcoholics *(Ref: http://www.who.int/tb/challenges/ltbi/en/)*

According to WHO guidelines, latent TB should be ruled out before treatment with TNF-alpha inhibitors, in patients of silicosis and patients undergoing hemodialysis among the provided options.

WHO Latent Tuberculosis Infection (LTBI) Guidelines

• **Latent Tuberculosis Infection (LTBI)** is a **state of persistent immune response to stimulation by Mycobacterium tuberculosis antigens without evidence of clinically manifested active TB.**
• The **lifetime risk of reactivation** for a person with documented LTBI is estimated to be **5–10%.**
 	
    • **Diagnosis: TST** (Tuberculin Skin Test) and **IGRAs** (Interferon- Gamma Release Assays) are the **main tests currently available for the diagnosis of LTBI.**
    • **Persons with LTBI have negative bacteriological tests:** the diagnosis is based on a **positive result of either a TST or IGRA test** indicating an **immune response to persons with LTBI have negative bacteriological tests.**
 	
• However these tests have limitations, as they cannot distinguish between latent infection with viable microorganisms and healed/treated infections; they also poorly predict who will progress to active TB.

Specific High-risk Populations	
• **HIV infection**^{Q}	• **Silicosis**^{Q}
• **Recent contact** with an infectious patient	• Being in prison
• **Initiation of an anti-tumor necrosis factor (TNF) treatment**^{Q}	• Being an **immigrant from high TB burden countries**
• **Receiving dialysis**^{Q}	• Being a homeless person
• Receiving an **organ or hematologic transplantation**	• Being an **illicit drug user**.

Treatment:

Currently available treatment options allow to reduce by at least 60% the risk of developing active TB:

• 6 month or 9 month isoniazid daily
• 3 month rifapentine plus isoniazid weekly
• 3 or 4 months isoniazid plus rifampicin daily
• 3 or 4 months rifampicin alone daily.

115. Ans. c. ANCA and evaluation for vasculitis *(Ref: Harrison 19/e p2182-2184, 18/e p2786, 2789)*

History of chronic sinusitis, nasopharyngeal ulcers, cavitary lung nodules and renal failure are suggestive of Wegener's Granulomatosis. Wegener's Granulomatosis is c-ANCA positive small vessel vasculitis^Q. c-ANCA levels are required for diagnosis.

"The histopathologic hallmarks of granulomatosis with polyangiitis (Wegener's) are necrotizing vasculitis of small arteries and veins together with granuloma formation, which may be either intravascular or extravascular. Lung involvement typically appears as multiple, bilateral, nodular cavitary infiltrates, which on biopsy almost invariably reveal the typical necrotizing granulomatous vasculitis. Upper airway lesions, particularly those in the sinuses and nasopharynx, typically reveal inflammation, necrosis, and granuloma formation, with or without vasculitis."– Harrison 19/e p2182

"The specificity of a positive antiproteinase-3 ANCA for granulomatosis with polyangiitis (Wegener's) is very high, especially if active glomerulonephritis is present. However, the presence of ANCA should be adjunctive and, with rare exceptions, should not substitute for a tissue diagnosis." – Harrison 19/e p2184

ANCA (Antineutrophilic cytoplasmic antibodies)	
• **ANCA** are **antibodies directed against certain proteins in cytoplasmic granules of neutrophils** & **monocytes.**	
• There are **two major categories**:	
C-ANCA (**Cytoplasmic protein 3** is the target antigen)	**P-ANCA** (**Perinuclear myeloperoxidase** is the major target antigen)
• **Wegner's Granulomatosis**[Q] **(90-95%)**	• **Microscopic PAN** (microscopic polyangitis)[Q] • **Churg-Strauss syndrome**[Q] • **Crescentic Glomerulonephritis**[Q] • **Good Pasteur's syndrome**[Q]

Wegener's Granulomatosis
• Characterized clinically by **granulomatous vasculitis** of the **upper & lower respiratory tracts** together with **glomerulonephritis** & variable degrees of **disseminated vasculitis** involving both **small arteries & veins.**   • **c-ANCA positive small vessel vasculitis**[Q]
Pathology:
• **Necrotizing vasculitis**[Q] of **small arteries & veins**[Q]   • **Intravascular** & **extravascular granuloma** formation[Q]   • Granulomas contain **multiple well defined multinucleated giant cells**[Q]   • **Bronchoalveolar lavage** fluid contains **high percentage of neutrophils** compared to other granulomatous diseases which contains increased number of Lymphocytes
Clinical Features:
• **Fever, skin manifestation** in the form of papules, vesicles, palpable purpura etc, **eye manifestations, joint manifestations, cardiac manifestations** & **nervous system manifestation**

Characteristic Triad of Wegener's Granulomatosis		
Vasculitis of upper respiratory tract[Q] **(ENT)**	**Vasculitis of Lower respiratory tract**[Q] **(Lung)**	**Vasculitis of Kidney**
• **MC (95%)** • **Otitis media**[Q] (conductive deafness) • Paranasal sinus pain & drainage • **Septal perforation**[Q] • **Sinusitis, subglottic stenosis**[Q] • **Strawberry gum & gum ulcers**[Q] • **Mucosal ulcerations of nasopharynx**	• **2nd MC (85-90%)** • **Cough, hemoptysis, dyspnea**[Q] • **Multiple bilateral cavitatory nodular infiltrates** & **cavitatory lesions** in the **lung**[Q]	• Seen in 80% patients • **Rapidly progressive renal failure**[Q] • **Crescentic glomerulonephritis**[Q] • Present with **hematuria, proteinuria & RBC cast in urine**[Q]

Less common Vasculitis associated with Wegener's Granulomatosis	
Organ involved	**Manifestations**
Skin (46%)	• **Palpable purpura, subcutaneous nodules**[Q], ulcers, vesicobullous lesions, splinter hemorrhages, digital ischemia & gangrene
Joints	• **Arthralgia & migratory arthritis**[Q]
Eyes (52%)	• **Orbital pseudotumors** behind the eye leading to proptosis & visual loss • Scleritis, keratitis, conjunctivitis & uveitis
Peripheral nerve	• **Mononeuritis multiplex**[Q]

Characteristic laboratory findings of Wegener's Granulomatosis	
• **Positive c-ANCA**[Q] • **Elevated ESR, RF**[Q] (mild elevation) • **Anemia, leukocytosis & thrombocytosis**[Q]	• **Hypergammaglobulinemia** (particularly **IgA class**)[Q] • **Hypocomplementemia** is **not seen** despite presence of circulating immune complexes[Q]

Treatment:

• **Treatment** of choice: **Cyclophosphamide**[Q]
• **Cyclophosphamide** is given in doses of **2 mg/kg per day** together with **glucocorticoids**[Q].

116. Ans. b. Chronic hepatitis recovery state *(Ref: Harrison 19/e p2017, 18/e p2550-2551)*

From the given serology profile and table given below it is clear that the patient has had hepatitis B infection in the remote past or is a low-level Hepatitis B carrier.

					Commonly Encountered Serologic Patterns of Hepatitis B Infection
HBsAg	**Anti-HBs**	**Anti-HBc**	**HBeAg**	**Anti-HBe**	**Interpretation**
+	–	IgM	+	–	• **Acute hepatitis B, high infectivity**
+	–	IgG	+	–	• **Chronic hepatitis B, high infectivity**[Q]
+	–	IgG	–	+	• **Late acute** or **chronic hepatitis B, low infectivity**[Q] • **HBeAg-negative** ('precoremutant') hepatitis B (chronic or rarely acute)
+	+	+	+/–	+/–	• HBsAg of one subtype and heterotypic anti-HBs (common) • Process of seroconversion from HBsAg to anti-HBs (rare)
–	–	IgM	+/–	+/–	• **Acute hepatitis B**[Q] • **Anti-HBc 'window'**[Q]
–	–	IgG	–	+/–	• **Low-level hepatitis B carrier**[Q] • **Hepatitis B in remote past**[Q]
–	+	IgG	–	+/–	• **Recovery from hepatitis B**[Q]
–	+	–	–	–	• **Immunization with HBsAg** (after vaccination) • **Hepatitis B in the remote past** (?) • False-positive

117. Ans. d. Decreased chest wall expansion *(Ref: Harrison 19/e p2170, 18/e p2775)*

History of back pain, which is more in the morning and relieved by bathing in warm water is characteristic of spondylo arthropathy, like ankylosing spondylitis. Ankylosing spondylitis leads to extra-parenchymal restrictive lung disease, associated with decreased chest wall expansion.

"Ankylosing Spondylitis: The initial symptom is usually dull pain, insidious in onset, felt deep in the lower lumbar or gluteal region, accompanied by low-back morning stiffness of up to a few hours' duration that improves with activity and returns following inactivity."– Harrison 19/e p2170

"Ankylosing Spondylitis: Initially, physical findings mirror the inflammatory process. The most specific findings involve loss of spinal mobility, with limitation of anterior and lateral flexion and extension of the lumbar spine and of chest expansion. Limitation of motion is usually out of proportion to the degree of bony ankylosis, reflecting muscle spasm secondary to pain and inflammation. Pain in the sacroiliac joints may be elicited either with direct pressure or with stress on the joints. In addition, there is commonly tenderness upon palpation at the sites of symptomatic bony tenderness and paraspinous muscle spasm."– Harrison 19/e p2170

See Q. No. 168 AIIMS May 2016

118. Ans. b. Ledipasvir *(Ref: Harrison 19/e p2049, 18/e p2556)*

Ledipasvir is an inhibitor of the hepatitis C virus NS5A protein. Ledipasvir is most commonly used in combination with sofosbuvir for treatment in chronic hepatitis C genotype 1 patients.

" Ledipasvir is an inhibitor of the hepatitis C virus NS5A protein. Sofosbuvir, on the other hand, is metabolized to the active uridine analog triphosphate, which acts as a RNA chain terminator when incorporated into the RNA via the NS5B polymerase."

Ledipasvir
• **Ledipasvir** is an **inhibitor of the hepatitis C virus NS5A protein**[Q]. • The **ledipasvir/sofosbuvir combination** is a **direct-acting antiviral agent** that **interferes with HCV replication and can be used to treat patients with genotypes 1a or 1b without PEG-interferon or ribavirin**. • On October 10, 2014 the **FDA approved the combination product ledipasvir/sofosbuvir** called **Harvoni**.
Mechanism of Action: • **Ledipasvir inhibits an important viral phosphoprotein, NS5A**, which is involved in viral replication, assembly & secretion

Contd...

Contd...

Clinical Uses:
• **Ledipasvir** is most commonly used in combination **with sofosbuvir** for **treatment in chronic hepatitis C genotype 1** patients[Q].
Side-effects:
• **MC side effects**: **Fatigue & headache**

Antiviral Therapy in Hepatitis C	
Indications for Antiviral Therapy in Hepatitis C	
• **Detectable HCV RNA** (with or without elevated ALT)	
• **Portal/bridging fibrosis or moderate to severe hepatitis** on liver biopsy	
Initial Recommended Treatment depends on the Type of Hepatitis C virus	
Genotype	**Recommended Treatment**
HCV genotype **1a**	• 12 weeks of **ledipasvir & sofosbuvir** OR 12 -24 weeks of **paritaprevir, ombitasvir, dasabuvir & ribavirin**
HCV genotype **1b**	• 12 weeks of **ledipasvir & sofosbuvir** OR 12 weeks of **paritaprevir, ombitasvir & dasabuvir**
HCV genotype **2**	• 12 to 16 weeks of **sofosbuvir & ribavirin**
HCV genotype **3**	• 12 weeks of **sofosbuvir, ribavirin & pegylated interferon**
HCV genotype **4**	• 12 weeks of **ledipasvir & sofosbuvir** OR **paritaprevir, ritonavir, ombitasvir & ribavirin**, OR 24 weeks of **sofosbuvir & ribavirin**
HCV genotype **5 or 6**	• **Sofosbuvir & ledipasvir**

119. **Ans. a. Obstructive jaundice** *(Ref: Harrison 19/e p280, 18/e p325)*

Absence of urinary urobilinogen is usually suggestive of obstructive jaundice.

"The conjugated bilirubin excreted into bile drains into the duodenum and passes unchanged through the proximal small bowel. Conjugated bilirubin is not taken up by the intestinal mucosa. When the conjugated bilirubin reaches the distal ileum and colon, it is hydrolyzed to unconjugated bilirubin by bacterial β-glucuronidases. The unconjugated bilirubin is reduced by normal gut bacteria to form a group of colorless tetrapyrroles called urobilinogens. About 80–90% of these products are excreted in feces, either unchanged or oxidized to orange derivatives called urobilins. The remaining 10–20% of the urobilinogens are passively absorbed, enter the portal venous blood, and are re-excreted by the liver. A small fraction (usually <3 mg/dL) escapes hepatic uptake, filters across the renal glomerulus, and is excreted in urine."– Harrison 19/e p280

Function test	Prehepatic jaundice	Hepatic jaundice	Post-hepatic (Obstructive) jaundice
Total bilirubin	**Normal/ increased**	**Increased[Q]**	**Increased[Q]**
Conjugated bilirubin	**Normal**	**Increased[Q]**	**Increased[Q]**
Unconjugated bilirubin	**Normal/ increased**	**Increased[Q]**	Normal
Urobilinogen	**Normal/ increased**	**Decreased[Q]**	**Decreased/ negative[Q]**
Urine color	Normal	Dark (urobilinogen + conjugated bilirubin)[Q]	Dark (conjugated bilirubin)[Q]
Stool color	Normal	**Normal/pale[Q]**	**Pale[Q]**
Alkaline phosphatase levels	Normal	**Increased[Q]**	**Increased[Q]**
Alanine transferase & aspartate transferase levels	Normal	**Increased[Q]**	**Increased[Q]**
Conjugated bilirubin in urine	**Absent[Q]**	**Present[Q]**	**Present[Q]**
Splenomegaly	**Present[Q]**	**Present[Q]**	**Absent[Q]**

Bilirubin metabolism and elimination
1. **Normal bilirubin production from heme** (0.2–0.3 gm/day) is derived **primarily from the breakdown of senescent circulating erythrocytes.**
2. **Extrahepatic bilirubin** is **bound to serum albumin** and **delivered to the liver.**
3. **Hepatocellular uptake**

Contd...

Contd...

Bilirubin metabolism and elimination
4. **Glucuronidation in the endoplasmic reticulum** generate **bilirubin monoglucuronides & diglucuronides**, which are **water soluble** and **readily excreted into bile**.
5. **Gut bacteria deconjugate the bilirubin and degrade it to colorless urobilinogens**. The **urobilinogens** and the **residue of intact pigments are excreted in the feces**, with **some reabsorption and excretion into urine**.

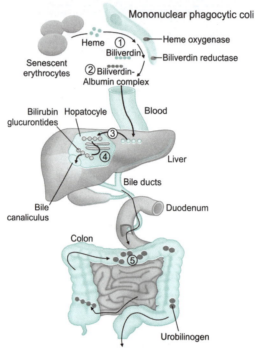

Fig. 30: Bilirubin metabolism and elimination

120. **Ans. a. Asterixis**   *(Ref: Harrison 19/e p1782, 2066, 1774, 18/e p199, 2259)*

The presence of asterixis on the motor examination is nonspecific but usually indicates a metabolic or toxic etiology of the delirium. In a drowsy and confused patient, bilateral asterixis is a certain sign of metabolic encephalopathy or drug intoxication.

> *"Hepatic encephalopathy is suggested by asterixis and can occur in chronic liver failure or acute fulminant hepatic failure."– Harrison 19/e p1782*

> *"In patients presenting with encephalopathy, asterixis is often present. Asterixis can be elicited by having patients extend their arms and bend their wrists back. In this maneuver, patients who are encephalopathic have a "liver flap"—i.e., a sudden forward movement of the wrist."– Harrison 19/e p2066*

> *"In a drowsy and confused patient, bilateral asterixis is a certain sign of metabolic encephalopathy or drug intoxication."– Harrison 19/e p1774*

Asterixis
• **Asterixis (flapping tremor)** is a **tremor of the hand when wrist is extended** (resemble a **bird flapping it's wings**^{Q}).
• Characterized by **inability to actively maintain a position**, demonstrated by **jerking movements of outstretched hands when bent upward at wrist**^{Q}.
• **Tremor is caused by abnormal function of the diencephalic motor centers in brain**, which regulate the muscles involved in maintaining position.
• **Asterixis is associated with** various encephalopathies especially due to faulty metabolism^Q.
• It can be **seen in any metabolic encephalopathy**, e.g. **chronic renal failure, severe congestive heart failure, acute respiratory failure** and of course commonly **decompensated liver failure**^{Q}.
• It can be a **sign of hepatic encephalopathy, damage to brain cells presumably due to the inability of the liver to metabolize ammonia to urea** (predominantly related to abnormal ammonia metabolism).

Contd...

Contd...

- Asterixis is **seen most often in drowsy or stuporous patients with metabolic encephalopathies, especially in decompensated cirrhosis or acute liver failure**[Q].
- **Asterixis can be prominent after receiving IV phenytoin** & **also if the patient is on narcotics.**

Description:
- **Brief, arrhythmic interruptions of sustained voluntary muscle contraction** causing **brief lapses of posture**
- **Frequency: 3–5 Hz**[Q]
- It is **bilateral, but may be asymmetric**[Q].

Asterixis is seen in	
• **Chronic renal failure**[Q] • **Severe congestive heart failure**[Q] • **Acute respiratory failure**[Q]	• **Hepatic encephalopathy**[Q] **(decompensated liver disease)** • **Wilson's disease**[Q]

121. **Ans. c. Breath sound**   *(Ref: Harrison 19/e p1573, 1719, 18/e p1972)*

Raised JVP, pulse pressure and muffled heart sounds along with pulsus paradoxus are seen in both cardiac tamponade and tension pneumothorax. These are differentiated by auscultation for breath sounds, which are normal in cardiac tamponade but absent in tension pneumothorax patients.

"Pericardial Tamponade: The three principal features of tamponade (Beck's triad) are hypotension, soft or absent heart sounds, and jugular venous distention with a prominent x-descent but an absent y-descent." – Harrison 19/e p1573

"Tension Pneumothorax: The positive pleural pressure is life-threatening both because ventilation is severely compromised and because the positive pressure is transmitted to the mediastinum, resulting in decreased venous return to the heart and reduced cardiac output. Difficulty in ventilation during resuscitation or high peak inspiratory pressures during mechanical ventilation strongly suggest the diagnosis. The diagnosis is made by physical examination showing an enlarged hemithorax with no breath sounds, hyperresonance to percussion, and shift of the mediastinum to the contralateral side." – Harrison 19/e p1719

Features	Cardiac Tamponade	Tension Pneumothorax
Presenting	**Shock**[Q] (Shortness of Breath may be seen)	**Respiratory Distress**[Q] (Shock my be the presenting feature but less common)
Neck Veins	**Distended**[Q]	**Distended**[Q]
Trachea	Midline	**Deviated**[Q]
Breath Sounds	Normal	**Decreased or absent on side of injury**[Q]
Percussion Note	Normal	**Hyper-resonant**
Heart Sound	**Muffled**[Q]	Normal

Pericardial Tamponade
• Pericardial tamponade must be differentiated from tension pneumothorax in the shocked patient with distended neck veins.   • It is most commonly the result of **penetrating trauma**[Q].   • Characterized by **Beck's Triad (MDH): Muffled** heart sounds, **Distended neck veins (jugular venous distention** with a **prominent X-descent** but an **absent Y-descent)** & **H**ypotension[Q]

Diagnosis:
- **Chest X-ray: Enlarged heart shadow**[Q]
- **Echocardiography:** ECHO is **diagnostic**[Q] showing fluid in the pericardial sac
- **Central line: Rising central venous pressure**[Q]

Treatment:
- **Needle pericardiocentesis** can **buy enough time to move to** the **operating room**[Q].
- **Treatment of choice: Surgical pericardiotomy**[Q]

122. **Ans. b. Hyperkalemia**   *(Ref: Harrison 19/e p2325, 18/e p2957)*

Hyperkalemia is seen in mineralocorticoid deficiency but not in isolated glucocorticoid deficiency. Fever is due to release of inflammatory mediators, which is suppressed by steroids, is seen in glucocorticoid deficiency.

Signs & Symptoms of Adrenal Insufficiency

Signs and Symptoms Caused by Glucocorticoid Deficiency	Signs and Symptoms Caused by Mineralocorticoid Deficiency (Primary Adrenal Insufficiency Only)
• **Fatigue,** lack of energy[Q] • **Weight loss,** anorexia[Q] • Myalgia, joint pain • **Fever**[Q] • **Normochromic anemia, lymphocytosis, eosinophilia**[Q] • Slightly increased TSH (due to loss of feedback inhibition of TSH release) • **Hypoglycemia**[Q] (more frequent in children) • **Low blood pressure, postural hypotension**[Q] • **Hyponatremia**[Q] (due to loss of feedback inhibition of AVP release)	• Abdominal pain, nausea, vomiting • Dizziness, postural hypotension • Salt craving • **Low blood pressure, postural hypotension**[Q] • **Increased serum creatinine**[Q] (due to **volume depletion**) • **Hyponatremia**[Q] • **Hyperkalemia**[Q]

Signs and Symptoms Caused by Adrenal Androgen Deficiency	Other Signs and Symptoms
• Lack of energy • **Dry and itchy skin**[Q] (in women) • **Loss of libido**[Q] (in women) • **Loss of axillary & pubic hair**[Q] (in women)	• **Hyperpigmentation (primary adrenal insufficiency only):** Due to excess of proopiomelanocortin [POMC]-derived peptides • **Alabaster-colored pale skin (secondary adrenal insufficiency only**[Q]**):** Due to deficiency of POMC-derived peptides

Adrenal Insufficiency (Addison's Disease)

• **Addison's disease** or **primary adrenocortical deficiency** is characterized by primary inability of adrenals to elaborate sufficient quantities of adrenal cortical hormones.
• **Addison's disease** is associated with **increased plasma rennin activity**[Q].

> • '**Elevated plasma rennin activity in Addison's disease** indicates the presence of **depleted intravascular volume** and **need for higher doses of fludrocortisone replacement'.**

Etiology:

MC cause of Addison's disease in developing countries	• *Tuberculosis*[Q]
MC cause of Addison's disease in developed countries	• *Autoimmune disease*[Q] *(Idiopathic atrophy)*

Manifestations of Addison's Disease

General features	Hyperpigmentation[Q]	Arterial Hypotension[Q]	Abnormal GI function
• **Asthenia**[Q] (weakness) is the **cardinal symptom** • **Personality changes excessive irritability & restlessness**[Q] • **Cardiac atrophy** may be seen, Addison's disease is associated with a **small heart**	• **Pigmentation** appears as a **diffuse brown, tan, or bronze darkening of skin**[Q] • This increased pigmentation is diffuse but may be **accentuated in the palmer crease, sites of friction & pressure**[Q] areas, oral mucosa, gums & conjunctival, areolae of nipples	• Addison's disease is associated with **both systolic & diastolic hypotension**[Q]. • Blood pressure may be in the range of 80/50 or less	• Anorexia[Q], nausea[Q], vomiting[Q] • **Diarrhea**[Q] • **Weight loss** • **Abdominal pain**[Q]

Abnormal Laboratory parameters in Addison's disease	
• *Hyponatremia*[Q] • *Hyperkalemia*[Q] • *Hypercalcemia*[Q]	• *Hypoglycemia*[Q] • *Decreased chloride*[Q] • *Decreased bicarbonate*[Q]

Contd...

AIIMS November 2015   1347

Contd...

Adrenal Insufficiency (Addison's Disease)
Diagnosis:
• The diagnosis of Adrenal insufficiency should be made only with ACTH stimulation testing: Cosyntropin stimulation test[Q]
• Addison's disease is associated with serum cortisol < 3 mg/dl[Q]
• Low plasma cortisol (<3 mg/dl) at 8:00 AM is diagnostic especially if accompanied by simultaneous elevationof plasma ACTH level (usually > 200 pg/ml)[Q].

123. **Ans. a. Broca's aphasia**   *(Ref: Harrison 19/e p279, 18/e p203, 3286)*

Naming and fluency is impaired in Broca's aphasia.

"Broca's Aphasia: Speech is nonfluent, labored, interrupted by many word-finding pauses, and usually dysarthric. It is impoverished in function words but enriched in meaning-appropriate nouns. Abnormal word order and the inappropriate deployment of bound morphemes (word endings used to denote tenses, possessives, or plurals) lead to a characteristic agrammatism. Speech is telegraphic and pithy but quite informative. Output may be reduced to a grunt or single word ("yes" or "no"), which is emitted with different intonations in an attempt to express approval or disapproval. In addition to fluency, naming and repetition are impaired.' - Harrison 19/e p279

	Comprehension	Repetition of spoken language	Naming	Fluency
Wernicke's	Impaired[Q]	Impaired[Q]	Impaired[Q]	Preserved or increased[Q]
Broca's	Preserved (except grammar)[Q]	Impaired[Q]	Impaired[Q]	Decreased[Q]
Global	Impaired[Q]	Impaired[Q]	Impaired[Q]	Decreased
Conduction	Preserved[Q]	Impaired[Q]	Impaired[Q]	Preserved[Q]
Nonfluent (motor) transcortical	Preserved[Q]	Preserved[Q]	Impaired	Impaired
Fluent (sensory) transcortical	Impaired	Preserved[Q]	Impaired	Preserved
Isolation	Impaired	Echolalia[Q]	Impaired	No purposeful speech
Anomic	Preserved[Q]	Preserved[Q]	Impaired	Preserved except for word-finding pauses[Q]
Pure word deafness	Impaired only for spoken language	Impaired	Preserved	Preserved
Pure alexia	Impaired only for reading	Preserved	Preserved	Preserved

Broca's Aphasia
• **Speech is nonfluent, labored, interrupted by many word-finding pauses**, and **usually dysarthric**.
• It is **impoverished in function words** but **enriched in meaning-appropriate nouns**.
• **Abnormal word order** and the **inappropriate deployment of bound morphemes** (word endings used to denote tenses, possessives, or plurals) lead to a **characteristic agrammatism**.
• **Speech is telegraphic & pithy but quite informative[Q]**.
• In the following passage, a patient with Broca's aphasia describes his medical history: "I see ... the dotor, dotor sent me ... Bosson. Go to hospital. Dotor ... kept me beside. Two, tee days, doctor send me home."
• **Output may be reduced to a grunt or single word** ("yes" or "no"), which is emitted with different intonations in an attempt to express approval or disapproval.
• **In addition to fluency, naming & repetition are impaired[Q]**.

Broca's Aphasia
- **Comprehension of spoken language is intact except for syntactically difficult sentences** with a passive voice structure or embedded clauses, indicating that **Broca's aphasia** is not just an "expressive" or "motor" disorder and that it also may **involve a comprehension deficit in decoding syntax.**   - Even when **spontaneous speech is severely dysarthric**, the **patient may be able to display a relatively normal articulation of words when singing**. This dissociation has been used to develop specific therapeutic approaches (**melodic intonation therapy**) for Broca's aphasia[Q].
Causes of Broca's Aphasia: - The cause is most often **infarction of Broca's area (inferior frontal convolution)** & **surrounding anterior perisylvian & insular cortex** due to **occlusion of superior division of middle cerebral artery**[Q]. - **Mass lesions, including tumor, intracerebral hemorrhage & abscess,** also may be responsible.
Associated features: - Patients with Broca's aphasia can be **tearful, easily frustrated & profoundly depressed.** - **Additional neurologic deficits**: Right facial weakness, hemiparesis or hemiplegia & **buccofacial apraxia** characterized by an inability to carry out motor commands involving oropharyngeal and facial musculature. - **Insight into their condition is preserved, in contrast to Wernicke's aphasia**[Q].
Prognosis: - When the cause of Broca's aphasia is **stroke, recovery of language function generally peaks within 2 to 6 months, after which time further progress is limited**. - **Speech therapy** is **more successful than in Wernicke's aphasia.**

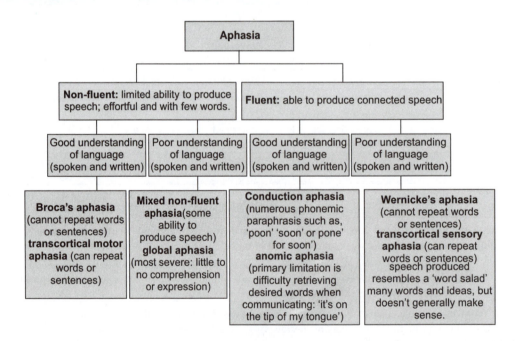

124. **Ans. a. Creatine kinase levels** (Ref: Harrison 19/e p462e-6, 18/e p3490–3491)

Symptoms of difficulty in climbing stairs and combing in a 9 years old boy, with swollen bilateral claves are highly suggestive of Duchenne muscular dystrophy (Pseudohypertrophic Muscular Dystrophy). Another evidence is that child uses his feet to stand up on his legs (Gower's sign). Next diagnostic step is creatine kinase levels.

AIIMS November 2015

1349

"Duchenne Muscular Dystrophy: By age 5 years, muscle weakness is obvious by muscle testing. On getting up from the floor, the patient uses his hands to climb up himself (Gower's maneuver). Contractures of the heel cords and iliotibial bands become apparent by age 6 years, when toe walking is associated with a lordotic posture. Loss of muscle strength is progressive, with predilection for proximal limb muscles and the neck flexors; leg involvement is more severe than arm involvement."– Harrison 19/e p462e-6

"Creatine kinase (CK) is the preferred muscle enzyme to measure in the evaluation of myopathies. Damage to muscle causes the CK to leak from the muscle fiber to the serum."

"Serum CK levels are invariably elevated to between 20 and 100 times normal. The levels are abnormal at birth but decline late in the disease because of inactivity and loss of muscle mass."– Harrison 19/e p462e-6

See Q. No. 159 AIIMS November 2016

125. Ans. a. Proptosis   *(Ref: Harrison 19/e p203, 18/e p233)*

Proptosis is not seen in benign intracranial hypertension.

"Characteristic features of Pseudotumor Cerebri: Elevated intracranial pressure (intracranial hypertension) with normal or Small sized ventricular system[Q], No focal neurological signs[Q], Papilledema[Q] (enlarged blind spot in visual fluid), Normal CSF findings[Q], Normal CT scan, MRI & isotope brain scan[Q], Excessive slow-wave activity on ECG[Q]."

Pseudotumor Cerebri (Idiopathic Intracranial Hypertension)
• **Benign self-limiting disorder** with a favorable outcome
• **Majority of patients** are **young, female & obese**[Q]
• It occurs **due to decreased CSF absorption**[Q]
• **Mostly idiopathic in nature** but seen in **hypervitaminosis, expired tetracyclines, OCPs & steroid use**[Q].

Causes of Pseudotumor Cerebri	
• **High doses of vitamin A**[Q]	• **Withdrawal of corticosteroid therapy**[Q]
• **Outdated Tetracycline**[Q]	• **Addison's disease**[Q]
• **Quinolones**[Q]	• **SLE**[Q]
• **Hypoparathyroidism**[Q]	

Clinical Features:
- Manifested by **headache, papilledema, normal CSF** and **normal ventricle size on imaging**.
- **No focal neurological signs**

Characteristic features of Pseudotumor Cerebri
Elevated intracranial pressure (intracranial hypertension) with:
• **Normal or Small sized ventricular system**[Q]
• **No focal neurological signs**[Q]
• **Papilledema**[Q] (enlarged blind spot in visual fluid)
• **Normal CSF findings**[Q]
• **Normal CT scan, MRI & isotope brain scan**[Q]
• **Excessive slow-wave activity on ECG**[Q]

Treatment:
- **Carbonic anhydrase inhibitor** (acetazolamide) **lowers ICP** by **reducing the production of CSF.**
- **Weight reduction is vital** but often unsuccessful.
- If acetazolamide and weight loss fail and **visual field loss is progressive**, a **shunt** should be performed without delay to prevent blindness.
- Occasionally, **emergency surgery** is required for **sudden blindness caused by fulminant papilledema.**

SURGERY

126. Ans. d. Calcium oxalate stone   *(Ref: Smith 17/e p249-254; Campbell 10/e p1296-1302)*

In the given image, which shows enveloped or bipyramidal crystals are seen in calcium oxalate (dihydrate) stones.

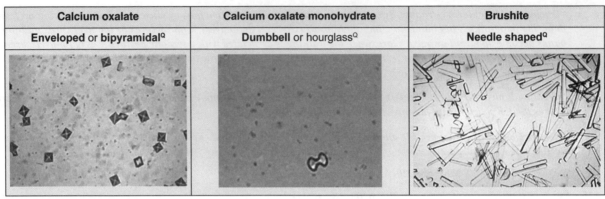

Calcium oxalate	Calcium oxalate monohydrate	Brushite
Enveloped or bipyramidal[Q]	Dumbbell or hourglass[Q]	Needle shaped[Q]

Struvite	Uric acid	Cystine
Coffin lid[Q]	Multifaceted, irregular plates or rosettes[Q]	Hexagonal or benzene ring[Q]

Types of Renal Calculi

1. **Calcium oxalate:**
   - MC type of **kidney stone (85%)**[Q]
   - Risk factors are **hypercalciuria, hypercalcemia, hyperoxaluria**
   - Have **hard, small & jagged surface**

2. **Uric acid stones:**
   - **5-10 %** of all kidney stones, **MC radiolucent urinary calculi**[Q], formed in **acidic urine**
   - Patients with uric acid stones may have **gout, myeloproliferative disorders** or **Lesch-Nehan syndrome (hyperuricemia)**

Uric Acid Stones Management
• Cornerstone of treatment: **Low purine diet, hydration & alkalization of urine**[Q]
• **Allopurinol**[Q] (Inhibits conversion of hypoxanthine & xanthine to uric acid)
• **Acetazolamide**[Q] (may be added if urine pH is <6.5)

3. **Struvite stones (Infection stones):**
   - Composed of **calcium, ammonium, magnesium phosphate (Triple phosphate stones)**[Q]
   - Tend to grow in **alkaline urine**[Q], especially with **Proteus** infection and **fill whole** of the **PCS**, forming **staghorn calculi**[Q]
   - Formed in **high urinary concentration** of **ammonia**
   - More common in **women**[Q] (increased susceptibility for UTI)
   - Most of the **stag horn calculi** are **silent**[Q] & cause **progressive destruction** of **renal parenchyma**[Q].
   - Increased tendency to form struvite calculi is seen in: **Foreign body** in the urinary tract (**Foley's catheter**) & **Neurogenic bladder**[Q]/Bladder dysfunction/Bladder outlet obstruction

Contd...

Contd...

Types of Renal Calculi

Struvite stones Management
• Complete stone removal +Treatment of a metabolic abnormality + Correction of any anatomic abnormalities contributing to stasis • **PCNL+ESWL (best treatment option)**[Q] • **Antibiotics** to prevent stone recurrences or growth after operative procedure • **Acetohydroxamic acid (irreversible inhibitor of urease)**[Q] decreases likelihood of precipitation • **Low calcium, low phosphorus diet.** • Upto **50%** of patient have **stone recurrences** or **UTI** over 10 years follow up

4. Cystine:
- **Extremely hard stone,** formed in **acidic urine**
- Relatively **resistant** to fragmentation by **ESWL**
- Occur in cystinuria with typical **"ground glass" appearance** with a **round smooth outline**[Q]
- Typical **benzene** or **hexagonal cystine crystals**[Q] in urine.

Cystine Stones Management
• **Stone removal** • To lower cystine concentration in urine (**Low methionine diet & alkalization**)[Q] • **Cystine complexing agents: D-Penicillamine**[Q] **& Alpha-mercaptopropionylglycine (MPG)**[Q]

5. Xanthine:
- Seen in **xanthinuria, radioluscent**[Q]
- Stones are **smooth, brick red colored, round** & show **lamination on cross section**[Q].
- **Management: High fluid intake** (most effective therapy) & **Allopurinol**[Q]

6. Indinavir:
- **A protease inhibitor** used in **AIDS patients,** resulting in **radioluscent calculi**[Q] in **6%** patients.

7. Silicate: Associated with **long term use of antacids** containing **silica**[Q]

8. Triamterene: Antihypertensive medication, leading to **radioluscent**[Q] stones

127. Ans. b. Hamartomatous polyps *(Ref: Sabiston 20/e p1372, 19/e p1342; Schwartz 10/e p1206, 9/e p1042-1043; Bailey 27/e p1250, 26/e p1161-1164)*

The given histology shows a large and pedunculated polyp with a firm lobulated contour. An arborizing network of connective tissue is seen with well-developed smooth muscle extending into the polyp and surrounding normal abundant glands lined by normal intestinal epithelium rich in goblet cells. This is typical of Peutz-Jegher's polyps, which are a type of hamartomatous polyp.

Histological Classification of Colorectal Polyps	
Neoplastic Polyps (Adenomatous polyps)	**Non-neoplastic polyps**
• **Tubular** • **Tubulovillous** • **Villous**	• **Hyperplastic** polyps • **Hamartomatous** polyps: **Juvenile polyps** & **PJS** • **Inflammatory** polyps

Non-neoplastic polyps

1. Hyperplastic Polyps
- **MC colorectal polyp**[Q]
- Account for **>90%** of all colorectal polyps, mostly found in the **rectosigmoid**[Q].
- Histologic appearance of these polyps is **serrated (saw-toothed appearance)**[Q]
- **No malignant potential**[Q]

Contd...

Contd...

Non-neoplastic polyps
4. **Hamartomatous Polyps** – A hamartomatous polyp is a **localized overgrowth** of normal, mature intestinal epithelial cells. – Usually **lined with normal epithelium** over a submucosal core. – **Juvenile polyps** are the **MC type** of colorectal **hamartomas**[Q]

Juvenile polyps
• **Juvenile polyps** are the **MC type** of **colorectal hamartomas**[Q] • Occur most commonly in **children <5 years** of age[Q]. • Up to **80%** of juvenile polyps occur as a **single lesion** of the **rectum**[Q] • Typical symptoms are **rectal bleeding, mucus discharge, diarrhea,** and abdominal pain[Q]. • Also called **retention polyps** due to the inflammatory obstruction of the crypt necks that leads to cystic dilation of the mucus-filled glands. • **No increased risk** of **cancer**[Q]

Peutz-Jeghers Syndrome (AD)
• PJS is also characterized by **hamartomatous polyps**[Q]. • Histological characteristics: **Arborization & Pseuoinvasion**[Q]

3. **Inflammatory Polyps**
   – **Inflammatory polyps** occur more frequently in **chronic ulcerative colitis**[Q], but are also seen in **Crohn's disease**[Q].
   – Inflammatory polyps have **no malignant potential**[Q] and require **no treatment**[Q] other than that of underlying colitis.

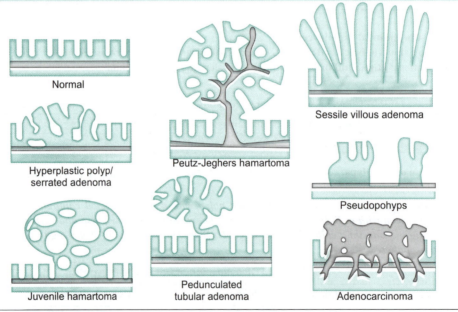

Peutz-Jeghers Syndrome (AD)
• **Hamartomatous** polyps (usually <100) throughout the GIT, **most common** in **jejunum**[Q] • Associated with **hypermelanotic macule** in the **perioral region, buccal mucosa**[Q]. • **Mucocutaneous pigmentation** usually occurs **during infancy** and most commonly noted in **perioral** and **buccal** region. 　• **Pigment spots** usually appear in **first few years** of life, reach a **maximum level** in **early adolescence** and **can fade in adulthood**[Q]. However, pigmentation on the **buccal mucosa remains throughout** the life[Q]. 　• The **pigmented macules** of PJS have **no malignant potential**[Q]. • **Polyposis** develops by **age 20**, occur most commonly in the jejunum (**jejunum**[Q] >colon >stomach).

Contd...

Peutz-Jeghers Syndrome (AD)
Histology:
• **Smooth muscle extends into the superficial epithelial layer in a tree like manner** known as **arborization**[Q].
• **Pseudoinvasion (epithelial cell trapping)**[Q] is noted in upto 10% of polyps >3 cm.
Genetics:
• It exhibits **autosomal dominant** inheritance
• Chromosome **19p13.3**[Q] encodes the serine threonine kinase **LKB1/STK11**[Q].
Clinical Features:
• **MC symptom** is **recurrent colicky abdominal pain**, as a **result of intermittent intussusception**[Q].
• **Lower abdominal pain associated with a palpable mass**[Q] has been reported to occur in one third of patients.
• **Hemorrhage as a result of autoamputation of the polyps** occurs less frequently and is most commonly manifested by anemia.
• **Extracolonic cancers** are common, occurring in **50-90%** of patients (**small intestine, stomach, pancreas, ovary, lung, uterus, and breast**)[Q].
Extra-intestinal Features:
• **Increased risk** for **extra-intestinal cancer** of the **pancreas, thyroid, breast** (may be bilateral), lung, gall bladder, biliary tract (**cholangiocarcinoma**)[Q].
• **Increased risk of gynecologic malignancies** of ovary (bilateral **sex cord tumors** with annular features) & **uterus** (**well-differentiated adenocarcinoma** of the cervix, known as **adenoma malignum**)[Q]
• In men there is increased risk of **feminizing Sertoli cell tumors** of **testis**[Q].

128. **Ans. a. Obstruction of sub-dermal lymphatics** *(Ref: Bailey 27/e p873, 874, 26/e p811, 25/e p840)*

Peau-d-orange is due to cutaneous lymphatic edema, caused by obstruction of subdermal lymphatics.

Peau-d-orange
• **Peau-d-orange is due to cutaneous lymphatic edema**, where the infiltrated skin is tethered by sweat ducts, it can not swell, leading to an appearance like **orange skin**[Q].
• Due to **obstruction** of **subdermal lymphatics** (**lymphatic permeation** by **tumor cells**[Q])
• Seen in **advanced breast cancer**[Q] (may be seen in **chronic abscess**[Q])

129. **Ans. d. Inadequate preoperative preparation** *(Ref: Schwartz 10/e p1534, 9/e p1355; Sabiston 20/e p304, 19/e p897; Bailey 27/e p815, 26/e p762)*

Thyrotoxic crisis (storm) is an acute exacerbation of hyperthyroidism. It occurs if a thyrotoxic patient has been inadequately prepared for thyroidectomy.

*"Thyrotoxic crisis (storm): This is an **acute exacerbation of hyperthyroidism. It occurs if a thyrotoxic patient has been inadequately prepared for thyroidectomy** and is now extremely rare. Very rarely, a thyrotoxic patient presents in a crisis and this may follow an unrelated operation. Symptomatic and supportive treatment is for dehydration, hyperpyrexia and restlessness. This requires the administration of intravenous fluids, cooling the patient with ice packs, administration of oxygen, diuretics for cardiac failure, digoxin for uncontrolled atrial fibrillation, sedation and intravenous hydrocortisone. Specific treatment is by carbimazole 10–20 mg 6-hourly, Lugol's iodine 10 drops 8-hourly by mouth or sodium iodide 1g i.v. Propranolol intravenously (1–2 µg) or orally (40 mg 6-hourly) will block β-adrenergic effects."*
—Bailey 27/e p815

Thyroid Storm (Thyrotoxic crisis)
• It is an **emergency** due to **decompensated hyperthyroidism**[Q].

Treatment of Thyroid Storm (Thyrotoxic crisis)
1. Non-selective beta--blocker (Propranolol):
– **Most valuable measure** in **thyroid storm**[Q].
– In thyroid storm most of the symptoms are because of adrenergic over activity due to **increased tissue sensitivity** to **catecholamines** in hyperthyroidism.
– This **increased sensitivity** is due to **increased** number of **beta receptors**[Q].
– Quick relief is obtained by blocking **beta**-receptors.

Contd...

Contd...

Thyroid Storm (Thyrotoxic crisis)
2. Propylthiouracil: – **Antithyroid drug of choice** for **thyroid storm**[Q]   – **Reduces hormone synthesis** as well as **peripheral conversion** of T_4 to T_3[Q]
3. Corticosteroids (Hydrocortisone):   – **Inhibits** both **release of thyroid hormone** from the gland and **peripheral conversion** of T_4 to T_3[Q]
4. Iodides (Potassium iodide or **Iopanoic acid):**   – Used to **inhibit** further **hormone release**[Q] from the gland.
5. Other Measures: – **Diltiazem**, if **tachycardia** is not controlled by propranolol alone**.   – **Rehydration, anxiolytics, external cooling** & appropriate antibiotics

130. **Ans. b. Periampullary carcinoma** *(Ref: Sabiston 20/e p1544, 19/e p1535-1544; Schwartz 10/e p1408, 9/e p1220-1225; Bailey 27/e p1234, 26/e p1138, Blumgart 5/e p919-925; Shackelford 7/e p1190-1196)*

A 60-year-old chronic smoker presented with progressive jaundice, pruritus and clay colored stools for 1 month. History of waxing and waning episodes was present. A CT scan revealed dilated main pancreatic duct and common bile duct (double duct sign). Most likely diagnosis is periampullary carcinoma, as history of waxing and waning episode is seen.

"The waxing and waning nature of jaundice is due to sloughing of ampullary cancer, resulting in transient resolution of the jaundice."

Carcinoma Pancreas

• **MC type** is **pancreatic ductal adenocarcinoma (PDAC)**[Q]
 • More common in **Men, African Americans**, mean age at diagnosis is **72 years**[Q]
 • Overall, **<5%** of individuals will **survive 5 years** beyond their diagnosis.
      • **Association** between risk of **pancreatic cancer**, **H. pylori** colonization, and **ABO** blood groups.
      • **Established risk factors**: Smoking (Tobacco) & Inherited susceptibility[Q]
 • **Hereditary risk factors:** Hereditary pancreatitis, HNPCC, Hereditary Breast Cancer associated with the BRCA2 mutation, Ataxia Telangiectasia, FAMMM, and Peutz-Jegher's syndrome. **(H3-AFP)**[Q]
      • **K-RAS2** oncogene is **activated** (by point mutation) in **>95%** of pancreatic cancers (**MC gene mutation**)[Q]

Pathology: • Macroscopically, ductal adenocarcinoma is a **scirrhous (scar forming)**[Q] **type** of carcinoma   • It is associated with **abundant desmoplastic stroma**[Q], in which the **neoplastic glands** are **widely scattered**[Q]
Clinical Features: • **MC symptom** for patients with PDACs in the periampullary region is **jaundice**[Q].   • **Pain** typically arising in the epigastrium and radiating to the back.   • **Weight loss** affecting more than 50% of individuals.   • For tumors of the **body & tail** of the pancreas, **pain** and **weight loss** become more common at presentation.

Presenting Symptoms of Periampullary Tumors	
Jaundice (75%)[Q]	Pruritus (11%)
Weight loss (51%)[Q]	Fever (3%)
Abdominal pain (39%)	Gastrointestinal bleeding (1%)
Nausea/vomiting (13%)	

- A **palpable distended gallbladder** in **1/3rd of patients** with periampullary PDAC (**Courvoisier Law**)[Q]
- With widespread disease, a left supraclavicular node (**Virchow's node**)[Q] may be palpable. Periumbilical lymphadenopathy may be palpable (**Sister Mary Joseph's node**)[Q].
- In cases of **peritoneal dissemination**, perirectal tumor involvement may be palpable via digital rectal examination, referred to as **Blumer's shelf**[Q].

Contd...

Carcinoma Pancreas

- The **waxing & waning nature of jaundice** is due to **sloughing of ampullary cancer, resulting in transient resolution of the jaundice**[Q].

Diagnosis:

- Tumor markers: CA19-9 (most sensitive)[Q] & CEA.
  - Individuals with **blood Lewis antigen-negative status (10-15%)** do **not** develop **elevation of** the **CA19-9**[Q].
- MDCT is **investigation of choice** for the evaluation of **lesions arising** in the **pancreas**[Q].
- For suspected periampullary pathology, a **three-phase (noncontrast, arterial,** and **portal venous)** CT scan with 3-mm slices and coronal and three-dimensional reconstruction should be routine.
  - **ERCP:** Reserved for cases requiring **therapeutic** or **palliative intervention**[Q]
  - **Double duct sign** on **ERCP** is highly suggestive of **pancreatic head cancer**[Q]
- EUS: For identifying lesions <2 cm[Q] that do not appear on CT scans
- **Tissue diagnosis** is **not necessary prior to** routine **resection**[Q].
- A suspicious lesion by imaging should be treated with resection.

Treatment:

- **Surgical resection** remains the **only potentially curative treatment** of pancreas cancer.

Tumors of **head** of the pancreas	**Pylorus preserving pancreaticoduodenectomy or Longmire-Traverso procedure** is preferr[e]d[Q]
Tumors of **body and tail** of the pancreas	**Distal pancreatectomy & en-bloc splenectomy**[Q]

- MC complication of pancreaticoduodenectomy is delayed gastric emptying[Q]
- MC cause of **death** following **pancreaticoduodenectomy** is **cardiopulmonary complications**[Q].
- Most important predictor of post-operative survival is R0 resection[Q].
- **Most important margin** in **pancreaticoduodenectomy** is **retroperitoneal** or **uncinate margin**[Q].

Palliative Therapy for Pancreatic Cancer	
Biliary obstruction	**ERCP** with **metal stent placement (Best)**[Q] Roux-en-Y hepaticojejunostomy
Gastric outlet obstruction	**Endoscopic stenting (Preferred)**[Q] Double bypass (Roux-en-Y hepaticojejunostomy + gastrojejunostomy)
Pain	**NSAIDs** or **opiates**[Q] **Celiac nerve block**[Q]

Chemotherapy:

- **Gemcitabine**[Q] is currently the standard of care for patients with **metastatic pancreatic cancer**.

Prognosis:

- **Five year** survival **after curative resection** (pancreaticoduodenectomy) approaches **15-20%**[Q]
- Overall, 5-year survival rate **with pancreatic cancer** is **5%**[Q].

Median survival in Carcinoma Pancreas	
Resectable disease (stage **I & II**)	**15-20** months[Q]
Locally advanced disease (stage **III**)	**6-10** months[Q]
Metastatic disease (stage **IV**)	**3-6** months[Q]

131. **Ans. a. Present in 3% of the population** *(Ref: Sabiston 20/e p1284, 19/e p1268-1270; Schwartz 10/e p1164, 9/e p1002-1004, 1435; Bailey 27/e p1252, 26/e p1169-1170; Shackelford 7/e p695-698)*
Meckel's diverticulum is present in 2% of the population and not 3%.

> *"A Meckel's diverticulum is a persistent remnant of the vitellointestinal duct and is present in about 2 per cent of the population. It is found on the antimesenteric side of the ileum, commonly at 60 cm from the ileocaecal valve and is classically 5 cm long. A Meckel's diverticulum contains all three coats of the bowel wall and has its own blood supply."*
> *– Bailey 26/e p1169*

Meckel's diverticulum

- **Most commonly** encountered **congenital anomaly** of the **small intestine**[Q]
- Occur **2%** of the **population**[Q].

Rule of two in Meckel's diverticulum	
• **2% prevalence**[Q] • **2 inch** in **length**[Q] • **2 feet** proximal to **ileocecal valve**[Q]	• Half of these who are **symptomatic** are **<2 years**[Q] of age

- **True**[Q] **diverticulum** as it has **all the 3 layers** of the intestine[Q].
- Located on the **antimesenteric border** of the **ileum 45 to 60 cm proximal** to the **ileocecal valve**
- Results from **incomplete closure** of **omphalomesenteric** or **vitellointestinal duct**[Q].
- An **equal incidence** among **men & women**[Q].
  - **MC heterotopic tissue**: Gastric mucosa (50%)[Q] >Pancreatic mucosa (5%) >colonic mucosa (rarely)

Clinical Features:

- **Most** are **entirely benign** & **incidentally discovered** during autopsy, laparotomy, or barium studies
  - **MC clinical presentation** is **GI bleeding (25-50%)**[Q]
  - **Hemorrhage**: MC symptomatic presentation in **children ≤2 years**[Q]

- **Hemorrhage** is manifested as **painless bright red blood** from the **rectum**, with **intermittent episodes**[Q] persisting without treatment.
- **Source** of the bleeding is a **chronic acid-induced ulcer** in the **ileum** adjacent to a Meckel's diverticulum that contains gastric mucosa.
- **Intestinal obstruction** (31%): Due to **volvulus**, **intussusception**, or, rarely, incarceration of the diverticulum in an inguinal hernia (**Littre's hernia**)[Q].

Complications of Meckel's diverticulum
• **MC complication** in **children & young adults**: Bleeding[Q]   • **MC complication** in **adults**: Intestinal obstruction[Q]

- **Diverticulitis** (10-20%) is **more common** in **adult patients**.
- Progression of the diverticulitis may lead to perforation and peritonitis.
  - When the **appendix** is found to be **normal** during exploration for suspected appendicitis, the **distal ileum** should be **inspected for** the presence of an **inflamed Meckel's diverticulum**[Q].

Diagnosis:

- **Most accurate diagnostic test** in **children**: Scintigraphy with sodium ^{99m}**Tc-pertechnetate**[Q].

^{99m}Tc-pertechnetate[Q] Scan
• The ^{99m}Tc-pertechnetate is **preferentially taken** up by the mucus-secreting cells of **gastric mucosa** & **ectopic gastric tissue** in the diverticulum[Q].   • (Sensitivity-85%, specificity-95% and an **accuracy-90%** in the pediatric age group)   • **Less accurate in adults** because of the **reduced prevalence** of **ectopic gastric mucosa**[Q]   • The **sensitivity & specificity** can be **improved by pentagastrin** and **glucagon** or H_2**-receptor antagonists (cimetidine)**[Q].

- In **adults** with normal nuclear medicine findings, **barium studies** should be performed.

Contd...

Contd...

Meckel's diverticulum
Treatment:
• **Symptomatic Meckel's diverticulum**: **Diverticulectomy** or **resection** of the **segment of ileum**[Q] bearing the diverticulum.
• **Segmental intestinal resection** is required **for bleeding** because the **bleeding site** usually is in the **ileum** adjacent to the diverticulum[Q].
• **Asymptomatic diverticula** found in **children** during laparotomy should be **resected**[Q].
• **Incidentally found Meckel's diverticulum** should be **removed at any age up to 80 years** as long as no additional conditions (e.g., peritonitis) made removal hazardous[Q].

132. Ans. a. The sac contains omentum only *(Ref: Sabiston 20/e p1097, 19/e p1114-1115; Schwartz 10/e p1503, 9/e p1307, 1316; Bailey 27/e p1031, 26/e p954-959; Schackelford 7/e p565-568)*

Gurgling sound on reduction in case of hernia indicates that the content is bowel, not omentum.

Content of Hernia	Name	Reduction
Omentum	**Omentocele**[Q]	• **Gurgles on reduction**[Q] • **First portion is more difficult to reduce than the last**[Q].
Intestine	**Enterocele**[Q]	• **Omentum is doughy**[Q] • **The last portion is more difficult to reduce than the first**[Q].

Indirect Inguinal Hernia
• **MC form of hernia** in both **males & females**[Q]
• **Indirect hernias** are **most common in** the **young**, whereas **direct hernias** are most common **in the old**[Q].
• In the **first decade** of life, inguinal hernia is **more common on** the **right side** in the male, due to **later descent of** the **right testis** and a **higher incidence of failure** of **closure of processus vaginalis**[Q].

Indirect Inguinal Hernia
• In **adult males, 65%** of **inguinal hernias** are **indirect** and **55%** are **right-sided**.
• **Hernia is bilateral in 12%** of cases[Q].
• **If both sides are explored** in an **infant presenting with one hernia**, the incidence of a **patent processus vaginalis on** the **other side** is **60%**[Q].

Types of Indirect Inguinal Hernia	
Bubonocele	• Hernia is **limited** to the **inguinal canal**[Q]
Funicular	• **Processus vaginalis** is **closed just above epididymis**[Q]. • **Contents** of the sac **can be felt separately from testis**, which lies below the hernia[Q].
Complete or scrotal	• **Testis** appears to **lie within** the **lower part of hernia**[Q].

Clinical Features:

• **Males** are **20 times more commonly affected** than females[Q].

• The patient complains of **pain in** the **groin** or **pain referred to the testicle** when performing **heavy work** or **taking strenuous exercise**.

• When asked to cough, a **small transient bulging** may be **seen & felt** together with an **expansile impulse**[Q].

• **Large hernias: Sensation** of **weight & dragging** on the mesentery may produce **epigastric pain.**

Content of Hernia	Name	Reduction
Omentum	**Omentocele**[Q]	• **Gurgles on reduction**[Q] • First portion is more difficult to reduce than the last[Q].
Intestine	**Enterocele**[Q]	• **Omentum is doughy**[Q] • The last portion is more difficult to reduce than the first[Q].

Treatment:

• **Surgery** is the **treatment of choice (open** or **laparoscopic)**[Q]

133. **Ans. a. Lateral cutaneous nerve of thigh** (Ref: Sabiston 19/e p1118; Schwartz 10/e p-1515, 9/e p1313-1315; Schackelford 7/e p562-565)

"Neuropathic groin pain is caused by damage to a nerve in the groin region and may be due to partial or complete division, stretching, contusion, crushing, suturing, or electrocautery. The nerves that are usually involved are the ilioinguinal nerve, iliohypogastric nerve, both the genital and femoral branches of the genitofemoral nerve, and the lateral femoral cutaneous nerve of the thigh. The first two are especially prone to injury during an open herniorrhaphy, while the latter (i.e. Lateral cutaneous nerve of thigh) are more likely damaged during laparoscopy. The genital and femoral branches of the genitofemoral nerve and the lateral cutaneous nerve of the thigh are most at risk when the surgeon staples below the iliopubic tract when lateral to the internal spermatic vessels. A burning, tingling pain along the lateral aspect of the thigh in the distribution of the lateral femoral cutaneous nerve is known as meralgia paresthetica, and is due to entrapment of that nerve; the affected skin area may be hyperaesthetic and/or pruritic, and patients may complain of the tactile hallucination of a sensation of small insects creeping under the skin (formication)." – Schwartz 10/e p1515

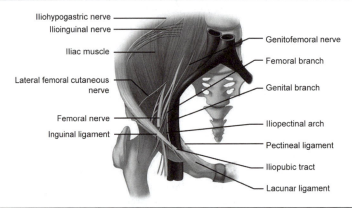

Complications of Groin Hernia Repairs
• **Neuropathic groin pain** is **caused by damage to a nerve in the groin region** and may be due to partial or complete division, stretching, contusion, crushing, suturing, or electrocautery.
• The **nerves that are usually involved** are the **ilioinguinal nerve, iliohypogastric nerve, both the genital and femoral branches of the genitofemoral nerve**, and the **lateral femoral cutaneous nerve of the thigh**.
• The **first two are especially prone to injury during an open herniorrhaphy**, while the **latter (i.e. Lateral cutaneous nerve of thigh) are more likely damaged during laparoscopy.**[Q]
• The **genital and femoral branches of the genitofemoral nerve** and the **lateral cutaneous nerve of the thigh are most at risk when the surgeon staples below the iliopubic tract** when lateral to the internal spermatic vessels[Q].
• A **burning, tingling pain along the lateral aspect of the thigh in the distribution of the lateral femoral cutaneous nerve** is known as **meralgia paresthetica**, and is **due to entrapment of that nerve**; the affected skin area may be hyperaesthetic and/or pruritic, and patients may **complain of the tactile hallucination** of a **sensation of small insects creeping under the skin** (formication).
• A femoral nerve injury is extremely rare and is almost always the result of a gross technical misadventure. Its rarity is fortunate because of the severe associated morbidity.

Landmarks in Laparoscopic Repair		
Triangle of Doom	**Triangle of Pain**	**Corona Mortis**
• Bounded **laterally** by **gonadal vessels**[Q] • **Medially** by **vas deferens**[Q] • **Apex** oriented superiorly at **internal ring**[Q] • Contain **external iliac vessels**[Q], deep circumflex iliac vein, the femoral nerve & genital branch of the genitofemoral nerve.	• Also known as **Electrical hazard zone**[Q] • Bounded **medially** by the **gonadal vessels**[Q] • **Superiorly** by the **iliopubic tract**[Q] • **Laterally** by **peritoneum**[Q] • This triangle **contains** from lateral to medial: • **Lateral femoral cutaneous nerve**[Q] (MC injured nerve during laparoscopic repair) • **Anterior femoral cutaneous**[Q] • **Femoral branch** of the **genitofemoral nerve**[Q] • **Femoral nerve**[Q]	• Also known as **Crown of death**[Q] • **Vascular connections** between the **obturator & external iliac** systems[Q] • **Aberrant obturator artery** arises from the **inferior epigastric** artery, **arches over** the **Coopers ligament** & **joins** the **normal obturator artery**[Q] to complete a vascular ring • **Significant hemorrhage**[Q] may occur **if accidentally cut** and it is **difficult to achieve** subsequent **hemostasis**

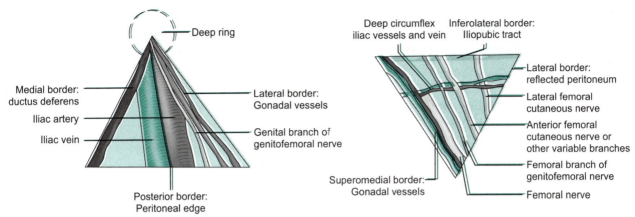

Triangle of Doom	Triangle of Pain
• Space of Retzius (Retropubic space)	• Extra-peritoneal space between pubic symphysis & urinary bladder[Q]
• Space of Bogros (Retroinguinal space)	• Extra-peritoneal space situated deep to inguinal ligament[Q]
	• Situated laterally & cranially to Retzius space[Q]

134. **Ans. a. Urine output** *(Ref: Harrison 19/e p1747, 18/e p2219; Sabiston 20/e p520, 19/e p72-84; Schwartz 10/e p169, 9/e p91-102; Bailey 27/e p17, 26/e p18, 25/e p13-16)*

"Ultimately, the goal of treatment is to restore cellular and organ perfusion. Ideally, therefore, monitoring of organ perfusion should guide the management of shock. The best measures of organ perfusion and the best monitor of the adequacy of shock therapy remains the urine output." – Bailey 26/e p18

Shock
• **Shock**: Inadequate delivery of **oxygen & nutrients** due to **poor tissue perfusion**[Q] to maintain normal tissue & cellular function
• **Mean arterial pressure <60 mm Hg** in previously normotensive patients
• **Systemic vascular resistance rises** leading to **decreased cutaneous blood flow**[Q] and **autoregulation is critical in sustaining cerebral & coronary blood flow**[Q].

Blalock Classification of Shock	
• Hypovolemic (MC)[Q]	• Cardiogenic
• Vasogenic	• Neurogenic

Monitoring in Shock
• The best management of shock is done by putting pulmonary catheter. PCWP is considered better guide than CVP for fluid titrations[Q] as it can also determine left ventricular preload.
• **Invasive arterial pressure** is **mandatory**[Q].
• **Blood gas analysis**[Q]. There is **metabolic acidosis** in shock.
• **Mixed venous oxygen saturation** is considered as **best guide for tissue perfusion** (i.e. cardiac output)
• **Urine output** is **best clinical guide of tissue perfusion**[Q].

135. **Ans. a. Minimum = 3, Maximum = 15** *(Ref: Harrison 19/e p1730; Sabiston 20/e p411, 19/e p1894; Schwartz 10/e p1712, 9/e p1522; Bailey 27/e p325, 26/e p312)*

In Glasgow Coma Scale (GCS), maximum score is 15 and minimum score is 3.

Glasgow Coma Scale (GCS)					
Eye Opening		**Verbal response**		**Best Motor response**	
Spontaneous	4	Oriented	5	Obeys commands	6
To loud voice	3	Confused, disoriented	4	Localizes pain	5
To pain	2	Inappropriate words	3	Flexion (withdrawal) to pain	4

Contd...

Contd...

Eye Opening		Verbal response		Best Motor response	
No response	1	Incomprehensible sounds	2	Abnormal flexion posturing	3
		No response	1	Extension posturing	2
				No response	1

- **Maximum score-15^Q, minimum score-3^Q.**
- **Best predictor of outcome: Motor response**^{Q}
- Patients scoring **3 or 4** have an **85% chance of dying** or **remaining vegetative**, while scores above **11** indicate only a **5-10% likelihood of death**^{Q}.

136. Ans. a. 16 Gauge *(Ref: Bailey 25/e p291)*

In a patient with massive bleeding, there is always a risk of patient going into shock and widest bore cannula available showed be used for cannulation. The ACLS guidelines recommend securing intravenous access with two large-bore cannulae (14–16G) in a patient needing resuscitation.

"Primary survey in Trauma: These include blood samples for full blood count (FBC), coagulation studies, plasma chemistry (urea and electrolytes and, sometimes, toxicology or other case-specific indices), transfusion screening (group and cross-match, etc.), 12-lead electrocardiography (ECG) monitoring and pulse oximetry, if available. The blood can be taken at the same time as securing intravenous access with two large-bore cannulae (14–16G)."– Bailey 25/e p291

"The sizes of needle-based instruments (such as Venflons and needles themselves) are measured in 'Gauge' (i.e. how many can be fitted into a tube of a fixed diameter). In Gauge, larger numbers, mean smaller diameter lumens. Catheters use the 'French' system. This is the circumference of the tube in millimeters, e.g. a 30 F catheter has a circumference of 30 mm. In French, larger numbers therefore mean larger diameter lumens."

Gauge	Color code	External Diameter	Length	Flow Rate
14G	Orange	2.1 mm	45 mm	240 ml/min
16G	Grey	1.8 mm	45 mm	180 ml/min
18G	Green	1.3 mm	32/45 mm	90 ml/min
Gauge	Color code	External Diameter	Length	Flow Rate
20G	Pink	1.1 mm	32 mm	60 ml/min
22G	Blue	0.9 mm	25 mm	36 ml/min
24G	Yellow	0.7 mm	19 mm	20 ml/min
26G	Violet	0.6 mm	19 mm	13 ml/min

OBSTETRIC AND GYNAECOLOGY

137. Ans. c. Endometriosis *(Ref: Shaw's 16/e p413-414, 15/e p471; Novak's 13/e p388)*

Lower abdominal pain and dysmenorrhea with chocolate cyst (Ovarian endometriosis) with blue-grey tattooing of the cyst is seen in given laparoscopic examination picture. This is highly suggestive of endometriosis.

"Chocolate Cyst: It is caused by endometriosis, and formed when a tiny patch of endometrial tissue (the mucous membrane that makes up the inner layer of the uterine wall) bleeds, sloughs off, becomes transplanted, and grows and enlarges inside the ovaries. As the blood builds up over months and years, it turns brown. When it ruptures, the material spills over into the pelvis and onto the surface of the uterus, bladder, bowel, and the corresponding spaces in between."

"The diagnosis of ovarian endometriosis is facilitated by careful inspection of all sides of both ovaries, which may be difficult when adhesions are present in more advanced stages of disease. With superficial ovarian endometriosis, lesions can be both typical and subtle. Larger ovarian endometriotic cysts (endometrioma) are usually located on the anterior surface of the ovary and are associated with retraction, pigmentation, and adhesions to the posterior peritoneum. These ovarian endometriotic cysts often contain a thick, viscous dark brown fluid ("chocolate fluid") composed of hemosiderin derived from previous intraovarian hemorrhage."– Novak's 13/e p388

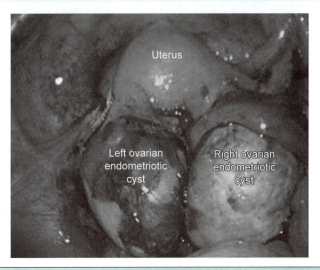

Endometriosis
• Presence of **ectopic functional endometrial tissue** is known as endometriosis. They contain **both gland & stroma** and respond to hormonal stimulation.
• **Prevalence** in general population: **10%**[Q]   • Prevalence among **infertile couple**: **30-40%**[Q]
Theories:
1. **Implantation theory** by Sampson   2. **Coelomic metaplasia** (Meyer & Ivanoff)
3. **Direct implantation**   4. **Metastatic theory**: **Halban's theory** of metastasis through vascular or lymphatic channel   5. **Histogenesis** by induction
Sites:
• **Ovary, Pouch of Douglas, uterosacral ligament, broad ligament**, peritoneum of bladder, sigmoid colon, intestinal coil.
Pathology:
• **Endometriotic implants** → Estrogen influence → Proliferation → No secretory change, **shedding of blood** → **Cystic structure** due to **pent up secretions** → **Fibrosis** due to blood[Q].
• **Powder Burn Appearance**[Q]: Appearance of endometriotic implant is **dark red, bluish or black cystic puckering due to fibrosis, small black dot**[Q]
• The **ovary** have **endometriotic cyst** of varying size, **bluish thickening of tunica albuginea**[Q]. The epithelial lining of cyst is columnar, adjacent to epithelium is a layer of large, polyhedral, Phagocytic cell laden with blood pigment hemosiderin, also known as **Pseudoxanthoma cells**[Q].
Clinical Features:
• **Dysmenorrhea, Pain, Infertility, Menstrual irregularity**[Q]   • **Dyspareunia** (specially when present in **pouch of Douglas**)[Q]
• **Pelvic Examination: Tenderness, nodule** in POD, **cobble stone feel**[Q] of uterosacral ligament, fixed retroverted uterus, bluish or blackish puckered spot in posterior fornix.
Diagnosis:
• **Laparoscopy** is **gold standard** for diagnosis of **endometriosis**[Q].   • **Powder burn** or **matchstick spots** are seen on laparoscopy[Q].

Contd...

Contd...

Endometriosis
Laparoscopic Findings
• **Unless disease** is **visible in** the **vagina** or **elsewhere**, laparoscopy is the **standard technique for visual inspection of pelvis** and **establishment of a definitive diagnosis**^{Q} • **Characteristic findings** include typical **"Powder burn or gun shot"** lesions on the **serosal surface** of peritoneum^Q. • In the presence of **ovarian endometrioma >3 cm in** diameter and **deeply infiltrative disease, histology** should be **obtained to identify endometriosis** and **to exclude rare instance of malignancy**^{Q}.
• CA-125 >35 U/mL may be used as **evidence of recurrence**^{Q}.
Complications:
• **Malignancy: MC type** is **endometroid adenocarcinoma**^{Q} • **Infertility**^{Q} • **Ureteric obstruction** & hydronephrosis

Treatment of Endometriosis	
Medical	**Surgical**
• **NSAIDs** in patients with **pelvic pain**, if the diagnosis of endometriosis has not been definitively (excision & biopsy) established. • **Achieve an anovulatory state by hormonal contraception:** Progestins (**Medroxyprogesterone acetate**), **danazol, gestrinone, or GnRH** • **GnRH** can be combined **with estrogen & progestogen** without loss of efficacy but with fewer hypoestrogenic symptoms.	• **Laparoscopic surgical approaches** include **excision of ovarian adhesions** & **of endometriomas**^{Q}. • **Endometriomas: Excision** is considered to be far superior in terms of permanent removal of the disease & pain relief. • **Operative laparoscopic surgery** can provide **pain relief & improved fertility**. • **Radical surgical options** could include **singular or bilateral oophorectomy**.

138. **Ans. b. Fetal distress** *(Ref: Williams 24/e p340)*

Late decelerations, typical of fetal distress can be seen in the given fetal tocography.

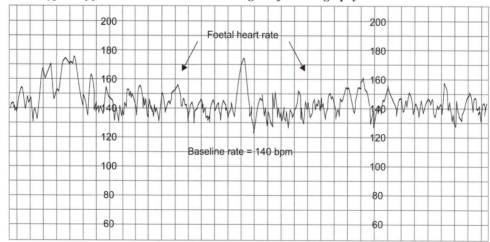

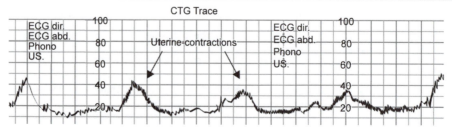

Methods of Monitoring Fetal Heart Rate
1. **Fetal stethoscope** (Pinard) & **Hand-held Doppler** (Sonicaid)
2. **Cardiotocograph (CTG)**

Cardiotocography (CTG)
• **CTG: Technical means of recording** (-graphy) **fetal heartbeat (cardio-)** & **uterine contractions (-toco-)** during pregnancy, typically in **third trimester.**
• The machine used to perform the monitoring is called a **Cardiotocograph,** more commonly known as an **Electronic Fetal Monitor (EFM).**
• Two separate transducers perform recordings, **one for** the measurement of **fetal heart rate** & **second one for uterine contractions.**

Types of measurement:

- Each of the transducers may be either external or internal.
- **External measurement** means taping or strapping the two sensors to the abdominal wall. This is called an indirect measure.
- **Internal measurement** (direct) requires a certain degree of cervical dilatation, as it involves inserting a pressure catheter into the uterine cavity, as well as attaching a scalp electrode to the childs head to adequately measure the electric activity of the fetal heart.

Interpretation:

- Includes description of **uterine activity** (contractions), baseline **fetal heart rate**, baseline **FHR variability**, presence of **accelerations**, periodic or episodic **decelerations**

  - The **3 primary mechanisms by which uterine contractions can cause a decrease in fetal heart rate** are **compression of fetal head, umbilical cord & uterine myometrial vessels[Q].**

Variability
• **Baseline variability** refers to the **variation of fetal heart rate from one beat to the next.**
• Variability occurs as a result of the interaction between nervous system, chemoreceptors, baroreptors & cardiac responsiveness.
• This is because a healthy foetus will constantly be adapting it's heart rate to respond to changes in it's environment.
• **Normal variability** is between **10-25 bpm**
• To calculate variability you look at how much the peaks & troughs of the heart rate deviate from baseline rate (in bpm)

Variability can be categorised as:	
Reassuring	**≥ 5 bpm[Q]**
Non-reassuring	**<5 bpm for between 40-90 minutes[Q]**
Abnormal	**<5 bpm for >90 minutes[Q]**

Accelerations
• **Abrupt increase in baseline heart rate of >15 bpm for > 15 seconds[Q]**
• The presence of accelerations is reassuring
• Antenatally there should be **at least 2 accelerations every 15 minutes[Q]**
• **Accelerations occurring alongside uterine contractions** is a **sign of a healthy foetus[Q]**

Decelerations
Decelerations: Abrupt decrease in baseline heart rate of >15 bpm for > 15 seconds

Types of deceleration	
Early deceleration	• Start **when uterine contraction begins** & recover when uterine contraction stops
	• Due to **increased foetal intracranial pressure** causing **increased vagal tone**
	• Resolves once the uterine contraction ends & intracranial pressure reduces
	• Considered to be **physiological** & not pathological

Contd...

Contd...

Cardiotocography (CTG)	
Variable deceleration	• Seen as a **rapid fall in baseline rate with a variable recovery phase** • Variable in their duration & may not have any relationship to uterine contractions • **Seen during labour** & in **patients with reduced amniotic fluid volume** • Variable decelerations are **usually caused by umbilical cord compression** • The **umbilical vein is often occluded first causing an acceleration in response** • Then the **umbilical artery is occluded causing a subsequent rapid deceleration** • **When pressure on the cord is reduced another acceleration occurs & then the baseline rate returns** • **Accelerations before & after a variable deceleration are known as the "shoulders of deceleration"** • Variable decelerations can sometimes resolve if the mother changes position • The **presence of persistent variable decelerations indicates the need for close monitoring**
Late deceleration	• **Begin at the peak of uterine contraction & recover after the contraction ends.** • Indicates there is **insufficient blood flow through the uterus & placenta, foetal hypoxia & acidosis** due to **reduced uteroplacental blood flow.** • If foetal blood pH is acidotic it indicates significant foetal hypoxia & the need for emergency C-section
Prolonged deceleration	• **A deceleration that last more than 2 minutes** • If it lasts between 2-3 minutes it is classed as non-reassuring • It it lasts longer than 3 minutes it is immediately classed as abnormal • **Action must be taken quickly**, e.g., Foetal blood sampling/emergency C-section

Sinusoidal Pattern
• A smooth, regular, wave-like pattern, frequency of around 2-5 cycles a minute, stable baseline rate around 120-160 bpm, no beat to beat variability • **It indicates severe foetal hypoxia**, severe foetal anaemia, foetal/maternal haemorrhage[Q] • **Management: Immediate C-section** is indicated for this kind of pattern. • **Significance:** This type of pattern is rare, however if present it is very serious. It is **associated with high rates of foetal morbidity & mortality. Outcome is usually poor.**

139. **Ans. a. Endometrial polyp**   *(Ref: Shaw's 16/e p103)*
   The HSG shows a well-defined filling defect characteristically seen in endometrial polyps.

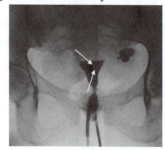

Endometrial Polyp
• Small, soft growths on the endometrium, also known as uterine polyps
Risk factors:
• **Obesity, tamoxifen, hypertension & cervical polyps**[Q]
Clinical Features:
• **Usually no symptoms** • **Symptoms:** Irregular menstrual bleeding, bleeding between menstrual periods, excessively heavy menstrual periods, vaginal bleeding after menopause & infertility

Contd...

Contd...

Endometrial Polyp
Diagnosis:
• **Ultrasound: Echogenic, smooth, intracavitary masses** outlined by the fluid (well-defined, homogenous, polypoid isoechoic lesion) 　　• **Hysterosalpingogram: Pedunculated or sessile-filling defects**[Q] within the uterine cavity.
Treatment:
• Small polyps: Wait & watch • Large polyps: Surgical removal, curettage

Hysterosalpingography
• Used for visualization of uterine cavity & fallopian tubes
• **Performed between** the **end of the menstrual period and ovulation**, usually the **10th day of the cycle**[Q]

Hysterosalpingography	
Indications	**Contraindications**
• To test **patency of fallopian tubes in infertility**[Q] • To **evaluate the result of tuboplasty**[Q] post-operatively • To **detect uterine abnormalities** such as **fibroid polyps** in menorrhagia, **septate & bicornuate uterus in habitual abortions**[Q] & **Asherman syndrome**[Q] • To study the **internal os in the habitual abortions**[Q]	• In the **post-ovulatory period**[Q] • In the **presence of genital infections**[Q] • If the **patient is sensitive to iodine**[Q]

140. **Ans. a. Can be fertile with surrogacy, b. Can be fertile with ovum donation, d. Gonadectomy is indicated for all patients** *(Ref: Shaw's 16/e p145)*

Swyer syndrome patients can be fertile with surrogacy, with ovum donation. Gonadectomy is indicated for all the patients due to risk of malignancy.

Swyer Syndrome
• **Swyer syndrome**, or **XY gonadal dysgenesis (Pure GD)**, is a type of **hypogonadism in a person** whose **karyotype is 46, XY**[Q]. • **Male individuals have female appearance**[Q] 　　• The person is **externally female with streak gonads**, and **left untreated, will not experience puberty**[Q].
Genetics basis:
• Chromosomal analysis shows a **male karyotype (46 XY).** • **Mutations in SRY gene** seen in 15-20% of patients • **Mutations in NR5A1 & DHH genes** are also known to be associated with this condition.
Clinical presentation:
• Classically presents as **sexually infantile phenotypic females with primary amenorrhoea**[Q]. • They are **usually raised as females**[Q]. • They **do not develop true breast tissue or undergo spontaneous menarche**[Q], and are thus brought to medical attention • **Gonads: Female external genitalia** but **uterus & fallopian tubes are underdeveloped. Streak gonads** present instead of functional gonads[Q]
Risk of Tumor:
• Risk of tumor development is **20-30%**[Q] • **MC tumor** seen is **gonadoblastoma**[Q] (**Dysgerminoma & embryonal carcinoma** also reported) 　　• Due to risk of tumours, **extensive search for rudimentary gonads is needed & bilateral gonadectomy is advisable**[Q].
Diagnosis:
• Due to the **inability of the streak gonads to produce sex hormones** (both estrogens & androgens), **most of the secondary sex characteristics do not develop**[Q]. • **Bilateral streak gonads, normally developed Mullerian structures, female appearing external genitalia, & hypergonadotropic hypogonadism**[Q]

Contd...

Contd...

Swyer Syndrome
• **Karyotype: XY chromosomes**[Q]
• **Imaging: Presence of a uterus but no ovaries**[Q] (the streak gonads are not usually seen by most imaging).
○ Although **an XY karyotype** can also indicate a person with complete androgen insensitivity syndrome, **absence of breasts**, **presence of a uterus & pubic hair** exclude the possibility. At this point it is usually possible for a physician to **make a diagnosis of Swyer syndrome**[Q].
Treatment:
• Treatment is required for **prevention of malignancy & osteoporosis, induction of puberty, fertility & psychological support.**
• **Management of puberty: Initiation of estrogen to induce development of secondary sexual characteristics & long term replacement therapy with estrogen & progesterone.**
○ Due to risk of tumours, extensive search for rudimentary gonads is needed & bilateral gonadectomy is advisable[Q].

141. Ans. b. Hypomenorrhea *(Ref: Shaw's 16/e p250; Novak's 13/e p351)*

Hypomenorrhea is seen in Asherman syndrome

*"Asherman's syndrome, which is **more common with secondary amenorrhea or hypomenorrhea, may occur in patients with risk factors for endometrial or cervical scarring, such as a history of uterine or cervical surgery, infections related to use of an intrauterine device, and severe pelvic inflammatory disease.** It is found in 39% of patients undergoing hysterosalpingography who have previously undergone postpartum curettage. **Infections such as tuberculosis and schistosomiasis may cause Asherman's syndrome but are rare in the United States."** – Novak's 13/e p351*

See Q. No. 148 AIIMS May 2016

142. Ans. a. Genital tuberculosis *(Ref: Shaw's 16/e p111)*

Most likely cause for beaded appearance of fallopian tubes with clubbed ends of fimbriae on HSG is genital Tuberculosis.

"Tubal occlusion in tuberculosis is considered the most common sign observed on an HSG and occurs most commonly in the region of isthmus and ampulla. Multiple constrictions along the course of fallopian tube can also form from scarring and give rise to 'beaded' appearance to the tubes. Scarring can also lead to a 'rigid pipe stem' appearance of the tubes."

"Hysterosalpingographic presentation of tubal TB vary from non-specific changes such as hydrosalpinx to specific pattern such as "beaded tube", "golf club tube", "pipestem tube", "cobble stone tube" and the "leopard skin tube"."

Genital Tuberculosis
• **Genital tuberculosis is almost always a secondary infection**[Q]
• **MC primary sites: Lungs >Lymph nodes >Abdomen**[Q]
• **MC Route of spread: Hematogenous**[Q]

Sites of Genital TB	% Involvement
Tubes	**90-100%**[Q]
Uterus	**50-60%**[Q]
Ovaries	**20-30%**[Q]
Vagina & Vulva	**1-2%**[Q]

Pathology:
• **MC site: Bilateral fallopian tubes**[Q]
• **In Fallopian tubes: MC affected part: Ampulla; MC** encountered **pathology** is **endosalpingitis**[Q]
• **2nd MC site of involvement: Uterus**[Q]
• **Cornu** of the uterus **is MC affected** as it is in **continuation with the fallopian tube & infection descends from the tubes**[Q]

Contd...

Contd...

Genital Tuberculosis
Clinical Features:
• **MC age group: 20-30 years (28 years specifically)**
• **MC symptom: Infertility**[Q]
• **Uterine TB can manifest in the form of**:
– **Asherman's syndrome (destruction of the endometrial lining** of uterine cavity with the **formation of intrauterine synechiae or adhesions)**[Q]
– **Pyometra** (pus-filled uterine cavity)
• If patient conceives spontaneously, **ectopic pregnancy** is the most likely outcome.
• **Menstrual abnormalities: Hypomenorrhea or amenorrhea due to Asherman's syndrome & polymenorrhea or menorrhagia**[Q]

Diagnosis:

Hysterosalpingography in TB
• **HSG is contraindicated in patients of genital TB** as it **can lead to reactivation or spreading of disease**[Q].

If unknowingly HSG is done in patients of TB, characteristic findings are	
• **Lead pipe appearance** of tube[Q]	• **Golf club tube**[Q]
• **Beaded appearance** of tube[Q]	• **Tobacco pouch appearance** of the fimbrial end of tube [Q]
• **Hydrosalpinx**[Q]	• **Uterus: Honeycomb appearance due to Asherman syndrome**[Q]
• **Corneal block**[Q]	
• **Intravasation** of dye[Q]	

• **Endometrial biopsy: Best time is 1-2 days before** or **12 hours after onset of menses**. In unmarried girls, menstrual blood can be collected within 12 hours of onset of menstruation.

• **PCR** done on endometrium or menstrual blood is **more sensitive than microscopy** & **bacteriological culture**.

Treatment:

• Genital tuberculosis falls in category 1. The treatment is ATT for 6 months

• **Surgery for restoration of fertility (corrective tuboplasty) is contraindicated in genital TB**[Q]

• **IVF after completion of ATT is the treatment of infertility.**

143. **Ans. a. Serum FSH > 40** *(Ref: Shaw's 16/e p66, 15/e p62)*

Serum FSH > 40 IU/L is diagnostic of menopause.

Criteria for Menopause	
• **Estrogen (E2): 10-20 pg/ml**[Q]	• **E2/E1 < 1**[Q]
• **Estrone (E1): 30-70 pg/ml**[Q]	• **Urine FSH > 40 IU/L**[Q]

	Normal Values of FSH in Females	Normal Values of LH in Females
Follicular Phase	2.5-10.2 mIU/mL	1.9-12.5 mIU/mL
Mid-cycle Peak	3.1-17.7 mIU/mL	8.7-76.3 mIU/mL
Luteal Phase	1.5-9.1 mIU/mL	0.5-16.9 mIU/mL
Postmenopausal	23.0-116.3 mIU/mL[Q]	10.0-54.7 mIU/mL[Q]

Menopause
• **Menopause**, also known as the **climacteric**, is the time in most women's lives when **menstrual periods stop permanently.**
• It is defined as the **time period that occurs after 12 consecutive months of amenorrhea**[Q].
• Menopause typically occurs between 45-55 years of age (**Average age: 51 years**)
• **Smoking** is the **greatest independent risk factor for earlier menstrual irregularity and earlier menopause.**
• **Smoking causes an earlier perimenopuase** and **menopause** by about **1-2 years.**

Contd...

1368   AIIMS ESSENCE

Contd...

Menopause
Laboratory diagnosis:
• **FSH and estrogen level** sometime can be **done to assess ovarian failure,** especially in case of premature ovarian failure or women seeking treatment for infertility.
• **A FSH level greater than 40 m IU/ml has been used to document ovarian failure associated with menopause[Q].**
• **Estrogen level may be normal, elevated depending on the stage of menopausal transition.**
• **After menopause estrogen level are extremely low[Q].**
• Estrogen level can be evaluated by some clinician to asses women's response to hormone replacement thrapy.
• **Usually serem estrodiol level of 50-100 pg/ml is desired while women on hormone replacement therapy.**

144. **Ans. a. Thelarche** *(Ref: Ghai 8/e p531-535; Nelson 20/e p2655)*

The first physical sign of puberty in girls is usually a firm, tender lump under the center of the areola of one or both breasts, occurring on average at about 10.5 years of age. This is referred to as thelarche.

Order of Signs of Puberty	
Males (TPAM)	**Females (TPM)**
• **Testicular enlargement (First sign)[Q]** • **Pubarche[Q]** • **Adrenarche[Q]** • **Moustache & Beard[Q]**	• **Thelarche (First sign)[Q]** • **Pubarche[Q]** • **Menarche[Q]**

Onset of Puberty	
Males	**Females**
• **Growth of testes (≥4 mL** in volume or **2.5 cm** in longest diameter) & **thinning of scrotum** are **first signs of puberty** (11-12 year)[Q]. • These are **followed by pigmentation of scrotum & growth of penis** & by **pubarche**[Q]. • **Appearance of axillary hair** usually occurs in mid-puberty[Q]. • In males, unlike in females, **acceleration of growth is maximal at genital stages IV-V** (typically between **13 & 14 years** of age)[Q]. • In males, **growth spurt occurs approximately 2 year later than in females** & growth **may continue beyond 18 years of age**[Q].	• **Breast development (thelarche)** is usually **first sign of puberty** (10-11 years of age) • Followed by the **appearance of pubic hair (pubarche)** 6-12 months later[Q]. • Interval to the onset of **menstrual activity (menarche)** is usually 2-2.5 years, but may be as long as 6 years[Q]. • **Peak height velocity occurs early** (at **breast stages II-III,** typically between 11-12 years of age) in girls and **always precedes menarche**[Q]. • **Mean age of menarche** is approximately **12.75 years**[Q].

145. **Ans. a. Any time as soon as she presents to the clinic irrespective of pregnancy** *(Ref: Williams 24/e p159, 1104; Nelson 20/e p2805, 19/e p2001)*

If a pregnancy is planned in high-risk women (previously affected child with neural tube defects), supplementation should be started with 4 mg (= 4000 microgram) of folic acid daily, beginning 1 month before the time of the planned conception.

"The U.S. Public Health Service has recommended that all women of childbearing age and who are capable of becoming pregnant take 0.4 mg of folic acid daily. If, however, a pregnancy is planned in high-risk women (previously affected child), supplementation should be started with 4 mg (= 4000 microgram) of folic acid daily, beginning 1 month before the time of the planned conception." – Nelson 20/e p2805

"A diet sufficient in folic acid prevents megaloblastic anemia. The role of folate deficiency in the genesis of neural- tube defects has been well studied. Since the early 1990s, nutritional experts and the American College of Obstetricians and Gynecologists (2013c) have recommended that all women of childbearing age consume at least 400 µg of folic acid daily. More folic acid is given in circumstances in which requirements are increased. These include multifetal pregnancy, hemolytic anemia, Crohn disease, alcoholism, and inflammatory skin disorders. There is evidence that women who previously have had infants with neural-tube defects have a lower recurrence rate if a daily 4-mg (= 4000 microgram) folic acid supplement is given preconceptionally and throughout early pregnancy." -Williams 24/e p1104]

AIIMS November 2015

Neural Tube Defects
• Result from failure of neural tube to close spontaneously between the 3rd & 4th week of in-utero development.
• **It leads to increased levels of AFP & acetylcholine esterase in amniotic fluid[Q].**
• Neural tube defects: Spina bifida occulta, meningocele & myelomeningocele

Etiological Factors for Neural Tube Defects	

• **Maternal diabetes[Q]**
 • **Zinc & folate deficiency[Q]**
 • **Trisomy 13 & 15[Q]**
	• Maternal exposure to:
	    – **Alcohol[Q]**
	    – **Valproate[Q]**
	    – **Carbamazepine[Q]**

Prevention:

- **Nutritional** and **environmental factors: Folate[Q]** is intricately involved in the prevention and etiology of NTDs.
- **Maternal periconceptional use** of folic acid supplementation **reduces** the **incidence** of **neural tube defects** in pregnancies at risk by at least **50%[Q].**
- To be effective, folic acid supplementation should be **initiated before conception** and **continued until** at least the **12th week of gestation** when neurulation is complete[Q].

  - **All women** of childbearing age and who are capable of becoming pregnant take **0.4 mg of folic acid** daily.
  - There is evidence that **women who previously have had infants with neural-tube defects have a lower recurrence rate if a daily 4 mg[Q] (= 4000 microgram) folic acid supplement is given preconceptionally and throughout early pregnancy**.

---

146. **Ans. b. Obstetric conjugate**   *(Ref: Williams 24/e p32; Dutta 7/e p89, 90)*

In the pelvic inlet, shortest anteroposterior diameter is obstetric conjugate (10 cm).

*"**Four** diameters of the pelvic inlet are usually described: anteroposterior, transverse, and two oblique diameters. Of these, distinct anteroposterior diameters have been described using specific landmarks. Most cephalad, the anteroposterior diameter, termed the **true conjugate, extends from the upper- most margin of the symphysis pubis to the sacral promontory**. The clinically important obstetrical conjugate is the shortest distance between the sacral promontory and the symphysis pubis. Normally, this measures 10 cm or more, but unfortunately, it cannot be measured directly with examining fingers. Thus, for clinical purposes, the obstetrical conjugate is estimated indirectly by subtracting 1.5 to 2 cm from the diagonal conjugate, which is determined by measuring the distance from the lowest margin of the symphysis to the sacral promontory."* – Williams 24/e p32

Diameters of the pelvic inlet		
Anteroposterior (AP) Diameter	**Transverse Diameter (13-13.5 cm)**	**Oblique Diameters (12 cm)**

• **True (anatomical) conjugate (11 cm):** Extends from **uppermost margin of symphysis pubis** to **sacral promontory[Q].**
 Obstetric conjugate (10 cm):
   – **Most important AP diameter of the pelvic inlet** as it is the one through which **fetus must pass[Q]**
   – **Smallest AP diameter[Q]**
   – Measured from **middle of sacral promontory to symphysis pubis[Q].**
   – **Pelvic inlet** is considered to be **contracted if OC <10 cm[Q]**
   – **OC can not be measured clinically,** can be estimated by **subtracting 1.5 cm from diagonal conjugate[Q]**
   – Diagonal conjugate (12.5 cm):
   – Measured from **tip of sacral promontory to the lower margin of pubic symphysis[Q]**
   – Out of three AP diameters, **only DC can be assessed clinically** during the **late pregnancy** or at the time of **labor[Q]**
	• **Distance between the farthest two points on the iliopectineal line[Q].**
	 • It is the **largest diameter of pelvic inlet[Q]**
	 • Lies **4 cm anterior to promontory & 7 cm behind the symphysis[Q]**
		• Two oblique diameters: Right & left
		 • **Right oblique diameter:** Passes from **right sacroiliac joint to left iliopubic eminence[Q]**
		 • **Left oblique diameter:** Passes from **left sacroiliac joint to right iliopubic eminence[Q]**

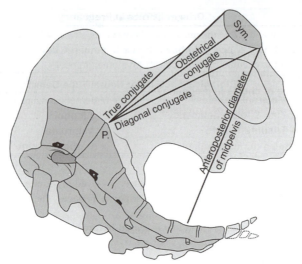

Fig. 31: Pelvic cavity and midpelvis

147. Ans. d. Corpus luteum *(Ref: Williams 24/e p169; Ganong 25/e p412, 24/e p414)*
Estrogen and progesterone in the first 2 months of pregnancy are produced by Corpus luteum.

> *"Detection of hCG in maternal blood and urine is the basis for endocrine assays of pregnancy. This hormone is a glycoprotein with high carbohydrate content. There are subtle hCG variants, and these differ by their carbohydrate moieties. The general structure of hCG is a heterodimer composed of two dissimilar subunits, designated α and β, which are noncovalently linked. The α-subunit is identical to those of luteinizing hormone (LH), follicle-stimulating hormone (FSH), and thyroid-stimulating hormone (TSH). HCG prevents involution of the corpus luteum, which is the principal site of progesterone formation during the first 6 weeks of pregnancy."– Williams Obstetrics 24/e p169*

> *"The enlarged corpus luteum of pregnancy secretes estrogens, progesterone, and relaxin. Progesterone and relaxin help maintain pregnancy by inhibiting myometrial contractions; progesterone prevents prostaglandin production by the uterus, which stops contractions from occurring. In humans, the placenta produces sufficient estrogen and progesterone from maternal and fetal precursors to take over the function of the corpus luteum after the 6th week of pregnancy. Ovariectomy before the 6th week thus leads to abortion, but ovariectomy thereafter has no effect on the pregnancy. The function of the corpus luteum begins to decline after 8 weeks of pregnancy, but it persists throughout pregnancy. hCG secretion decreases after an initial marked rise, but estrogen and progesterone secretion increase until just before parturition."- Ganong 25/e p412*

148. Ans. d. Alpha-methyldopa *(Ref: Williams 24/e p100; Goodman Gillman 12/e p773, 774; Katzung 13/e p176, 12/e p176)*
Drug of choice for hypertension in pregnancy is methyldopa.

> *"Methyldopa is a centrally acting antihypertensive agent. It is a prodrug that exerts its antihypertensive action via an active metabolite. Although used frequently as an antihypertensive agent in the past, methyldopa's significant adverse effects limit its current use largely to treatment of hypertension in pregnancy, where it has a record for safety."–Goodman Gillman 12/e p773*

> *"Methyldopa is a preferred drug for treatment of hypertension during pregnancy based on its effectiveness and safety for both mother and fetus. The usual initial dose of methyldopa is 250 mg twice daily, and there is little additional effect with doses >2 g/day."– Goodman Gillman 12/e p774*

> *"Methyldopa was widely used in the past but is now used primarily for hypertension during pregnancy. It lowers blood pressure chiefly by reducing peripheral vascular resistance, with a variable reduction in heart rate and cardiac output."-Katzung 12/e p176*

Antihypertensives in Pregnancy	
Safe	**Contraindicated**
• Labetalol[Q] • Alpha methyldopa[Q] • Calcium channel blockers[Q] • Hydralazine • Sodium nitroprusside	• ACE inhibitors[Q] • Reserpine • Loratidine

Drug of Choice in Pregnancy

Condition	Drug of Choice
DOC for malaria in pregnancy	Chloroquine[Q]
DOC for anticoagulation in pregnancy	Heparin[Q]
Antihypertensive of choice in pregnancy	Alpha-methyldopa[Q]
Antihypertensive of choice for hypertensive crisis in pregnancy	Labetalol[Q]
DOC for nausea in pregnancy	Doxylamine & pyridoxine[Q]
Analgesic of choice during pregnancy	Acitoaminophen[Q]
Anti-epileptic of choice during pregnancy	Phenobarbitone[Q]

149. Ans. c. Cordocentesis   *(Ref: Williams 24/e p300; Ghai 8/e p341-344)*

A G3P2, pregnant comes to your clinic at 18 weeks of gestation for genetic counselling. She has a history of two kids born with thalassemia major. The recommended test for this patient is Cordocentesis, since this patient is presenting at 18 weeks, a quick method to diagnose thalassemia antenatally is needed as the legal age of abortion is only till 20 weeks. Fetal karyotyping takes 7–10 days when done through CVS or amniocentesis as the shredded cells are to be cultured. Cordocentesis is a much quicker method to achieve the same.

"Fetal blood karyotyping can be accomplished within 24 to 48 hours. Thus, it is significantly quicker than the 7- to 10-day turnaround time with amniocentesis or CVS."– Williams 24/e p300

Cordocentesis (Percutaneous Umbilical Blood Sampling/PUBS)

- **Cordocentesis** was initially described for **fetal transfusion of red blood cells** in the setting of anemia from alloimmunization.

Indications of Cordocentesis
- Fetal anemia assessment[Q]
- Assessment & treatment of platelet alloimmunization[Q]
- Fetal karyotype determination in cases of mosaicism identified following amniocentesis or CVS[Q]

- **Fetal blood karyotyping** can be accomplished **within 24 to 48 hours**. Thus, it is **significantly quicker than the 7- to 10-day turnaround time with amniocentesis or CVS**[Q].

Complications of Cordocentesis
Fetal-maternal bleeding[Q] (40%)	Fetal bradycardia (5-10%)
Cord vessel bleeding (20 to 30%)	Procedure-related fetal loss (1.4%)

Amniocentesis

- Deliberate puncture of the fluid sac per abdomen
- **MC performed invasive test** for prenatal diagnosis of genetic disease[Q]
- **Commonest indication** is **maternal age**[Q]
- Performed at **14-20 weeks**, (**14-16 weeks** is mentioned in Dutta)[Q]
- Two samples of around **30 ml**[Q] is taken
- **Pregnancy loss is high** in **early amniocentesis**[Q]

Amniocentesis

Indications of Amniocentesis	
Diagnostic	**Therapeutic**
Early months (12-14 weeks)[Q]: antenatal diagnosis of chromosomal and genetic disorders	**First half:** induction of abortion by instillation of chemicals, repeated decompression in acute hydramnios
Later months (16-18 months)[Q]: Fetal maturity, degree of fetal hemolysis in Rh sensitized mother, meconium staining of liquor, amniography or fetography	**Second half:** Decompression in unresponsive cases of chronic hydramnios, to give intrauterine fetal transfusion, amnioinfusion

Contd...

Contd...

Chorionic Villus Sampling
• Performed **for prenatal diagnosis of genetic disorders**[Q]
• **Transcervical** between **10-12 weeks**[Q] & transabdominal from **10 weeks to term**[Q]
• A few **villi** are collected from **chorionic frondosum**[Q] under ultrasonic guidance with the help of a long malleable polyethylene catheter introduced transcervically along the extraovular space.

Chorionic Villus Sampling	
Advantages	**Disadvantages**
• **Early diagnosis, early termination, lesser complications**[Q] (as compared to amniocentesis) • Villi are good source of DNA	• Increased pregnancy loss[Q] (as compared to amniocentesis) • **Severe limb reduction defect (Oro-mandibular limb deformity, when CVS is performed before 9 weeks)**[Q]

• **NTD cannot be detected by CVS**[Q].
• **Transabdominal CVS can be performed in 2nd and 3rd trimester**[Q].

Techniques for Prenatal Diagnosis				
Fetal tissues	**Technique**	**Timing (weeks)**	**Studies done on Tissue**	**Risk**
Amniotic fluid	a. **Conventional** Amniocentesis b. **Early** amniocentesis	15-16 11-14	AFP/ACHE/hCG	**Abortion, needle puncture injuries, placental abruption, chorio amniocentesis abruption,** preterm labour.
Amniocytes	a. **Conventional** Amniocentesis b. **Early** amniocentesis	15-16 11-14	**Cell culture for karyotypes, enzyme assay, DNA studies, FISH**	–
Chorionic Villi	a. **Transvaginal** b. **Transabdominal**	8-11 12-24	**Biochemical chromosomal, DNA**	**2% fetal loss, limb defects, mosaicism** and **maternal bleeding**
Fetal blood	a. **Fetoscopic aspiration** b. **Cordocentesis**	18-20 16-20	**Coagulation factor Immunoglobulin antibodies estimation; DNA and enzyme study; karyotype, FSH**	**1% fetal loss, Rhesus sensitization,** fetal infection, PROM
Fetal liver	a. **Fetoscopic biopsy** b. **Percutaneous biopsy**	18-20	Enzyme assay as in OTC deficiency	–
Fetal skin	a. **Fetoscopic biopsy** b. **Percutaneous biopsy**	18-20	Histopathology	–
Fetal muscle	a. **Fetoscopic biopsy** b. **Percutaneous biopsy**	18-20	Histopathology	–
Maternal serum	Maternal blood	12-14	AFP/UE3 hCG	Nil
Fetal cells in maternal circulation	Flow cytometry, PCR1 monoclonal antibodies	1st trimester	Fish fetal sexing DNA testes	Nil
Pre-implantation embryo biopsy	IVF Biopsy of blastocysts	4-8 cell stage blastocyst	DNA, PCR enzyme assay	–

150. Ans. a. NST with amniotic fluid index *(Ref: Williams 24/e p342, 343)*

Modified Biophysical profile consists of NST with amniotic fluid index.

"*Modified Biophysical Profile: Because the biophysical profile is labor intensive and requires a person trained in sonography, Clark and coworkers (1989) used an* **abbreviated biophysical profile** *as a first-line screening test in 2628 singleton pregnancies. Specifically, a vibroacoustic nonstress test was performed twice weekly and combined with amnionic fluid index determination for which < 5 cm was considered abnormal. This abbreviated biophysical profile required approximately 10 minutes to perform, and they concluded that it was a superb antepartum surveillance method because there were no unexpected fetal deaths. The American College of Obstetricians and Gynecologists and the American Academy of Pediatrics (2012) have concluded that the modified biophysical profile test is as predictive of fetal well-being as other approaches to biophysical fetal surveillance.*" *– Williams 24/e 343*

| AIIMS November 2015 | 1373 |

Biophysical Profile

- **Manning** proposed **combined use of 5 fetal biophysical variables as a more accurate means of assessing fetal health than a single element**[Q].
- Typically, these tests **require 30 to 60 minutes** of examiner time[Q].
- 5 fetal biophysical components assessed: **(1) heart rate acceleration, (2) breathing, (3) movements, (4) tone, and (5) amniotic fluid volume**[Q].
- **Normal variables** were assigned a **score of 2 each**, and **abnormal variables** were given a **score of 0**[Q].
- **Highest score possible for a normal fetus is 10**[Q].

Components and Scores for the Biophysical Profile		
Component	**Score 2**	**Score 0**
Non stresstest	≥ 2 acceleration of ≥ 15 beats/min for ≥ 15 sec within 20-40 min	0 or 1 acceleration within 20-40 minutes
Fetal breathing	≥ 1 episode of rhythmic breathing lasting ≥ 30 sec within 30 min	< 30 sec of breathing within 30
Fetal movement	≥ 3 discrete body or limb movements within 30 min	< 3 discrete movements
Fetal tone	≥ 1 episode of extremity extension and subsequent return to flexion	0 extension/flextion events
Amniotic fluid volume	A pocket of amniotic fluid that measure at least 2 cm in two planes perpendicular to each other (2 x 2 cm pocket)	Largest single vertical pocket ≤ 2

Interpretation of Biophysical Profile Score		
Biophysical profile Score	**Interpretation**	**Recommended Management**
10	**Normal**, non-asphyxiated fetus	- No fetal indication for intervention, repeat test weekly except in diabetic patients & Post-term pregnancy (twice weekly)
8/10 (Normal AFV) 8/8 (NST not done)	**Normal**, non-asphyxiated fetus	- No fetal indication for intervention; repeat testing as per protocol
8/10 (Decreased AFV)	**Chronic fetal asphyxia** suspected	- **Deliver**
6	**Possible fetal asphyxia**	- If amniotic fluid volume abnormal, deliver - If normal fluid at ≥ 36 weeks with favourable Cervix, deliver - If repeat test ≤ **6, deliver** - If repeat test > **6**, observe, and repeat as per protocol
4	**Probable fetal asphyxia**	- Repeat testing same day; if biophysical profile score ≤ **6, deliver**
0 to 2	**Almost certain fetal asphyxia**	- **Deliver**

151. **Ans. b. Pre-menstrual tension** *(Ref: Williams 24/e p701; Goodman Gilman 12/e p1184, 1190)*

Pre-menstrual tension is not a non-contraceptive use of levonorgestrel.

*"Emergency contraception: With progestin-only regimens, 1.5 mg of levonorgestrel is taken, either as a single, one-time 1.5 mg dose or as two tablets, each containing 0.75 mg levonorgestrel. With these regimens, the **first dose is ideally taken within 72 hours of unprotected coitus but may be given up to 120 hours.**"_ Williams 24/e p714*

*"In addition, progestins are **highly efficacious in decreasing the occurrence of endometrial hyperplasia** and **carcinoma caused by unopposed estrogens**; when used in this setting, there appears to be less irregular uterine bleeding with sequential rather than continuous administration. **Local intrauterine application via a hormone- releasing intrauterine device (IUD) containing levonorgestrel** can be used to decrease estrogen-induced endometrial hyperplasia while reducing untoward effects (e.g. unfavorable lipid profiles and incidence of breast cancer) of systemically administered progestins."*
– Goodman Gilman 12/e p1184

*"In postmenopausal women with an intact uterus, a progestin is included **to prevent endometrial cancer**. Medroxyprogesterone acetate is used in the U.S., but micronized progesterone is preferred; norethindrone and norgestrel/ levonorgestrel are also commonly used. Women without a uterus are administered estrogen alone. **Postmenopausal hormone therapy and contraception are the most frequent uses of progestins**."_ Goodman Gilman 12/e p1190*

Premenstrual syndrome (PMS) or Perimenstrual Syndrome
• Consistent pattern of **emotional & physical symptoms** occurring on **during the luteal phase of the menstrual cycle** that are of "**sufficient severity to interfere with some aspect of life**"
• **Criteria: At least 5 of the following symptoms** must be present at some point during the **ten day immediately before the onset of menses**, and must not be present for at least one week between the onset menses & ovulation.

Emotional & Behavioral symptoms	Physical sings & symptoms
• Tension or anxiety, depressed mood • Crying spells • Mood swings & irritability or anger • Appetite changes, insomnia	• Joint or muscle pain, headache, fatigue • Weight gain related to fluid retention, abdominal bloating • Brest tenderness, acne flare-ups, constipation or diarrhoea

Treatment:

- **Conservative:** Elimination of caffeine from diet, smoking cessation, counselling change, regular exercise, stress management, dietary changes, adequate sleep
- **Ovulation inhibition: OCPs & GnRH anonists**
- **Medication: Antidepressants** (SSRI: Fluxetine, paroxetine, sertraline), NSAIDs, Diuretics.

152. Ans. a. Desogestrel   *(Ref: Williams 24/e p714)*

Desogestrel is not used as post-coital contraceptive.

Emergency (Post-coital) Contraceptives
• It can be **started up to five days (120 hours) after unprotected intercourse** but **greatest protection** occurs if it is given **within 72 hours** of unprotected sex^Q.
• **Levonorgestrel 1.5 mg single dose (Method of choice^Q)**
Mechanism of Action:
• **Prevents ovulation**
• **Prevents fertilization** (by affecting sperm mobility and thickness of cervical mucus)
• **Prevents implantation by affecting endometrial lining**

Drugs used for Emergency Contraception	
Drug	**Dose**
Levonorgestrel	• **0.75 mg stat and after 12 hours^Q**
Ethinyl estradiol 50 µg + Norgestrel 0.25 mg	• **2 tab stat and 2 after 12 hours^Q**
Conjugated estrogen	• 15 mg BD × 5 days
Ethinyl estradiol	• 2.5 mg BD × 5 days
Mifepristone	• **10 mg single dose^Q**
Copper IUDs^Q	• Insertion of an IUCD within **maximum period of 5-7 days after accidental unprotected exposure^Q**. • It **prevents implantation** but is **not suitable for women with multiple sex partners** and **for rape victims^Q**
Centchroman	• **2 tablets (60 mg) to be taken twice at an in interval of 12 hours within 24 hours of intercourse^Q**
Ulipristal	• It is a **synthetic progesterone receptor modulator, delays ovulation^Q**. • Dose = 30 mg • **Effective as levonorgestrel if taken within 72 hours^Q** • **More effective than levonorgestrel between 72 and 120 hours^Q**

153. Ans. d. Selective progesterone receptor modulator   *(Ref: Harrison's 19/e p2391; Goodman Gilman 12/e p1185)*

Ulipristal, a derivative of 19-norprogesterone, functions as a selective progesterone receptor modulator (SPRM), act as a partial agonist at progesterone receptors.

*"Ulipristal, a derivative of 19-norprogesterone, functions as a selective progesterone receptor modulator (SPRM), acting as a partial agonist at progesterone receptors. It has a dimethyl- aminophenol group at the 11β position, as does mifepristone, with an additional acetoxy group at the C17. Unlike mifepristone, **ulipristal appears to be a relatively weak glucocorticoid antagonist**."– Goodman Gilman 12/e p1185*

Ulipristal acetate
• **Ulipristal acetate** (trade name **EllaOne** in the European Union, **Ella** in US for contraception & **Esmya** for uterine fibroid) is a **selective progesterone receptor modulator**[Q] (SPRM).
Pharmacological Actions:
• **Most relevant action**: **Inhibition of ovulation** (due to **progesterone regulation at many levels**, including **inhibition of LH release** through hypothalamus & pituitary & **inhibition of LH-induced follicular rupture within ovary**)[Q]
• A **30 mg dose of ulipristal** can **inhibit ovulation when taken up to 5 days after intercourse**[Q].
• In **high doses**, ulipristal has **anti-proliferative effects in the uterus**[Q].
Medical Uses
• **Emergency contraception**:
– **30 mg tablet** is used **within 120 hours (5 days)** after an unprotected intercourse or contraceptive failure[Q].
– **Prevent about 60% of expected pregnancies** (prevents more pregnancies than emergency contraception with levonorgestrel)[Q]
• **Treatment of uterine fibroids**:
– Used for **preoperative treatment of moderate to severe symptoms of uterine fibroids** in adult women of reproductive age in a daily dose of a 5 mg tablet[Q].
Side-Effects:
• Self-limited **headache & abdominal pain.**
Contraindications:
• **Severe liver diseases** because of its **CYP-mediated metabolism**[Q].
• **Pregnancy: Embryotoxic in animal studies** (Before taking the drug, a pregnancy must be excluded)

154. **Ans. c. 600 mcg**   *(Ref: Williams 24/e p785)*
The approved dose of misoprostol in emergent management of postpartum hemorrhage is 600 µg.

*"**Misoprostol:** Derman (2006) compared a **600 µg oral dose given at delivery against placebo** and found that the **drug decreased hemorrhage incidence from 12 to 6 percent** and that of severe hemorrhage from 1.2 to 0.2 percent." - Williams 24/e p785*

Misoprostol
• **Misoprostol** (*Cytotec*) is a **synthetic prostaglandin E1 analogue** has been **found to be effective in prevention & treatment of atony & postpartum hemorrhage**[Q].
• Derman (2006) compared a **600 µg oral dose given at delivery against placebo** and found that the **drug decreased hemorrhage incidence from 12 to 6 percent** and that of **severe hemorrhage from 1.2 to 0.2 percent**[Q].
• In another study, however, 400 microgram misoprostol administered rectally was not more effective than intravenous oxytocin in preventing postpartum hemorrhage.

155. **Ans. b. 28 weeks**   *(Ref: Williams 24/e p312; COGT 11/e p353; FERNANDO ARIAS 4/e p374)*
Best time to give anti-D to a pregnant patient is 28 weeks.

*"**In the United States, anti-D immune globulin is given prophylactically to all Rh D-negative, unsensitized women at approximately 28 weeks, and a second dose is given after delivery if the infant is Rh D-positive** (American College of Obstetricians and Gynecologists, 2010). Before the 28-week dose of anti-D immune globulin, repeat antibody screening is recommended to identify individuals who have become alloimmunized (**American Academy of Pediatrics and American College of Obstetricians and Gynecologists 2012**). Following delivery, anti-D immune globulin should be given within 72 hours. Importantly, if immune globulin is inadvertently not administered following delivery, it should be given as soon as the omission is recognized, because there may be some protection up to 28 days postpartum (Bowman, 2006). **Anti-D immune globulin is also administered after pregnancy-related events that could result in fetomaternal hemorrhage."** – Williams 24/e p312*

1376   AIIMS ESSENCE

Prevention of Rh-D Alloimmunization
• **Rh-D immunoglobulin** is given by IM injection, used to prevent the immunological condition known as **Rh disease** (or **hemolytic disease of newborn**)[Q].
• It contains **IgG anti-D (anti-RhD) antibodies that take out any fetal RhD-positive erythrocytes,** which have **entered the maternal blood stream from fetal circulation, before the maternal immune system can react to them,** thus **preventing maternal sensitization**[Q].
Indication:
• **Rh –ve mother with Rh +ve father to prevent hemolytic disease of the fetus**[Q]
Dose:
• **IM dose of anti-D immune globulin: 1500 IU protects haemorrhage of 30 mL blood/15 mL of fetal red cells**[Q].
Prophylaxis:
• **Given prophylactically to all Rh D-negative unsensitized women at approximately 28 weeks, and a second dose is given after delivery if the infant is Rh D-positive**[Q].
• Before the 28-week dose of anti-D immune globulin, repeat antibody screening is recommended to identify individuals who have become alloimmunized.
• **Following delivery, anti-D immune globulin should be given within 72 hours**[Q].
Special cases:
• In 1% of pregnancies, **volume of fetomaternal haemorrhage exceeds 30 mL**, **higher dose of Anti D Immunoglobulin is required.** Example: Abdominal trauma, placental abruption, placenta previa, intrauterine manipulation, multifetal gestation, or manual placenta removal.

PEDIATRICS

156. Ans. c. Meningocele *(Ref: Ghai 8/e p576)*

The given image shows a skin covered, brilliantly transilluminant defect in the back in a newborn. This is typical of a meningocele.

Neural Tube Defects
• Result from failure of neural tube to close spontaneously between the 3rd & 4th week of in-utero development.
• It leads to increased levels of AFP & acetylcholine esterase in amniotic fluid[Q].
• Neural tube defects: Spina bifida occulta, meningocele & myelomeningocele

Spectrum of Neural Tube Defects includes
• **Spina bifida (meningocele, meningomyelocele, spina bifida occulta)**
• **Anencephaly (absence of brain calvaria,** total or partial)
• **Encephalocele (herniation of brain & meninges** through defect in calvaria)
• **Craniorhachischisis** (anencephaly associated with **continuous bony defect of spine & exposure of neural tissue)**
• **Iniencephaly (dysraphism of occipital region** accompanied by retroflexion of neck & trunk)
• Others (dermal sinus, tethered cord, syringomyelia, diastematomyelia, and lipoma involving the conus medullaris).

Etiological Factors for Neural Tube Defects	
• **Maternal diabetes**[Q]	• **Maternal exposure to:**
• **Zinc & folate deficiency**[Q]	– **Alcohol**[Q]
• **Trisomy 13 & 15**[Q]	– **Valproate**[Q]
	– **Carbamazepine**[Q]

Contd...

Contd...

Neural Tube Defects

Prevention:

- **Nutritional** and **environmental factors: Folate**[Q] is intricately involved in the prevention and etiology of NTDs.
- **Maternal peri-conceptional use** of folic acid supplementation **reduces** the **incidence** of **neural tube defects** in pregnancies at risk by at least **50%**[Q].
- To be effective, folic acid supplementation should be **initiated before conception** and **continued until** at least the **12th week of gestation** when neurulation is complete[Q].

- **All women** of childbearing age and who are capable of becoming pregnant take **0.4 mg of folic acid** daily.
- There is evidence that **women who previously have had infants with neural-tube defects have a lower recurrence rate if a daily 4 mg**[Q] **(= 4000 microgram) folic acid supplement is given preconceptionally and throughout early pregnancy**.

Risk of Recurrence	
1st affected child	3.5%[Q]
2nd affected child	10%[Q]
3rd affected child	25%[Q]

Spina Bifida Occulta

- **Midline defect of vertebral bodies without protrusion of the spinal cord or meninges**[Q]
- Usually **asymptomatic** & **lack neurological signs**

Clinical Features:

- Associated with **patch of hair, a lipoma, discoloration of skin,** or **dermal sinus in the midline** of the **lower back**[Q]

Diagnosis:

- **X-ray spine: Defect in closure of posterior vertebral arches and laminae,** typically involving **L5 & S1**[Q].

Meningocele

- **Herniation** of **meninges** through a **defect** in the **posterior vertebral arches**[Q].
- **Spinal cord** is **usually normal** & assumes a **normal position** in the spinal canal
- There may be **tethering, syringomyelia,** or **diastematomyelia**.

Clinical Features:

- A **fluctuant midline mass,** that may transilluminate occurs along the vertebral column, in the **lower back**[Q].
- Most meningoceles are **well covered with skin** and pose no threat to the patient.

- **Anterior meningocele:** Projects into **pelvis** through a **defect in** the **sacrum**[Q].
- Symptoms of **constipation** & **bladder dysfunction** develop due to the increasing size of the lesion[Q].

Diagnosis:

- **Plain roentgenograms** demonstrate a defect[Q].

Treatment:

- **Asymptomatic children** with **normal neurologic findings** and **full-thickness skin** covering the meningocele may have surgery delayed[Q].
- Patients with **leaking CSF** or a **thin skin** covering should undergo **immediate surgical treatment** to prevent meningitis[Q].

Myelomeningocele

- **Most severe form of dysraphism** involving the vertebral column
- **Incidence**: **1/4,000** live births[Q]
- **MC site** of myelomeningocele: **Lumbosacral region (75%)**[Q]

Contd...

Myelomeningocele	
Drugs increasing the risk of myelomeningocele	
• **Trimethoprim**[Q]	• **Phenobarbital**[Q]
• **Carbamazepine**[Q]	• **Primidone**[Q]
• **Phenytoin**[Q]	• **Valproic acid**[Q]

Clinical Features:

• Produces **dysfunction of skeleton, skin**, **gastrointestinal** & **genitourinary tracts**, in addition to the **peripheral nervous system** & **CNS**[Q].

• **Extent** & **degree** of the **neurologic deficit** depend on the **location** of the myelomeningocele, as well as the **associated lesions**.

Location	Manifestation
Low sacral region	• **Bowel** and **bladder incontinence** associated with **anesthesia** in the **perineal area** but with no impairment of motor function.
Midlumbar region	• Flaccid paralysis of lower extremity, absence of deep tendon reflexes, lack of response to touch & pain
Thoracic region	• **Increasing neurologic deficit** as the myelomeningocele **extends higher** into the thoracic region.
Upper thoracic & cervical region	• **Very minimal neurological deficit** & no hydrocephalus

Anencephaly
• **Absence of a major portion of the brain, skull, and scalp** that occurs during embryonic development.
◦ It is **a cephalic disorder** that **results from a neural tube defect** that occurs when the **rostral (head) end of the neural tube fails to close**, usually between the 23rd and 26th day following conception.
• **Largest part of the brain consisting mainly of the cerebral hemispheres**, including the neocortex, which is responsible for cognition.
• The **remaining structure is usually covered only by a thin layer of membrane-skin, bone, meninges, etc. are all lacking.**

157. **Ans. a. High-dose dexamethasone** *(Ref: Ghai 8/e p376, 398; Nelson 20/e p2032-2034)*

A 2-year-old child with fever and barking cough for last 2 days presented to the pediatric emergency at 2.30 AM. On examination, respiratory rate is 36/min, temperature of 39°C and stridor heard only on crying. No other abnormality is found. The clinical picture described is diagnostic of laryngotracheobronchitis or croup of mild severity. Hence, high-dose dexamethasone will be the treatment of choice.

"The effectiveness of oral corticosteroids in viral croup is well established. Corticosteroids decrease the edema in the laryngeal mucosa through their anti-inflammatory action. Oral steroids are beneficial, even in mild croup, as measured by reduced hospitalization, shorter duration of hospitalization, and reduced need for subsequent interventions such as epinephrine administration. Most studies that demonstrated the efficacy of oral dexamethasone used a single dose of 0.6 mg/kg; a dose as low as 0.15 mg/kg may be just as effective. Intramuscular dexamethasone and nebulized budesonide have an equivalent clinical effect; oral dosing of dexamethasone is as effective as intramuscular administration." - Nelson 20/e p2034.

"The indications for the administration of nebulized epinephrine include moderate to severe stridor at rest, the possible need for intubation, respiratory distress, and hypoxia." - Nelson 20/e p2034

"A helium-oxygen mixture (Heliox) may be effective in children with severe croup for whom intubation is being considered. Children with croup should be hospitalized for any of the following: progressive stridor, severe stridor at rest, respiratory distress, hypoxia, cyanosis, depressed mental status, poor oral intake, or the need for reliable observation." – Nelson 20/e p2034

Acute Laryngotracheobronchitis or Croup

- **Viral infection** of **upper respiratory tract** (glottis & subglottic region)
- **Causative organisms: Parainfluenza type I**[Q], RSV, Influenza, Adenovirus, Rhinovirus
- **Age: 1-5 years**[Q]

Clinical Features:

- Most patients initially have **upper respiratory tract infection** with some combination of **rhinorrhea, pharyngitis** and **mild cough** and **low-grade fever for 1-3 days**[Q].
  - After this upper airway obstruction becomes apparent, child develops **characteristic barking cough, hoarseness & inspiratory stridor**[Q].
  - **Symptoms** are characteristically **worse at night** & often **recur with decreasing intensity for several days** and **resolve completely within a week**[Q].

- **Agitation & crying greatly aggravates** the **signs & symptoms**[Q].
- The child may prefer to **sit up in bed** or be **held upright**.
- Croup is a disease of upper airway and alveolar **gas exchange is usually normal**[Q].

Diagnosis:

- It is a **clinical diagnosis** and **doesn't require a radiograph of the neck.**[Q]
  - **Radiograph** of the neck may show the **typical subglottic narrowing or "steeple sign" of croup on PA view**[Q].

Treatment:

- **Cornerstone of Treatment: Glucocorticoids & nebulized epinephrine**[Q]

Glucocorticoids	Nebulized epinephrine
• Glucocorticoids are useful in **mild, moderate & severe croup**[Q]. • **Dexamethasone** is **most effective** corticosteroid[Q].	• Useful in **moderate to severe distress**[Q] • By adrenergic stimulation causes **constriction of precapillary arterioles & decreases capillary hydrostatic pressure leading to fluid resorption from the interstitium & improvement in laryngeal mucosal edema**[Q].

- **Antibiotics** are **not indicated**[Q]
  - **Heliox** (mixture of **oxygen & helium**) has low viscosity & low specific gravity, which **allow for greater laminar airflow through respiratory tract,** considered in the treatment of children with severe croup[Q].

Assessment of Severity of Acute Laryngotracheobronchitis			
	Mild	**Moderate**	**Severe**
General appearance	Happy, feeds well, interested in surroundings	**Irritable** but can be comforted by parents	**Restless or agitated or altered sensorium**
Stridor	**Stridor on coughing**, no stridor at rest	Stridor at rest worsens when agitated	**Stridor at rest worsens when agitated**
Respiratory distress	No distress	**Tachypnea & chest retractions**	**Marked tachypnea with chest retractions**
Cyanosis	Absent	Absent	**May be present**
Oxygen saturation in room air	> 92%	> 92%	< 92%

158. **Ans. b. ORS only** *(Ref: Ghai 8/e p293-294, 296)*

The infant is suffering from acute diarrhea and treatment includes oral rehydration therapy, zinc supplementation and continued breastfeeding.

Low lactose diet is required in management of persistent diarrhea. Antibiotics are required in management of dysentery, i.e. blood in stools.

"Routine use to probiotics in acute diarrhea is not recommended. It was recommended till the previous edition of the book, but the latest data shows no added advantage of probiotics in children." - Ghai 8/e p296

Acute Diarrhea Management

- The **cornerstone of acute diarrhea management** is **rehydration by using oral rehydration solutions (ORS)**.

Principles of Acute Diarrhea Management

1. Correction of **dehydration, electrolytes & hypoglycemia**[Q]
2. **Evaluation for infections** using appropriate investigations and their management[Q]
3. **Nutritional therapy**[Q]

Acute Diarrhea Management

Physiological Basis for Oral Rehydration Therapy

- In most cases of acute diarrhea, **sodium & chloride are actively secreted from the gut mucosa** due to pathogen-induced dysfunction of several actively functioning absorption pumps.
- However, **glucose dependent sodium pump remains intact** and **functional transporting one molecule of glucose** and **dragging along a molecule of sodium** and **one of water across intestinal mucosa** resulting in repletion of sodium and water losses.

  - The **glucose dependent sodium & water absorption** is the **principle behind replacing glucose** and **sodium in 1:1molar ratio in the WHO oral rehydration solution (ORS)**[Q].
  - **Use of low osmolality ORS causes reduction of stool output, decrease in vomiting** and **decrease in the use of unscheduled IV fluids without increasing the risk of hyponatremia**.
  - For this reason, the **recommendation for use of standard WHO ORS** (having osmolarity of **311** mmol/l) **was changed to low osmolarity WHO ORS** (having osmolality of **245** mmol/l)[Q]

Home available fluids for Acute Diarrhea

Fluids that contain salt (preferable)	• **Oral rehydration solution** • Salted drinks (e.g. Salted rice water or salted yoghurt drink) • Vegetable or chicken soup with salt
Fluids that do not contain salt (acceptable)	• Plain water, water in which a cereal has been cooked (e.g. unsalted rice water), unsalted soup, yoghurt drinks without salt, green coconut water, weak unsweetened tea, unsweetened fresh fruit juice
Unsuitable home available fluids	• Commercial carbonated beverages, commercial fruit juices, sweetened tea

Zinc Supplementation

- It is helpful in **decreasing severity** & **duration of diarrhea** and also **risk of persistent diarrhea**[Q].
- Zinc is recommended to be supplemented as **sulphate, acetate or gluconate formulation**, at a **dose of 20 mg** of elemental zinc per day for children **>6 months** for a period of **14 days**[Q].

Composition of WHO Recommended ORS			
Constituent	g/l	Osmole or ion	mmol/l
Sodium chloride	2.6	Sodium	75[Q]
Glucose, anhydrous	13.5	Chloride	65
Potassium chloride	1.5	Glucose, anhydrous	75
Trisodium citrate, dihydrate	2.9	Potassium	20[Q]
		Citrate	10
Total osmolarity			245[Q]

	Standard ORS solution	Low Osmolar ORS solution
Glucose	111	75
Sodium	90	75
Chloride	80	65
Potassium	20	20
Citrate	10	10
Total osmolarity	311[Q]	245[Q]

159. **Ans. a. Iron and Vitamin C**   *(Ref: Ghai 8/e p153)*

Human breast milk has enough of all nutrients except Vitamin D and Vitamin K. It is also slightly deficient in Vitamin C and iron.

Comparing Human and Animal Milks (per cup)			
Nutrient	Human Milk	Cow's Milk	Goat's Milk
Calories	**172**	146	168
Protein (g)	2.5	7.9	**8.7**
Fat (g)	10.8	7.9	**101**
Saturated fat (g)	4.9	4.6	**6.5**
Polyunsaturated fat (g)	**1.2**	0.5	0.4
Carbohydrate (g)	**17.0**	11.0	10.9
Folate (mcg)	12	12	2
Monounsaturated fat (g)	**4.1**	2.0	2.7
Vitamin C (mg)	**12.3**	0	3.2
Sodium (mg)	42	98	**122**
Iron (mg)	**0.07**	0.07	**0.12**
Calcium (mg)	79	276	**327**

Breast Milk

- Contains **bacterial and viral antibodies**, including relatively **high concentrations of secretory immunoglobulin A** that **prevent microorganisms from adhering to the intestinal mucosa[Q]**.
- **Macrophages** in human milk may synthesize **complement, lysozyme,** and **lactoferrin[Q]**.
  - In addition, breast milk contains **lactoferrin** an **iron-binding whey protein** has an **inhibitory effect on the growth of Escherichia coli** in the intestine[Q].
  - Human milk also contains **bile salt-stimulated lipase**, which **kills Giardia lamblia** and **Entamoeba histolytica[Q]**.

Contd...

Contd...

Breast Milk
• Most of the protein is **lactalbumin** & **lactglobulin**, which is **easily digested**.
• Human milk contains certain amino acids like **taurine & cysteine,** which are necessary **for neurotransmission and neuromodulation**[Q]. These are lacking in cow's milk and formula.
• **Breast milk is rich in PUFA**, necessary **for myelination of nervous system**, also contains **omega-2 & 6 fatty acids**[Q], important for formation of prostaglandins and cholesterol, required as a base for steroid hormones.

WHO Guidelines for India
• *WHO recommends, in developing countries, **exclusive breastfeeding till 6 months age**[Q]*
• *WHO recommends, in developing countries, **breastfeeding till minimum 2 years age**[Q]*

Nutritional Importance of Breast milk	
Energy content of breast milk	*65 Kcal/ 100 ml[Q]*
Protein content of breast milk	*1.1 grams/ 100 ml[Q]*

Mean output of breast milk per day	
Months of lactation	**Mean output (ml)**
0 – 2	*530*
3 – 4	*640*
5 – 6	**730[Q]**
7 – 8	*660*
9 – 10	*600*
11 – 12	*525*

Nutritive values of milk (per 100 gm)		
	Cow's milk	*Human milk*
Lactose (gm)	*4.4*	*7.4*
Proteins (gm)	*3.2*	*1.1*
Fat (gm)	*4.1*	*3.4*
Calcium (mg)	*120*	*28*
Iron (mg)	*0.2*	*1.0*
Water (gm)	*87*	*88*
Energy (Kcal)	*67*	*65*

- **Human milk** is **richer in carbohydrate (lactose), iron & water content**
- **Cow's milk** is **richer in fat, protein, calcium & energy content**[Q]
- **Human milk proteins: More cystine & taurine**; less methionine; **better digested than cow's milk proteins**[Q]
- **Human milk fats: Higher levels of PUFAs, esp., linoleic acid & linoleic acid**; better digested and absorbed; **low calcium content** but **better absorbed than cow's milk**[Q]

• **Human milk is richer in Vitamin A & C; richer in copper, cobalt & selenium; richer in iron & higher bioavailability; high calcium/phosphorus ratio; Human milk has lesser sodium**[Q]

Contd...

Contd...

Breast Milk	
Comparative contents of nutrients in different types of milk	
Fat content of milk	• ***Buffalo** > Goat > Cow > **Human**[Q]*
Protein content of milk	• ***Buffalo** > Goat > Cow > **Human**[Q]*
Energy content of milk	• ***Buffalo** > Goat > Cow > **Human**[Q]*
***Lactose content of milk*[Q]**	• ***Human > Buffalo > Goat > Cow*[Q]**

Colostrum
• **Most suitable food immediately after birth** of the baby
• Regular milk comes 3-6 days after birth
• Also known as '***Beestings***', '***First milk***' or '***Immune Milk***'[Q]
• **High in carbohydrates, protein & antibodies** and **low in fat**
• **Contains all five immunoglobulins** found in all mammals, IgA, IgD, IgE, IgG & IgM[Q]

Few occasions when breastfeeding might harm the infant[Q]
• **Infants** with **classic galactosemia**
• **Mother** has **untreated pulmonary tuberculosis**
• **Mother** is taking **certain medications that suppress the immune system**
• **Mother** has had unusually excessive **exposure to** heavy metals such as **mercury**
• **Mother** has **HIV**
• **Mother** uses potentially harmful substances such as **cocaine, heroin, & amphetamines.**

160. **Ans. d. Height for age** *(Ref: Ghai 8/e p97)*

Height for age is not a criterion for severe acute malnutrition in a 6-month old child.

Severe Acute Malnutrition
• Severe acute malnutrition (SAM) among children 6–59 months of age is defined by World Health Organization (WHO) and UNICEF as any of the following:
1. **Weight-for-height below –3 standard deviation** (SD or Z scores) of the median WHO growth reference[Q]
2. **Visible severe wasting**[Q]
3. **Presence of bipedal edema**[Q]
4. **Mid-upper arm circumference below 11.5 cm**[Q]
• This classification is used to **identify children at high risk of death.**
• **Children having SAM require urgent attention & management in the hospital.**
• **In a child below 6 months of age, mid-upper arm circumference cannot be used, and SAM should be diagnosed in the presence of 1, 2 or 3**[Q].

161. **Ans. b. Weight for height < –2 SD** *(Ref: Ghai 8/e p96)*

Under nutrition is defined in terms of Weight for Height, i.e. < –2 SD. Weight for Height < –3 SD is severe under nutrition.

Indicators of Malnutrition		
Indicator	*Parameter*	*Interpretation*
Stunting	*Low height for age*	*Chronic malnutrition*[Q]
Wasting	*Low weight for height*	*Acute malnutrition*[Q]
Under weight	*Low weight for age*	*Both acute & chronic malnutrition*[Q]

WHO Classification of Malnutrition		
	Moderate malnutrition	**Severe malnutrition (type)**
Symmetrical edema	No	Yes (edematous malnutrition)
Weight-for-height	SD score from –2 to –3	SD score < –3 (severe wasting)
Height-for-age	SD score from –2 to –3	SD score < –3 (severe stunting)

162. Ans. a. Neonatal Pulmonary alveolar proteinosis *(Ref: Nelson 20/e p852, 2119)*

The clinical history of respiratory distress and no response to surfactant therapy in a newborn and a family history of sibling death points towards a diagnosis of neonatal pulmonary alveolar proteinosis.

Pulmonary Alveolar Proteinosis
• **Pulmonary alveolar proteinosis** is a disorder characterized by **intra-alveolar accumulation of pulmonary surfactant[Q]**. • **Two clinically distinct forms of pulmonary alveolar proteinosis are seen:** • **Fatal form:** Presenting shortly after birth (congenital PAP) • **Gradually progressive form:** Presenting in older infants & children.
Pathology • **Disruption of pulmonary surfactant metabolism[Q].** • Main surface tension lowering agent in surfactant is phospholipids i.e. **primary dipalmityol phosphatidyl choline[Q].** • DPCC needs **"surfactant protein"** for **efficient dispersion,** which enables the formation of a phospholipid monolayer on the alveolar surface[Q]. • **Surfactant proteins** present in the body: **Protein A & B[Q]**

• In **pulmonary alveolar proteinosis,** there is **absence of protein B[Q]**
      • In the **absence of protein B,** the **rapid spread & absorption of the phospholipid (DPCC) does not take place** so they **cannot form a phospholipid monolayer on the alveolar surface[Q].**
      • This in turn leads to **failure of expansion of alveoli** leading to **poor cardiorespiratory adaptation at birth.**

Clinical manifestation: • Immediately apparent in the **newborn period & rapidly leads to respiratory failure[Q].** • Clinically and radiographically **indistinguishable from more common disorders** of the newborn **that lead to respiratory failure** including **pneumonia, generalized bacterial infection, respiratory distress syndrome** and **total anomalous pulmonary venous return with obstruction[Q].**
Pulmonary Alveolar Proteinosis
Diagnosis • **Gold standard for diagnosis: Lung biopsy[Q]**
• On histopathological examination **distal air spaces** are **filled with a granular, eosinophilic material that stains positively with periodic-acid Schiff regent & is diastase resistant[Q].**
Treatment • **Untreated alveolar proteinosis** in newborns in **rapidly fatal** and **no successful medical therapy has been developed[Q].** • **Repeated bronchoalveolar lavage** is a temporizing measure. • **Lung transplantation** is the **only therapeutic option** but its use is limited by concerns about **disease recurrence[Q].** • Recent trials have suggested that **subcutaneous administration of recombinant GM-CSF may improve pulmonary function in some adults** with later-onset primary alveolar proteinosis.

ORTHOPEDICS

163. Ans. a. Hallux valgus *(Ref: Apley's 9/e p603, 604)*

The given picture shows hallux valgus in which outward or lateral deviation of great toe occurs.

"Hallux valgus is the commonest of the foot deformities (and probably of all musculoskeletal deformities). In people who have never worn shoes the big toe is in line with the first metatarsal, retaining the slightly fan- shaped appearance of the forefoot. In people who habitually wear shoes the hallux assumes a valgus position; but only if the angulation is excessive is it referred to as 'hallux valgus'."- Apley's 9/e p603

Hallux Valgus

- **Outward or lateral deviation of great toe** (lateral deviation of proximal phalanx on metatarsal head)
- **MC foot deformity (and probably of all musculoskeletal deformities)**[Q]
- Occurs due to **improper shoe wearing** in majority of patients

Elements of deformity:

- **Lateral deviation & rotation of hallux with prominence of medial side of head of 1st metatarsal (bunion)**[Q]

Secondary Changes:

- **Contracture of lateral joint capsule, attenuation of medial joint capsule**[Q]
- A **medial eminence** of varying size; **pronation of the hallux** as the deformity becomes more severe
- **Medial deviation of first metatarsal**, giving rise to an **increase in intermetatarsal angle**[Q]. This leads to an **uncovering of the sesamoids**, which are anchored in their lateral-ward position by the adductor hallucis.

Clinical Features:

- More common in **women** between **50-70 years of age**
- **MC complaints: Pain over bunion**, worries about cosmesis & difficulty fitting shoes.
  - **Great toe is in valgus** & **bunion** varies in appearance **from a slight prominence over medial side of first metatarsal head to a red and angry-looking bulge that is tender**[Q].

X-ray:

- **Standing views**: Degree of metatarsal & hallux angulation[Q]
  - Lines are drawn along middle of 1st & 2nd metatarsals & proximal phalanx of great toe
  - **Normally intermetatarsal angle is <9° & valgus angle at MTP joint <15°**[Q]
  - **Any greater degree of angulation should be regarded as 'hallux valgus'**[Q]

Treatment:

- **Conservative management especially in adolescents & young patients, as surgical correction is associated with recurrence rate of 20-40% in this age group.**
- **Relief of pain is good after surgery**

164. **Ans. b. Thomas test**   *(Ref: Apley's 9/e p495)*

The given image demonstrates Thomas test in which both hips are flexed simultaneously to their limit, thus completely obliterating the lumbar lordosis; holding the 'sound' hip firmly in position (and thus keeping the pelvis still), the other limb is lowered gently; with any flexion deformity the knee will not rest on the couch.

"The assessment of hip movements is difficult because any limitation can easily be obscured by movement of the pelvis. Thus, even a gross limitation of extension, causing a fixed flexion deformity, can be completely masked simply by arching the back into excessive lordosis. Fortunately it can be just as easily unmasked by performing Thomas' test: both hips are flexed simultaneously to their limit, thus completely obliterating the lumbar lordosis; holding the 'sound' hip firmly in position (and thus keeping the pelvis still), the other limb is lowered gently; with any flexion deformity the knee will not rest on the couch. Meanwhile the full range of flexion will also have been noted; the normal range is about 130 degrees."_ Apley's 9/e p495.

Thomas Test

- **Thomas test** is a test **used to rule out hip flexion contracture & psoas syndrome**. Often associated with **runners, dancers & gymnasts**, who **complain of hip 'stiffness'** and reported **'snapping' feeling** when flexing at the waist.
- Even a gross limitation of extension in hip, causing a fixed flexion deformity, can be completely masked simply by arching the back into excessive lordosis. Fortunately, it can be just as easily unmasked by performing Thomas test.

Contd...

Contd...

Thomas Test
Steps of Performing Thomas Test
• The patient lies supine on examination table & brings one knee in direction to the chest/flexes hip, while other leg remains extended.   • **Step 1:** The patient lies supine on examination table. Clinician passes the palm of his hand beneath the patient's spine to **identify lumbar lordosis.**   • **Step 2:** The 'normal' hip is flexed till thigh just touches abdomen to obliterate lumbar lordosis.   • **Step 3:** Measure angle between affected thigh & table to reveal the fixed flexion deformity of the hip.
The Thomas test is said to be positive if the patient's:
• **Opposite/contralateral hip flexes without knee extension: Tight iliopsoas**   • **Hip abducts during the test: Tight tensor fasciae latae**   • **Knee extension occurs: Tight rectus femoris**   • **Lateral rotation of tibia: Tight biceps femoris**
• **Hip flexion contracture** is **physiologic in first 3 months** of life and, **if it is absent in this period**, it may be **a sign of developmental dysplasia of hip.**

Straight Leg Raising Test (SLRT)	• **SLRT** also called **Lasègue's sign**, is done **to determine whether a patient with low back pain has an underlying herniated disk, often located at L5.** • With the patient lying down on his or her back on an examination table or exam floor, the examiner lifts the patient's leg while the knee is straight. • A variation is to lift the leg while the patient is sitting. However, this reduces the sensitivity of the test. • In order to make this test more specific, the ankle can be dorsiflexed and the cervical spine flexed. This increases the stretching of the nerve root and dura.
Vascular Sign of Narath	• **Tests for presence of the head of the femur.** • **Palpate the femoral artery pulse bilaterally to evaluate volume, intensity, and position.** • **If very readily palpated: possible unreduced anterior hip dislocation.** • **If palpated with great difficulty or not felt at all, it implies femoral head displaced from the hip joint due to hip dislocation, most commonly posterior hip dislocation.**
Trendelen-burg's Test	• **Trendelenburg's sign** is found in people with **weak or paralyzed abductor muscles of the hip** namely **gluteus medius & gluteus minimus**. • The gluteus medius is very important during the stance phase of the gait cycle to maintain both hips at the same level. • One leg stance accounts for about 60% of the gait cycle. Furthermore, during the stance phase of the gait cycle, there is approximately three times the body weight transmitted to the hip joint. • The hip abductors' action accounts for two thirds of that body weight. • **Trendelenburg's sign is said to be positive if, when standing on one leg, pelvis drops on the side opposite to the stance leg to reduce load by decreasing lever arm.** • By reducing the lever arm, this decreases the work-load on the hip abductors. The muscle weakness is present on the side of the stance leg. • **Trendelenburg's sign** can occur when there is **presence of a muscular dysfunction** (weakness of the gluteus medius or minimus) or **when someone is experiencing pain.** • The body is not able to maintain the center of gravity on the side of the stance leg. Normally, the body shifts the weight to the stance leg, allowing the shift of the center of gravity and consequently stabilizing or balancing the body. • However, in this scenario, when the patient/person lifts the opposing leg, the shift is not created and the patient/person cannot maintain balance leading to instability.

165. **Ans. d. Supracondylar Fracture** *(Ref: Apley's 9/e p371, 760)*
The given picture shows cubitus varus or gun-stock deformity. The most common cause is malunion of a supracondylar fracture.

AIIMS November 2015

"Cubitus Varus ('Gun-Stock' Deformity): The deformity is most obvious when the elbow is extended and the arms are elevated. The most common cause is malunion of a supracondylar fracture. The deformity can be corrected by a wedge osteotomy of the lower humerus but this is best left until skeletal maturity."– Apley's 9/e p371

"Cubitus Valgus: The normal carrying angle of the elbow is 5–15 degrees of valgus; anything more than this is regarded as a valgus deformity, which is usually quite obvious when the patient stands with arms to the sides and palms facing forwards. The commonest cause is longstanding non-union of a fractured lateral condyle; the deformity may be associated with marked prominence of the medial condylar outline. The importance of cubitus valgus is the liability to delayed ulnar palsy; years after the causal injury the patient notices weakness of the hand, with numbness and tingling of the ulnar fingers. The deformity itself needs no treatment, but for delayed ulnar palsy the nerve should be transposed to the front of the elbow. Great care is needed in performing the operation. Excessive dissection of the nerve or rough handling can impair nerve function."– Apley's 9/e p371

See Q. No. 173 AIIMS November 2016

166. **Ans. d. Galeazzi's fracture**   *(Ref: Apley's 9/e p771)*

In the given X-ray, a transverse or short oblique fracture is seen in the lower third of the radius, with angulation or overlap. The distal radio-ulnar joint is subluxated or dislocated. This is classically seen in Galeazzi's fracture.

"Galeazzi's fracture's X-ray: A transverse or short oblique fracture is seen in the lower third of the radius, with angulation or overlap. The distal radio-ulnar joint is subluxated or dislocated."– Apley's 9/e p771

See Q. No. 164 AIIMS May 2016

167. **Ans. a. Lateral cutaneous nerve of thigh**   *(Ref: Apley's 9/e p292)*

The lateral cutaneous nerve can be compressed as it runs through the inguinal ligament just medial to the anterior superior iliac spine. The patient complains of numbness, tingling or burning discomfort over the anterolateral aspect of the thigh (meralgia paraesthetica).

"The lateral cutaneous nerve can be compressed as it runs through the inguinal ligament just medial to the anterior superior iliac spine. The patient complains of numbness, tingling or burning discomfort over the anterolateral aspect of the thigh (meralgia paraesthetica). Testing for sensibility to pinprick will reveal a patch of numbness over the upper outer thigh. If the symptoms are troublesome the nerve can be released."– Apley's 9/e p292

Meralgia paresthetica
• **Meralgia paresthetica** is a common disorder characterized by **pain & paresthesias occurring along the course** of lateral femoral cutaneous nerve of thigh[Q].
Course:
• This **nerve enters beneath the inguinal ligament 1 cm medial to anterior superior iliac spine** & supplies sensation to anterolateral aspect of thigh[Q].
Etiology:
• **Direct pressure or constriction** of the nerve at its point of exit into the thigh • More common in **joggers & gymnasts**[Q] • Rarely due to an **intra-abdominal or pelvic mass** (**retroperitoneal course** of nerve).
Clinical Features:
• **Hypersensitivity, burning, tingling & pain** that **occurs with activity or direct pressure** over the nerve by rest & hip flexion. • **Pain** may be **aggravated by passive extension of hip.** • A **slight decrease in sensation over the anterolateral aspect of thigh** • **Pain** may be **reproduced with pressure on nerve medial to anterior superior iliac spine.**
Treatment:
• **Painful symptoms often subside spontaneously** over a variable length of time, but numbness may be permanent. • **Weight loss & avoidance of constricting garment** • Injection of local anesthetic • Surgical release or even removal of the nerve

Contd...

Entrapment Syndrome	Nerve Involved
Carpal tunnel syndrome	• Median nerve[Q] (at wrist)
Pronator teres syndrome	• Median nerve (proximally compressed beneath ligament of Struthers, bicipital aponeurosis or origins of pronator teres or flexor digitorum superficialis)[Q]
Cubital tunnel syndrome	• Ulnar nerve (between two heads of flexor carpi ulnaris or arcade of Struthers)[Q]
Guyon's canal syndrome	• Ulnar nerve[Q] (at wrist)
Thoracic outlet syndrome	• Lower trunk of brachial plexus, (C_8 & T_1) & subclavian vessels (between clavicle & first rib)[Q]
Meralgia paraesthetica	• Lateral cutaneous nerve of thigh[Q]
Tarsal tunnel syndrome	• Posterior tibial nerve[Q] (behind & below medial malleolus)
Morton's metatarsalgia	• Interdigital nerve compression[Q] (usually of 3rd, 4th toe)

168. **Ans. c. Improper use of crutches**   *(Ref: Apley's 9/e p282)*

Improper use of crutches causes radial nerve palsy mostly rather than axillary nerve injury.

> *"Radial Nerve Injury: Very high lesions may be caused by trauma or operations around the shoulder. More often, though, they are due to chronic compression in the axilla; this is seen in drink and drug addicts who fall into a stupor with the arm dangling over the back of a chair ('Saturday night palsy') or in thin elderly patients using crutches ('crutch palsy'). In addition to weakness of the wrist and hand, the triceps is paralysed and the triceps reflex is absent."* – Apley's 9/e p282

Axillary Nerve Injury

- Axillary nerve (C5, 6) arises from the **posterior cord** of the brachial plexus & **runs along subscapularis & across axilla just inferior to shoulder joint**[Q].
- It **emerges behind humerus, deep to deltoid; after supplying teres minor, it divides into a medial branch** which **supplies posterior part of deltoid & a patch of skin over muscle & an anterior branch** that **curls round the surgical neck of humerus to innervate the anterior two-thirds of deltoid**[Q].

Etiology of Axillary Nerve Injury

• **Brachial plexus injury**[Q] • **Shoulder dislocation**[Q] • **Fractures of the humeral neck**[Q]	• **Iatrogenic injuries occur in transaxillary operations** on shoulder & **lateral deltoid-splitting incisions**[Q].

Clinical features:

- **Shoulder 'weakness', deltoid is wasted**[Q].
- Although **abduction** can be initiated (by supraspinatus), it **cannot be maintained**.
- **Retropulsion** (extension of shoulder with arm abducted to 90°) **is impossible**.
- **Small area of numbness over deltoid ('sergeant's patch')**[Q].

Motor	Sensory
• **Deltoid muscle palsy**[Q] • **Loss of round contour of shoulder**[Q] (flattened appearance of shoulder) with hollow inferior to acromian • **Weakness of abduction (15° to 90°)**[Q] • **Teres minor palsy**[Q]	• **Lateral cutaneous nerve of arm**[Q] • **Sensory loss over lower half of deltoid (regimental batch area)**[Q]

Treatment:

- **Nerve injury associated with fractures or dislocations recovers spontaneously in about 80%** of cases.
- If the **deltoid shows no sign of recovery by 8 weeks**, EMG should be performed; if the tests suggest denervation then the **nerve should be explored**.
- **Excision of the nerve ends & grafting** are usually necessary; a **good result** can be expected **if the nerve is explored within 3 months of injury**.

OPHTHALMOLOGY

169. **Ans. c. Lateral geniculate body** *(Ref: Walsh and Hoyt's Clinical Neuro-Ophthalmology 6/e p122)*

Key-hole shaped visual field defects are typically seen in the lesions involving lateral geniculate body but keyhole shaped defect (not visual field defect) is seen in the coloboma of Iris.

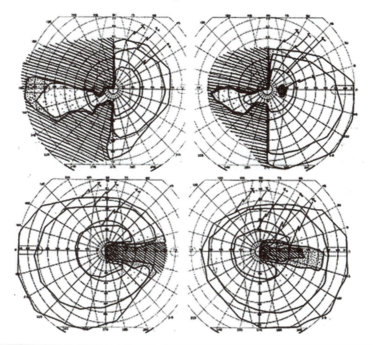

"Foveola Sparing: Complete anopia with foveola sparing (also known as keyhole vision, tunnel vision or bitemporal hemianopia) is to be expected in the case of bilateral embolisms or lesions affecting both lobes of the occipital region. The involved axons terminate at the perigeniculate nucleus (PGN) after passing through the optic chiasm. The PGN is usually identified as a small section of the morphologically identified lateral geniculate nucleus (LGN). The functional significance of the PGN is generally greater than that of the LGN. Physicians often struggle with patients who report 20/20 vision (or any vision at all) over a small field after total lobectomies (both hemispheres). The reason is this small field represents the foveola as projected to the PGN as part of the high performance precision optical system (POS) of vision. It is in the PGN that information is extracted from the neural signals in order to both identify fine detail and to steer the eyes. The POS is fundamental to the human ability to read efficiently."

"Macular Sparing: Macular sparing has no physical relationship to the observed macula. The phenomenon relates to the survival of the neurons of the external portions of the occipital area upon the functional loss of the neurons of one or both walls of the occipital lobes facing the longitudinal fissure. Therefore, the designation macular sparing is an anachronism."

*"A coloboma is a **hole in one of the structures of the eye**, such as the **iris, retina, choroid, or optic disc**. The hole is present from birth and can be caused when a gap called the choroid fissure, which is present during early stages of prenatal development, fails to close up completely before a child is born. The classical description in medical literature is of a **key-hole shaped defect**. A coloboma can occur in one eye (unilateral) or both eyes (bilateral). **Most cases of coloboma affect only the iris.** The effect a coloboma has on the vision can be mild or more severe depending on the size and location of the gap."*

170. **Ans. b. Candida** *(Ref: Ryan's Retina 5/e p733)*

Candidemia is the most common fungal infection seen in patients with HIV.

"Candidemia is the most common fungal infection seen in patients with HIV. Candida albicans, an important nosocomial pathogen, is the most common Candida species. It is the most commonly cause of keratitis, conjunctivitis and endogenous fungal endophthalmitis." – Ryan's Retina 5/e p733.

AIIMS ESSENCE

"Candida yeasts reach the eye most commonly by hematogenous spread to the choroid or rarely from direct inoculation following ocular trauma or surgery. With Candidemia, the organisms typically cause one or more foci of chorioretinitis which may progress to involve the vitreous, where it is then termed endophthalmitis. Predisposing conditions include diabetes, intravenous drug use, prolonged hospitalization, history of major surgery, bacterial sepsis requiring broad-spectrum systemic antibiotics, hyperalimentation, chronic indwelling catheters, and immunosuppression secondary to organ transplantation, chemotherapy or acquired immunodeficiency syndrome (AIDS). "

"Eyes with Candida endophthalmitis have acute, progressive inflammation in the vitreous cavity. Involvement of the retina and uvea usually is mild, though foci of retinal damage from invasion of the organisms can be seen. Regarding the distribution of fungi, yeasts are mainly localized to the vitreous abscess with the presence of few organisms in the retina. Retinal vessel wall invasion is not seen in Candida endophthalmitis."

"Cryptococcosis is the most common systemic fungal disease in HIV-infected persons. CNS is the most commonly involved organ, presenting with meningitis."

ENT

171. Ans. b. Stapes defect with fixation of footplate and lenticular process involvement   *(Ref: Nelson 20/e p3071)*

Most common type of congenital ossicular dysfunction is stapes defect with fixation of footplate and lenticular process involvement.

Congenital Stapes Anomalies with Normal Eardrum
• **Incus & stapes anomalies > isolated stapes anomalies > anomalies in all 3 ossicles[Q].**
• **Among stapes anomalies: Stapes footplate fixation only > Mobile stapes footplate with other anomalies > Stapes footplate fixation with other anomalies > Isolated stapes defect[Q].**
• A nonprogressive & conductive hearing loss with normal eardrum, but no history of trauma & infection, is highly suggestive of a congenital ossicular malformation.

Congenital Stapes Anomalies with Normal Eardrum
• **Among ossicular anomalies, stapes anomaly** is the **most common.**
• **Footplate fixation (Stapes super-structure)** is the **most common anomaly,** mostly with **involvement of long apophysis/ lenticular process of incus.**

Teunissen and Cremers' Classification of Congenital Malformations of Ear		
Class	**Malformations**	**%**
1	• **Ankylosis or isolated congenital fixation of the stapes** • (Footplate or superstructure fixation)	30.6%
2	• **Stapes ankylosis associated with other malformations of ossicular chain like:** deformities of incus and/or malleus, or aplasia of long apophysis of the incus or bone fixation of malleus and/or incus	**38.1%**
3	• **Congenital anomalies of the ossicular chain with mobile stapes footplate like:** disruption of ossicular chain, epitympanic or tympanic fixation	21.6%
4	• **Congenital aplasia or severe dysplasia of oval & round windows**	9.7%

172. Ans. b. Meniere's disease   *(Ref: Dhingra 7/e p115, 6/100-104, 5/e pg 112-113; Logan-Turner 10th/335; Scott-Brown 7/e p3570)*

Among the given options, only Meniere's disease involves the vestibular system of inner ear. Hence, a neurotherapy, i.e. direct nerve stimulation, is going to be useful only in Meniere's disease.

Meniere's Disease
• **Meniere's disease** is also known as **endolymphatic hydrops[Q]**
• **Disorder of** the **inner ear** where the **endolymphatic system is distended due to increased volume of endolymph[Q].**

Contd...

AIIMS November 2015

Contd...

Meniere's Disease

Cardinal symptoms of Meniere's Disease	
• Episodic vertigo[Q] • Fluctuating hearing loss[Q]	• Tinnitus[Q] • Sense of fullness or pressure[Q] in the involved ear

Tullio phenomenon
• **Loud sounds** or **noise produce vertigo**[Q] • Due to **distended saccule lying against the stapes footplate**. • Some cases of Meniere's Disease show **Tullio phenomenon**[Q] • Also seen when there are **three functioning windows** in the ear, e.g. **fenestration of horizontal canal** in the presence of mobile stapes.

- **Displacusis** may be seen in Meniere's disease.

  - **Displacusis:** Condition in which the **pitch of single tone** is **heard as two different pitches** by the two ears[Q].
  - This causes **distortion of sound**[Q].

- Patients with Meniere's disease **cannot tolerate loud sounds** due to **recruitment phenomenon**[Q], they are thus **poor candidates for hearing aids.**

Investigations for Meniere's Disease			
Pure tone audiometry	**Speech audiometry**	**Special audiometry tests**	**Electrocochleography**
• In early stages, **lower frequencies** are **affected** and the **curve** is of **rising type.** • When **higher frequencies** are **involved** curve becomes **flat** or **falling type.**	• **Discrimination score** is usually **55-85%** between the attacks but **discrimination ability** is **much impaired during & immediately following an attack.**	• They indicate **cochlear nature of disease** and thus help to differentiate from retrocochlear lesions e.g. acoustic neuroma.	• **Electrocochleography is diagnostic** • Ratio of Summating Potential (SP) to Action Potential (AP) is >30%.

Management of Meniere's Disease		
Medical	**Surgical**	**Others**
Medical management is the mainstay of treatment: • **Vestibular sedatives** to relieve vertigo (Promethazine, Diazepam) • **Vasodilators:** Carbogen, histamine drip, nicotinic acid (in chronic phase) • **Intratympanic Gentamicin therapy:** Gentamicin is **vestibulotoxic.**	Surgical treatment when medical management fails: • **Decompression of endolymphatic Sac** • **Shunt** between endolymphatic sac & subarachnoid space • **Sacculotomy (Fick's operation)**	• Intermittent low pressure pulse therapy (Meniett device) using a myringotomy and a ventilation tube.

173. **Ans. c. Evoked OAE** *(Ref: Nelson 20/e p3075-3079; Dhingra 7/e p29-30, 5/e p116)*
Evoked otoacoustic emission (OAE) is recommended for neonatal screening of hearing.

Neonatal/Infantile Hearing Screening

• **American Academy of Pediatrics** endorses the goal of **universal detection of hearing loss in infants before 3 months of age**, with appropriate intervention no later than 6 months of age.
• The **recommended hearing screening techniques** are either **otoacoustic emissions (OAE)** testing or auditory brainstem evoked responses (ABRs).
    • **ABR test** is an **auditory evoked electrophysiologic response** that correlate highly with hearing.
    • **OAE tests**, used successfully in most universal newborn screening programs, are quick, easy to administer & inexpensive, and they provide a sensitive indication of the presence of hearing loss.

Contd...

AIIMS ESSENCE

Contd...

Neonatal/Infantile Hearing Screening
• Results of OAE are relatively easy to interpret.
• **OAE tests elicit no response if hearing is worse than 30-40 dB**, no matter what's the cause.
• **Children who fail OAE tests undergo an ABR for a more definitive evaluation.**
• Screening methods such as observing behavioural responses to uncalibrated noisemakers or using automated systems such as the Crib-o-gram or the auditory response cradle are not recommended.

Otoacoustic Emissions
• During normal hearing, **OAEs originate from the hair cells in the cochlea**
• **OAEs travel through the middle ear to the external auditory canal, where they can be detected using miniature microphones.**
• **Transient evoked OAEs (TEOAEs) may be used to check the integrity of the cochlea.**
• In neonatal period, detection of OAEs can be accomplished during natural sleep.
• **TEOAEs can be used as screening tests in infants and children for hearing at the 30 dB level of hearing loss.**
• **If a hearing loss is suspected based on the absence of OAEs, ears should be examined for evidence of pathology, and then ABR testing should be used for confirmation & identification of type, degree & laterality of hearing loss.**

Types of Otoacoustic Emissions (OAE)		
Spontaneous OAE (SOAEs)	**Sounds emitted without an acoustic stimulus** (i.e, spontaneously).	• SOAE are seen in **25-80% of neonates with normal hearing** & absence of SOAEs is not necessarily abnormal
Transient evoked OAE (TEOAEs)	**Sounds emitted in response to an acoustic stimuli of very short duration**; usually clicks but can be tone-bursts	• TOAEs commonly are **used to screen infant hearing, to validate behavioural or electrophysiologic auditory thresholds & to assess cochlear function**
Distortion product OAE (DPOAEs)	**Sounds emitted in response to 2 simultaneous tones of different frequencies**	• Particularly useful for **early detection of cochlear damage as** they are for **ototoxicity & noise-induced damage.**
Sustained-frequency OAE (SFOASEs)	**Sounds emitted in response to a continuous tone**	• SPOAEs are responses recorded to a continuous tone.

• Advantages of using OAE as a screening test: Less time consuming & cost lower than ABR
• Infants who fail the OAE test are then screened using ABR.

174. **Ans. b. Schwabach's test**   *(Ref: Dhingra 7/e p23, 5/e p25-27)*

Lateralization of Weber's test to right implies either right-sided conductive deafness or left sided sensorineural deafness. Now in conductive deafness bone conduction is better than air conduction in Rinnie's test, hence the patient probably has sensorineural deafness involving the left ear, as per the findings of Rinnie's and Weber tests. In such a case, Schwabach's test should be performed to see the absolute bone.

Tuning Fork Tests	
• **Qualitative test** (as they **indicate the type of hearing loss**).	
• **Most common used tuning fork: 512 Hz**[Q] (because of Longer tone decay & distinct sound)	
Air conduction (AC)	**Bone conduction (BC)**
• AC is tested by **placing tuning fork ½-1 inch in front of external acoustic meatus**	• BC is tested by **placing tuning fork on mastoid bone or on forehead.**
• It **indicates integrity of tympano-ossicular chain**[Q].	• It **indicates integrity of inner ear**[Q].

Contd...

Contd...

Tuning Fork Tests

Rinne Test

- **In this test, AC is compared with BC of the patient.** Tuning fork is struck and placed in front of external auditory meatus. When the patient stops hearing, move it on to the mastoid bone and ask the patient if he/she still hears and then reverses the process. The object is to find out whether the patients hears longer by air or by bone conduction. **Rinne test will be negative in conductive deafness of more than 15dB.**[Q]

Interpretation of Rinne Test

- Normally, **AC is 2 times better than BC: Positive Rinne**[Q]
- In **conductive deafness, BC>AC: Negative Rinne**[Q]
- In **SNHL, AC>BC: Low Positive Rinne**[Q]
- In **severe SNHL, BC>AC: False negative Rinne** (Due to **transcranial transmission of sounds to the normal ear**)[Q]

Weber's Test

- In this test vibrating **tuning fork is placed in the middle of forehead** and the patient is asked about the **lateralization of sound to left or right ear or in which the sound is heard better.**
- It is a **very sensitive test**[Q] and even less than 5 dB difference in 2 ears hearing level will be **indicated** by this test.
- **Weber test readily detects false negative Rinne**[Q].

Weber's Test

Conductive Deafness	Sensorineural Hearing Loss (SNHL)	Normal Ear
- **Sound is lateralized to the deaf ear**[Q] - In **bilateral conductive loss, sound is lateralized to the more deaf ear**[Q] - **Centrally heard if both ears are equally deaf**[Q]	- **Sound is lateralized to better hearing ear**[Q] - **Heard centrally if both ears are equally bad**[Q].	- **No lateralization** of sound occurs.

Absolute bone conduction (ABC) Test

- In this test, **bone conduction of the patient is tested after occluding the external auditor meatus** and **compared with the BC of the examiner** if he has a normal hearing.
- The test **detects SNHL**[Q].
- If **both patient & examiner hear equally** either **hearing is normal** in-patient or there is **conductive deafness**[Q].
- **If patient ceases to hear before examiner (ABC is reduced), it indicates SNHL**[Q].

Schwabach's Test

- **Bone conduction of the patient & examiner is compared, but meatus is not occluded.**
- **Schwabach is shortened in SNHL**[Q] **& lengthened in conductive hearing loss**[Q].
- **Other Tuning Fork Tests: Bing test, Stenger's test**[Q], **Teel's test**[Q], **Lombard's test**[Q]
- These tests are **done for those patients who feign deafness but actually are normal subjects.**

Tuning Fork Tests and their Interpretation

Test	Normal	Conductive Deafness	Sensorineural Deafness
Rinne	AC > BC[Q] (Rinnie positive)	BC > AC[Q] (Rinnie negative)	AC > BC[Q]
Weber	Not lateralized[Q]	Lateralized to poorer ear[Q]	Lateralized to better ear[Q]
Absolute Bone Conduction	Same as examiner's[Q]	Same as examiner's[Q]	Reduced[Q]
Schwabach	Equal[Q]	Lengthened[Q]	Shortened[Q]

SKIN

175. Ans. b. Lichen planus *(Ref: Fitzpatrick 7/e p244-255; Rooks 8/e p41.1-41.20; Roxburgh 18/e p154-158)*

History of burning sensation on eating spicy food and on examination bilateral white lacy streaks (Wickham's striae) in buccal mucosa and amalgamated third molar is highly suggestive of Lichen planus.

Lichen Planus
• It is **self-limiting papulosquamous**[Q] inflammatory disorder of skin of **unknown origin**[Q]
• Typical lesion is **pruritic, polygonal, purple, plain topped papule & plaques**[Q] which often has **whitish lacy pattern on its surface (Wickham's striae)**[Q]

Etiology:

- **Etiology is unknown**[Q]
- Cutaneous eruptions resembling LP (**lichenoid eruptions**) may be caused by:
  1. **Drugs,** e.g. gold, antimalarials (Chloroquine), thiazide diuretics, penicillamine, phenothiazines & rarely NSAIDs
  2. **Contact sensitizer**
  3. **Hepatitis C infection**[Q]
  4. **Graft versus host reaction** (chronic)

Pathology:

- **Immunological attack** on the **basal layer of epidermis** causing **dense continuous infiltration of lymphocytes & histiocytes** along **dermoepidermal junction**[Q] (**subepidermally lichenoid band**)
- This results in **vacuolar degeneration and necrosis of basal keratinocytes (basal epidermal cell)**[Q]

As a consequence of this lymphocytic infiltration & basal cell degeneration
• Epithelial connective tissue interface weakness resulting in formation of **histological cleft** known as **Max. Joseph space**[Q].
• Redefinition of normal smoothly undulating configuration of dermoepidermal interface to a more **angulated zigzag contour (saw toothing)**[Q]
• A nucleate, necrotic basal cells may become incorporated into inflamed papillary dermis and form eosinophilic – **cytoid, colloid or Civatte bodies**[Q].

- Show changes of chronicity, namely **epidermal hyperplasia**, thickening of granular cell layer (**hypergranulosis**) & stratum corneum (**hyperkeratosis**)

Characteristic Histopathology in Lichen Planus
• **Basal epidermal cell degeneration**[Q] causing saw tooth profile & eosinophilic **cytoid bodies (civatte body)**[Q]
• **Epidermal thickening** especially of granular cell layer
• **Subepidermal-Lichenoid Band**[Q] due deposition of lymphocytes & histiocytes
• **Max Joseph histological cleft**[Q].

Clinical Features		
Cutaneous lesions	**Mucosal lesions**	**Nail changes**
• **Typical lesion:** Pink (purple or **violaceous**[Q]), **plain topped (flat), polygonal, pruritic papule**[Q], which often has a **whitish lacework pattern** on its surface **(Wickham's striae)**[Q] • Lesions have a **predilection for wrist, shins, lower back** & **genitalia** • **Face** is generally **not involved.** • **Isomorphic or Koebner's phenomenon** is positive	• **Commonly involves mucous membranes**[Q], particularly the **buccal mucosa** • A **white lacework pattern in buccal mucosa is MC type of lesion**[Q] • But the tongue & else where in the mouth may also be involved with **white lace work, whitish macule or punctate type of lesions**[Q].	• **Pterygium formation (diagnostic):** **Wing shaped projection of proximal nail fold onto nail bed, splitting** & **destroying nailplate**[Q]. • **Onychorrhexia:** Slight roughness of nail plate with longitudinal ridges and brittleness. • **Thinning**[Q], tenting & distal splitting of nail plates • **Anychia:** Complete loss of nail plate
• **Genital mucosal lesions** are **annular shaped**[Q] • **Scalp involvement** leads to **cicatricial (scarring) alopecia**[Q].		

Contd...

Lichen Planus		
Clinical variants of Lichen Planus		
• Annular	• Lichen planus pemphigoides	• **Follicular (Lichen planopilaris[Q])**
• **Hypertrophic[Q]**	• Lichen planus **pigmentosus[Q]**	• Lichen planus follicularis decalvans
• Atrophic	• Erythrodermic	• Actinic
• Ulcerative	• Linear	
• Bullous		
• Inverse		

Course & Complications:

• A **chronic self-limiting disease,** mostly showing spontaneous remissions in 6 months to 2 years duration.
• As lesions heal, they flatten and often leave hyperpigmented patch[Q].
• Nail & hair loss is irreversible
• Very rarely chronic ulcerative lesions may develop malignant changes (**squamous cell carcinoma**)[Q].

Treatment:

• **Steroids are main stay of treatment[Q],** initially given topically followed by systemic.

176. Ans. a. Aspergillus *(Ref: Neena Khanna 4/e p285)*

The lesions in the given picture are suggestive of Tinea cruris, also known as Jack itch, which is a dermatophytosis of the groin region caused by usually Trichophyton rubrum (not the aspergillus).

"Dermatophytes include a group of fungi (ring worm), that under moist conditions have the ability to infect & survive only on dead keratin, that is the superficial topmost layer of skin, hair & nails. It belongs to 3 genera Microsporum, Epidermophyton, & Trichophyton."

177. Ans. c. Isotretinoin *(Ref: Fitzpatrick 7/e p624-625, Rooks 8/e p58.39-58.51; Harrison 19/e p357-359, 18/e p409-412)*

In the given picture, patient is having localized vitiligo. Isotretinoin is used in management of acne and it should always be avoided in a young female because of teratogenic potential.

Guidelines for Treatment of Vitiligo		
Disease extent	**Type of lesions**	**Treatment**
Localized disease	**New lesions**	• **Topical steroids**
	Old lesion	• **Topical PUVA** (Psoralens with UVA)/PUVA sol
Extensive disease	**New lesions**	• **Oral steroids + PUVA/PUVA sol** or Narrow band UV-B (NB-UVB)
	Rapid increase	• **Oral steroids + PUVA/PUVA sol/NB-UVB**
	Generalized lesions	• **Monobenzyl ether of hydroquinone**

Drugs used in treatment of Vitiligo
• **Topical clobetasol** is a topical steroid
• **Topical tacrolimus** is an immunosuppressant
• **Topical methoxasalen** is a psoralen

Vitiligo
• Vitiligo is a **depigmenting disease of autoimmune etiology**
• **Selective destruction of melanocytes by autoimmune mechanism[Q]**
• **Skin biopsy** specimen shows **absence of melanocytes**.
• Occur at any age; Both sexes are affected equally
• **Associated with other autoimmune disorders**

Associated disease with Vitiligo	
• **Hashimoto thyroiditis (MC)[Q]**	• **Addison's disease[Q]**
• **Graves disease[Q]**	• **MEN[Q]**
• **Diabetes[Q]**	• **Pernicious anemia[Q]**

Contd...

Contd...

Vitiligo

Clinical features:
 • **Depigmented macule** is the **hallmark of vitiligo[Q]**
 • **Typical macule of vitiligo** has a **chalky or milky white color[Q]**
 • **Trichrome vitiligo**: Sometime **three shades** (white, light brown & dark brown) **are seen in the same lesion** and represents the different stages of evolution
 • **Macules** have a **scalloped margin,** which may be hypopigmented, normal color or hyperpigmented.
      • **Leukotrichia[Q]**: In the **older lesions,** the **hair may lose their pigment**
      • **Koebner's (isomorphic) phenomenon[Q]**: Damage to normal skin results in depigmentation

Sites of lesions: • Occurs in any part of the body   • **Areas subjected to repeated friction & trauma[Q]** are frequently affected, e.g., the dorsal aspect of hands and feet, knees and elbows.

Patterns of vitiligo	Characteristic Features
1. Vitiligo vulgaris	• **MC type of vitiligo[Q]** • **Widespread & symmetrical involvement** of **face, extremities & trunk**
2. Segmental vitiligo	• **Occurs along a nerve segment** • **Common on face** along the branches of **trigeminal nerve[Q]** • Not associated with autoimmune diseases • **Stable course,** i.e. lesions increase initially (6-12 months) and then remain static. • **Leukotrichia** on the depigmented areas as well as away from vitiliginous areas frequently seen. **Margins are feathery.** • Distant lesions are uncommon • **Response to treatment less than satisfactory.**
3. Acrofacial vitiligo	• **Involves acral areas** (palms, soles & periungual areas) & **facial areas** (around eyes & lips) • **Resistant to therapy**
4. Lip-tip vitiligo	• **Lips, tips of penis, vulva & nipples** are involved
5. Vitiligo universalis	• **Widespread vitiligo** associated with **multiple endocrinopathies.**

Treatment: • **Photochemotherapy with psoralens with UVA exposure (PUVA) forms the mainstay therapy** in vitiligo.   • **Topical corticosteroids are the 1st line of treatment for children**. It is indicated **for new lesions**.

Poor Prognostic Factors for Vitiligo	
• **Leukotrichia (depigmented hair)** • **Acrofacial lesion** • **Long standing vitiligo**	• **Lesions on resistant areas** (bony prominences, nipples, areola, genitals, non-hairy areas & mucosa

178. Ans. a. Oral isotretinoin *(Ref: Fitzpatrick 6/e p672-686; Rooks 8/e p42.17-42.70; Roxburgh 18/e p159-172)*

In the given picture patient is suffering from severe nodulocystic acne with pus filled lesions. Oral therapy with Isotretinoin is indicated is such a patient.

Isotretenoin
• **Doc for nodulocystic acne / severe acne**[Q].
• Side effects:
1. **Rash (MC)**[Q]
2. **Teratogenic (contraindicated in pregnancy)**[Q]
3. **Hypertriglyceridemia (on prolonged use)**[Q]

Treatment options for Acne					
Drug/Acne	**Mild**		**Moderate**		**Severe**
	Comedonal	**Papular/Pustular**	**Papular/Pustular**	**Nodular**	**Nodular/ Conglobate**
1st Choice	**Topical retinoid**	**Topical retinoid** + Topical antimicrobial	**Topical retinoid** + Oral antibiotic ± BPO	Topical **retinoid +** Oral antibiotic ± BPO	**Oral isotretinoin**
Alternatives for **Females**	**Topical retinoid**	**Topical retinoid** + Topical antimicrobial	**Oral antiandrogen** + topical retinoid ± **topical** antimicrobial	**Oral anti- androgen** + topical retinoid ± **oral** antibiotic	**High dose oral antiandrogen** + topical retinoid ± topical antimicrobial

179. **Ans. b. Poxvirus** *(Ref: Neena Khanna 4/e p274)*

The lesions in the given picture on the forehead are pearly white papules, with a history of transmission to daughter, most likely to be Molluscum contagiosum, which is caused by the poxvirus.

See Q. No. 181 AIIMS May 2016

180. **Ans. a. TT** *(Ref: Neena Khanna 4/e p266)*

The patient has presented with a single anesthetic patch and single enlarged nerve, and a well-defined granuloma can be seen on the skin biopsy. These findings are typical of Tuberculoid leprosy.

See Q. No. 186 AIIMS May 2016

181. **Ans. d. TEN** *(Ref: Neena Khanna 4/e p83, 174)*

A 28-year-old patient of neurocysticercosis develops generalized peeling of skin all over except palms and soles starting one month after taking anti-epileptics. Most probable diagnosis is toxic epidermal necrolysis. Toxic epidermal necrolysis (TEN), also known as Lyell's syndrome, is a rare, life-threatening skin condition that is usually caused by a reaction to drugs.

Epidermal Necrolysis (EN)		
• Also known as **Stevens-Johnson syndrome-toxic epidermal necrolysis (SJS-TEN) complex**.		
• **EN is almost always due to drugs**[Q].		
Epidermal Necrolysis (EN)		
Etiology of Epidermal Necrolysis		
Drugs	**Miscellaneous**	**Idiopathic**
• **Anticonvulsants: carbamazepine, phenytoin barbiturates, lamotrigine**[Q] • **Chemotherapeutic agents: sulfonamides, penicillin**[Q] • **NSAIDs: Butazones, oxicams** • Others: **Allopurinol, nevirapine**[Q]	• **SLE, GVHD** • Lymphoreticular malignancies • Infections (**Mycoplasma pneumoniae, herpes virus infection**)	• 5% of patients

Contd...

Morphology:

- Consists of **deeply erythematous** (often purpuric) **irregular lesions** that rapidly coalesce.
- Either develop **bullae or peel-off in sheets** either spontaneously or when pressure is applied (**positive Nikolsky's sign^Q**)
- On peeling, leave large areas of **denuded skin** that **heal with hyperpigmentation**.

Based on total body surface area (BSA) of skin detached, EN classified into	
SJS	<10% BSA
SJS/TEN overlap (Stevens-Johnson syndrome-Toxic Epidermal Necrolysis)	10-30% BSA
TEN	> 30% BSA^Q

Sites:

- **Symmetrical involvement** of **face, truck** and **proximal part of extremities; Spares distal part of extremities**.
- **Mucous membranes: Mouth & eyes frequently**, other mucosae less frequently affected; manifest as **hemorrhagic crusts** & **white pseudomembrane of the lips**

Complications:

- **EN is an emergency, associated with high mortality** due to:
  - **Infections:** Including sepsis
  - **Fluid & electrolyte imbalance**
  - **Pulmonary involvement:** Interstitial syndrome
  - **Renal failure:** A direct nephrotoxic effect of the drug or due to hypotension
  - **Ophthalmic complications:** Acute complications and late sequelae like dry eyes, symblepharon

Investigations:

- **Biopsy: Subepidermal split with necrotic epidermis^Q**
- Provocation: Causative drug can be identified by provocation test, but this is controversial

Treatment:

- General measures: Withdrawal of suspected drug with supportive care
- Specific therapy: Use of steroids is controversial. **IVIg & cyclosporine** are promising modalities.

Fixed Drug Eruption

- **Adverse cutaneous drug reaction appearing soon after ingestion^Q** (from 30 min to 8 hours) of offending agent in previously sensitized individuals.

Drugs Implicated in Fixed Drug Eruption	
• **Phenolpthalein^Q** (present in some laxatives)	• **Sulphonamides^Q (Cotrimoxazole, dapsone)**
• **Barbiturates^Q**	• **Tertracycline^Q**
• **Metronidazole^Q**	• **Salicylates & phenacetin^Q**
• **Fluoroquinolones^Q**	

Characteristic Features:

- **Mucocutaneous junction (lip, glans) is most frequently involved, genital skin (glans) is the most commonly involved site^Q.**

  - **Most commonly lesions are solitary^Q** but they may be multiple.
  - Lesions **evolve from macules to papules to vesicles & bullae then erode^Q.**
  - Lesions **heal by hyperpigmentation^Q**

Contd...

Contd...

- **Usually asymptomatic**[Q] but may be pruritic, painful, or burning (when eroded)
- Lesions persist if the drug is continued and resolve days to weeks after drug is continued

> - *FDE occurs repeatedly at the same (i.e. fixed) site within hours, every time drug is taken and heals by residual grayish or slate colored hyperpigmentation*[Q].

Diagnosis:
- Diagnosis is **confirmed by provocation.**
- **Rechallenging the patient to the suspected offending drug** is the **only known test to possibly discern the causative agent.**

Treatment:
- The main goal of treatment is to **identify the causative agent and avoid it.**
- **Symptomatic treatment: Systemic antihistamines** and **topical corticosteroids** may be all that are required.

182. **Ans. a. Chronic atrophic candidiasis**   *(Ref: Neena Khanna 4/e p294)*

Chronic erythematous (atrophic) candidiasis appears as a red, raw-looking lesion instead of a white patch seen in all other types.

Types of Oral Candidiasis	
Pseudomembranous	• Classic form of oral candidiasis commonly **referred to as thrush.** • Characterized by a **coating or individual patches of pseudomembranous white slough** that can be **easily wiped away to reveal erythematous &** sometimes **minimally bleeding mucosa beneath.** • Chronicity of this subtype generally **occurs in immunocompromised states,** (leukemia, HIV) or in persons who use **corticosteroids topically** or by aerosol. • Acute & chronic pseudomembranous candidiasis are indistinguishable in appearance.
Erythematous	• **Erythematous (atrophic) candidiasis** is where the condition **appears as a red, raw-looking lesion.** • Some sources consider denture-related stomatitis, angular stomatitis, median rhomboid glossitis & antibiotic-induced stomatitis as subtypes of erythematous candidiasis, since these lesions are commonly erythematous/atrophic. • It may **precede the formation of a pseudomembrane,** be left when the membrane is removed, or arise de novo. • On the tongue, there is loss of the lingual papillae, leaving a smooth area on the tongue. • **Usually occurs on the dorsum of the tongue in persons taking long-term corticosteroids or antibiotics,** but occasionally it can occur after only a few days of using a topical antibiotic. This is usually termed **'antibiotic sore mouth/ stomatitis'** because it is commonly **painful as well as red.** • Chronic erythematous candidiasis is usually **associated with denture wearing.**
Hyperplastic	• This variant is also sometimes termed **'plaque-like candidiasis'** or **'nodular candidiasis'** or **'candidal leukoplakia'.** • **MC appearance of hyperplastic candidiasis** is a **persistent white plaque that does not rub off.** • Usually **chronic & found in adults.** • **MC site of involvement** is the **commissural region of the buccal mucosa,** usually on both sides of mouth. • It can be clinically indistinguishable from true leukoplakia, but tissue biopsy shows candidal hyphae invading the epithelium.

Contd...

Contd...

Types of Oral Candidiasis	
Chronic multifocal oral candidiasis	• This is an uncommon form of chronic (more than one month in duration) candidal infection involving multiple areas in the mouth, without signs of candidiasis on other mucosal or cutaneous sites. • The **lesions are variably red and/or white.** • There is an **absence of predisposing factors such as immunosuppression,** and it occurs in **apparently healthy individuals, normally elderly males.** • Smoking is a known risk factor.
Chronic mucocutaneous candidiasis	• Chronic candidal lesions on the skin, in the mouth and on other mucous membranes (i.e. a secondary oral candidiasis). These include lo**calized chronic mucocutaneous candidiasis, diffuse mucocutaneous candidiasis** (Candida granuloma), **candidiasis–endocrinopathy syndrome and candidiasis thymoma syndrome.** • About 90% of people with chronic mucocutaneous candidiasis have candidiasis in the mouth.

ANESTHESIA

183. Ans. b. Lumbar puncture *(Ref: Harrison 19/e p443e-1, 18/e p46)*

The given needle in the question is used for lumbar puncture.

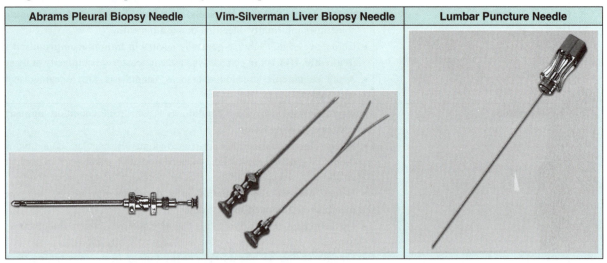

| Abrams Pleural Biopsy Needle | Vim-Silverman Liver Biopsy Needle | Lumbar Puncture Needle |

184. Ans. a. Laryngoscopy *(Ref: Miller 7/e p1587; Lee 13/e p210)*

This is an image of a laryngoscope with curved blade. Laryngoscope is used in direct laryngoscopy.

Laryngoscope
• **Laryngoscope** is an instrument **used to visualize the larynx & surrounding structures** either **by displacing the soft tissue away from the line of vision or by optical aids**[Q]. • The **main purpose** of a laryngoscope is **to aid the intubation**[Q]. • Laryngoscopes, by bringing the esophagus and larynx under view, are helpful in passing the nasogastric tube, oral suctioning, throat packing and removing oral foreign body[Q].
Laryngoscope Blades: • **Commonly used straight blade: Magill Blade**[Q] **(used in infants)** • **Commonly used curved blade: Macintosh blade**[Q]

Contd...

Head & Neck Position for Laryngoscopy:
- Extension at atlanto-occipital joint & flexion at cervical spine[Q]
  - Teeth most vulnerable to damage during laryngoscopy: Upper incisor[Q]

185. **Ans. d. Above esophagus** *(Ref: Miller 7/e p1584; Lee 13/e p206)*

The arrow in the given picture shows the internal gastric tube (drainage tube) kept just above the esophageal opening to aspirate GI secretions.

*"The **LMA Pro-Seal** is a reusable supraglottic airway device that incorporates a gastric drainage tube placed lateral to the main airway tube and which ends at the tip of the mask. The gastric drainage tube is designed to separate the gastrointestinal and respiratory tracts, allowing regurgitated fluid to pass up the drain tube and bypass the glottis, thereby protecting the airway from soiling in the event of passive regurgitation."*

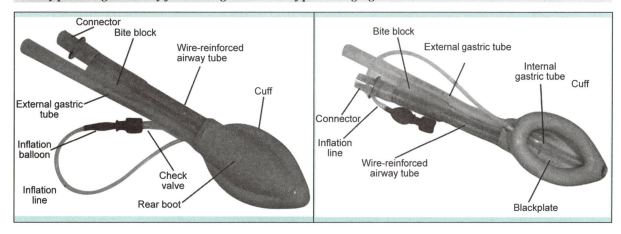

ProSeal Laryngeal Mask Airway

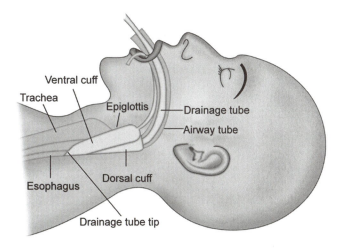

Laryngeal Mask Airway (LMA)
• Provide **an airway intermediate between the face-mask and tracheal tube in terms of anatomical position, invasiveness, security to protect the airway**[Q], and facilitate gas exchange.
• Also known as **Brain mask** (after the name of its inventor **Archies Brain**).

Contd...

1402   AIIMS ESSENCE

Laryngeal Mask Airway (LMA)
• **Consists of 3 components**: an **inflatable mask, mask inflation** line and **airway tube**.
• It is **very effective in maintaining a patent airway in spontaneously breathing patient**.
• It is used **in place of a face mask or ETT during administration of an anesthetic to facilitate ventilation & passage of ETT in a patient with difficult airway**[Q] and to aid in ventilation during fiber optic bronchoscopy (FOB) as well as placement of bronchoscope.
• **LMA partially protects the larynx from pharyngeal secretions** but not gastric regurgitation.
• It is **avoided in bronchospasm** or **high airway resistance**.
• It is available in **7 different sizes**[Q] (i.e. 1, 1.5, 2, 2.5, 3, 4, 5).
• The **flexible LMA** differs from standard LMA in that it has a flexible wire reinforced tube available in sizes 2, 2.5, 3, 4, and 5.
• It allows a tracheal tube to be passed in order to intubate trachea[Q].

LMA PRO-SEAL
• **LMA PRO-SEAL** is another advanced form of classic LMA that has a **double lumen**.
• The **airway tube is wire reinforced to prevent collapse** and has built in bite block (to reduce airway obstruction due to biting).
• The drainage tube passes lateral to the airway tube and allows passage of orogastric tube, drainage of gastric content and prevents gastric insufflation.
• The cuff allows a higher seal than classical LMA.

Laryngeal Mask Airway (LMA)	
Indications	**Contraindications**

• **To facilitate ventilation & passage of ETT in patient with a difficult airway**[Q] & to aid in ventilation during fiber optic bronchoscopy as well as placement of bronchoscope
• **Difficult airway management during cardiopulmonary resuscitation**[Q]**:**
  – **Difficult intubation**[Q] is anticipated
  – **In emergency** where **intubation & mask ventilation is not possible**
  – **For minor surgeries**, where anesthetist wants to avoid intubation
  – As a **conduit for bronchoscopes**, small size tubes, gum elastic bougies.
  – For **extra & intraocular surgeries** including retinopathy surgery in ex-premature infants
  – LMA have **little effect on intraocular pressure (absence of face mask may facilitate eye examination**[Q]**)**
  – **Mouth opening <1.5 cm**
	• **Oropharyngeal abscess or mass**[Q]
	• **Conditions with high risk of aspiration:**
	  – **Hiatus hernia**
	  – **Pregnancy**
	• **Full stomach patients who are vulnerable to go in bronchospasm**[Q]
	• **Pharyngeal pathology** (e.g. abscess)
	• **Pharyngeal obstruction**
	• **Full stomach (e.g. pregnancy, hiatus hernia)** as it **partially protects larynx from pharyngeal secretions but not gastric regurgitation**[Q]
	• Low pulmonary compliance (e.g. obesity)
	• Peak inspiratory pressure > 20 cm of H_2O.

Laryngeal Mask Airway (LMA)	
Advantages	**Disadvantage**
• **Easy to insert** • **Does not require any laryngoscope, visualization, & muscle relaxants**[Q] • **Does not require any specific position of cervical spine**, so **can be used in cervical injuries**	• **Does not prevent aspiration** so should not be used for full stomach patients. • **High incidence of laryngospasm & bronchospasm**.

186. **Ans. a. Increase muscle relaxant**   *(Ref: Miller 7/e p1427)*

    A cleft in capnograph is due to patients' own respiratory effort because of inadequate muscle relaxation. Increasing the dose of muscle relaxant will solve this problem.

    See Q. No. 190 AIIMS November 2016

187. **Ans. c. Black body with white shoulder**   *(Ref: Anaesthetic Equipments & Procedures, Practical Approach/p37, 38)*

    The color of a medical oxygen cylinder is a black body with a white shoulder.

Color Identification of Medical Gas Cylinders			
Name of gas	Body	Shoulder	Pin index
Air	Grey[Q]	White & black quarter[Q]	1, 5[Q]
Carbon dioxide (Conc. >7.5%)	Grey[Q]	Grey[Q]	1, 6[Q]
Oxygen	Black	White[Q]	2, 5[Q]
Carbon dioxide (Conc. <7.5%)	Grey[Q]	Grey[Q]	2, 6[Q]
Nitrous oxide	Blue[Q]	Blue[Q]	3, 5[Q]
Cyclopropane	Orange[Q]	Orange[Q]	3, 6[Q]
Entonox (50% O_2 + N_2O)	Blue[Q]	Blue & white quarter[Q]	7[Q]
Helium	Brown[Q]	Brown[Q]	-
Mix of oxygen & helium (He <80.5%)	Brown[Q]	White[Q]	2, 4[Q]
Mix of oxygen & helium (He >80.5%)	Brown[Q]	White[Q]	4, 6[Q]
Nitrogen	Black[Q]	Black[Q]	1, 4[Q]

188. **Ans. b. Distal esophagus**   *(Ref: Miller's 7/e p1550)*

Though pulmonary artery is the gold standard site for core temperature measurement, esophagus has similar reliability and is the most commonly used site in the anesthetic practice for temperature monitoring.

Core-Temperature Monitoring

• **Most accurate site to obtain core body temperature** is **hypothalamus**. It is located in the base of the brain and acts as the body's thermostat. But **access to the hypothalamus is quite inconvenient.**
• The **body temperature** is best described as an **estimate of the average temperature of the core portions of the body** as reflected by the **temperature of the blood in the major vessels.**
    • **Pulmonary artery is an ideal site** because, **in heart, the blood is mixed from viscera & skin.**
    • **The truest, accessible, core temperature ('Gold Standard') is measurement of pulmonary artery temperature with a thermistor catheter.**[Q]
• **Other core accessible sites** are the **esophagus, tympanic membrane and urinary bladder**. Similar **thermistor catheters can be placed in the esophagus and bladder for core temperature measurement. These sites are used when accurate knowledge of core temperature is critical.**
• However, none of these sites are convenient for routine acute care temperature measurement.
    • **Core thermal compartment is composed of highly perfused tissues whose temperature is uniform & high in comparison to the rest of body.**
    • **Temperature in this compartment** can be **evaluated in the pulmonary artery, distal part of esophagus, tympanic membrane, or nasopharynx.**

Esophagus
• **Proper placement** is in the **lower 1/3 of the esophagus which will allow the sensor to be closer to the heart and aorta,** and that it **will accurately reflect the core temperature**[Q]. • It also **indicates changes in core temperature significantly faster than peripheral sites**[Q]. • **Temperature probes incorporated into esophageal stethoscopes must be positioned at the point of maximal heart sounds, or even more distally, to provide accurate readings**[Q]. • Even during rapid thermal perturbations, such as cardiopulmonary bypass, these temperature-monitoring sites remain reliable.

Sites for Core Temperature Measurement	
Gold standard site for core temperature measurement	• **Pulmonary artery**[Q]
Most accurate for brain temperature	• **Tympanic membrane**[Q]
Best for brain temperature	• **Nasopharynx**[Q]
Best site & most commonly used for core body temperature	• **Lower end of esophagus**[Q]

189. **Ans. a. Ligamentum flava**   *(Ref: Gray's 40/e p729, Snell's 9/e p705)*

While performing a lumbar puncture, a snap is felt just before entering into the epidural space. This is due to piercing of ligamentum flava.

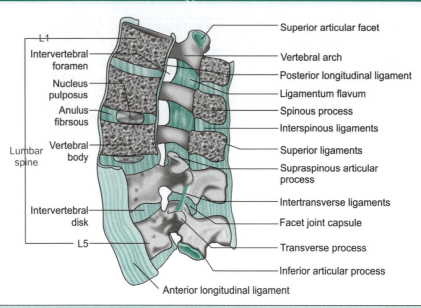

Lumbar Puncture
• The **depth** to which the needle will have to pass varies from **2.5 cm** or less in a **child** to as much as **10 cm in obese adults**. • In **caudal anesthesia, needle pierces skin & fascia & sacrococcygeal membrane** that fills in the sacral hiatus.   • The **membrane** is **formed of dense fibrous tissue** & represents **fused supraspinous & interspinous ligaments** as well as **ligamentum flavum. A distinct feeling of 'give' is felt when the ligament is penetrated**[Q].

During lumbar puncture, the needle passes through the following anatomic structures before it enters the subarachnoid space:
• Skin[Q] • Subcutaneous tissue[Q] • Supraspinous ligament[Q] • Interspinous ligament[Q] • Ligamentum flavum[Q] • Dura mater[Q] • Arachnoid mater[Q]

190. **Ans. a. General anesthesia with IV induction by ketamine**   *(Ref: Williams 24/e p518; Morgan 4/e p197-199)*

This patient of placenta previa is in labor and has bled into shock. She should be delivered by cesarean section under general anesthesia. General anesthesia is preferred as it is a more controllable modality and there is a significant risk of hypotension associated with spinal anesthesia. Ketamine is the preferred agent in cases of acute shock.

"Ketamine stimulates sympathetic system causing tachycardia and hypertension, so it is intravenous anaesthetic of choice for shock."

Ketamine
• **Phencyclidine derivative**[Q], contains **benzthonium chloride**[Q] as preservative • **Strong analgesic**, but not a muscle relaxant (rather it **increases the muscle tone**)[Q] • Primary site of action is **thalamoneocortical projection**[Q], inhibits cortex (unconsciousness) and thalamus (analgesia) and stimulates limbic system (emergence reaction and hallucination) • Produces **dissociative anaesthesia**[Q], individual is in **cataleptic state**

• Acts on **NMDA receptor**[Q], dose is **2 mg/kg I.V.**[Q] • Onset of action in 30 to 60 seconds, elimination half life is **2-3 hours** • Early regain of consciousness because of **redistribution**[Q]

Ketamine		
Systemic Effects of Ketamine		
CNS	**CVS**	**Respiratory system**
• Increases brain oxygen consumption and metabolic rate, **intracranial tension is highly raised**[Q] • **Emergence reactions**[Q] (vivid dreaming, illusion, etc) is seen. • **Hallucinations:** both auditory and visual (**mainly auditory**[Q]), incidence is **30-40%**, **hallucination is MC side effects of Ketamine**[Q], these hallucinations and emergence reactions can be **decreased by** giving **benzodiazepines**[Q] along with ketamine.	• Ketamine **stimulates sympathetic system** causing **tachycardia** and **hypertension**, so it is **intravenous anaesthetic of choice for shock**[Q]. • **Benzodiazepines attenuate this hemodynamic response**[Q] (tachycardia, hypertension and increased oxygen demand of myocardium) of Ketamine.	• **Stimulates respiration, potent bronchodilator & is intravenous anaesthetic of choice for asthmatics**[Q] • **Pharyngeal and laryngeal reflexes are preserved**[Q] • Tracheobronchial and salivary secretions are increased
Eye	**GIT**	**Muscular system**
• **Increased intraocular tension**[Q]	• **Increased intragastric pressure & salivary secretions**	• **Increases muscle tone**[Q]

Advantages & uses of Ketamine

• Induction agent of choice for:
     – **Asthmatics, shock**[Q]
     – **Constrictive Pericarditis, cardiac tamponade**[Q] (in theses conditions cardiac output is dependent on tachycardia and Ketamine causes tachycardia)
     – **Right to left shunt like TOF**[Q] (Ketamine by causing hypertension increases the afterload there by decreasing the right to left shunt fraction)
 • Can be used as **sole agent** for minor procedures, safely used in **remote places**
 • Preferred agent for patients with **full stomach (pharyngeal and laryngeal reflexes are preserved)**[Q]

Contraindications of Ketamine
• **Head injury, intracranial space occupying lesion, eye injury**[Q] (increases ICT, IOT)   • **Ischemic heart disease, vascular aneurysm & hypertension**[Q] (increases myocardial oxygen demand & hypertension)   • **Psychiatric diseases & drug addicts**[Q] (more incidence of hallucination & emergence reaction)

191. **Ans. d. Glycopyrrolate** *(Ref: Miller 7/e p293; KDT 7/e p386, 117)*

Glycopyrrolate is most commonly used as pre-anesthetic medication. Glycopyrrolate is an anticholinergic drug used for reducing secretions in the mouth, throat, airway, and stomach before surgery. It is used before and during surgery to block certain reflexes and to protect against certain side effects of some medicines.

Action	Atropine	Glycopyrrolate
Antisecretory	++	+++[Q]
Tachycardia	+++[Q]	++
CNS effects	+[Q]	-[Q]
Bronchodilation	++	++

Glycopyrrolate
• **Glycopyrrolate** is an **anticholinergic drug used for reducing secretions in mouth, throat, airway & stomach before surgery**[Q].   • **Potent & rapidly acting antimuscarinic lacking central effects**[Q].   • **Antisecretory action is more marked than atropine, while tachycardia is less marked** after IM injection[Q]

Contd...

Pharmacokinetics:
• A **synthetic quaternary ammonium derivative of atropine, glycopyrrolate, does not diffuse through the blood-brain barrier,** and is **frequently used to limit the anticholinergic effects to periphery**[Q].
• Glycopyrrolate has a **longer duration of action than atropine**[Q].
Therapeutic Uses:
• It is **used before & during surgery to block certain reflexes** and **to protect against certain side effects of some medicines**[Q].

RADIOLOGY

192. Ans. d. Osteoclastoma   *(Ref: Apley 9/e p202)*

A 20-year old male patient presents with pain on movement. X-ray of knee joint shows lytic lesion on the upper end of tibia. In the given X-ray, epiphyseal lytic lesion in tibia with a 'soap bubble' appearance is characteristic of osteoclastoma. The tumour always abuts against the joint margin in osteoclastoma.

*"X-ray (Giant-cell Tumour): Radiolucent area situated eccentrically at the end of a long bone & bounded by subchondral bone plate. The **centre** sometimes has a **soap-bubble appearance** due to ridging of the surrounding bone. **Appearance of a 'cystic' lesion in mature bone, extending right up to the subchondral plate, is so characteristic that the diagnosis is seldom in doubt."- Apley 9/e p202*

Simple Bone Cyst	Admantinoma	Multiple Myeloma
• **Fills the medullary cavity but does not expand the bone**[Q] • X-rays: **Well-defined radiolucent cyst, often trabeculated & eccentrically placed**[Q]. • In a growing tubular bone it is **always situated in the metaphysis**[Q].	• **X-ray** shows a typical **bubble-like defect in the anterior tibial cortex**; sometimes there is **thickening of the surrounding bone**[Q].	• X-rays: The 'classical' lesions are **multiple punched-out defects with 'soft' margins (lack of new bone) in the skull, pelvis and proximal femur, a crushed vertebra, or a solitary lytic tumour in a large-bone metaphysis**[Q].

193. Ans. b. Hydropneumothorax   *(Ref: Sutton Radiology 7/e p92)*

The air fluid level seen on the left side in the given X-ray is suggestive of a diagnosis of hydropneumothorax.

Hydropneumothorax
• Hydropneumothorax is defined as the **presence of both air & fluid within the pleural space** surrounding the lung.
Etiology:
• Iatrogenic: Introduction of air during **pleural fluid aspiration** in effusion   • Presence of a gas-forming organism   • **Thoracic trauma**   • **Bronchopleural fistula**

Contd...

Hydropneumothorax
Signs (4S):
• Straight line dullness; Shifting dullness; Succussion splash; Sound of coin[Q]
X-ray Findings:
• An **upright chest X-ray** will show **air fluid levels**.
• **Horizontal fluid level** is usually **well-defined** & extends across the whole length of hemithorax.

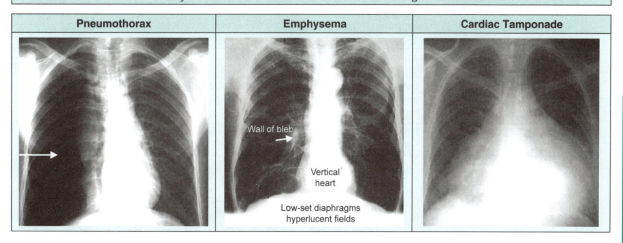

194. Ans. a. Spondylolisthesis (Ref: Apley's 9/e p484-486; Turek 6/e p503)

The given X-ray is showing a forward displacement of the arrow-marked vertebra on lower one, suggestive of spondylolisthesis.

> *"Spondylolisthesis means forward translation of one segment of the spine upon another. The shift is nearly always between L4 and L5, or between L5 and the sacrum. Normal discs, laminae and facets constitute a locking mechanism that prevents each vertebra from moving forwards on the one below. Forward shift (or slip) occurs only when this mechanism has failed."- Apley's 9/e p484*

Spondylolisthesis
• **Spondylolisthesis** means **forward translation of one segment of the spine upon another**.
• Shift is nearly **always between L4 & L5**, or **between L5 & sacrum**[Q].

Types of Spondylolisthesis	
• Dysplastic (20%)	• Post-traumatic
• **Lytic or isthmic (50%)**[Q]	• Pathological
• Degenerative (25%)	• Postoperative (iatropathic)

Pathology:
• In **lytic type of spondylolisthesis, pars interarticularis on both sides is disrupted**, as in an ununited fracture (spondylolysis), **leaving posterior neural arch separated from vertebral body anteriorly**; gap is occupied by fibrous tissue[Q].

> • With stress, vertebral body & superior facets in front of gap may subluxate or dislocate forwards, carrying superimposed vertebral column with it (spondylolisthesis)[Q]

Clinical Features:
• **Children:** It is usually painless but **unduly protruding abdomen** & **peculiar stance**.
• **Adults: Backache** is the **usual presenting symptom**; **Sciatica** may occur in one or both legs.
• **Lumbar spine** is **on a plane in front of sacrum** & **looks too short**.

	Spondylolisthesis

X-rays:

- **Lateral views: Forward shift of the upper part of spinal column on the stable vertebra below**; elongation of the arch or defective facets may be seen.
- **Gap in the pars interarticularis is best seen in the oblique views (Beheaded scotty dog sign & inverted Napoleon hat sign[Q])**

Treatment:

- **Conservative treatment is suitable for most patients.**
- **Operative treatment:** If the **symptoms are disabling** & interfere significantly with work & recreational activities; if the **slip is >50% & progressing**; if **neurological compression** is significant.

	Spondylolisthesis	Spondylosis
Definition	Forward displacement of a vertebra, especially 5th lumbar vertebra, most commonly occurring after a break or fracture[Q]	Degenerative changes in the spine[Q]
Oblique ("Scotty Dog") view	Beheaded scotty dog sign & inverted Napoleon hat sign[Q]	Scotty dog wearing a collar sign[Q]
Lateral view		

PSYCHIATRY

195. Ans. a. Haloperidol *(Ref: Niraj Ahuja 7/e p79)*

Haloperidol is the only antipsychotic mentioned in the options, which can be used in pregnant patients suffering from bipolar disorders.

Treatment of Acute Mania (Hypomania)

- Most **mood stabilizers & antipsychotics** have **acute antimanic effects**, but **lithium[Q] or valproate[Q] is drug of choice.**
- Since **response takes 7-14 days**, an **antipsychotic is often required with effect within days** in controlling acute manic symptoms.
- **Haloperidol[Q] (older antipsychotic) should not be used with lithium** due to **risk of neurotoxicity syndrome**.
- **High potency benzodiazepines (Clonazepam & lorazepam)** may be **used temporarily to treat hyperactivity, agitation & insomnia.** Its most useful role is as an adjunct to mood stabilizers because the later drug can take several days to become effective. **Their safety & benign side effect profile make them ideal adjunct to mood stabilizers (Lithium, carbamazepine or valproate).**
- Mania with impaired judgment, loss of insight, hyperactivity & diminished behavior need hospitalization. **ECT may be used for severe cases, refractory mania**, or for patients with **medical complication as well as extreme exhaustion.**

Contd...

Contd...

Treatment of Bipolar Disorders in Pregnancy
• **Lithium & anticonvulsants are withdrawn due to risk of fetal malformations** but may be restarted in later pregnancy.
• **Antidepressants & (older) antipsychotics** may be used. **Olanzapine is safe.**
• Medications are **withdrawn at the time of delivery** to avoid effects on fetus but **restarted again as soon as possible thereafter, as risk of relapse is increased in postpartum.**

> • **DOC for acute mania in pregnancy & lactation: Atypical antipsychotics >typical antipsychotics.**

196. Ans. d. Guilt *(Ref: Niraj Ahuja 7/e p164)*

Beck's cognitive triad involves negative thoughts about the self (the self is worthless) , the world/environment (i.e. the world is unfair, helpless), and the future (the future is hopeless).

"Beck's cognitive triad represents three types of negative thoughts present in depression, as proposed by Aaron Beck in 1976. The triad forms part of his cognitive theory of depression. The triad involves negative thoughts about: The self (i.e. the self is worthless) ; The world/environment (i.e. the world is unfair, helpless), and The future (i.e. the future is hopeless)."

DSM IV Criteria for Major Depressive Episode
A. Five (or more) of the following symptoms have been present during the same 2-week period and represent a change from previous functioning; at least one of the symptoms is either (1) depressed mood or (2) loss of interest or pleasure. Note: Do not include symptoms that are clearly due to a general medical condition, or mood-incongruent delusions or hallucinations.
1. **Depressed mood most of the day, nearly everyday**, as indicated by either **subjective report** (e.g. feels sad or empty) or **observation made by others** (e.g. appears tearful).
2. **Markedly diminished interest or pleasure in all, or almost all, activities** most of the day, nearly everyday
3. **Significant weight loss when not dieting or weight gain** (e.g. a change of more than 5% of body weight in a month) or **decrease or increase in appetite**
4. **Insomnia or hypersomnia nearly everyday**
5. **Psychomotor agitation or retardation**
6. **Fatigue or loss of energy** nearly everyday
7. **Feelings of worthlessness or excessive or inappropriate guilt** (which may be delusional)
8. Diminished ability to think or concentrate, or indecisiveness
9. **Recurrent thoughts of death** (not just fear of dying), **recurrent suicidal ideation**.
B. The symptoms **do not meet criteria for a mixed episode.**
C. The symptoms cause **clinically significant distress or impairment in social, occupational, or other important areas of functioning.**
D. The symptoms are **not due to the direct physiological effects of a substance** (e.g. a drug of abuse, a medication) or **a general medical condition** (e.g. hypothyroidism).
E. The symptoms are **not better accounted for by bereavement,** i.e. after the loss of a loved one, the **symptoms persist for longer than 2 months** or are **characterized by marked functional impairment, morbid preoccupation with worthlessness, suicidal ideation, psychotic symptoms, or psychomotor retardation.**

197. Ans. a. Sodium bicarbonate   *(Ref: Harrison 19/e p172)*

A young female on antidepressants presents to the emergency with altered sensorium and hypotension. ECG reveals wide QRS complexes and right axis deviation. The clinical features and ECG findings typically suggest a diagnosis of tricyclic antidepressant poisoning. Antidote for TCA poisoning is sodium bicarbonate administered IV 100 mEq (1–2 mEq/kg), and repeated every few minutes until BP improves and QRS complexes begin to narrow. Hemodialysis should not be used since TCAs are highly protein-bound with large volume of distribution.

Tricyclic Antidepressant Overdose

- **TCA overdose** is **caused by excessive use** or **overdose of a TCA drug**.
- It is a **commonly used antidepressant** & **in children prescribed for bed-wetting**[Q].

Pathophzysiology:

- Most of the toxic effects of TCAs are caused by four major pharmacological effects:
    - Anticholinergic effects[Q]
    - **Excessive blockade of norepinephrine reuptake** at the preganglionic synapse[Q]
    - Direct alpha adrenergic blockade[Q]
    - **Block sodium membrane channels with slowing of membrane depolarization**, thus having **quinidine-like effects on the myocardium**[Q].

Signs and Symptoms:

- **Peripheral ANS**, **CNS & heart** are the **main systems that are affected** following overdose.
- Initial or **mild symptoms typically develop within 2 hours** and include **tachycardia, drowsiness, a dry mouth, nausea & vomiting, urinary retention, confusion, agitation & headache**[Q].

    - **More severe complications** include **hypotension, cardiac rhythm disturbances, hallucinations & seizures**[Q].
    - **ECG abnormalities are frequent; MC is sinus tachycardia & intraventricular conduction delay** resulting in **prolongation of the QRS complex & PR/QT intervals**[Q].

- **Seizures, cardiac dysrhythmias & apnea** are the **most important life-threatening complications**[Q].

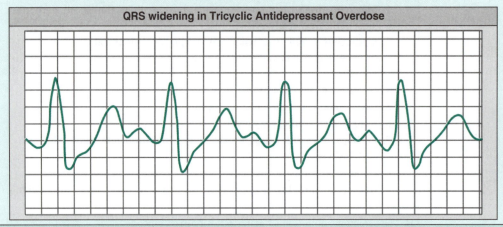

Treatment

- **Initial treatment**: **Gastric decontamination**[Q] of the patient.
- This is achieved by **administering activated charcoal lavage**, which **adsorbs the drug in the GIT** either orally or via a nasogastric tube. **Activated charcoal** is **most useful if given within 1-2 hours of ingestion**[Q].

    - Other decontamination methods, such as **stomach pumps, ipecac-induced emesis, or whole bowel irrigation** are **not recommended in TCA poisoning**[Q].

Contd...

Tricyclic Antidepressant Overdose
• **Supportive therapy** is given if necessary, including respiratory assistance, maintenance of body temperature, etc.

> • **Administration of IV sodium bicarbonate**[Q] as an antidote has been shown to be an effective treatment for resolving the metabolic acidosis and cardiovascular complications of TCA poisoning.

- If **sodium bicarbonate therapy fails to improve cardiac symptoms**, conventional antiarrhythmic drugs, such as **phenytoin & magnesium can be used to reverse any cardiac abnormalities**.
- **Hypotension** is initially **treated with fluids along with bicarbonate to reverse metabolic acidosis** (if present).
- If the patient remains **hypotensive despite fluids**, then further measures, such as the **administration of epinephrine, norepinephrine, or dopamine** can be used to increase blood pressure.
- **Seizures often resolve without treatment** but administration of a benzodiazepine or other anticonvulsive may be required for persistent muscular over activity.

> • There is **no role for physostigmine in the treatment of tricyclic toxicity** as **it may increase cardiac toxicity and cause seizures**[Q].

- In cases of **severe TCA overdoses that are refractory to conventional therapy**, **intravenous lipid emulsion therapy has been reported to improve signs & symptoms** in moribund patients suffering from toxicities involving several types of lipophilic substances. Therefore, **lipids may have a role in treating severe cases of refractory TCA overdose.**

> • **Tricyclic antidepressants are highly protein-bound** and have a **large volume of distribution.** Therefore, **removal of these compounds from the blood with hemodialysis, hemoperfusion or other techniques** is **unlikely to be of any significant benefit**[Q].

---

198. Ans. c. 2 years *(Ref: Niraj Ahuja 7/e p67)*

Multiple randomized trials have found that maintenance of antipsychotic medication reduces the risk of relapse over a period of up to two years.

"A meta-analysis of 6493 patients with schizophrenia in 65 randomized trials of 7 to 12 months duration found that patients who continued on an antipsychotic experienced a lower relapse rate compared to patients withdrawn from an antipsychotic and receiving placebo (27 versus 64 percent; number needed to treat to benefit = 3, 95% CI 2–3). Other studies of up to two years have found similar results."

"Although the current consensus is that antipsychotic should be prescribed for 1-2 years after 1st episode of schizophrenia. Gitlan et al found that withdrawing the antipsychotic leads to relapse at rate of 80 % after one years of medication free and relapse at rate of 98% after 2 years of medication free."- Maudsley Prescribing Guidelines in Psychiatry 12/e p31

Treatment Duration for Schizophrenia		
• **1st episode: 1–2 years**[Q]	• **2nd episode: 2–5 years**[Q]	• **3rd/Recurrent: Lifetime**[Q]

199. Ans. d. Impaired cognition *(Ref: Kaplan 10/e p1191-1197; Niraj Ahuja 7/e p163-165)*

According to DSM-V, intellectual disability should be ruled out prior to a diagnosis of pervasive developmental defects.

"The diagnostic category pervasive developmental disorders (PDD), as opposed to specific developmental disorders (SDD) is characterized by delays in the development of multiple basic functions including socialization and communication."

Pervasive Developmental Disorders

- The diagnostic category **pervasive developmental disorders (PDD),** as opposed to specific developmental disorders (SDD) **are characterized by delays in the development of multiple basic functions including socialization and communication.**

Pervasive Developmental Disorders are

- **Pervasive developmental disorder** not otherwise specified (PDD-NOS), **(includes atypical autism): Most common**
- **Autism**
- **Asperger syndrome**
- **Rett syndrome**
- **Childhood disintegrative disorder (CDD).**

  - **The first three of these disorders are commonly called the autism spectrum disorders.**

- **Onset of PDD occurs during infancy,** but the condition is usually **not identified until the child is around three years old.**
- Parents may begin to question the health of their child when developmental milestones are not met, including **age-appropriate motor movement & speech production**.

DSMV: Diagnostic Criteria Autism Spectrum Disorder 299.00 (F84.0)

A. **Persistent deficits in social communication and social interaction across multiple contexts**, as manifested by:
- **Deficits in social-emotional reciprocity**
- **Deficits in nonverbal communicative behaviors used for social interaction**
- **Deficits in developing, maintaining, and understanding relationships.**

B. **Restricted, repetitive patterns of behavior, interests, or activities**, as manifested by at least two of the following:
- Stereotyped or repetitive motor movements, use of objects, or speech
- **Insistence on sameness, inflexible adherence to routines,** or ritualized patterns or verbal-nonverbal behavior
- **Highly restricted, fixated interests** that are abnormal in intensity or focus
- **Hyper- or hyporeactivity to sensory input or unusual interests** in sensory aspects of the environment

C. **Symptoms must be present in the early developmental period**

DSMV: Diagnostic Criteria Autism Spectrum Disorder 299.00 (F84.0)

D. Symptoms cause **clinically significant impairment in social, occupational**, or other important areas of current functioning.

E. These disturbances are **not better explained by intellectual disability** (intellectual developmental disorder) or **global developmental delay.**

- **Intellectual disability & autism spectrum disorder frequently co-occur;** to make comorbid diagnoses of autism spectrum disorder and intellectual disability, **social communication should be below that expected for general developmental level.**

- **Note:** Individuals with a well-established DSM-IV diagnosis of autistic disorder, Asperger 's disorder, or pervasive developmental disorder not otherwise specified should be given the diagnosis of autism spectrum disorder. **Individuals, who have marked deficits in social communication, but whose symptoms do not otherwise meet criteria for autism spectrum disorder, should be evaluated for social (pragmatic) communication disorder.**

Autistic Disorder (Kanner's Autism)

- It is characterized by **qualitative impairment in reciprocal social interaction, delayed and aberrant communication skills & a restricted repertoire of activities and interests**[Q].
- By definition, the **onset is before the age of 3 years**[Q].

Contd...

AIIMS November 2015 1413

Contd...

Autistic Disorder (Kanner's Autism)
• More common in boys[Q]   • Developmental milestones are normal[Q].   • Temporal lobe is believed to be critical area.

Clinical Features			
Autism (marked impairment in reciprocal social and interpersonal interaction)	**Marked impairment in language and non-verbal communication**	**Abnormal behavioral characteristics**	**Mental retardation**
• **Absent social smile** • **Lack of eye-to-eye-contact** • **Lack of awareness** of others existence or feelings; treats people as furniture • **Lack of attachment to parents** and **absence of separation anxiety.** • **No or abnormal social play**; prefers solitary games. • **Marked impairment in making friends** • **Lack of imitative behaviour** • **Absence of fear in presence of danger**	• **Lack of verbal or facial response** to sounds or voices; might be thought as deaf initially. • In **infancy, absence of communicative sounds like babbling.** • **Absent or delayed speech** • **Abnormal speech patterns and content.** Presence of **echolalia, perseveration, poor articulation** and pronominal reversal is common. • Remote memory is usually good. • **Abstract thinking is impaired.**	• **Mannerisms** • **Stereotyped behaviour** such as **head-banging, body-spinning, lining-up objects, rocking, clapping, twirling,** etc. • **Ritualistic & compulsive behaviour.** • Resistance to even the slightest change in the environment. • Attachment may develop to inanimate objects. • **Hyperkinesis** is commonly associated.	• Only about 25% of all children with autism have an **IQ >70.** • **>50%** of these children have **moderate to profound mental retardation.** • There appears to be a correlation between severity of mental retardation, absence of speech & epilepsy in autism.

Treatment of Autism		
Behaviour Theory	**Psychotherapy**	**Pharmacotherapy**
• Development of a regular routine with as few changes as possible. • Structured classroom training, aiming at learning new material & maintenance of acquired learning.	• **Parental counseling & supportive psychotherapy** can be very useful in allaying parental anxiety and guilt, and helping their active involvement in therapy.	• **Haloperidol** decreases dopamine levels in brain, decreases hyperactivity & behavioral symptoms.

Treatment of Autism		
Behaviour Theory	**Psychotherapy**	**Pharmacotherapy**
• Positive reinforcements to teach self-care skills. • Speech therapy and/or sign language teaching. • **Behavioral techniques to encourage interpersonal interactions.**	• However, **overstimulation** of child **should be avoided during treatment.**	• **Risperidone**, for treatment of autism in children aged 5 and above. • Anticonvulsants are used for the treatment of generalized or other seizures

200. Ans. a. Psychoeducation *(Ref: Niraj Ahuja 7/e p67-68)*

In the question patient symptoms of bipolar disorder are well controlled by medication, which implies pharmacotherapy is efficient and added psychotherapy is necessary only to keep the patient compliant to the medication. In such a case, psychoeducation of the patient about adherence to strict treatment is most crucial psychotherapy modality in preventing relapse.

Psychoeducation

- **Psychoeducation** refers to the **education offered to individuals with a mental health condition** & their families to help empower them & deal with their condition in an optimal way.
  - Frequently psychoeducational training involves **individuals with schizophrenia, clinical depression, anxiety disorders, psychotic illnesses, eating disorders, and personality disorders**, as well as patient training courses in **context of the treatment of physical illnesses.**
- **Family members** are also **included.**
- A **goal** is for the **consumer to understand** and **be better able to deal with the presented illness.**
  - Also, the **patient's own capabilities, resources & coping skills are strengthened & used to contribute to their own health & well-being on a long-term basis.**
- Since it is often difficult for the patient and their family members to accept the patient's diagnosis, **psychoeducation** also has the **function of contributing to the destigmatization of psychological disturbances** and **to diminish barriers to treatment.**
  - The **relapse risk is in this way lowered**; patients & family members, who are **more well-informed about the disease, feel less helpless**[Q].

Important elements in psychoeducation are:

- **Information transfer** (symptomatology of the disturbance, causes, treatment concepts, etc.)
- **Emotional discharge** (understanding to promote, exchange of experiences with others concerning, contacts, etc.)
- **Support of a medication or psychotherapeutic treatment, as cooperation is promoted between the mental health professional and patient (compliance, adherence).**
- **Assistance to self-help** (e.g. training, as crisis situations are promptly recognized and what steps should be taken to be able to help the patient).

Supportive Psychotherapy

- It is a **psychotherapeutic approach** that **integrates psychodynamic, cognitive-behavioral, & interpersonal conceptual models & techniques.**
- The objective of the therapist is **to reinforce the patient's healthy & adaptive patterns of thought behaviors in order to reduce the intrapsychic conflicts that produce symptoms of mental disorders.**
- Unlike in psychoanalysis, in which the analyst works to maintain a neutral demeanor as a 'blank canvas' for transference, in supportive therapy, the therapist engages in a fully emotional, encouraging, and supportive relationship with the patient as a method of furthering healthy defense mechanisms, especially in the context of interpersonal relationships.
  - This therapy has been used for patients suffering from severe cases of addiction as well as bulimia nervosa, stress and other mental illnesses.
- **Supportive psychotherapy is used as an initial therapy, to be reduced and not to be prolonged, in situations or periods where there is a lack of means for a systematic approach or behaviorism.** Examples of such situations include:
  - **Critical negotiations**
  - **Volatile but unavoidable everyday life or decisive situations**
  - **Compromises** (to introduce at least minimal operational, efficient relationship conditions) in long-term, engaged relationships, based on lasting agreements

Insight-oriented Psychotherapy

- It relies on **conversation between the therapist & client.**
- It **helps people through understanding & expressing feelings, motivations, beliefs, fears and desires**.
- As insight-oriented psychotherapy is a **client-centered therapy**, it is **assumed that the client is healthy & his/her problem is a result of faulty thinking.**
- During the therapy, the patient talks about what is on his/her mind and the therapist looks for patterns in situations in which the patient might feel stress or anxiety.
- Patients typically wish to explore their anxiety more deeply because of a belief that deeper exploration will lead to change.

Insight-oriented psychotherapy can refer to:

- **Psychoanalysis,** a method of treatment of mental disorders by using **talk-therapy** to discover and process unconscious thoughts and desires.
- **Psychodynamic psychotherapy,** a **more-brief & less intensive type of talk therapy** that uses psychoanalytic theory & methods.

AIIMS MAY 2015

Multiple Choice Questions

ANATOMY

1. **Which of the following cranial nerve nucleus is located deep to facial colliculus?**
   (AIIMS May 2015, November 2014)
   a. Abducent nerve
   b. Glossopharyngeal nerve
   c. Facial nerve
   d. Trigeminal nerve

2. **Lower two parts of sternal body is fused by:**
   a. 8 years
   b. 10 years
   c. 12 years
   d. 14 years

3. **Oogonia at the time of birth, is present in which of the following stage of meiosis?**
   a. Prophase I
   b. Metaphase I
   c. Anaphase I
   d. Telophase I

4. **All of the following are branches of external carotid artery except?**
   a. Superior thyroid artery
   b. Transverse cervical artery
   c. Ascending pharyngeal artery
   d. Superior thyroid artery

5. **Which of the following muscle is not inserted to the greater tubercle of humerus?**
   a. Supraspinatus
   b. Infraspinatus
   c. Teres minor
   d. Subscapularis

6. **Card test is done for which of the following muscle?**
   a. Palmar interossei
   b. Dorsal interossei
   c. Lumbricals
   d. Adductor pollicis

7. **In which of the following microvilli are not present?**
   a. Gallbladder
   b. Duodenum

   c. Collecting duct
   d. Proximal convoluted tubule

8. **Independent assortment of maternal and paternal chromosome occurs at which stage of spermatocyte maturation:**
   (AIIMS May 2015, November 2013)
   a. Spermatogonia to primary spermatocyte
   b. Primary spermatocyte to secondary spermatocyte
   c. Secondary spermatocyte to spermatids
   d. Spermatid to spermatozoa

9. **Which of the following is not a support of the uterus?**
   a. Urogenital diaphragm
   b. Pelvic diaphragm
   c. Perineal body
   d. Rectovaginal septum

10. **All of the following are derived from mesonephros except:**
    a. Paroophoron
    b. Vas deferens
    c. Epididymis
    d. Glomerulus

11. **Which of the following is not a content of mesorectal fascia?**
    (AIIMS May 2015, May 2014, November 2013)
    a. Inferior rectal vein
    b. Superior rectal vein
    c. Pararectal lymph node
    d. Inferior mesenteric plexus

12. **Reticular fibers of collagen tissues are present in all of the following except:**
    a. Thymus
    b. Spleen
    c. Bone marrow
    d. Lymph node

13. **Sensory supply of cornea is by:**
    a. Infraorbital nerve
    b. Supraorbital nerve
    c. Infratrochlear nerve
    d. Nasolacrimal nerve

14. **All of the following have general visceral efferent fibers except:**
    a. Facial nerve
    b. Olfactory nerve

c. Oculomotor nerve
d. Glossopharyngeal nerve

PHYSIOLOGY

15. In a study to detect extracellular fluid volume, 10 gm mannitol was injected by intravenous route and after waiting for adequate time for equilibration of levels, concentration was measured as 50 mg/100 ml. In this time, 10% mannitol was excreted. What is the calculated volume of ECF?
    a. 10 Litres
    b. 18 Litres
    c. 42 Litres
    d. 52 Litres

16. If the interstitial hydrostatic pressure is 2 mm Hg, interstitial oncotic pressure is 7 mm Hg and capillary hydrostatic pressure is 25 mm Hg. What should be the capillary oncotic pressure to allow a net filtration pressure of 3 mm Hg?
    a. 20
    b. 21
    c. 23
    d. 27

17. The clot formed is not stable unless extensive cross-linking occurs. This extensive cross-linking of blood clot is done by:
    a. Plasmin
    b. Thrombin
    c. HMWK
    d. Factor XIII

18. In the following diagram, left ventricular pressure is equal to diastolic blood pressure indicated by which point?

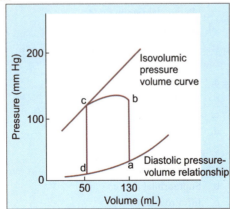

    a. a
    b. b
    c. c
    d. d

19. Which of the following site doesn't contain brown adipose tissues?
    a. Scapula
    b. Subcutaneous tissue
    c. Around blood vessel
    d. Around adrenal cortex

20. Adrenergic beta-receptors having lipolysis property in fat cells is:
    a. Alpha-1   b. Alpha-2
    c. Beta-1   d. Beta-3

21. What is the rise of blood flow if the radius of blood vessel is increased by 50%?
    a. 5 times   b. 10 times
    c. 20 times   d. 100 times

22. Which of the following is true regarding alpha and gamma motor neurons during initiation of voluntary movements?
    a. Alpha motor neurons are activated first followed by gamma motor neurons
    b. Gamma motor neurons are activated first followed by alpha motor neurons
    c. Both are activated together
    d. Only alpha motor neurons get activated

23. Which of the following is secreted by beta cells of pancreas along with insulin?
    a. Somatostatin
    b. Amylin
    c. Pancreatic polypeptide
    d. Glucose like peptide

24. In the given image, wave B represents:

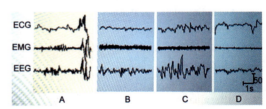

    a. REM
    b. NREM
    c. Quiet wakefulness
    d. Awake

BIOCHEMISTRY

25. A 10-year old boy presented with muscle weakness and fatigue with increased lead in the blood. Which of the following enzyme production in the liver is increased?

a. ALA synthase

b. Heme oxygenase

c. Ferrochelatase

d. Porphobilinogen deaminase

26. **A 7-year old boy presented with severe abdominal pain. On examination, he had xanthomas. Blood sample was taken for work-up, blood sample had milky appearance of plasma. Which of the following lipoprotein is increased?**

a. LDL

b. HDL

c. Chylomicron

d. Chylomicron remnants

27. **A child was brought to the hospital was found to have hypoglycemia, hepatomegaly and accumulation of highly branched glycogen called limit dextrins. He is likely to be suffering from:**

a. McArdle's disease

b. Anderson's disease

c. von-Gierke's disease

d. Cori's disease

28. **Which of the following types of collagen is present in basement membrane?**

a. Type I

b. Type III

c. Type IV

d. Type V

29. **What does forward scatter in flow cytometry used to assess?**

a. Cell death

b. Cell size

c. Cell granules

d. Cell fluorescence

30. **Which of the following enzyme is common between glycogenesis and glycogenolysis?**

(AIIMS May 2015, May 2014)

a. Glycogen synthase

b. Glycogen phosphorylase

c. Glucan transferase

d. Phosphoglucomutase

31. **A 48-year old lady presented with bony pain and hepatosplenomegaly. On examination of biopsy specimen from spleen, crumpled tissue paper appearance is seen. Which of the following product is likely to have accumulated?**

a. Ganglioside

b. Sulfatide

c. Sphingomyelin

d. Glucocerebroside

32. **Which of the following is used by RBCs in the fasting state?**

a. Glucose

b. Alanine

c. Ketone body

d. Fatty acid

33. **RNAi causes the following in a gene:**

a. Knock in

b. Knock out

c. Knock down

d. Knock up

34. **In gene studies, the specific site to which the enzyme CRE recombinase binds is:**

a. RE site

b. LoxP site

c. INT site

d. FRT site

35. **On laboratory investigations in a patient, LDL was highly elevated but the level of LDL receptors was normal. Which of the following is most probable cause?**

a. Phosphorylation of LDL receptors

b. Lipoprotein lipase deficiency

c. Apo B-100 mutation

d. Cholesterol Acyl Co-A transferase deficiency

36. **Find out the value of LDL, if total cholesterol level is 300 mg/dL, HDL level is 25 mg/dL and triglycerides level is 150 mg/dL:**

a. 55   b. 95

c. 125   d. 245

37. **Which of the following enzyme dysfunction leads to lactic acidosis in thiamine deficiency?**

a. Pyruvate carboxylase

b. Phosphofructokinase

c. Phosphoenol pyruvate carboxykinase

d. Pyruvate dehydrogenase

PATHOLOGY

38. **The phenomenon where subsequent generations are at the risk of earlier and more severe disease is known as:**

a. Mosaicism

b. Imprinting

c. Pleiotropy

d. Anticipation

39. A 10-year old boy was presented with a mass in abdomen. On imaging, the para-aortic lymph nodes were enlarged. On biopsy, starry sky appearance was seen. What is the underlying abnormality?
   a. p53 gene mutation
   b. Rb gene mutation
   c. Translocation involving BCR-ABL gene
   d. Translocation involving Myc gene

40. After an incised wound, new collagen fibrils are seen along with a thick layer of growing epithelium. The approximate age of the wound is:
   a. 4–5 days
   b. About 1 week
   c. 12–24 hours
   d. 24–72 hours

41. A 45-year old patient presented with fever, night sweats and weight loss. On X-ray, a mass was seen in apical lobe. On histopathology, caseous necrosis was present. What is the name of underlying process?
   a. Enzymatic degeneration
   b. Acute decrease in blood supply
   c. Decreased supply of growth factor
   d. Hypersensitivity reaction with modified macrophages, lymphocytes and giant cells

42. Which of the following abnormality is seen in the given karyotype?

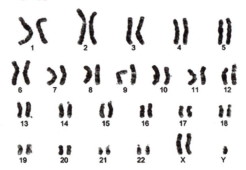

   a. High pitched cry
   b. Round face with protruding tongue
   c. Short stature with webbed neck
   d. Gynecomastia with long thin limbs

43. Inheritance of ABO blood group is:
   a. X-linked inheritance
   b. Recessive inheritance
   c. Mitochondrial inheritance
   d. Codominance

44. Most common nephropathy associated with malignancy is:
   a. Focal segmental glomerulosclerosis (FSGS)
   b. Minimal change disease
   c. IgA nephropathy
   d. Membranous glomerulonephritis

45. Oil red 'O' stain is used for:
   a. Glutaraldehyde fixed specimen
   b. Alcohol fixed specimen
   c. Formalin fixed specimen
   d. Frozen specimen

46. Which of the following is responsible for adhesion of platelets to the vessel wall? *(AIIMS May 2015, November 2013)*
   a. Factor IX
   b. Von Willebrand factor
   c. Fibrinogen
   d. Fibronectin

47. Lymphatic spread is most commonly seen in which type of thyroid malignancy:
   a. Papillary carcinoma
   b. Follicular carcinoma
   c. Medullary carcinoma
   d. Anaplastic carcinoma

48. This image was taken by attaching the camera to the microscope. What is the requirement for such a microscope?

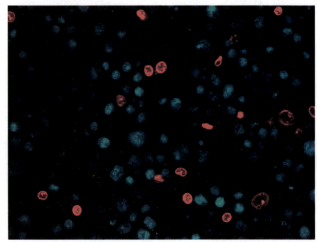

   a. Dark field condenser
   b. Phase shifter
   c. Dichroic mirror
   d. Cathode ray tube

49. In Langerhans Cell Histiocytosis, the characteristic abnormality seen is:
   a. Foamy macrophages
   b. Giant cell
   c. Plasma cell
   d. Birbeck's granules

PHARMACOLOGY

50. Nitroglycerin is effective as sublingual medication because it is:
a. Ionic and lipid soluble
b. Ionic and less lipid soluble
c. Nonionic and highly lipid soluble
d. Nonionic and less lipid soluble

51. What is the rationale behind xenobiotic metabolism by CYP enzymes?
a. Increase in water solubility
b. Increase in lipid solubility
c. Conversion to an active metabolite
d. Makes it suitable to evaporate through skin surface

52. Which of the following is a protease inhibitor?
a. Abacavir
b. Nevirapine
c. Saquinavir
d. Enfuvirtide

53. Which of the following does not act by increasing insulin secretion?
a. Rosiglitazone
b. Repaglinide
c. Exenatide
d. Sitagliptin

54. All of the following drugs cause amorphous whorl like corneal deposits except:
a. Chloroquine
b. Amiodarone
c. Indomethacin
d. Chlorpromazine

55. Best antihypertensive drug used in pulmonary hypertension is:
a. Digoxin   b. Furosemide
c. Amlodipine   d. Bosentan

56. Which of the following drugs cause Heterochromia iridis?
a. Latanoprost
b. Prednisolone
c. Timolol
d. Olopatadine

57. Which of the following diuretic can be given in mild to moderate hypertension?
a. Potassium sparing diuretic
b. Osmotic diuretic
c. Thiazide diuretic
d. Loop diuretic

58. Methacholine acts at which receptor?

(AIIMS May 2015, May 2014)
a. M1
b. M2
c. M3
d. M4

59. All of the following drugs can cause hearing loss except:
a. Vancomycin
b. Kanamycin
c. Metronidazole
d. Quinine

60. What is the type of inhibition of acetylcholinesterase caused by organophosphates?
a. Competitive and reversible
b. Noncompetitive and irreversible
c. Uncompetitive and reversible
d. Competitive and irreversible

MICROBIOLOGY

61. Which of the following structure is disrupted by Vibrio cholerae?
a. Hemi desmosome
b. Gap junctions
c. Zona occludens
d. Zona adherens

62. Adult stage of filarial worms responsible for diseases in all of the following except:
a. Brugia malayi   b. Onchocerca volvulus
c. Mansonella ozzardi   d. Wuchereria bancrofti

63. Reverse transcriptase is a RNA dependent DNA polymerase. Which of the following uses reverse transcriptase?
a. Hepatitis A virus
b. Hepatitis B virus
c. Hepatitis C virus
d. Hepatitis E virus

64. Which of the following causes tropical spastic paresis?
a. HIV
b. HBV
c. HTLV
d. EBV

65. IgE receptor is present on:
a. Mast cell
b. Promonocyte
c. B cell
d. NK cell

66. **Which of the following malignancy is not caused by Human Papilloma Virus (HPV) infection?**
   a. Carcinoma base of tongue
   b. Cervical carcinoma
   c. Tonsillar carcinoma
   d. Nasopharyngeal carcinoma

67. **A child was admitted to the hospital with *H. influenza* meningitis. Cefotaxime is preferred over ampicillin because:**
   a. Cefotaxime is more bioavailable
   b. Cefotaxime is more active against altered penicillin binding protein
   c. Drug of choice is trimethoprim sulfamethoxazole but cannot be given
   d. Cefotaxime is more active against beta-lactamase

FORENSIC MEDICINE

68. **A bomb blast took place in Delhi following which 2 persons died. All of the following are true about their injuries except:**
   a. Injuries occurred due to burns air blast
   b. Force of explosion decreases rapidly
   c. Force of explosion is directional
   d. Bruise, laceration, fractures are triad of main explosive injuries seen

69. **In judicial hanging, the knot is placed at:**
   a. Below the chin
   b. Angle of the jaw
   c. The back of the neck
   d. Choice of hangman

70. **Sweating is not present in:**
   a. Heat syncope
   b. Heat cramp
   c. Heat stroke
   d. Heat fatigue

71. **Acrid smell or pear smell is seen in:**
   a. Ether
   b. Paraldehyde
   c. Nitrobenzene
   d. Carbolic acid

72. **According to the 2013 amendment the age for sexual consent is:**
   a. 15 years
   b. 16 years
   c. 18 years
   d. 20 years

73. **A person was advised by his orthopedic surgeon to get regular dressing of his wound done. But the patient did not give much care. During follow-up, patient was repeatedly told to get the dressing done timely but patient didn't do the dressing himself, saying that he was busy. Finally the wound enlarged and the underlying bone developed osteomyelitis. Which of the following statement is true regarding above-mentioned situation?**
   a. Doctor is guilty under "Last clear chance" doctrine
   b. Doctor is not guilty under "Contributory negligence"
   c. Doctor is punishable under avoidable negligence
   d. Doctor is guilty as he prescribed wrong medicines

74. **Segmentation of blood in blood vessel after death is known as:**
   a. Kevorkian sign
   b. Rokitansky sign
   c. Kennedy phenomenon
   d. Tache noir

75. **Rat hole is associated with which injury?**
   a. Bomb injury
   b. Burn injury
   c. Postmortem artifact
   d. Bullet injury

76. **A man fell down from a height of 35 feet. Eyewitnesses say that he landed on his feet. Which of the following injury is possible?**
   a. Gutter fracture skull with cervical spine injury
   b. Pond fracture skull with cervical spine injury
   c. Depressed fracture skull with cervical spine injury
   d. Ring fracture of foramen magnum with lumbar spine injury

77. **The high court has the power to stay the execution of a pregnant woman according to which section of Criminal Procedure Code?**
   a. 416 CrPC
   b. 417 CrPC
   c. 418 CrPC
   d. 419 CrPC

78. **Mr. X fired his gun at Mr. Y who moved and escaped with the bullet only grazing his thigh. There was only a little bleeding without any significant injury. Mr. X is liable for arrest under which section of Indian Penal Code:**
   a. 302
   b. 304
   c. 324
   d. 326

79. Two bodies are found outside the car following an accident. The doctor conducting the autopsy was able to decide who was driver based on all of these features except:
   a. Whiplash injury
   b. Steering wheel imprint
   c. Sparrow foot marks
   d. Seat belt abrasion over left shoulder

PSM

80. Screening is not useful in which carcinoma:
   a. Carcinoma prostate
   b. Carcinoma colon
   c. Carcinoma breast
   d. Testicular tumor

81. In a group of 100 people, the average GFR is 85 ml/min with a standard deviation of 25. What is the range for 90% confidence interval?
   a. 81-89
   b. 80-90
   c. 75-95
   d. 70-100

82. "Nikshay" is a newly launched central government software. It is used for tracking:
   a. Tuberculosis
   b. High-risk pregnancies
   c. High-risk newborns
   d. Malaria

83. A 10-year boy with dog bite unprovoked comes to you. Appropriate action is:
   a. Give cell culture derived vaccine
   b. Withhold vaccine and observe dog for 10 days
   c. Kill dog and send brain for biopsy
   d. No further action is necessary

84. Haddon matrix is related to:
   a. Injury prevention
   b. Communicable diseases
   c. Maternal and child mortality
   d. Hypertensive disorders

85. In a study, two groups of newborns are checked for their weights based on whether their mothers received food supplements or not. The appropriate test which can be used for comparing the data is:
   a. Chi square test
   b. Paired T-test
   c. Student's T-test
   d. Fischer exact test

86. A researcher wants to do a study of blood levels of lipids among people who smoke and those who do not. But he is now concerned that the smokers might differ from non-smokers in their diet, exercise, etc as well. This concern is known as:
   a. Recall bias
   b. Information bias
   c. Selection bias
   d. Interviewer bias

87. Regarding Japanese encephalitis vaccine, what is not true?
   a. Not given for infants less than 6 months
   b. Two primary doses given to children in the one to three year age group
   c. Booster doses are given after 1 year and repeated every 3 years
   d. In endemic areas vaccination is given to cover children between one to nine years age group

88. Human Developmental Index is a composite measure, which uses?
   a. Life expectancy at age one, literacy and infant mortality
   b. Freedom, spice and right to express oneself
   c. Life expectancy at birth, infant mortality and quality of life
   d. Life expectancy at birth, knowledge and decent standard of living

89. Data about recent trends of immunization in the community can be found by:
   a. Sample registration system
   b. District level health survey
   c. Rural survey
   d. Census data

90. Food safety and standards authority of India comes under which ministry:
   a. Rural statistics
   b. Ministry of health and family and welfare
   c. Ministry of consumer affairs food and public distribution
   d. Ministry of agriculture

91. In a survey of sleep apnea scores among 10 people, the highest sample of 58 was entered by mistake as 85. This will affect the result as:
   a. Increased mean, decreased median
   b. Increased mean, increased median
   c. Increased mean, no change in median
   d. No change in mean, increased median

92. The blood pressure data of 200 persons were collected. The first quartile BP of the data was 94 mm Hg and third quartile was 110 mm Hg. How many patients have blood pressures between the 3rd and 4th quartile?

a. 25
b. 50
c. 100
d. 200

93. Window period is defined as the time taken from:

a. Entry of pathogen to appearance of first clinical symptoms
b. Exposure to laboratory detection of disease
c. Entry in cell to expulsion of first viral particle
d. Entry to maximum communicability

94. Tuberculin test is a cheap and easily available test. In which of the following situations there is high failure in the interpretation of the test?

a. High percentage of immunized people
b. HIV cases are less
c. High prevalence of disease
d. Environmental mycobacterium infections are less

95. There has been a gradual increase in number of non-communicable disease cases as compared to previous years. This trend is called:

a. Seasonal
b. Cyclical
c. Periodical
d. Secular

96. Sensitivity measures:

a. True positive
b. True negative
c. False positive
d. False negative

MEDICINE

97. A man comes with aphasia. He is unable to name things and repetition is poor. However comprehension, fluency and understanding written words is unaffected. He is probably suffering from:

a. Anomic aphasia
b. Broca's aphasia
c. Transcortical sensory aphasia
d. Conduction aphasia

98. Which of the following is not a part of Duke's Criteria for infective endocarditis?

a. Splenomegaly
b. Fever > 100.4 Celsius
c. IV drug user
d. Blood culture positive

99. A middle-aged man comes after a road traffic accident with bleeding from the scalp. He is unconscious. A card in his pocket reveals that he is a known diabetic on Tab Glimepiride + Metformin 2 tablets twice daily. What should be the next step in management?

a. Send blood for tests, start IV glucose and send to CT
b. Start normal saline and send to CT
c. Dextrose solution, CT scan
d. Airway, CT scan, Blood sugar if <70 start dextrose

100. A girl comes with symptoms of involuntary movements. Sydenham's chorea and acute rheumatic fever is suspected. Other major criteria of Rheumatic fever (arthritis, skin rashes, subcutaneous nodules and carditis) were absent. No evidence of sore throat. Best investigation to prove rheumatic etiology is:

(AIIMS May 2015, November 2014)

a. Antistreptolysin S
b. Antistreptolysin O
c. Throat culture
d. PCR for M protein

101. A person is HBsAg positive, but Anti- HBc Ab is negative. What should be the next step?

a. Repeat test after 6 months
b. Check HBV DNA load
c. Check HBeAg, if positive start interferon
d. Reassure patient that he does not have any disease

102. Which of the following is false about Transfusion-Related Acute Lung Injury?

a. Develops within 24 hours
b. Mostly seen after sepsis and cardiac surgeries
c. It's a cause of noncardiogenic pulmonary edema
d. Plasma is more likely to cause it than whole blood

103. Which of the following is not an autoimmune disorder?

a. Ulcerative colitis
b. Grave's disease
c. Rheumatoid arthritis
d. SLE

104. Which of the following statements is true regarding H1N1 Influenza?

a. Pregnant woman with sore throat can be started immediately on oseltamivir without diagnostic testing under category B
b. People on long-term steroids cannot receive Oseltamivir
c. Category B concerns with low risk cases
d. Category B patients have to undergo immediate testing

105. Hyperdynamic circulation is seen in all except:

a. Anemia
b. Beriberi
c. Cor pulmonale
d. AV fistula

AIIMS May 2015

106. **Which of the following do not usually cause reduction in Diffusion Lung Capacity of Carbon Monoxide?**
   a. Emphysema
   b. Asthma
   c. Pulmonary vascular obstruction
   d. Interstitial lung disease

107. **Hypertensive hemorrhage is most commonly seen in:**
   a. Basal ganglia
   b. Thalamus
   c. Brain stem
   d. Cerebrum

SURGERY

108. **A pregnant lady was stabbed in the right side of the chest. She is shouting and yelling for help on entering the casualty. On examination she has tachycardia and BP was 90/60 mm Hg, breath sounds are decreased on the right side. What is the first consideration for | her?**
   a. Oropharyngeal airway
   b. Establish IV line and start normal saline
   c. Needle decompression on right side of the chest
   d. Immediate tracheostomy

109. **Bleeding from a Mallory Weiss tear occurs usually from:**
   a. Phrenic vein
   b. Left gastric artery
   c. Short gastric arteries
   d. Coronary vein

110. **In esophageal cancer prognosis is best determined by:**
   a. Cellular differentiation
   b. Age of patient
   c. T stage
   d. Length of involvement

111. **Best blood product to be given in a patient of multiple clotting factor deficiency with active bleeding:**
   a. Whole blood
   b. Packed RBCs
   c. Fresh frozen plasma
   d. Cryoprecipitate

112. **A young lady with symptoms of hyperthyroidism with elevated T4 and TSH levels were 8.5. Further examination reveals bitemporal hemianopia. Next step of management:**
   a. Start antithyroid drugs, and do urgent MRI brain
   b. Start beta-blockers
   c. Conservative management
   d. Start antithyroid drugs and wait for symptoms to resolve

113. **A 60-year-old lady comes with blood stained discharge from the nipple with family history of breast cancer. Next best step for her will be:**
   a. Ductoscopy
   b. Sonomammogram
   c. Nipple discharge cytology
   d. MRI

114. **A lady who is 9 weeks pregnant comes with a 2.5 cm mass in the upper outer quadrant of left breast. Ultrasound failed to show any abnormality. The ideal management will be to:**
   a. Aspirate the cyst and reassure
   b. Finger guided core biopsy
   c. Call patient one month after delivery
   d. Do mammography

115. **Oncotype Dx test is done to for the following in breast cancer:**
   a. Chemotherapy in hormone receptor positive patients
   b. Hormone therapy in hormone positive
   c. Chemotherapy in hormone receptor negative patients
   d. Herceptin in Her-2-neu +ve

116. **A 3-year-old child comes with hydrocele of the hernia sac. Management will include:**
   a. Herniotomy
   b. Herniorrhaphy
   c. Observation only
   d. Operate after 5 years of age

117. **Most commonly performed shunt for hydrocephalus is:**
   a. Ventriculoperitoneal
   b. Ventriculopericardial
   c. Ventriculopleural
   d. Lumboperitoneal

118. **During laparoscopic inguinal hernia repair a tack was accidently placed below and lateral to the iliopubic tract. Postoperatively the patient complained of pain and soreness in the thigh. This is due to the involvement of:** *(AIIMS November 2015, May 2015)*
   a. Obturator nerve
   b. Genital branch of genitofemoral nerve
   c. Ilioinguinal nerve
   d. Lateral cutaneous nerve of thigh

119. **In a female who had Steroid Resistant ITP it was decided to perform splenectomy. On day 3 post laparoscopic surgery patient had fever. Which of the following scenarios is most likely?**
   a. Left lower lobe consolidation
   b. Port site infection
   c. Intra-abdominal collection
   d. Urine for pus should be sent

120. **Which is the best incision preferred for diaphragmatic surgery?** *(AIIMS May 2015, May 2014)*
    a. Circumferential
    b. Radial
    c. Vertical
    d. Transverse

121. **Best diagnostic investigation for acute appendicitis in children is:** *(AIIMS May 2015, November 2014, May 2013)*
    a. MRI
    b. CECT
    c. USG
    d. X-ray

122. **Investigation of choice to rule out biliary atresia in a 2-month-old child is:**
    a. Hepatic scintigraphy
    b. ERCP
    c. USG
    d. CT scan

123. **Physiological changes seen in laparoscopy include all except:**
    a. Increased ICP
    b. Decreased FRC
    c. Increased CVP
    d. Increased pH

124. **Which is not true regarding the basis of functional divisions of Liver?**
    a. Based on portal vein and hepatic vein
    b. Divided into 8 segments
    c. There are three major and three minor fissures
    d. 4 sectors

125. **In a patient with thrombocytopenia, what is the target platelet count after transfusion to perform an invasive procedure?**
    a. 30,000
    b. 40,000
    c. 50,000
    d. 60,000

126. **Most commonly performed and acceptable method of bariatric surgery is:**
    a. Biliopancreatic diversion
    b. Biliopancreatic diversion with ileostomy
    c. Laparoscopic gastric banding
    d. Roux-en-Y gastric bypass

OBS AND GYNAE

127. **Which of the following antihypertensive drug is not used in pregnancy?** *(AIIMS May 2015, 2014)*
    a. Enalapril
    b. Labetalol
    c. Nifedipine
    d. Hydralazine

128. **What are the cut-off values in 2 hours oral glucose tolerance test for fasting and at 1 hour and 2 hours after meals respectively?**
    a. 92, 182, 155
    b. 92, 180, 153
    c. 95, 180, 155
    d. 92, 180, 155

129. **A mother comes with history of antenatal fetal death due to neural tube defect in first child. What is the amount of folic acid you will prescribe during pre-conceptional counseling?**
    a. 4 micrograms/day
    b. 40 micrograms/day
    c. 400 micrograms/day
    d. 4000 micrograms/day

130. **A 32-year-old P2L2 lady comes five days after unprotected sexual intercourse. What will be your advice for contraception in this lady?**
    a. Copper IUCD
    b. Levonorgestrel 0.75 mg
    c. Two tablets of high dose OCP, repeated after 24 hours
    d. Laparoscopic tubectomy

131. **A G6+0+0 lady with h/o recurrent missed abortions at 14–16 weeks comes to you with a missed abortion at 12 weeks. Which of the following tests is not warranted?**
    a. Lupus anticoagulant
    b. VDRL for husband and wife
    c. Anticardiolipin antibody
    d. Fetal karyotype

132. **What is the level of proteinuria to diagnose severe preeclampsia?**
    a. 20 mg
    b. 200 mg
    c. 300 mg
    d. 3000 mg

133. **A 16-year old girl was brought with primary amenorrhea. Her mother mentioned that she started developing breast at the age of 12. She was prescribed OCPs 2 years back by a doctor with no effect. She was having normal stature and was a football player. On examination, breasts were well developed (Tanner's stage 5) and pubic hair was minimal (Tanner's stage 1). What is the most probable diagnosis?**
    a. Premature ovarian failure
    b. Turner's syndrome
    c. Müllerian agenesis
    d. Androgen insensitivity

134. **Drug not given in PCOD in a 30-year-old lady with infertility?** *(AIIMS May 2015, November 2013)*
    a. Clomiphene
    b. Tamoxifen
    c. OCPs
    d. Metformin

AIIMS May 2015

135. **Drug of choice for hypertension in pregnancy:**
    (AIIMS November 2015, May 2015)
    a. Enalapril
    b. Verapamil
    c. Methyldopa
    d. Furosemide

136. **A lady with abdominal mass was investigated. On surgery, she was found to have bilateral ovarian masses with smooth surface. On microscopy they revealed mucin-secreting cells with signet ring shapes. Most probably diagnosis is:**
    a. Krukenberg tumor
    b. Dysgerminoma
    c. Mucinous adenocarcinoma of the ovaries
    d. Dermoid cyst

137. **A lady underwent vaginal hysterectomy for Carcinoma cervix. Following the surgery after her urethral catheter was removed, she complained of urinary incontinence. On examination she had normal voiding as well as continuous incontinence. Methylene blue dye was instilled in her bladder through her urethra and she was given oral Phenazopyridine dye. After some time her pads were checked and it showed yellow staining at the top most pad, while the middle or bottom pads were unstained. She is likely to have:**
    a. Vesicovaginal fistula
    b. Ureterovaginal fistula
    c. Urethrovaginal fistula
    d. Vesicouterine fistula

138. **In Galactorrhoea—amenorrhea syndromes, which is the investigation you should advise (apart from serum prolactin)?**
    a. TSH
    b. LH
    c. hCG
    d. Urinary ketosteroids

139. **Dose of dexamethasone given to mother in anticipated preterm delivery:**
    a. 12 mg 12 hourly 2 doses
    b. 12 mg 24 hourly 4 doses
    c. 6 mg 24 hourly 2 doses
    d. 6 mg 12 hourly 4 doses

140. **Dose of Carbetocin used for PPH is:**
    a. 50 microgram IV
    b. 100 microgram IM
    c. 150 microgram IV
    d. 200 microgram IV

141. **A young lady with 6 weeks amenorrhea had nausea and vomiting with severe abdominal pain. Her BP was 100/80 mm Hg. Examination revealed a 5 × 5 cm adnexal mass. What is the plan of management?**
    a. Plan for immediate laparoscopic surgery
    b. Send beta-hCG

    c. Methotrexate
    d. Give IV fluids, keep NPO and observe for 4—5 days

142. **According to the 2010 WHO criteria what are the characteristics of normal semen analysis?**
    a. Volume 2.0 mL, count 20 million, morphology 4% progressive motility 32%
    b. Volume 1.5 mL, count 15 million, morphology 4% progressive motility 32%
    c. Volume 2.0 mL, count 15 million, morphology 40% progressive motility 32%
    d. Volume 1.5 mL, count 20 million, morphology 4% progressive motility 32%

143. **Earliest diagnosis of pregnancy can be established safely by:** *(AIIMS May 2015, November 2013)*
    a. USG for fetal cardiac activity
    b. Fetal cardiac Doppler study
    c. hCG levels
    d. MRI pelvis

144. **A 10-year-old girl presents with a mass in lower abdomen involving umbilical and the hypogastrium. On examination it is cystic and mobile and the examiner is unable to insinuate fingers between the mass and the pelvic bone. What is the likely diagnosis?**
    a. Duplication of small intestine
    b. Omental cyst
    c. Ovarian cyst
    d. Mesenteric cyst

PAEDIATRICS

145. **A 10-year-old child presented with edema, oliguria and frothy urine. He has no past history of similar complaints. On examination, his urine was positive for 3+ proteinuria, no RBCs/WBCs and no casts. His serum albumin was 2.5 gm/L and serum creatinine was 0.5 mg/dL. The most likely diagnosis is:**
    a. Minimal change disease
    b. IgA nephropathy
    c. Interstitial nephritis
    d. Membranous nephropathy

146. **Initial fluid of choice for diarrhea in an infant is:**
    a. Salt water
    b. Sugar water
    c. ORS
    d. Dextrose

147. **A male child with coarse facial features, macroglossia, thick lips presents with copious mucous discharge from nose at 10 months of age. The child was absolutely normal at birth. On examination he was found to have enlarged Liver and Spleen. Diagnosis is:**

a. Hurler's syndrome

b. Beckwith-Weidman syndrome

c. Hypothyroidism

d. Proteus syndrome

148. **A 1-month-old child presented with conjugated bilirubinemia and intrahepatic cholestasis. On Liver biopsy staining with PAS, red colored granules were seen inside the hepatocytes. Probable diagnosis is:**

a. Congenital hepatic fibrosis

b. Wilson's disease

c. Alpha-1 antitrypsin deficiency

d. Hemochromatosis

149. **An infant at 7 months of age presented with history of vomiting and failure to thrive. Patient improved with administration of intravenous glucose and came out of coma within 24 hours. After one month he returned with similar complaints. On evaluation he is found to have raised blood ammonia and No ketones. Also, he has high urinary glutamine, alanine and uracil. Which is the likely enzyme defect is this patient?**

a. Ornithine transcarbamoylase

b. CPS1

c. Arginase

d. Argininosuccinate lyase

150. **In a child, surgery was done for biliary stricture with hepatojejunal anastomosis. Postoperative bilirubin level after 2 weeks was 6 mg/dL from a preoperative level 12mg/dL. The reason for this could be:**

a. Normal lowering of bilirubin takes time

b. Anastomotic stricture

c. Delta bilirubin

d. Mistake in lab technique

ORTHOPAEDICS

151. **Jersey finger is caused by rupture of:**

a. Flexor digitorum superficialis

b. Flexor digitorum profundus

c. Extensor digiti minimi

d. Extensor indicis proprius

152. **Shenton line is seen in X-ray of:**

a. Shoulder

b. Elbow

c. Knee

d. Hip

153. **Judet view of X-ray is for:**

a. Calcaneum

b. Scaphoid

c. Shoulder

d. Pelvis

154. **Removal of vertebral disc can be done by all these approaches except:**

a. Laminotomy

b. Laminectomy

c. Laminoplasty

d. Hemilaminectomy

155. **Which of the following tractions is not used in lower limb?**

a. Gallows

b. Bryant

c. Dunlop

d. Perkin

156. **In Osteoporosis which of these is seen?**

a. Normal calcium, normal ALP

b. Decreased calcium, increased ALP

c. Decreased calcium, decreased ALP

d. Normal calcium, decreased ALP

157. **A young patient is diagnosed to have irreparable tear of the rotator cuff. Treatment of choice will be:**

a. Tendon transfer

b. Total shoulder replacement

c. Reverse c shoulder replacement

d. Acromioplasty

158. **Investigation of choice in stress fracture:**

a. CT scan

b. MRI

c. X-ray

d. Bone scan

159. **Most metabolically active layer in the bone is:**

a. Periosteum

b. Endosteum

c. Cancellous bone

d. Cortical bone

OPHTHALMOLOGY

160. **The most common mode of spread of retinoblastoma:**

a. Optic nerve invasion

b. Lymphatics

c. Vascular

d. Direct invasion

161. **Cherry red spot after trauma is seen in children due to:**

a. CRAO

b. CRVO

c. Berlin's edema

d. Niemann-Pick's disease

162. **A person presents with painful unilateral dimness of vision. He gives a history of persistence of after images. What is the likely diagnosis?**

a. Papilledema
b. Ocular ischemic syndrome
c. Retrobulbar neuritis
d. CRVO

163. **High molecular weight proteins in cataractous lens seen only in humans:**
    a. HM 1 and 2
    b. HM 2 and 3
    c. HM 2 and 4
    d. HM 3 and 4

164. **Cherry red spot and Hollenhorst plaque are seen in:**
    a. CRAO
    b. CRVO
    c. Branch RAO
    d. Branch RVO

165. **Universal marker of limbal epithelial stem cells:**
    a. Elastin
    b. Keratin
    c. Collagen
    d. ABCG2

166. **Which of the following stain is used for diagnosis of Granular dystrophy of cornea?**
    a. Colloidal iron
    b. Congo red
    c. PAS
    d. Masson trichrome

167. **Right trochlear nerve palsy can lead to all except:**
    a. Diplopia on upward gaze and adduction
    b. Right head tilt
    c. Exotropia
    d. Hyperopia

168. **Which of the following is not an indication for evisceration?**
    a. Malignancy
    b. Panophthalmitis
    c. Severe globe trauma
    d. Expulsive hemorrhage

169. **Multifocal ERG is useful to assess the function of:**
    a. Rods
    b. Macular cones
    c. Ganglion cells
    d. Retinal pigment epithelium

170. **As compared to blood, vitreous humor has high concentration of:**
    a. Sodium   b. Potassium
    c. Glucose   d. Ascorbate

171. **True statements regarding Direct Ophthalmoscopy are all except:**
    a. Image is virtual and erect
    b. 2 disk diameter field of vision
    c. Magnification is 5 times
    d. Self-illuminated device

ENT

172. **Kashima operation is done for:**
    a. Recurrent cholesteatoma
    b. Bilateral vocal cord palsy
    c. Atrophic rhinitis
    d. Choanal atresia

173. **Eustachian tube function is best assessed by:**
    a. Tympanometry
    b. VEMP
    c. Rhinomanometry
    d. Politzer test

174. **Topical treatment for recurrent respiratory papillomatosis includes:**
    a. Acyclovir
    b. Cidofovir
    c. Ranitidine
    d. Zinc

175. **The main vessel involved in bleeding from Juvenile nasopharyngeal angiofibroma:**
    a. Facial artery
    b. Ascending pharyngeal artery
    c. Internal maxillary artery
    d. Anterior ethmoidal artery

SKIN

176. **A child came with similar lesions as shown in the picture over elbows and shaft of penis. What is the diagnosis?** *(AIIMS May 2015, May 2014)*

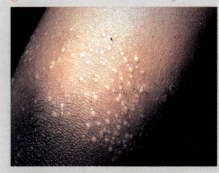

   a. Lichen planus
   b. Scabies
   c. Lichen nitidus
   d. Lichen scrofulosorum

177. A 26-year-old man from Bihar comes with juicy looking papules over face and back of neck, which were hypopigmented and normoaesthetic. History revealed an episode of prolonged fever in childhood. Diagnosis:

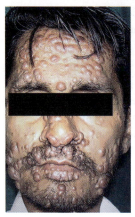

a. Tuberculoid leprosy
b. Lepromatous leprosy
c. Post Kala Azar dermal leishmaniasis
d. Histoid Hansen's

178. The patient came with history of bullae involving >30 % body surface area along with erosions of the lips and other mucosae for the past 7 days. What is the most probable underlying etiology?

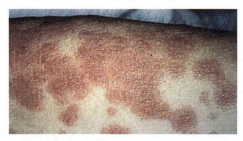

a. Bacterial infection
b. Viral infection
c. Drugs
d. Malignancy

179. A 7 months pregnant lady with diabetes mellitus comes with the following lesions all over the body, mainly on the trunk. Which of these drugs can be appropriately used in the treatment?

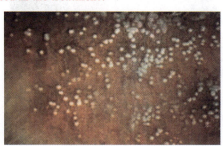

a. Azathioprine
b. Cyclosporine
c. Retinoids
d. Methotrexate

180. A 25-year-old girl presented with erythematous papules on the face as seen in the figure. The lesions were exacerbated on excessive sweating, sun exposure and emotional disturbance. What is the diagnosis?
 (AIIMS May 2015, November 2014)

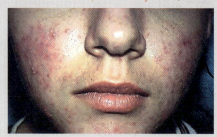

a. SLE   b. Acne rosacea
c. Acne vulgaris d. Photodermatitis

181. A lady came with complaints of a bluish lesion over left side of forehead and left eye. An irregular bluish lesion in left superior conjunctive and forehead is seen. What is the diagnosis?

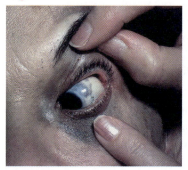

a. Nevus of Ota
b. Nevus of Ito
c. Becker's nevus
d. Mongolian spot

182. A man with Leprosy came with the following lesion on the shin. What is the correct classification?

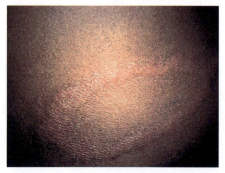

a. LL b. BL
c. BT d. BB

183. A lady came with unilateral white skin lesions with leukotrichia as shown in the picture. What is likely diagnosis?

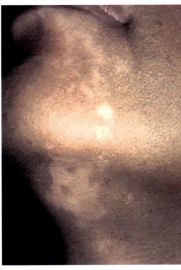

a. Piebaldism
b. Segmental vitiligo
c. Focal vitiligo
d. Waardenburg syndrome

184. A patient came with itchy tense blisters on normal skin as well as over urticarial plaques, as shown in the image. What is the diagnosis?
(AIIMS May 2015, November 2014)

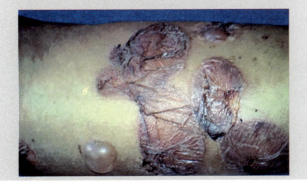

a. Pemphigus vulgaris
b. Bullous pemphigoid
c. Linear IgA disease
d. Dermatitis herpetiformis

185. A patient presented with a vesicle on shin. Microscopy of Tzanck smear showed giant cells. Causative agent is:
a. Vaccinia virus
b. Varicella zoster
c. Mycobacterium
d. Molluscum contagiosum

ANAESTHESIA

186. Which of the following combinations can be used for day care surgery?
a. Ramifentanil, midazolam, propofol
b. Fentanyl, midazolam, thiopentone sodium
c. Morphine, midazolam, propofol
d. Morphine, diazepam, ketamine

187. Which anesthetic agent can cause pain on IV administration?
a. Ketamine
b. Propofol
c. Thiopentone
d. Midazolam

188. A patient with history of coronary artery disease presents with pulse rate of 48/min and low BP. Patient has decreased myocardial contractility on Echo. Which of these anesthetic agents is contraindicated?
a. Fentanyl
b. Etomidate
c. Ketamine
d. Dexmedetomidine

189. Muscle relaxant that can be used in a patient with high serum bilirubin of 6.0 and serum creatinine of 4.5 mg/dL?
a. Atracurium
b. Vecuronium
c. Pancuronium
d. Mivacurium

RADIOLOGY

190. Best noninvasive investigation to check for viability of myocardium is:
a. FDG-18 PET CT
b. MIBG scintigraphy
c. Echocardiogram
d. Thallium scintigraphy

191. Patient with history of tachyarrhythmias is on implantable cardioverter defibrillator. He develops shock. Best method to know the position and integrity of ICD is: *(AIIMS May 2015, November 2012)*
a. CECT
b. MRI
c. USG
d. Plain radiograph

192. Expansion of the contrast filled space in myelography is seen in:
a. Intramedullary tumor
b. Intradural extramedullary tumor
c. Spinal dysraphism
d. Extradural tumor

PSYCHIATRY

193. Which of these is not a part of catatonia?

   a. Akathisia   b. Ambivalence

   c. Ambitendency   d. Akinesia

194. Feeling of uncertainty and excessive sense of responsibility is seen in:

   a. Obsessive compulsive disorder

   b. Phobia

   c. Personality disorder

   d. Generalized anxiety disorder

195. A smoker is worried about the side effects of smoking. But he does not stop smoking thinking that he smokes less as compared to others and takes a good diet. This thinking is called as:

   a. Self-exemption

   b. Self-protection

   c. Cognitive behaviour

   d. Distortion

196. A person with histrionic, shy, anxious avoidant personality comes under which cluster?

   a. A   b. B

   c. C   d. D

197. A man comes with history of abnormal excessive blinking and grunting. He says he has no control over his symptoms, which have risen in frequency of late. This has started affecting his social life making him depressed. Which of the following medications should be used in him?

   a. Risperidone

   b. Imipramine

   c. Carbamazepine

   d. Methylphenidate

198. A person with violent behavior and agitation was diagnosed to have Schizophrenia and was receiving haloperidol. Following this he developed rigidity and inability to move his eyes. Which of the following drugs should be added to his treatment intravenously for this condition?

   a. Diazepam

   b. Resperidone

   c. Promethazine

   d. Haloperidol

199. Key symptom in alcohol withdrawal syndrome is:

   a. Sleep disturbance

   b. Visual hallucinations

   c. Tremors

   d. Delirium

200. A woman comes to the psychiatrist with history of spending a lot of time in washing her hands. She is distressed about it but says that she cannot stop the practice and spends a lot of time on it. This has started affecting her social life as well. What is the best mode of treatment for her?

   a. Cognitive behavioral therapy

   b. Exposure and response prevention

   c. Systematic desensitization

   d. Pharmacological agents

Explanations

ANATOMY

1. **Ans. a. Abducent nerve** *(Ref: Gray's 41/e p318, 40/e p240; Netter Collection of Medical Illustrations 2013/Vol. 7/e p178)*
   Abducent nerve nucleus is located deep to facial colliculus.

   > *"Facial colliculus is situated in the pons. It overlies the abducent nucleus. The facial nerve originates from its nucleus and goes around the abducent nerve. This is called as neurobiotaxis."*- Gray's 40/e p240

   > *"On each side of the median sulcus is a **longitudinal elevation, the medial eminence**, lateral to which lies sulcus limitans. Its **superior part is the locus ceruleus**, coloured bluish-grey from the patch of deeply pigmented nerve cells. Also **lateral to the upper part of the medial eminence is a slight depression**, the superior fovea, and **just below and medial in this fovea is a rounded swelling, the facial colliculus**, which **overlies the nucleus of the abducens (VI) nerve** and the facial (VII) nerve fibers encircling in the motor nucleus of the facial nerve lies more deeply in the pons. Inferolateral to the superior fovea is the upper part of the vestibular area, which overlies parts of the nuclei of the vestibulococchlear (VIII) nerve."*
   > Netter Collection of Medical Illustrations 2013/Vol. 7/e p178

   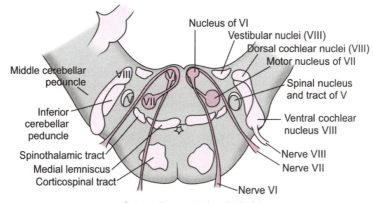

   Fig. 1: Cut section at the level of mid pons.

2. **Ans. d. 14 years** *(Ref: BDC 6/Vol. 1/e p203; Gray's 40/e p918; Parikh 6/e p2.9)*
   Lower two parts of sternal body is fused by 14 years.

   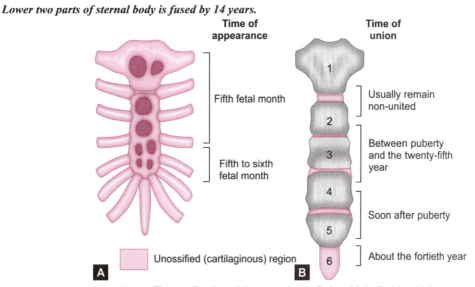

   Fig. 2: The ossification of the sternum. A, Before birth. B, After birth.

"The four middle pieces of sternum fuse with one another from below upwards between 14 and 25 years of age."—Parikh 6/e p2.9

Sternum Development & Ossification

- The sternum develops by fusion of two sternal plates formed on either side of the midline.
- Fusion of the two plates takes place in a craniocaudal direction.
  - Manubrium is ossified from 2 centers appearing in 5th fetal month.
  - 1st & 2nd sternebrae ossify from one center appearing in 5th fetal month[Q].
  - 3rd & 4th sternebrae ossify from paired centers, which appear in 5th & 6th months[Q].
  - These fuse with each other from below upwards during puberty.
  - Fusion is complete by 25 years of age[Q].
- Centre for the xiphoid process appears during the 3rd year. It fuses with the body at 40 years[Q].

Xiphoid unites with body	40 years[Q]
Manubrium unites with body	60 years[Q]
Pieces of body unite between	14–25 years[Q]

3. **Ans. a. Prophase I** *(Ref: Langman's 12/e p22; Gray's 41/e p19)*

Oogonia at the time of birth, is present in Prophase I.

"Meiosis I of ootidogenesis begin during embryonic development, but halts in the diplotene stage of prophase I until puberty."-Langman's 12/e p22

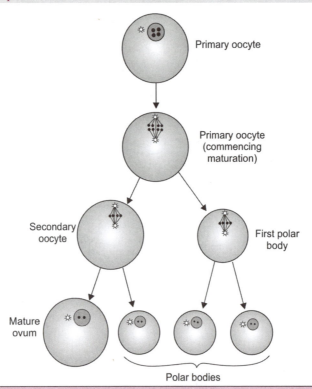

Human Oogenesis

- Oogenesis starts with the **process of developing oogonia**, which occurs via the **transformation of primordial follicles into primary oocytes**, a process called **oocytogenesis**[Q].
- Oocytogenesis is complete either before or shortly after birth.
- **Primary oocytes** reach their **maximum development at ~20 weeks of gestational age**, when approximately **7 million primary oocytes** have been created; however, **at birth**, this number has already been **reduced to approximately 1–2 million**[Q].

Contd...

Contd...

Human Oogenesis

- In fact, a **primary oocyte** is, by its biological definition, **a cell whose primary function is to divide by the process of meiosis**. However, although **this process begins at prenatal age**, it **stops at prophase I**. After menarche, these cells then continue to develop, although only a few do so every menstrual cycle.

  - **Meiosis I of ootidogenesis begin during embryonic development, but halts in the diplotene stage of prophase I until puberty^Q.**

Cell Type	Ploidy	Process	Process Completion
Oogonium	Diploid	Oocytogenesis (mitosis)	Third trimester (forming oocytes)
Primary oocyte	Diploid	Ootidogenesis (meiosis 1) (Folliculogenesis)	Halted in prophase I until puberty^Q
Secondary oocyte	Haploid	Ootidogenesis (meiosis 2)	Halted in metaphase II until fertilization^Q
Ovum	Haploid		

4. **Ans. b. Transverse cervical artery** *(Ref: Gray's 41/e p453, 797)*

   Transverse cervical artery is not a branch of external carotid artery.

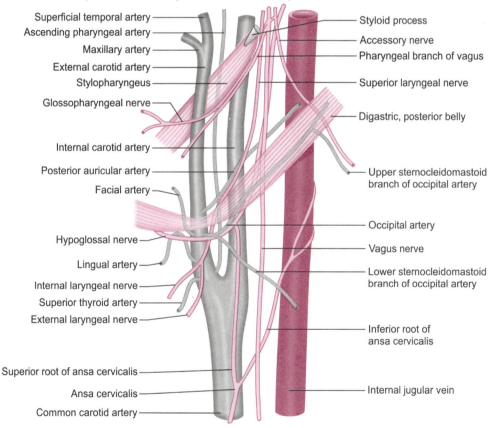

Fig. 3: The branches of the external carotid artery.

Common Carotid Artery

- **Right CCA** arises **from brachiocephalic trunk**.
- **Left CCA** arises directly **from arch of aorta**.
- **CCA** usually **bifurcates at the level of upper border of the lamina of thyroid cartilage (upper border of C4 vertebra)** into external & internal carotid^Q.

Contd...

Contd...

Common Carotid Artery

- **CCA** along with **vagus nerve & internal jugular vein** is **enclosed by carotid sheath** overlapped by anterior margin of sternocleidomastoid.
- Therefore **carotid pulse** can be **felt along the anterior margin of sternocleidomastoid at the level of laryngeal prominence**[Q].
- **CCA** can be **compressed against anterior tubercle of transverse process of C6 vertebra** as carotid tubercle (**Chassaignac tubercle**), at cricoid cartilage level[Q].

Branches of External Carotid Artery		Branches of Internal Carotid Artery	
Anterior	Superior thyroid artery[Q] Lingual artery Facial artery	**Cervical part**	No branch
		Petrous part	Caroticotympanic branch[Q] Pterygoid branch[Q]
Posterior	Occipital artery[Q] Posterior auricular[Q]	**Cavernous part**	Meningeal branch[Q] Hypophyseal branch[Q] Cavernous branch[Q]
Medial	Ascending pharyngeal artery[Q]	**Cerebral part**	Ophthalmic artery[Q] Posterior communicating artery[Q] Anterior choroidal artery[Q] Anterior cerebral artery[Q] Middle cerebral artery[Q]
Terminal	Maxillary artery[Q] Superficial temporal artery		

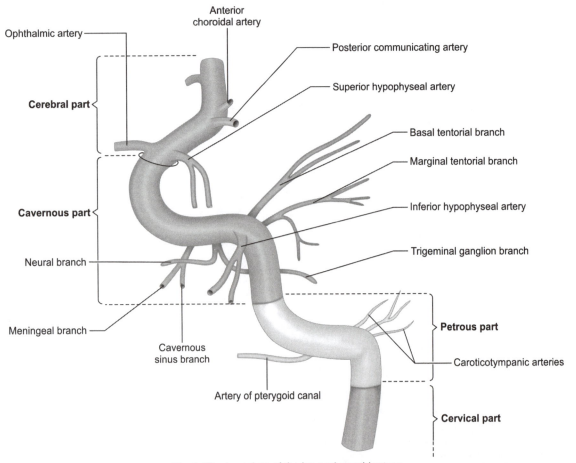

Fig. 4: The branches of the internal carotid artery

5. **Ans. d. Subscapularis** *(Ref: Gray's 41/e p823, 40/e p797)*

Subscapularis muscle is not inserted to the greater tubercle of humerus.

"The **subscapularis muscle** forms the largest component of the posterior wall of the axilla. It **originates from, and fills, the subscapularis fossa** and **inserts on the lesser tubercle of the humerus.**"—Gray's 41/e p823

"**Supraspinatus, Infraspinatus and Teres minor are inserted to greater tubercle of humerus.**"

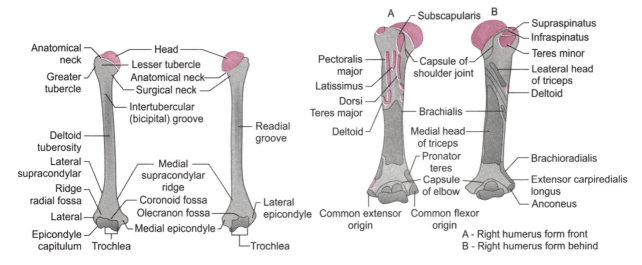

Attachments on the Humerus				
Upper Part (All are insertions)				**Lower Part (All are origins)**	
Bicipital Groove (Intertubercular sulcus)				**Medial**	**Lateral**
Attachments	**Content**				
• Pectoralis major[Q] • Lattisimus dorsi[Q] • Teres major[Q] (Lady between two majors)	• Ascending branch of anterior circumflex humeral artery[Q] • Biceps long tendon with its double tubular synovial sheath[Q]			• Pronator teres[Q] • Common flexor origin[Q]	• Brachioradialis[Q] • Extensor carpi radialis longus[Q] • Common extensor origin[Q] • Anconeus[Q]
Greater Tubercle	**Lesser Tubercle**				
• Supraspinatus[Q] • Infraspinatus[Q] • Teres minor[Q]	• Subscapularis[Q]				

6. **Ans. a. Palmar interossei** *(Ref: Apley's 9/e p291)*

Card test is done for palmar interossei.

Nerve	Test	Muscle
Ulnar nerve	Book test[Q]	Adductor pollicis[Q]
	Card test[Q]	Palmar interossei[Q]
	Froment's sign[Q]	Flexor pollicis substitutes for adductor pollicis[Q]
	Igawa test[Q]	Dorsal interossei[Q]

Contd...

Contd...

Nerve	Test	Muscle
Median Nerve	Ape thumb[Q]	Thenar muscles[Q]
	Pen test[Q]	Adductor pollicis brevis[Q]
	Pincer grasp (Kiloh Nevin sign)[Q]	Flexor digitorum profundus + Flexor pollicis longus[Q] (Anterior interosseus nerve)
	Pointing index (Ochsner clasp/ Benediction test)[Q]	Flexor digitorum superficialis + Lateral half of Flexor digitorum profundus[Q]
Radial Nerve	Thumb & finger drop[Q]	Extensors[Q] (Posterior interosseus nerve)
	Wrist drop[Q]	Extensors of wrist[Q]

7. **Ans. c. Collecting duct**   *(Ref: Gray's 40/e p17-19)*

Microvilli are not present collecting duct.

"Microvilli are finger-like cell surface extensions usually 0.1 mm in diameter and up to 2 mm long. When arranged in regular parallel series, they constitute a striated border, as typified by the absorptive surfaces of the epithelial enterocytes of the small intestine. When they are less regular, as in the gallbladder epithelium and proximal kidney tubules, the term brush border is used."

Classification of Epithelium	
Type	**Location**
Simple columnar epithelium (without cilia & microvilli)	• Lining of **stomach & large intestine**[Q] • **Cervical canal**[Q]
Columnar epithelium with striated border (regularly arranged microvilli)	• **Lining of small intestine**[Q]
Columnar epithelium with brush border (Irregularly placed microvilli)	• **Gallbladder**[Q]
Ciliated columnar epithelium (cilia on surface for propulsion of fluid)	• **Uterus and fallopian tubes**[Q] • **Eustachian tube** • **Central canal of spinal cord & ventricles of brain** • **Respiratory epithelium**
Simple cuboidal epithelium	• **Thyroid follicles** • **Germinal epithelium** of ovary • Ducts of glands • **Proximal & distal convoluted tubules of kidney (cuboidal with microvilli)**[Q]
Simple squamous epithelium (pavement epithelium)	• **Endothelium of heart & blood vessels** • **Mesothelium** of serous cavity (**peritoneum & pleura**) • **Lung alveoli** • **Loop of henle & parietal layer of Bowman's capsule**[Q]
Pseudostratified columnar epithelium	• **Larynx (except vocal cord), trachea, bronchi** • **Olfactory epithelium**[Q] • **Epididymis & parts of male urethra**
Stratified squamous keratinized	• Epidermis of skin • Vestibule of nose, external auditory meatus and ducts of sebaceous glands.
Stratified squamous non-keratinized	• Epithelium of oral cavity, tongue, esophagus, oropharynx, laryngopharynx, • Part of anal canal, vagina, cornea & conjunctiva
Stratified columnar epithelium	• Large ducts of glands
Stratified cuboidal epithelium	• **Ducts of sweat glands, salivary gland, pancreas & seminiferous tubules**[Q]
Transitional epithelium	• **Urinary passage** (from minor calyces, renal pelvis, ureter, urinary bladder) and **proximal portion of urethra**[Q]

8. **Ans. b. Primary spermatocyte to secondary spermatocyte**   *(Ref: Gray's 41/e p1275, Langman 12/e p26)*

Independent assortment of maternal and paternal chromosome occurs when primary spermatocyte converts into secondary spermatocyte.

> "In spermatogenesis, independent assortment of paternal and maternal chromosomes occurs during meiosis I, in which primary spermatocyte (2n) is converted into two secondary spermatocytes (1n)."

Meiosis
• In spermatogenesis, **independent assortment** of paternal and maternal chromosomes **occurs during meiosis I,** in which **primary spermatocyte (2n)** is **converted into** two **secondary spermatocytes (1n)**[Q].
• **Meiosis I** separates pairs of homologous chromosomes, reduces the **cell from diploid to haploid**[Q].
• **Meiosis II** separates each chromosome into two chromatids[Q].

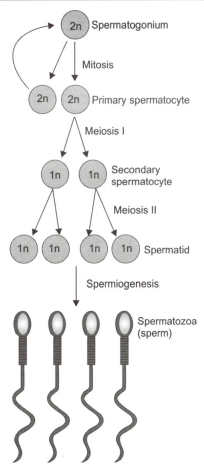

Stages of Spermatogenesis		
Cell type	**Ploidy/ Chromosomes in Human**	**Process entered by Cell**
Spermatogonium	Diploid (2N)/46	Spermatocytogenesis (mitosis)
Primary spermatocyte	Diploid (2N)/46	Spermatidogenesis (meiosis 1)
Two secondary spermatocytes	Haploid (N)/23	Spermatidogenesis (meiosis 2)
Four spermatids	Haploid (N)/23	**Spermiogenesis**[Q]
Four functional spermatozoids	Haploid (N)/23	**Spermiation**[Q]

9. **Ans. d. Rectovaginal septum** *(Ref: Shaw's 16/e p8-9; 15/e p331)*
   Rectovaginal septum is not a support of the uterus.

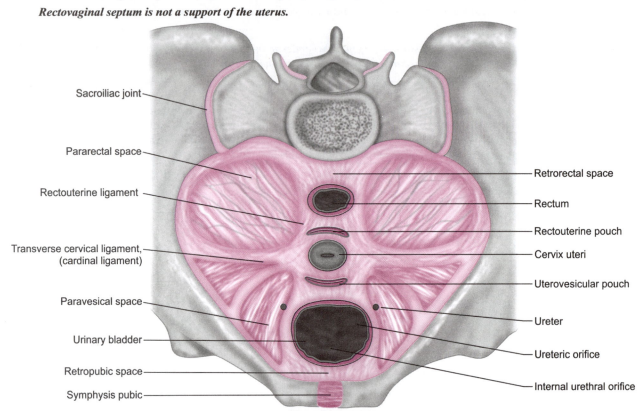

Fig. 5: Supporting ligaments of the pelvis showing the transverse cervical ligaments

Supports of the Uterus	
Primary Supports	**Secondary Supports** (Formed by peritoneal Ligaments)
• Muscular or Active support: – Pelvic diaphragm^Q – Perineal body^Q – Urogenital diaphragm^Q • Ligamentous (Fibromuscular or Mechanical) support: – Transverse cervical ligaments of Mackenrodt or Cardinal ligament^Q – Uterosacral ligament^Q – Round ligament of uterus^Q – Pubocervical ligament^Q – Uterine axis^Q	• Broad ligament • Uterovesical fold of peritoneum • Rectovaginal fold of peritoneum

10. **Ans. d. Glomerulus** *(Ref: I.B. Singh 4/e p260)*
    Glomerulus is not derived from mesonephros.

Embryonal structure	Fate	
	Female	**Male**
Genital ridge	Ovary^Q	Testis^Q
Genital swelling	Labia majora^Q	Scrotum^Q
Genital fold (fold of Urogenital sinus)	Labia minora^Q	Ventral aspect of penis Penile urethra
Genital tubercle	Clitoris^Q	Glans penis^Q

AIIMS May 2015

Genital Ducts			
Mesonephric / Wolffian duct (Main genital duct of males[Q])		**Paramesonephric /Mullerian duct** (Main genital duct of females[Q])	
Males	Females	Males	Females
I. Structure formed: "PUT A DEEP Semen"	I. Structure formed: "PUT"	Remnants:	Structures formed:
1. **P**osterior wall of prostate urethra, cranial to openings of ejaculatory duct 2. **U**reteric buds[Q] forming ureter, pelvis, calyces, & collecting tubule 3. **T**rigone of bladder[Q] 4. **A**ppendix of epididymis[Q] (not testis) 5. **D**uctus deferens[Q] 6. **E**pididymis[Q] 7. **E**jaculatory ducts[Q] 8. **P**rostate (mesodermal part) 9. **S**eminal vesicles[Q] II. Remnants: "SIP" 1. **S**uperior aberrant ductule (epigenital tubule) 2. **I**nferior aberrant ductule 3. **P**aradidymis[Q] (para-genital tubule)	1. **P**osterior wall of female urethra 2. **U**reteric buds[Q] forming ureter, pelvis, calyces, & collecting tubule 3. **T**rigone of bladder[Q] II. Remnants: "PEG" 5. **P**aroophoron[Q]: In males it is equivalent to paradidymis[Q] 6. **E**poophoron /**G**artner's duct[Q]: In males it is equivalent to ductus deferens[Q].	1. Appendix of testis[Q] 2. Prostatic utricle[Q]	1. Uterine tube[Q] 2. Uterus[Q] 3. Part of vagina

11. **Ans. a. Inferior rectal vein** *(Ref: Grays 41/e p1147, 40/e p1151-1153)*
Inferior rectal vein is not enclosed in mesorectal fascia.

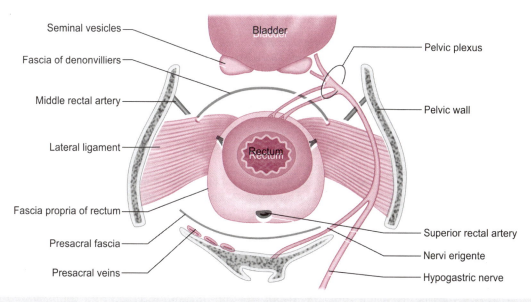

"*Mesorectum is enclosed by **mesorectal fascia** which is **derived from the visceral peritoneum**, and is also known as **visceral fascia of mesorectum, fascia propria of rectum** or **presacral wing of hypogastric sheath**. **Upper rectum** is derived from the embryological hind gut, it is **surrounded by mesorectum** and **its contents** namely **superior rectal artery** and its **branches, superior rectal vein** and **tributaries, lymphatic vessels** and **nodes along superior rectal artery, branches from inferior mesenteric plexus to innervate rectum** and loose adipose connective tissue down to the level of levator ani (pelvic floor).*"

Mesorectal Fascia
• Mesorectum is enclosed by **mesorectal fascia,** which is **derived from the visceral peritoneum[Q],** and is also known as **visceral fascia of mesorectum, fascia propria of rectum or presacral wing of hypogastric sheath[Q].** • **Upper rectum** is derived from the embryological hind gut, it is **surrounded by mesorectum[Q].**

Contents of Mesorectal fascia
• **Superior rectal artery** and its **branches[Q]** • **Superior rectal vein** and **tributaries[Q]** • **Lymphatic vessels** and **nodes** along superior rectal artery[Q] • **Branches from inferior mesenteric plexus to innervate rectum[Q]** • **Loose adipose connective tissue[Q]** down to the level of levator ani (pelvic floor)

12. **Ans. a. Thymus**   *(Ref: Gray's anatomy 41/e p38, 40/e p75, 47)*

Reticular fibers of collagen tissues are present in Spleen, Bone marrow & Lymph node but not in thymus.

"Reticular fibers: Reticulin is a type of fiber in connective tissue composed of type III collagen secreted by reticular cells. Reticular fibers crosslink to form a fine meshwork which acts as a supporting mesh in soft tissues such as liver, bone marrow and the tissues and organs of the lymphatic system."

Fibers of Connective Tissue		
Collagen	**Reticular Fibers**	**Elastic Fibers**
• **Most abundant, tough, thick, fibrous, non-branching** protein	• Composed of **type III collagen** secreted by reticular cells. • Present in **liver, bone marrow, lymph node, spleen[Q]**	• **Thin branching fibers that allow stretch[Q]** • **Composed of microfibrils & protein elastin[Q]** • Present in **lungs, bladder, skin & major vessels (aorta & pulmonary trunk)**

Collagen types:

Type 1	Ubiquitous[Q]
Type 2	Cartilage[Q] Intervertebral disc[Q]
Type 3	Hollow organs[Q]
Type 4	Basement membrane[Q]

13. **Ans. d   Nasolacrimal nerve**   *(Ref: BDC 7/e/Vol-III/p301; 6/e Vol. III p296, 368)*

Cornea is richly supplied by nerves, which originate from small ophthalmic division of trigeminal nerve, mainly by long ciliary nerve[Q] (a branch of Nasociliary nerve). There is probably printing mistake. There is no such nerve called nasolacrimal nerve. This is probably Nasociliary nerve.

*"Cornea is **richly supplied by nerves[Q]** (without myelin sheaths and Schwann cell sheath) which originate from **small ophthalmic division of trigeminal nerve, mainly by long ciliary nerve[Q] (a branch of Nasociliary nerve).** Due to its dense nerve supply, the cornea is extremely sensitive structure."*

Ophthalmic Nerve Division		
Frontal[Q]	**Lacrimal[Q]**	**Nasociliary[Q]**

1. **Supratrochlear:**
  – Upper eyelid
  – Conjunctiva
  – Lower part of forehead
2. **Supraorbital:**
  – Frontal air sinus
  – Upper eyelid
  – Forehead
  – Scalp till vertex
	• Lateral part of upper eyelid
	• Conveys secretomotor fibres from zygomatic nerve to lacrimal gland
		1. **Long ciliary: Sensory to eyeball[Q]**
		2. **Branch to ciliary ganglion.**
		3. **Infratrochlear:**
		  – Both eyelids, side of nose
		  – Lacrimal sac
		4. **Anterior ethmoidal:**
		  – Middle and anterior ethmoidal sinuses
		  – Medial internal nasal
		  – Lateral internal nasal
		  – External nasal: Skin of ala of vestibule and tip of nose
		5. **Posterior ethmoidal:**
		  – Sphenoidal air sinus
		  – Posterior ethmoidal air sinuses[Q]

14. Ans. b. Olfactory nerve   *(Ref: Gray's 41/e p390, 562, BDC 6/e Vol III p351)*

Olfactory nerve does not have general visceral efferent fibers.

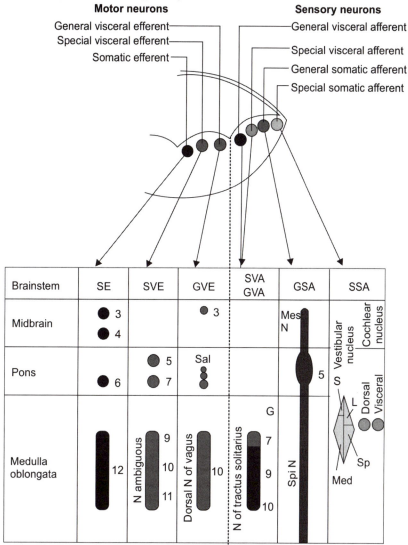

Functional Division of Cranial Nerve Nuclei	
Sensory / Afferent	**Motor / Efferent**

1. General Somatic
– **Sensory nucleus of trigeminal** (descending & mesencephalic nucleus of Vth nerve)
– Receive sensation of face
	1. General Somatic
	– Supply striated muscle derived from somites & involved in tongue & eye movements i.e.
	    – **Hypoglossal nucleus of 12th**[Q]
	    – **Oculomotor nucleus of 3rd**[Q]
	    – **Trochlear nucleus of 4th**[Q]
	    – **Abducent nucleus of 6th**[Q]

2. General Visceral – **Nucleus of tractus solitarius**[Q] – Receive taste from tongue & epiglottis	**2. General Visceral** – **Edinger Westphal nucleus**[Q] of 3rd – **Superior salivatory nucleus**[Q] of 7th – **Inferior salivatory nucleus**[Q] of 9th – **Dorsal motor nucleus**[Q] of 10th (Vagus)

Contd...

Contd...

Functional Division of Cranial Nerve Nuclei	
Sensory / Afferent	**Motor / Efferent**
3. Special somatic – **4 vestibular nucleus** – **2 cochlear nucleus** – Receive stimuli from ear	3. Special Visceral or Branchial component – Innervate muscles derived from branchial arches i.e. **Masticatory nucleus^Q of 5th** **Facial nucleus of 7th** **Nucleus ambigus^Q of 9th, 10th, 11th** **Spinal accessory nucleus of 12th**

Nerve	Components	Nucleus	Location of nucleus in brainstem
I (olfactory)	**SVA**	–	–
II (optic)	**SSA**	–	–
III (Oculomotor)	**GSE** **GVE**	Oculomotor nucleus **Edinger-Westphal Nucleus**	**Superior colliculus** (midbrain)
IV (Trochlear)	**GSE**	Trochlear nucleus	**Inferior colliculus** (midbrain)
V (Trigeminal)	**GSA** **GSA** **GSA** **SVE**	Spinal nucleus Main sensory nucleus Mesencephalic nucleus Motor nucleus	Pons, medulla, C1, C2 segment Pons Pons Pons
VI (Abducent)	**GSE**	Abducent nucleus	**Facial colliculus** (Pons)
VII (Facial)	**SVE** **SVA** **GVE**	Motor nucleus **Nucleus of Tractus Solitarius** **Superior Salivatory Nucleus**	**Pons**
VIII (Vestibulocochlear)	**SSA** **SSA**	Vestibular Nucleus Cochlear Nucleus	**Pons, medulla**
IX (Glossopharyngeal)	**SVE** **GVE** **GVA, SVA, GSA**	Motor **Inferior Salivatory Nucleus** **Nucleus of Tractus Solitarius**	**Medulla**
X (Vagus)	**GVE, SVE** **GVA, SVA, GSA**	Motor, Parasympathetic **Nucleus of Tractus Solitarius**	**Medulla**
XI (Accessory)	**SVE** **SVE**	Motor Spinal nucleus	**Medulla** **Upper five cervical segments**
XII (Hypoglossal)	**GSE**	Motor	**Medulla**

(SVA: **Special visceral afferent; SVE: Special visceral efferent; GVA: General visceral afferent; GVE: General visceral efferent)**

PHYSIOLOGY

15. **Ans. b. 18 Litres** *(Ref. Ganong 25/e p3, 24/e p2)*

> Out of 10 gm mannitol, 10% was excreted.
> Hence, amount of mannitol distributed in ECF = 10-1= 9 gm
> Given concentration of mannitol in ECF = 50 mg/100 ml
> **Volume of ECF = Amount/Concentration = 9 g/50 mg × 100 ml = 18 L**

See Q. No. 20 AIIMS November 2015.

16. **Ans. d. 27** *(Ref: Ganong 25/e p677, 24/e p679)*

Control of GFR
• The **factors governing filtration across the glomerular capillaries are the same as those governing filtration across all other capillaries**, that is, the **size of the capillary bed**, the **permeability of the capillaries**, and the **hydrostatic and osmotic pressure gradients across the capillary wall.**

Contd...

Contd...

- For each nephron:

$$GFR = K_f [(P_{GC} - P_T) - (\pi_{GC} - \pi_T)]$$

- where K_f, the glomerular ultrafiltration coefficient, is the product of the glomerular capillary wall hydraulic conductivity (i.e. its permeability) and the effective filtration surface area.
- P_{GC} is the mean hydrostatic pressure in the glomerular capillaries = **25**
- P_T the mean hydrostatic pressure in the tubule (Bowman's space) = **2**
- π_{GC} the oncotic pressure of the plasma in the glomerular capillaries
- π_T the interstitial colloid oncotic pressure = **7**
- In this question, GFR, 3 = $K_f[(25-2) - (\pi_{GC} -7)] = K_f[23 - \pi_{GC} +7] = K_f[30 - \pi_{GC}]$
- π_{GC} = **27 mm Hg**

17. **Ans. d. Factor XIII**   *(Ref: Robbins 9/e p 119; Ganong 25/e p564, 24/e p565, 577)*

    Extensive cross-linking of blood clot is done by factor XIII.

    *"The loose aggregation of platelets in the temporary plug is bound together and converted into the definitive clot by **fibrin**. Fibrin formation involves a cascade of enzymatic reactions and a series of numbered clotting factors. The **fundamental reaction is conversion of the soluble plasma protein fibrinogen to insoluble fibrin**. The process involves the release of two pairs of polypeptides from each fibrinogen molecule. The remaining portion, **fibrin monomer, then polymerizes with other monomer molecules to form fibrin**. The fibrin is initially a loose mesh of interlacing strands. It is **converted by the formation of covalent cross-linkages to a dense, tight aggregate (stabilization)**. This latter reaction is **catalyzed by activated factor XIII and requires Ca^{2+}.**"* -Ganong 24/e p564

    "Conversion of fibrinogen into cross-linked fibrin: Thrombin directly converts soluble fibrinogen into fibrin monomers that polymerize into an insoluble clot, and also amplifies the coagulation process, not only by activating factor XI, but also be activating two critical co-factors, factors V and VIII. It also stabilizes the secondary hemostatic plug by activating factor XIII, which covalently cross-links fibrin." -Robbins 9/e p119

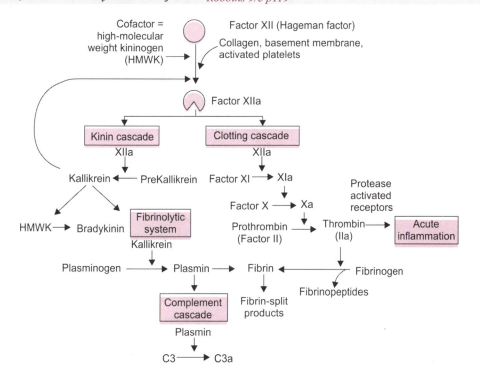

System for Naming Blood Clotting Factors	
Factors	Names
I	**Fibrinogen**
II	**Prothrombin**
III	**Thromboplastin**
IV	**Calcium**^{Q}
V	**Proaccelerin**^{Q}, labile factor, accelerator globulin
VII	**Proconvertin**, SPCA, stable factor
VIII	Antihemophilic factor (AHF), **antihemophilic factor A**^{Q}, antihemophilic globulin (AHG)
IX	Plasma thromboplastic component (PTC), Christmas factor, **antihemophilic factor B**^{Q}
X	**Stuart-Prower factor**^{Q}
XI	Plasma thromboplastic antecedent (PTA), **antihemophilic factor C**^{Q}
XII	**Hageman factor**^{Q}, glass factor
XIII	Fibrin-stabilizing factor, **Laki-Lorand factor**
HMW-K	High-molecular-weight kininogen, **Fitzgerald factor**
Pre-Ka	Prekallikrein, Fletcher factor
Ka	Kallikrein
PL	Platelet phospholipid

Factor VI is not a separate entity and has been dropped.

18. **Ans. b. b** *(Ref: Ganong 25/e p546, 24/e p542)*

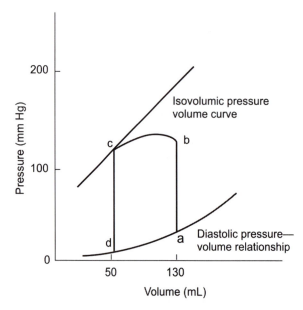

Fig. 6: Normal pressure—volume loop of the left ventricle.
During diastole, the ventricle fills and pressure increases from d to a. Pressure then rises sharply from a to b during isovolumetric contraction and from b to c during ventricular ejection. At c, the aortic valves close and pressure falls during isovolumetric relaxation from c back to d.

Ventricular Systole
• **At the start of ventricular systole, the AV valves close**. Ventricular muscle initially shortens relatively little, but intraventricular pressure rises sharply as the myocardium presses on the blood in the ventricle. This period of **iso-volumetric (isovolumic, isometric) ventricular contraction** lasts about 0.05 s, until the pressures in the left and right ventricles exceed the pressures in the aorta (80 mm Hg; 10.6 kPa) and pulmonary artery (10 mm Hg) and the aortic and pulmonary valves open.
• **During isovolumetric contraction, the AV valves bulge into the atria, causing a small but sharp rise in atrial pressure.**
• **When the aortic and pulmonary valves open**, the phase of **ventricular ejection** begins. Ejection is rapid at first, slowing down as systole progresses. The intraventricular pressure rises to a maximum and then declines somewhat before ventricular systole ends. Peak pressures in the left and right ventricles are about 120 and 25 mm Hg, respectively. Late in systole, pressure in the aorta actually exceeds that in the left ventricle, but for a short period momentum keeps the blood moving forward.
• The **AV valves are pulled down by the contractions of the ventricular muscle**, and **atrial pressure drops**. The amount of blood ejected by each ventricle per stroke at rest is 70–90 mL.
• The **end-diastolic ventricular volume** is about **130 mL**. Thus, about 50 mL of blood remains in each ventricle at the end of systole **(end-systolic ventricular volume)**, and the **ejection fraction,** the percentage of the end-diastolic ventricular volume that is ejected with each stroke, is **about 65%**.
• The **ejection fraction** is a **valuable index of ventricular function**. It can be **measured by injecting radionuclide-labeled red blood cells** and **imaging the cardiac blood pool at the end of diastole and the end of systole** (equilibrium radionuclide angiocardiography), or **by computed tomography**.

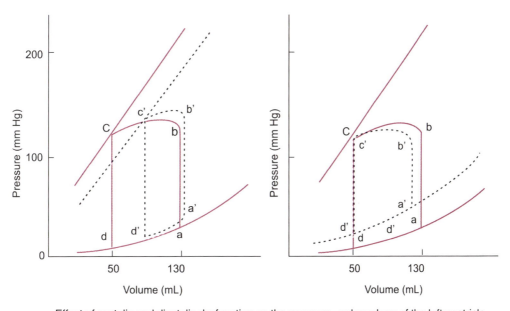

Fig. 7: Effect of systolic and diastolic dysfunction on the pressure–volume loop of the left ventricle.

In both panels the solid lines represent the normal pressure–volume loop and the dashed lines show how the loop is shifted by the disease process represented.

Left	Right
Systolic dysfunction shifts the isovolumic pressure–volume curve to the right, decreasing the stroke volume from b–c to b–c.	Diastolic dysfunction increases and diastolic volume and shifts the diastolic pressure–volume relationship upward and to the left. This reduces the stroke volume from b–c to b–c.

19. **Ans. a. Scapula** *(Ref: Ghai 7/e p115; Ganong 25/e p26, 24/e p38; Guyton 13/e p909)*
   Scapula doesn't contain brown adipose tissues. Brown fat is located between the scapula.

*"**Brown fat**, which is some-what **more abundant in infants** but is **present in adults as well**, is **located between the scapulas, at the nape of the neck, along the great vessels in the thorax and abdomen**, and in other scattered locations in the body. **In brown fat depots, the fat cells as well as the blood vessels have an extensive sympathetic innervation**. This is in contrast to white fat depots, in which some fat cells may be innervated but the principal sympathetic innervation is solely on blood vessels. In addition, ordinary lipocytes have only a single large droplet of white fat, whereas **brown fat cells contain several small droplets of fat**. Brown fat cells also contain many mitochondria. In these mitochondria, an **inward proton conductance that generates ATP** takes places as usual, but in addition there is a **second proton conductance that does not generate ATP**. This "short-circuit" conductance depends on a 32-kDa uncoupling protein (UCP1). It **causes uncoupling of metabolism and generation of ATP**, so that **more heat is produced**."* -Ganong 25/e p26

Locations of Brown Adipose Tissues	
Visceral Brown Fat	**Subcutaneous Brown Fat**
• **Perivascular:** Aorta, common carotid artery, brachiocephalic artery, paracardial mediastinal fat, epicardial coronary artery & cardiac veins, internal mammary artery and intercostal artery & vein • **Perivisvus:** Heart, trachea and major bronchi at lung hilum, esophagus, greater omentum & transverse mesocolon • **Around solid organs:** Thoracic, paravertebral, pancreas, kidney, adrenal, liver & hilum of spleen	• **Between anterior neck muscles & supraclavicular fossa**[Q] • **Under the clavicles**[Q] • **In the axilla**[Q] • **Anterior abdominal wall**[Q] • **Inguinal fossa**[Q]

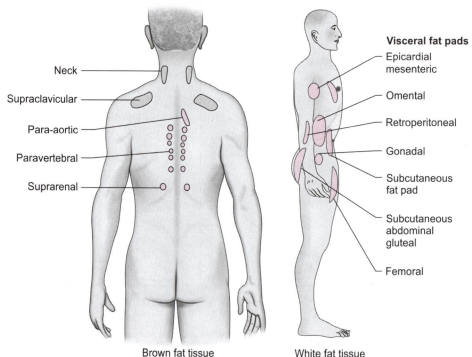

Brown Fat
• A **newborn baby** is **more prone to develop hypothermia** because of **large surface area per unit of body weight**. • In infants, **brown fat is an important site of thermogenesis**. It results in the so-called **non-shivering thermogenesis**[Q]. • **Brown fat** is located around the **adrenal glands, kidney, nape of neck, interscapular and axillary region**[Q]. • Metabolism of brown fat leads to **heat production**[Q].   • Blood flowing through the brown fat becomes warm and through circulation, transfers heat to other parts of the body. This mechanism oh heat production is known as non-shivering thermogenesis[Q].

AIIMS May 2015

20. Ans. c. >d Beta-1 >Beta-3 *(Ref: Miller 7/e p267, 268; Guyton 13/e p778; Ganong 25/e p260, 24/e p260; Goodman Gilman 12/e p199)*

Adrenergic beta-receptors having lipolysis property in fat cells is Beta-1 >Beta-3. According to the text and tables given in Miller and Guyton, its beta-1 and in Ganong and Goodman Gilman, its beta-3. Beta-1 is seen in white adipose tissues and triggered by catecholamines and sympathetic stimuli for lipolysis, which is then used for Calorigenesis, but not for non-shivering thermogenesis. Beta-3 adrenergic receptor is limited to brown adipose tissues, which is limited in adults. It's triggered by catecholamines and sympathetic stimuli for lipolysis, which is used mainly for non-shivering thermogenesis. Hence, beta-1 would be the preferred answer.

Adrenergic Receptors and Function	
Alpha Receptor	**Beta Receptor**
• Vasoconstriction[Q]	• Vasodilation (β2)[Q]
• Iris dilation[Q]	• Cardio-acceleration (β1)[Q]
• Intestinal relaxation[Q]	• Increased myocardial strength (β1)[Q]
• Intestinal sphincter contraction[Q]	• Intestinal relaxation (β2)[Q]
• Pilomotor contraction[Q]	• Uterus relaxation (β2)[Q]
• Bladder sphincter contraction[Q]	• Bronchodilation (β2)[Q]
• Inhibits neurotransmitter release (α2)[Q]	• Calorigenesis (β2)[Q]
	• Glycogenolysis (β2)[Q]
	• Lipolysis (β1)[Q]
	• Bladder wall relaxation (β2)[Q]
	• Thermogenesis (β3)[Q]

"The β_1-receptor mechanism is thought to primarily be involved in cardiac effects and release of fatty acids and renin, whereas β_2-receptors are primarily responsible for smooth muscle relaxation and hyperglycemia."- Miller 7/e p268

"Activation of β_3 receptors produces a vigorous thermogenic response as well as lipolysis."-Goodman Gilman 12/e p199

Responses Elicited in Effector Organs by Stimulation of Sympathetic and Parasympathetic Nerves				
Effector Organ	**Adrenergic (A) Response**	**Receptor Involved**	**Cholinergic (C) Response**	**Dominant Response (A or C)**
Heart				
Rate of contraction	**Increase**[Q]	β_1[Q]	**Decrease**[Q]	C
Force of contraction	**Increase**[Q]	β_1[Q]	**Decrease**[Q]	C
Blood vessels				
Arteries (most)	Vasoconstriction	α_1[Q]		A
Skeletal muscle	**Vasodilation**[Q]	β_2[Q]		A
Veins	Vasoconstriction	α_2[Q]		A
Bronchial tree	Bronchodilation	β_2[Q]	Bronchoconstriction	C
Splenic capsule	**Contraction**[Q]	α_1[Q]		A
Uterus	**Contraction**[Q]	α_1[Q]	Variable	A
Vas deferens	**Contraction**[Q]	α_1[Q]		A
Prostatic capsule	**Contraction**[Q]	α_1[Q]		A
GIT	**Relaxation**[Q]	α_2[Q]	**Contraction**[Q]	C
Eye				
Radial muscle, iris	**Contraction (mydriasis)**[Q]	α_1[Q]		A
Circular muscle, **iris**			Contraction (miosis)	C
Ciliary muscle	**Relaxation**[Q]	β[Q]	**Contraction**[Q] (accommodation)	C
Kidney	Renin secretion	β_1[Q]		A

Contd...

Contd...

Urinary bladder				
Detrusor	Relaxation[Q]	β[Q]	Contraction[Q]	C
Trigone and sphincter	Contraction[Q]	α_1[Q]	Relaxation[Q]	A, C
Ureter	Contraction[Q]	α_1[Q]	Relaxation[Q]	A
Insulin release from pancreas	Decrease[Q]	α_2[Q]		A
Fat cells	Lipolysis[Q]	β_1[Q]		A
Liver glycogenolysis	Increase	α_1		A
Hair follicles, smooth muscle	Contraction (piloerection)	α_1		A
Nasal secretion			Increase	C
Salivary glands	Increase secretion	α_1[Q]	Increase secretion[Q]	C
Sweat glands	Increase secretion	α_1[Q]	Increase secretion[Q]	C

21. **Ans. a. 5 times** *(Ref: Ganong 25/e p573, 24/e p575)*

Poiseuille Hagen Formula

- Mathematic expression of the relationship between the flow in a long narrow tube, the viscosity of the fluid, and the radius of the tube:

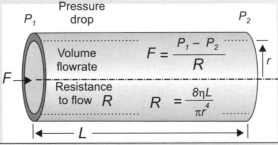

$$F = (P_A - P_B) \times (\pi/8) \times (1/\eta) \times (r^4/L)$$
Where
F = flow
$P_A - P_B$ = pressure difference between two ends of the tube
η = viscosity
r = radius of tube
L = length of tube
Because flow is equal to pressure difference divided by resistance (R),
$R = 8\eta L/\pi r^4$

- Because **flow varies directly and resistance inversely with the fourth power of the radius, blood flow, and resistance in vivo are markedly affected by small changes in the caliber of the vessels**. Thus, for example, flow through a vessel is doubled by an increase of only 19% in its radius; and when the radius is doubled, resistance is reduced to 6% of its previous value.
- This is why **organ blood flow is so effectively regulated by small changes in the caliber of the arterioles** and why variations in arteriolar diameter have such a pronounced effect on systemic arterial pressure.

In this question, $F = k r^4$
r" = r + 50% of r = 1.5r
Hence, $F" = k (1.5 r)^4 = 5.1 k r^4$
which implies flow is around 5 times the original flow.

22. **Ans. c. Both are activated together** *(Ref: Ganong 25/e p232, 24/e p232; Guyton 13/e p699)*

In response to descending excitatory input to spinal motor circuits, both α- and γ-motor neurons are activated.

"In response to descending excitatory input to spinal motor circuits, both α- and γ-motor neurons are activated. Because of this "α–γ coactivation," intrafusal and extrafusal fibers shorten together, and spindle afferent activity can occur throughout the period of muscle contraction. In this way, the spindle remains capable of responding to stretch and reflexively adjusting α-motor neuron discharge."–Ganong 25/e p232

*"Role of the muscle spindle in voluntary motor activity: To understand the importance of the gamma efferent system, one should recognize that 31 percent of all the motor nerve fibers to the muscle are the small type A gamma efferent fibers rather than large type A alpha motor fibers. Whenever signals are transmitted from the motor cortex or from any other area of the brain to the alpha motor neurons, in most instances the gamma motor neurons are stimulated simultaneously, an effect called **coactivation of the alpha and gamma motor neurons**. This effect causes both the extrafusal skeletal muscle fibers and the muscle spindle intrafusal muscle fibers to contract at the same time."*–Guyton 13/e p699

23. **Ans. b. Amylin** *(Ref: Katzung 13/e p723, 12/e p763; Guyton 12/e p939; Sabiston 20/e p943, 19/e p946)*

Amylin is produced by pancreatic beta cells, packaged within beta-cell granules in a concentration 1-2% that of insulin and co-secreted with insulin in a pulsatile manner and in response to physiologic secretory stimuli.

*"**Amylin** is a 37-amino-acid peptide originally **derived from islet amyloid deposits in pancreas** material from **patients with long-standing type 2 diabetes or insulinomas**. It is **produced by pancreatic beta cells**, packaged within beta-cell granules in a concentration 1–2% that of insulin and **co-secreted with insulin in a pulsatile manner** and in response to physiologic secretory stimuli. The **physiologic effect of amylin** may be to **modulate insulin release by acting as a negative feedback on insulin secretion**. At pharmacologic doses, amylin reduces glucagon secretion, slows gastric emptying by a vagally medicated mechanism, and **centrally decreases appetite**."*-Katzung 13/e p723

Islet Cells	Content
Alpha cells	Glucagon, pancreastatin[Q], glicentin[Q], (PG)
Beta cells	Insulin, amylin[Q], pancreastatin[Q] (IAP)
D cells	Somatostatin
D₂ cells	VIP
G cells	Gastrin
PP cells	Pancreatic polypeptide

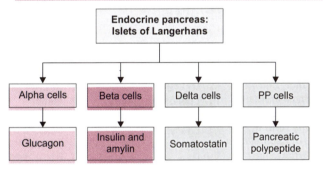

24. **Ans. b. NREM** *(Ref: Ganong 25/e p274, 24/e p274; Guyton 12/e p764)*

EEG in "B" shows high amplitude, low frequency waves as compared to waves A and C and EOG and EMG are nearly flat when compared to A. In C also they are flat. In NREM stage-4 delta waves are seen. So high amplitude, low frequency (delta waves) are seen in NREM.

In quiet wakefulness and awake state, alpha waves (high frequency, low amplitude) are seen.
In REM sleep, beta waves (high frequency, low amplitude) are seen.

Alert wakefulness (beta waves)	
Quiet wakefulness (alpha waves)	
REM sleep (beta waves)	
Stage 1 sleep (low voltage and spindles)	

Contd...

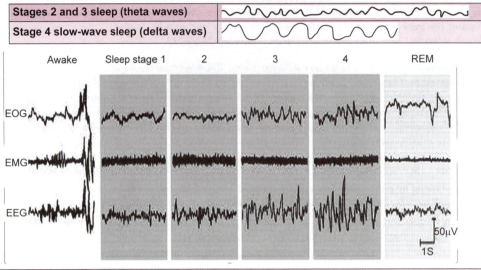

Contd...

Stages 2 and 3 sleep (theta waves)	
Stage 4 slow-wave sleep (delta waves)	

EEG Patterns In Sleep				
	Beta (β) Wave	**Alpha (α) Wave**	**Theta Wave**	**Delta Wave**
Seen in	• **Parietal & frontal**[Q] **region** • **Patients awake, at rest with eyes open**[Q]	• Recorded from **parieto occipital region**[Q]. • Related to decreased level of attention • Seen in **awake patient at rest with eyes closed**[Q] **& mind wandering**	• Seen in **hippocampus**[Q] **in children**[Q] **& drowsiness** • Found over **parietal & temporal areas.**	• Seen in deep **NREM sleep**[Q] **& infant**[Q]
Frequency	>14 Hz[Q]	8-13 Hz	4-7 Hz	3-5 Hz (minimum)[Q]
Amplitude	Low amplitude	High amplitude	High amplitude[Q]	Large amplitude (Maximum)[Q]
Characteristic Feature:	• **Low-voltage, high frequency desynchronized** electrical activity • Can be **produced by any form of sensory stimulation** or **mental concentration**, such as solving arithmetic problems alpha rhythm gets replaced by beta, therefore beta rhythm known as **alpha block** • **Beta rhythm** is also known as **arousal** or **alerting response**, because it is **correlated with the aroused, alert state**	Frequency of alpha rhythm is decreased by: • **Old age** • **Low blood glucose** • **Low body temperature** • **Low** levels of adrenal **glucocorticoids** • **High arterial PaCO$_2$** • **Sleep**	Recorded in: • **Newborn infants** • **Stage 1** of **NREM sleep** • **Emotional stress** in adults particularly **disappointment & frustration** • Many brain disorders • **Accentuated in children** when they are **crying**	• **High-voltage, low frequency synchronized** electrical activity. • **Evoked by overbreathing** • Seen in **pathological states** in which **thalamocortical transmission is blocked**, such as **coma.** • Presence of **intracranial tumor** act as a source of delta wave activity. • In **metabolic encephalopathy, Delta waves** are seen predominantly **due to a decrease in the consciousness.**

Contd...

Contd...

EEG Pattern In Sleep	
Non Rapid Eye Movement (NREM) Sleep	**Rapid Eye Movement (REM) Sleep**
Also known as **Slow wave sleep or Orthodox sleep**[Q] (**70-80% of total sleep**[Q])	Also known as **Paradoxical sleep**[Q] (**20-30%** of total sleep)
Stage I: • First & lightest stage of sleep. • Predominantly **theta waves**[Q] **Stage II:** Characterized by- • **Sleep spindles**[Q] • **K-complex (easily evoked)**[Q] **Stage III:** (deep sleep transition) • **Delta wave first appear**[Q] • **K-complex** (with strong stimuli only) **Stage IV:** (Cerebral sleep) • Predominant **delta activity**[Q]	• Light phase of sleep, but **arousal is difficult**[Q] • Mixed frequency, **low amplitude**[Q] waves on EEG. Predominantly β- like activity. • Also known as **Desynchronized**[Q] or paradoxical sleep (because EEG is rapid) • **Dreaming is seen**[Q] • Active sleep
Sleep disorder during NREM IV	**Sleep disorder of REM (3N)**
1. Sleep walking (**Somnambulism**)[Q] 2. Sleep talking (**Somniloquy**)[Q] 3. **Night terror**[Q] (Pavor nocturnes) 4. **Bruxism**[Q] (tooth grinding) 5. **Nocturnal enuresis**[Q] (bed wetting)	1. Night mares[Q] 2. **Narcolepsy**[Q] : The hallmark of this disorder being decreased sleep latency. 3. Nocturnal penile tumescene[Q]

BIOCHEMISTRY

25. **Ans. a. ALA synthase**   *(Ref: Harper 30/e p325-328, 28/e p272,278,563)*

    *High levels of lead can affect heme metabolism by combining with SH groups in enzymes such as Ferrochelatase and ALA dehydratase (zinc containing enzyme). This affects porphyrin metabolism. Elevated levels of protoporphyrin are found in red blood cells and elevated levels of ALA and Coproporphyrin are found in urine. It appears that **heme, probably acting through an aporepressor molecule, acts as a negative regulator of the synthesis of ALA synthase**. Thus, the **rate of synthesis of ALA synthase increases greatly in the absence of heme** and **is diminished in its presence**.*

    > *"ALA synthase occurs in both hepatic (ALAS1) and erythroid (ALAS2) forms. The rate-limiting reaction in the synthesis of heme in liver is that catalyzed by ALAS1, a regulatory enzyme. It appears that **heme, probably acting through an aporepressor molecule, acts as a negative regulator of the synthesis of ALAS1**. Thus, the **rate of synthesis of ALAS1 increases greatly in the absence of heme** and **is diminished in its presence**."* –Harper 28/e p563

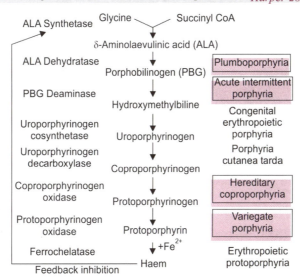

26. **Ans. c. Chylomicron** *(Ref: Harrison 19/e p2438-2447, 18/e p3148)*

Severe abdominal pain, xanthomas and milky appearance of plasma suggest either type I or type V hyperlipoproteinemia. In both of these conditions, levels of chylomicrons are elevated.
See Q. No. 35 AIIMS May 2015

Types of Xanthoma in Hyperlipoproteinemia	
Types of Xanthoma	Hyperlipoproteinemia
Eruptive xanthoma	Type I, III, IV^Q
Plain xanthoma	Type III^Q
Tendinous xanthoma	Type IIa^Q
Tuberous xanthoma	Type II, III, IV^Q
Xanthelesma palpebrum	Type II, III^Q

See Q. No. 37 AIIMS November 2016

27. **Ans. d. Cori's disease** *(Ref: Harrison 19/e p433 e-2, 18/e p3200, 3201; Harper 30/e p179, 28/e p335, 27/166)*

A child was brought to the hospital was found to have hypoglycemia, hepatomegaly and accumulation of highly branched glycogen called limit dextrins. He is likely to be suffering from Cori's disease.

Type IIIa Glycogen Storage Disease or Cori's Disease or Forbes Disease:
- Caused by a **deficiency of glycogen debranching enzyme**.
- **Childhood:** Hepatomegaly, growth retardation, muscle weakness, fasting hypoglycemia,
- Accumulation of characteristic branched polysaccharide (limit dextrins)

See Q. No. 160 AIIMS May 2016

28. **Ans. c. Type IV** *(Ref: Robbins 9/e p20-23, 8/e p95)*

Type IV collagens are the **main components of the basement membrane, together with laminin.**

*"The **basement membrane** is synthesized by contributions from the overlying epithelium and underlying mesenchymal cells, forming a flat lamellar "chicken wire" mesh (although labeled as a membrane, it is quite porous). The **major constituents are amorphous nonfibrillar type IV collagen and laminin.**"* –Robbins 9/e p21.

*"**Type IV collagens** have **long but interrupted triple-helical domains and form sheets instead of fibrils**; they are the **main components of the basement membrane, together with laminin.**"* –Robbins 9/e p23

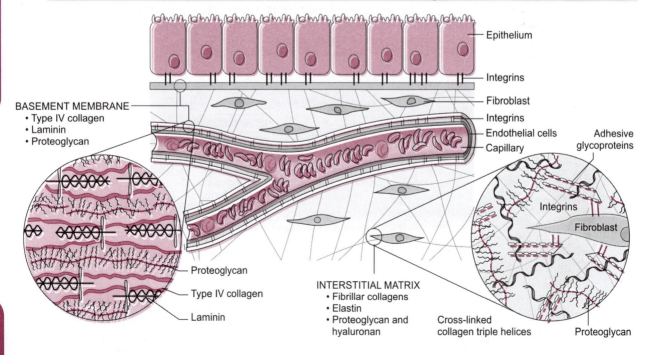

AIIMS May 2015

Main Types of Collagens, Tissue Distribution, and Genetic Disorders		
Collagen Type	Tissue Distribution	Genetic Disorders
Fibrillar Collagens		
I	Ubiquitous in hard & soft tissues (**Bone, cornea & myofibrils**[Q])	**Osteogenesis imperfecta**; **Ehlers-Danlos syndrome**-arthrochalasias type I
II	Cartilage, **intervertebral disc**[Q], **vitreous**[Q]	Achondrogenesis type II, spondyloepiphysea dysplasia syndrome
III	Hollow organs, soft tissues, **granulation tissue**[Q]	**Vascular Ehlers-Danlos syndrome**
V	**Soft tissues, blood vessels**[Q]	**Classical Ehlers-Danlos syndrome**
IX	**Cartilage, vitreous**[Q]	**Stickler syndrome**
Basement Membrane Collagens		
IV	**Basement membranes, eye lens**[Q]	**Alport syndrome**
Other Collagens		
VI	Ubiquitous in microfibrils	Bethlem myopathy
VII	**Anchoring fibrils at dermal-epidermal junctions**[Q]	**Dystrophic epidermolysis bullosa**
IX	**Cartilage, intervertebral discs**[Q]	Multiple epiphyseal dysplasias
XVII	**Transmembrane collagen in epidermal cells**[Q]	**Benign atrophic generalized epidermolysis bullosa**
XV & XVIII	**Endostatin-forming collagens, endothelial cells**[Q]	**Knobloch syndrome** (type XVIII collagen)

29. **Ans. b. Cell size** *(Ref: Hematology: Clinical Principles and Applications/p456)*
   Forward scatter in flow cytometry is used to assess cell size.

Flow Cytometry
• Flow cytometry is a **technique for counting, examining**, and **sorting microscopic particles suspended in a stream of fluid.**
• It allows **simultaneous multi-parametric analysis** of the physical and/or chemical characteristics **of single cells flowing through an optical and/or electronic detection apparatus.**
• Flow cytometry **measures optical & fluorescence characteristics of single cells.**

Parts of Flow cytometer:

• A flow cytometer is made up of **three main systems: fluidics, optics, and electronics**.

Fluidics System	Optics System	Electronics System
The fluidics system **transports particles in a stream to the laser beam for interrogation.**	The optics system **consists of lasers to illuminate the particles** in the sample stream and **optical filters to direct the resulting light signals to the appropriate detectors.**	**The electronics system converts the detected light signals into electronic signals** that can be processed by the computer. For some instruments equipped with a sorting feature, the electronics system is also **capable of initiating sorting decisions to charge and deflect particles.**

The direction of light scattered by the cell correlates to:	
• Forward Scatter (FS) for cell size[Q]	• Side Scatter (SS) for density of the cell[Q] (Granularity, vacuoles & membrane size)

• **Live cells** will have **more forward scatter (FS) than dead and apoptotic cells.**
• **Granulocytes or monocytes** have **more granularity or vacuoles** and the will have **more side scattering (SS).**

Clinical Applications in Flow Cytometry	
• **Imunophenotyping of leukemia & lymphoma**	• **PNH-diagnostics**
• **DNA & cell cycle analysis**	• **Immune-deficiencies**
• **Minimal residual disease**	• **Platelet Function Analysis**

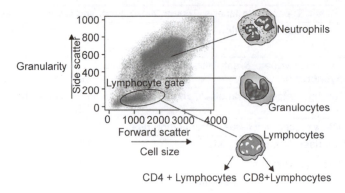

30. **Ans. d. Phosphoglucomutase** *(Ref: Harper's 29/e p180; Harper 30/e p176, 177, 28/e p158, 333)*
    Phosphoglucomutase enzyme is common between glycogenesis and glycogenolysis.

    > "The combined action of phosphorylase and these other enzymes leads to the complete breakdown of glycogen. The **reaction catalyzed by phosphoglucomutase is reversible**, so that **glucose 6-phosphate can be formed from glucose 1-phosphate**. In liver (and kidney), but not in muscle, glucose 6-phosphatase hydrolyzes glucose 6-phosphate, yielding glucose that is exported, leading to an increase in the blood glucose concentration." *–Harper 30/e p177*

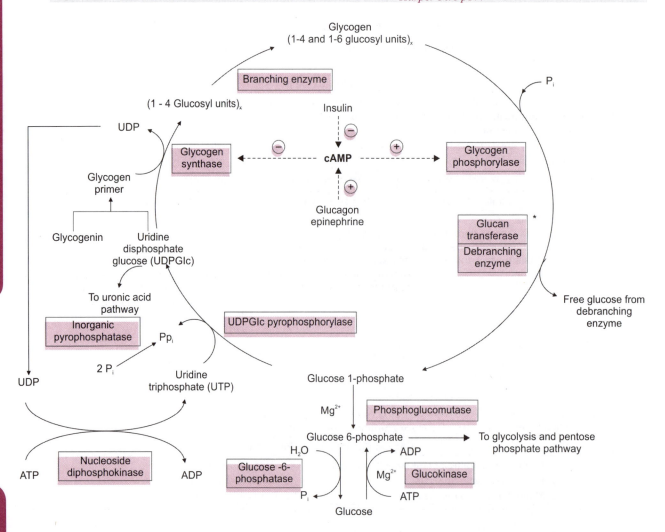

Glucotransferase:
- Both the **branching enzyme** involved **in glycogenesis** and **debranching enzyme involved in glycogenolysis** are **involved in transfer of glucose residues from one chain to another**;
- Also known as **'glucan transferase'** or **'glucotransferase'**.

Glycogen phosphorylase is an enzyme of glycogenolysis.
Glycogen synthase is an enzyme of glycogenesis.

Glucotransferase
• Both the **branching enzyme** involved **in glycogenesis** and **debranching enzyme involved in glycogenolysis** are **involved in transfer of glucose residues from one chain to another**; also known as **'glucan transferase'** or **'glucotransferase'**[Q].
• When a growing chain is at least 11 glucose residues long, **branching enzyme transfers a part of the 1 → 4 chain (at least 6 glucose residues) to a neighboring chain to form a 1 → 6 linkage**, establishing a **branch point**[Q].
• The branches grow by **further additions of 1 → 4 glucosyl units** and further branching.
• The **debranching enzyme** has **two distinct catalytic sites** in a single polypeptide chain.
• One is a **glucan transferase,** that **transfers a trisaccharide unit from one branch to the other, exposing the 1 → 6 glycosidase** that **catalyzes hydrolysis of the 1 → 6 glycoside bond to liberate free glucose**[Q].

31. Ans. d. Glucocerebroside   *(Ref: Harrison 19/e p432-e5; Robbin's 9/e p151-154, 8/e p153; Nelson 20/e p708, 19/e p487, 488, 500)*

Clinical history of bone pain and hepatosplenomegaly with crumpled tissue paper appearance on biopsy is highly suggestive of Gaucher's disease. Gaucher's Disease is caused by deficiency of tissue enzyme Glucocerebrocidase, which splits glucose from glucosyl ceramide. So there is accumulation of Glucocerebroside.

*"**Gaucher's Disease is** caused by **deficiency of** tissue enzyme **Glucocerebrocidase**[Q], which splits glucose from glucosyl ceramide. **Enzyme replacement therapy** is done with **natural or recombinant glucocerebrocidase**[Q]."*

Gaucher's Disease (AR)
• **MC lysosomal storage disorder, autosomal recessive**[Q] in inheritance,
• Caused by **deficiency of** tissue enzyme **Glucocerebrocidase**[Q], which splits glucose from glucosyl ceramide
• Glucosyl ceramide, a cerebrocide, accumulates in the cell of reticuloendothelial system

Histopathology

- The **cerebrocide laden cells are large** and have **eccentric nuclei**; the **cytoplasm appears like crumpled silk** or **tissue paper (Gaucher's Cells)**[Q]
- With the electron microscope, the fibrillary cytoplasm can be resolved as **elongated, distended lysosomes containing the stored lipid in stacks of bilayers**[Q].
- In patients with cerebral involvement, **Gaucher's cells** are **seen in** the **Virchow-Robin spaces**[Q], and arterioles are surrounded by swollen adventitial cells.

- **Figure: Gaucher disease involving the bone marrow.**
- **Gaucher cells (A,** Wright stain; **B,** Hematoxylin and eosin) are **plump macrophages** that characteristically have the **appearance in the cytoplasm of crumpled tissue paper** due to accumulation of glucocerebroside.

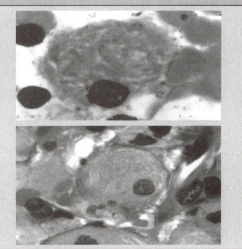

Clinical features:
- **Spleen** is always **markedly enlarged** with signs of **hypersplenism**[Q]
- **Liver is enlarged** and the **marrow cavity is widened**[Q], due to deposits of Gaucher's cells
- **Expansion of bone**[Q] is prominent, especially at the lower end of the femur and humerus
  - **Pancytopenia & thrombocytopenia secondary to hypersplenism**[Q].
  - **Pathologic fracture & bone pain** occur if there has been **extensive expansion of the marrow space**[Q].

Clinical variants of Gaucher's Disease		
Type 1 **(Chronic non-neuronopathic)**	**Type 2** **(Acute neuronopathic)**	**Type 3** **(Chronic neuronopathic)**
• Chronic illness with prominent visceral involvement without neurological signs	• Starts early, death before 2 years, prominent neurological symptoms	• Both visceral & neurological manifestations occur

Treatment:

- **Enzyme replacement therapy** is done with **natural or recombinant glucocerebrocidase[Q]**.
- **OGT-918[Q]** slows the rate of accumulating glycolipids and is under trial.

> • **Chitotriosidase[Q]**, an enzyme synthesized by macrophages, is **markedly elevated in patients with Gaucher's disease**. It is reasonably **specific biomarker[Q] for Gaucher's disease** because levels are only slightly elevated in other disorders affecting macrophages.

32. **Ans. a. Glucose** *(Ref: Harper 30/e p146, 150, 28/e p141)*

Glucose is used by RBCs in the fasting state.

Organ	Fed	Fasting	Starvation
Brain	**Glucose**	**Glucose**	**Ketone bodies[Q]**
Heart	**Fatty acids[Q]**	**Fatty acids[Q]**	**Ketone bodies[Q]**
Liver	**Glucose**	**Fatty acids[Q]**	**Amino acids[Q]**
Muscles	**Glucose**	**Fatty acids[Q]**	Fatty acids & ketone bodies
Adipose tissue	**Glucose**	**Fatty acids[Q]**	Fatty acids & ketone bodies
RBCs	**Glucose**	**Glucose**	

33. **Ans. b. Knock down** *(Ref: Robbins 9/e p5)*

RNAi causes Knock down in a gene.

> *"Small interfering RNAs (siRNAs): Another species of gene-silencing RNA, called small interfering RNAs (siRNAs), works in a manner quite similar to that of miRNA. siRNAs are becoming powerful tools for studying gene function and may in the future be used therapeutically to silence specific genes, such as oncogenes, whose products are involved in neoplastic transformation."-Robbins 9/e p5*

Small interfering RNAs (siRNAs)
• **Short RNA sequences introduced experimentally into cells**
• Another **species of gene-silencing RNA,** works in a manner quite similar to that of miRNA.
• **Synthetic siRNAs targeted against specific mRNA** have become useful laboratory tools **to study gene function** (so called **"knockdown technology"[Q]**)

> • **siRNAs** are becoming **powerful tools for studying gene function** and may in the future be **used therapeutically to silence specific genes**, such as **oncogenes,** whose products are involved in neoplastic transformation[Q].

Knock out	• **Targeted gene is completely removed from the DNA sequence by replacing it with an artificial piece of DNA[Q]**
Knock down	• **Gene** is not completely removed but **its expression is suppressed by using RNA interference technology[Q]**
Knock in	• **Segment of a gene is inserted into a DNA sequence[Q]**

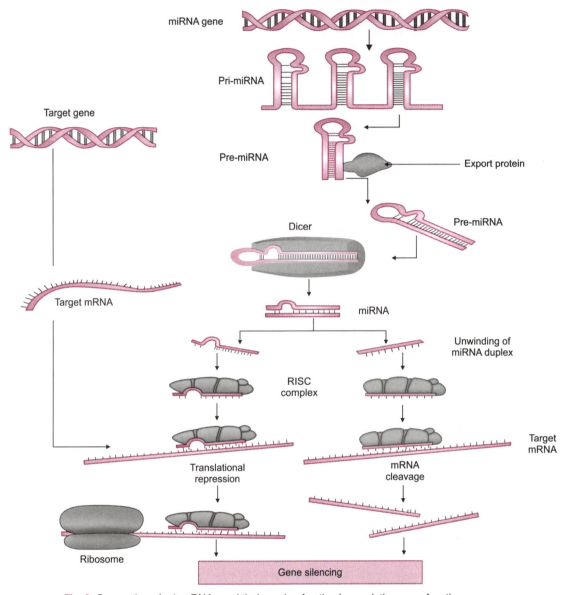

Fig. 8: Generation of microRNAs and their mode of action in regulating gene function.
(Pri-miRNA, primary microRNA transcript; pre-miRNA, precursor microRNA; RISC, RNA-induced silencing complex)

34. **Ans. b. LoxP site**   *(Ref: https://en.wikipedia.org/wiki/Cre-Lox_recombination)*

    In gene studies, the specific site to which the enzyme CRE recombinase binds is LoxP site.

    > "In the field of genetics, **Cre-Lox recombination** is known as a site-specific recombinase technology and is widely used to carry out deletions, insertions, translocations and inversions at specific sites in the DNA of cells."—*https://en.wikipedia.org/wiki/Cre-Lox_recombination*

Site-specific Recombinase Technology
• In the field of genetics, **Cre-Lox recombination** is known as a site-specific recombinase technology and is widely used to carry out **deletions, insertions, translocations** and **inversions at specific sites in the DNA of cells.**
• It **allows the DNA modification** to be targeted to a specific cell type or be triggered by a specific external stimulus. It is implemented both in eukaryotic & prokaryotic systems.

Contd...

AIIMS ESSENCE

- The system consists of a single enzyme, **Cre-recombinase** that **recombines a pair of short target sequences** called the *Lox* **sequences**. This system can be implemented without inserting any extra supporting proteins or sequences.
- The **Cre enzyme** and the **original *Lox* site** called the *LoxP* **sequence** are **derived from bacteriophage P1.**
- The **Cre protein** is a **site-specific DNA recombinase**, that is, it can **catalyze the recombination of DNA between specific sites in a DNA molecule.** These sites, known as **loxP sequences**, contain specific binding sites for Cre that surround a directional core sequence where recombination can occur.
- The **Cre protein** (encoded by the locus originally named as 'Causes recombination', with 'cyclization recombinase'
- *Lox P* **(locus of X-over P1)** is a **site on the bacteriophage P1 consisting of 34 bp.**

Flp-FRT Recombination

- **Flp-FRT recombination** is another **site-directed recombination technology**, increasingly **used to manipulate an organism's DNA** under controlled conditions in vivo.
- It is **analogous to Cre-*lox* recombination** but **involves the recombination of sequences between short flippase recognition target (*FRT*) sites** by the **recombinase (Flp)** derived from the 2 μm plasmid of baker's yeast **Saccharomyces cerevisiae.**

35. **Ans. c. Apo B-100 mutation**   *(Ref: Harrison 19/e p2438-2447, 18/e p3148)*

Highly elevated levels of LDL with normal level of LDL receptors is seen in Type IIa Familial hyper-cholesterolemia characterized by mutation in ligand region of apoB-100.

*"Familial Defective apoB-100 (FDB), also known as **autosomal dominant hypercholesterolemia (ADH) type 2,** is a dominantly inherited disorder that clinically resembles heterozygous familial hypercholesterolemia (FH) with **elevated LDL-C levels and normal TGs.** FDB is **caused by mutations in the gene encoding apoB-100, specifically in LDL receptor-binding domain of apoB-100.** Several different mutations have been identified, but a single mutation predominates: substitution of glutamine for arginine at position 3500. The **mutation results in a reduction in the affinity of LDL binding to the LDL receptor, so LDL is removed from the circulation at a reduced rate.** FDB is **characterized by elevated plasma LDL-C levels with normal TGs; tendon xanthomas** can be seen, although not as frequently as in FH, and there is an **associated increase in risk of CHD."-Harrison 19/e p2442***

Familial Defective apoB-100 (FDB)

- Also known as **autosomal dominant hypercholesterolemia (ADH) type 2**
- Clinically resembles heterozygous familial hypercholesterolemia (FH) with **elevated LDL-C levels and normal TGs**. FDB is **caused by mutations in the gene encoding apoB-100, specifically in LDL receptor-binding domain of apoB-100^Q.**

Characteristic Features:

- The **mutation results in a reduction in the affinity of LDL binding to the LDL receptor, so LDL is removed from the circulation at a reduced rate.** FDB is **characterized by elevated plasma LDL-C levels with normal TGs; tendon xanthomas** can be seen, although not as frequently as in FH, and there is an associated **increase in risk of CHD^Q.**

Diagnosis:

- The **apoB-100 gene mutations** can be **detected directly through sequencing of the receptor-binding region of the apoB gene** or **genotyping for the most common mutation**, but genetic diagnosis is not generally performed because there is no direct implication for clinical management.

Treatment:

- As with FH, patients are **treated with statins first** and, if necessary, with additional classes of LDL-lowering drugs.

Classification of Hyperlipoproteinemias

Phenotype	I	IIa	IIb	III	IV	V
	Familial lipoprotein lipase deficiency	Familial hyper-cholesterolemia	Familial combined hyperlipidemia	Familial dysbeta-lipoproteinemia	Familial hypertriglyc-eridemia	Combined hyperlipidemia

Contd...

Contd...

Phenotype	I	IIa	IIb	III	IV	V
Defect	Defect in LPL, or apo C-11[Q]	Defective LDL receptors or mutation in ligand region of apoB-100[Q]	Unknown	Deficiency in remnant clearance by the liver, due to abnormality in apo E	Apo A-V & unknown	Apo A-V & unknown
Lipoprotein elevated	Chylomicrons[Q]	LDL[Q]	LDL & VLDL[Q]	Chylomicron & VLDL remnants[Q]	VLDL[Q]	Chylomicrons & VLDL[Q]
Triglycerides	++++[Q]	—	++	++ to +++	++	++++[Q]
Xanthomas	Eruptive[Q]	Tendon, tuberous[Q]	None	Palmar, tuberoeruptive[Q]	None	Eruptive[Q]
Coronary	0	+++[Q]	+++[Q]	+++[Q]	+/–	+/–
Peripheral atherosclerosis	0	+	+	++	+/–	+/–

36. Ans. d. 245 *(Ref: Harrison 19/e p2446; Clinical Laboratory Medicine by Kenne 2/e p319)*

*"Plasma lipid and lipoprotein levels should be measured in all adults, preferably after a 12-h overnight fast. **In most clinical laboratories, the total cholesterol and TGs in the plasma are measured enzymatically, and then the cholesterol in the supernatant is measured after precipitation of apoB-containing lipoproteins to determine the HDL-C. The LDL-C is then estimated using the following equation: LDL-C = total cholesterol – (TG/5) – HDL-C** (The VLDL cholesterol content is estimated by dividing the plasma TG by 5, reflecting the ratio of TG to cholesterol in VLDL particles.) **This formula (the Friedewald formula) is reasonably accurate if test results are obtained on fasting plasma and if the TG level does not exceed ~200 mg/dL; by convention it cannot be used if the TG level is >400 mg/dL."** -Harrison 19/e p2446*

Friedewald Equation

- The **ultra centrifugal measurement of LDL** is **time consuming & expensive** and **require specialist equipment**.
- For this reason, **LDL-cholesterol is most commonly estimated from quantitative measurements of total and HDL-cholesterol and plasma triglycerides** using the empirical relationship of Friedewald et al.
- **Total cholesterol = LDL + HDL + Triglycerides/5**

  - **Total cholesterol = LDL + HDL + Triglycerides/5**
  - 300 = LDL + 25 + 150/5
  - **LDL = 300 – (25 + 30) = 245 mg/dl**

Limitations of Friedewald Equation

- **Friedewald Equation should not be** used under the following circumstances:
  - When **chylomicrons are present**
  - When **plasma triglyceride** concentration **exceeds 400 mg/dL**
  - In patients with **dysbeta-lipoproteinemia (type III hyperlipoprteinemia)**

37. Ans. d. Pyruvate dehydrogenase *(Ref: Harper 30/e p172, 198, 555, 556; 28/e p321,473)*

In thiamine deficiency, pyruvate cannot be converted to acetyl Co-A as thiamine pyrophosphate is a coenzyme for pyruvate dehydrogenase, which catalyzes the conversion of pyruvate to acetyl Co-A. Hence, excess of pyruvate is metabolized to lactate by lactate dehydrogenase. This results in lactic acidosis.

*"Pyruvate, formed in the cytosol, is transported into the mitochondrion by a proton symporter. Inside the mitochondrion, it is **oxidatively decarboxylated to acetyl-CoA by a multienzyme complex** that is associated with the inner mitochondrial membrane. This **pyruvate dehydrogenase complex** is analogous to the alpha-ketoglutarate dehydrogenase complex of the citric acid cycle. Pyruvate is decarboxylated by the pyruvate dehydrogenase component of the enzyme complex to a hydroxyethyl derivative of the thiazole ring of enzyme-bound thiamin diphosphate, which in turn reacts with oxidized lipoamide, the prosthetic group of dihydrolipoyl transacetylase, to form acetyl lipoamide. **Thiamin is vitamin B1 and in deficiency, glucose metabolism is impaired,** and there is **significant (and potentially life-threatening) lactic and pyruvic acidosis."** –Harper 28/e p321*

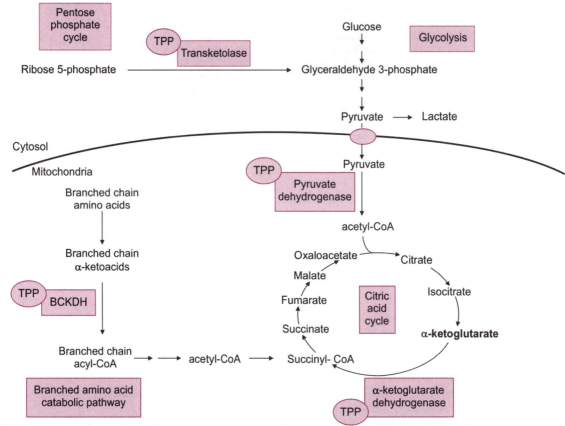

BCKDH, branched chain α-ketoacid dehydrogenase complex; CoA, coenzyme, A; TPP, thiamin pyrophosphate

Thiamin (Vitamin B1)
• **Thiamin diphosphate (TDP)**[Q] also known as **Thiamin pyrophosphate (TPP)**[Q] is **biologically active & storage form of vitamin B1,** formed by **transfer of pyrophosphate group from ATP.**
Physiological Role: • **Thiamin** has a **central role in energy yielding metabolism** and especially of **carbohydrates.** • **Thiamin requirements increase in excess intake of carbohydrates** and its **deficiency leads to decreased energy production.**

Thiamin diphosphate	• Thiamin diphosphate is the coenzyme for:
	1. 3 multienzyme complexes that catalyze oxidative decarboxylation reactions:
	   – Branched-chain ketoacid dehydrogenase[Q] involved in the metabolism of **leucine, isoleucine & valine**
	   – Alpha-ketoglutarate dehydrogenase[Q] in the **citric acid cycle**
	   – Pyruvate dehydrogenase[Q] in carbohydrate metabolism
	2. Transketolase[Q] reaction in the **pentose phosphate pathway**

Thiamin triphosphate	• **Thiamin triphosphate** has a **role in nerve conduction;** it phosphorylates, and so **activates a chloride channel**[Q] in the **nerve membrane**

Contd...

| AIIMS May 2015 | 1461 |

Contd...

Thiamin (Vitamin B1)

Thiamine Deficiency Diseases:

• **Chronic peripheral Neuritis, Beriberi & Wernicke Encephalopathy with Korsakoff's Psychosis**

Beriberi	Wernicke Encephalopathy with Korsakoff's Psychosis
• **Wet beriberi:** Patients present with an **enlarged heart, tachycardia, high-output congestive heart failure**, peripheral edema & peripheral neuritis[Q].	• Alcoholic patients with **chronic thiamin deficiency** also may have **CNS manifestations** known as *Wernicke's encephalopathy*[Q].
• **Dry beriberi:** Symmetric peripheral neuropathy of the motor and sensory systems, with diminished reflexes. **Neuropathy affects the legs most markedly**[Q]	• *Wernicke's encephalopathy*: Consists of **horizontal nystagmus, ophthalmoplegia** (due to weakness of one or more extraocular muscles), **cerebellar ataxia, & mental impairment**[Q].
• **Infantile beriberi:** Occurs in infants born to thiamin deficiency mothers and show tachycardia, vomiting, convulsions & death.	• When there is an **additional loss of memory** and a **confabulatory psychosis**, the syndrome is known as *Wernicke-Korsakoff syndrome*[Q].

PATHOLOGY

38. **Ans. d. Anticipation**   *(Ref: Robbins 9/e p168-171)*

The phenomenon where subsequent generations are at the risk of earlier and more severe disease is known as anticipation.

*"Anticipation: This refers to the observation that **clinical features** of fragile X syndrome **worsen with each successive generation**, as if the mutation becomes increasingly deleterious as it is transmitted from a man to his grand- sons and great-grandsons."-Robbins 9/e p169*

1st generation

CAGCAGCAGCAGCAG

2nd generation

CAGCAGCAGCAGCAGCAGCAGCAGCAG

3rd generation

CAGCAGCAGCAGCAGCAGCAGCAGCAGCAGCAGCAG

Diagram showing anticipation.

Anticipation

• **Anticipation:** A phenomenon whereby the **symptoms of a genetic disorder become apparent at an earlier age as it is passed onto the next generation.** In most cases, an **increase of severity of symptoms** is also noted.

• Anticipation is **common in trinucleotide repeat disorders**, such as **Huntington's disease and myotonic dystrophy**, where a dynamic mutation in DNA occurs.

• All of these diseases have neurological symptoms.

• The **clinical features worsen with each successive generation**, as if the **mutation becomes increasingly deleterious as it is transmitted from a man to his grandsons and great-grandsons.**

Diseases showing anticipation			
Autosomal dominant	**Autosomal Recessive**	**X-linked**	**Without Expression Type**
• **Several spinocerebellar ataxias**[Q] • **Huntington's disease: CAG**[Q] • **Myotonic dystrophy: CTG**[Q] • **Dyskeratosis congenita**[Q]	• **Freidreich's ataxia: GAA**[Q] (Freidreich's ataxia does not usually exhibit anticipation because it is an autosomal recessive disorder.)	• **Fragile X syndrome: CGG**[Q]	• Crohn's disease • Behcet's disease

39. **Ans. d. Translocation involving myc gene**   *(Ref: Robbins 9/e p597)*

Starry eye pattern on biopsy is highly suggestive of Burkitt lymphoma. All forms of Burkitt lymphoma are associated with translocations of the c-MYC gene on chromosome 8.

*"Burkitt lymphoma: **The tumor exhibits a high mitotic index and contains numerous apoptotic cells**, the nuclear remnants of which are phagocytosed by interspersed benign macrophages. These **phagocytes** have **abundant clear cytoplasm**, creating a characteristic **"starry sky" pattern**."-Robbins 9/e p597*

*"**All forms of Burkitt lymphoma are associated with translocations of the c-MYC gene on chromosome 8**. The translocation partner is usually the IgH locus [t(8;14)] but may also be the Ig κ [t(2;8)] or γ [t(8;22)] light-chain loci." -Robbins 9/e p597*

Burkitt lymphoma

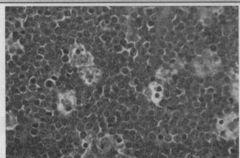
A, At low power, **numerous pale tingible body macrophages** are evident, producing a **"starry sky" appearance**.

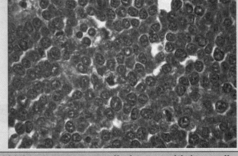
B, At high power, **tumor cells have multiple small nucleoli** and **high mitotic index**. The lack of significant variation in nuclear shape and size lends a **monotonous appearance**.

Burkitt Lymphoma

- Accounts for about **30% of childhood NHLs** in the United States
- **Mature B cell lymphoma (CD34+ & Ig+)**^{Q}
- **Very aggressive** but **responds well to intensive chemotherapy**.
- Most children & young adults can be cured.

Types of Burkitt Lymphoma

African (Endemic)	Sporadic (Nonendemic)	HIV Associated
• Seen in **children** or young adults • MC site: Mandible^Q • EBV infection: 100%^{Q}	• Seen in children or young adults • Most commonly occurs as **ileocecal mass** or peritoneal mass^Q • EBV infection: 20–30%	• 25% patients are latently infected by EBV • Involve **LN** or **bone marrow** • EBV infection: 25-40%

Morphology:
- **The tumor exhibits a high mitotic index and contains numerous apoptotic cells**^{Q}, the nuclear remnants of which are phagocytosed by interspersed benign macrophages.
- These **phagocytes** have **abundant clear cytoplasm**, creating a characteristic **"starry sky" pattern**^{Q}.

Immunophenotype:
- **Express surface IgM, CD19, CD20, CD10, and BCL6**, a phenotype consistent with a germinal center B-cell origin^Q.
- **Burkitt lymphoma** almost always **fails to express the anti-apoptotic protein BCL2**^{Q}.

Molecular Pathogenesis:
- **All forms of Burkitt lymphoma are associated with translocations of the c-MYC gene on chromosome 8**^{Q}.
- The **translocation partner is usually the IgH locus [t(8;14)]** but may also be the Ig κ [t(2;8)] or γ [t(8;22)] light-chain loci^Q.

Clinical Features:
- *Most tumors manifest at extranodal sites*.
- **Endemic Burkitt lymphoma** often presents as a **mass involving the mandible**
- **Sporadic Burkitt lymphoma** most often appears as a **mass involving the ileocecum & peritoneum**^{Q}.

Treatment:
- **Treatment** should begin **within 48 hours of diagnosis**
- Involves the use of **intensive combination chemotherapy regimens** incorporating **high doses of cyclophosphamide**.
- **Prophylactic therapy to the CNS is mandatory**.

Contd...

Translocation	Gene (Chromosome)	Malignancy
(9;22) (q34;q11)[Q]	ABL-BCR	Chronic myeloid leukemia[Q]
(11;14)(q13;q32)[Q]	BCL1-IgH	Mantle cell lymphoma[Q]
(8;21)[Q] (15;17)[Q] (16;16)[Q]	RUNX1-RUNX1T1 PML-RARA CBFB-MYH11	Acute myeloid leukemia[Q]
(11;22)(q24;q12)	FLI1-EWS	Ewing's sarcoma[Q]
(8;14)(q24;q32)	MYC-IgH	Burkitt's lymphoma[Q] B cell acute lymphocytic leukemia[Q]
Inv (2p13;p11.2-14)	REL-NRG	Non-Hodgkin's lymphoma
(1;3)(p34;p21)[Q]	TAL1-TCTA[Q]	Acute T cell leukemia[Q]

40. **Ans. a. 4–5 days** *(Ref: Robbins 9/e p107)*
    The approximate age of the wound in an incised wound, when new collagen fibrils are seen along with a thick layer of growing epithelium is 4-5 days.

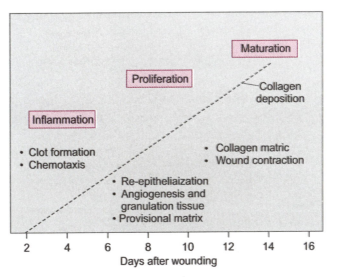

Healing of Clean Uninfected Wound	
Day	**Features of Wound**
Day 0	• Presence of **blood clot** in the incision/scab
Day 1 (within 24 hours)	• **Neutrophilic infiltration + blood clot**[Q]
Day 2 (24-48 hours)	• Neutrophils + blood clot + **continuous thin epithelial layers**[Q]
Day 3	• Macrophages replace neutrophils[Q] • Appearance of **granulation tissue**[Q] • **Deposition of type III collagen** but they do not bridge the incision
Day 5	• Abundant granulation tissue[Q] • **Collagen fibrils bridge the incision**[Q] • **Neovascularization** is maximum, full epithelial thickness with surface keratinization[Q]
End of 2nd week	• **Accumulation of collagen, fibroblast proliferation** • Disappearance of leucocyte inflammation
1 month	• **Replacement** of collagen type III with collagen type I (has greater tensile strength)[Q] • Dermal appendages are lost[Q]

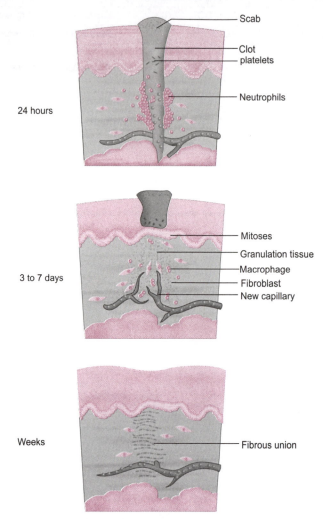

Fig. 9: Wound healing and scar formation—Healing of wound that caused little loss of tissue: note the small amount of granulation tissue, and formation of a thin scar with minimal contraction.

41. **Ans. d. Hypersensitivity reaction with modified macrophages, lymphocytes and giant cells** *(Ref: Robbins 9/e p208, 375,376; Anananarayan 10/e p169, 9/e p162)*

   Clinical features like fever, night sweats and weight loss and X-ray finding of mass in apical lobe with histopathological findings of caseous necrosis are highly suggestive of tuberculosis. The underlying process is type IV hypersensitivity, which is characterized by presence of modified macrophages, lymphocytes & giant cells.

   Schematic illustration of the events that give rise to the formation of granulomas in cell-mediated (type IV) hypersensitivity reactions.

Tuberculosis
Antigenic property:
• **Group specificity** is due to **polysaccharide**[Q] while **type specificity** is due to **protein antigen**[Q].
• Antibodies are not useful for diagnosis and immunity.
Pathogenecity:
• **Macrophages** are the **primary cells infected**[Q] by **M. tuberculosis**.

Contd...

Contd...

Tuberculosis
• M. tuberculosis replicated within the macrophages (phagosome) by **blocking fusion of phagosome and lysosome**[Q].   • It is due to **escape of killing by macrophages**[Q] and **induction of type IV hypersensitivity**.
• Factors contributing in pathogenesis: **Cord factor, Lipoarabinomannan, Complement system, M. tuberculosis heat shock proteins.**
• **Risk of acquiring infection** is determined mainly by **exogenous factors**[Q] while **risk of developing disease** depends largely on **endogenous factors**[Q].   • Most potent risk factor- **HIV coinfection**[Q]

Clinical Features:

Pulmonary TB		Extrapulmonary TB
Primary disease	**Post primary disease**	• **MC site: Lymph node**[Q] (MC cervical & supraclavicular) • Involvement of **genitourinary tract** (sterile pyuria in acidic urine) • Skeletal TB (**MC site spine**, hip, knee) • TB meningitis (**paresis of cranial nerves** especially ocular, is frequent finding)[Q] • GI TB (MC site terminal ileum & caecum)[Q] • **Tuberculous pericarditis** (MC cause of chronic constrictive pericarditis)[Q]
• Usually localized in **middle & lower zones**[Q] • Primary focus is usually **peripheral** in **subpleural** region and is accompanied by draining lymphatics, **inflamed regional LNs** which are collectively called **Primary complex / Ghon's focus**[Q]. • **Occult hematogenous dissemination to apex** of lung (**Simons Focus**[Q])	• Also called **adult type** or **reactivation** or **secondary** tuberculosis or **chronic pulmonary TB** • Usually localized to **apical & posterior segments of upper lobe** due to high O_2 concentration (**Puhl's lesion**[Q]) • MC hematologic finding: **mild anemia & leukocytosis** • **Infraclavicular lesion** is called **Assman's Focus**[Q]	

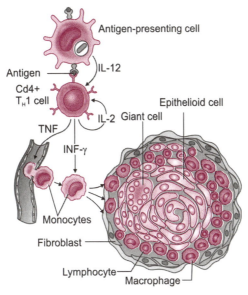

Fig. 10: Mechanisms of granuloma formation.

42. **Ans. d. Gynecomastia with long thin limbs** *(Ref: Harrison 19/e p2350; Robbins 9/e p166,167; Nelson 20/e p622)*
Given karyotype shows 2X chromosomes and 1Y chromosome. So this is a case of Klinefelter syndrome (47, XXY). Gynecomastia with long thin limbs is seen in Klinefelter syndrome.

> *"Klinefelter's syndrome is characterized by small testes, infertility, gynecomastia, tall stature/increased leg length, and hypogonadism in phenotypic males."* -Harrison 19/e p2350

Condition	Seen in
High pitched cry	Cri-du-chat syndrome
Round face with protruding tongue	Down syndrome (Trisomy 21)
Short stature with webbed neck	Turner syndrome (45, X)
Gynecomastia with long thin limbs	Klinefelter's syndrome (47, XXY)

Important chromosomal abnormalities	
Involving autosomes	Involving sex chromosomes
• **Down** syndrome (Trisomy 21) • **Edward** syndrome (Trisomy 18) • **Patau** syndrome (Trisomy 13)	• **Klinefelter's** syndrome (47, XXY) • **Turner** syndrome (45, X)

> *"Clinical Features of Klinefelter's Syndrome: Small testes, azoospermia, decreased facial and axillary hair, decreased libido, tall stature and increased leg length, decreased penile length, increased risk of breast tumors, thromboembolic disease, learning difficulties, speech delay and decreased verbal IQ, obesity, diabetes mellitus, metabolic syndrome, varicose veins, hypothyroidism, systemic lupus erythematosus, epilepsy."* -Harrison 19/e p2350

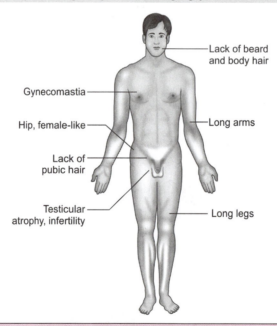

Klinefelter's Syndrome
• Defined classically by a **47, XXY karyotype**[Q] with variants demonstrating additional X & Y chromosomes.   • MC chromosomal disorder associated with **male hypogonadism & infertility**   • **Incidence: 1 in 1000 men**, but approximately **75% of cases are not diagnosed**.
Pathophysiology: • **Classic form of KS (47, XXY)** occurs after **meiotic nondisjunction** of the **sex chromosomes during gametogenesis** (40% during spermatogenesis, 60% during oogenesis).   • **Mosaic forms of KS (46, XY/47,XXY)** are thought to **result from chromosomal mitotic nondisjunction within the zygote** and occur in at least 10% of individuals with this condition.

Contd...

Contd...

Klinefelter's Syndrome

Clinical Features:

- Characterized by **small testes, infertility, gynecomastia, tall stature/increased leg length** & **hypogonadism in phenotypic males**[Q].
- **CVS: Mitral valve prolapse**[Q] & **varicose veins**[Q]
- **Developmental delay, speech difficulties**, and **poor motor skills** may be features but are variable, especially in adolescence.

> - **Testicular Biopsy: Seminiferous tubule hyalinization & azoospermia**[Q].
> - Plasma concentrations of **FSH & LH are increased** in most adults with 47,XXY, and **plasma testosterone is decreased** (50–75%), reflecting **primary gonadal failure**[Q].

- **Estradiol is often increased**, likely because of **chronic Leydig cell stimulation by LH** and **aromatization of androstenedione** by adipose tissue; the **increased ratio of estradiol-to-testosterone results in gynecomastia**[Q].

43. **Ans. d. Codominance**   *(Ref: Robbins 9/e p140)*

    Inheritance of ABO blood group is Codominance.

    > *"Although Mendelian traits are usually described as dominant or recessive, in some cases both of the alleles of a gene pair contribute to the phenotype—a condition called codominance. Histocompatibility and blood group antigens are good examples of codominant inheritance."-Robbins 9/e p140*

    > *Codominance is a relationship between two versions of a gene. Individuals receive one version of a gene, called an allele, from each parent. If the alleles are different, the dominant allele usually will be expressed, while the effect of the other allele, called recessive, is masked. In Codominance, however, neither allele is recessive nor are the phenotypes of both alleles are expressed, e.g., ABO blood group, where in AB blood group both A and B are dominant."*

    > *Codominance: When both alleles of a gene pair contribute to the phenotype. E.g., Blood group AB.*

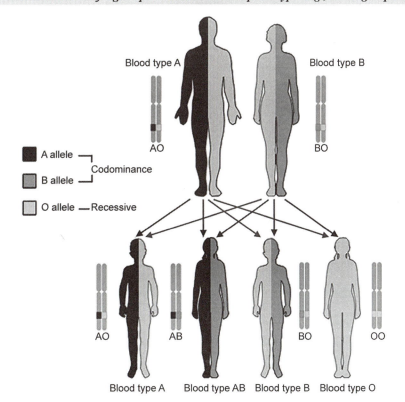

Contd...

ABO Blood Group System
• **A** and **B** **antigens** of the ABO blood group system are **glycoproteins present on the RBC membrane.**
• **H substance** is the **immediate precursor on which A and B antigens are added.**
• **H substance** is **formed by the addition of fucose to the glycolipid or glycoprotein backbone.**
• The **subsequent N-acetyl glucosamine creates the A antigen**, while the **addition of galactose produces the B antigen.**

Bombay phenotype
• Individuals with the **rare Bombay phenotype (hh) do not express the H antigen** (also called the H substance), **the antigen, which is present in blood group O**[Q].
• As a result of the **absence of the H antigen** they **cannot make either the A antigen** or the **B antigen**[Q].
• These individuals **have antibodies not only against A and B antigens** but also **against the H antigen**[Q].

44. **Ans. d. Membranous glomerulonephritis**   *(Ref: Robbins 9/e p917-918; Harrison 19/e p1843)*

Most common nephropathy associated with malignancy is membranous glomerulonephritis.

> *"In 25-30% of cases, **membranous glomerulonephritis is associated with a malignancy (solid tumors of the breast, lung, colon)**, infection (hepatitis B, malaria, Schistosomiasis), or rheumatologic disorders like lupus or rarely rheumatoid arthritis."-Harrison 19/e p1843*

Electron-dense deposits along the epithelial side of the basement membrane *with* effacement of foot processes overlying deposits.

See Q. No. 42 AIIMS May 2016

45. **Ans. d. Frozen specimen**   *(Ref: Netter's Essential Histology 2/e p479)*

Oil red 'O' stain is used for frozen specimen.

For Connective Tissue and Lipids	
Name of stain	**Elements stained**
Trichrome Stain	**Collagen**[Q]
Verhoeff-Van Gieson stain (Best for Elastin)	**Elastic fibers**[Q]
Luna stain	Elastin & Mast cells
Silver Methenamine stain	**Reticulin**[Q]
Oil red 'O' stain (on Fresh specimen) Sudan black (on fixed specimen)	**Fat**[Q]
Mallory's PTAH stain	Muscle striations
Martius scarlet blue (MSB)	**Fibrin**[Q]
PAS, Silver Methenamine stain	**Basement membrane**[Q]
Bielschowsky (silver stain)	**Neurofibrillary tangles senile plaques**[Q]
Luxol fast blue	**Myelin**[Q]

46. **Ans. b. von-Willebrand factor**   *(Ref: Robbins 9/e p116, 660)*

von-Willebrand factor is responsible for adhesion of platelets to the vessel wall.

> *"Endothelial injury allows* platelets *to contact the underlying extracellular matrix; subsequent* adhesion occurs through interactions with *von Willebrand factor (vWF), which is a product of normal endothelial cells and an* essential cofactor for platelet binding to matrix elements."- Robbins 9/e p116*

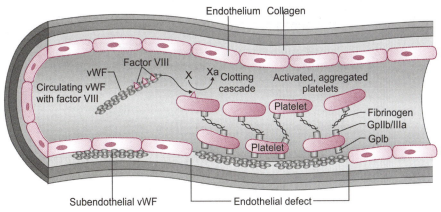

Fig. 11: Structure and function of factor VIII–von-Willebrand factor (vWF) complex.

Factor VIII is synthesized in the liver and kidney, and vWF is made in endothelial cells and megakaryocytes. The two associate to form a complex in the circulation. vWF is also present in the subendothelial matrix of normal blood vessels and the α-granules of platelets. Following endothelial injury, exposure of subendothelial vWF causes adhesion of platelets, primarily via the glycoprotein Ib (GpIb) platelet receptor. Circulating vWF and vWF released from the α-granules of activated platelets can bind exposed subendothelial matrix, further contributing to platelet adhesion and activation. Activated platelets form hemostatic aggregates; fibrinogen (and possibly vWF) participates in aggregation through bridging interactions with the glycoprotein IIb/IIIa (GpIIb/IIIa) platelet receptor. Factor VIII takes part in the coagulation cascade as a cofactor in the activation of factor X on the surface of activated platelets.

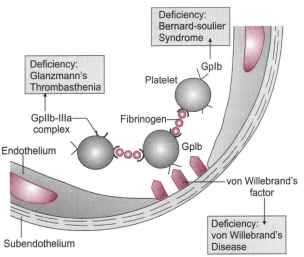

Fig. 12: Platelet adhesion and aggregation.

von-Willebrand factor functions as an adhesion bridge between subendothelial collagen and the glycoprotein Ib (GpIb) platelet receptor. Aggregation is accomplished by fibrinogen bridging GpIIb-IIIa receptors on different platelets. Congenital deficiencies in the various receptors or bridging molecules lead to the diseases indicated in the colored boxes. ADP, adenosine diphosphate.

Platelet Adhesion

- Certain **proteins** are **expressed on the platelet surface** that subsequently **regulate collagen-induced platelet adhesion**, particularly **under flow conditions**, and include **glycoprotein (GP)-IV, GP-VI,** and the **integrin-alfa2, & beta1.**
  - The **GPIb-IX-V complex** binds to the **exposed von-Willebrand factor**, causing **platelets to adhere**.
  - **von-Willebrand factor–bound GPIb-IX-V** promotes a **calcium-dependent conformational change in the GPIIb/IIIa receptor**, transforming it from an **inactive low-affinity state to an active high-affinity receptor for fibrinogen**[Q].

Contd...

Contd...

Platelet Adhesion
Factors Promoting Platelet Aggregation

Factors Promoting Platelet Aggregation	
• **ADP**[Q]	• **Fibrinogen**[Q]
• **Epinephrine**[Q]	• **Thrombospondin**[Q]
• **Thromboxane**-A2[Q]	• Collagen
• Serotonin	• Immune complex
• **von-Willebrand factor**[Q]	• **Thrombin**[Q]

47. Ans. a. Papillary carcinoma *(Ref: Robbin's 9/e p1096, 8/e p1121-1122, Schwartz 10/e p1542; 9/e p1361-1363; Sabiston 20/e p902-904, 19/e p906-909; Bailey 27/e p818, 26/e p765-768)*

Papillary Carcinoma of Thyroid

- Accounts for **80%** of all thyroid malignancies in **iodine-sufficient areas**[Q]
- **MC thyroid cancer** in **children** and **individuals** exposed to **external radiation**[Q].
- More often in **women, 30-40** years.

Pathology:

- **Grossly: Hard** and **whitish** and **remain flat** on sectioning with a blade with macroscopic **calcification, necrosis**, or **cystic changes**
  - **Multifocality**[Q] is **common** (up to **85%** of cases) on **microscopic examination**.
  - **Multifocality** is associated with an **increased risk** of **cervical nodal metastases**[Q], **rarely invade adjacent structures** such as the trachea, esophagus, and RLNs.
- **Rarely encapsulated**[Q] (PCT are **seldom encapsulated**)
- **Other variants: Tall cell**[Q], **insular**[Q], columnar, diffuse sclerosing, clear cell, **trabecular**, and poorly differentiated types; account for about **1%**; associated with a **worse prognosis**.

Histological characteristics of Papillary Carcinoma Thyroid

- **Papillary projections**[Q]: PTC contains branching papillae of cuboidal epithelial cells
- **Orphan Annie eye nuclei:**
  - The nuclei contain finely dispersed chromatin, which imparts an **optically clear** or **empty appearance**, giving rise to term **ground glass** or **Orphan Annie eye nuclei**[Q].
  - **Invaginations** of cytoplasm in cross-sections: **Intranuclear inclusions**[Q] **(pseudo-inclusion)** or **intranuclear grooves**[Q].
  - **Diagnosis** of PTC is **based on** these **nuclear characteristics**[Q] even in the absence of papillary structures.
- **Psammoma bodies**[Q]: **Microscopic, calcified deposits** representing clumps of sloughed cells

Clinical Features:

- Most patients are **euthyroid** and present with a **slow-growing painless mass**[Q] in the neck.
- Dysphagia, dyspnea & dysphonia are associated with locally advanced invasive disease.
- **Lymph node metastases** are **common**[Q], especially in **children** and **young adults**, and may be the presenting complaint.
  - **"Lateral aberrant thyroid"** almost always denotes a **cervical lymph node** that has been **invaded by metastatic cancer**[Q].
- **Distant metastases** are **uncommon** at initial presentation, but may ultimately develop in up to **20%** of patients.
- The **MC sites of metastasis: Lungs**[Q] >bone >liver >brain.

Diagnosis:

- **Diagnosis is** established by **FNAC** of the **thyroid mass** or **lymph node**[Q].
- Once thyroid cancer is diagnosed on FNAC, a **complete neck ultrasound** to evaluate the **contralateral lobe** and for **LN metastases** in the central & lateral neck compartments.

- **Treatment: Total** or **near-total thyroidectomy**[Q]
- During thyroidectomy, **enlarged central neck nodes** should be **removed**[Q].
- **Biopsy-proven lymph node metastases** detected clinically or by imaging in the lateral neck in patients with papillary carcinoma are managed with **modified radical neck dissection**.

Prognosis:

- PTC have an **excellent prognosis** with a **>95% 10-year survival rate**[Q].

48. **Ans. c. Dichroic mirror** *(Ref: Molecular Fluorescence: Principles and Applications by Bernard Valeur, Mario Nuno Berberan Santos 2nd edition)*

> *"Typical components of a fluorescence microscope are a light source (xenon are lamp or mercury-vapor lamp are common; more advanced forms are high-power LEDs and lasers), the excitation filter, the dichroic mirror (or dichroic beam splitter), and the emission filter."*

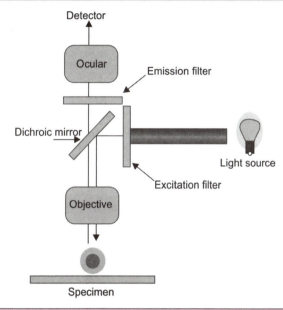

Fluorescence Microscope
• An **optical microscope** that **uses fluorescence & phosphorescence** instead of, or in addition to, reflection and absorption to, study properties of organic or inorganic substances. • The **"fluorescence microscope"** refers to any microscope that **uses fluorescence to generate an image**, whether it is a more simple set up like an epifluorescence microscope, or a more complicated design such as a confocal microscope, which uses optical sectioning to get better resolution of the fluorescent image.
Principle: • The **specimen is illuminated with light of a specific wavelength**, which is **absorbed by the fluorophores**, causing them to emit light of longer wavelengths (i.e., of a different color than the absorbed light). • The illumination light is separated from the much weaker emitted fluorescence through the use of a spectral emission filter. • **Typical components of a fluorescence microscope** are a **light source** (xenon are lamp or mercury-vapor lamp are common; more advanced forms are high-power LEDs and lasers), **the excitation filter**, **the dichroic mirror** (or **dichroic beam splitter**), and the **emission filter**.   • The **filters** and the **dichroic are chosen to match the spectral excitation** and emission characteristics of the **fluorophore used to label the specimen**. In this manner, the distribution of a single fluorophore (color) is imaged at a time. **Multi-color images of several types of fluorophores must be composed by combining several single-color images.** • Most fluorescence microscopes in use are **epifluorescence microscopes**, where **excitation of the fluorophore** and **detection of the fluorescence are done through the same light path** (i.e. through the objective). These microscopes are **widely used in biology** and are the basis for more advanced microscope designs, such as the confocal microscope and the total internal reflection fluorescence microscope (TIRF).
Limitations: • Unlike transmitted and reflected light microscopy techniques **fluorescence microscopy only allows observation of the specific structures**, which have been labeled for fluorescence.

49. **Ans. d. Birbeck's granules** *(Ref: Robbins 9/e p621,622, 8/e p631,632; Harrison 19/e p135 e-9, 18/p2883)*
In Langerhans Cell Histiocytosis, the characteristic abnormality seen is Birbeck's granules.

*"Regardless of the clinical picture, the **proliferating Langerhans cells have abundant, often vacuolated cytoplasm and vesicular nuclei containing linear grooves or folds**. The **presence of Birbeck granules in the cytoplasm is characteristic**. Birbeck granules are **pentalaminar tubules**, often with a **dilated terminal end producing a tennis racket-like appearance**, which **contain the protein langerin**. In addition, the tumor cells also **typically express HLA-DR, S-100, and CD1a**."*— Robbins 9/e p622

"Langerhans cells (LCs) are specialized DCs that reside in mucocutaneous tissue and upon activation become specialized for antigen presentation to T cells. LC histiocytosis (LCH; also known as histiocytosis X) represents neoplastic proliferation of LCs (S-100+, CD1a+, and Birbeck granules on electron microscopy)."—Harrison 19/e p135 e-9

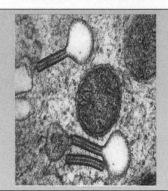

Histiocytosis-X (Langerhans Cell Histiocytosis)

- **Histiocytosis** is an **"umbrella" designation** for a variety of **proliferative disorders of dendritic cells** or **macrophages**[Q].
- It is a spectrum of **proliferations of** a **special type of immature dendritic cell** called the **Langerhans cell**[Q].

Pathology:

- **Proliferating Langerhans cells** have abundant, often **vacuolated cytoplasm** and **vesicular nuclei containing linear grooves** or folds.
- The presence of **Birbeck granules**[Q] in the cytoplasm is **characteristic**.
  - Birbeck granules: **Pentalaminar tubules**, often with a dilated terminal end producing a **tennis racket–like appearance**[Q], which contain the **protein langerin**[Q].

Clinical Variants of Langerhans Cell Histiocytosis

Letterer-Siwe Disease	Eosinophilic Granuloma	Hand-Schuller-Christian Disease
• Occurs **most frequently before 2 years of age**[Q] • **Cutaneous lesions** resembling a **seborrhoeic eruption**[Q] caused by **infiltrates of Langerhans cells** over the **front & back** of the **trunk** & on **scalp**. • Most of those affected have **concurrent hepatosplenomegaly**[Q], **lymphadenopathy**[Q], **pulmonary lesions & destructive osteolytic bone lesions**[Q]. • **Extensive infiltration of** the marrow often leads to **anemia, thrombocytopenia**, and a **predisposition to recurrent infections**, such as **otitis media & mastoiditis**[Q].	• Characterized by **proliferations of Langerhans cells** admixed with variable numbers of **eosinophils, lymphocytes, plasma cells & neutrophils**[Q]. • Typically **arises within** the **medullary cavities of bones**, most commonly the **calvarium, ribs**, and **femur**[Q]. • **Unifocal lesions most commonly affect** the **skeletal system in older children** or **adults**[Q]. • **Bone lesions** can be **asymptomatic** or cause **pain, tenderness**, and, in some instances, **pathologic fractures**[Q].	• **Calvarial bone defects, diabetes insipidus & exophthalmos** is referred as **Hand-Schuller-Christian triad**[Q].

Letterer-Siwe Disease	Eosinophilic Granuloma	Hand-Schuller-Christian Disease
• Course of **untreated disease** is **rapidly fatal**. • With **intensive chemotherapy**[Q], 50% of patients survive 5 years.	• **Involvement of** the **posterior pituitary stalk** of the hypothalamus leads to **diabetes insipidus** in about 50% of patients.	

Diagnosis:

Light Microscopy	Electron Microscopy	Immunohistochemistry
• **Langerhans cell** (large mononuclear cells with few cytoplasmic vacuoles) is the **'sin qua non'** (essential) of **diagnostic lesion**[Q]	• **Birbeck granules (Tennis racket appearance**[Q]	• **CD1a, S-100** or **langerin (CD-207)** demonstration on the surface of LCH cells[Q]

AIIMS May 2015

PHARMACOLOGY

50. Ans. c. Non-ionic and highly lipid soluble   *(Ref: Goodman Gillman 12/e p22; KDT 7/e p6)*

Nitroglycerine is effective as sublingual medication because it is non-ionic and highly lipid soluble.

> *"Sublingual Administration. Absorption from the oral mucosa has special significance for certain drugs despite the fact that the surface area available is small. Venous drainage from the mouth is to the superior vena cava, bypassing the portal circulation and thereby protecting the drug from rapid intestinal and hepatic first-pass metabolism. For example, nitroglycerin is effective when retained sublingually because it is non-ionic and has very high lipid solubility. Thus, the drug is absorbed very rapidly. Nitroglycerin also is very potent; absorption of a relatively small amount produces the therapeutic effect."*-Goodman Gillman 12/e p22

Systemic Routes of Drug Administration			
1. Oral	• **Most common** & **most convenient**		
2. Sublingual	• **Avoid first pass metabolism**, used in emergencies • Drug should be **nonionic** having **very high lipid solubility^Q** • Example: **Nitroglycerine, Isosorbide dinitrate & Nifedipine**		
3. Rectal	• Drug is **absorbed into external hemorrhoidal veins, bypasses liver**, but not that absorbed into internal hemorrhoidal veins. • **First pass metabolism** occurs, but **less than oral route** (Avoid first pass metabolism by 50%) • **Example: Diazepam in children for febrile seizures**		
4. Cutaneous	• Transdermal for **highly lipid soluble drugs** • **Example: Nitroglycerine, Nicotine, Hyoscine, Fentanyl & Estrogen**		
5. Inhalational	• Drug delivery can be controlled like IV Infusion • Drugs used in asthma: Salbutamol, Ipratropium, Monteleukast, Inhalational steroids& Inhalational anesthetics		
6. Nasal	• Example: Nafarelin (GnRH agonist), Calcitonin, Desmopressin, Influenza vaccine		
7. Parenteral	**Intravenous**	• **Emergency use**, increased risk of adverse effect, not suitable of oily solutions, or poorly soluble substance best for steady state plasma concentration.	
	Subcutaneous	• Suitable **for some poorly soluble suspensions**, appropriate for self administration (Example: **Insulin**)	
	Intradermal	• The drug is injected into skin raising a bleb (e.g. **BCG vaccine, sensitivity testing**). • It produces local tissue necrosis and irritation	
	Intramuscular	• Suitable for **oily solutions** and some irritating substances	

Nanotherapy
• **Nanotherapy: Novel method for drug delivery** • Nanoparticles are offering **new opportunities for diagnosis**, **targeted drug delivery** and **imaging of clinical effect**

51. Ans. a. Increase in water solubility   *(Ref: Goodman Gillman 12/e p124,125; Katzung 13/e p56, 12/e p53,54)*

Rationale behind xenobiotics metabolism by CYP enzymes is to increase water solubility.

> *"The body removes xenobiotics by xenobiotic metabolism. This consists of the deactivation and the excretion of xenobiotics, and happens mostly in the liver. Excretion routes are urine, feces, breath, and sweat. Hepatic enzymes are responsible for the metabolism of xenobiotics by first activating them (oxidation, reduction, hydrolysis and/or hydration of the xenobiotic), and then conjugating the active secondary metabolite with glucuronic acid, sulfuric acid, or glutathione, followed by excretion in bile or urine. An example of a group of enzymes involved in xenobiotic metabolism is hepatic microsomal cytochrome P450."*

> *"Phase I reactions include oxidation (especially by the cytochrome P450 group of enzymes, also called mixed-function oxidases), reduction, deamination, and hydrolysis. These enzymes are found in high concentrations in the smooth endoplasmic reticulum of the liver. Of the drugs metabolized by phase I cytochrome P450s, approximately 75% are metabolized by just two: CYP3A4 or CYP2D6."*

Xenobiotic Metabolism

- **Xenobiotic metabolizing enzymes** have historically been grouped into those that carry out *phase 1 reactions*, which include **oxidation, reduction, or hydrolytic reactions**, and the *phase 2 reactions*, in which **enzymes catalyze the conjugation of the substrate** (the phase 1 product) with a second molecule.
- The **phase 1 enzymes** lead to the **introduction of functional groups such as –OH, –COOH, –SH, –O–, or NH$_2$**.
  - The **addition of functional groups does little to increase the water solubility of the drug**, but can **dramatically alter the biological properties of the drug**.
  - Reactions carried out by **phase 1 enzymes** usually **lead to the inactivation of a drug**.
- However, in certain instances, metabolism, usually the **hydrolysis of an ester or amide linkage, results in bioactivation of a drug**. Inactive drugs that undergo metabolism to an active drug are called *prodrugs*. **Examples** are the anti-tumor drug **cyclophosphamide**, which is bioactivated to a cell-killing electrophilic derivative; and **clofibrate**, which is converted in the cell from an ester to an active acidic metabolite.
- The **phase 1 oxidation reactions** are **carried out by CYPs, flavin-containing monooxygenases (FMO), and epoxide hydrolases (EH).**
  - **Phase 2 enzymes facilitate the elimination of drugs** and the **inactivation of electrophilic and potentially toxic metabolites produced by oxidation**.
  - While **many phase 1 reactions result in the biological inactivation of the drug, phase 2 reactions produce a metabolite with improved water solubility, a change that facilitates the elimination of the drug from the tissue, normally via efflux transporters.**
- The **phase 2 enzymes include several superfamilies of conjugating enzymes**. Among the more important are the **glutathione- S-transferases (GST)**, **UDP-glucuronosyltransferases** (UGT), **sulfotransferases (SULT)**, *N*-acetyltransferases (NAT), and methyltransferases (MT).
- These **conjugation reactions usually require the substrate to have oxygen** (hydroxyl or epoxide groups), **nitrogen, or sulfur atoms** that serve as acceptor sites for a hydrophilic moiety, such as **glutathione, glucuronic acid, sulfate, or an acetyl group**.

52. **Ans. c. Saquinavir**   *(Ref: Goodman Gillman 12/e p1648; Katzung 13/e p852-853, 12/e p870; KDT 7/e p810)*

Saquinavir is a protease inhibitor.

"Saquinavir, the first approved HIV protease inhibitor, is a peptidomimetic hydroxyethylamine."-Goodman Gillman 12/e p1648

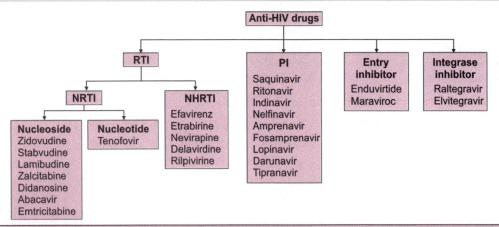

Anti-Retroviral Therapy

- There are **five classes of drugs**, which are **usually used in combination**, to treat HIV infection.
- Use of these drugs in combination can be termed **anti-retroviral therapy (ART), combination anti-retroviral therapy (cART)** or **highly active anti-retroviral therapy (HAART)**
- Anti-retroviral (ARV) drugs are broadly classified by the phase of the retrovirus life cycle that the drug inhibits.
- Typical combinations include **2 NRTIs as a "backbone"** along with **1 NNRTI, PI or INSTI as a "base"**.

Name of Group	Examples	Mechanism
Entry inhibitor **(Fusion inhibitors)**	**Maraviroc[Q]** **Enfuvirtide[Q]**	• **Interfere with binding, fusion & entry of HIV-1 to host cell by blocking a target.** • **Maraviroc** works by **targeting CCR5**, a co-receptor located on human helper T-cells
Nucleoside Reverse Transcriptase Inhibitors (NRTI) & Nucleotide Reverse Transcriptase Inhibitors (NtRTI)	**Zidovudine, Abacavir, Lamivudine, Emtricitabine & Tenofovir (NtRTI)**	• Nucleoside & nucleotide analogues which **inhibit reverse transcription** • Both act as **competitive substrate inhibitors**
Non-Nucleoside reverse transcriptase inhibitors (NNRTI)	**1st generation: Nevirapine & Efavirenz[Q]** **2nd generation: Etravirine & Rilpivirine[Q]**	• **Inhibit reverse transcriptase** by binding to an allosteric site of the enzyme • **NNRTIs** act as **non-competitive inhibitors of reverse transcriptase.** • **HIV-2** is **naturally resistant to NNRTIs.**
Integrase inhibitors (Integrase Nuclear Strand Transfer Inhibitors or **INSTIs**)	**Raltegravir[Q]** **Elvitegravir[Q]** **Dolutegravir[Q]**	• **Inhibit** the viral enzyme **integrase**, which is responsible for integration of viral DNA into the DNA of the infection cell.
Protease inhibitors	Lopinavir, Indinavir, Nelfinavir, Ritonavir, Amprenavir; **Darunavir & Atazanavir** (1st line)	• **Block** the **viral protease enzyme** necessary to produce mature virions upon budding from the host membrane.

53. Ans. a. Rosiglitazone *(Ref: Harrison 19//e p2057; 18/e p2998, KDT 7/p270, 6/e p269,270; Goodman Gillman 12/e p1260; Katzung 13/e p738, 12/e p757)*

Rosiglitazone does not act by increasing insulin secretion. Rosiglitazone is an oral antihyperglycemic agent that acts primarily by decreasing insulin resistance.

"Rosiglitazone is an oral antihyperglycemic agent that acts primarily by decreasing insulin resistance. It deceases insulin resistance in the muscles, adipose tissues and in the liver resulting in increased insulin dependent glucose disposal and decreased hepatic glucose output."

"Pioglitazone and rosiglitazone are insulin sensitizers and increase insulin-mediated glucose uptake by 30-50% in patients with type 2 diabetes. Although adipose tissue seems to be the primary target for PPARγ agonists, both clinical and preclinical models support a role for skeletal muscle, the major site for insulin-mediated glucose disposal, in the response to thiazolidinediones. In addition to promoting glucose uptake into muscle and adipose tissue, the thiazolidinediones reduce hepatic glucose production and increase hepatic glucose uptake."-Goodman Gillman 12/e p1260

"Thiazolidinediones (Tzds) act to decrease insulin resistance. Tzds are ligands of peroxisome proliferator-activated receptor- gamma, part of the steroid and thyroid superfamily of nuclear receptors. These PPAR receptors are found in muscle, fat, and liver."-Katzung 13/e p738

Anti-hyperglycemic Drugs			
Oral		**Parenteral**	
Insulin Secretagogues (Increase Insulin Secretion)		**Insulin**	
Sulfonylureas	• **1st Generation:** – Tolbutamide, Chlorpropamide • **2nd Generation:** – Glibenclamide, Glipizide – Gliclazide, Glimepiride	**Ultra short acting**	• Lispro, Aspart, Glulisine
		Short acting	• Regular (Crystalline zinc) • Semi lente
		Intermediate Acting	• NPH, Lente
Meglitinides	• **Repaglinide, Nateglinide[Q]**	**Long Acting**	• Glargine, Detemir
Dipeptidyl Peptidase-4 inhibitors	• **Sitagliptin, Vildagliptin[Q]** • **Saxagliptin, Alogliptin[Q]** • **Linagliptin[Q]**	**Newer generation**	• Albulin, Inhaled insulin
		• **GLP-1analogs: Exenatide[Q], Liraglutide[Q]** • **Amylin analogues: Pramlintide[Q]**	

Oral	Parenteral
Other Mechanisms	
Overcome insulin resistance	• Biguanides: Metformin[Q] • Thiazolidinediones
Alpha-glucosidase inhibitors	• Acarbose, Miglitol[Q] • Vaglibose[Q]
Sodium glucose Contransporter-2 (SGLT-2) inhibitors	• Dapaglifozin • Serglifozin • Remoglifozin • Canaglifozin

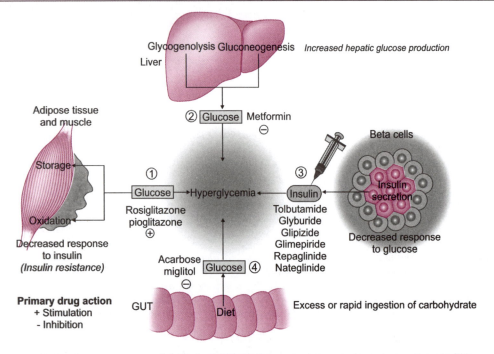

Rosiglitazone
• **Belongs to Thiazolidinedione's;** Other drugs of this group are **Troglitazone, Pioglitazone**. • It is an **oral antihyperglycemic** agent that acts primarily by **decreasing insulin resistance**[Q]   • **Rosiglitazone deceases insulin resistance** in the **muscles, adipose tissues** and in the liver resulting in **increased insulin dependent glucose disposal** and **decreased hepatic glucose output**[Q]
Mechanism of action: • Potent and **highly selective agonist for peroxisome proliferator activated receptor gamma (PPARg)**[Q] • **PPAR receptors** are found in tissues important for insulin action such as **adipose tissue, skeletal muscle** and **liver** (highest level in **adipose tissue**).   • **Activation of (PPARγ) nuclear receptors** modulates the **transcription of** a number of **insulin responsive genes** involved in the **control of glucose & lipid metabolism**[Q]. • **Rosiglitazone appears to reduce insulin resistance** by **enhancing fatty acids storage** and possibly by **increasing adiponectin levels**[Q]

Contd...

Contd...

Rosiglitazone
Metabolism: • **Extensively metabolized in liver by hydroxylation & oxidation**[Q] • **Liver function** should be **monitored in patients receiving thiazolidinedione's** even though **pioglitazone & rosiglitazone rarely** have been **associated with hepatotoxicity.** • **Thiazolidinedione's should not be used** in patients with **NYHA class III or IV failure.**
• **Main side effect** of all thiazolidinedione's is **water retention** leading to **edema.** • Sometimes there is **significant water retention leading to decompensation of potentially previously unrecognized heart failure**
• **Thiazolidinedione's** should be **prescribed with both caution** and **patient warnings** about the **potential for water retention/weight gain especially in patients with decreased ventricular function.**
Adverse Effect: • Rosiglitazone increases the risk of **angina & MI**

54. Ans. d. Chlorpromazine *(Ref: Goodman Gillman 12/e p1793; Parsons 22/e p220, 21/e p214)*

Amorphous whorl like corneal deposit suggests a case of vortex keratopathy. All the mentioned drugs cause this condition except chlorpromazine.

*"The cornea, the conjunctiva, and even the eyelids can be affected by systemic medications. **One of the most common drug deposits found in the cornea** is from the cardiac medication **amiodarone**. It deposits in the **inferior and central cornea** in a **whorl-like pattern termed cornea verticillata**. It appears as fine tan or brown pigment in the epithelium. Fortunately, the **deposits seldom affect vision**, and therefore, this rarely is a cause to discontinue the medication. The **deposits disappear slowly if the medication is stopped**. Other medications, including indomethacin, atovaquone, chloroquine, and hydroxychloroquine, can cause a similar pattern."–Goodman Gillman 12/e p1793*

*"The **phenothiazines**, including **chlorpromazine and thioridazine**, can cause **brown pigmentary deposits in the cornea, conjunctiva, and eyelids**. The deposits generally are found **in Descemet's membrane** and the **posterior cornea**. They typically **do not affect vision**. The ocular deposits generally **persist after discontinuation of the medication** and **can even worsen**, perhaps because the **medication deposits in the skin are slowly released and accumulate in the eye**."–Goodman Gillman 12/e p1793*

*"**Cornea verticillata**: This is a **whorl-like opacity in the corneal epithelium** seen in patients on **long-term treatment with medication** such as **amiodarone, chloroquine, phenothiazines and indomethacin**. It is also seen in patients with **Fabry disease** and its carrier state. The condition is **generally asymptomatic, harmless and reversible on stopping the drug**. The whorl-like pattern shows the direction of migration of corneal epithelial cells. Occasionally the condition has been known to cause glare and surface discomfort which responds to topical lubricants."–Parsons 22/e p220*

Systemic Agents with Ocular Side-effects	
Drugs	**Ocular Side-effects**
• **Amiodarone**[Q] • **Indomethacin**[Q] • **Atovaquone**[Q] • **Chloroquine**[Q] • **Hydroxychloroquine**[Q]	• Deposits in the **inferior and central cornea** in a **whorl-like pattern termed cornea verticillata**[Q]. • Appears as **fine tan or brown pigment** in the epithelium. • Deposits **seldom affect vision** • Deposits **disappear slowly** if the medication is stopped.
• **Chlorpromazine**[Q] • **Thioridazine**[Q]	• **Brown pigmentary deposits in the cornea, conjunctiva,** and **eyelids**. The deposits generally are **found in Descemet's membrane** and the **posterior cornea**. They typically **do not affect vision**. • **Ocular deposits generally persist** after discontinuation of the medication and **can even worsen**, perhaps because the **medication deposits in the skin are slowly released and accumulate in the eye.**

Contd...

Contd...

Drugs	Ocular Side-effects
Gold treatments for arthritis[Q]	• **Gold deposition in the cornea and conjunctiva**, which are termed **chrysiasis** and are **gold to violet in color**. • These **deposits usually disappear with discontinuation of the medication**. • The **deposits generally do not affect vision** and are not a reason to stop gold therapy.
Tetracyclines[Q]	• **Yellow discoloration** of the **light-exposed conjunctiva[Q]**.
Systemic minocycline[Q]	• **Blue-gray scleral pigmentation** that is **most prominent in the interpalpebral zone[Q]**.

55. Ans. d. Bosentan *(Ref: Harrison 19/e p1659, 18/e p2079)*

Bosentan is a non-specific antagonist of endothelin receptors (both ET-A & ET-B). It is FDA approved drug for the treatment of pulmonary arterial hypertension. Calcium channel blockers (amlodipine) have not been approved for the treatment of PAH by the US FDA.

> *"Treatment of Pulmonary Arterial Hypertension: Endothelin receptor antagonists (ERAs) target endothelin-1 (ET-1), a potent endogenous vasoconstrictor and vascular smooth muscle mitogen that is elevated in PAH patients. Endothelin levels are increased coincident with increased PVR and mPAP and decreased CO and 6MWD.*
> *ERAs block the binding of ET-1 to either endothelin receptor A (ET-A) and/or B (ET-B). ET-A receptors found on pulmonary artery smooth muscle cells mediate vasoconstriction. In the normal pulmonary vasculature, ET-B receptors are found on endothelial cells and mediate vasodilation via production of prostacyclin and nitric oxide as well as ET-1 clearance. **Three ERAs approved for use in the United States are bosentan and macitentan both, nonselective receptor antagonists, and ambrisentan, a selective ET-A receptor antagonist.**"—Harrison 19/e p1659*

Idiopathic Pulmonary Arterial Hypertension (IPAH)
• Formerly referred to as **primary pulmonary hypertension, is uncommon** • **Female predominance[Q]** • **Most patients presenting in** the **4th & 5th decades** • **Familial IPAH** accounts for **up to 20%** of cases of IPAH and is characterized by **autosomal dominant inheritance** and incomplete penetrance.

Natural History:
- **Disease typically is diagnosed late in its course[Q]**.
- **Before current therapies**, a **mean survival of 2-3 years from the time of diagnosis[Q]** was reported.
- **Functional class** remains a **strong predictor of survival**, with patients who are in New York Heart Association (NYHA) functional class IV having a mean survival of <6.

Treatment of Pulmonary Arterial Hypertension	
Calcium Channel Blockers	• Patients **who respond to short-acting vasodilators** at the time of cardiac catheterization **should be treated with CCBs**. • **Not effective in patients who are not vasoreactive**. • **Not approved for the treatment of PAH** by the **US FDA[Q]**.
Endothelin-Receptor Antagonists	• **Bosentan & ambrisentan** are **approved** for the **treatments of PAH[Q]**. • **Bosentan is contraindicated** in patients who are on **cyclosporine or glyburide concurrently[Q]**.
Phosphodiesterase-5 Inhibitors	• **Sildenafil and tadalafil** are **approved for the treatment of PAH[Q]**. • **MC side effect is headache**. • **Neither drug should be given to patients** who are **taking nitro vasodilators**.
Prostacyclins	• **Iloprost is approved via inhalation for PAH[Q]**. • **Epoprostenol** is approved as a **chronic IV treatment of PAH**. • **Treprostinil, an analogue of epoprostenol**, is **approved for PAH** and may be given intravenously, subcutaneously, or via inhalation. • The **intravenous prostacyclins** have the **greatest efficacy** as treatments for PAH and are often **effective in patients who have failed all other treatments**.
Lung Transplantation	• Lung transplantation is considered for patients who, **while on an intravenous prostacyclin, continue to manifest right heart failure**.

FDA-Approved Therapies for Pulmonary Arterial Hypertension		
Group	**Drugs**	**Indication**
Prostacyclin derivative	Epoprostenol[Q]	• Treatment of **PAH** to **improve exercise capacity**
	Iloprost[Q]	• Treatment of **PAH** to improve a composite endpoint consisting of exercise tolerance, symptoms (NYHA Class), and lack of deterioration
	Treprostinil[Q]	• Treatment of **PAH** to **improve exercise ability**
Non-selective endothelin receptor antagonist	Bosentan[Q]	• Treatment of **PAH** to **improve exercise capacity** and to **decrease clinical worsening**
	Macitentan[Q]	• Treatment of **PAH** to **improve exercise capacity** and **delay clinical worsening**
Endothelin receptor antagonist	Ambrisentan[Q]	• Treatment of **PAH** to **improve exercise capacity** and **delay clinical worsening**
PDE5 inhibitor	Sildenafil[Q]	• Treatment of **PAH** to **improve exercise capacity** and **delay clinical worsening**
	Tadalafil[Q]	• Treatment of **PAH to improve exercise ability**
Soluble guanylyl cyclase stimulator	Riociguat[Q]	• Treatment of **PAH to improve exercise capacity** and **delay clinical worsening**

56. **Ans. a. Latanoprost** *(Ref: Katzung 13/e p328, 12/e p328)*

Latanoprost causes heterochromia iridis.

*"Latanoprost, a stable long-acting PGF2-alpha derivative, was the first prostanoid used for glaucoma. The success of latanoprost has stimulated development of similar prostanoids with ocular hypotensive effects, and **bimatoprost**, **travoprost**, and **unoprostone** are now available. These drugs act at the FP receptor and are administered as drops into the conjunctival sac once or twice daily. Adverse effects include irreversible brown pigmentation of the iris and eyelashes, drying of the eyes, and **conjunctivitis**."-Katzung 13/e p328, 12/e p328*

*"Acquired Heterochromia: Heterochromia that is acquired is usually due to injury, inflammation, the use of **certain eye drops** that damages the iris, or tumors. **Prostaglandin analogues (latanoprost, isopropyl unoprostone, travoprost, and bimatoprost)** are used topically to lower intraocular pressure in glaucoma patients. A **concentric heterochromia** has developed in some patients applying these drugs."*

Heterochromia of Iris

- **Congenital anomaly** characterized by **variations in the iris colour**
- **Heterochromia iridium**: **Colour of one iris differs** from the other.
- **Heterochromia iridis**: **One sector of the iris differs** from the remainder of iris.

Causes of Heterochromia iridis	
• **Waardenburg syndrome**[Q] • **Fuch's heterochromic iridocyclitis**[Q] • **Horner syndrome**[Q] • Melanosis oculi	• **Drugs: Prostaglandin analogues (Latanoprost**[Q]**)** • Iris melanoma

57. **Ans. c. Thiazide diuretic** *(Ref: Harrison 19/e p1623, 18/e p2054)*

Thiazide diuretic can be given in mild to moderate hypertension.

"Low-dose thiazide diuretics may be used alone or in combination with other antihypertensive drugs. Thiazides inhibit the Na⁺/Cl⁻ pump in the distal convoluted tubule and hence increase sodium excretion. In the long term, they also may act as vasodilators. Thiazides are safe, efficacious, inexpensive, and reduce clinical events. They provide additive blood pressure–lowering effects when combined with beta blockers, angiotensin-converting enzyme inhibitors (ACEIs), or angiotensin receptor blockers (ARBs)."-Harrison 19/e p1623

AIIMS ESSENCE

*"Two potassium-sparing diuretics, amiloride and triamterene, act by inhibiting epithelial sodium channels in the distal nephron. These agents are **weak antihypertensive agents** but may be **used in combination with a thiazide to protect against hypokalemia**."-Harrison 19/e p1623*

*"The **main pharmacologic target for loop diuretics** is the Na⁺-K⁺-2Cl⁻ cotransporter in the thick ascending limb of the loop of Henle. Loop diuretics generally are reserved for hypertensive patients with reduced glomerular filtration rates (reflected in serum creatinine >220 μmol/L [>2.5 mg/ dL]), **CHF, or sodium retention and edema** for some other reason, such as **treatment with a potent vasodilator, e.g., minoxidil**."-Harrison 19/e p1623*

Diuretics in Hypertension

- **Low-dose thiazide diuretics** may be **used alone or in combination with other antihypertensive drugs. Thiazides inhibit the Na⁺/Cl⁻ pump in the distal convoluted tubule** and hence increase sodium excretion. In the long term, they also may act as vasodilators.

  - **Thiazides are safe, efficacious, inexpensive, and reduce clinical events.** They provide additive blood pressure–lowering effects when combined with beta blockers, angiotensin-converting enzyme inhibitors (ACEIs), or angiotensin receptor blockers (ARBs)ᵠ.

- In contrast, addition of a diuretic to a calcium channel blocker is less effective.
- Usual doses of hydrochlorothiazide range from 6.25–50 mg/d. Owing to an increased incidence of metabolic side effects (hypokalemia, insulin resistance, increased cholesterol), higher doses generally are not recommended.

- **Chlorthalidone** is a diuretic structurally similar to hydrochlorothiazide, and like hydrochlorothiazide, it **blocks sodium-chloride cotransport** in the **early distal tubule**. However, **chlorthalidone has a longer half-life** (40–60 h vs. 9–15 h) and an antihypertensive potency ~1.5–2.0 times that of hydrochlorothiazide. Potassium loss is also greater with chlorthalidone.

  - Two potassium-sparing diuretics, **amiloride and triamterene**, act by **inhibiting epithelial sodium channels in the distal nephron.** These agents are **weak antihypertensive agents** but may be **used in combination with a thiazide to protect against hypokalemia**ᵠ.

- The **main pharmacologic target for loop diuretics** is the **Na⁺-K⁺-2Cl⁻ cotransporter in the thick ascending limb of the loop of Henle**.

  - **Loop diuretics generally are reserved for hypertensive patients with reduced glomerular filtration rates** (reflected in serum creatinine >220 μmol/L [>2.5 mg/ dL]), **CHF, or sodium retention and edema** for some other reason, such as **treatment with a potent vasodilator, e.g., minoxidil**ᵠ.

Drug of Choice in Hypertension

Condition	Drug of Choice
Hypertension	• **Thiazides**ᵠ
Hypertension with **BPH**	• **Prazosin**ᵠ
Hypertension with **diabetes mellitus**	• **ACE inhibitors**ᵠ
Hypertension with **ischemic heart disease (angina)**	• **Beta-blockers**ᵠ
Hypertension with **chronic kidney disease**	• **ACE inhibitors**ᵠ
Hypertension in **pregnancy**	• **Alpha-methyldopa**ᵠ
Hypertensive emergencies	• **Nicardipine + Esmolol**ᵠ
Hypertensive emergencies in **cheese reaction**	• **Phentolamine**ᵠ
Hypertensive emergencies in **clonidine withdrawal**	• **Phentolamine**ᵠ
Hypertensive emergencies in **aortic dissection**	• **Nitroprusside + Esmolol**ᵠ
Hypertensive emergencies in **pregnancy**	• **Labetalol**ᵠ

---

58. **Ans. b. M2** *(Ref: Goodman Gillman 13/e p107, 12/e p; Katzung 13/e p107, 12/e p100; KDT 7/e p101)*

Methacholine is a M2 receptor agonist.

	M_1	M_2	M_3
Location and function	**Autonomic ganglia:** Depolarization (late EPSP)[Q] **Gastric glands:** Histamine release and **acid secretion**[Q] **CNS:** Learning, memory and **motor functions**[Q]	**SA node:** Hyperpolarization, ↓ rate of impulse generation[Q] **AV node:** ↓ velocity of conduction **Atrium:** Shortening of APD, ↓ **contractility**[Q] **Ventricle:** ↓ contractility (slight as receptors are sparse) **Cholinergic nerve endings:** ↓ ACh release[Q] **CNS:** Tremors, analgesia **Visceral smooth muscles:** Contraction[Q]	**Visceral smooth muscles: Contraction**[Q] **Iris:** Constriction of pupil[Q] **Ciliary muscles: Contraction**[Q] **Exocrine glands: Secretion**[Q] **Vascular endothelium:** Release of NO → **Vasodilation**[Q]
Nature	**Gq-protein coupled**	**Gi/Go protein coupled**	**Gq-protein coupled**
Transducer mechanism	**IP$_3$/DAG** → ↑ cytosolic calcium; ↑ PLA$_2$ → PG synthesis	**K$^+$ channel opening, ↓ cAMP**	**IP$_3$/DAG** →↑ cytosolic calcium; ↑PLA$_2$ → PG synthesis
Agonists (Relatively selective)	**Oxotremorine,** MCN-343A	**Methacholine**[Q]	**Bethanechol**
Antagonists (Relatively selective)	Pirenzepine, Telenzepine	**Methoctramine, Tripitramine**	**Darifenacin, Solefenacin**

59. Ans. c. Metronidazole *(Ref: Goodman Gillman 12/e p1512,1542,1407; Katzung 13/e p802, 12/e p824)*

Metronidazole does not cause hearing loss.

"All aminoglycosides are ototoxic and nephrotoxic. Ototoxicity and nephrotoxicity are more likely to be encountered when therapy is continued for more than 5 days, at higher doses, in the elderly, and in the setting of renal insufficiency. Concurrent use with loop diuretics (e.g, furosemide, ethacrynic acid) or other nephrotoxic antimicrobial agents (eg, vancomycin or amphotericin) can potentiate nephrotoxicity and should be avoided if possible. Neomycin, kanamycin, and amikacin are the most ototoxic agents. Streptomycin and gentamicin are the most vestibulotoxic. Neomycin, tobramycin, and gentamicin are the most nephrotoxic."—Katzung 13/e p802

"Vestibular and auditory dysfunction can follow the administration of any of the aminoglycosides, and ototoxicity may become a dose-limiting adverse effect. Aminoglycoside induced ototoxicity results in irreversible, bilateral high-frequency hearing loss and temporary vestibular hypofunction."—Goodman Gillman 12/e p1512

"Auditory impairment, sometimes permanent, may follow the use of vancomycin or teicoplanin. Ototoxicity is associated with excessively high concentrations of these drugs in plasma (60-100 µg/mL of vancomycin)."—Goodman Gillman 12/e p1542

"The fatal oral dose of quinine for adults is ~2-8 g. Quinine is associated with a triad of dose-related toxicities when given at full therapeutic or excessive doses. These are cinchonism, hypoglycemia, and hypotension. Hearing and vision are particularly affected. Functional impairment of the eighth nerve results in tinnitus, decreased auditory acuity, and vertigo. Visual signs consist of blurred vision, disturbed color perception, photophobia, diplopia, night blindness, constricted visual fields, scotomata, mydriasis, and even blindness."—Goodman Gillman 12/e p1407

Drugs causing Ototoxicity	
Antibiotics	• **Aminoglycosides**[Q] • **Vancomycin**[Q]
Chemotherapeutic drugs	• **Cisplatin**[Q]
Diuretics	• **Ethacrynic acid**[Q] • **Furosemide**[Q]
Others	• **Quinine**[Q] • **Salicylates**[Q]

Aminoglycosides Side-Effects		
	Maximum	**Minimum**
Ototoxicity	• **Amikacin**[Q] **(Auditory)** • **Streptomycin**[Q] **(Vestibular)**	• **Netilmycin**[Q]
Nephrotoxicity	• **Neomycin >Gentamicin**[Q]	• **Streptomycin**[Q]
Neuromuscular Blockade	• **Neomycin >Streptomycin**[Q]	• **Tobramycin**[Q]

60. **Ans. d. Competitive and irreversible** *(Ref: Goodman Gillman 12/e p242; Katzung 13/e p115, 12/e p106; KDT 7/e p99)*

The type of inhibition of acetyl cholinesterase caused by organophosphates is competitive & irreversible.

"Organophosphates cause irreversible inhibition of Acetyl-cholinesterase while that caused by carbamates is reversible. Both bind at the esteratic site of the enzyme causing competitive inhibition."

*"Thus, the terms **reversible and irreversible** as applied to the **carbamoyl ester** and **organophosphate anti-ChE agents**, respectively, reflect only quantitative differences in rates of decarbamoylation or dephosphorylation of the conjugated enzyme. Both chemical classes **react covalently with the active center serine** in essentially the same manner as does ACh."*
—*Goodman Gillman 12/e p242*

Anticholinesterases			
Reversible		**Irreversible**	
Carbamates	**Acridine**	**Organophosphate**	**Carbamates**
• **Physostigmine** • **Neostigmine** • **Pyridostigmine** • **Edrophonium** • **Rivastigmine** • **Donepezil** • **Galantamine**	• **Tacrine**	• **Dyflos (DFP)** • **Echothiophate** • **Parathion** • **Malathion** • **Diazinon (TIK -20)** • **Tabun** • **Sarin** • **Soman**	• **Carbaryl** • **Propoxur**

MICROBIOLOGY

61. **Ans. c. Zona occludens** *(Ref: Sleisenger and Fordtran's textbook of Gastrointestinal and Liver Disease 10/e p1903)*

Zona occludens is disrupted by Vibrio cholerae.

*"**Vibrio cholerae** also produces **additional toxins** that may contribute to disease, including the **zonula occludens toxin (ZOT)** that **alters intestinal permeability by acting on intestinal epithelial cells tight junctions,** and the **accessory cholera endotoxin (ACE)."**—Sleisenger & Fordtran's textbook of Gastrointestinal and Liver Disease 10/e p1903*

Cholera Toxin
• **Vibrio cholerae** secretes **enterotoxin** protein, which is **actually encoded by a *bacteriophage (CT Xf)* resident in V. cholerae**[Q]. • **Enterotoxin is made up of 1 A subunit** (composed of **1A1 & 1 A2** peptide joined by disulfide link) and **5 B subunits**[Q].   • **Vibrio cholerae** also produces **additional toxins** that may contribute to disease, including the **zonula occludens toxin (ZOT)** that **alters intestinal permeability by acting on intestinal epithelial cells tight junctions,** and the **accessory cholera endotoxin (ACE).**

Contd...

AIIMS May 2015

Cholera Toxin	
Cholera Toxin	
B Subunit Pentamer	**Monomeric A Subunit**
• B subunit serves as a **landing pad** and it **binds (attaches) the holotoxin to the ganglioside GM1** present in plasma membrane of **mucosal cell (enterocyte) in intestine**[Q]	• A subunit contains **enzymatic activity**. A subunit then dissociates and **A$_1$ peptide passes (translocated) across cell membrane** into cytoplasm. • A$_1$ interacts with ARF **(ADP ribosylation factor)** and forms **ARF-A1 complex.** • ARF-A1 complex catalyzes **ADP ribosylation**[Q] **(using NAD$^+$ as donor)** of Gsα (GTP binding regulatory component) of **adenylate cyclase** up regulating the activity of this enzyme • **Chronically (persistently) activated adenyl cyclase** results in **elevation of C-AMP**, which **activates protein Kinase A (PKA)**. This in turn via **phosphorylation of CFTR (cystic fibrosis transmembrane regulator protein) and of Na$^+$ - H$^+$ exchanger** leads to **enhancement of Cl$^-$ secretion and inhibition of Na$^+$ absorption**[Q]. • Thus massive amounts of NaCl accumulate inside intestine lumen, attracting more water by osmosis and contributing to **characteristic watery (liquid) stools of cholera**[Q].

Toxin	Mode of Action
Pertussis Toxin	• **Inhibits adenyl cyclase (through Gi α subunit)**[Q]
Heat stable enterotoxin (ST) by **enterotoxigenic E. coli**	• **Persistent activation of _gaunylate cyclase_ & elevation of intracellular _Cyclic -GMP_**[Q]
Cholera Toxin **Heat labile enterotoxin (LT)** produced by enterotoxigenic strains of E. coli	• **ADP ribosylation (activation) of Gsα subunit** leads to persistent chronic activation of adenyl cyclase → **elevated c-AMP → activates PKA → Phosphorylation of CFTR & Na$^+$ - H$^+$ exchanger – ↓ Na$^+$ absorption & Cl$^-$ secretion → watery diarrhoea**[Q]

62 Ans. b. Onchocerca volvulus   *(Ref: Harrison 19/e p1420, 1422; Jawetz 27/e p733)*
Adult stage of Onchocerca volvulus filarial worms does not cause any illness or disease.

"Onchocerciasis primarily affects the skin, eyes, and lymph nodes. In contrast to the pathology in lymphatic filariasis, the damage in onchocerciasis is elicited by microfilariae and not by adult parasites."-Harrison 19/e p1420

"The distribution of M. ozzardi is restricted to Central and South America and certain Caribbean islands. Adult worms are rarely recovered from humans. Microfilariae circulate in the blood without periodicity. Although this organism has often been considered nonpathogenic, headache, articular pain, fever, pulmonary symptoms, adenopathy, hepatomegaly, pruritus, and eosinophilia have been ascribed to M. ozzardi infection. The diagnosis is made by detection of microfilariae in peripheral blood. Ivermectin is effective in treating this infection."-Harrison 19/e p1422

With Onchocerca, it is the microfilariae released from the female worms that cause the most severe damage. Migrating microfilariae, exclusively found in the interstitial fluids of the skin and subdermal tissues (not the bloodstream), cause changes in skin pigment and loss of elastic fibers, leading to "hanging groin," other skin changes, and severe pruritus, sometimes intractable and intolerable. Far more serious is the blindness that affects millions, mainly in Africa (primarily men). Visual loss develops over many years from an accumulation of microfilariae in the vitreous humor, since the microfilariae are not blood borne and can concentrate and remain in the fluids of the eye. Visual clouding, photophobia, and ultimately retinal damage result in incurable blindness."-Jawetz 27/e p733

Filariasis					
Organism	Periodicity	Vector	Location of Adult	Microfilarial Location	Sheath
Wuchereria bancrofti	Nocturnal	**Culex Anopheles Aedes**[Q]	Lymphatic tissue	Blood	+
Brugia malayi	Nocturnal	Mansonia, Anopheles Coquillettidia	Lymphatic tissue	Blood	+

Contd...

Contd...

Organism	Periodicity	Vector	Location of Adult	Microfilarial Location	Sheath
B. timori	Nocturnal	Anopheles[Q]	Lymphatic tissue	Blood	+
Loa loa	Diurnal	Chrysops[Q] (deer flies)	Subcutaneous tissue	Blood	+
Onchocerca volvulus	None	Simulium[Q] (black flies)	Subcutaneous tissue	Skin, eye	−
Mansonella ozzardi	None	Culicoides[Q] (midges)	Undetermined site	Blood	−
M. streptocerca	None	Culicoides[Q]	Subcutaneous tissue	Skin	−

63. **Ans. b. Hepatitis B virus**   *(Ref: Ananthanarayan 10/e p548, 9/e p544, 8/e p540; Harrison 19/e p2005; Robbins 9/e p831-832)*
    Hepatitis B virus uses reverse transcriptase.

    "Hepatitis B virus: A polymerase (Pol) that exhibits both DNA polymerase activity and reverse transcriptase activity. Genomic replication occurs via an intermediate RNA template, through a unique replication cycle: DNA → RNA → DNA."—Robbins 9/e p832

    "The third of the HBV genes is the largest, the P gene, which codes for the DNA polymerase; as noted above, this enzyme has both DNA-dependent DNA polymerase and RNA-dependent reverse transcriptase activities."—Harrison 19/e p2005

Hepatitis B virus Genes & Antigens	
Gene	Antigen Produced
C gene	HBcAg (Hepatitis B core antigen)[Q]
C & Pre C genes	HBeAg (Hepatitis B e antigen)[Q]
S gene	HBsAg (Hepatitis B surface antigen): large, middle & small HBsAg[Q]
P gene	DNA polymerase (pol) & reverse transcriptase[Q]
X gene	HBxAg: virus replication & transcriptional transactivator[Q]

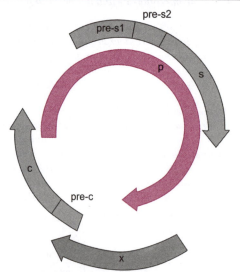

Fig. 13: Compact genomic structure of HBV

64. **Ans. c. HTLV**   *(Ref: Ananthanarayan 10/e p571, 574, 9/e p567; Harrison 19/e p697)*
    HTLV causes tropical spastic paresis.

    "HTLV-1 is also the cause of tropical spastic paraparesis—a neurologic disorder that occurs somewhat more frequently than lymphoma and with shorter latency and usually from transfusion-transmitted virus."—Harrison 19/e p697

"*HTLV-1 has been established as the causative agent of adult T-cell Leukemia-Lymphomas (ATL) as well as nervous system degenerative disorder called tropical spastic paraparesis.*"

Tropical Spastic Paraparesis
• Caused by HTLV[Q] • Affects **females** disproportionately
Pathology: • **Spinal cord**: **Symmetric degeneration** of the lateral columns, including the **corticospinal tracts**; some cases involve the posterior columns as well. • **Spinal meninges & cord parenchyma**: Inflammatory infiltrate with **myelin destruction**.

Clinical Features:
• Onset is **insidious; weakness or stiffness in one or both legs, back pain & urinary incontinence**[Q].
• The disease generally takes the **form of slowly progressive & unremitting thoracic myelopathy**[Q]
  • Patients display **spastic paraparesis or paraplegia with hyperreflexia, ankle clonus & extensor plantar responses**.
  • **Cognitive function is usually spared**; cranial nerve abnormalities are unusual.

Diagnosis: • MRI: Lesions in both the **white matter & paraventricular regions of the brain & spinal cord**[Q].

65. **Ans. a. Mast cell**   *(Ref: Ananthanarayan 10/e p100, 9/e p162, 163)*

IgE receptor is present on Mast cell.

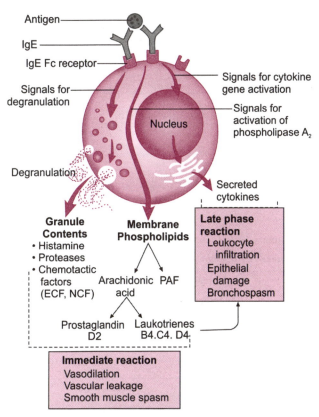

Fig. 14: Mast cell mediators

"IgE molecules are bound to surface receptors on mast cells and basophils. These cells carry large number of such receptors called Fc ER receptors, analogous to TCR receptors on T cell surface. IgE molecules attach to these receptors by their Fc end. Following exposure to the shocking dose, the antigen molecules combine with the cell bound IgE, bridging the gap between adjacent antibody molecules."—Ananthanarayan 10/e p101

Upon activation, mast cells release various classes of mediators that are responsible for the immediate and late-phase reactions. ECF, eosinophil chemotactic factor; NCF, neutrophil chemotactic factor (neither of these is biochemically defined); PAF, platelet-activating factor.

IgE
• **IgE molecules are bound to surface receptors on mast cells and basophils**[Q].
• Exhibits **unique properties such as heat lability** (inactivated at 56°C in one hour)
• **Affinity for the surface of tissue cells** (particularly mast cells) of the same species (homocytotropism).
• It **mediates the Prausnitz-Kustner reaction.**
• Normal serum contains only traces but **greatly elevated levels are seen in atopic** conditions (**type 1 allergic conditions such as asthma, hay fever and eczema.**)
• Children living in insanitary conditions, with a **high load of intestinal parasites**, have **high serum levels of IgE.**
• **IgE is chiefly produced in the linings of the respiratory and intestinal tracts**[Q].   • It is **responsible for the anaphylactic type of hypersensitivity**[Q]
• The physiological role of IgE appears to be **protection against pathogens by mast cell degranulation and release of inflammatory mediators**
• It is also believed to have a **special role in defense against helminthic infections**

Property	IgG	IgA	IgM	IgD	IgE
1. Percentage of total serum Ig	75-85% **(commonest)**[Q]	7-15%	5-10%	0.3%	0.019% **(least)**[Q]
2. Molecular weight (kDa)	150 **(Lightest)**[Q]	160	950 **(Heaviest)**[Q]	175	190
3. Usual molecular form	**Monomer**[Q]	Monomer **Dimer**[Q]	**Pentamer**[Q]	Monomer	Monomer
4. Subclasses	G_1, G_2, G_3, G_4 **(four)**[Q]	A_1, A_2 **(Two)**[Q]	None	None	None
5. Serum half life (Days)	**23**[Q] **(Maximum half life)**	6	5	3	**2.5**[Q] **(Shortest)**
6. Complement activation	**Classical**[Q] **(++)**	**Alternate**[Q]	**Classical**[Q] **(+++)**[Q]	**Alternate**[Q]	None
7. Placental transport	+	–	–	–	–
8. Present in milk	+	+	–	–	–
9. Selective secretion by seromucous glands	–	+	–	–	–
10. Heat stability (56°C)	+	+	+	+	–

66. **Ans. d. Nasopharyngeal carcinoma** *(Ref: Ananthanarayan 10/e p557, 9/e p553)*

Nasopharyngeal carcinoma is caused by Ebstein-Barr virus, not by HPV.

Human infections caused by HPV	
Diseases	**Serotype**
Skin warts (**Plantar wart**[Q], common wart, flat wart & **Epidermodysplasia verruciformis**[Q])	1, 2, 3, 4
Papilloma (Laryngeal, Oral)[Q]	6, 11
Condyloma acuminatum (genital wart)[Q]	6, 11
Oral squamous cell carcinoma[Q]	16, 18
Cervical intraepithelial neoplasia (CIN)[Q]	6, 11
Carcinoma cervix[Q]	16, 18, 31, 33, 35, 42-44

Oncogenic DNA virus	Oncogenic RNA virus
• *Human papilloma virus*[Q]	• *Hepatitis C virus*[Q]
• *Epstein-Barr virus*[Q]	• *Human T-cell leukemia virus type-1*[Q]
• *Hepatitis B virus*[Q]	• *Helicobacter pylori*[Q]

Infectious Agent	Lymphoid Malignancy
Epstein-Barr virus	• *Burkitt's lymphoma*[Q]
	• *Post-organ transplant lymphoma*[Q]
	• *Primary CNS diffuse large B cell lymphoma*[Q]
	• *Hodgkin's disease*[Q]
	• *Extranodal NK/T cell lymphoma, nasal type*[Q]
HTLV-I	• *Adult T cell leukemia/lymphoma*[Q]
HIV	• *Diffuse large B cell lymphoma*[Q]
	• *Burkitt's lymphoma*[Q]
Hepatitis C virus	• *Lymphoplasmacytic lymphoma*[Q]
Helicobacter pylori	• *Gastric MALT lymphoma*[Q]
Human herpes virus 8	• *Primary effusion lymphoma*[Q]
	• *Multicentric Castleman's disease*[Q]

Suspected Carcinogens	
Carcinogens	**Associated Cancer or Neoplasm**
Alkylating agents	**Acute myeloid leukemia, bladder** cancer[Q]
Androgens	**Prostate** cancer[Q]
Aromatic amines (dyes)	**Bladder** cancer[Q]
Arsenic	Cancer of the **lung, skin**[Q]
Asbestos	Cancer of the **lung, pleura, peritoneum**[Q]
Benzene	Acute myelocytic leukemia[Q]
Chromium	**Lung** cancer[Q]
Diethylstilbestrol (prenatal)	**Vaginal** cancer (clear cell)[Q]
Epstein-Barr virus	**Burkitt's lymphoma**, nasal T cell lymphoma[Q]
Estrogens	Cancer of the **endometrium, liver, breast**[Q]
Ethyl alcohol	Cancer of the **breast, liver, esophagus, head & neck**[Q]
Helicobacter pylori	Gastric cancer, gastric MALT lymphoma[Q]
Hepatitis B or C virus	**Liver** cancer[Q]
Human immunodeficiency	**Non-Hodgkin's lymphoma, Kaposi's sarcoma,** virus **squamous cell carcinomas**[Q] (especially of the urogenital tract)
Human papilloma virus	Cancers of the **cervix, anus, oropharynx**[Q]
Human T cell lymphotropic /lymphoma virus type 1 (HTLV-1)	Adult T cell leukemia[Q]
Immunosuppressive agents (azathioprine, cyclosporine, glucocorticoids)	Non-Hodgkin's lymphoma[Q]
Ionizing radiation (therapeutic or diagnostic)	**Breast, bladder, thyroid, soft tissue, bone, hematopoietic**[Q], and many more
Nitrogen mustard gas	Cancer of the **lung, head & neck, nasal sinuses**[Q]
Nickel dust	Cancer of the **lung, nasal sinuses**[Q]
Diesel exhaust	**Lung** cancer[Q] (miners)
Phenacetin	Cancer of the **renal pelvis & bladder**[Q]
Polycyclic hydrocarbons	Cancer of the **lung, skin**[Q] (especially SCC of scrotal skin)
Radon gas	**Lung** cancer[Q]
Schistosomiasis	**Bladder** cancer (squamous cell)[Q]
Sunlight (ultraviolet)	**Skin** cancer (squamous cell and melanoma)[Q]
Tobacco (including smokeless)	Cancer of the **upper aerodigestive tract, bladder**[Q]
Vinyl chloride	Liver cancer (angiosarcoma)[Q]

AIIMS ESSENCE

67. Ans. d. Cefotaxime is more active against beta-lactamase

(Ref: Ananthanarayan 10/e p333, 335, 9/e p327, 8/e p 331; Harrison 19/e p1011, 18/e p1228; Nelson 19/e p941,942)

"Cefotaxime or ceftazidime is the drug of choice for the treatment of Hemophilus meningitis. Ampicillin and cotrimoxazole were popular for respiratory infections, but as plasmid-borne resistance to these drugs is now common, thus amoxicillin-clavulanate or clarithromycin is more effective. Plasmid for beta lactamase production makes them resistant."—Ananthanarayan 10/e p335

"Antibiotic Resistance: Most H. influenzae isolates are susceptible to ampicillin amoxicillin, but about a third produce a beta-lactamase and are therefore resistant beta-Lactamase-negative ampicillin-resistant (BLNAR) isolates have been identified that manifest resistance by production of a beta-lactam-insensitive cell wall synthesis enzyme called PBP3. Amoxicillin-clavulanate is uniformly active against H. influenzae clinical isolates except for the rare BLNAR isolates. Among macrolides azithromycin is active against about 99% of H. influenza isolates; in contrast, the activity of erythromycin and clarithromycin against H. influenzae clinical isolates is poor. H. influenzae resistance to 3rd-generation cephalosporins has not been documented. Resistance to trimethoprim-sulfamethoxazole is infrequent (≈10%), and resistance to quinolones is believed to be rare."

"Initial therapy for meningitis due to Hib should consist of a cephalosporin such as ceftriaxone or cefotaxime.

Administration of glucocorticoids to patients with Hib meningitis reduces the incidence of neurologic sequelae. Many infections caused by non-typable strains of H. influenzae, such as otitis media, sinusitis, and exacerbations of COPD, can be treated with oral antimicrobial agents. Approximately 20–35% of non-typable strains produce β-lactamase (with the exact proportion depending on geographic location), and these strains are resistant to ampicillin. Several agents have excellent activity against non-typable H. influenzae, including amoxicillin/clavulanic acid, various extended-spectrum cephalosporins, and the macrolides, azithromycin and clarithromycin. In addition to β-lactamase production, alteration of penicillin- binding proteins—a second mechanism of ampicillin resistance—has been detected in isolates of H. influenzae."—Harrison 19/e p1011

"Clinically, meningitis caused by H. influenzae type b cannot be differentiated from meningitis caused by Neisseria meningitidis or Streptococcus pneumoniae. Antimicrobial therapy should be administered intravenously for 7-14 days for uncomplicated cases. Cefotaxime, ceftriaxone, and ampicillin cross the blood-brain barrier during acute inflammation in concentrations adequate to treat H. influenzae meningitis. Intramuscular therapy with ceftriaxone is an alternative in patients with normal organ perfusion."—Nelson 19/e p941

Hemophilus influenzae (Pfeiffer's bacillus)
Morphology:
• **Non-motile, non-sporing, oxidase positive**, gram negative bacilli[Q]
• Capsulated coccobacilli shows **pleomorphism**[Q]
• Stained by **Loeffler's methylene blue**[Q] or **Dilute carbol fuschin**[Q]
• Divided into 8 biotypes on the basis of **indole production, urease** and **ornithine decarboxyalse activity**[Q]
Culture:
• **Fildes agar** is the best for primary isolation[Q]
• On **Levinthal's medium**[Q], capsulated strains show distinctive iridesecence
• Requires **both X factor** (heat stable hemin) and **V factor** (heat labile coenzyme present in RBC), so heated or boiled blood agar is superior to plain agar[Q]
• Shows **"Satellitism"**[Q] (dependence on V factor) when **S. aureus is streaked across the blood agar.**
Antigenic properties:
• Hemophilus influenzae is the **first free living organism whose complete genome is sequenced**[Q]
• There are three major surface antigen- the **capsular polysaccharide**, the **outer membrane protein**, and **lipo-oligosaccharide**[Q]
• Major antigenic determinant is **capsular polysaccharide**[Q] based on which, it is typed into six capsular types
• Most isolates from **acute invasive infections belong to type b**[Q]
• **Type b capsule** has **unique structure containing pentose sugar** (ribose and ribitol) in the form of **polyribosyl ribitol phosphate** (PRP)[Q] instead of hexose and hexosamines

Contd...

AIIMS May 2015

Contd...

Types of Hemophilus influenzae	
Invasive	**Non-invasive**
• **Bacillus acts as a primary pathogen**, causing **acute invasive infections**[Q].	• **Bacillus spreads by local invasion along mucosal surfaces**[Q]
• **Bacilli spread through blood**, being protected from phagocytes by their **capsule**[Q].	• **Causes secondary or superadded infections**, usually of the **respiratory tract**[Q].
• **Meningitis** is the most important infection in this group,	• These include **otitis media, sinusitis and exacerbations of chronic bronchitis and bronchiectasis**[Q].
• **Others:** Laryngoepiglottits, conjunctivitis, bacteremia, pneumonia, arthritis, endocarditis and pericarditis.	
• Usually seen in **children**	• Usually seen in **adults**[Q]
• Caused by the **capsulated strains, type b accounting for most cases**.	• Caused by **non-capsulated strains**[Q]

Clinical Features:

• **Meningitis & respiratory tract infection** are the **most common presentation**[Q].

Meningitis
• Most frequently caused by **biotype-1**[Q]
• Occur in **children**[Q] due to absence of PRP antibodies
• **Subdural effusion**[Q] is the **MC complication**
• **DOC** is **ceftriaxone** or **cefotaxime**[Q]

• Hemophilus influenzae is called Pfeiffer's bacillus but **Pfieffer's phenomenon (bacteriolysis in vivo) is associated with V. cholera**[Q] (cholera vibrios were lysed when injected intraperitoneally into specifically immunized guinea pigs)

Organism	Drug of Choice
• **Streptococcus pneumoniae, S. viridans, Hemolytic streptococci group A, B, C, G** • **Staphylococcus (non-penicillinase producing)** • **Actinomyces, Bacillus cereus, Clostridium** • **Neisseria meningitidis** • **Treponema pallidum, T. pertenue**	**Penicillin G**[Q]
• **MRSA, Coagulase negative Staphylococcus** • **Enterococcus faecium**	**Vancomycin**[Q]
• **Enterococcus faecalis, Listeria**	**Ampicillin**[Q]
• **Bacillus anthracis** • **Borrelia burgdorferi, B. recurrentis** • **Chlamydia & Rickettsiae**	**Doxycycline**[Q]
• **Corynebacterium**	**Erythromycin**[Q]
• **Hemophilus ducreyi & Mycoplasma**	**Azithromycin**[Q]
• **Nocardia**	**Cotrimoxazole**[Q]
• **E. coli, Klebsiella, Proteus** • **Salmonella**	**Ceftriaxone**[Q]
• **Serratia, Enterobacter, Acinetobacter**	**Carbapenems**[Q] **(SEA)**
• **Bacteroides**	**Metronidazole**[Q]

FORENSIC MEDICINE

68. **Ans. d. Bruise, laceration, fractures are triad of main explosive injuries seen** *(Ref: Reddy 34/e p226, 33/e p239,240; Sabiston 19/e p612,613; Bailey 26/e p430, 25/e p422,423)*

Marshall's triad is diagnostic of explosive injury. Marshall's triad includes bruises, abrasions & puncture lacerations, not the fracture.

AIIMS ESSENCE

"*Marshall's* triad is diagnostic of explosive injury. Marshall's triad includes bruises, abrasions & puncture lacerations."

See Q. No. 86 AIIMS November 2015.

69. Ans. b. Angle of the jaw *(Ref: Reddy 34/e p315, 316, 33/e p346)*

In judicial hanging, the knot is placed at angle of the jaw.

"*Judicial Hanging: Placement of knot beneath the chin (submental position) is thought to be **most effective, ensuring a quicker death**. However, in **India & UK**, left sub aural (below angle of jaw) knot* is preferred for hanging."

Hanging
• A form of **violent asphyxia** as a result of **suspension of body by a ligature round the neck**
• **Constricting force: Weight of the body**

Types of Hanging			
According to Knot Ligature		According to Degree Suspension	
Typical Hanging	**Atypical Hanging**	**Complete Hanging**	**Partial Hanging**
Knot at the **nape of neck** on the **back**[Q]	• Knot at any site other than nape of neck • **MC site: Near one side of mastoid process** or **near angle of mandible**[Q]	• Body is **fully suspended**[Q] • No part of the body touches ground • **Constricting force: Body weight**[Q]	• **Lower part of body** is in **touch with ground**[Q] • **Constricting force: Weight of head**[Q]

Judicial Hanging
• Placement of knot beneath the chin (submental position) is thought to be **most effective, ensuring a quicker death**[QQ].
• However, in **India & UK**, left sub aural (below angle of jaw) knot is **preferred for hanging**.
• Rope is looped around the neck & person is allowed to **drop for 5-7 meters** according to the weight, age and build of the person.
• **Sudden stop** causes **fracture dislocation** usually at level of **C2-C3** or **C3-C4 vertebra**[Q], and rupture of brain stem between pons & medulla.
• **Death is instantaneous** but the heart-beat may continue for 15-20 minutes and spasmodic muscle jerking may occur for considerable time.

70. Ans. c. Heat stroke *(Ref: Reddy 34/e p296, 297, 33/e p319; Parikh 6/e p3.81)*

Sweating is not present in Heat stroke.

"*Heat stroke (hyperpyrexia, sunstroke, systemic hyperthermia): This is attributed to an **impaired functioning of the heat regulating mechanism** caused by **failure of cutaneous circulation** and **sweating**. It is due to prolong exposure to the sun's infrared rays, and/or to hot atmosphere.*"

Heat stroke (Heat hyperpyrexia/Sun stroke/ Thermic Fever)	Heat cramps (Miner's cramps/ Stoker's cramp/ Firemen's cramp)	Heat exhaustion (Heat collapse/Heat syncope/Heat prostration)
• It is **due to failure of heat regulating mechanism**[Q] • Caused by **failure of cutaneous circulation & sweating**[Q]. • Occurs due to **exposure to heat** in **open & humid environment**[Q]. • **All signs of shock** are present • There is **sudden collapse with loss of consciousness**. • Dry skin, hot flushes with **absence of sweating**[Q]	• These are **painful spasm** of voluntary muscles, which follow strenuous work in a hot atmosphere. • Caused by **loss of water & salt in profuse sweating**[Q].	• Collapse without any elevation of body temperature. • Occurs due to **exposure to high temperature in closed environment** • **Precipitated by muscular exercise & unsuitable clothing.** • There is **extreme exhaustion with peripheral vascular collapse with scanty** sweating[Q]

AIIMS May 2015

71. Ans. b. Paraldehyde *(Ref: Reddy 34/e p349, 33/e p507)*

Acrid smell or pear smell is seen in paraldehyde and chloral hydrate[Q] poisoning

*"Paraldehyde is a **clear colorless liquid** with an **ethereal odour and acrid taste**. It is used as a hypnotic by mouth rectum or parenterally as a basal anesthetic."*

Characteristic Odours produced by Toxins	
Odour	**Toxins**
Acrid (Pear smell)	• **Paraldehyde[Q], Chloral hydrate[Q]**
Bitter almonds	• **Cyanide[Q]**
Burnt rope	• **Marijuana (Cannabis)[Q]**
Disinfectant	• **Phenol** (Carbolic acid), Creosote
Garlic	• **Phosphorus[Q]**, Tellurium, Thallium • Dimethyl sulfoxide (DMSO)
Fish or raw liver (Musty)	• **Zinc phosphide[Q], Aluminum phosphide[Q]**
Kerosene like	• **Organophosphate**
Mint	• Methylsalicylate (Oil of Wintergreen), Menthol
Mothballs	• Naphthalene, Camphor, p-dichlorobenzene
Pepper	• **o-chlorobenzylidene malonitrile (Tear gas)**
Rotten eggs	• **Hydrogen sulphide[Q], Carbon disulphide[Q]** • **Mercaptans. Disulfiram[Q], N-acetylcysteine[Q]**
Shoe polish	• **Nitrobenzene**
Vinegar	• **Acetic acid[Q]; Hydrofluoric acid**

72. Ans. c. 18 years *(Ref: http://indiacode.nic.in/acts-in-pdf/132013.pdf; https://en.wikipedia.org/wiki/Criminal_Law_(Amendment)_Act,_2013)*

According to the 2013 amendment, the age for sexual consent is 18 years.

"The age of consent in India has been increased to 18 years, which means any sexual activity irrespective of presence of consent with a woman below 18 years of age will constitute rape."

*"Section 375 Sexual Assault: Sexual assault means **with or without the complainant's consent**, when such complainant is **under eighteen years of age."***

The Criminal Law (Amendment) Act, 2013	
• The Bill was passed by the Lok Sabha on 19 March 2013, and by the Rajya Sabha on 21 March 2013, making certain changes from the provisions in the Ordinance.	
• The Bill received Presidential assent on 2 April 2013 and came into force from 3 April 2013.	
• **The changes made in the Act in comparison with the Ordinance is listed as follows:**	

Offence	Changes
Acid attack	• Fine shall be just and reasonable to meet medical expenses for treatment of victim, while in the Ordinance it was fine up to Rupees 10 lakhs.
Sexual harassment	• "Clause (v) any other unwelcome physical, verbal or non-verbal conduct of sexual nature" has been removed. • Punishment for offence under clause (i) and (ii) has been reduced from five years of imprisonment to three years. **The offence is no longer gender-neutral, only a man can commit the offence on a woman.**

Contd...

Contd...

Offence	Changes
Voyeurism	• The offence is no longer gender-neutral, only a man can commit the offence on a woman.
Stalking	• The offence is **no longer gender-neutral, only a man can commit the offence on a woman**. The definition has been reworded and broken down into clauses, The exclusion clause and the following sentence has been removed "or watches or spies on a person in a manner that results in a fear of violence or serious alarm or distress in the mind of such person, or interferes with the mental peace of such person, commits the offence of stalking". • Punishment for the offence has been changed; A man committing the offence of stalking would be liable for imprisonment up to three years for the first offence, and shall also be liable to fine and for any subsequent conviction would be liable for imprisonment up to five years and with fine.
Trafficking of person	• "Prostitution" has been removed from the explanation clause
Rape	• The word **sexual assault has been replaced back to rape**. The offence is **no longer gender-neutral**, only a man can commit the offence on a woman. • The clause related to touching of private parts has been removed.

73. **Ans. a. Doctor is guilty under "Last clear chance" doctrine** *(Ref: Reddy 34/e p38, 33/e p40)*

Last Clear Chance Doctrine: In our case the doctor could have saved the patient (plaintiff) by his action of dressing the wound properly the second time he must have been cured without developing osteomyelitis (defendant-in this case doctor), so he is partly guilty for the outcome (osteomyelitis).

Contributory negligence
• **Contributory negligence** is any **unreasonable conduct, or absence of ordinary care on the part of the patient,** or **his personal attendant,** which **combined with the doctor's negligence,** contributed to the injury complained of, as a direct, proximate cause and without which the injury would not have occurred.

• These include:
   – **Failure to give the doctor accurate medical history.** If the patient provides incomplete or inadequate information, it could result in misdiagnosis, mistreatment and harm.
   – **Failure to cooperate** with his doctor in carrying out all reasonable and proper instructions
   – **Refusal to take the suggested treatment**
   – **Leaving the hospital against the doctor 's advice**
   – **Failure to seek further medical assistance if symptoms persist**
• As such, the doctor's negligence is not the direct, proximate cause (actual or legal cause) of the injury suffered by the patient. Proximate cause means, that which in natural and continuous sequence unbroken by any efficient intervening cause produces the injury, and without which the result would not have occurred. If the doctor and the patient are negligent at the same time, it is a good defense for the doctor.
• **The doctor cannot plead contributory negligence, if he fails to give proper instructions.** Liability of the doctor: The extent of contributory negligence may vary and with it will vary the doctor's liability, from complete no liability to a substantial liability for damages.
• **Normally, contributory negligence is only a partial defense,** and the Court has right to fix liability between the parties (doctrine of comparative negligence), and damages awarded may be reduced accordingly. The burden of proof lies entirely on the doctor.
• If a patient consent's to take the risk of the injurious event actually taking place, he cannot claim damages. If a doctor is not negligent, but if a patient is negligent which results in injury, it is called negligence of the patient.

Contd...

Last Clear Chance Doctrine

- If the **doctor fails to prevent damage resulting from the negligent act of the patient, even after getting clear time, he cannot plead contributory negligence in civil cases**.
- **The elements of proof for the last clear chance doctrine are:**
  - The **plaintiff placed themselves in a situation of risk or danger through their own negligence**
  - The plaintiff **could not avoid the danger**
  - The **defendant recognized the danger, and thus acquired a duty to avoid it**
  - The **defendant failed to avoid the danger**
  - The **plaintiff was injured as a result of the defendant's failure**
    - In our case the **doctor could have saved the patient (plaintiff) by his action of dressing the wound properly the second time he must have been cured without developing osteomyelitis** (defendant-in this case doctor), so **he is partly guilty for the outcome (osteomyelitis).**

Avoidable Consequences Rule

- It is the **negligence of the patient, which aggravated the damage already caused by negligence of the doctor**, which could have been avoided if the patient was not negligent afterwards.
- In such case the **doctor cannot plead contributory negligence in civil cases.**
- **Good Samaritan doctrine: One who assists another who is in serious danger cannot be charged with contributory negligence**, unless the assistance is reckless or rash.

Limitations to Contributory negligence

Last Clear Chance Doctrine	Avoidable Consequences Rule
• Under this rule, a **person who has negligently placed himself in a position of danger may recover damages, if the doctor discovered the danger while there was still time to avoid the injury or failed to do so.**	• This is applicable where the **negligence of the injured person occurs after that of the doctor being sued and increases the severity of injury.** • In such cases, the patient is not guilty of contributory negligence, since his actions were not a cause of the injury.

---

74. **Ans. a. Kevorkian sign** *(Ref: Reddy 34/e p145, 33/e p154)*

Segmentation of blood in blood vessel after death is known as Kevorkian sign.

"Fragmentation or segmentation (trucking or shunting) of the blood columns (Kevorkian sign) in the retinal vessels appear within minutes after death, and persist for about an hour."- Reddy 34/e p145

Postmortem changes in the Body

- The postmortem changes take place in the body after death and **help in estimation of the approximate time since death.**
- These changes can be divided into following signs:

Immediate Signs of Death (Due to somatic death)

Permanent & complete cessation of functions of lung	• There is complete cessation of respiration for **>5 minutes** **Tests for confirming cessation of respiration are:** • **Feather test:** No movement of feather if held in front of nose. • **Mirror test:** Mirror held in front of nose does not show vapors and blurring. • **Winslow's test: No movement of reflection of light shone on mirror/ surface water in bowl, kept on chest**[Q].

AIIMS ESSENCE

Contd...

Permanent & complete cessation of functions of heart & flat ECG	• There is **complete stoppage of heartbeat for >3 minutes with flat ECG.** **Tests for confirming cessation of circulation are:** • **Magnus test (ligature test):** Fingers fail to show congestion & swelling to a ligature applied at their base[Q]. • **Diaphanous test (transillumination test): Failure to show redness in finger web spaces** on transillumination from behind. • **Icard's test: Failure to produce yellowish green discoloration of skin** on injection of fluorescein dye[Q]. • **Fingernail test: No blanching & filling** applying pressure and release of pressure.
Permanent & complete cessation of functions of brain function & flat EEG	• There is complete cessation of function, which leads to insensibility, unresponsiveness to external stimuli or internal needs, loss of muscle tone and flat EEG.

Early Signs (Due to molecular or cellular death)	
Skin	Loss of translucency and elasticity, skin becomes greyish white, lips become dry hard and brownish.
Eye	The changes in eye are: • **Abolition of pupillary & corneal reflexes[Q]** • **Cornea** becomes **hazy & opaque[Q]** • **Tache noire de salerotica: Cellular debris & mucus form yellow triangles** at each side of iris/cornea. • **Decrease in IOP causes flaccidity of eyeball.** Normal IOP is 14-25 mmHg. It is 12 mmHg immediately after death, 3 mmHg at 3 hours after death and 0 at 2 hours after death. • **Increased in level of potassium[Q], ascorbic acid[Q] & lactic acid[Q]** in vitreous humor. • **Potassium: Most useful component of vitreous humor for determining the time since death[Q]** • **Retinal Vessels: Fragmentation or segmentation** (trucking or shunting) of **the blood columns (Kevorkian sign) in the retinal vessels appear within minutes after dea**th, and persists for about an hour. • This occurs all over the body due to loss of blood pressure but it can be seen only in retina by ophthalmoscope.
Algor mortis	**Cooling of body**
Livor mortis	**Postmortem lividity or postmortem staining**
Muscular changes	Primary relaxation, Rigor mortis, secondary relaxation

Late Signs (Decomposition or Decay after molecular Death)
• **Putrefaction, Adipocere & Mummification**

75. **Ans. d. Bullet injury** *(Ref: Reddy 34/e p207, 33/e p219; Parikh 6/4.43)*

Rat hole is associated with Bullet injury.

*"**Intermediate range shotgun wounds:** At a distance of 60–90 cm, **single irregular circular aperture** 4 to 5 cm with **irregular and lacerated edges** is produced. The shots are **scattered after entering the wound** and **cause much damage to the internal tissues**. At a distance of 1.5 meters, the shot mass enters the body in one mass, producing a round defect. The margins are abraded. **At a distance of 2 meters, the shot mass begins to spread. The wound of entry is irregular**, with **ragged margins (rat hole)** about 5 cm in a diameter with a **few satellite perforations at the margins of the main defect**."*

See Q. No. 81 AIIMS May 2016

76. **Ans. d. Ring fracture of foramen magnum with lumbar spine injury** *(Ref: Reddy 34/e p231, 33/e p247; Parikh's 6/4.94-4.97)*

*"**Ring fracture:** This term is commonly used to signify **any fracture around the foramen magnum.** Technically it means a **fissured fracture** about 3.5 cm outside the foramen magnum at the back, **involving middle ear sideways** and **roof of nose anteriorly**. It is **rare** and usually **requires a lot of force to produce**. It results from **fall from a height on feet or buttocks**, sudden violent turn of head on spine, severe blow on the vertex which drives the skull downwards on the vertebral column or heavy blow directed underneath the occiput or chin."*

AIIMS May 2015

Ring or Foramen Fractures
• It is **fissured fracture**, which **encircles the skull** in such a manner that **the anterior third is separated at its junction with the middle and posterior third**.
• But usually the term is applied to a fracture, which **runs at about 3 to 5 cm outside the foramen magnum at the back and sides of the skull**, and **passes forwards through the middle ears** and **roof of the nose,** due to which the **skull is separated from the spine**.
• They are **rare** and **occur after falls from a height on to the feet or buttocks.**[Q]

Skull-vault fracture	
Type of fracture	**Description**
Diastatic fracture (sutural fractures)	• **Separation of sutures**[Q] • Occurs only in young persons due to **blow with blunt weapon** or from **cerebral edema**[Q]
Fissured fracture	• A linear fracture or crack involving the outer or inner table or both. • Fracture only involving inner table cannot be detected on X-ray. It can be detected at autopsy
Depressed fracture	• Caused by a **heavy weapon** with a **small striking surface** e.g., hammer • Its **shape** may indicate the **type of weapon** with which it is produced. It is therefore called as **signature fracture**[Q].
Comminuted fracture	• It has **stellate appearance** when there is no displacement of fragments. • Also called **spider web fracture**[Q]
Pond fracture	• Occurs in children due to elasticity of their bones • Also called **indented fractures**[Q]
Gutter fracture	• When a part of thickness of bone is removed to form a gutter e.g., **glancing oblique bullet wounds**[Q]
Elevated fracture	• Result from a blow of **moderately heavy sharp edge weapon** e.g., axe which **elevate one end of bone above the surface while other end may dip down to injured dura**[Q]
Ring fracture	• Any fracture around the foramen magnum[Q]

77. **Ans. a. 416 CrPC**   *(Ref: Reddy 33/e p392; Textbook on the Indian Penal Code by Krishna Deo Gaur 4/e p594; the-indian-penal-code-pdf-d74214920)*

The high court has the power to stay the execution of a pregnant woman according to section 416 of Criminal Procedure Code.

*"Section 416 in the Code of Criminal Procedure, 1973: Postponement of capital sentence pregnant woman. If a woman sentenced to death is found to be **pregnant, the High Court** shall **order** the **execution of the sentence to be postponed,** and may, if it thinks fit, **commute the sentence to imprisonment for life."***

See Q. No. 83 AIIMS November 2016

78. **Ans. c. 324**   *(Ref: Reddy 34/e p275, 33/e p292)*

In this case, a dangerous weapon was used for causing hurt it comes under section 324 of IPC.

Section	Deals with
302 IPC	**Punishment for murder**[Q]
304A IPC	• **Causing death by negligence, punishment up to 2 years (medical negligence)**
304B IPC	• **Dowry death**[Q], **punishment 7 years to life imprisonment**
324 IPC	• **Voluntarily causing hurt by dangerous weapons or means**
326 IPC	• Voluntarily causing **grievous hurt by dangerous weapons or means**

See Q. No. 83 AIIMS November 2016

79. **Ans. c. Sparrow foot marks**   *(Ref: Reddy 34/e p263, 33/e p281)*

Sparrow footmarks occur in both driver as well as passengers. It does not differentiate between driver and passenger.

> *"Sparrow foot marks: Multiple punctuate lacerations of the face are produced **due to the shattering of the windscreen glass into multiple small cubical fragments with relatively blunt edges (Windshield glass injury)**.*

Motor Vehicle Injuries	
Car (Four-wheeler) Injuries	
Sparrow foot marks[Q]	• **Multiple punctuate lacerations on face** are produced **due to shattering of windscreen glass into multiple small blunt edged fragments**.
Whiplash injury[Q]	• **Acute hyperflexion followed by hyperextension of neck** due to violent acceleration or deceleration force. • **Applied to (front seat) passenger** (passenger >Driver)
Steering wheel impact type injury[Q]	• Occurs **due to sudden stop of car, throwing forward the driver** • **Throat crushed across top of steering wheel** or **horn ring** (Occurs in driver)
Seat belt syndrome[Q]	• Contusion, laceration, perforation & avulsions of small intestine, omentum, & mesentery • There may be **rupture of abdominal aorta, spleen, liver, pancreas, caecum;** hematoma of lower abdomen; and fracture of lumbar vertebra. • **Seat belt injury: Left shoulder in passenger & right shoulder in driver**
Hinge fracture	• **Skull base fracture** running along the petrous ridges through sella turcica, i.e. **transverse fracture through middle cranial fossa**
Ladder tears	• **Multiple transverse intimal tears in aorta**, adjacent to main rupture.
Motor cycle (Two-wheelers) Injuries	
Motorcyclist fracture	• **Hinge fracture of base of skull**, dividing it into anterior & posterior half
Under running (Tail gating)	• Motorcyclist may drive into the back of large vehicle (e.g. truck) due to its sudden and unexpected stoppage.
Ring fracture (Foramen magnum fracture)[Q]	• **Fissured fracture of skull** which **encircles foramen magnum** in such a way that anterior 1/3rd is separated from posterior 2/3rd at its junction.
Bicycle spoke injury[Q]	• It occurs when a rider or passenger on a bicycle slips from seat and his foot or leg passes through the space of wheel.

PSM

80. **Ans. d. Testicular tumor**   *(Ref: Harrison 19/e p481, 18/e p662)*

   Screening is not useful in testicular tumor.

Screening Recommendations for Asymptomatic Subjects		
Cancer Type	Test or Procedure	ACS: American Cancer Society
Breast	Self-examination	Women ≥20 years: Breast self-exam is an option
	Clinical examination	Women 20–39 years: Perform every 3 years Women ≥40 years: Perform annually
	Mammography	Women ≥40 years: **Screen annually for as long as the woman is in good health**
	Magnetic resonance imaging (MRI)	Women with **>20% lifetime risk** of breast cancer: Screen with **MRI plus mammography annually** Women with **15–20% lifetime risk** of breast cancer: Discuss option of **MRI plus mammography annually** Women with **<15% lifetime risk** of breast cancer: **Do not screen annually with MRI**

Contd...

Contd...

Cervical	Pap test (cytology)	Women **21–29 years**: Screen **every 3 years** Women **30–65 years**: Acceptable approach to screen with cytology **every 3 years** Women **<21 years: No screening** Women **>65 years: No screening following adequate negative prior screening**
	HPV test	Women **30–65 years**: Preferred approach to screen with **HPV and cytology co-testing every 5 years** Women **<30 years: Do not use HPV testing** Women **>65 years: No screening following adequate negative prior screening** Women **after total hysterectomy** for noncancerous causes: **Do not screen**
Colorectal	Sigmoidoscopy	Adults **≥50 years**: Screen every **5 years**
	Fecal occult blood testing (FOBT)	Adults **≥50 years**: Screen every **5 years**
	Colonoscopy	Adults **≥50 years**: Screen every **10 years**
	Fecal DNA testing	Adults ≥50 years: Screen, but interval uncertain
	Fecal immunochemical testing (FIT)	Adults **≥50 years**: Screen **every year**
	CT colonography	Adults **≥50 years**: Screen **every 5 years**
Lung	Low-dose computed tomography (CT) scan	Men and women, 55–74 years, with ≥30 pack-year smoking history, still smoking or have quit within past 15 years: Discuss benefits, limitations, and potential harms of screening; only perform screening in facilities with the right type of CT scanner and with high expertise/specialists
Ovarian	CA-125 Transvaginal ultrasound	There is **no sufficiently accurate test proven effective in the early detection of ovarian cancer.** For women at high risk of ovarian cancer and/or who have unexplained, persistent symptoms, the combination of CA-125 and transvaginal ultrasound with pelvic exam may be offered.
Prostate	Prostate-specific antigen (PSA)	**Starting at age 50**, men should talk to a doctor about the pros and cons of testing so they can decide if testing is the right choice for them. If African American or have a father or brother who had prostate cancer before age 65, men should have this talk starting at age 45. How often they are tested will depend on their PSA level.
	Digital rectal examination (DRE)	As for PSA; if men decide to be tested, they should have the PSA blood test with or without a rectal exam
Skin	Complete skin examination	Self-examination monthly; clinical exam as part of routine cancer-related checkup

81. **Ans. a. 81-89**   *(Ref: Park 24/e p888, 22/e p793; Essentials of Biostatistics 2/e p170)*

Range for 90% confidence interval in the given question is 81-89.

Confidence Intervals
The Lower Limit and Upper Limit estimates for the Statistic are given as: • **Lower Limit: statistic – C x SE (statistic)** • **Upper Limit: statistic + C x SE (statistic)** **Standard Error, SE = {Standard Deviation / $\sqrt{n}$}** • **n = sample size**

Confidence coefficient
C = Confidence coefficient = 1.65 for **90%** confidence interval = **1.96** for **95%** confidence interval = **2.58** for **99%** confidence interval = **3.29** for **99.9%** confidence interval

Contd...

Confidence Intervals

In this question: **n = 100; SD = 25**
SE = 25/√100 = **2.5**

Now for 90% Confidence Interval
Lower limit = 85 – (1.65 x 2.5) = 85 – 4 = 81
Upper limit = 85 + (1.65 x 2.5) = 85 + 4 = 89
Hence, 90% CI will be 81–89.

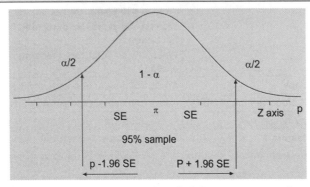

82. Ans. a. Tuberculosis *(Ref: Park 24/e p448, 23/e p429; http://nikshay.gov.in; www.nhp.gov.in)*

"Nikshay" is newly launched central government software. It is used for tracking tuberculosis.

"NIKSHAY, the web based reporting for monitoring RNTEP has been a notable achievement initiated in 2012. It has enabled capture and transfer of individual patient data from the remotest health institutions of the country."

Revised National Tuberculosis Control Programme: New Initiatives
1. The RNTCP has completed the feasibility study of introducing GeneXpert in RNTCP in 18 tuberculosis units in 12 states. RNTCP is currently using CB NAAT for the diagnosis of tuberculosis and MDT-TB in high-risk population like HIV positive and pediatric groups. **Cartridge based nucleic acid amplification test (CBNAAT):** The **second generation NAAT-based TB diagnostics** offer the prospect of **very high sensitivity,** approaching that of **liquid culture-the gold standard for TB diagnosis.**
2. **Nikshay: TB surveillance using case based, web based IT system** • Central TB division in collaboration with National Informatics Centre has undertaken the initiative to develop a **case based web based application Nikshay.** This software was launched in May 2012 and has following functional components: – **TB patient registration** and **details of diagnosis, DOTS provider, HIV status, follow-up, contact tracing, outcomes.** – **Details of solid and liquid culture and DST, LPA, CBNAAT details** – **Referral & transfer of patients** – **Private health facility registration and TB notification** – Mobile application for TB notification – SMS alerts to patients on registration – SMS alerts to programme officers – **Automated periodic reports: Case finding, sputum conversion, treatment outcome**
3. **TB Notification:** – In order to **ensure proper diagnosis and management of TB cases,** and **to reduce TB transmission** and the **emergence** and **spread of MDR-TB,** it is essential to have complete information of all TB cases. – According to Government of India notification dated 7th May 2012, it is now **mandatory for all healthcare providers to notify every TB case to local authorities** every month in a given format.
4. **Ban on TB Serology:** – The serological tests are based on antibody response, which is highly variable in TB and may reflect remote infection rather than active disease. – **Currently available serological tests** are having **poor specificity** and **should not be used for the diagnosis of pulmonary or extrapulmonary TB.** – Their **import, manufacturing, sale distribution** and **uses** are **banned by Government of India.**

AIIMS May 2015

83. Ans. a. Give cell culture derived vaccine *(Ref: Park's 24/e p297, 23/e p279, 22/e p253)*

The most appropriate course of action for this case is to give post-exposure prophylaxis with cell-culture derived vaccine.

Post-Exposure Prophylaxis

• The vast majority of patients requiring anti-rabies treatment are those who were bitten by a suspected rabid animal.
• **Aim: To neutralize the inoculated virus before it can enter the nervous system[Q].**
• **Every instance of human exposure should be treated as a medical emergency.**
 	
  • It is now well established that **irrespective of the class of wound**, the **combined administration of a single dose of rabies immunoglobulin** if indicated, with a course of **vaccine**, together with **local treatment of the wound** is the **best specific prophylactic treatment after exposure of a man to rabies[Q].**
 	
• Since their development more than four decades ago, **concentrated and purified cell-culture vaccine (CCV)** and **embryonated egg-based vaccine (EEV)** have **proved to be effective and safe in preventing rabies[Q].**
• These vaccines are **intended for pre-exposure** as well as **post-exposure prophylaxis**.
 	
  • **Post-exposure prophylaxis** may be **discontinued** if the **suspected animal** is proved by appropriate examination to be **free of rabies** or in the case of domestic dogs, cats or ferrets, the animal **remains healthy throughout a 10 days** observation period **starting from the date of bite.**

Categories of contact with suspected Rabid animal	Post-exposure prophylaxis measures
I. **Touching or feeding** animals **Licks on intact skin**	• **None[Q]**
II. **Nibbling of uncovered skin** **Minor scratches or abrasions** without bleeding	• **Immediate vaccination** and **local treatment of the wound[Q]**
III. **Single or multiple transdermal bites** or **scratches** **Licks on broken skin** **Contamination of mucous membrane with saliva from licks** **Contact with bats**	• **Immediate vaccination** and **administration of rabies immunoglobulin** and **local treatment of the wound[Q]**

84. Ans. b. Injury prevention *(Ref: http://en.wikipedia.org/wiki/Haddon_Matrix)*

Haddon matrix is related to injury prevention.

*"The **Haddon Matrix** is the **most commonly used paradigm in the injury prevention field**. The matrix looks at **factors related to personal attributes, vector or agent attributes and environmental attributes before, during and after an injury or death**. By utilizing this framework, one can then think about evaluating the relative importance of different factors and design interventions."*

Example of a typical Haddon Matrix			
Phase		**Human Factors**	**Vehicles and Equipment Factors**	**Environment Factors**
Pre-crash	Crash prevention	Information attitudes Impairment police Enforcement	Road worthiness Working lights Good brakes Driving skills Speed control	Road design and layout Speed limits Pedestrian facilities
Crash	Injury prevention during crash	Use of seat-belts Impairment	Seat-belts present Other safety devices Crash-protective Design	Crash protective road side objects
Post-crash	Life-sustaining	First-aid skills Access to medical help	Ease of access Fire-risk	Rescue facilities

Steps in using the Haddon Matrix	
Step 1	Use community data to **determine injury problem** that requires an intervention
Step 2	Brainstorm potential **ideas for interventions** and fill them into the cells of Haddon's Matrix
Step 3	**Make decisions about best intervention options** based upon effective strategies and practical to implement in your local situation

85. Ans. c. Student's T-test   *(Ref: Park 22/e p795; Biostatistics by Mahajan 7/e p134)*

In this question we are comparing a parametric quantitative variable (weight) in two groups of people who are unrelated. Hence, Student's t-test will be used.

	Parametric tests	**Non-parametric tests**
Based on	Gaussian Normal distributions	Non-normal distributions
Type of data	Quantitative	Qualitative
Compares	Means (+ SD)	Percentage, proportions & fractions
Examples	• **Students (paired) t-test:** Comparing means (+ SD) in paired data (in same group of individuals before and after an intervention) • **Students (unpaired) t-test:** Comparing means (+ SD) in two different groups of individuals • **ANOVA F-test:** Comparing means (+ SD) in more than two different group of individuals	• **Sign test:** Comparing percentage, proportions & fractions in paired data (in same group of individuals before and after an intervention) • **Chi-square test (χ^2-test):** Comparing percentage, proportions & fractions in two or more different group of individuals • **Fischer's test:** A variant of Chi-square test when **sample size <30** • **Wilcoxan test (signed rank):** Comparing percentage, proportions & fractions in matched paired data • **Wilcoxan test (rank sum):** Comparing percentage, proportions & fractions in two unpaired samples

Student t-test	

- **Student t-test** is used when the **outcome variable is normally distributed in the population (for quantitative data)** e.g., blood pressure, blood glucose

Paired t-test	**Unpaired t-test (Independent t-test)**
• **Comparing means (+ SD) in paired data (in same group of individuals before and after an intervention)** • **Example:** Blood sugar level in a sample of 10 patients is measured before giving and after giving the oral hypoglycemic. In this condition, **paired t-test is used (before & after)**	• **Comparing means (+ SD) in two different groups of individuals** • **Example:** Blood sugar concentration is measured in two different groups (A group of 10 patients and other group of 8 patients). To test the significance of difference between the means of the two groups, unpaired t-test is used.

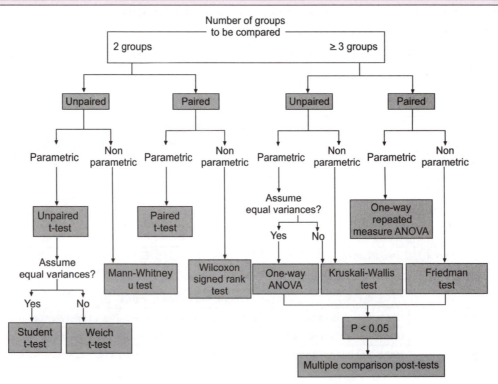

Chi-square Test (χ^2 Test)
• A 'non-parametric test' of significance[Q]
• Used to 'test significance of association between 2 or more qualitative characteristics'[Q]
• Used to compare proportions in 2 or more groups[Q]
• Used for non-Normal (non-Gaussian) distributions

Applications of Chi-square test		
• Test of proportions	• Test of association	• Test of goodness of fit

Essential requirements for calculation of Chi-square test		
• Random sample	• Qualitative data	• Lowest expected frequency not < 5

86. Ans. c. Selection bias *(Ref: Park 24/e p78, 88, 23/e p73, 22/e p71; en.wikipedia.org/wiki/Bias_(statistics); http://sphweb. bumc.bu.edu/otlt/mph-modules)*

Groups to be compared are differentially susceptible to the outcome of interest, even before the experimental maneuver is performed is known as selection bias. In the given question, researcher is concerned that the smokers might differ from non-smokers in their diet, exercise, etc. This concern is known as selection bias.

Some Important Types of Biases in Epidemiological Studies	
Interviewer bias	• Interviewer devotes more time of interview with cases as compared to controls[Q]
Memory/ Recall bias	• Cases are more likely to remember exposure more correctly than controls[Q]
Selection bias (Susceptibility bias)	• Groups to be compared are differentially susceptible to the outcome of interest, even before the experimental manoeuvre is performed[Q]
Information bias (Observer or misclassification bias)	• Connective type of bias in which **proportion of subjects are misclassified on exposure or diseases** • Occurs due to **people's curiosity and confusion of goals when trying to choose a course of action** • It includes reporting, recall, interviewer & attention bias[Q].

Bias
• **Bias** is **any 'systematic error'** in an epidemiological study, occurring during data collection, compilation, analysis and interpretation[Q]

Predominantly Biases are of 3 Types		
Subject bias	**Investigator bias**	**Analyzer bias**

• **Error introduced by study subjects.**
• Examples:
  – **Hawthorne effect**
  – **Recall bias**[Q]
	• **Error introduced by investigator**
	• **Selection bias**[Q]
		• **Error introduced by analyzer**

Some Important Types of Biases in Epidemiological Studies	
Apprehension bias	• Certain levels (**pulse, blood pressure**) may alter systematically from their usual levels when the subject is apprehensive
Attention bias (Hawthorne effect)	• Study **subjects may systematically alter their behaviour** when they know **they are being observed**[Q]
Berkesonian bias (Admission rate bias)	• **Bias due to hospital cases** and **controls being systematically different from each other**[Q]
Interviewer bias	• Interviewer devotes more time of interview with cases as compared to controls[Q]
Lead time bias (Zero time shift bias)	• Bias of over-estimation of survival time, due to backward shift in starting point, as by screening procedures[Q]
Memory/ Recall bias	• Cases are more likely to remember exposure more correctly than controls[Q]
Neymann Bias (Prevalence-incidence bias)	• Bias due to missing of fatal cases, mild/ silent cases and cases of short duration of episodes from the study[Q]
Selection bias (Susceptibility bias)	• Groups to be compared are differentially susceptible to the outcome of interest, even before the experimental manoeuvre is performed[Q]

Contd...

Bias		
Minimization of Biases in Epidemiological Studies by Blinding		
Type	**Method**	**Minimizes**
Single blinding	**Study subjects** are **not aware** of the treatment they are receiving	**Subject bias**
Double blinding	**Study subjects** as well as **investigator** are **not aware** of the treatment study subjects are receiving	**Subject bias + Investigator bias**
Triple blinding	**Study subjects, investigator as well as analyzer** are **not aware** of the treatment study subjects are receiving	**Subject bias + Investigator bias + Analyser bias**

87. **Ans. d. In endemic areas vaccination is given to cover children between one to nine years age group** *(Ref: Park 24/e p303, 22/e p261; Indian Journal of Pediatrics; Vol. 51, October 15, 2015 p785)*

In endemic areas, Japan Encephalitis vaccine is given to cover children between 1-15 years, not 1 to 9 years.

Japanese Encephalitis Vaccine:

- **In endemic areas, vaccine is given to cover children between 1-15 years**
- **2 primary doses** 4 weeks apart, **booster after 1 year** and **3 years** until the age of 10-15 years
- **Booster after 1 year** and **then repeated every 3 years**
- **Minimum age: According to US-FDA-2 months**

See Q. No. 91 AIIMS November 2015

88. **Ans. d. Life expectancy at birth, knowledge and decent standard of living** *(Ref: Park 24/e p17, 23/e p17)*

The Human Development Index (HDI) is a composite statistic of life expectancy, education, and income indices used to rank countries into four tiers of human development.

Human Development Index (HDI)

- The **Human Development Index (HDI)** is a **composite statistic of life expectancy**, **education**, and **income indices** used to rank countries into four tiers of human development.
- Published on 4 November 2010 (and updated on 10 June 2011), starting with the 2010 Human Development Report the HDI combines three dimensions:
  - **A long and healthy life: Life expectancy at birth**[Q]
  - **Education index: Mean years of schooling** and **Expected years of schooling**[Q]
  - **A decent standard of living: GNI per capita**[Q] (PPP US$)

Index	Minimum value	Maximum Value
Life expectancy at birth[Q]	25	85
Adult literacy rate[Q] **(%)**	0	100
Combined gross enrollment ratio[Q] **(%)**	0	100
Gross domestic product[Q] **(per capita US$)**	100	40,000

	Human Development Index (HDI)	**Physical Quality of Life Index (PQLI)**
Components	1. **Longevity**[Q] (Life expectancy at birth) 2. **Income**[Q] (Real GDP per capita in PPP US$) 3. **Knowledge**[Q] (Mean years of schooling- Gross enrolment ratio and literacy rate)	1. **Life expectancy at 1 year**[Q] 2. **Infant mortality rate**[Q] **(IMR)** 3. **Literacy rate**[Q]
Range	**0 to +1**	**0 to 100**
Value of India	0.519	65

89. **Ans. b. District level health survey** *(Ref: Park's 22/e p786)*

Data about recent trends of immunization in the community can be found by District level health survey.

*"District Level Health Survey: The **Ministry of Health and Family Welfare** (MoHFW), Government of India **conducts** the **District Level Household and facility Survey (DLHS)**. It is a household survey at the district level and in DLHS-3, the survey covered 611 districts in India. The total number of households representing a district varies from 1000 to 1500 households. The **DLHS-3** is designed to provide **information on family planning, maternal** and **child health, reproductive health** of ever married women and adolescent girls, **utilization of maternal** and **child healthcare services** including **immunization at the district level for India.** In addition, DLHS-3 also provides **information on newborn care, postnatal care within 48 hours**, role of ASHA in enhancing the reproductive and child health care and coverage of Janani Suraksha Yojana (JSY). An **important component of DLHS-3** is the **integration of Facility Survey of health institution** (Sub centre, Primary Health Centre, Community Health Centre and District Hospital) **accessible to the sampled villages**. The **focus of DLHS-3** is to **provide health care** and **utilization indicators at the district level for the enhancement of the activities under National Rural Health Mission (NRHM).**"-Park's 22/e p786*

District Level Health Survey Objectives
• Coverage of **ante-natal, natal** and **post-natal checkups** and **child immunization** • Proportion of **institutional/safe deliveries** • **JSY beneficiaries** • **Contraceptive prevalence rates** • **Unmet need for contraceptives**- spacing and limiting • **Awareness about RTI/ STI and HIV/AIDS**   • Ministry of Health and Family Welfare (MOHFW), Government of India, has included the **Clinical, Anthropometric and Biochemical (CAB) component for data collection** in the **District Level Household Survey (DLHS)-4.**

90. **Ans. b. Ministry of health and family welfare** *(Ref: Park's 24/e p697, 23/e p660, 22/e p613; www.fssai.gov.in)*

Food safety and standards authority of India comes under Ministry of health and family and welfare.

The Food Safety and standards Authority of India (FSSAI)
• It has been established under **Food Safety and Standards Act, 2006.** • FSSAI has been created **for laying down science-based standards for articles of food** and **to regulate their manufacture, storage, distribution, sale and import to ensure availability of safe** and **wholesome food** for human consumption.
Establishment of the Authority
• **Ministry of Health and Family Welfare**, Government of India is the **administrative ministry for the implementation of FSSAI.** • The chairperson is in the rank of secretary to Government of India

Programme	Ministry
Vitamin A prophylaxis	• **Ministry of health and Family welfare**[Q]
Prophylaxis against nutritional anemia	• Ministry of health and family welfare[Q]
Iodine deficiency disorders control programme	• **Ministry of health and Family welfare**[Q]
Special nutrition programme	• Ministry of Social Welfare[Q]
Balwadi nutrition	• **Ministry of Social Welfare**[Q]
ICDS programme	• **Ministry of Social Welfare**[Q]
Mid-day meal programme	• Ministry of education
Mid-day meal scheme	• **Ministry of Human Resources Development**[Q]
Employees State Insurance (ESI)	• **Ministry of Labour**[Q]
Biomedical Waste Management	• **Ministry of Environment and Forests**[Q]

91. Ans. c. Increased mean, no change in median *(Ref: Park 24/e p885, 23/e p847, 22/e p786)*

The value of median is not affected by abnormal very high or very low value. But mean is unduly influenced by abnormal values (either very high or very low) in the distribution.

See Q. No. 106 AIIMS May 2016.

92. Ans. b. 50 *(Ref: Biostatistics by Mahajan 7/e p45)*

Fifty patients have blood pressures between the 3rd and 4th quartile in the given question.

Quartile

• In descriptive statistics, the **quartiles of a ranked set of data values** are the **three points** that **divide the data set into four equal groups, each group comprising a quarter of the data.**
• A quartile is a type of quantile.
• The **first quartile (Q1)** is defined as the **middle number between the smallest number and the median of the data set.**
• The **second quartile (Q2)** is the **median of the data.**
• The **third quartile (Q3)** is the **middle value between the median** and the **highest value of the data set.**
 	
  • **First quartile** (designated **Q1**) also called the **lower quartile** or the **25th percentile** (splits off the lowest 25% of data from the highest 75%).
  • **Second quartile** (designated **Q2**) also called the **median** or the **50th percentile** (cuts data set in half).
  • **Third quartile** (designated **Q3**) also called the **upper quartile** or the **75th percentile** (splits off the highest 25% of data from the lowest 75%).
 	
• **Interquartile range** (designated **IQR**) is the **difference between** the **upper** and **lower quartiles. (IQR = Q3 - Q1)**
• In the given question, **between every two quartiles one/ fourth of the total number of patients are present**, i.e. **200/4 = 50 patients.**

93. Ans. b. Exposure to laboratory detection of disease *(Ref: Park 24/e p104-106, 23/e p99, 22/e p95)*

Window period is defined as the time taken from Exposure to laboratory detection of disease.

*"**Window** Period: Time between first infection & when the test can reliably detect that infection."*

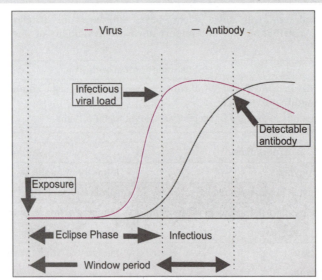

Disease Transmission: Definitions	
Window period	• **Time between first infection** & when the **test can reliably detect that infection** • In **antibody-based testing**, the window period is dependent on the **time taken for sero-conversion**
Incubation period^Q	• **Time interval between invasion by an infectious agent** and **appearance of the first sign or symptom** of the disease in question

AIIMS May 2015

Disease Transmission: Definitions	
Median incubation period[Q]	• Time required for **50% of cases to occur following exposure**
Generation time[Q]	• Time taken for a person **from receipt of infection to develop maximum infectivity** • **Roughly equal to the incubation period** of the disease
Latent period[Q]	• Period **from disease initiation to disease detection,** • Used in **non-infectious diseases** as **equivalent of incubation period**
Serial interval[Q]	• **Gap in onset between primary case** (first case in the community) and **secondary case** (case developing through infection from the primary case) • By collecting information on series of secondary cases with serial intervals, one can guess the incubation period of a disease
Period of communicability[Q]	• Time during which an **infectious agent may be transferred directly/indirectly from an infected person to another person**, from infected animal to man or from an infected person to animal, including arthropods • An important measure of communicability is secondary attack rate

94. **Ans. a. High percentage of immunized people**   *(Ref: Park's 24/e p195-196, 23/e p186)*

High failure in the interpretation of tuberculin test occurs when high percentage of immunized people are there in the population, due to high coverage of BCG.

"In countries with a high coverage of BCG, which also produces tuberculin hypersensitivity, tuberculin test has lost its sensitivity as an indicator of the true prevalence of infection. The true prevalence rates of infection maybe exaggerated by infection with atypical mycobacteria as well as the 'boosting effect' of a second dose of tuberculin producing a larger reaction than the first."

Limitations of Tuberculin Testing
• The **validity of tuberculin test**, like all medical tests, is **subject to variability**. It is **limited by lack of specificity**. • Apart from **errors associated with the mode of administration**, **reading of results** and the **test material used**, there are other factors such as cross-reactions due to sensitization by other mycobacteria which should be taken into account.   • **"In countries with a high coverage of BCG, which also produces tuberculin hypersensitivity, tuberculin test has lost its sensitivity as an indicator of the true prevalence of infection. The true prevalence rates of infection maybe exaggerated by infection with atypical mycobacteria** as well as the **'boosting effect' of a second dose of tuberculin** producing a larger reaction than the first." • It is often assumed that **delayed hypersensitivity** as measured by tuberculin testing is a **correlate of the protective immune response**. But evidence indicates that this hypersensitivity is irrelevant to the ability of the host to combat the disease. • **Despite these limitations**, the **tuberculin test continues to be the only tool for measuring the prevalence of TB**. • It has been aptly said that **tuberculin test 'must be approached with respect, administered with care, read with deliberation** and **interpreted with sentient discrimination'.**

Tuberculin Test		
• **Purified protein derivative (PPD)** has replaced the old tuberculin (OT) antigen[Q]. • Discovered by **Von Pirquet**[Q] • WHO advocates **'PPD-RT with Tween-80'**[Q] • Dosage: First strength (1 TU), Intermediate strength (5 TU), second strength (250 TU) • **Tuberculin test conversion** is defined as an **increase of 10 mm or more within a 2-year period,** regardless of age • **Tuberculin test** is the **only way of estimating the prevalence of infection in a population**[Q]		
Tuberculin Test in Use		
Mantoux Intradermal Test	• **More precise test of tuberculin sensitivity**[Q]	
Heaf Test	• **Quick, easy, reliable & cheap, preferred for testing large groups**[Q]	
Tine Multiple Puncture Test	• Unreliable, not recommended	

Contd...

Contd...

Tuberculin Test

Mantoux Test

- **Mantoux test is a test of prognostic significance,** has **limited validity due to lack of specificity**[Q]
- **Dose: 1 TU of PPD in 0.1 ml** injected **intradermally** on **forearm**[Q]
- WHO advocates **'PPD-RT with Tween-80'**
- Reading: Result read after 72 hours

Mantoux Test: Only induration is measured	
Induration	**Interpretation**
>9 mm	Positive (Past or current infection with TB)[Q]
6-9 mm	Doubtful (M. tuberculosis or atypical mycobacteria)[Q]
<6 mm	Negative[Q]

Mantoux Test	
False Positive	**False Negative**
• **Faulty technique of injection**	• Pre-allergic phase
• Using degraded tuberculin	• High grade fever
• Too deep injection	• **Measles & chicken pox**
• **Other Mycobacterium infection**	• **Whooping cough**
• **Repeated tuberculin testing**	• Malnutrition
• **Prior BCG vaccination**	• **HIV/AIDS**
	• Use of **anti-allergic drugs & immunosuppressants**

Results of Tuberculin Test

- Results of tuberculin test must be interpreted carefully
- The **persons medical risk factors determine at which increment** (5 mm, 10 mm or 15 mm) **of induration,** the **result is considered positive.**

5 mm or more is positive in	10 mm or more is positive in	15 mm or more is positive in
• **Immunocompromised patients** (HIV positive, transplant recipients)	• **Recent arrivals (< 5 years)** from **high prevalence countries**	• Persons with **no known risk factors for TB**
• **Recent contacts of TB case**	• **IV drug abusers**	
• Persons with nodular or fibrotic changes on chest X-ray, consistent with **old healed TB**	• Residents & employees of **high-risk congregate settings (prisons, nursing homes, hospitals)**	
	• **Mycobacteriology lab personnel**	
	• **High risk patients** (DM, immunocompromised patients)	
	• **Children <4 years**	
	• Children & adolescents exposed to adults in high risk categories	

95. **Ans. d. Secular**   *(Ref: Park's 24/e p69, 23/e p66, 22/e p63)*
    Trend of gradual increase in number of non- communicable disease cases as compared to previous years is called secular.

    *"The term **secular trend** implies **changes in the occurrence of disease over a long period of time,** generally **several years or decades.** There may be **progressive increase** or **decrease in the occurrence** of disease."*

Time Distribution of Disease

I. Short term fluctuation:
  – **Best known short-term fluctuation** in the occurrence of a disease is an **epidemic**
  – **Three types of epidemics:**
    - **Common-source epidemics: Single exposure or point source epidemics** and **continuous or multiple exposure epidemics**

Contd...

Contd...

Time Distribution of Disease

Single Exposure or Point Source Epidemics	Continuous or Multiple Exposure Epidemics
• **Exposure to the disease agent is brief & essentially simultaneous (single exposure)** • **Epidemic curve rises & falls rapidly**[Q] • Because **disease agent enters into all exposed persons at same time, all resultant cases** develop **within one incubation period** of the disease[Q] • **Exposure is single** with **no further exposure: No secondary wave** (no secondary case)[Q] • **Epidemic tends to be explosive**[Q] (clustering of cases within a narrow interval of time) • **Mostly due to exposure to an infectious agent** • Example: **Food poisoning, Bhopal gas tragedy, Chernobyl tragedy**[Q]	• **Exposure** from the common (same) source is **prolonged**[Q] **(continuous, repeated or intermittent)** • Exposure is not at the same time or place. • For example, a prostitute may be a common source in a gonorrhea outbreak, but since she will infect her clients over a period of time there may be **no explosive rise in number of case**[Q] • Because disease agent enters into exposed person at different time, **outbreaks continue over more than incubation period.** • Example: **Gonorrhea epidemic by prostitute**[Q], outbreak of **Legionnaire's disease** in 1976 in Philadelphia (USA).

2. **Propagated epidemics:**
   - Most often of **infectious origin, results from person to person transmission**.
   - **Source of disease agent** is **not common to all cases. Every new case becomes the source for others**

     • Shows a **gradual rise** and **tails off over a much longer period of time**[Q]
     • **Speed of spread depends upon herd immunity**[Q], opportunities for contact & secondary attack rate
     • More likely to occur where **large number of susceptible are aggregated**, or where there is a **regular supply of new susceptible individuals** (e.g. birth, immigrants) **lowering herd immunity**

   - Transmission continues until the number of susceptible is depleted or susceptible individuals are no longer exposed to infected persons or intermediary vectors
   - Epidemic continues over **more than one incubation period**
   - **Secondary waves are seen**
   - Example: **Epidemic of polio & hepatitis A**[Q]

3. **Slow (modern) epidemics:**

II. Periodic fluctuation:

Seasonal Trends	Cyclical Trends
• Due to **environmental condition** • Occurs in **communicable disease** and few non-communicable • Example: **Measles more common in spring**[Q]	• Due to **herd-immunity development** • Occurs in **cyclic spread over short period of time**, may be week/mon/year • Example: **Influenza pandemic at interval of 7-10 years**[Q]

III.   Long term or secular trends:
   - The term secular trend implies **changes in the occurrence of disease over a long period of time**, generally **several years or decades.**
   - There may be **progressive increase** or **decrease in the occurrence** of disease
   - **Example:**
   - **CHD, lung cancer & DM (non-communicable disease)**[Q] have shown a **consistent upward trend in developed countries**
   - **TB, typhoid fever, diphtheria and polio** have shown a **declined trend in developed countries**

96. **Ans. a. True positive**   *(Ref: Park's 24/e p149, 23/e p125, 22/e p131)*

   Sensitivity measures true positive cases.

   *"The term **sensitivity** was introduced as a **statistical index of diagnostic accuracy**. It has been defined as the **ability of a test to identify correctly all those who have the disease, that is 'true positive'.**"*

Assessment & Value of A Diagnostic Test

	Condition Present	Condition Absent
Positive Test	a (True positive)	b (False positive)
Negative Test	c (False negative)	d (True negative)

Sensitivity	Proportion of persons with the condition who test positive: a /(a + c)^Q
Specificity	Proportion of persons without the condition who test negative: d /(b + d)^Q
Positive predictive value (PPV)	Proportion of persons with a positive test who have the condition: a /(a + b)^Q
Negative predictive value (NPV)	Proportion of persons with a negative test who do not have the condition: d /(c + d)^Q

Predictive Value

- Prevalence, sensitivity, and specificity determine predictive value^Q
- PPV = Prevalence × Sensitivity /(Prevalence × Sensitivity) + (1 − Prevalence) (1 − Specificity)^Q
- NPV = (1 − Prevalence) (Specificity) /(1 − Prevalence)(Specificity) + (1 − Sensitivity)(Prevalence)^Q

MEDICINE

97. Ans. d. Conduction aphasia *(Ref: Harrison 19/e p176, 18/e p302)*

This is a typical case of conduction aphasia with normal comprehension and fluency but impaired naming and repetition.

"Conduction aphasia results from damage to the arcuate fasciculus. The connection between the Wernicke's (language comprehension) and Broca's (Language production) areas is lost. The hallmark of conduction aphasia is the inability to repeat words. Comprehension and the expression of language are intact but patients cannot transfer the understood word to Broca's area to be expressed. Conduction aphasia results in meaningful fluent speech and relatively good comprehension but very poor repetition."-Harrison 19/e p176

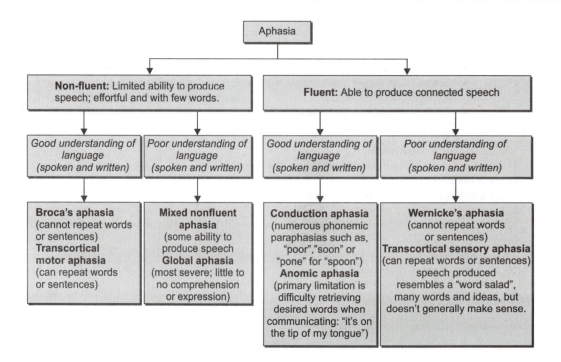

Contd...

Transfusion-Related Acute Lung Injury (TRALI)
Etiopathogenesis:
• TRALI usually **results from the transfusion of donor plasma** that **contains high-titer anti-HLA class II antibodies** that **bind recipient leukocytes.**
• The **leukocytes aggregate in the pulmonary vasculature** and **release mediators** that **increase capillary permeability.**
Clinical Features:
• The recipient develops **symptoms of hypoxia (PaO₂/FIO₂ <300 mmHg)** and **signs of non-cardiogenic pulmonary edema,** including **bilateral interstitial infiltrates on chest X-ray**, either during or within 6 hours of transfusion.
Diagnosis:
• Testing the **donor's plasma for anti-HLA antibodies can support this diagnosis**.
Treatment:
• Treatment is **supportive**, and patients usually **recover without sequelae.**

103. **Ans. a. Ulcerative colitis** *(Ref: Harrison 19/e p377, 18/e p2723)*

Ulcerative colitis is not an autoimmune disorder.

Autoimmune Diseases		
Organ Specific		**Organ Nonspecific (Systemic)**
• Grave's disease	• **Vitiligo**	• **Systemic lupus erythematosus**[Q]
• Hashimoto's thyroiditis	• Autoimmune hemolytic anemia	• **Rheumatoid arthritis**[Q]
• Autoimmune polyglandular syndrome	• Autoimmune thrombocytopenic purpura	• **Systemic necrotizing vasculitis**[Q]
• **Type 1 diabetes mellitus**	• **Pernicious anemia**[Q]	• **Granulomatosis with polyangitis (Wegener's)**[Q]
• **Insulin-resistant diabetes mellitus**	• **Myasthenia gravis**[Q]	• **Antiphospholipid syndrome**[Q]
• Immune-mediated infertility	• **Multiple sclerosis**[Q]	• **Sjogren's syndrome**[Q]
• Autoimmune Addison's disease	• **Guillain-Barre syndrome**[Q]	
• **Pemphigus vulgaris**[Q]	• **Stiff-man syndrome**	
• **Pemphigus foliaceus**[Q]	• **Acute rheumatic fever**	
• **Dermatitis herpetiformis**[Q]	• **Sympathetic ophthalmia**[Q]	
• Autoimmune alopecia	• **Goodpasture's syndrome**[Q]	

104. **Ans. a. Pregnant woman with sore throat can be started immediately on oseltamivir without diagnostic testing under category B** *(Ref: http://www.mohfw.nic.in/WriteReadData/l892s/ 804456402Categorisation.pdf)*

Regarding H1N1 Influenza, pregnant woman with sore throat can be started immediately on oseltamivir without diagnostic testing under category B.

Guidelines on categorization of Influenza a H1N1 cases during screening for home isolation, testing treatment, and hospitalization (Revised on 05.10.09)		
• In order to prevent and contain outbreak of Influenza-A H1N1 virus for screening, testing and isolation following guidelines are to be followed:		
• At first **all individuals seeking consultations for flu like symptoms should be screened at healthcare facilities** both Government and private or **examined by a doctor** and these will be **categorized as under**:		
Category- A	**Category-B**	**Category-C**
• Patients with **mild fever + cough / sore throat** with or without body ache, headache, diarrhea and vomiting will be categorized as Category-A.	1. In addition to all the signs & symptoms mentioned under Category-A, if the patient has **high-grade fever & severe sore throat**, may require **home isolation & Oseltamivir.**	• In **addition to** the above signs and **symptoms of Category-A & B**, if the patient has **one or more of the following:**
• They **do not require Oseltamivir** and should be treated for the symptoms mentioned above. The patients should be monitored for their progress and reassessed at 24-48 hours by the doctor.	2. In addition to all the signs and symptoms mentioned under Category-A, individuals having **one or more of the following high risk conditions** shall be **treated with Oseltamivir:**	– **Breathlessness, chest pain, drowsiness, fall in blood pressure, sputum mixed with blood, bluish discoloration of nails**

Contd...

Contd...

Category- A	Category-B	Category-C
• **No testing of the patient for H1N1 is required.**	– **Children** with **mild illness** but with **pre-disposing risk factors** – **Pregnant women** – Persons aged **65 years or older** – Patients with **lung** diseases, **heart** disease, **liver** disease, **kidney** disease, **blood disorders, diabetes, neurological** disorders, **cancer** and **HIV/AIDS**.	– Children with **influenza like illness,** who had a severe disease as manifested by the **red flag signs (Somnolence, high & persistent fever, inability to feed well, convulsions, shortness of breath, difficulty in breathing**, etc).
• Patients should **confine themselves at home** and avoid mixing up with public and high-risk members in the family.	– Patients on long-term **cortisone therapy.** • No tests for H1N1 is required for Category-**B1 & B2** • All patients of Category-**B1 & B2** should **confine themselves at home** and avoid mixing with public and high-risk members in the family.	– **Worsening of underlying chronic conditions.** All these patients mentioned above in **Category-C require testing, immediate hospitalization and treatment.**

Influenza

Causative agent:
- **Orthomyxovirus** (3 types: A, B, C)
  - **Type A: MC cause of outbreaks/ epidemics[Q]; Only cause of pandemics[Q]**
  - **Type B**
  - **Type C: Not circulating currently**

Incubation period	*18-72 hours[Q]*
Period of infectivity	*1-2 days before to 1-2 days after onset of symptoms[Q]*

Currently circulating influenza viruses in world

- H_1N_1 *(Type A): Cause of Swine flu[Q]*
- H_2N_2 *(Type A)*
- H_3N_2
- H_5N_1 *(Type A): Cause of Avian influenza (Bird flu)[Q]*
- H_7N_9
- *Type B*

Cyclical trends in Influenza[Q]

Type A epidemics	Every **2–3 years[Q]**
Type B epidemics	Every **4–7 years[Q]**
Type A pandemics	Every **10–15 years[Q]**

Antigenic variations in Influenza: (MC in Type A[Q])

	Antigenic shift[Q]	Antigenic drift[Q]
Occurs due to	**Genetic recombination / reassortment / rearrangement**	**Point mutation[Q]**
Nature	**Sudden**	**Gradual / insidious**
May lead to	**Epidemics/ Pandemics[Q]**	**Sporadic cases**

Vaccines for Influenza

Killed vaccines	Live attenuated vaccines
• **2 doses, 3–4 weeks apart, 0.5 ml** (for **age >3 years), subcutaneous** • **70-90% protective efficacy; duration 3-6 months** • **Rarely** associated with Guillain-Barre Syndrome[Q] (GBS)	• **Stimulate local + systemic immunity** • Antigenic variations presents difficulties in manufacture

Contd...

Contd...

Influenza

Newer vaccines[Q] for Influenza

Split-virus vaccine	Neuraminidase-specific vaccine	Recombinant vaccine
• Also known as 'Sub-virion vaccine' • **Highly purified** • **Lesser side effects** • **Less antigenic**: multiple injections required • **Useful for children**	• **Sub-unit vaccine containing N-antigen** • **Permits subclinical infection: Long lasting immunity**	• Antigenic properties of virulent strain transferred to a less virulent strain

Contraindications to Inactivated Influenza vaccines

- *Severe allergy to chicken eggs[Q]*
- *History of hypersensitivity/anaphylactic reactions previously[Q]*
- *Development of Guillain-Barre Syndrome (GBS) within 6 weeks of vaccine[Q]*
- *Infants less than 6 months age[Q]*
- *Moderate-to-severe illness with fever[Q]*

H1N1 Influenza Pandemic

- *New Nomenclature:* Influenza A (H1N1) pdm09[Q]
- *WHO declaration of Influenza pandemic: 11 June 2009*
- *World is now post-pandemic except India & New Zealand (locally intense transmission)*

Incubation period	2–3 days[Q]
Duration of isolation	*For 7 days after onset of illness or 24 hours after resolution of fever/respiratory symptoms whichever is longer[Q]*

H1N1 Influenza Pandemic: Case definitions

Suspected case	Probable case	Confirmed case
Acute febrile respiratory illness (>38° C): • **Within 7 days of contact[Q]** • **Within 7 days of travel** to area having cases or residence in such an area	Acute febrile respiratory illness: • **Positive for Influenza A[Q]** • Individual with compatible illness	Acute febrile respiratory illness with Laboratory confirmed Influenza (H1N1) 2009 virus at WHO-approved laboratory by one of the following tests: • **Real time PCR** • **Viral culture** • **4-fold rise** in Influenza A **(H1N1) neutralizing antibodies**

H1N1 Influenza Pandemic Clinical Features

Uncomplicated influenza	Complicated/severe influenza	Progressive disease
• **Influenza like illness** (Fever, cough, sore throat, rhinorrhea, headache, muscle pain) • **GIT illness (diarrhea without dehydration)**	• **Pneumonia** • **CNS involvement** • **Severe diarrhea** • **Secondary complications** • Exacerbation of chronic diseases	• **Oxygen impairment** /cardiopulmonary insufficiency • **CNS complications** • **Invasive secondary bacterial infection** • **Severe dehydration**

Risk factors of severe disease[Q]

• **Infants & children <2 years** • **Pregnant females** • **COPD** • **Chronic cardiac disease** • **Metabolic disorders** • **Children on aspirin therapy**	• **Chronic renal/hepatic/neurological/hemoglobinopathies/** immunosuppression (including **HIV**) **disorders** • **Persons aged > 65 years** • **Morbid obesity**

Contd...

Contd...

H1N1 Influenza Pandemic

Laboratory diagnosis:
- *Most timely and sensitive detection:* RT-PCR test[Q]
- *Samples:* Nasopharyngeal + throat swabs (Tracheal/bronchial aspirates in lower respiratory tract infection cases)[Q]
  - *Point-of-care/Rapid diagnostic tests: Not recommended*

Treatment:

Antiviral therapy for H1N1 Influenza Pandemic	
Severe/progressive clinical illness	Oseltamivir[Q] (if not available or resistance, use **Zanamivir**)
High risk of severe/ complicated illness	Oseltamivir or Zanamivir
Not high risk or **Uncomplicated confirmed/suspected illness**	No need of treatment

Drug	Dosage
Oseltamivir	75 mg BD × 5 days
Zanamivir 2 inhalations	(2 × 5 mg) BD × 5 days

Chemoprophylaxis:
- **Oseltamivir** is the **drug of choice**[Q] (given for **10 days** post-exposure).

Priority groups (in order) for Influenza vaccines	
• Pregnant women[Q] • Age >6 months with chronic medical conditions • 15-49 years healthy young adults	• Healthy young children • Healthy adults 49–65 years • Healthy adults > 65 years

H_1N_1 (Swine flu) Vaccine	
H_1N_1 Inactivated vaccine	**H_1N_1 Live attenuated vaccine**

• *Single IM injection*
 • *Strain:* A/California/7/2009 (H1N1) V like strain[Q]
 • *Storage temperature:* +2° to +8° C
 • *Contraindications:*
    – History of **anaphylaxis/ severe reaction/ Guillain-Barre Syndrome**
    – **Infants < 6 months**
    – **Moderate-to severe illness with fever**
 • *Protective immunity:* Develops after 14 days (Not 100%)
	• *Nasal spray*
	 • *Side effects:*
	    – Rhinorrhea
	    – Nasal congestion
	    – Cough, sore throat
	    – Fever
	    – Wheezing
	    – Vomiting

105. Ans. c. Cor Pulmonale *(Ref: Harrison 19/e p1501, 18/e p1901)*

Hyperdynamic circulation is seen in anemia, beriberi & AV fistula, but not in Cor pulmonale.

"Conditions that lead to a high cardiac output (e.g., arteriovenous fistula, anemia) are seldom responsible for the development of HF in a normal heart; however, in the presence of underlying structural heart disease, these conditions can lead to overt HF."—Harrison 19/e p1501

Etiologies of Heart Failure			
Depressed Ejection Fraction (< 40%)		**Preserved Ejection Fraction (> 40–50%)**	**High-Output States**

• **Coronary artery disease:**
    – Myocardial infarction
    – Myocardial ischemia
	• **Non-ischemic dilated cardiomyopathy:**
	    – Familial/genetic disorders
		• **Pathologic hypertrophy:**
		    – Primary (hypertrophic cardiomyopathies)
		    – Secondary (hypertension)
			• **Metabolic disorders:**
			    – **Thyrotoxicosis**[Q]

Contd...

Depressed Ejection Fraction (< 40%)		Preserved Ejection Fraction (> 40–50%)	High-Output States

• **Chronic pressure overload:**
  – Hypertension
  – Obstructive valvular disease
• **Chronic volume overload:**
  – Regurgitant valvular disease
  – **Intracardiac** (left-to-right) **shunting**
  – Extracardiac shunting[Q]
• **Chronic lung disease:**
  – **Cor pulmonale**[Q]
  – Pulmonary vascular disorders
	– Infiltrative disorders
	• **Toxic/drug-induced damage:**
	  – Metabolic disorder
	  – Viral
	• **Chagas' disease**
	• **Disorders of rate & rhythm:**
	  – Chronic bradyarrhythmias
	  – Chronic tachyarrhythmias
		• **Aging**
		• **Restrictive cardiomyopathy:**
		  – Infiltrative disorders (amyloidosis, sarcoidosis)
		  – Storage diseases (hemo-chromatosis)
		• **Fibrosis**
		• **Endomyocardial disorders**
			• **Nutritional disorders (beriberi)**[Q]
			• **Excessive blood flow requirements:**
			  – Systemic AV shunting[Q]
			  – Chronic anemia[Q]

106. Ans. b. Asthma   *(Ref: Harrison 19/e p306 e-5, 18/e p2092)*

DLCO is normally or mildly elevated during an episode of acute asthma.

*"During an **episode of acute asthma**, luminal narrowing due to smooth muscle constriction as well as inflammation and thickening within the small- and medium-sized bronchi raise frictional resistance and reduce airflow. "Scooping" of the flow-volume loop is caused by reduction of airflow, especially at lower lung volumes. Often, airflow obstruction can be reversed by inhalation of β -adrenergic agonists acutely or by treatment with inhaled steroids chronically. **TLC usually remains normal** (although elevated TLC is sometimes seen in long-standing asthma), but **FRC may be dynamically elevated. RV is often increased due to exaggerated airway closure at low lung volumes, and this elevation of RV reduces FVC**. Because central airways are narrowed, Raw is usually elevated. **Mild arterial hypoxemia is often present due to perfusion of relatively under ventilated alveoli distal to obstructed airways** (and is responsive to oxygen supplementation), but **DLCO is normal or mildly elevated**."-Harrison 19/e p306 e-5*

Parameter	Restriction due to increased lung elastic recoil (Pulmonary fibrosis)	Restriction due to chest wall abnormality (moderate obesity)	Restriction due to respiratory muscle weakness (Myasthenia gravis)	Obstruction due to airway narrowing (Acute asthma)	Obstruction due to elastic recoil (Severe emphysema)
TLC	60%	95%	75%	**100%**	130%
FRC	60%	65%	100%	**104%**	220%
RV	60%	100%	120%	**120%**	310%
FVC	60%	92%	60%	**90%**	60%
FEV1	60%	92%	60%	**35% pre b. d.** **75% post b. d.**	35% pre b. d. 38% post b. d.
R_{aw}	1.0	1.0	1.0	**2.5**	1.5
DLCO	60%	95%	80%	**120%**	40%

(b.d., bronchodilator; DLCO, diffusion capacity of lung for carbon monoxide; FEV1, forced expiratory volume in 1 sec; FRC, functional residual capacity; FVC, forced vital capacity; R_{aw}, airways resistance; RV, residual volume; TLC, total lung capacity)

Diffusing Capacity of the Lung for Carbon Monoxide (DLCO)
• This test uses a **small (and safe) amount of carbon monoxide to measure gas exchange across the alveolar membrane** during a 10-second breath hold.

Contd...

Contd...

Diffusing Capacity of the Lung for Carbon Monoxide (DLCO)
• Carbon monoxide in exhaled breath is analyzed to determine the **quantity of CO absorbed by crossing the alveolar membrane** and **combining with hemoglobin in red blood cells.**
• This **'single-breath diffusing capacity'** [diffusion capacity of the lung for carbon monoxide (DLCO)] value **increases with the surface area available for diffusion** and the **amount of hemoglobin within the capillaries**, and varies **inversely with alveolar membrane thickness.**
• Thus, **DLCO decreases in diseases that thicken or destroy alveolar membranes** (e.g., **pulmonary fibrosis, emphysema**), **curtail the pulmonary vasculature** (e.g., **pulmonary hypertension**), or **reduce alveolar capillary hemoglobin** (e.g., **anemia**).
• **Single-breath diffusing capacity may be elevated in acute congestive heart failure, asthma, polycythemia, and pulmonary hemorrhage.**

107. Ans. a. Basal ganglia *(Ref: Harrison 19/e p2582, 18/e p3294)*

Hypertensive hemorrhage is most commonly seen in basal ganglia.

"Hypertensive intracerebral hemorrhage usually results from spontaneous rupture of a small penetrating artery deep in the brain. The most common sites are the basal ganglia (especially the putamen), thalamus, cerebellum, and pons. The small arteries in these areas seem most prone to hypertension-induced vascular injury."—Harrison 19/e p2582

Intracerebral (Parenchymal) Hemorrhage	Subarachnoid Hemorrhage
• **MC type** of **intracranial hemorrhage**[Q]	• **2nd MC cause** of intracranial hemorrhage[Q]
• **MC cause** is **hypertension**[Q], causing rupture of small perforating arteries or arterioles[Q]	• **MC cause: Trauma >**Spontaneous rupture of **Berry aneurysm**[Q]
• **MC site**: **Basal ganglia (Putamen**[Q])	• **MC site** of Berry aneurysm is **anterior circulation** of **"circle of Willis"**[Q]

SURGERY

108. Ans. c. Needle decompression on right side of the chest *(Ref: Sabiston 20/e p425, 1635, 19/e p1599; Schwartz 10/e p163, 9/e p138; Bailey 27/e p919, 26/e p354)*

This case is a classical description of tension pneumothorax of right hemithorax with decreased breath sounds and shock. Since patient is shouting it means her airway is clear. Immediate decompression with large bore needle in mid clavicular line in 2nd intercostal space is the urgent treatment for this patient followed by insertion of IV line and fluid administration.

See Q. No. 131 AIIMS May 2016.

109. Ans. b. Left gastric artery *(Ref: Harrison 19/e p277, 18/e p2436; Sabiston 20/e p1145, 19/e p1167,1222; Schwartz 10/e p1020, 9/e p875,941; Bailey 27/e p1128, 26/e p994; Shackelford 7/e p768)*

Bleeding from a Mallory-Weiss tear occurs usually from left gastric artery.

"Mallory-Weiss tears are characterized by arterial bleeding. Most Mallory-Weiss tears stop bleeding spontaneously and supportive treatment is all that is required. If bleeding continues, infusion of vasoactive substances into the celiac artery or into the left gastric artery often obviates the need for operation."

Mallory Weiss Syndrome
• Mallory-Weiss tears are related to **forceful vomiting, retching, coughing,** or **straining**[Q]
• **Forceful contraction** of the **abdominal wall** against an **unrelaxed cardia**, resulting in **mucosal laceration** of the **proximal cardia**[Q] as a result of the increase in intragastric pressure.
• Results in **disruption** of **gastric mucosa** high on the **lesser curve** at **cardia (just below GE junction)**[Q]
• Results in **disruption** of **gastric mucosa** high on the **lesser curve** at **cardia** (just below GE junction)
• Tear is **partial thickness**, extending through the **mucosa & submucosa**[Q]

Contd...

Contd...

Mallory Weiss Syndrome

Clinical Features:

- Classically, seen in **alcoholic patients**[Q] after a period of **intense retching** and **vomiting** after binge drinking.
- Cause of up to **15%** of all **severe upper GI bleeds**[Q]

  - **Arterial bleeding**, usually **painless** and are **rarely**[Q] associated with **massive bleeding**.

- The overall **mortality rate** is **3-4%**, with the **greatest risk** for massive hemorrhage in **alcoholic** patients with **preexisting portal hypertension**[Q].

Diagnosis:

- Usually diagnosed by **history**
- **Endoscopy** is used to **confirm the diagnosis**[Q].
- **Most tears** occur along the **lesser curvature**[Q].

Treatment:

- **Supportive therapy** is often all that is necessary because **90%** of **bleeding episodes** are **self-limited**, and the **mucosa** often **heals within 72 hours**[Q].

Persistent Bleeding in Mallory Weiss Syndrome is managed by

- **Endoscopic electrocoagulation**[Q] or endoscopic therapy with injection
- **Angiographic embolization**[Q]
- Surgery consists of laparotomy and **high gastrotomy** with **oversewing of the linear tear**[Q], if above maneuvers fails.

- **Recurrent bleeding** from a Mallory-Weiss tear is **uncommon**[Q].

- Remember: A **Sengstaken-Blakemore tube** will **not stop bleeding** in Mallory-Weiss syndrome, as the **bleeding is arterial** and the pressure in the balloon is not sufficient to overcome the arterial pressure and is **contraindicated**[Q].

110. **Ans. c. T stage** *(Ref: Sabiston 20/e p1029, 19/e p1049-1064; Schwartz 10/e p1005, 9/e p862-870; Bailey 27/e p1088, 26/e p1004-1013; Shackelford 7/e p416-434)*

Long-term survival following esophagectomy depends on a number of factors such as the depth of tumor invasion (T), the number of involved lymph nodes (N), and on the location of the tumor in the esophagus. In esophageal cancer prognosis is best determined by T stage, among the options provided.

Carcinoma Esophagus

- **MC esophageal cancer worldwide: Squamous cell carcinoma**[Q]
- **MC esophageal cancer in United States** (Western countries): **Adenocarcinoma**[Q]
- More common in **males**[Q]
- **MC site of CA esophagus: Middle 1/3rd (Overall)**[Q]
- **Chemotherapy regimen: Epirubicin + Cisplatin**[Q] + **5-FU**

Squamous cell carcinoma	Adenocarcinoma
• Rarely seen before the age of 30 years	• Seen infrequently before the age of 40 years
• **Highest mortality rates** seen in **men** between **60-70 years**[Q] of age.	• **Increases in incidence** with **age**[Q]
• Predominantly affects **African American men**[Q]	• Disease affecting **white men**[Q]
• **MC site: Middle 1/3rd**[Q]	• **Barrett's esophagus: 40-fold**[Q] increased risk for adenocarcinoma
• Obesity is protective	• **MC site: Lower 1/3rd**[Q]
• **H. pylori CAG-A strain** is a **risk factor**[Q]	• **Obesity** is a **risk factor**
• Usually appears as an **exophytic lesion** with a **large fungating mass**[Q]	• **H. pylori CAG-A strain** is a **protective**
• More sensitive to **chemoradiotherapy**[Q]	• Polypoid (5-10%), flat (10-15%), fungating (20-25%), or **infiltrative (40-50%)**[Q]
• Treated aggressively with **nonsurgical therapy**[Q]	• **Not as sensitive to chemoradiotherapy**
	• Treated by a more **aggressive surgical approach**[Q]

Contd...

Contd...

Carcinoma Esophagus
Pathology: • Esophageal cancer asserts **aggressive biologic behavior**. • With **only two layers** to the **esophageal wall**, tumors **rapidly infiltrate through** the **muscular wall into surrounding structures**[Q]. • The **rich vascular** and **lymphatic supply** facilitates spread to **regional lymph nodes**[Q].
Clinical Features: • **Early-stage cancers: Asymptomatic** or **mimic symptoms** of **GERD**. <p align="center">• **MC symptom: Dysphagia >Weight loss**[Q]</p>• **Most patients** with esophageal cancer **present with dysphagia** & **weight loss**, symptoms that usually indicate advanced disease. • **Choking, coughing**, and **aspiration** from a **tracheoesophageal fistula** (In advanced cases)[Q] • **Hoarseness** and **vocal cord paralysis** from **direct invasion** into the **recurrent laryngeal nerve** (In **advanced cases**)[Q] • **MC site of metastasis: Liver**[Q] **>lung >bone**

Diagnosis:
• **Barium swallow: First investigation done**[Q] in suspected case of **CA esophagus** (classic finding of an **apple core lesion**[Q])
 	
    • **Endoscopy** with **biopsy: Investigation of choice** for **diagnosis of CA esophagus**[Q].
    • **Endoscopic Ultrasound: Investigation of choice** for **staging of CA esophagus, best for T staging & LN metastasis**[Q].
 	
• **CECT (abdomen & chest):** Assess the length of the tumor, thickness of the esophagus and stomach, **regional LN status** and **metastasis to liver & lungs**[Q].

Treatment of CA Esophagus	
High grade dysplasia (Tis) or T1a	• **Endoscopic Mucosal Resection**[Q]
Localized Esophageal Cancer	• **T1**: Vagal sparing or transhiatal or **minimal invasive esophagectomy** with limited LN dissection[Q] • **T2 & T3: Neo-adjuvant chemoradiation + Surgery**[Q] • **Cervical SCC** or **Non-ideal candidate** for resection: **Definitive chemoradiation**[Q]
Locally Advanced Cancer	• **Chemoradiation**[Q] (± Surgical resection in T4a)
Metastatic Disease	• **Definitive chemoradiation**[Q] (for involved distant LN or metastatic disease)
Malignant TEF	• **Coated SEMS**[Q] (self expanding metallic stents)

• **Post-operative chemoradiation** is **reserved** for **GE junction tumors**[Q]
• **Extent of Resection:** An in-situ **margin of 10 cm**[Q] should be the goal

Prognosis:

Long-term survival following esophagectomy depends on
• **Depth** of **tumor invasion** (T)[Q] • **Number** of **involved lymph nodes** (N)[Q] • **Location**[Q] of the tumor in the esophagus

• **Prognosis is better** for **tumors of** the **cervical esophagus** & tumors **located at GE junction**[Q], in comparison to tumors located in the thoracic esophagus.

---

111. **Ans. c. Fresh frozen plasma** *(Ref: Harrison 19/e p138 e-3, 18/e p953; Sabiston 20/e p79-80, 19/e p588)*

Best blood product to be given in a patient of multiple clotting factor deficiency with active bleeding is fresh frozen plasma.

"FFP contains stable coagulation factors and plasma proteins: fibrinogen, antithrombin, albumin, as well as proteins C and S. Indications for FFP include correction of coagulopathies, including the rapid reversal of warfarin; supplying deficient plasma proteins; and treatment of thrombotic thrombocytopenic purpura."—Harrison 19/e p138 e-3

AIIMS May 2015

Fresh-frozen Plasma (FFP)

- **FFP** is produced from the **separation of plasma** from **donated blood**[Q].
- **Stored at -18⁰C** and has a **shelf life** of **1 year**[Q].
- **Each unit** contains **400 mg of fibrinogen** and **1 unit activity of each** of the **clotting factors**[Q].
  - **Most labile clotting factors (V & VIII)** may be **diminished**[Q] proportional to shelf life.
- **FFP contains stable coagulation factors & plasma proteins: fibrinogen, antithrombin, albumin, proteins C & S**[Q].

Indications for FFP	
Correction of coagulopathies: – **Rapid reversal of warfarin**[Q] – **Supplying deficient plasma proteins**[Q]	Treatment of **thrombotic thrombocytopenic purpura**[Q]

- Patients who are **IgA-deficient** and **require plasma support** should receive **FFP from IgA-deficient donors to prevent anaphylaxis.**
  - **FFP should not be** routinely **used to expand blood volume**[Q].
  - **FFP**: An **acellular component** & **does not transmit intracellular infections**, e.g., CMV.

Characteristics of Selected Blood Components

Component	Volume (mL)	Content	Clinical Response
Whole Blood	450 ml ± 45	• No elements removed • Contains **RBCs, WBCs, plasma & platelets (WBCs & platelets** may be **non-functional**[Q])	• Not for routine use • Used for **acute massive bleeding, open heart surgery** & neonatal total exchange
Packed RBCs	180–200	• **RBCs** with variable **leukocyte** content & **small** amount of **plasma**	• Increase **Hb 1 gm/dL & hematocrit 3%**[Q]
Platelets	50–70	• 5.5 x 10¹⁰/RD unit	• Increase platelet count **5000–10,000/μL**[Q]
FFP	200–250	• **Plasma proteins: Coagulation factors**, proteins C & S, antithrombin[Q]	• Increases **coagulation factors about 2%**
Cryoprecipitate	10–15	• Cold-insoluble plasma proteins, fibrinogen, factor VIII, vWF[Q]	• Topical fibrin glue, also **80 IU factor VIII**[Q]

Cryoprecipitate

- **Cryoprecipitate** is a source of **fibrinogen**[Q], **factor VIII**[Q] and **von Willebrand factor (vWF)**[Q].
- It is **ideal for supplying fibrinogen** to the volume-sensitive patient.
- **Stored at ≤-18°C**
  - **1 unit** of cryoprecipitate contains **80-145 units of Factor VIII & 250 mg of fibrinogen**[Q].
  - Cryoprecipitate is **pooled from many donors**, so there are **maximum chances of disease transmission** among all blood products[Q].
- Cryoprecipitate may also **supply vWF** to patients with **dysfunctional (type II)** or **absent (type III) von Willebrand disease.**

---

112. Ans. a. Start anti-thyroid drugs, and do urgent MRI brain *(Ref: Harrison 19/e p2274, 18/e p2880; Sabiston 20/e p982, 19/e p1890; Schwartz 10/e p1533, 9/e p1541; Bailey 27/e p811, 26/e p614-616)*

Hyperthyroidism with elevated T4 and TSH levels and bitemporal hemianopia is highly suggestive of TSH-secreting adenoma. MRI should be done to confirm the diagnosis of (TSH-secreting) pituitary adenoma.

"TSH-producing macroadenomas are rare but are often large and locally invasive when they occur. Patients usually present with thyroid goiter and hyperthyroidism, reflecting overproduction of TSH. Diagnosis is based on demonstrating elevated serum free T4 levels, inappropriately normal or high TSH secretion, and MRI evidence of a pituitary adenoma."
—Harrison 19/e p2274

TSH-Secreting Adenomas

- **TSH-producing macroadenomas** are rare but are often **large** and **locally invasive** when they occur.
- **Patients** usually **present with thyroid goiter** and **hyperthyroidism**, reflecting **overproduction of TSH**.

Clinical Features:

- **Patients** usually **present with thyroid goiter** and **hyperthyroidism**, reflecting **overproduction of TSH**.
- **Neurologic deficits** by **mass effect** on the **chiasm** with consequent **bitemporal hemianopsia[Q]**.

Diagnosis:

- **Diagnosis is based on demonstrating elevated serum free T4 levels, inappropriately normal or high TSH secretion, and MRI evidence of a pituitary adenoma.**
- **Presence of a pituitary mass** and **elevated alpha subunit levels** are suggestive of a **TSH-secreting tumor.**

Treatment:

- **Initial therapeutic approach: Remove or debulk the tumor mass surgically**, usually using a **transsphenoidal approach**.
- **Total resection** is **not often achieved** as most of these **adenomas** are **large & locally invasive**.
- Normal circulating thyroid hormone levels are achieved in about two-thirds of patients after surgery.

> - **Thyroid ablation** or **antithyroid drugs (methimazole & propylthiouracil) can be used to reduce thyroid hormone levels.**
> - **Somatostatin analogue treatment** effectively normalizes **TSH** and **alpha subunit hypersecretion, shrinks the tumor mass in 50% of patients**, and **improves visual fields in 75% of patients; euthyroidism is restored in most patients.**

Pituitary adenoma

- Pituitary adenomas arise primarily from the **anterior pituitary gland[Q]**
- **MC cause** of **hyperpituitarism: Pituitary adenoma[Q]**
- Classified as either **functional** (secreting) or **nonfunctional** (nonsecreting) tumors
- Former presenting **earlier with symptoms** caused **by physiologic effects** and the latter presenting when of **sufficient size** to cause **neurologic deficits** by **mass effect** on the **chiasm** with consequent **bitemporal hemianopsia[Q]**.
- Incidence is increased in **MEN-1[Q]**

> - **Pituitary adenoma** can be **differentiated from hyperplasia by reticulin stain[Q]**
> - **Absence of reticulin stain** in **pituitary adenoma[Q]**

Clinical Features:

- Occur commonly in the **third** and **fourth decades** and affect **both sexes equally[Q]**.
- **MC functional tumor** is **prolactinoma[Q]**, which causes **amenorrhea** and **galactorrhea** in women[Q].

Diagnosis:

- **MRI** is **IOC for pituitary tumors[Q]**
- Typically, the **pituitary gland enhances rapidly** owing to lack of blood-brain barrier.
- **Microadenoma** may appear as a **nonenhancing area within the gland**.
- Diagnostic workup includes a **full endocrinologic profile** and a **formal visual fields test[Q]**.

Treatment:

- **Dopamine agonist, bromocriptine[Q]**, can **shrink prolactinomas** in **75%** of patients with **macroadenomas** in **6-8 weeks**, but only as long as therapy is maintained.
- Bromocriptine may also work on **GH-secreting tumors** with tumor **shrinkage in <20%.**
- **Octreotide[Q]** can **reduce GH levels** in 71% of patients, with a **significant reduction** in tumor **volume** in **30%** of cases.

Indications of Surgery as an initial treatment	
- **GH-secreting tumors[Q]**	- **Primary Cushing's disease[Q]**
- Any **adenoma** causing **acute visual deterioration[Q]**	- **Nonprolactin-secreting macroadenomas** causing symptoms by **mass effect[Q]**

Contd...

Pituitary adenoma
• **Surgical approach** of choice: **Sublabial** or **intranasal trans-sphenoidal**[Q] approach
• **Recurrence rate: 12%** (**most** recurrences occur **4-8 years after surgery**)
• **Radiosurgery** can also be used either as **primary therapy**, as an **adjuvant therapy** after subtotal resection, or **for recurrent disease**.
• The **main dose-limiting structure** is proximity to the **optic chiasm** and **optic nerves** (within 3-5 mm). In this case, **fractionated EBRT** may be indicated as an adjuvant therapy.

113. Ans. d. MRI *(Ref: Schwartz 10/e p527, 9/447-450; Harrison 19/e p526; Sabiston 20/e p828, 19/830-832; Bailey 27/e p861-862, 26/799-801)*

A 60-year-old lady comes with blood stained discharge from the nipple with family history of breast cancer. Next best step for her (high risk female) will be MRI for screening of breast cancer.

*"There is **current interest in the use of MRI to screen the breasts of high-risk women** and of women with a newly diagnosed breast cancer. In the first case, women who have a strong family history of breast cancer or who carry known genetic mutations require screening at an early age, but mammographic evaluation is limited because of the increased breast density in younger women. In the second case, an MRI study of the contralateral breast in women with a known breast cancer has shown a contralateral breast cancer in 5.7% of these women."-Schwartz 10/527*

*"However, the ACS suggests that **younger women who are BRCA1 or BRCA2 carriers or untested first-degree relatives of women with cancer; women with a history of radiation therapy to the chest between ages 10 and 30 years; women with a lifetime risk of breast cancer of at least 20%; and women with a history of Li-Fraumeni, Cowden, or Bannayan-Riley-Ruvalcaba syndromes may benefit from MRI screening**, where the higher sensitivity may outweigh the loss of specificity."-Harrison 19/e p526*

Investigations in CA Breast	
Mammography	• **Initial investigation** for symptomatic breast in **women >35 years** & for **screening**[Q] • **IOC for microcalcification**[Q]
Sonomamogram (Ultrasound Breast)	• **Breast ultrasound** that produces **picture of internal structures of the breast** • **Initial investigation for palpable lesions** in **women <35 years**[Q] **(dense breast)** • **Not useful in screening** • **Useful in distinguishing cysts from solid lesions** • Used to localize impalpable areas of breast pathology
Ductoscopy	• It **uses a microendoscope for direct visualization of ductal system** of the breast and **aspiration of lavage fluid** to be used in cytological analysis • Ductoscopy allows a **targeted approach** to the diagnosis of intraductal breast diseases • Ductoscopy can serve as an adjunct to established techniques of breast imaging but is not a substitute • **Perforation of the lactiferous sinus** in the immediate retroareolar space is a **common complication**
PET scan	• **IOC for detecting recurrences** in **scarred breast**[Q] • Useful in multifocal disease and in helping detect axillary involvement

Indications for Breast MRI
1. **Lobular carcinoma**[Q]: Difficult to detect and measure by conventional method because of multifocal and infiltrating growth pattern.
2. **Staging of primary breast cancer**[Q]
3. **Occult primary tumour** with malignant axillary lymphadenopathy and **normal mammogram** and **breast USG**[Q].
4. **Screen younger women** with **high familial risk** of breast cancer[Q]
5. Assessing the **integrity of breast implant**[Q]

AIIMS ESSENCE

114. Ans. b. Finger guided core biopsy *(Ref: Schwartz 10/e p554, 9/467; Sabiston 20/e p2058-2059, 19/2035-2037; Bailey 27/e p881, 26/818, 25/846)*

Most breast lesions in pregnancy are benign but biopsy should be done to rule out malignancy. Core-needle biopsy with or without ultrasound guidance is a safe and reliable method for obtaining tissue.

*"Fewer than 25% of the breast nodules developing during pregnancy and lactation will be cancerous. **Ultrasonography and needle biopsy are used in the diagnosis of these nodules. Open biopsy may be required. Mammography is rarely indicated because of its decreased sensitivity during pregnancy and lactation**; however, the fetus can be shielded if mammography is needed."-Schwartz 10/e p554*

"Because of the changes in the breast tissue with pregnancy, imaging modalities may be difficult to interpret. If used with appropriate shielding, mammography carries a limited risk to the fetus. Mammography has a high false-negative rate due to the increased density of the fibroglandular breast tissue, however, so it has limited usefulness in the evaluation of the pregnant patient. Ultrasonography can safely be performed as an initial evaluation or in conjunction with mammography. Ultrasound is able to distinguish solid from cystic lesions in 97% of patients and is helpful in guiding fine-needle aspiration or biopsy. Although MRI does not use ionizing radiation, the two main risks to the fetus from the magnetic field and electromagnetic radiation are heating and cavitation. With other reliable imaging modalities available, MRI is not currently recommended for breast imaging in the pregnant patient. Tissue diagnosis is essential. Core-needle biopsy with or without ultrasound guidance is a safe and reliable method for obtaining tissue. Fine-needle aspiration may be a reliable alternative to core-needle or open biopsy."-Sabiston 19/e p2058

Breast Cancer during Pregnancy
• Occurs in **1 of every 3000**[Q] pregnant women • **MC non-gynecologic malignancy** associated with **pregnancy**[Q]. • **Ductal carcinoma** is **MC type,** accounting for **75-90%**[Q] of breast cancer in pregnancy.
Clinical Features: • Presents as **painless palpable mass**[Q] with or without nipple discharge • **Axillary LN metastases** in upto **75%** patients • Approx. **<25% nodules** developing during **pregnancy** and **lactation** will be **cancerous**[Q] • **Present at a later stage** of disease because breast changes occurring in hormone-rich environment of pregnancy obscure early cancer.
Diagnosis: • **USG** and **needle biopsy**[Q] are **used for diagnosis** • **Mammography** is rarely indicated due to its **decreased sensitivity** during **pregnancy** & **lactation**

Treatment: Mainstay of therapy is **surgical resection.**

Stage I & II	**Mastectomy** with **axillary dissection**[Q]
LABC	**NACT after 1st trimester + MRM in 2nd trimester + RT after delivery**[Q]

LABC in Pregnancy
• **MRM** can be performed during **first and second** trimester (increased risk of spontaneous abortion after first-trimester anesthesia), **chemotherapy after first trimester** & **radiotherapy after delivery**. • **Chemotherapy** during **first trimester** carries a risk of **spontaneous abortion** & **12%** risk of **birth defects, given after first trimester.** • No evidence of teratogenecity by chemotherapy during second and third trimester. • Breast cancer in pregnancy have **prognosis stage by stage similar** to that of non-pregnant patient • **Elective termination of pregnancy** to receive appropriate therapy without the risk for fetal malformation is **no longer routinely recommended** because no improvement in survival has been demonstrated.

115. Ans. a. Chemotherapy in hormone receptor positive patients *(Ref: Harrison 19/e p528; http://www.oncotypedx.com/ http://education.nccn.org/node/11346. http://www.cancercare.on.ca/common/pages/UserFile.aspx?fileld=291504)*

Oncotype DX may be used to guide chemotherapy decisions among certain women with:
• **Node-negative**[Q]
• **Hormone receptor-positive**[Q]
• **HER2-negative breast cancer**[Q]

Contd...

Oncotype DX

- **Oncotype DX** is a **genomic test that predicts the likelihood of a cancer recurrence**, the **likelihood of benefit from chemotherapy**, and the **likelihood of survival in patients with newly diagnosed breast cancer** that **has not spread to the lymph nodes (nodenegative)** and is **hormone receptor-positive**.
- Oncotype DX evaluates the **activity of 21 genes** from a sample of the patient's cancer **to determine the patient's Recurrence Score.**
- The **Recurrence Score** ranges from **0 to 100**, with a **higher score indicating a greater risk of recurrence**.
- The **Oncotype DX diagnostic tests help individualize treatment planning for breast, colon and prostate cancer patients.**

Oncotype DX may be used to guide chemotherapy decisions among certain women with:		
• **Node-negative**[Q]	• **Hormone receptor-positive**[Q]	• **HER2-negative breast cancer**[Q]

For Breast Cancer	For Colon Cancer	For Prostate Cancer
• The Oncotype DX® Breast Cancer Assay can help physicians and patients **decide on the best course of treatment.** • For invasive breast cancer, the Oncotype DX Breast Cancer Assay **predicts chemotherapy benefit** and the **likelihood of distant breast cancer recurrence.** • The **Oncotype DX Breast Cancer Assay for DCIS** patients **predict the risk of local recurrence.** • Even when traditional measures seem conclusive, Oncotype DX Recurrence Score can lead to a different approach.	• The Oncotype DX® Colon Cancer Assay quantifies **recurrence risk in stage II** and **stage III colon cancer**, beyond traditional qualitative measures. • This enables an **individualized approach to treatment planning.** • The Oncotype DX test measures a group of cancer genes in the tumor, **providing a quantitative Recurrence Score** result beyond traditional measures so physicians and patients can have a **more complete discussion of recurrence risk.**	• The Oncotype DX Prostate Cancer Assay harnesses the power of genomics to provide a **more precise** and **accurate assessment of risk based on individual tumor biology.** • Using a minimal tissue sample from a needle biopsy, the test builds on traditional clinical pathologic factors to provide additional, clinically relevant insight into the underlying prostate tumor biology, enabling physicians and their patients **to make treatment decisions** with greater confidence.

The Oncotype DX, PAM50, and Mamma Print are multigene tests that are being used clinically for early-stage breast cancer to predict recurrence risk and guide adjuvant chemotherapy decisions.

Name of test	Brief description	Scoring/Measurement	Tissue needed
Oncotype DX	A genomic test that uses a **21-gene assay** to provide an **individual, quantitative assessment of the likelihood of disease recurrence.**	Recurrence Score, a number between **0 and 100** that **correlates to a specific likelihood of breast cancer recurrence within 10 years** of initial diagnosis	**Fixed-tissue blocks**
Mamma Print	A unique **70-gene assay** that has the ability to **identify which early-stage breast cancer patients** are **at risk of distant recurrence following surgery, independent of Estrogen Receptor status** and any **prior treatment.**	**Low risk or high risk**	**Paraffin embedded or fresh tissue**
PAM50	A **50-gene test** in development that is designed to be performed in local routine hospital pathology laboratories and has been optimized **to separate intrinsic disease subtypes that are used to generate a ROR score**	**Risk of Recurrence (ROR) score**	**Fixed-tissue blocks**

116. Ans. a. Herniotomy *(Ref: Sabiston 20/e p1884, 19/e p1120-1126; Schwartz 10/e p1635, 9/1318-1331; Bailey 27/e p125, 1503, 26/e p111, 1382; Schackelford 7/e p568-579)*

Management of hydrocele of the hernia sac (congenital hydrocele) in a 3 years old child is herniotomy.

"A patent processus vaginalis may allow only peritoneal fluid to track down around the testis to form a hydrocoele. Hydrocoeles are unilateral or bilateral, asymptomatic, non-tender scrotal swellings. They may be tense or lax, but typically transilluminate. The majority resolve spontaneously as the processus continues to obliterate, but surgical ligation is recommended in boys older than three years of age."-Bailey 27/e p125

"In congenital hydrocele, the processus vaginalis is patent and connects with the peritoneal cavity. The communication is usually too small to allow herniation of intra-abdominal contents. Pressure on the hydrocele does not always empty it but the hydrocele fluid may drain into the peritoneal cavity when the child is lying down; thus, the hydrocele may be intermittent. Ascites should be considered if the swelling are bilateral. Congenital hydroceles are treated by herniotomy if they do not resolve spontaneously." -Bailey 27/e p1503

Herniotomy	• Ligation of hernial sac[Q]
Herniorrhaphy	• Herniotomy with **posterior wall repair** using in-situ structures[Q]
Hernioplasty	• Herniotomy with **strengthening of posterior wall** using exogenous material like **mesh**[Q]

Management of Inguinal Hernia

• **Objectives** of treatment: **Treatment of hernia sac** and **Inguinal floor reconstruction**

Management of Inguinal Hernia	
Treatment of Hernia Sac	**Inguinal Floor Reconstruction**
• Basic operation is **inguinal herniotomy**, which entails **dissecting out** & **opening** the **hernial sac, reducing any contents** and then **transfixing the neck** of the sac and **removing the remainder**[Q]. • **Direct sacs** are usually too broad for ligation and should not be opened but instead are simply **inverted into peritoneal cavity**[Q].	• **Management of the hernia sac is sufficient for children** and **young adults**[Q] • **Reconstruction** (repair or strengthening) of the inguinal floor is **necessary in all adult hernias to prevent recurrence**[Q]. • **Types of repair:** 1. Primary **tissue repair**[Q] 2. **Anterior tension-free mesh repair**[Q] 3. **Pre-peritoneal repairs: Open** & **laparoscopic** approach[Q]

Inguinal Floor Reconstruction		
Primary Tissue Repair	**Anterior Tension-Free Mesh Repair**	**Laparoscopic and Pre-Peritoneal Repairs**

• **Posterior wall** of inguinal wall is **strengthened by approximation of tissues with sutures**[Q].
• There is **no use of prosthetic material**[Q].
• **Advantages: Simplicity** of the repair & **absence of** any **foreign body** in groin
• **Disadvantage: Higher recurrence rates** due to **tension** on the repair and **slower return to unrestricted physical activity**[Q].
• **Types:**
  – **Bassini repair**[Q]
  – Halsted repair
  – **McVay**[Q] (Cooper ligament) repair
  – **Shouldice repair**[Q]
  – Darn repair
	• Current practice in hernia management employ **synthetic mesh** to **bridge the defect**
	• **Recurrence** is **very low**
	• **Types:**
	• **Lichtenstein repair**[Q]: Mesh is used to reconstruct the inguinal floor.
	• **Patch and plug repair**[Q]: **Plug** of mesh is **inserted into** the hernia **defect** and sutured in place. Then another piece of **mesh** is **placed over** the inguinal floor.
		• Pre-peritoneal space is reached by either trans-abdominal laparoscopy (**TAPP**) or by totally extra-peritoneal repair (**TEP**).
		• Both techniques are similar in actual repair but differ in the manner by which the preperitoneal space is accessed.
		• **TAPP (Trans-abdominal Pre-Peritoneal)**[Q]: Peritoneal space is reached by conventional laparoscopy and pre-peritoneum overlying the inguinal floor is dissected away as a flap.
		• **TEP (Totally Extra-Peritoneal)**[Q]: Pre-peritoneal space is accessed without entering the peritoneal cavity

Gibbon's hernia	• Hernia with hydrocele[Q]
Berger's hernia	• Hernia into pouch of Douglas[Q]
Beclard's hernia	• Femoral hernia through opening of saphenous vein[Q]
Amyand's hernia	• Inguinal hernia containing appendix[Q]
Ogilive's hernia	• Hernia through the defect in conjoint tendon just lateral to where it inserts with the rectus sheath[Q]
Stammer's hernia	• Internal hernia occurring through window in the transverse mesocolon after retrocolic gastrojejunostomy[Q]
Peterson hernia	• Hernia under Roux limb after Roux-en-Y gastric bypass[Q]

117. **Ans. a. Ventriculoperitoneal**   *(Ref: Bailey 27/e p655, 26/e p608; Nelson 20/e p2817, 19/e p2008-2011)*

Most common shunt used for hydrocephalus is ventriculoperitoneal shunt.

*"**Therapy for hydrocephalus** depends on the cause. **Medical management**, including the use of **acetazolamide** and **furosemide**, can provide **temporary relief by reducing the rate of CSF production**, but long-term results have been disappointing. **Most cases of hydrocephalus require extracranial shunts, particularly a ventriculoperitoneal shunt.** Endoscopic third ventriculostomy (ETV) has evolved as a viable approach and criteria have been developed for its use, but the procedure might need to be repeated to be effective."-Nelson 20/e p2817, 19/e p2011*

Management of Hydrocephalus

- **Acute hydrocephalus** is **an emergency** since the condition can **progress over minutes or hours to coma** and **death**.
- It may be relieved by addressing the underlying pathology, for instance by **excision of a tumour responsible for an obstructive hydrocephalus**.
- **Most often**, however, **temporary ventricular drainage is required**, either as an emergency in an obtunded or deteriorating patient, or as a precaution during definitive surgery considering the possibility for postoperative swelling.

External ventricular drain:

- EVDs are an effective **temporary measure to relieve hydrocephalus**.
- Most commonly they are **inserted freehand to the right of midline**, anterior to the coronal suture, so that the **catheter tip rests adjacent to the foramen of Monro in the lateral ventricle**.
- The catheter is then connected to a drain set such that CSF drains when the ventricular pressure exceeds a threshold typically set at 10–20 mmHg. Intrathecal antibiotics may also be delivered through the EVD.

Ventriculoperitoneal shunts:

- **Ventriculoperitoneal (VP) shunting** comprises insertion of a ventricular catheter, which may be antibiotic impregnated, **into the frontal or occipital horn of the lateral ventricle**, while a **distal catheter is tunnelled subcutaneously to the abdomen**.
- Ventriculoatrial and ventriculopleural shunting is also possible.
- A shunt valve, with an opening pressure, which may be high, medium or low, is inserted at the junction of these catheters.
- Selection of the shunt valve is a balance and must be tailored to each patient: high pressure valves may fail to allow adequate CSF drainage, whereas low pressure valves can overdrain.

Shunt complications

- **Over drainage** can result in **low-pressure headaches**, which are **typically worse on standing**.
- **Collapse of the ventricles** can cause **accumulation of fluid in the subdural space, a subdural hygroma**, or bleeding producing a **subdural hematoma**.
- **Shunts are vulnerable to infection and to blockage[Q]**, so that 15–20 percent require replacement within three years.
- 75% of infection presents within one month, a result of introduction at the time of insertion.

  - **Risk factors** include **very young patients, open myelomeningocele, long operation time** and **staff movement in and out of theatre**.

- **Majority of blockages** are **attributable to cellular and proteinaceous debris especially due to infection**, but choroid plexus adhesion or blood clot may also be responsible.

Contd...

Management of Hydrocephalus
Endoscopic third ventriculostomy: • This procedure is **especially useful in obstructive hydrocephalus due to aqueduct stenosis**. • A **neuroendoscope is inserted into the frontal horn of the lateral ventricle** and then into the **third ventricle via the foramen of Monro**. • The floor of the ventricle is then opened between the mamillary bodies and the pituitary recess. • Free drainage between the third ventricle and the adjacent subarachnoid cisterns is then possible, without the infection risk posed by implanted tubing.

118. **Ans. d. Lateral cutaneous nerve of thigh** *(Ref: Sabiston 20/e p1105, 19/e p1118; Schwartz 10/e p1515, 9/e p1313-1315; Schackelford 7/e p562-565)*

"**Neuropathic groin pain** is **caused by damage to a nerve in the groin region** and may be due to partial or complete division, stretching, contusion, crushing, suturing, or electrocautery. The **nerves that are usually involved** are the **ilioinguinal nerve, iliohypogastric nerve, both the genital and femoral branches of the genitofemoral nerve, and the lateral femoral cutaneous nerve of the thigh**. The first two are especially prone to injury during an open herniorrhaphy, while the **latter (i.e. Lateral cutaneous nerve of thigh) are more likely damaged during laparoscopy.**[Q] The **genital and femoral branches of the genitofemoral nerve and the lateral cutaneous nerve of the thigh are most at risk when the surgeon staples below the iliopubic tract** when lateral to the internal spermatic vessels. A **burning, tingling pain along the lateral aspect of the thigh in the distribution of the lateral femoral cutaneous nerve is known as meralgia paresthetica, and is due to entrapment of that nerve**; the affected skin area may be hyperaesthetic and/or pruritic, and patients may complain of the tactile hallucination of a sensation of small insects creeping under the skin (formication)."*-Schwartz 9/e p1313*

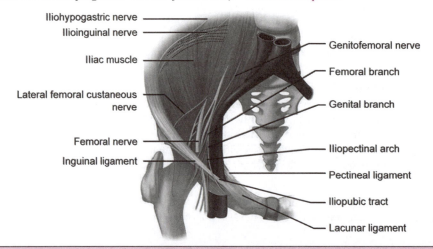

Complications of Groin Hernia Repairs

• **Neuropathic groin pain** is **caused by damage to a nerve in the groin region** and may be due to partial or complete division, stretching, contusion, crushing, suturing, or electrocautery.
• The **nerves that are usually involved** are the **ilioinguinal nerve, iliohypogastric nerve, both the genital and femoral branches of the genitofemoral nerve, and the lateral femoral cutaneous nerve of the thigh**.
   • The **first two are especially prone to injury during an open herniorrhaphy, while the latter (i.e. Lateral cutaneous nerve of thigh) are more likely damaged during laparoscopy.**[Q]
   • The **genital and femoral branches of the genitofemoral nerve** and the **lateral cutaneous nerve of the thigh are most at risk when the surgeon staples below the iliopubic tract** when lateral to the internal spermatic vessels.[Q]
• A **burning, tingling pain along the lateral aspect of the thigh in the distribution of the lateral femoral cutaneous nerve** is known as **meralgia paresthetica**, and is **due to entrapment of that nerve**; the affected skin area may be hyperaesthetic and/or pruritic, and patients may **complain of the tactile hallucination** of a **sensation of small insects creeping under the skin** (formication).
• A femoral nerve injury is extremely rare and is almost always the result of a gross technical misadventure. Its rarity is fortunate because of the severe associated morbidity.

Landmarks in Laparoscopic Repair		
Triangle of Doom	**Triangle of Pain**	**Corona Mortis**

• Bounded **laterally** by the **gonadal vessels**[Q]
• **Medially** by the **vas deferens**[Q]
• **Apex** oriented superiorly at the **internal ring**[Q]
• Contain **external iliac vessels**[Q], deep circumflex iliac vein, the femoral nerve & genital branch of the genitofemoral nerve.
	• Also known as **Electrical hazard zone**[Q]
	• Bounded **medially** by the **gonadal vessels**[Q]
	• **Superiorly** by the **iliopubic tract**[Q]
	• **Laterally** by **peritoneum**[Q]
	• This triangle **contains** from lateral to medial:
	  – Lateral femoral cutaneous nerve[Q] (MC injured nerve during laparoscopic repair)
	  – Anterior femoral cutaneous[Q]
	  – Femoral branch of the genitofemoral nerve[Q]
	  – Femoral nerve[Q]
		• Also known as **Crown of death**[Q]
		• **Vascular connections** between the **obturator & external iliac** systems[Q]
		• **Aberrant obturator artery** arises from the **inferior epigastric** artery, arches over the **Cooper's ligament** & **joins** the **normal obturator artery**[Q] to complete a vascular ring
		• **Significant hemorrhage**[Q] may occur **if accidentally cut** and it is **difficult to achieve** subsequent **hemostasis**

Space of Retzius (Retropubic space)	• Extra-peritoneal space between **pubic symphysis and urinary bladder**[Q]
Space of Bogros (Retroinguinal space)	• Extra-peritoneal space situated **deep to inguinal ligament**[Q] • Situated **laterally and cranially to Retzius space**

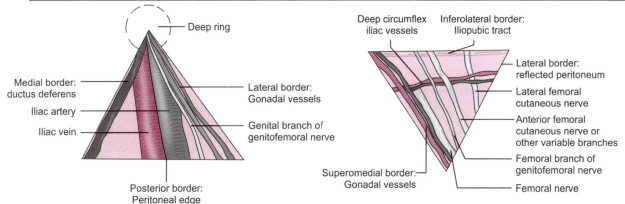

119. Ans. a. Left lower lobe consolidation *(Ref: Sabiston 20/e p1567, 19/1558-1559; Schwartz 10/e p1444, 9/1260-1262; Bailey 27/e p1186, 26/1096; Shackelford 7/e p1674-1676)*

Fever on postoperative day 3 after laparoscopic splenectomy suggests left lower lobe consolidation.

> *"**Left lower lobe atelectasis is the most common complication after OS**; **pleural effusion** and **pneumonia** also can occur. Hemorrhage can occur intraoperatively or postoperatively, presenting as subphrenic hematoma. Transfusions have become less common since the advent of LS, although the indication for operation influences the likelihood of transfusion as well. Subphrenic abscess and wound infection are among the perioperative infectious complications."* -Schwartz 10/e p1444

Complications of Splenectomy	
Pulmonary Complications: • **Left lower lobe atelectasis: MC complication**[Q] • Pleural effusion • Pneumonia **Hemorrhagic Complications:** • Subphrenic hematoma **Infectious Complications:** • Subphrenic abscess • Wound infection **Pancreatic Complications:** • Pancreatitis • Pseudocyst • Pancreatic fistula	**Thromboembolic Complications:** • DVT • Portal vein thrombosis • **DVT prophylaxis** is **routinely recommended**[Q]. • In patients with **hemolytic anemia** or **myeloproliferative disorders** and **splenomegaly**, **thrombotic risk** is **heightened**, particularly the risk of **portal vein thrombosis**[Q]. • Patients undergoing splenectomy for **malignancy** or **myeloproliferative disorders** should be strongly considered for **perioperative pharmacoprophylaxis**, either **LMWH** or **unfractionated heparin**[Q].

Contd...

Overwhelming Postsplenectomy Infection (OPSI)
• OPSI is the **MC fatal late complication** of **splenectomy**.
• **Infection may occur** at **any time after splenectomy**[Q]
• In one recent series, **most infections occurred more than 2 years after splenectomy** and **42% occurred more than 5 years after splenectomy**[Q].
Clinical Features:
• OPSI **typically begins with** a **prodromal phase** characterized by **fever, rigors** and chills and other **nonspecific symptoms**, including sore throat, malaise, myalgias, diarrhea, and vomiting.
• Many patients have no identifiable focal site of infection and present only with high-grade primary bacteremia.
• **Progression of** the **illness is rapid**, with the **development of hypotension, disseminated intravascular coagulation, respiratory distress, coma**, and **death within hours of presentation**[Q].
• **Despite antibiotics** and **intensive care**, the **mortality rate** is between **50-70% for florid OPSI**[Q].
• **Most frequently involved organism** in OPSI is **S. pneumoniae**[Q] (**50-90%** of cases)
• Other organisms involved in OPSI: **H. influenzae, N. meningitidis, Streptococcus** and **Salmonella spp**[Q].
• **Risk for OPSI** is **greater** in **splenectomy for malignancy** or **hematologic conditions** than for those who underwent splenectomy for trauma[Q].
• **Risk is greater for young children**[Q] (**<4 years** of age).

120. **Ans. a. Circumferential**   *(Ref: Sabiston and Spencer's Surgery of Chest 8/chapter 7)*

Circumferential incision is generally taken for diaphragmatic surgery.

Diaphragmatic incisions		
Circumferential incisions	**Incisions in the central tendon**	**Transverse radial incision**
• **Circumferential incisions** in the periphery result in **little loss of function**[Q].	• Do not interrupt any major branch of the nerve itself.	• Made from the midaxillary line centrally
• Must be **at least 5 cm lateral to the edge of the central tendon** to avoid the posterolateral and anterolateral branches of the phrenic nerve.	• **Provide excellent visualization of the abdomen from the thorax**, and vice versa.	• **Relatively safe**
• **Difficult to correctly realign after a long operation.**	• **Easy to open & to close.**	• **May result in segmental diaphragmatic paralysis** if the incision transects the crural or posterolateral branches of the phrenic nerve.
• **Placement of surgical clips on each side of the muscular incision** can greatly facilitate the correct spatial orientation on closing.		

121. **Ans. c. USG**   *(Ref: Ghai 8/e p 287; Sabiston 20/e p1299, 19/e p1279-1282; Schwartz 10/e p1256, 9/e p1074-1078; Bailey 27/e p1307, 26/e p1201-1210; Shackelford 7/e p2019-2023)*

Best diagnostic investigation for acute appendicitis in children is USG.

"Abdominal ultrasound detects a dilated (< 6 mm) tubular, aperistaltic structure which is not compressible and is surrounded by fluid. Ultrasound has a sensitivity of 85-90% and specificity of 95-100% for diagnosing appendicitis. Computed tomography may be done occasionally if the diagnosis is in doubt."-Ghai 8/e p287

Acute Appendicitis
• **Acute appendicitis** is the **MC general surgical emergency**[Q]
• Worldwide, **perforated appendicitis** is the **leading general surgical cause** of **death**[Q].
Pathophysiology:
• **Obstruction of the lumen**[Q] is believed to be the **major cause** of **acute appendicitis**[Q].
• **Obstruction of the lumen** may be **caused by inspissated stool** (fecalith[Q] or appendicolith[Q]), **lymphoid hyperplasia**[Q], **vegetable matter** or **seeds**[Q], **parasites**, or a **neoplasm**[Q].

Contd...

Contd...

Acute Appendicitis

- Obstruction of the appendiceal lumen contributes to **bacterial overgrowth** and **continued secretion of mucus** leads **to intraluminal distention** and **increased wall pressure. Luminal distention** produces the **visceral pain** sensation experienced by the patient as **periumbilical pain**[Q].

- Subsequent impairment of lymphatic and **venous drainage** leads to **mucosal ischemia**.

Bacteriology:
- **MC bacteria isolated** in **perforated appendicitis: Bacteroides fragilis**[Q] (80%) >**E. coli**[Q] (77%).

Clinical Features:
- **Diagnosis** can be **made primarily** on the basis of the **history** and **physical examination** in **most cases**[Q].
- **Typical presentation**: Periumbilical pain followed by **anorexia** and **nausea**.

- The **pain** then **localizes to** the **right lower quadrant** as the inflammatory process progresses to involve the parietal peritoneum overlying the appendix.
- This **classic pattern of migratory pain** is the **most reliable symptom** of **acute appendicitis**[Q].
- A **bout of vomiting** may occur. **Fever ensues, followed by** the development of **leukocytosis**.
- **Occasional patients** have **urinary symptoms** or **microscopic hematuria**

- **Tenderness** is **directly over** the **appendix, at McBurney's point**[Q].
- **Rectal** and **pelvic examinations** are **most likely** to be **negative (Tenderness on P/R examination in pelvic appendix)**[Q]

Dunphy's sign[Q]	• **Pain** on **coughing**[Q]
Rovsing's sign[Q]	• **Pain in** the **right lower quadrant** during **palpation of** the **left lower quadrant**[Q]
Obturator sign[Q]	• **Pain** on **internal rotation** of the **hip**[Q] • Suggestive of **pelvic appendix**[Q]
Iliopsoas sign[Q]	• **Pain on extension** of the **right hip**[Q] • Suggestive of **retrocecal appendix**[Q]

Diagnosis:

Laboratory Studies

- **WBC count** is **elevated**, with **more than 75% neutrophils** in most patients[Q].
- **Normal WBC count** and **differential** is found in **10%** of **patients** with acute appendicitis[Q].
- **High WBC count (>20,000/mL)** suggests **complicated appendicitis** with **gangrene** or **perforation**[Q].
- **Microscopic hematuria** is **common in appendicitis (gross hematuria** may **indicate** the presence of a **kidney stone)**[Q]

Ultrasound:
- USG has a **sensitivity of 85%** and a **specificity >90%** for the diagnosis of acute appendicitis in patients of abdominal pain.
- **Characteristic findings**: Appendix ≥7 mm diameter, a **thick-walled, non-compressible luminal structure** seen in cross section (**target lesion**), or the **presence of an appendicolith**[Q].
- Commonly used in **children** & **pregnant patients**[Q] with equivocal clinical findings suggestive of acute appendicitis.

Plain X-ray:
- A **calcified appendicolith** is **visible** in only **10-15%** of patients with acute appendicitis.
- **Failure of the appendix to fill during** a **barium enema** has been **associated with appendicitis**[Q] (this finding lacks sensitivity and specificity because up to 20% of normal appendices do not fill).

Contd...

Contd...

Acute Appendicitis
CT Scan
<ul><li>**CT scan**: **Sensitivity** of **90%** and a **specificity** of **80-90%** for the diagnosis of **acute appendicitis** in patients with abdominal pain[Q].</li><li>**Classic findings** on CT: **Distended appendix >7 mm** in diameter and **circumferential wall thickening** and **enhancement** (appearance of a **halo** or **target**)[Q]</li><li>**CT detects appendicoliths** in **50%** of patients with appendicitis.</li><li>**Most valuable for older patients** and in patients with atypical symptoms.</li></ul>
Treatment: <ul><li>Most patients are managed by prompt **appendectomy**[Q].</li></ul>

122. **Ans. a. Hepatic scintigraphy** *(Ref: Nelson 20/e p1934, 19/e p1385; Sabiston 20/e p1880, 19/e p1852-1853; Schwartz 10/e p1628, 9/1438-1440; Bailey 27/e p1196, 26/e p1104-1105; Blumgart 5/e p595-603; Shackelford 7/e p1390-1396)*

Investigation of choice to rule out biliary atresia in a 2- month-old child is Hepatic scintigraphy. Hepatobiliary scintigraphy with technetium-labeled iminodiacetic acid derivatives (HIDA scan) is used to differentiate biliary atresia from non-obstructive causes of cholestasis.

> *"Hepatobiliary scintigraphy with technetium-labeled iminodiacetic acid derivatives (HIDA scan) is used to differentiate biliary atresia from non-obstructive causes of cholestasis. The hepatic uptake of the agent is normal in patients with biliary atresia but excretion into the intestine is absent. Although the uptake may be impaired in neonatal hepatitis, excretion into the bowel will eventually occur. Obtaining a follow-up scan after 24 hours is of value to determine the patency of the biliary tree. The administration of phenobarbital (5 mg/kg/day) for 5 days before the scan is recommended because it may enhance biliary excretion of the isotope. Hepatobiliary scintigraphy is a very sensitive but not specific test for biliary atresia. It fails to identify other structural abnormalities of the biliary tree or vascular anomalies."*
> *-Nelson 20/e p1934*

Biliary Atresia
<ul><li>Characterized by **progressive obliteration** of the **extrahepatic** and **intrahepatic** bile ducts[Q].</li><li>**Etiology** is **unknown; Incidence 1 in 12,000** live births[Q].</li><li>Presently, there is **no medical therapy** to **reverse** the **obliterative process**[Q]<ul><li>Patients who are **not offered surgical treatment** uniformly develop biliary cirrhosis, portal hypertension, and **death** by **2 years of age**[Q].</li></ul></li><li>**MC indication** for **pediatric liver transplantation**[Q]</li></ul>
Pathology: <ul><li>**Bile duct proliferation**, **severe cholestasis** with **plugging**, and **inflammatory cell infiltrate** are the **pathologic hallmarks** of this disease[Q].</li><li>Over time, these changes **progress to fibrosis** with **end-stage cirrhosis**[Q].</li><li>Positive for neural cell adhesion molecule (**CD56**) staining.</li></ul>

Variants of biliary atresia
1. Patency to the level of CBD
2. Patency to the level of common hepatic duct
3. Left and right hepatic duct at porta involved, solid porta hepatis (90%)

Clinical Features:
<ul><li>Infants with biliary atresia present with **jaundice at birth** or **shortly thereafter**[Q].</li><li>Infants with biliary atresia characteristically have **acholic, pale gray stools**, secondary to obstructed bile flow.</li><li>With passage of time, **progressive failure to thrive** and, if untreated, develop **stigmata of liver failure** and **portal hypertension** (splenomegaly & esophageal varices)</li><li>**Associated malformations** in **25%**: **Polysplenia, malrotation, preduodenal portal vein**, and **intrahepatic vena cava**[Q].</li></ul>

Contd...

Contd...

Biliary Atresia
Diagnosis: • USG of the liver and GB is important in the evaluation of the infant with cholestasis. <ul><ul><li>**USG: GB is shrunken** and **CBD** is **not visible**[Q]. A **triangle cord sign**[Q] found on ultrasound has a **predictive accuracy** of **95%**, the **gallbladder ghost triad**[Q] in which the **gallbladder** is **short** (<1.9 cm) and **irregular** and **lacks an echogenic inner lining** also got good sensitivity.</li></ul></ul>• **Next diagnostic step:** Percutaneous **liver biopsy**[Q] if the hepatic synthetic function is normal (diagnostic accuracy 90%). • **Hepatobiliary scintigraphy**: In cases in which the USG and biopsy findings are inconclusive (**absent excretion into the intestine**)[Q] <ul><ul><li>*Hepatobiliary scintigraphy with technetium-labeled iminodiacetic acid derivatives (HIDA scan) is used to differentiate biliary atresia from non-obstructive causes of cholestasis*[Q]</li></ul></ul>
Treatment: • **Exploratory laparotomy**: If the needle biopsy or abdominal ultrasound is consistent with BA • **Intraoperative cholecystocholangiography: To confirm** the **diagnosis**, demonstration of the **fibrotic biliary remnant** and definition of **absent proximal** and **distal bile duct patency**[Q] <ul><ul><li>**Treatment of choice: Kasai hepatoportoenterostomy**[Q] **(Roux-en-Y hepaticojejunostomy)**</li></ul></ul>
Postoperative Management: • **Ursodeoxycholic acid** (facilitate bile flow) + **Methylprednisolone** (anti-inflammatory agent) + **TMP-SMX** (antimicrobial prophylaxis)[Q] <ul><ul><li>**Cholangitis** is the **MC** postoperative **complication**[Q].</li></ul></ul>
Prognosis: • About **30%** of infants undergoing hepatoportoenterostomy **before 60 days** of age will have a **long-term successful outcome** and **not require liver transplantation**[Q]. • **Liver transplantation** in the patients who develop **progressive hepatic fibrosis** with resultant **portal hypertension** and progressive cholestasis[Q]. • **Serum bilirubin** at **3 months** after surgery seems to be **strongly predictive** of **long-term survival**[Q].

123. Ans. d. Increased pH *(Ref: Bailey 27/e p87, 26/e p94; http://www.laparoscopyhospital.com/physiological-changes-laparoscopy.html)*

Metabolic acidosis (decrease pH) from CO_2 absorption is the primary derangement with laparoscopy.

Laparoscopy
• In laparoscopic surgeries, a rigid endoscope is introduced through a sleeve into the peritoneal cavity. • **Needle used** for pneumoperitoneum: **Veress needle**[Q] • **Most commonly used gas: CO_2**[Q] • **Flow of gas: 1L/min**[Q] • **Intra-abdominal pressure: 12-15** mm Hg[Q] • **Trocar** is inserted **at or just below** the **umbilicus**[Q] penetrating **skin, superficial** and **deep fascia, fascia transversalis** and **parietal peritoneum.**[Q] <ul><ul><li>Use of **carbon dioxide** and **helium as insufflants** causes **locoregional hypoxia** and may also **change pH**. The CO_2 can diffuse into the **blood** and **cause decrease in pH**.</li><li>**Post-laparoscopy shoulder pain** is due to CO_2 **retention** causing **irritation of diaphragm** and **referred pain to** the **shoulder** through **phrenic nerve**[Q].</li></ul></ul>

Contd...

AIIMS ESSENCE

Contd...

Laparoscopy

Gases used in Pneumoperitoneum
• **First pneumoperitoneum** was created by **filtered room air**[Q].
• CO_2 and N_2O are now **preferred** because of **increased risk of gas embolism with room air**[Q].
• CO_2: 200 times **more diffusible than** O_2, **rapidly cleared** from the body and lungs, **doesn't support combustion**[Q]
• N_2O: 68% as **rapidly absorbed in blood** as CO_2, have **mild analgesic effect**, used **for short operative procedures** like sterilization or drilling[Q].
• For prolonged laparoscopic procedures, N_2O should not be preferred because it **supports combustion** better than air[Q].

Physiological Effects of Laparoscopy	
Cardiovascular	• ↑ **Intra-abdominal pressure leads to** ↑ **CVP**, ↑ **PCWP**, ↑**SVR** and ↑ **MAP** which further ↓ **Preload** and ↑ **Afterload**, ultimately **decreasing cardiac output**[Q].
Pulmonary	• **Cephalad shift of diaphragm decreases FRC, chest wall compliance** and **tidal volume increasing the work of breathing**[Q]. • **Hypercapnia** leading to **increase in respiratory rate** further adds to this.
Renal	• **Increased IAP decreases renal flow, decreasing GFR and reduced urine output**. • Raised pCO_2 leads to **RAAS stimulation**. No long-term change in GFR/UO.
Gastrointestinal	• **Decreased perfusion to intestines and stomach** (as a result of increase IAP) **decreases pH** • **Decreased portal and hepatic flow** leads to **elevation of LFTs**.
Peripheral vascular	• Incidence of **DVT, PE is generally lower** post-laparoscopic procedures probably secondary to improved prophylaxis • Risk is **increased with longer procedures** and **reverse Trendelenberg position**.

Advantages of minimal access surgery	**Limitations of minimal access surgery**
• **Decrease in wound size**[Q] • **Reduction in wound infection, dehiscence, bleeding, herniation** and **nerve entrapment**[Q] • **Decrease in wound pain**[Q] • **Improved mobility**[Q] • Decreased wound trauma • **Decreased heat loss**[Q] • **Improved vision**[Q] • Faster recovery and shorter hospital stay	• Reliance on remote vision and operating • **Loss of tactile feedback** • **Dependence on hand-eye coordination** • Difficulty with hemostasis • Reliance on new techniques • Extraction of large specimens.

124. **Ans. b. Divided into 8 segments** *(Ref: Gray's 40/e p1165, 1166,1178; Sabiston 20/e p1484, 19/e p/1413-1417; Schwartz 10/e p1265, 9/e p1095; Bailey 27/e p1154, 26/e p1065-1067; Blumgart 5/e p31-37; Shackelford 7/e p1426-1430)*

All of the given options are true. If we have to choose one answer, most preferred option is 'liver is divided into 8 segments', because sometimes segment IX is described. Segment IX is a recent subdivision of segment I, and describes that part of the segment that lies posterior to segment VIII.

"Current understanding of the functional anatomy of the liver is based on Couinaud's division of the liver into eight (subsequently nine) functional segments, based upon the distribution of portal venous branches and the location of the hepatic veins in the parenchyma (Couinaud 1957)."—Gray's 40/e p1165

"Segment IX is a recent subdivision of segment I, and describes that part of the segment that lies posterior to segment VIII."—Gray's 40/e p1166

Functional Anatomical Divisions of Liver

- Current understanding of the **functional anatomy of the liver** is **based on Couinaud's division of the liver into eight (subsequently nine) functional segments,** based upon the distribution of **portal venous branches** and the location of the **hepatic veins** in the parenchyma **(Couinaud 1957).**

  - **Segment IX** is a **recent subdivision of segment I,** and describes that **part of the segment that lies posterior to segment VIII**[Q].

- The liver is **divided into four portal sectors** by the **four main branches of the portal vein.** These are **right lateral, right medial, left medial and left lateral** (sometimes the term posterior is used in place of lateral and anterior in place of medial).
- The **three main hepatic veins lie between these sectors as intersectorial veins.** These **intersectoral planes** are also called **portal fissures (scissures). The fissures containing portal pedicles** are called **hepatic fissures.**
- **Each sector** is sub-divided **into segments (usually two)** based on their **supply by tertiary divisions of the vascular biliary sheaths.**

Fissures of the liver:

- **Three major fissures,** not visible on the surface, run through the liver parenchyma and **harbor the three main hepatic veins (main, left and right portal fissures)**[Q].
- **Three minor fissures** are visible as **physical clefts of the liver surface (umbilical, venous and fissure of Gans)**[Q].

Major Fissures of the Liver		
Main portal fissure	**Left portal fissure**	**Right portal fissure**
- **Extends from the tip of the GB back to the midpoint of IVC** and **contains the middle (main) hepatic vein.** - **Separates liver** into **right and left hemi-livers.** - Segments V and VIII lie to the right and segment IV to the left of the fissure.	- Divides left hemi-liver into medial (anterior) and lateral (posterior) sectors. - Extends from the **mid point of the anterior edge of the liver** between **falciform ligament** and **left triangular ligament** to the point, which marks the confluence of the left and middle hepatic veins. - **Contains left hepatic vein** - Separates the left anterior and left posterior sectors: **segment III lies anteriorly** and **segment II posteriorly.**	- **Divides right hemi-liver into lateral (posterior) and medial (anterior) sectors.** - **Plane of right fissure** is the **most variable** amongst the main fissures and runs approximately diagonally through the gross right lobe from the lateral end of the anterior border to the confluence of the left and middle hepatic veins. - The fissure **divides right anterior sector to its left (segments V and VIII)** from **right posterior sector to its right (segments VI and VII)** - **Contains right hepatic vein** - **Right fissure marks the thickest point** of liver parenchyma, which is commonly **transected during liver resection.**

Minor Fissures of the liver		
Umbilical fissure	**Venous fissure**	**Fissure of Gans**
- Umbilical fissure **separates segment III from segment VI** within left anterior sector and **contains** a main branch of left hepatic vein **(umbilical fissure vein).** - It is **marked by attachment of falciform ligament** and sometimes covered by a ridge of liver tissue extending between the segments: it is **often avascular** and can be **divided safely with diathermy** during a surgical approach. - It **contains umbilical portion of left portal vein** and the **final divisions of left hepatic duct** and **left hepatic artery branches.**	- Venous fissure is a **continuation of umbilical fissure** on under surface of liver - **Contains ligamentum venosum** - It **lies between caudate lobe** and **segment IV.** - The deeper continuation of this plane is the dorsal fissure.	- **Fissure of Gans lies on undersurface of right lobe of liver** behind GB fossa. - **Contains portal pedicle** to **right posterior sector**

Contd...

Contd...

Functional Anatomical Divisions of Liver

Sectors and segments of the liver:
- The sectors of the liver are made up of between one and three segments: right lateral sector = segments VI and VII; right medial sector = segments V and VIII; left medial sector = segments III and IV (and part of I); left lateral sector = segment II.
  - **Segments are numbered in an ante-clockwise spiral centered on the portal vein** with the **liver viewed from beneath**, starting with segment I up to segment VI, and then back clockwise for the most cranial two segments VII and VIII.

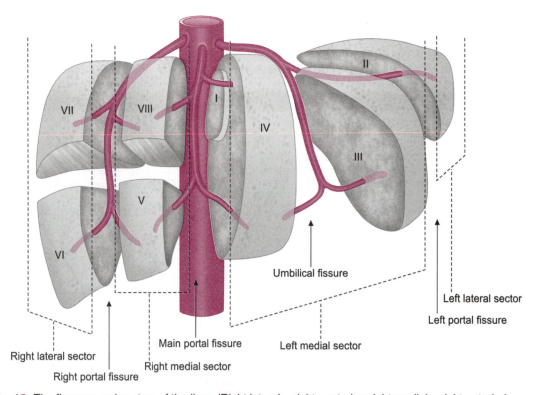

Fig. 15: The fissures and sectors of the liver. (Right lateral = right posterior; right medial = right anterior)

Segmental Nomenclature	
I	Caudate lobe[Q] (sometimes subdivided into left and right parts called segment IX)
II	Left **lateral superior** segment
III	Left **lateral inferior** segment
IV	Left medial segment or **Quadrate lobe**[Q]
V	Right **anterior inferior** segment
VI	Right **posterior inferior** segment
VII	Right **posterior superior** segment
VIII	Right **anterior superior** segment

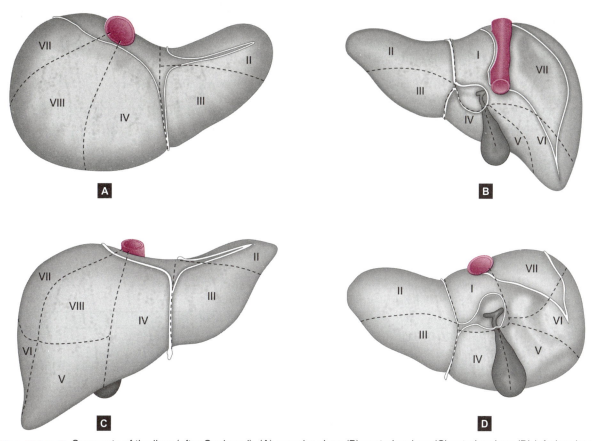

Figs. 16A to D: Segments of the liver (after Couinaud). (A) superior view; (B) posterior view; (C) anterior view; (D) inferior view.

125. **Ans. c. 50,000** *(Ref: Bailey 27/e p22-23, 26/e p23; Nelson 20/e p2374)*
In a patient with thrombocytopenia, target platelet count after transfusion to perform an invasive procedure is 50, 000.

Management of coagulopathy	

- Correction of coagulopathy is **not necessary if there is no active bleeding or haemorrhage** is not anticipated (not due for surgery).
- However, coagulopathy following or during massive transfusion should be anticipated and managed aggressively.

Blood Product	Standard Guidelines
FFP	• If prothrombin time (PT) or partial thromboplastin time (PTT) > 1.5 times normal[Q]
Cryoprecipitate	• If fibrinogen < 0.8 g/L[Q]
Platelets	• If platelet count <50 × 10⁹/mL[Q]

- However, in the presence of non-surgical haemorrhage these tests take time to arrange and may underestimate the degree of coagulopathy.
- Treatment should then be instituted on the basis of clinical evidence of non-surgical bleeding.
- There are **pharmacological adjuncts to blood component therapy**, although their indications and efficacy are yet to be established.
- Antifibrinolytics such as **tranexamic acid** and **aprotinin** are the **most commonly administered**.
- **Recombinant factor VIIa** is also under investigation **for the treatment of non-surgical haemorrhage.**

Guidelines for Pediatric Platelet Transfusion
Children and Adolescents:
1. Maintain PLT count **>50×10⁹/L with bleeding**
2. Maintain PLT count **>50×10⁹/L with major invasive procedure; >25×10⁹/L with minor**
3. Maintain PLT count **>20×10⁹/L and marrow failure WITH hemorrhagic risk factors**
4. Maintain PLT count **>10×10⁹/L and marrow failure WITHOUT hemorrhagic risk factors**
5. Maintain PLT count at any level with PLT dysfunction PLUS bleeding or invasive procedure

126. **Ans. d. Roux-en-Y gastric bypass** *(Ref: Sabiston 20/e p1187, 19/e p363; Schwartz 10/e p1112, 9/952; Harrison 19/e p2398)*

Most commonly performed and acceptable method of bariatric surgery is Roux-en-Y gastric bypass.

> *"The **three restrictive-malabsorptive bypass procedures** combine the elements of **gastric restriction and selective malabsorption**. These procedures are **Roux-en-Y gastric bypass, biliopancreatic diversion, and biliopancreatic diversion with duodenal switch**. Roux-en-Y is the most commonly undertaken and most accepted bypass procedure. It may be performed with an open incision or by laparoscopy."*-Harrison 19/e p2398

Bariatric Surgery

- **Indication for Bariatric Surgery:**
  - Patients that have a BMI of **35 Kg/m²** or more **with comorbidity**[Q]
  - Those with a BMI of **40 Kg/m²** or greater regardless of comorbidity[Q]

New Guidelines for Asia
• **Overweight if the BMI is 23 Kg/m² or more**[Q] (International Standard is 25).
• **Obese if the BMI is 25 Kg/m² or more**[Q] (I.S. is 30).
• An Indian qualifies for **bariatric surgery** for obesity if the BMI is **32.5 Kg/m² (I.S. 35) with comorbidity**[Q] or **37.5 Kg/m²** without comorbidity(I.S. 40)[Q].

Bariatric Operation	Mechanism of Action
• **Vertical banded gastroplasty** • Laparoscopic adjustable **gastric banding**	**Restrictive**[Q]
• **Roux-en-Y gastric bypass (RYGB): MC performed and most accepted procedure**	**Largely Restrictive**[Q]/Mildly Malabsorptive
• **Biliopancreatic diversion** • **Duodenal switch**	**Largely Malabsorptive**[Q]/ Mildly Restrictive

Biliopancreatic Diversion
• When the bile is diverted from the intestinal tract so that only the **distal 50 to 100 cm of ileum** is **used for bile reabsorption**, the procedure is termed a biliopancreatic diversion.
• **Most effective bariatric surgery**[Q], especially valuable in patients with **severe morbid obesity** or in those who have **failed to maintain weight loss** following gastric bypass surgery or restrictive procedures[Q].
• **Main side effect** with BPD: Patients usually have an increase of **2-4 bowel movements**/day, which in general are **more malodorous**, suggesting fat malabsorption.

Duodenal Switch Operation
• It involves a greater curvature **sleeve gastrectomy** with maintenance of the **continuity of** the antrum, pylorus and **first portion** of the duodenum.
• This allows for a **lower marginal ulcer** rate and a lower incidence of **dumping syndrome**.

Components of Duodenal Switch Operation	
• **Sleeve gastrectomy**[Q]	• **Cholecystectomy**[Q]
• **Duodenoileostomy**[Q]	• **Appendectomy**[Q]
• **Jejunoileal bypass**[Q]	

Contd...

Conduction aphasia

- Conduction aphasia results from damage to the arcuate fasciculus[Q].
- The **connection between the Wernicke's (language comprehension) and Broca's (Language production) areas is lost[Q]**.
  - The **hallmark of conduction aphasia** is the **inability to repeat words[Q]**.
- **Comprehension and the expression of language are intact** but patients cannot transfer the understood word to Broca's area to be expressed.
  - **Conduction aphasia results in meaningful fluent speech** and **relatively good comprehension but very poor repetition[Q]**.

	Comprehension	Repetition of spoken language	Naming	Fluency
Wernicke's	Impaired	Impaired	Impaired	Preserved or increased[Q]
Broca's	Preserved (except grammar)[Q]	Impaired	Impaired	Decreased
Global	Impaired	Impaired	Impaired	Decreased
Conduction	Preserved[Q]	Impaired	Impaired	Preserved[Q]
Nonfluent (motor) transcortical	Preserved[Q]	Preserved[Q]	Impaired	Impaired
Fluent (sensory) transcortical	Impaired	Preserved[Q]	Impaired	Preserved
Isolation	Impaired	Echolalia[Q]	Impaired	No purposeful speech
Anomic	Preserved[Q]	Preserved[Q]	Impaired	Preserved except for word-finding pauses[Q]
Pure word deafness	Impaired only for spoken language	Impaired	Preserved	Preserved
Pure alexia	Impaired only for reading	Preserved	Preserved	Preserved

98. **Ans. a. Splenomegaly** *(Ref: Harrison 19/e p819, 18/e p1055; Nelson 20/e p2266)*

Splenomegaly is not a part of Duke's Criteria for infective endocarditis.

Criteria for the Clinical Diagnosis of Infective Endocarditis		
Major Criteria		**Minor Criteria**
1. Positive blood culture for IE	**2. Evidence of endocardial involvement**	1. Predisposition: **predisposing heart condition** or **injection drug use**

• **Typical microorganism for infective endocarditis from two separate blood cultures:**[Q]
  – Viridans streptococci, *Streptococcus gallolyticus*, HACEK group, *Staphylococcus aureus*, *or*
  – Community-acquired enterococci in the absence of a primary focus, *or*
• Persistently positive blood culture, defined as recovery of a microorganism consistent with infective endocarditis from:
  – Blood cultures drawn >12 h apart; *or*
  – All of 3 or a majority of ≥ 4 separate blood cultures, with first and last drawn at least 1 h apart
• **Single positive blood culture for *Coxiella burnetii*** or phase I IgG antibody titer of >1:800
	• **Positive echocardiogram:**
	  – **Oscillating intracardiac mass** on valve or supporting structures or in the path of regurgitant jets or in implanted material
	  – **Abscess**, *or*
	  – **New partial dehiscence of prosthetic valve**, *or*
	• New valvular regurgitation (increase or change in preexisting murmur not sufficient)
		2. Fever ≥38.0°C (≥100.4°F)
		3. **Vascular phenomena:** major arterial emboli, septic pulmonary infarcts, mycotic aneurysm, intracranial hemorrhage, conjunctival hemorrhages, **Janeway lesions**
		4. **Immunologic phenomena:** glomerulonephritis, Osler's nodes, Roth's spots, rheumatoid factor
		5. **Microbiologic evidence: positive blood culture** but not meeting major criterion as noted previously or serologic evidence of active infection with organism consistent with infective endocarditis

AIIMS ESSENCE

- **Definite endocarditis** is defined by **documentation of two major criteria, of one major criterion** and **three minor criteria, or of five minor criteria**.
- **Transesophageal echocardiography** is recommended **for assessing possible prosthetic valve endocarditis** or **complicated endocarditis**.
- Excluding single positive cultures for coagulase-negative staphylococci and diphtheroids, which are common culture contaminants, and organisms that do not cause endocarditis frequently, such as gram-negative bacilli.
- *Note:* **HACEK**, *Haemophilus* spp., *Aggregatibacter actinomycetemcomitans*, *Cardiobacterium hominis*, *Eikenella corrodens*, *Kingella* spp.

99. Ans. d. Airway, CT scan, Blood sugar if <70 start dextrose *(Ref: Harrison 19/e p2435, 18/e p3008; ATLS 9/e 2013; 72(5): p1363-1366)*

First testing of blood sugar is necessary before giving glucose as the patient may also be dehydrated and be in diabetic ketoacidotic coma rather then hypoglycemia. A NCCT head is advisable in emergency situations as administration of glucose can lead to cerebral edema.

Hypoglycemia: Approach to the Patient
• **Hypoglycemia** is suspected in patients with **typical symptoms;** in the presence of **confusion, an altered level of consciousness,** or a **seizure;** or in a **clinical setting in which hypoglycemia is known to occur.** • **Blood should be drawn,** whenever possible, **before the administration of glucose to allow documentation of a low plasma glucose concentration.** • Convincing documentation of hypoglycemia requires the **fulfillment of Whipple's triad.** • Thus, the **ideal time to measure the plasma glucose level** is **during a symptomatic episode**. • A **normal glucose level excludes hypoglycemia** as the cause of the symptoms. • A **low glucose level confirms that hypoglycemia** is the cause of the symptoms, provided the latter resolve after the glucose level is raised. • When the cause of the hypoglycemic episode is obscure, additional measurements, while the glucose level is low and before treatment, should include plasma insulin, C-peptide, proinsulin and beta-hydroxybutyrate levels, as well as screening for circulating oral hypoglycemic agents, and symptoms should be assessed during and after the plasma glucose concentration is raised.
Diagnosis of the Hypoglycemic Mechanism: • In a patient with documented hypoglycemia, a plausible hypoglycemic mechanism can often be deduced from the history, physical examination, and available laboratory data. • **Drugs, particularly those used to treat diabetes or alcohol, should be the first consideration,** even in the absence of known use of a relevant drug, given the possibility of surreptitious, accidental, or malicious drug administration. • Other considerations include evidence of a **relevant critical illness**, less commonly **hormone deficiencies**, and **rarely a non beta-cell tumor** that can be pursued diagnostically. • Absence of these mechanisms, in an otherwise seemingly well individual, one should consider endogenous hyperinsulinism and proceed with measurements and assessment of symptoms during spontaneous hypoglycemia or under conditions that might elicit hypoglycemia.

Urgent Treatment:
• Oral treatment with **glucose tablets** or **glucose-containing fluids**, **candy, or food** is appropriate if the patient is able and willing to take these.
     • A reasonable initial dose is 20 g of glucose. If the **patient is unable or unwilling**, because of neuroglycopenia, **to take carbohydrates orally, parenteral therapy is necessary**.
     • IV glucose (25 g) should be given and followed by a glucose infusion guided by serial plasma glucose measurements.
• If **intravenous therapy is not practical, subcutaneous or intramuscular glucagon** (1.0 mg in adults) can be used, particularly in patients with **Type I DM**. Because it **acts by stimulating glycogenolysis**, glucagon is **ineffective in glycogen-depleted individuals** (e.g., those with alcohol-induced hypoglycemia). It also stimulates insulin secretion and is therefore less useful in T2DM.

100. Ans. b. Antistreptolysin O *(Ref: Harrison 19/e p2149, 18/e p2755; Ghai 8/e p 435)*
ASLO is a marker for recent streptococcal infection. Best investigation to prove rheumatic etiology is Antistreptolysin O.

AIIMS May 2015

"Supporting evidence of a preceding streptococcal infection within the last 45 days: Elevated or rising anti-streptolysin O or other streptococcal antibody, or A positive throat culture, or Rapid antigen test for group A streptococcus, or Recent scarlet fever."

World Health Criteria for the diagnosis of Rheumatic Fever and Rheumatic Heart Disease		
Major Criteria	**Minor Criteria**	**Supporting evidence of a preceding streptococcal infection within the last 45 days**
1. Carditis[Q] 2. Migratory polyarthritis[Q] 3. Syndenham's chorea[Q] 4. Subcutaneous nodules[Q] 5. Erythema marginatum[Q]	• Clinical: Fever, polyarthralgia[Q] • Laboratory: Elevated ESR or leukocyte count[Q] • ECG: Prolonged P-R interval @1992 *Revised Jones criteria do not include elevated leucocyte count as a laboratory minor manifestation (but do include elevated C-reactive protein)*	• Elevated or rising anti-streptolysin O or other streptococcal antibody[Q], or • A positive throat culture[Q], or • Rapid antigen test for group A streptococcus[Q], or • Recent scarlet fever @1992 *Revised Jones criteria do not include recent scarlet fever as supporting evidence of a recent streptococcal infection*

Diagnostic Categories	Criteria
Primary episode of rheumatic fever	*Two major or one major two minor manifestations plus evidence of preceding group A streptococcal infection*
Recurrent attack of rheumatic fever in a patient without established rheumatic heart disease	*Two major or one minor manifestations plus evidence of preceding group A streptococcal infection*
Recurrent attack of rheumatic fever in a patient with established rheumatic heart disease	*Two minor manifestations plus evidence of preceding group A streptococcal infection*

101. Ans. b. Check HBV DNA load   *(Ref: Harrison 19/e p2032, 18/e p2551)*

As the person is HBsAg positive, but Anti- HBc Ab is negative, this is a case of chronic Hepatitis B. HBV-DNA load should be done before initiating treatment.

"Chronic HBV infection can occur in the presence or absence of serum hepatitis Be antigen (HBeAg), and generally, for both HBeAg-reactive and HbeAg negative chronic hepatitis B, the level of HBV DNA correlates with the level of liver injury and risk of progression."-Harrison 19/e p2032

Simplified Diagnostic Approach in Patients Presenting with Acute Hepatitis Serologic Tests of Patient's Serum				
HBsAg	**IgM Anti-HAV**	**IgM Anti-Hbc**	**Anti-HCV**	**Diagnostic Interpretation**
+	–	+	–	**Acute hepatitis B**
+	–	–	–	**Chronic hepatitis B**
+	+	–	–	**Acute hepatitis A superimposed on chronic hepatitis B**
+	+	+	–	**Acute hepatitis A and B**
–	+	–	–	**Acute hepatitis A**
–	+	+	–	**Acute hepatitis A and B** (HBsAg below detection threshold)
–	–	+	–	**Acute hepatitis B** (HBsAg below detection threshold)
–	–	–	+	**Acute hepatitis C**

Serology of Hepatitis B	
Hbs Ag	• Indicates that the **person is infected with the virus**[Q]. • The infection **may manifest as 'disease' either acute or chronic**, or be **just present as in carrier state**[Q]

Contd...

Serology of Hepatitis B

Anti-Hbs Ag	• With the development of antibody to Hbs Ag i.e. Anti Hbs Ag, the Hbs Ag antigen disappears from the serum: – **Patient is immune** (with immunization Antibody develops and Hbs Ag disappears) – **Patient is protected** w • Anti Hbs Ag indicates good immunity[Q] • Anti Hbs Ag indicates protection against Hepatitis B[Q]
Hbc Ag	• It is a **hidden component of the viral core** and is **not detectable at all**[Q]
Anti-Hbc Ag	• Antibodies to Hbc Ag **develop early in the course of disease**[Q] • Anti-Hbc Ag is the **first antibody to appear after an acute infection** and **persists in serum even during the recovery phase**[Q] | Acute infection | Antibody of IgM type[Q] | | Chronic infection | Antibody of IgG type[Q] |
Hbe Ag	• Denotes **high infectivity**[Q] and **active disease**[Q]
Anti-Hbe Ag	• Denotes **low infectivity**[Q]

Scheme of typical clinical and laboratory features of acute viral hepatitis B	Sequential

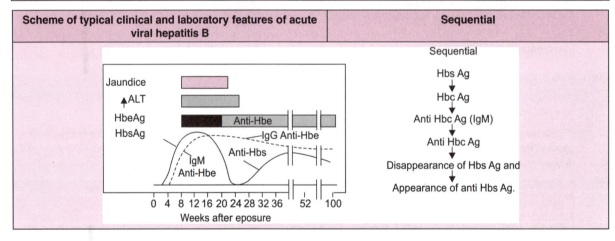

102. **Ans. a. Develops within 24 hours** *(Ref: Harrison 19/e 138e-5, 18/e p1217)*

Transfusion-Related Acute Lung Injury usually occurs either during or within 6 hours of transfusion.

*"The recipient develops **symptoms of hypoxia ($PaO_2/FIO_2 < 300$ mmHg)** and **signs of non-cardiogenic pulmonary edema**, including **bilateral interstitial infiltrates on chest X-ray**, either during or within 6 h of transfusion."*
-Harrison 19/e 138e-5

Transfusion-Related Acute Lung Injury (TRALI)

- **TRALI is the MC cause of transfusion related fatalities**[Q]
- The **implicated donors** are frequently **multiparous women**.
- The **transfusion of plasma from male** and **nulliparous women donors reduces the risk of TRALI**.

Recipient factors that are associated with increased risk of TRALI	
• Smoking[Q] • Chronic alcohol use[Q] • Shock[Q] • Liver surgery (transplantation)[Q]	• Mechanical ventilation with >30 cmH_2O pressure support[Q] • Positive fluid balance[Q]

Contd...

Contd...

Bariatric Surgery
Perioperative Mortality in Bariatric Surgery
• **MC cause of death** within 30 days of bariatric surgery: **Pulmonary embolism**[Q] (36%) > **Cardiac complications** (24%) > **Anastomotic leaks** (20%) • **MC cause of death** in immediate post-operative period: **Peritonitis** secondary to **anastomotic leak**[Q] (leak **most commonly** occurs at the **gastrojejunostomy**)

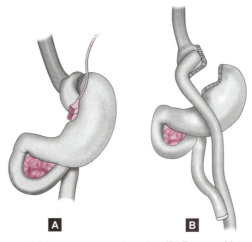

Figs. 17A and B: (A) Laparoscopic adjustable gastric banding (B) Roux-en-Y gastric bypass (RYGB)

Obesity according to BMI	
Category	**BMI**
Underweight	<18.5[Q]
Normal	18.5–24.9[Q]
Overweight	25.0–29.9[Q]
Obesity (Class I)	30–34.9[Q]
Severe obesity (Class II)	35–39.9[Q]
Morbid obesity (Class III)	40–49.9[Q]
Superobesity	> 50[Q]

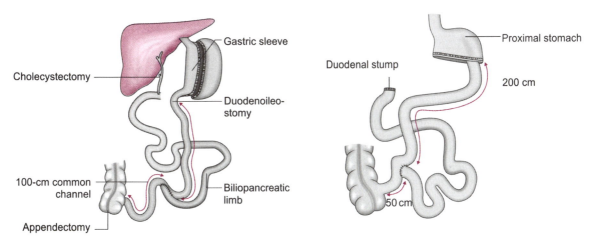

Configuration of the duodenal switch   Configuration of biliopancreatic diversion

OBS AND GYNAE

127. Ans. a. Enalapril   *(Ref: Williams 24/e p1006; Goodman and Gilman 12/e p736; Dutta 7/e p228; Katzung 13/e p185, 12/e p299)*

Enalapril is the antihypertensive drug, which is not used in pregnancy.

*"Angiotensin-Converting Enzyme Inhibitors: These drugs **inhibit the conversion of angiotensin-I to the potent vasoconstrictor angiotensin-II**. They can **cause severe fetal malformations when given in the second and third trimesters**. These include **hypocalvaria** and **renal dysfunction**. Some preliminary studies have also suggested **teratogenic effects**, and because of this, they are **not recommended during pregnancy**. Angiotensin-receptor blockers act in a similar manner. But, instead of blocking the production of angiotensin-II, **they inhibit binding to its receptor**. They are **presumed to have the same fetal effects as ACE inhibitors and thus are also contraindicated**."-Williams 24/e p1006*

*"**ACE inhibitors** inhibit the conversion of angiotensin-I to the potent vasoconstrictor angiotensin-II. They **can cause severe fetal malformations** that include **hypocalvaria** when **given in the second and third trimesters**. Because of this, they are **not recommended during pregnancy**. Angiotensin-receptor blockers act in a similar manner, but instead of blocking the production of angiotensin-II, they inhibit binding to its receptor. They are **presumed to have the same fetal effects as ACE inhibitors** and are **also contraindicated**."-Goodman and Gilman 12/e p736*

*"ACE inhibitors not only block the conversion of ANG I to ANG II but also inhibit the degradation of other substances, including bradykinin, substance P, and enkephalins. The action of ACE inhibitors to inhibit bradykinin metabolism contributes significantly to their hypotensive action and is apparently **responsible for** some adverse side effects, including **cough and angioedema**. These drugs are **contraindicated in pregnancy because they cause fetal kidney damage**." -Katzung 13/e p185*

Antihypertensives to be avoided in Pregnancy (Mnemonic: SAAND)
• **Sodium nitroprusside**[Q]
• **ACE inhibitors**[Q]
• **ARBs**[Q]
• **Non-selective beta blockers**[Q]
• **Diuretics**[Q]

128. Ans. b. 92, 180, 153   *(Ref: Williams 24/e p1137)*

Cut-off values in 2 hours oral glucose tolerance test for fasting and at 1 hour and 2 hours after meals respectively.

Diagnosis of Gestational Diabetes by Oral Glucose Tolerance Testing[a]		
Time	**75-gm Glucose**[b]	
Fasting	92 mg/dL[Q]	5.1 mmol/L
1-hour	180 mg/dL[Q]	10.0 mmol/L
2-hours	153 mg/dL[Q]	8.5 mmol/L

[a]The test should be performed in the morning after an overnight fast of at least 8 hours but not more than 14 hours and after at least 3 days of unrestricted diet (>150 gm carbohydrate/day) and physical activity. The subject should remain seated and should not smoke during the test.

[b]Two or more of the venous plasma glucose concentration indicated below must be met or exceeded for a positive diagnosis.

129. Ans. d. 4000 micrograms/day   *(Ref: Williams 24/e p1104; Nelson 20/e p2805, 20/e p2805, 19/e p2001)*

If a pregnancy is planned in high-risk women (previously affected child with neural tube defects), supplementation should be started with 4 mg (= 4000 microgram) of folic acid daily, beginning 1 month before the time of the planned conception.

"The U.S. Public Health Service has recommended that all women of childbearing age and who are capable of becoming pregnant take 0.4 mg of folic acid daily. If, however, a pregnancy is planned in high-risk women (previously affected child), supplementation should be started with 4 mg (= 4000 microgram) of folic acid daily, beginning 1 month before the time of the planned conception."-Nelson 20/e p2805

AIIMS May 2015

*"A diet sufficient in folic acid prevents megaloblastic anemia. The role of folate deficiency in the genesis of neural- tube defects has been well studied. Since the early 1990s, **nutritional experts and the American College of Obstetricians and Gynecologists (2013c) have recommended that all women of childbearing age consume at least 400 μg of folic acid daily.** More folic acid is given in circumstances in which requirements are increased. These include multifetal pregnancy, hemolytic anemia, Crohn disease, alcoholism, and inflammatory skin disorders. There is evidence that **women who previously have had infants with neural tube defects have a lower recurrence rate if a daily 4-mg (= 4000 microgram) folic acid supplement is given preconceptionally and throughout early pregnancy.*"-Williams 24/e p1104*

See Q. No. 156 AIIMS November 2015.

130. **Ans. a. Copper IUCD**   *(Ref: Dutta 8/e p615, 7/e p551)*

In this 32-year old P2L2 lady, who comes five days after unprotected sexual intercourse, copper-containing IUCD is the best contraceptive.

Copper IUCD:
- Insertion of an IUCD within **maximum period of 5-7 days after accidental unprotected exposure.**
- It **prevents implantation** but is **not suitable for women with multiple sex partners** and **for rape victims**

See Q, No. 152 AIIMS November 2015.

131. **Ans. b. VDRL for husband and wife**   *(Ref: Williams 24/e p358-359; Dutta 8/e p343, 7/e p167)*

Though VDRL is a simple test, mostly performed in initial work up of all cases of multiple abortions, in this case all abortions are by 16th week while in syphilis, usually there is a improvement in the duration of pregnancy (Kassowitz Law).

*"**Kassowitz law: If a woman with untreated syphilis has series of pregnancies, the likelihood of infection of the fetus in later pregnancies becomes less.**"*

*"There are **many putative causes of recurrent abortion**, however, **only three are widely accepted: parental chromosomal abnormalities, antiphospholipid antibody syndrome,** and a **subset of uterine abnormalities.** Other suspected but not proven causes are alloimmunity, endocrinopathies, environmental toxins, and various infections. Infections seldom cause even sporadic loss. Thus, most are unlikely to cause recurrent miscarriage, especially since maternal antibodies usually have developed."-Williams 24/e p358*

Causes and Specific Treatment of Recurrent Miscarriage		
Cause	**Diagnosis**	**Treatment**
Genetic Causes		
Recurrent aneuploidy	**Fetal karyotyping**	Not available
Parental balanced translocation	**Parental karyotyping**	Genetic counseling
Endocrine cause		
Thyroid function	Thyroid function tests, thyroid antibodies	Treat hypo- or hyperthyroidism
Diabetes	Blood sugar fasting and post prandial	Treat diabetes with insulin
Inadequate luteal phase	Luteal phase < 10 days progesterone levels, 15 mmol/L on 21 day in five consecutive cycles. Endometrial biopsy	Natural micronized progesterone clomiphene low dose FSH
Polycystic ovarian disease (rare cause)	Elevated serum LH and free testosterone	Laparoscopic diathermy to ovaries in selected resistant cases
Anatomical Causes		
Fibroids (rare cause)	Ultrasound or hysterosalpingogram (HSG)	Myomectomy in selected cases
Uterine anomalies	Transvaginal scan or HSG	Resection of septum hysteroscopically or on laparotomy
Asherman's syndrome	Hysteroscopy	**Synechiolysis** (Resection of synechia)
Cervical incompetence (mid trimester abortion)	HSG or transvaginal ultrasound	Cervical circlage (**McDonald or Shirodkar suture**) during pregnancy

AIIMS ESSENCE

Contd...

Immunological Causes		
Antiphospholipid antibody syndrome (APLA)	Anti-phospholipid antibodies	Low dose aspirin 75 mg daily and injection heparin 5000 units SC twice daily or low molecular weight heparin 40 mg IM daily from the time of appearance of fetal heart activity up to 34 weeks
Disorders of materno-fetal immune status	Autoimmune antibodies	The benefit of immunotherapy is not yet proven

132 **Ans. c. 300 mg** *(Ref: Hypertension in pregnancy (ACOG Taskforce on hypertension in pregnancy)-Obstetrics and gynaecology, Vol-122, No.5, November 2013; William's 24/e p181; Danforth 10/e p264)*

In 2013, the American College of Obstetricians and Gynecologists removed proteinuria (if other severe preeclampsia features are present) as an essential criterion for diagnosis of preeclampsia. Massive proteinuria (5 gm/24 hours) and fetal growth restriction was also removed because massive proteinuria has a poor correlation with outcome and fetal growth restriction is managed similarly whether or not preeclampsia is diagnosed. Hence in absence of diagnostic requirement of 5 gm a s massive proteinuria for severe eclampsia , general definition of proteinuria (>300 mg) will suffice, provided that other criteria of severe preeclampsia are present.

Diagnostic Criteria for Preeclampsia	
Blood pressure	• ≥140 mm Hg systolic or ≥90 mm Hg diastolic on **two occasions at least 4 hours apart after 20 weeks of gestation** in a woman with a previously normal blood pressure[Q] • ≥160 mm Hg systolic or ≥110 mm Hg diastolic, hypertension can be confirmed within a short interval (minutes) to facilitate timely antihypertensive therapy[Q]
AND	
Proteinuria	• ≥300 mg per 24 hour urine collection[Q] (or this amount extrapolated from a timed collection) Or • **Protein/creatinine ratio ≥0.3 mg/dL**[Q] • **Dipstick reading of 1+**[Q] (used only if other quantitative methods not available)

• **Or in the absence of proteinuria, new-onset hypertension with the new onset of any of the following:**

Thrombocytopenia[Q]	Platelet count <100,000/microliter[Q]
Renal insufficiency[Q]	Serum creatinine concentrations >1.1 mg/dL or a doubling of the serum creatinine concentration in the absence of other renal disease[Q]
Impaired liver function[Q]	Elevated blood concentrations of liver transaminases to twice normal concentration[Q]
Pulmonary edema[Q]	
Cerebral or visual symptoms[Q]	

Severe Preeclampsia (Old Definition)
• **Severe preeclampsia** is defined as the **presence of 1 of the following symptoms** or **signs in the presence of preeclampsia:** • **SBP of 160 mm Hg or higher or DBP of 110 mm Hg or higher on 2 occasions at least 6 hours apart**[Q] • **Proteinuria of more than 5 gm**[Q] **in a 24-hour collection** or more than 3+ on 2 random urine samples collected at least 4 hours apart • **Pulmonary edema or cyanosis**[Q] • **Oliguria** (<400 ml in 24 hours)[Q] • **Persistent headaches**[Q] • **Epigastric pain and/or impaired liver function**[Q] • **Thrombocytopenia**[Q] • **Oligohydramnios, decreased fetal growth, or placental abruption**[Q]

Contd...

AIIMS May 2015

Contd...

Severe Features of Preeclampsia (Any of these findings) ACOG-2013
(Note: Oliguria & Massive proteinuria is removed)

- **Systolic blood pressure ≥ 160 mm Hg or diastolic blood pressure ≥110 mm Hg on two occasions at least 4 hours apart** while the patient is on bed rest[Q] (unless antihypertensive therapy is initiated before this time)
- **Thrombocytopenia (platelet count <100,000/microliter)**[Q]
- Impaired liver function as indicated by abnormally elevated blood concentrations of liver enzymes (to twice normal concentration), severe persistent right upper quadrant or epigastric pain unresponsive to medication and not accounted for by alternative diagnoses, or both[Q]
- **Progressive renal insufficiency** (serum **creatinine concentration >1.1 mg/dL** or a doubling of the serum creatinine concentration in the absence of other renal disease)[Q]
- **Pulmonary edema**[Q]
- **New-onset cerebral or visual disturbances**[Q]

---

133. Ans. d. Androgen insensitivity *(Ref: : Shaw's 16/e p141, 15/e p111-112; Novaks 14/1037-1038; Dutta Gynae 6/e p424)*

Most likely diagnosis in a 16-year old girl who presents with primary amenorrhea, normal sexual development, normal breasts (Tanner stage 5) but minimal pubic hair (Tanner stage 1) is androgen insensitivity syndrome.

"Androgen Insensitivity Syndrome: Because the testes produce normal amounts of mullerian-inhibiting factor (MIF), also known as mullerian-inhibiting substance (MIS) or anti-mullerian hormone/factor (AMH/AMF), affected individuals do not have fallopian tubes, a uterus, or a proximal (upper) vagina. Most cases are identified in the newborn period by the presence of inguinal masses, which later are identified as testes during surgery. Some patients are first seen in the teenage years for evaluation of primary amenorrhea. In addition, adolescent patients have no pubic and axillary hair, with otherwise scanty body hair, and lack acne, although breast is normal as a result of conversion of testosterone to estradiol."

Turner's syndrome	• **All secondary sexual characters** are **absent.**
Mullerian agenesis	• Patient presents with **primary amenorrhea with well-developed secondary sexual characters** (breast and pubic hair).
Premature ovarian failure	• Patient presents with **secondary amenorrhea**

Classification of Sexual Maturity States in Girls		
SMR Stage	Pubic Hair	Breasts
1	**Preadolescent**	**Preadolescent**
2	**Sparse, lightly pigmented, straight**, medial border of labia	Breast and papilla elevated as **small mound; diameter of areola increased**
3	**Darker, beginning to curl**, increased amount	**Breast and areola enlarged**, no contour separation
4	**Coarse, curly, abundant**, but less than in adult	Areola and papilla form **secondary mound**
5	**Adult feminine triangle**, spread to medial surface of thighs	**Mature, nipple projects**, areola part of general breast contour

134. Ans. b. Tamoxifen *(Ref: Jeffcott 6/e p205; Shaw's 16/e p431-434, 15/e p371, 14/331-332, 13/353-354; Novak's 15/e p1076; Dutta Gynae 6/e p470)*

Drug not given in PCOD in a 30-year-old lady with infertility is tamoxifen.

Polycystic Ovarian Syndrome/Stein Levinthal's Syndrome	
Diagnostic Criteria for PCOS	
Major	**Minor**
1. Chronic anovulation[Q] 2. Hyperandrogenemia[Q] 3. Clinical signs of hyperandrogenemia[Q] 4. Other etiologies excluded[Q]	1. Insulin resistance[Q] 2. Perimenarchal onset of hirsutism and obesity[Q] 3. Elevated LH to FSH ratio[Q] 4. Intermittent anovulation with hyperandrogenemia[Q]

Clinical Features:

- Seen mostly in **15-25 years of age**[Q]

  - It includes **chronic non-ovulation** and **hyperandrogenemia** associated with normal or **raised estrogen (E_2), raised LH, low FSH/LH ratio.**[Q]
  - The raised E_2 level causes negative feedback to pituitary resulting in **diminished FSH, but raised LH**[Q].

- The involvement of the adrenal gland is seen in raised androstenedione, dehydroepiandrosterone, testosterone and 17 alpha-hydroxyprogesterone.
- Much of the **testosterone** is **secreted by** the **ovarian stroma**[Q].

Appearance:

- Macroscopically, the **ovaries** are often **bilaterally enlarged**, with **thick capsule**[Q].
- The surface may be **lobulated** but the **peritoneal surface** is **free from adhesions**.

  - **Multiple cyst 0.5 to 1 mm** and at times **up to 20 mm** in size are **localized along the surface of the ovary** giving a **"necklace" appearance on ultrasound**[Q].

- Theca cell hyperplasia is seen which produces excess testosterone secretion.

  - **Ultrasound** shows several **"subcapsular cysts" of varying size, diagnostic of PCOS**[Q].
  - **Laparoscopic evaluation** is not only **diagnostic**, but also **therapeutic**[Q].

Treatment:

- **Weight loss**[Q] of more than 5% of previous weight is important. Cigarette **smoking** should be **avoided**[Q]

  - **Estrogen best given with progesterone** with no androgenic properties.

- **Dexamethasone 0.5 mg** at bedtime also reduces androgen production.

  - **Hirsutism** is treated with **cyproterone acetate** or **spironolactone**.
  - **Infertility** is **treated with Clomiphene, 80% ovulate and 40% conceive.** However, **abortion rate of 25-40%** is **due to corpus luteal phase defect** manifested **by Clomiphene**[Q].

- In Clomiphene failed group, **ovulation** can be **induced with FSH or GnRH analogues**[Q].

  - **Metformin treats the root cause of PCOS**[Q], rectifies endocrine and metabolic functions and improves fertility and is **drug of choice**[Q].

- **Surgery (laparoscopic multiple puncture of cyst)** is reserved for those in whom:
- Medical therapy fails
- Hyperstimulation occurs
- Use of GnRH analogue is a cost constraint

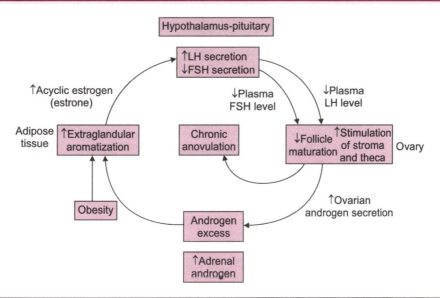

Consequences of Polycystic Ovarian Syndrome	
Short-Term Consequences	**Long-Term Consequences**

• **Menstrual dysfunction**[Q] (Irregular menses):
  – **Amenorrhea, Oligomenorrhea**
  – *Episodic menomectorrhagia*
• **Hyperandrogenism**[Q]:
  – ***Hirsutism***[Q], Acne, Androgenic alopecia
• **Infertility**[Q]
• **Obesity**[Q]
• **Insulin resistance**[Q] (Acanthosis nigricans)
• **Dyslipidemia**[Q] (Androgenic lipoprotein profile):
  – *Increased LDL and TG*
  – *Increased Total cholesterol: HDL ratio*
  – *Decreased HDL*
• **Metabolic syndrome**[Q]: Characterized by insulin resistance, obesity, androgenic dyslipidemia and hypertension
• **Obstructive sleep apnea**[Q] (Related to central obesity and dyslipidemia)
	• **Diabetes mellitus**[Q]: Increased risk of impaired glucose tolerance and type 2 DM in PCOS patients
	• **Cardiovascular diseases**[Q]: Greater prevalence of **atherosclerosis** and **cardiovascular disease** with an increased risk of **myocardial infarction**
	• **Cancer:**
	• **Endometrial carcinoma**[Q] (3 fold increase risk)
	• **Ovarian cancer**[Q]
	
	  • Women with PCOS are associated with a definite increased risk of **endometrial cancer**. An increased risk of **ovarian cancer** and **breast cancer** has also been suggested.

135. **Ans. c. Methyldopa**   *(Ref: Williams 24/e p100; Dutta 8/e p265, 7/e p228; Goodman Gillman 12/e p773, 774; Katzung 12/e p176)*
Drug of choice for hypertension in pregnancy is methyldopa.

*"Methyldopa is a **centrally acting antihypertensive agent**. It is a **prodrug** that exerts its antihypertensive action via an active metabolite. Although used frequently as an antihypertensive agent in the past, methyldopa's significant adverse effects limit its **current use largely to treatment of hypertension in pregnancy, where it has a record for safety.**"*
-Goodman Gillman 12/e p773

*"**Methyldopa is a preferred drug for treatment of hypertension during pregnancy based on its effectiveness and safety for both mother and fetus**. The usual initial dose of methyldopa is 250 mg twice daily, and there is little additional effect with doses >2 g/day."-Goodman Gillman 12/e p774*

*"**Methyldopa** was widely used in the past but is **now used primarily for hypertension during pregnancy**. It **lowers blood pressure chiefly by reducing peripheral vascular resistance**, with a variable reduction in heart rate and cardiac output."*
-Katzung 12/e p176

Antihypertensives in Pregnancy	
Safe	**Contraindicated**
• Labetalol[Q]	• ACE inhibitors[Q]
• Alpha methyldopa[Q]	• Reserpine
• Calcium channel blockers[Q]	• Loratidine
• Hydralazine	
• Sodium nitroprusside ±	

Drug of Choice in Pregnancy	
Condition	**Drug of Choice**
DOC for malaria in pregnancy	• Chloroquine[Q]
DOC for anticoagulation in pregnancy	• Heparin[Q]
Antihypertensive of choice in pregnancy	• Alpha-methyldopa[Q]
Antihypertensive of choice for hypertensive crisis in pregnancy	• Labetalol[Q]
DOC for nausea in pregnancy	• Doxylamine and pyridoxine[Q]
Analgesic of choice during pregnancy	• Acitoaminophen[Q]
Anti-epileptic of choice during pregnancy	• Phenobarbitone[Q]

136. Ans. a. Krukenberg tumor *(Ref: Robbins 9/e p1034; 8/e p1050)*

*"A classic **metastatic gastrointestinal carcinoma involving the ovaries** is termed **Krukenberg tumor**, characterized by **bilateral metastases composed of mucin-producing, signet-ring cancer cells**, most **often of gastric origin.**" -Robbins 9/e p1034*

Metastatic Tumors of Ovary
• **MC metastatic tumors of the ovary are derived from tumors of müllerian origin**: the **uterus, fallopian tube, contralateral ovary**, or **pelvic peritoneum**[Q].
• **MC extra-müllerian tumors metastatic to the ovary: CA breast** and **GI tract**, including colon, stomach, biliary tract, and pancreas[Q].
• Also included in this group are the rare cases of pseudo-myxoma peritonei, derived from appendiceal tumors.
• A classic **metastatic gastrointestinal carcinoma involving the ovaries** is termed **Krukenberg tumor**, characterized by **bilateral metastases composed of mucin-producing, signet-ring cancer cells**, most **often of gastric origin**[Q].

Krukenberg Tumor
• Refers to a **metastatic bilateral ovarian malignancy** whose **primary site is GIT or breast**[Q]
• Tumor is having **smooth surfaces, slightly bossed, freely movable in the pelvis.**
• **Most often of gastric origin (70%)**[Q;] CA colon, appendix, breast (invasive lobular carcinoma), pancreas and gallbladder are other primary sites.
Pathology:
• **No tendency to from adhesions** and there is **no infiltration through the capsule**[Q].
• **Tumor retains the shape of the normal ovary with peculiar solid waxy consistency**[Q].
• Composed of **cellular or myxomatous stroma with scattered mucin-producing, signet-ring cancer cells**[Q]

137. Ans. b. Ureterovaginal fistula *(Ref: Shaw's 16/e p223-224, 15/e p184; William Gynae 1st/e p573)*

In this patient methylene blue dye was instilled in bladder and she was given oral phenazopyridine dye. Pad showed yellow staining at the top portion, but not the middle or bottom portions. She is likely to have Ureterovaginal fistula.

"Ureterovaginal fistula: Upper most swabs soaked with urine but unstained with dye. The urine, which is being brought by ureters is clear, i.e. does not have any dye. Through the fistula it will reach vagina and uppermost cotton swab will be wet with urine but will not have any colour, (as dye is in bladder and not ureter)."

Methylene Blue 3 Swab Test

- The **three-swab test helps to differentiate between vesicovaginal, ureterovaginal and urethrovaginal fistula.**
- **Procedure of 3 swab test:**
  - A red rubber catheter is introduced into the bladder through the urethra.
  - **3 cotton swabs are placed in the vagina as follows:** (One at **vault**, one at the **middle**, one **just above the introitus**).
  - **Methylene blue dye is instilled into the bladder** through catheter and **swabs are removed for inspection.**

Observation	Interpretation
• **Upper most swabs soaked with urine but unstained with dye.** The urine, which is being brought by, ureters is clear, i.e. does not have any dye. **Through the fistula it will reach vagina and uppermost cotton swab will be wet with urine but will not have any colour, (as dye is in bladder and not ureter)**	Ureterovaginal fistula[Q]
• Upper and lower swab remain dry but the **middle swab soaked with dye**	Vesicovaginal fistula[Q]
• The **upper two swab remain dry** but **lower one soaked with dye**	Urethrovaginal fistula[Q]

Important Points about Fistula	
• **MC urinary fistula**	**Vesicovaginal**[Q]
• **MC cause of vesicovaginal fistula in India**	**Obstructed labour**[Q]
• **MC cause of ureterovaginal fistula**	**Injury to ureter after gynecological operations** especially **Wertheim's hysterectomy**[Q]
• **MC cause of Vesicouterine fistula**	**Cesarean section**[Q]
• **MC cause of Rectovaginal fistula**	**Cesarean perineal tear**[Q]

138. Ans. a. TSH *(Ref: Harrison 19/e p2 p2267)*

In Galactorrhea - amenorrhea syndromes, apart from serum prolactin, TSH should be advised.

"Galactorrhea: Basal, fasting morning PRL levels (normally <20 µg/L) should be measured to assess hypersecretion. Both false-positive and false-negative results may be encountered. In patients with markedly elevated PRL levels (>1000 µg/L), reported results may be falsely lowered because of assay artifacts; sample dilution is required to measure these high values accurately. Falsely elevated values may be caused by aggregated forms of circulating PRL, which are usually biologically inactive (macroprolactinemia). Hypothyroidism should be excluded by measuring TSH and T4 levels."- Harrison 19/e p2267

Galactorrhea

- **Galactorrhea, the inappropriate discharge of milk-containing fluid from the breast**, is considered abnormal if it **persists longer than 6 months after childbirth** or **discontinuation of breast-feeding**[Q].
- Postpartum galactorrhea associated with amenorrhea is a self-limiting disorder usually associated with moderately elevated PRL levels.
- Galactorrhea may occur spontaneously, or it may be elicited by nipple pressure.

Characteristic features:
- In both men and women, galactorrhea may vary in color and consistency (transparent, milky, or bloody) and arise **either unilaterally or bilaterally**.
- Mammography or ultrasound is indicated for bloody discharges (particularly from a single nipple), which may be caused by breast cancer.
- **Galactorrhea is commonly associated with hyperprolactinemia**[Q].
- **Acromegaly is associated with galactorrhea in about one-third of patients**[Q].

Contd...

AIIMS ESSENCE

Contd...

Galactorrhea
Laboratory Investigation:
• **Basal, fasting morning PRL levels** (normally < 20 µg/L) should be measured to assess hypersecretion. Both false-positive and false-negative results may be encountered.
• In patients with markedly elevated PRL levels (> 1000 µg/L), reported results may be falsely lowered because of assay artifacts; sample dilution is required to measure these high values accurately.
• Falsely elevated values may be caused by aggregated forms of circulating PRL, which are usually biologically inactive (macroprolactinemia).
• **Hypothyroidism should be excluded by measuring TSH and T$_4$ levels**[Q]
Treatment:
• Treatment of galactorrhea usually involves managing the underlying disorder (e.g., **replacing T$_4$ for hypothyroidism, discontinuing a medication, treating prolactinoma**).

139. Ans. d. 6 mg 12 hourly 4 doses *(Ref: Dutta 8/e p367, 7/e p316; Nelson 20/e p 852)*

Dose of dexamethasone given to mother in anticipated preterm delivery is 6 mg 12 hourly 4 doses.

"A single course of antenatal corticosteroids is recommended to women with pregnancies 24-34 weeks of gestation that are at risk for preterm delivery. Antenatal steroids decrease the risk of RDS, death, grade III and IV IVH (Intra-ventricular hemorrhage), PVL (Peri-ventricular leukomalacia) and NEC (Necrotizing enterocolitis) in the neonate. For prevention of RDS, antenatal glucocorticoids act synergistically with postnatal exogenous surfactant therapy, so they should be given even though surfactant therapy is so effective. Postnatal growth is not adversely affected. Antenatal steroids do not increase the risk of maternal death, chorioamnionitis, or puerperal sepsis. Betamethasone (12 mg, 2 doses, 24 hours apart) and dexamethasone (6 mg, 12 hourly, 4 doses) have been used antenatally."

Antenatal Corticosteroids
• Maternal administration of glucocorticoids is advocated where the pregnancy is <34 weeks.

Antenatal steroids reduce	
• **Incidence and mortality of RDS**[Q]	• **NEC** (Necrotizing enterocolitis)[Q]
• **Overall neonatal mortality**[Q]	• **Neurodevelopmental impairment**[Q]
• **IVH** (Intra-ventricular hemorrhage)[Q]	• **PVL** (Peri-ventricular leukomalacia)[Q]

• **For prevention of RDS, antenatal glucocorticoids act synergistically with postnatal exogenous surfactant therapy,** so they should be given even though surfactant therapy is so effective.

• Postnatal growth is not adversely affected. **Antenatal steroids do not increase the risk of maternal death, chorioamnionitis, or puerperal sepsis.**

• **Betamethasone (12 mg, 2 doses, 24 hours apart) and dexamethasone (6 mg, 12 hourly, 4 doses) have been used antenatally**[Q].

Steroid	Dose
Betamethasone (Steroid of choice)	**12 mg IM 12 hours apart (two doses)**[Q]
Dexamethasone	**6 mg IM every 12 hours (four doses)**[Q]

140. Ans. b. 100 microgram IM *(Ref: Goodman Gillman 12/1851; Dutta 8/e p477, 7/e p412; Williams 24/e p547, 595)*

Carbetocin (long acting Oxytocin) 100 microgram IM is very useful to prevent post-partum hemorrhage.

"Carbetocin (long acting Oxytocin) 100 microgram is very useful to prevent post-partum hemorrhage, recently developed with longer half life, used to control postpartum hemorrhage and bleeding after giving birth, particularly following cesarean section."

"Uterotonics are the most important factor to decrease postpartum blood loss. Choices include oxytocin (Pitocin), misoprostol (Cytotec), carboprost (Hemabate) and the ergots, namely ergometrine (Ergotrate) and methylergometrine (Methergine). Also, carbetocin (Duratocin), a long-acting oxytocin analogue, is available and effective for hemorrhage prevention during cesarean delivery."-Williams 24/e p547

"Carbetocin, a longer-acting derivative of oxytocin, is under evaluation in clinical trials to prevent or treat postpartum hemorrhage; a dose of 100 µg is given intravenously."-Goodman Gillman 12/e p1851

*"Carbetocin: It can be **administered intravenously** or **intramuscularly**, resulting in different pharmacokinetic action. In both cases, the **recommended dose for an average adult female is 100 microgram, administered slowly over a minute**. Contractile effects of the uterus are apparent within two minutes and can be observed for approximately one hour, though maximum binding occurs about 30 minutes after intramuscular injection. Administration is performed immediately following parturition to minimize risk of postpartum hemorrhage by inducing uterine contractions, increasing muscle tone and thickening the blood."*-http://en.wikipedia.org/wiki/Carbetocin

Uterine Stimulants		
Hormones of posterior pituitary	**Ergot alkaloids**	**Prostaglandins**
• Oxytocin • Desamino-oxytocin (buccal formulation of oxytocin) • Carbetocin (longer half life)^Q	• **Ergometrine** (Ergonovine) • Mehtylergometrine	• PGE2 (dinoprostone)^Q • PGF2-alpha (dinoprost)^Q • 15-methyl PGF2-alpha (Carboprost)^Q

Carbetocin
• **Long acting oxytocin analogue** • **Mechanism of action: Binds to oxytocin receptors present on smooth musculature of the uterus**, resulting in rhythmic contractions of the uterus, increased frequency of existing contractions and increased uterine tone^Q.
Pharmacokinetics:
• Bioavailability is 80% following IM injection • Half-life: 40 minutes
• Dosage and Action:
• **100 microgram in 1 ml slow injection over one minute**^{Q}
Uses:
• **PPH** and bleeding during pregnancy^Q

141. **Ans. a. Plan for immediate laparoscopic surgery** *(Rer: Dutta 8/e p215, 7/e p180-182; Williams 24/e p385)*

In this patient the size of adnexal mass is 5 × 5 cm so expectant management cannot be done. But since the patient is hemodynamically stable, laparoscopic surgery will be the management of choice.

"Ectopic Pregnancy: Laparoscopy is the preferred surgical treatment for ectopic pregnancy unless a woman is hemodynamically unstable."-Williams 24/e p385

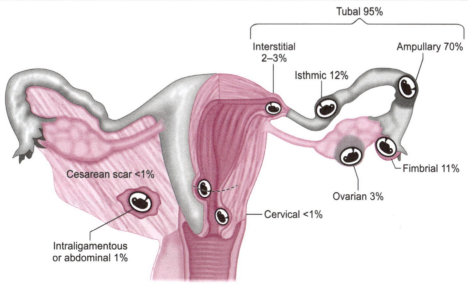

Ectopic Pregnancy

- Definition: Fertilized ovum implanted and developed outside the normal uterine cavity.
- **MC site of ectopic pregnancy: Tubal[Q] (97%)**
- **Rarest** ectopic pregnancy: **Primary abdominal[Q]**

  - **MC site** of ectopic pregnancy **in fallopian tube: Ampulla[Q] (Ampulla >Isthmus >Infundibulum >Interstitium)**
  - **Least common site** of ectopic pregnancy **in fallopian tube: Interstitial part[Q]**

Etiology:

- **PID: PID** is the **MC cause of ectopic pregnancy[Q]. Chlamydia** is the **MC cause of PID[Q]**
- **IUCD failure: Highest rate** with **progesterone[Q]; Lowest rate** with **levonorgestrel[Q]**
- **Prior tubal damage either from a previous ectopic pregnancy** or from **tubal surgery** to relieve infertility or for sterilization confers the **highest risk for ectopic pregnancy.**

Risk factors for Ectopic Pregnancy		
High Risk	**Moderate Risk**	**Slight Risk**
• **Tubal corrective surgery** • **Tubal sterilization** • **Previous ectopic pregnancy** • **Artificial reproductive technology** • **PID**	• Infertility • Contraceptive failure • Previous genital infection • Multiple partners	• Previous pelvic or abdominal surgery • Smoking • Douching • Intercourse before 18 years

Clinical Features:

- **Classical triad: Abdominal pain (100%) + Amenorrhea (75%) + Vaginal bleeding[Q] (70%)**
- **Classical triad** is seen only in **50% cases[Q]**
- **Amenorrhea is usually of short period (<6 week)**
- Abdominal pain is acute, agonizing and colicky, located in lower abdomen
- **Vaginal bleeding** may be **slight and continuous**
- **Danforth sign: Shoulder pain** due to **large intraperitoneal hemorrhage** (observed in **10%** patients)[Q]

Site of Ectopic Pregnancy	Name of Criteria
Primary abdominal pregnancy	• **Studiford's criteria[Q]**
Ovarian pregnancy	• **Spigelberg's criteria[Q]**
Cervical pregnancy	• **Rubin's criteria[Q]**

Diagnosis:

Ultrasound

- **Diagnostic feature** on USG: **Absence of intrauterine pregnancy** with a **positive pregnancy fluid** in **pouch of Douglas[Q]**
- **Blob sign: Adnexal mass** clearly **separated** from **ovary[Q]**
- **Bagel's sign:** Typical **intact tubal ring[Q]**
- **Color Doppler USG: Ring of fire** pattern[Q]

Combination of quantitative hCG and Sonography

- **Lowest level of beta-hCG at which gestational sac is visible:**
  - **For TAS: 6000 IU/L**
  - **For TVS: 1000-2000 IU/L**

- **Beta-hCG >1500 IU/L** with **empty uterine cavity** is suggestive of ectopic pregnancy[Q]
- **Failure to double** the value of **beta-hCG by 48-hours** with **empty uterine cavity: Ectopic[Q]**

Serum Progesterone	
>25 ng/mL	**Viable intrauterine** pregnancy[Q]
<5 ng/mL	**Ectopic or abnormal** intrauterine pregnancy[Q]

Contd...

Contd...

Ectopic Pregnancy

- **Culdocentesis:** Reserved for emergency situation when USG is not possible; positive culdocentesis means hemoperitoneum.

Laparoscopy
• Direct visualization of pelvis especially the tube, feasible in hemodynamically stable patient
• **Gold standard for diagnosis of ectopic pregnancy**

Management:

- Expectant management

Medical Therapy		Surgical Therapy (Laparoscopically or by microsurgical laparotomy)

Systemic Medical Therapy (Methotrexate): Criteria	Salpingocentesis	• **Salpingostomy:**
		  – **Procedure of choice in hemodynamically stable patient**, who whishes to retain the fertility
		  – **Recommended surgical procedure for ampullary ectopic pregnancy**
		• **Salpingotomy:** Not done nowadays
		• **Segmental resection and anastomosis: Done in isthmic pregnancy**
		• **Fimbrial expression:** Done in distal ampullary pregnancy

1. **<6 weeks** pregnancy[Q]
2. **Hemodynamic stability**[Q]
3. Tubal diameter **<3.5 cm**[Q]
4. **No fetal cardiac activity**[Q]
5. **Beta-hCG <15,000** mIU/mL[Q]
	• Local injection of drug in gestational sac
	• Drugs used are:
	  – Methotrexate[Q]
	  – Potassium chloride[Q]
	  – Actinomycin D[Q]
	  – PGF-2-alpha[Q]
	  – Hyperosmolar glucose[Q]	

• **Salpingectomy** is done when **whole of the tube is damaged;** Contralateral tube is normal; Future fertility is not desired.		

Recurrence:

- **Recurrence of ectopic pregnancy** in **10-12% cases**

142. **Ans. b. Volume 1.5 ml, count 15 million, morphology 4% progressive motility 32%** *(Ref: Dutta 6/e p222)*

According to the 2010 WHO criteria, the characteristics of normal semen analysis are: Volume 1.5 ml, count 15 million, morphology 4% and progressive motility 32%.

Semen Characteristics	WHO 1999	WHO 2010
Volume (ml)	≥ 2 ml	≥ 1.5 ml[Q]
Sperm count	≥ 20 million/ml	≥ 15 million/ml[Q]
Total sperm count	≥ 40 million per ejaculate	≥ 39 million per ejaculate[Q]
Total motility	≥ 50%	≥ 40%[Q]
Progressive motility	≥ 25%	≥ 32%[Q]
Vitality	≥ 75%	≥ 58%[Q]
Morphology (Normal form)	14%	≥ 4%[Q]
Leukocyte count (10⁴/ml)	<1	<1[Q]

Semen Analysis (WHO 2010)

- Semen analysis is the **cornerstone of male factor infertility evaluation**.
- Semen sample should be **collected after at least 3 days of abstinence** and is **best evaluated within 1 hour of ejaculation**
- Two specimens should be collected within 2-3 weeks intervals, if markedly different, additional specimens should be collected.
- Assisted reproductive technologies such as in vitro fertilization (IVF) require that **motile sperm be isolated from seminal plasma within 1 hour if ejaculation** to protect sperm from the inhibitory effects of seminal plasma on fertilization.

Contd...

Contd...

Semen Analysis (WHO 2010)

Common Indications for Semen Analysis
• As a part of **couple's infertility investigation**   • **After vasectomy to verify that the procedure was successful**   • **Testing human donors** for sperm donation

Semen Characteristics	
Volume	• **Lower reference limit: 1.5 ml** • **Low volume:** Due to **partial or complete blockage of seminal vesicles**
Count	• Over **15 million sperm per ml** is considered normal
Liquefaction	• Process when the gel formed by proteins from the seminal vesicle is broken up and the semen becomes more liquid • In the nice guidelines, a liquefaction time <60 minutes is within normal range • Semen analysis should be done after liquefaction with thorough mixing
Morphology	• **≥ 4%** (or 5th centile) of the observed sperm should have normal morphology.
pH	• **7.2–7.8** • **Acidic ejaculate: When one or both of the seminal vesicles are blocked** • **Basic ejaculate: Seen in infection**

143. **Ans. a. USG for fetal cardiac activity** *(Ref: Williams 24/e p196; Ultrasound Obstet Gynecol 2011; 37:625-628; Dutta 8/e p77-78, 7/e p68)*

Earliest diagnosis of pregnancy can be established safely by ultrasound for the fetal cardiac activity.

*"An **intrauterine gestational sac is reliably visualized with transvaginal sonography by 5 weeks**, and **an embryo with cardiac activity by 6 weeks**. The embryo should be visible transvaginally once the mean sac diameter has reached 20 mm— otherwise the gestation is anembryonic. **Cardiac motion is usually visible with transvaginal imaging when the embryo length has reached 5 mm**. If an embryo less than 7 mm is not identified to have cardiac activity, a subsequent examination is recommended in 1 week (American Institute of Ultrasound in Medicine, 2013a)."-Williams 24/e p196*

Most accurate and safest method to diagnose viable pregnancy at 6 weeks is USG for fetal cardiac activity.

USG for fetal cardiac activity: At 6 weeks it is routine to detect fetal cardiac activity by ultrasound (and Doppler is not indicated).

Doppler is most sensitive but not safe in early pregnancy.

Doppler examination of fetal vessels in early pregnancy should not be performed without a clinical indication - Ultrasound Obstet Gynecol 2011; 37:625-628

Week 6 – Gestational Age (Fetal age 4 weeks)
• **5 ½ to 6 ½ weeks** is usually a very **good time to detect either a fetal pole** or even a **fetal heart-beat by vaginal ultrasound**.
<blockquote>• The **fetal pole is the first visible sign of a developing embryo.**   • The **fetal pole now allows for crown to rump measurements** (CRL) to be taken, so that pregnancy dating can be a bit more accurate.</blockquote>
• The fetal pole may be seen at a crown-rump length (CRL) of 2-4 mm, and the **heartbeat may be seen as a regular flutter** when the **CRL has reached 5 mm.**
• If a **vaginal ultrasound** is done and no fetal pole or cardiac activity is seen, **another ultrasound scan** should be done in **3–7 days.**

AIIMS May 2015

Human Chorionic Gonadotrophin

- hCG is a **glycoprotein**
- It consists of a hormone **non-specific α** and a **hormone specific β subunit**[Q]
- It is chemically and functionally similar to pituitary luteinizing hormone
- The α subunit is biochemically similar to LH, FSH and TSH whereas β subunit is relatively unique to hCG
- Have **highest carbohydrate content (30%)** of any human hormone

Functions of Human Chorionic Gonadotrophin

• **Rescue and maintenance of corpus luteum till 6 weeks of pregnancy**[Q] • **Stimulates both adrenal and placental steroidogenesis**[Q] • **Stimulates maternal thyroid**[Q] because of its thyrotrophic activity	• **Immunosuppressive activity**[Q] which may inhibit the maternal process of immunorejection of the fetus as the homograft • **Stimulates Leydig cells of the male fetus**[Q] to produce testosterone in conjunction with fetal pituitary gonadotrophins

Levels of hCG:

- Production by **syncytiotrophoblast**[Q]
- **Half life=24 hours, Doubling time=48** hours (2 days)[Q]

  - By **radio immunoassay** detected in **maternal serum** or **urine** as early as **8-9 days** following **ovulation**[Q]
  - **Maximum blood and urine level 100-200 IU/ml** between **60-70 days of pregnancy**[Q]
  - **Disappears** from circulation **within 2 weeks following delivery**[Q]

High levels of hCG is detected in

• **Multiple pregnancy**[Q] • **Hydatidiform mole or Choriocarcinoma**[Q] • **Down's syndrome**[Q]	• **Erythroblastosis fetalis**[Q] resulting from maternal D-Ag isoimmunization

- **hCG is decreased in ectopic pregnancy** and **impending spontaneous abortion.**

---

144. Ans. c. Ovarian cyst *(Ref: Shaw's 16/e p83, 448, 15/e p79, 385)*

As described in the examination, the swelling is typically arising from the pelvis, as the hand cannot be insinuated between mass and pelvic bone. Among the given options, only ovarian cyst arises from pelvis.

Swellings Arising from the Pelvis: Abdominal Palpation

- The **sensitive ulnar border of the left hand** is used **from above downwards to palpate swellings arising from the pelvis.**
- The **upper and lateral margins of such swellings can be felt but the lower border cannot be reached**, i.e. the **hand cannot be insinuated between the mass and the pelvis.**

PAEDIATRICS

145. Ans. a. Minimal change disease *(Ref: Harrison 19/e p184, 18/2345)*

*A 10-year old child presents with **edema, oliguria and frothy urine** with no past history of similar complaints. On examination, **urine is positive for 3+ proteinuria, no RBCs/WBCs and no casts**, with serum albumin 2.5 g/L and **serum creatinine 0.5 mg/dL**, the most likely diagnosis is **minimal change disease**.*

Minimal Change Disease:

- **Peak Age of onset** is between **6-8 years of age** (usually **<10 years**)
- Type of **onset: Insidious**
- **Nephrotic syndrome** is the **typical presentation**
- **Peripheral edema is the hallmark of Nephrotic syndrome** occurring when **serum albumin** levels become **< 3 gm/dl**
- **Laboratory findings:** Proteinuria and hypoalbuminemia

Minimal Change Disease

- **MC cause of Nephrotic syndrome in children (80% in children; 20% in adults)**[Q]
- **Peak Age of onset** is between **6-8 years of age**[Q] (usually < 10 years)
- Type of **onset: Insidious**

Contd...

Minimal Change Disease
Clinical Features: • **Presenting Feature: Peripheral edema**[Q] • **Nephrotic syndrome** is the **typical presentation**[Q] • **Peripheral edema is the hallmark of Nephrotic syndrome** occurring when **serum albumin** levels become **< 3 gm/dl**[Q] • **Initially dependent edema,** generalized edema later • May develop **pleural effusion, pulmonary edema, ascites** • **Hematuria: 20-30%** • **Hypertension: Very rare** • Renal failure: **Does not usually progress to renal failure**
Laboratory Findings (Features of Nephrotic syndrome): • **Proteinuria**[Q] • **Hypoalbuminemia**[Q] • **Hyperlipidemia/Hypercholesterolemia**[Q] (Increased hepatic production of lipids) • **Hypercoagulability**

Renal pathology (Biopsy)	
Investigation	Observation
Light microscopy[Q]	No abnormality hence the term minimal change
Electron microscopy[Q]	Fusion of foot processes
Immunofluorescence[Q]	Absence of immuno-globulin or complement

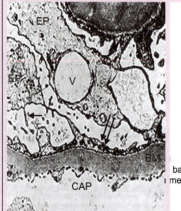
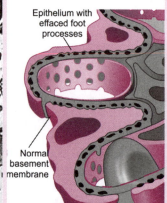

Treatment:
• **Corticosteroids** are the **mainstay for treatment of MCD**[Q]
Prognosis: • Prognosis is **good** • **Response to steroids is excellent**[Q] • **Does not progress to renal failure**[Q]

146. **Ans. c. ORS**   *(Ref: Ghai 8/e p293-294)*

The cornerstone of acute diarrhea management is rehydration by using oral rehydration solutions (ORS). Initial fluid of choice for diarrhea in an infant is ORS.

See Q. No. 158 AIIMS November 2015

147. **Ans. a. Hurler's syndrome**   *(Ref: Nelson 20/e p739)*

A male child with coarse facial features, macroglossia, thick lips presents with copious mucous discharge from nose at 10 months of age. The child was absolutely normal at birth. On examination he was found to have enlarged Liver and Spleen. Diagnosis is Hurler's syndrome.

> *"Hurler's syndrome (type 1 mucopolysacharidoses) is an AR disorder characterized by deficiency of alpha L-iduronidase resulting in accumulation of dermatan > heparin sulfate. It presents with Gortesque gargoyle facies (coarse and heavy face, enlarged head due to hydrocephalus caused by meningeal deposits, low forehead and ears, eyes wide set, wide nose, poorly formed and widespread teeth, open mouth, enlarged tongue and everted lips) and hepatosplenomegaly. Short neck, thora-columbur kyphosis, gibbus deformity with motor delays, flexion contracture of joints, short stature, genu valgum, flat feet, broad-short hand, radially curved little finger and carpal tunnel syndrome in children are other skeletal manifstations."*

AIIMS May 2015

1555

Mucopolysaccharidoses (MPS)								
Disorder	Enzyme Deficiency	Stored Material	Neurologic	Liver Spleen Enlargement	Skeletal Dysplasia	Ophthalmologic	Hematologic	Unique Features
MPS I H, **Hurler** MPS I H/S, Hurler/Scheie MPS I S, Scheie	alpha-L-Iduronidase	**Dermatan sulfate** **Heparan sulfate**	**Mental retardation** **Mental retardation** **None**	+ + +	+ + + +	Corneal clouding	Vacuolated lymphocytes	Coarse facies; cardiovascular involvement; joint stiffness
MPS II, Hunter	Iduronate sulfatase	**Dermatan sulfate** **Heparan sulfate**	**Mental retardation, less in mild form**	+ + +	+ + + +	Retinal degeneration, no corneal clouding	Granulated lymphocytes	**Coarse facies; cardiovascular involvement; joint stiffness;** distinctive **pebbly skin lesions**
MPS III, **Sanfilippo**	A: Heparan-N-sulfatase B: N-Acetyl-alpha-glucosaminidase C: Acetyl-CoA: alpha-glucosaminide N-acetyltransferase D: N-Acetylglucosamine-6-sulfate sulfatase	Heparan sulfate	Severe mental retardation	+	+	None	Granulated lymphocytes	Mild coarse facies
MPS IV, **Morquio**	A: N-Acetyl-galactosamine-6-sulfate sulfatase B: beta-Galactosidase	Keratan sulfate Chondroitin-6 sulfate	None	±	+ + + +	Corneal clouding	Granulated lymphocytes	Distinctive skeletal deformity; odontoid hypoplasia; aortic valve disease
MPS VI, **Maroteaux-Lamy**	Arylsulfatase B	Dermatan sulfate	None	+ +	+ + + +	Corneal clouding	Granulated neutrophils and lymphocytes	Coarse facies; valvular heart disease
MPS VII	beta-Glucuronidase	Dermatan sulfate Heparan sulfate	Mental retardation, absent in some adults	+ + +	+ + +	Corneal clouding	Granulated neutrophils	Coarse facies; vascular involvement; hydrops fetalis in neonatal form

148. **Ans. c. Alpha-1 Antitrypsin deficiency**   *(Ref: Harrison 19/e 367-e2; Nelson 20/e p2052; Robbin's 9/e p815)*

One-month-old child with conjugated bilirubinemia and intrahepatic cholestasis suggests neonatal cholestasis syndrome. The biopsy from liver is PAS positive. So most probable diagnosis would he Alpha-l Antitrypsin deficiency.

"α1AT deficiency is characterized by the presence of round- to-oval cytoplasmic globular inclusions in hepatocytes, which on routine hematoxylin and eosin stains are acidophilic, but are strongly periodic acid–Schiff (PAS)-positive and diastase-resistant."-Robbin's 9/e p815

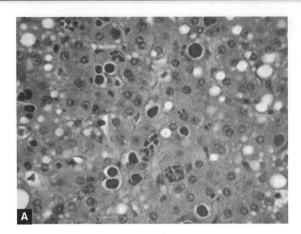
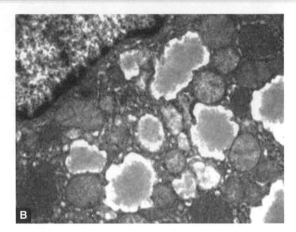

Figs. 18A and B: α1-Antitrypsin deficiency. (A) Periodic acid–Schiff (PAS) stain of the liver, highlighting the characteristic red cytoplasmic granules. (B) Electron micrograph showing the dilatation of the endoplasmic reticulum.

Alpha-1 Anti-Trypsin Deficiency (AR)
• **α1-Antitrypsin deficiency** is an **autosomal recessive disorder of protein folding** marked by **very low levels of circulating α1-Antitrypsin (α1AT)**. <ul><li>Gene is located on **chromosome 14**[Q]</li><li>MC genotype is **PiMM**, occurring in **90%** of individuals (the "wild-type")[Q]</li><li>MC clinically significant mutation is **PiZ**; homozygotes for the **PiZZ protein have circulating α1AT levels that are only 10% of normal.** These individuals are at **high risk for developing clinical disease**[Q].</li></ul>
• Because of its **early presentation with liver disease**, α1AT deficiency is the **most commonly diagnosed inherited hepatic disorder in infants and children.**

Pathology:

- **Major function of this protein: Inhibition of proteases, particularly neutrophil elastase, cathepsin G,** and **proteinase 3**, which are normally released from neutrophils at sites of inflammation.
- **α1AT deficiency** leads to the development of **pulmonary emphysema**, because the **activity of destructive proteases is not inhibited**.
- It also **causes liver disease** as a consequence of hepatocellular **accumulation of the misfolded protein**.
- **Cutaneous necrotizing panniculitis** also occurs in a minor subset of patients.

Morphology
• Characterized by the **presence of round- to-oval cytoplasmic globular inclusions in hepatocytes,** which on routine hematoxylin and eosin stains are **acidophilic**, but **are strongly periodic acid–Schiff (PAS)-positive and diastase-resistant**[Q].

Clinical Features:

- **Neonatal hepatitis with cholestatic jaundice** appears in **10-20% of newborns** with the deficiency.
- In **adolescence**, presenting symptoms may be related to **hepatitis, cirrhosis** or **pulmonary disease**.
- Disease may remain silent until **cirrhosis** appears in **middle to later life.**
- **HCC** develops in **2-3% of PiZZ adults**, usually, but not always, in the setting of cirrhosis.

Diagnosis:

- **Diagnosis is confirmed by blood tests** showing **reduced levels of serum AAT, accompanied by Pi determinations.**
- **Liver biopsy:** To determine **stage of hepatic fibrosis** and shows **characteristic PAS-positive, diastase-resistant globules in the periphery of the hepatic lobule**[Q].

Treatment:

- The treatment, indeed the **cure, for severe hepatic disease** is **orthotopic liver transplantation**.
- In patients with **pulmonary disease** the single most important preventive measure is **avoidance of cigarette smoking**, because **smoking markedly accelerates emphysema** and the **destructive lung disease associated with α1AT deficiency**[Q].

149. Ans. a. Ornithine transcarbamoylase (Ref: Nelson 20/e p670, Harper 30/e p295, 356, 30/e p295, 356, 28/e p242-246)

The recurrent symptoms with raised ammonia levels point towards the diagnosis of a Urea cycle defect. The most common urea cycle defect is due to deficiency of the enzyme Ornithine transcarbamoylase.

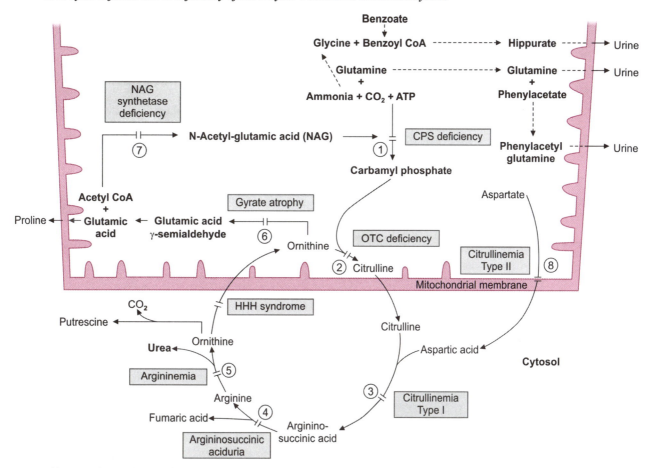

Fig. 19: Urea cycle: pathways for ammonia disposal and ornithine metabolism. Reactions shown with *interrupted arrows* are the alternate pathways for the disposal of ammonia. Enzymes: *(1)* carbamyl phosphate synthetase (CPS), *(2)* ornithine transcarbamylase (OTC), *(3)* argininosuccinic acid synthetase (AS), *(4)* argininosuccinic acid lyase (AL), *(5)* arginase, *(6)* ornithine 5-aminotransferase, *(7)* N-acetylglutamate (NAG) synthetase, *(8)* citrin. HHH syndrome, hyperammonemia-hyperornithinemia-homocitrullinemia.

Ornithine Transcarbamoylase (OTC) Deficiency
• **X-linked partially dominant disorder**
• **Hemiazygous males** are **more severely affected than heterozygous females**.
• **MC** form of all the **urea cycle disorders**[Q]
• **OTC Gene** is mapped to the **X chromosome (Xp21.1)**[Q]
Clinical Features:
• **Mild forms** characteristically have **episodic manifestations,** which may occur at any age (usually after infancy).
• **Episodes of hyperammonemia** (manifested by **vomiting** and **neurologic abnormalities** such as **ataxia, mental confusion, agitation, combativeness** and **frank psychosis**) are separated by periods of wellness[Q].
• These episodes **usually occur after ingestion of a high-protein diet** or as a **result of a catabolic state** such as infection.
• **Hyperammonemic coma, cerebral edema,** and **death** may occur during one of these attacks.
• **Gallstones** have been seen in the survivors; the mechanism remains unclear

Contd...

Ornithine Transcarbamoylase (OTC) Deficiency

Diagnosis:

- **Major laboratory finding** during the acute attack is **hyperammonemia** accompanied by **marked elevations** of plasma concentrations **of glutamine and alanine** with **low levels of citrulline and arginine**[Q].
- **Blood level of urea** is **usually low**[Q].

- A marked increase in the urinary excretion of Orotic acid differentiates it from Carbamoyl Phosphate Synthase deficiency[Q].
- Orotate may precipitate in urine as a pink colored gravel or stones[Q].

Treatment of Acute hyperammonemia

- Provide adequate calories, fluid, and electrolytes intravenously (10% glucose, NaCl and intravenous lipids 1 g/kg/24 hour).
- Give priming doses of the following compounds: **Sodium benzoate, Sodium phenyl acetate** and **Arginine hydrochloride**
- Continue infusion of sodium benzoate, sodium phenyl acetate, and arginine following the above priming doses. These compounds should be added to the daily intravenous fluid.
- Initiate **peritoneal dialysis** or **hemodialysis if above treatment fails** to produce an appreciable decrease in plasma ammonia.

- **Citrulline** is used **in place of arginine** in patients with OTC deficiency.
- **Liver transplantation** is a **successful treatment for patients with OTC deficiency.**

150. **Ans. c. Delta bilirubin**   *(Ref: Harrison 19/e p280, 18/e p325)*

"Delta Bilirubin: Part of the direct-reacting bilirubin fraction includes conjugated bilirubin that is covalently linked to albumin. This albumin-linked bilirubin fraction (delta fraction, or biliprotein) represents an important fraction of total serum bilirubin in patients with cholestasis and hepatobiliary disorders. By virtue of its tight binding to albumin, the clearance rate of albumin-bound bilirubin from serum approximates the half-life of albumin, 12-14 days, rather than the short half-life of bilirubin, about 4 hours."-Harrison 19/e p280

Delta Bilirubin

- **Part of the direct-reacting bilirubin fraction** includes **conjugated bilirubin** that is **covalently linked to albumin.** This **albumin-linked bilirubin fraction** (*delta fraction,* or *biliprotein*) represents an **important fraction of total serum bilirubin** in patients with **cholestasis** and **hepatobiliary disorders.**
- **Albumin-bound conjugated bilirubin is formed in serum when hepatic excretion of bilirubin glucuronides is impaired** and the **glucuronides are present in serum in increasing amounts.**

    - By virtue of its **tight binding to albumin**, the **clearance rate of albumin-bound bilirubin from serum** approximates the **half-life of albumin, 12-14 days**, rather than the short half-life of bilirubin, about 4 hours[Q].

- The **prolonged half-life of albumin-bound conjugated bilirubin explains two previously unexplained enigmas in jaundiced patients with liver disease.**
- That **some patients with conjugated hyperbilirubinemia do not exhibit bilirubinuria during the recovery phase** of their disease because the **bilirubin is covalently bound to albumin** and therefore **not filtered by the renal glomeruli.**
- That the **elevated serum bilirubin level declines more slowly than expected** in some patients who otherwise appear to be recovering satisfactorily.

    - **Late in the recovery phase of hepatobiliary disorders, all the conjugated bilirubin may be in the albumin-linked form.** Its **value in serum falls slowly because of the long half-life of albumin**[Q].

ORTHOPAEDICS

151. Ans. b. Flexor digitorum profundus *(Ref: Bailey 26/e p465)*

Jersey finger is caused by rupture of Flexor digitorum profundus.

"*Rugger jersey finger* – where there is **injury to the flexor profundus tendon**."-Bailey 26/e p465

"*Jersey finger is an injury to an FDP tendon at its point of attachment to the distal Phalanx. This injury often occurs in American football when a player grabs another player's jersey with the tips of one or more fingers while that player is pulling or running away.*"

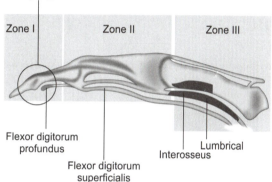

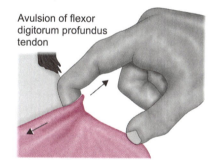

Caused by violent traction on flexed distal phalanx, as in catching on jersey of running football player

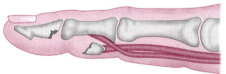

Flexor digitorum protundus tendon may be torn directly from distal phalanx or may avulse small or large bone fragment. Tendon usually retracts to about level of proximal interphalangeal joint. where it is stopped at its passage through flexor digitorum superficialis tendon; occasionally, it retracts into palm. Early open repair of tendon and its torn fibrous sheath indicated

Jersey finger
• **Jersey finger** is an **injury to an FDP tendon** at its **point of attachment to the distal Phalanx**[Q].
Mechanism of Injury: • This injury often occurs in **American football** when a **player grabs another player's jersey with the tips of one or more fingers while that player is pulling or running away**[Q].   • The **force of this action hyperextends the tip of the finger at the DIP joint** while the **proximal portion of the finger is flexed**[Q].   • This action can **partially or completely rupture the FDP tendon at or near its attachment point on the distal phalanx**[Q].

AIIMS ESSENCE

Contd...

Jersey finger
Clinical Features:
• A **pop or rip felt in the finger** at the time of the injury. Pain when moving the injured finger and the inability to bend the last joint. Tenderness, swelling and warmth of the injured finger.
• Bruising after 48 hours. Occasionally a lump felt in the palm of the finger.
Management:
• The **Leddy and Packer Classification** breaks Jersey finger tendon injuries **based on the degree of tendon injury, retraction,** and presence of a concomitant fracture[Q].
• **Conservative management for partial tears.**
• **Primary tendon repair within 10 days** or **repair of fracture fragment (6 weeks).**

152. Ans. d. Hip   *(Ref: Apley 9/e p354)*

Shenton's line is seen in X-ray of hip.

"Shenton's line is an imaginary line drawn along the inferior border of the superior pubic ramus (superior border of the obturator foramen) and along the inferomedial border of the neck of femur. This line should be continuous and smooth. It is breached in fracture neck of femur, head of femur, superior pubic rami and dislocation of hip."-

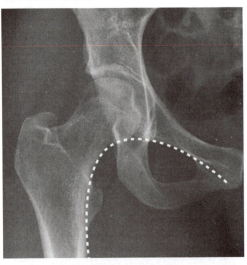

Fig. 20: Shenton's line

Radiological Features of Congenital Dislocation of Hip (Developmental Dysplasia of Hip)
In Von Rosen's view (both hips abducted, internally rotated and extended) following parameters are seen
1. **Hilgenreiner's (H) line: Horizontal line** through tri-radiate cartilages[Q] 2. **Perkin's line: Vertical line** drawn at the **outer border of acetabulum** and is **perpendicular to H-line**[Q]. 3. **Acetabular index:** Angle formed by **junction of H line and line drawn along acetabular surface**[Q].	4. **Shenton's line: Smooth curve** formed by **inferior border of neck of femur with superior margin of obturator foramen**[Q]. 5. **Center-Edge Angle of Wilberg:** Angle between **Perkin's line** and a **line drawn from lateral lip of acetabulum** through the center of femoral head[Q].

153. Ans. d. Pelvis   *(Ref: Maheshwari 5/e p38, 369)*

Judet's view of X-ray is for acetabular (pelvic) fracture.

"Judet's views are standard radiographic projections which are employed in patients with acetabulum fractures. Judet views are basically 45° oblique of the affected hip. The 45° angle is best achieved by rolling the patient. They are generally only performed as a supplementary view. In cases of acute injury, they can be useful in demonstrating or confirming acetabular fractures."

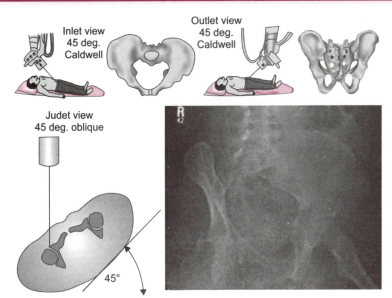

View	Done for
Ahlback view	• Knee (Weight-bearing AP view of knee in full extension)
Ball's method	• Pelvimetry
Brattstrom/Skyline view	• **Patella**
Butterfly views	• Elongated views of the rectosigmoid segments of large intestine.
Bett's/Clement's view	• **Trapezium**
Caldwell view	• **Frontal sinuses (Occipito-frontal view of skull)**
Capitellum/Berquist view	• Fracture of radial head
Colcher-Sussman Projection	• Pelvimetry
Danelius-Miller method	• Hip (Routine horizontal beam view)
Ferguson's view	• **Sacroiliac joints**
Friedman method	• **Femoral head, neck and upper femur**
Frog-leg position	• Bilateral hips
Fuchs method	• **Styloid process (Temporal bone)**
Garth's view	• **Shoulder instability**
Hayes' view	• **Superior-inferior SI joints**
Hill-Sachs view[Q]	• **Shoulder (AP view in marked internal rotation)**
Hobb's view	• Sternoclavicular joints
Judet view[Q]	• **Acetabulum (Hip)**
Kite view[Q]	• **Clubfoot**
Law's view	• **Petrous temporal bone**
Lowestein's view	• Hip (Routine frog lateral view)
May view	• Zygomatic arch
Risser method	• **Bilateral iliac crests**
Rhese view	• **Optic foramen**
Stenver method	• **Petrous temporal bone**
Stryker's view[Q]	• **Humeral head**
Tile's view	• Pelvic inlet and outlet
Town's view[Q]	• **Petrous pyramids, Arcuate eminence, Superior semicircular canal**
Velpeau view	• Shoulder
Waters' view[Q]	• **Maxillary sinuses**[Q]
'Y' view	• Shoulder

154. Ans. c. Laminoplasty *(Ref: Maheshwari 5/e p257)*
Removal of vertebral disc can be done by all these approaches except laminoplasty.

> "Laminoplasty describes the process of increasing the space available for the spinal cord by reconstruction of the laminar arch via a posterior approach."

Operative Management of Prolapsed Intervertebral Disc

- **Indications for operative treatment: 1.** Failure of conservative treatment; **2.** Cauda equina syndrome; **3.** Severe sciatic tilt

Methods of Removal of Disc	
Fenestration	The **ligamentum flavum** bridging the two adjacent laminae is **excised** and the spinal canal at the level exposed.
Laminotomy	In addition to fenestration, a **hole is made in the lamina** for wider exposure.
Hemi-laminectomy	The **whole of the lamina on one side is removed**
Laminectomy	The **laminae on both sides, with the spinous process are removed**. Such a wide exposure is **required for a big, central disc producing cauda equina syndrome**.

155. Ans. c. Dunlop *(Ref: Maheshwari 5/e p27)*
Dunlop traction is used for supracondylar fracture of humerus, not for lower limb.

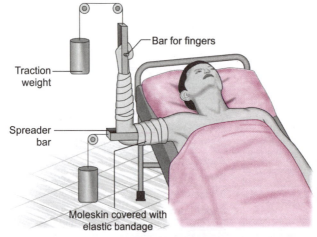

Uses of Tractions	
Name	**Use**
Bryant's Traction[Q]	Fracture **shaft of femur** in children **<2 years**
Gallow's Traction[Q]	Fracture **shaft of femur** in children **<2 years**
Russel's Traction[Q]	Fracture **shaft of femur** in **older children**
Perkin's Traction[Q]	Fracture **shaft of femur** in **adults**
90°-90° Traction[Q]	Fracture **shaft of femur** in **children**
Agnes-Hunt Traction	Correction of **Hip deformity**
Well-Leg Traction	Correction of **adduction or abduction deformity of hip**
Dunlop Traction[Q]	**Supracondylar fracture of humerus**
Smith's Traction[Q]	**Supracondylar fracture of humerus**
Calcaneal Traction	**Open fractures of ankle or leg**
Metacarpal Traction	**Open forearm fractures**
Head-Halter Traction	**Cervical spine injuries**
Crutchfield Traction[Q]	**Cervical spine injuries**
Halo-Pelvic Traction	**Scoliosis**

AIIMS May 2015

156. Ans. a. Normal calcium, normal ALP *(Ref: Harrison 19/e p2493, 18/e p3120; Apley 9/e p131-133)*
Serum calcium, phosphate and alkaline phosphatase are normal in osteoporosis.

Osteoporosis
• Osteoporosis is the **MC metabolic bone disease**.
• Osteoporosis is a **state of decreased mass per unit volume** (low bone density) of a normally mineralized bone.

Causes of Osteoporosis		Drugs Causing Osteoporosis
• **Immobilization**	• **Hyperprolactinemia**	• **Glucocorticoids[Q], Cytotoxic drugs[Q]**
• Senility	• **Osteogenesis imperfecta**	• Aromatase inhibitors
• **Post-menopausal[Q]**	• **Marfan's syndrome**	• **Lithium[Q],** Aluminium
• Cushing's disease,	• **Hypophosphatasia**	• **Cyclosporin[Q],** Excessive alcohol
• **Cushing's syndrome**	• **Homocystinuria**	• **Heparin[Q], Aromatase inhibitors**
• **Hyperparathyroidism**	• **Ehler's Danlos syndrome**	• **Excessive thyroxine[Q]**
• **Type 1 DM**	• **Multiple myeloma**	• **GnRH agonists**
• Acromegaly		

Clinical features:

• Osteoporosis is an **asymptomatic disorder** unless complications (predominantly fractures) occur
• **MC symptom of osteoporosis** is **back pain** secondary to vertebral compression fracture

Sites of Osteoporotic (Fragile) Fractures
• **MC site: Fracture vertebrae (Dorsolumbar pine** is the **MC site)[Q]**
• Colle's fracture; Fracture neck femur

• **Serum calcium, phosphate** and **alkaline phosphatase** are normal in osteoporosis[Q]

Diagnosis:

• **At least 30% of the bone mass must be lost before it becomes apparent on X-ray.**

Osteoporosis: X-ray findings
• **Loss of vertical height** of a vertebra **due to collapse[Q]**
• **Cod-fish appearance**: The disc bulges into the adjacent vertebral bodies so that the **disc becomes biconvex[Q]**.
• **Ground glass appearance** of the bones, conspicuous in bones like the **pelvis.**

Measurement of Bone Mass
• Noninvasive techniques for estimating skeletal mass or density: Dual-Energy X-ray Absorptiometry (DEXA), single-energy X-ray absorptiometry (SEXA), quantitative CT, and ultrasound (US).
• **Dual energy X-ray Absorptiometry (DEXA)** is the **gold standard for the screening (estimation) of bone density and bone mass and for diagnosis of osteoporosis[Q].**

Drugs useful in Osteoporosis		
Inhibit Bone Resorption	Stimulates Bone Formation	Both action
• **Bisphosphonates:** Alendronate, Risedronate, **Etidronate[Q]**	• **Teriparatide[Q]**	• **Strontium ranelate[Q]**
• Calcium receptor agonist: **Cinacalcet**	• Calcium	
• **Calcitonin[Q]**	• **Calcitriol[Q]**	
• SERMs: Tamoxifen, Raloxifene	• Fluoride	
• **Gallium nitrate[Q]**		
• **RANKL Inhibitors**: Donesumab		

157. Ans. a. Tendon transfer *(Ref: Apley 9/e p347,348)*

Treatment of choice for irreparable tear of the rotator cuff in a young patient is tendon transfer.

"Massive full thickness tears that cannot be reconstructed are treated by subacromial decompression and debridement of degenerate cuff tissue; the relief of pain may allow reasonable abduction of the shoulder by the remaining muscles. Other methods to reconstruct irreparable tears in the younger patient include supraspinatus advancement, latissimus dorsi transfer, rotator cuff transposition, fascia lata autograft and synthetic tendon graft."-Apley 9/e p348

AIIMS ESSENCE

"Debridement and partial repair can be considered for some patients, whereas reconstruction of the rotator cuff is most useful in young active patients for whom functional restoration is important. Latissimus dorsi muscle transfer is the preferred treatment active disabled patient with a posterosuperior irreparable cuff defect and good deltoid function. Anterosuperior irreparable defects can be treated with pectoralis and teres major tendon transfers but with less predictable results. A hemiarthroplasty can be considered for patients with severe disability, arthritis, and glenohumeral stability; however, in patients with unstable glenohumeral arthritis, the reverse ball prosthesis will provide more predictable pain relief and return of function, at least in the short term."-http://www.orthoontheweb.com/pdfs/Irreparable_Rotator_Cuff_Tears_JBJS_2006.pdf

"Every year, thousands of conventional total shoulder replacements are successfully done for patients with shoulder arthritis. This type of surgery, however, is not as beneficial for patients with large rotator cuff tears who have developed a complex type of shoulder arthritis called "cuff tear arthropathy". For these patients, conventional total shoulder replacement may result in pain and limited motion, and reverse total shoulder replacement may be an option."

Treatment of Rotator Cuff Injuries
• The **indications for surgical treatment** are **essentially clinical**.
• If **symptoms do not subside after 3 months of conservative treatment**, or if they **recur persistently after each period of treatment**, an operation is advisable.
• **Indications: Partial rotator cuff tear** and **full thickness tear** in a **younger patient**.
• The object is to **decompress the rotator cuff** by **excising the coracoacromial ligament, undercutting the anterior part of the acromion process** and, if necessary, reducing **any bony excrescences at the acromioclavicular joint**.
• This can be achieved by **open surgery** or **arthroscopically**.

Open Acromioplasty	• Through an anterior incision the deltoid muscle is split and the part arising from the anterior edge of the acromion is dissected free, **exposing** the **coracoacromial ligament, acromion** and **acromioclavicular joint**. • **Coracoacromial ligament is excised** and the **anteroinferior portion of the acromion is removed** by an undercutting osteotomy.
Arthroscopic Acromioplasty	• **Arthroscopic acromioplasty** has now **become the gold standard** and allows **earlier rehabilitation** than open acromioplasty because detachment of the deltoid is not performed. • It allows **good visualization of both sides of the rotator cuff** and the **identification of partial and full thickness tears**.
Open Repair of Rotator Cuff	• **Indications for open repair of the rotator cuff: Chronic pain, weakness of the shoulder** and **significant loss of function**. • The **younger** and **more active** the patient, the **greater is the justification for surgery**. The operation always includes an **acromioplasty**.

	• **Massive full thickness tears that cannot be reconstructed** are **treated by subacromial decompression** and **debridement of degenerate cuff tissue**. • Other methods **to reconstruct irreparable tears in the younger patient** include **supraspinatus advancement, latissimus dorsi transfer, rotator cuff transposition, fascia lata autograft and synthetic tendon graft**. • **Acute rupture of the rotator cuff in patients over 70 years** usually becomes **painless**; although movement is restricted, **operation is contraindicated**.
Arthroscopic Repair of Rotator Cuff	• Since the 1990s the **repair of full thickness tears** has undergone a **transition from open techniques to arthroscopically assisted (mini open) repairs** and **now full arthroscopic techniques**. • **Advantages: Less soft-tissue damage, faster rehabilitation and a better cosmetic appearance**.

158. **Ans. b. MRI** *(Ref: bApley's 9/e p724-725)*

Investigation of choice in stress fracture is MRI.

"The earliest changes, particularly in 'spontaneous' undisplaced osteoarticular fractures, are revealed by MRI. This investigation should be requested in older patients (possibly with osteoporosis) complaining of sudden onset of pain over the anteromedial part of the knee."-Apley's 9/e p725

Stress Fracture
• A **stress or fatigue fracture** is one occurring **in the normal bone** of a healthy patient, due to **small repetitive stresses** of two main types: **bending and compression**. • Commonly occurs in **athletes** or **new military recruits**[Q]. • **March fracture: Fatigue** or **stress fracture of metatarsals** often encountered in **military personnel**[Q].
Sites affected:
• **MC bones affected: Metatarsals >Fibula >Tibia**[Q]
Clinical features:
• History of **unaccustomed and repetitive activity** or **one of a strenuous physical exercise** programme. • A **common sequence of events** is: *pain after exercise – pain during exercise – pain without exercise*. • Affected site may be swollen or red. It is sometimes **warm and usually tender**; the callus may be palpable. **'Springing' the bone** (attempting to bend it) is often **painful.**
Imaging:
• **X-Ray:** Plain X-rays taken a **few weeks later** may show a **small transverse defect in the cortex** and/or **localized periosteal new-bone formation**.

MRI
• **The earliest changes, particularly in 'spontaneous' undisplaced osteoarticular fractures, are revealed by MRI**[Q]. • This investigation **should be requested in older patients (possibly with osteoporosis) complaining of sudden onset of pain over the anteromedial part of the knee**[Q].

Treatment:
• **Most stress fractures need no treatment** other than an **elastic bandage** and **avoidance of the painful activity** until the lesion heals

> • An **important exception** is **stress fracture of the femoral neck**. This should be **suspected in all elderly people** who **complain of pain in the hip** for which no obvious cause can be found.
> • If the **diagnosis is confirmed by bone scan**, the **femoral neck should be internally fixed with screws as a prophylactic measure.**

159. **Ans. b. Endosteum > a. (Periosteum)** *(Ref: Osteoporosis and Bone Densitometry Measurements edited by Giuseppe Guglielmi/ p72)*

Most metabolically active layer in the bone is endosteum. In children, periosteum is very active but endosteum is the most active layer in the bone (overall).

"Most metabolically active bone areas are those immediate contact with bone marrow. Most metabolically active component of bone is endosteal surface of cortex, with trabecular bone is next most metabolically active area. The endosteal surface has a total area of approximately 0.5 m², with higher remodelling activity than the periosteal surface, likely as a result of greater biomechanical strain or greater cytokine exposure from the adjacent bone marrow compartment."-http://cjasn. asnjournals.org/content/3/Supplement_3/S131.full

"There are two surfaces at which the bone is in contact with soft tissue: an external surface (periosteum) and an internal surface (endosteum). These surfaces are lined with layers of osteogenic or bone-building cells. The endosteum is more active metabolically because of the structural differences in compact and trabecular bone. Between 80 and 90% of the volume of compact bone is calcified, whereas only 15-20% of the trabecular bone is calcified. Trabecular bone is in close contact with bone marrow, blood vessels, and connective tissue. The endosteal bone surface is 70% of the interface with soft tissues such as muscles. The strength of compact bone helps it fulfill its mostly mechanical function, and trabecular bone is more mutable and metabolically active.

"Separating the trabeculae from the marrow is an endosteum. Under electron microscopy, the endosteal layer has a rich supply of osteoclasts and osteoblasts. Trabecular bone is more metabolically active than compact bone. Consequently, metabolic bone studies are best carried out on this component of bone."-Bone Pathology by Khurana (2009)/p6

1566

AIIMS ESSENCE

OPHTHALMOLOGY

160. **Ans. a. Optic nerve invasion**   *(Ref: Kanski 7/e p510-517; Yanoff and Duker 4/e p793)*

The most common mode of spread of retinoblastoma is by optic nerve invasion. Direct extension by continuity to the optic nerve and brain is common.

"Retinoblastoma is a primary malignant intraocular neoplasm that arises from immature retinoblasts within the developing retina. It is the most common primary intraocular malignancy of childhood in all-racial groups. The neoplasm has strong tendencies to invade the brain via the optic nerve and metastasize widely."-Yanoff and Duker 4/e p793

Retinoblastoma
• Retinoblastoma is common congenital malignant tumor **arising from** the **neurosensory retina**[Q] • **MC congenital intraocular tumor of childhood**[Q] • Occurring **1 in 15,000-20,000** live births • Though congenital, usually seen between **1-2 years of age**[Q] • **Bilateral in 25-30% cases** • **90% are sporadic**; 10% are familial

Genetics:
- **Rb gene** is located on chromosome **13q14**[Q]
- Rb gene is a tumor suppressor gene, deletion or inactivation of this protective gene by two mutations (**Knudson's two hit hypothesis**) results in retinoblastoma[Q]

Pathology:
- **Origin:** Arises as malignant proliferation of the immature retinal neural cells called **retinoblasts**
- Characterized by **Flexner-Wintersteiner rosettes (highly specific for retinoblastoma), Homer-Wright rosettes, pseudorosettes** and **fleurettes formation**[Q]
- Presence of areas **of hemorrhage and necrosis**

Clinical Features:

Quiescent stage	Glaucomatous/ Inflammatory stage	Stage of Extra-ocular extension	Stage of Distant Metastasis
• **MC presenting feature: Leukocoria** (amaurotic cat's eye appearance)[Q] • **2nd MC presenting feature: Squint (convergent)**[Q] • **Nystagmus** is a rare feature, noted in bilateral cases • Defective vision is very rare • **Endophytic** retinoblastoma: **Cottage cheese appearance**[Q] • **Exophytic** retinoblastoma: **Exudative retinal detachment** appearance[Q]	• Untreated retinoblastoma during quiescent stage may present with **severe pain, redness** and **watering**[Q]	• Due to progressive enlargement of tumor, the **globe bursts through the sclera**, usually **near the limbus** • Followed by **rapid fungation** and involvement of extra-ocular tissues resulting in **marked proptosis**[Q]	• **Lymphatic spread** first occurs in **preauricular lymph nodes**[Q] • **Direct extension** by continuity to the **optic nerve** and **brain** is common[Q] • Metastasis by bloodstream involves cranial and other bones

Diagnosis:
- **X-ray orbit: Calcification in 75% cases**[Q]
- **Raised LDH in aqueous humor**
- **CT: Extension to optic nerve, orbit and CNS**

Treatment:

Tumor destructive therapy	Enucleation is treatment of choice when
• For **early stage** (tumor **involves less than half of retina** and **optic nerve is not involved**) • **Primary systemic chemotherapy** (Vincristine, carboplatin and etoposide) followed by **local therapy** (cryotherapy, laser photocoagulation, thermotherapy)	• Tumor involves more than half of retina • Optic nerve is involved • Glaucoma is present and anterior chamber is involved • **Eye-ball is enucleated along with maximum length of optic nerve** taking special care not to perforate the eye ball.

Retinoblastoma

Indications of Palliation (Chemotherapy, surgical debulking, EBRT)
• Retinoblastoma with **orbital extension** • Retinoblastoma with **intracranial extension** • Retinoblastoma with **distant metastasis**

Poor prognostic factors		
• Optic nerve involvement[Q]	• Undifferentiated tumor cells[Q]	• Massive choroidal invasion[Q]

• **Reese-Ellsworth classification** to **predict survival of** the **eye** with retinoblastoma[Q]

---

161. Ans. c. Berlin's edema *(Ref: Kanski 7/e p882; Parson's 22/e p392, 21/e p382, 20/e p367; Yanoff and Duker 4/e p671)*

Cherry red spot after trauma is seen in children due to Berlin's edema.

Commotio retinae (Berlin's Edema) is of common occurrence following a blow on the eye. It manifests as milky white cloudiness involving a considerable area of posterior pole with a 'cherry-red spot' in the foveal region. It may appear after some days or may be followed by pigmentary changes."-Khurana 5/e p434

"Commotio retinae most frequently affect the temporal fundus. If the macula is involved, a 'cherry-red spot' may be seen at the fovea."-Kanski 7/e p882

Berlin's Edema (Commotio Retinae)
• **Most commonly involves temporal fundus** occasionally involves **macula with a "cherry-red spot"**[Q]. • Subsequent macular change will include **progressive pigmentary degeneration** and **macular-hole formation**[Q]. • Commotio retinae are a **contrecoup injury to the retina**. • It can **occur centrally or peripherally**, and **when it involves the macula, it is called Berlin's edema.** • The **retina appears normal** on examination although the patient may complain of decreased vision.

• The **affected area becomes white** and **opaque usually hours after the trauma.**
   • Berlin's "edema" is not a true edema[Q].
   • **Swelling and disorganization of the outer retinal layers causes the opaqueness** and there is **no intercellular fluid**[Q].

Clinical Features:
• This **occurs in blunt trauma to eye** (e.g. **Tennis ball injury to eye**). • The visual acuity in commotion retinae varies from 20/20 to 20/400 and **does not always correlate with the degree of retinal opacification.**
Course and Prognosis:
• Berlin's edema is **usually self-limited** and **resolves without sequelae** • There is **no known intervention that alters its course and prognosis.**

---

162. Ans. c. Retrobulbar neuritis *(Ref: Yanoff and Duker 4/e p879)*

Most likely diagnosis in the patient who presents with painful unilateral dimness of vision and history of persistence of after images is retrobulbar neuritis.

*"Loss of vision in patients with **acute demyelinating optic neuritis** is **usually abrupt**, occurring over several hours to days. Visual loss is usually monocular, although occasionally both eyes are affected simultaneously, particularly in children. Mild pain in or around the eye is present in more than 90% of patients. Such pain may precede or occur concomitantly with visual loss, is usually exacerbated by eye movement, and generally lasts no more than a few days. The **presence of pain, particularly on eye movement**, is a helpful (although not definitive) clinical feature that **differentiates acute demyelinating optic neuritis from nonarteritic anterior ischemic optic neuropathy (AION).** Color vision and contrast sensitivity are impaired in almost all cases, often out of proportion to visual acuity.*

Contd...

Contd...

*Visual field loss, which maybe **diffuse** (48%) or **focal** (i.e. nerve fiber bundle defects, central or cecocentral scotomas, hemianopic defects), is also common in acute optic neuritis. An **afferent pupillary defect (APD)** is detected in almost all unilateral cases of optic neuritis. The optic disk appears normal in approximately two thirds of adults with acute demyelinating optic neuritis (retrobulbar optic neuritis), while disk swelling is present in about one third of adult cases (papillitis)."-Yanoff and Duker 4/e p879*

Causes of Loss of Vision

Sudden Painless Loss of Vision	Sudden Painful Loss of Vision	Gradual Painless Loss of Vision	Gradual Painful Loss of Vision
• **CRAO** • Massive vitreous hemorrhage • Retinal detachment (involving macular area) • **Ischemic CRVO**	• **Acute congestive glaucoma** • **Acute iridocyclitis** • Chemical and mechanical injuries to eyeball • **Retrobulbar neuritis**	• Progressive pterygium • Corneal dystrophy • **Senile cataract** • **Optic atrophy** • **Refractive errors** • **ARMD**	• **Chronic iridocyclitis** • **Corneal ulceration**

Optic Neuritis

- It is an **inflammatory or demyelinating disorder** of the **optic nerve**
- Typically affects the patients between **18-45 years of age**

Etiology:

- **Multiple sclerosis,** Vitamin B1, B6 and B12 deficiency, Leber's hereditary optic neuritis
- **Drugs: Quinine^Q, chloroquine^Q, ethambutol^Q, digitalis^Q**
- **Tobacco, alcohol (ethanol and methanol)^Q**
- Giant cell arteritis, Takayasu arteritis, PAN, SLE

Types of Optic Neuritis

Papillitis	Neuroretinitis	Retrobulbar neuritis	Perineuritis
• It **involves** the **optic disc** (optic nerve head)	• Involves **peripapillary retina** • **Exudation in macular area** leads to **macular star formation^Q**	• Involves **posterior part of optic nerve** which is not visualized	• **Peripheral fibers of optic nerve** are involved causing **constriction of visual field**

Clinical features:

- Predominant symptom: **Loss of vision,** which **typically deteriorates over hours to days** and reaches a trough **about 1 week after the onset.**
- **Monocular sudden, progressive and profound loss of vision^Q**
- **Deep orbital, retroocular or brow pain** especially when the eye is moved superiorly due to attachment of some fibers of superior rectus to duramater **(especially seen in retrobulbar and perineuritis)^Q**.
- **Visual impairment** is accompanied by **loss of colour vision (typically red desaturation)** and **reduced perception of light intensity.**

Pulfrich phenomenon	Altered perception of moving objects^Q
Uhthoff sign	Worsening of symptoms with exercise or an increase in body temperature^Q

Clinical signs of Optic Neuritis

• Variable degree of **decreased visual acuity^Q** • **Decreased colour vision^Q** • **Abnormal contrast sensitivity^Q** • **Decreased stereoacuity^Q**	• **Visual field defects**: Central, centrocaecal, arcuate or **sectorial^Q** • **Altitudinal focal pattern defects** or a **generalized non-specific depression in retinal sensitivity.**

- **Perimetry: Visual function depression over the entire field** but is **more marked in the central 20°** with varied pat terns of field defects.
- **Lack of sustained constriction of the pupil to light,** if it can be proved beyond dispute, is of **great diagnostic significance**.
- **Presence of a relative afferent pupillary defect** or **Marcus Gunn pupil** is of **greater diagnostic significance,** indicating a defect in the afferent limb of the pupillary light reflex due to a **pathological lesion in the optic nerve^Q**.
- **Prolonged latency** is seen on testing the **visual evoked potentials (VEP)^Q**.

Optic Neuritis
Ophthalmoscopy
• **Disc could be normal in retrobulbar neuritis** • It may be **hyperemic and swollen** with or without peripapillary **flame-shaped haemorrhage in papillitis**. • It may be **inflamed with involvement of the neighboring retina** showing a **stellate pattern of retinal exudates in neuroretinitis**[Q]. • **Papillitis**: The **disc is at first hyperemic; later the margins become** blurred, swelling and edema ensue which spread onto the retina, the retinal veins become tortuous and extensively distorted, exudates may accumulate upon the disc and there are fine vitreous opacities.

163. **Ans. d. HM 3 and 4** *(Ref: The Eye 3/e p305-307; Biochemistry of Eye by David R/p28)*

High molecular weight proteins in cataractous lens seen only in humans are HM 3 and 4.

"HM3 and HM4 are insoluble high molecular weight proteins and found in cataractous lens."

Cataract Lens
• **The most general effect is the change in the amount of soluble and insoluble lens proteins.** • **Resnik first isolated the high molecular weight fraction from lens proteins. There are four fractions known till now: HM1, HM2, HM3, HM4**

High Molecular (HM) Weight Proteins		
HM1	Large aggregate isolated from alpha-crystalline preparations of gel chromatography	• **Soluble kind**
HM2	Directly isolated from total soluble fractions	• **Soluble kind**
HM3	Disulphide bonded aggregate	• **Insoluble, found in cataractous lens**[Q]
HM4	Aggregates held together by covalent bonds and not disulphide bonds	• **Insoluble, found in cataractous lens**[Q] • **Occurs exclusively in nuclear cataract**[Q]

164. **Ans. a. CRAO** *(Ref: Parson's 22/e p320-321, 21/e p313,314; Kanski 7/e p559-562; Yanoff and Duker 4/e p522)*

Cherry red spot and Hollenhorst plaque are seen in both CRAO and BRAO. But the incidence of CRAO is more common than BRAO.

Central Retinal Artery Occlusion (CRAO)		
• Main circulation to retina is by **central retinal artery,** its **occlusion** causes **severe ischemia to retina** • **MC cause: Atherosclerosis-related thrombosis** at the level of **lamina cribrosa**[Q]		

Retinal Artery Occlusions		
• **Central retinal artery involvement (60%)**[Q]	• **Branch retinal artery involvement (35%)**[Q]	• **Cilioretinal artery involvement (5%)**

Etiology		
Thrombosis (80%)	**Embolism (20-40%)**	**Systemic Vasculitis**
• **Atherosclerosis related thrombosis** at the level of **lamina cribrosa (MC cause)**[Q] • Systemic coagulopathies or Thrombophilic disorders: – Protein C deficiency – Protein S deficiency – Anti-thrombin III deficiency	• **Origin of emboli** is mostly an **atheromatous plaque** at the **carotid bifurcation** and less often an aortic arch. • **Cardiac embolism** from **valvular heart disease,** vegetations of SABE • **Oncogenic embolism:** Leukemia, lymphoma and metastatic tumors. • **Procedure induced emboli:** Angiography, angioplasty • **Orbital inflammations: Orbital mucormycosis**	• **SLE** • **Polyarteritis nodosa** • **Temporal arteritis** • Wegner's granulomatosis • Kawasaki's syndrome • Inflammatory bowel disease • Dermatomyositis • Behcet's syndrome

Clinical Features:
• **Sudden painless loss of vision**[Q] within few minutes the eye may become totally blind

Contd...

Central Retinal Artery Occlusion (CRAO)
Fundoscopy
• **Larger retinal arteries are constricted** and look like thin threads while smaller vessels are scarcely visible • **Retina loses its transparency** becoming opaque or **milky white** • **Cherry red spot at fovea**[Q] • Attenuation of arteries but the veins are little altered except on the disc • **Cattle trucking or segmentation of blood columns of venous blood**[Q]

Treatment:
- **Ocular massage** using 3 mirror contact lens for 10 seconds followed by 5 seconds of release, is the **most effective method**[Q]
- Sublingual **isosorbide dinitrate** or inhalation of **amyl nitrate to produce vasodilation**
- Lowering of intraocular pressure by **IV acetazolamide** and **mannitol or oral glycerol**

Prognosis:
- **Prognosis is poor**[Q], mostly resulting in **blindness due to retinal and optic atrophy**; some eyes develop **rubeosis iridis**[Q].

165. **Ans. d. ABCG2** *(Ref: Indian J Med Res. 2008 Aug;128(2):149-56. PMID:19001678; http://www.stembook.org/node/588)*

Universal marker of limbal epithelial stem cells is ABCG2.

> *"The limbal epithelial cells cultured over intact HAM expressed the stem cell associated markers (ABCG2, p63) and showed reduced expression of the differentiation markers (Cnx43 and K3/K12) when compared to limbal epithelial cells cultured over denuded HAM, which expressed more differentiation markers at the end of three weeks." -Indian J Med Res. 2008 Aug;128(2):149-56. PMID:19001678*

Limbal Stem Cell Marker	ABCG2
Corneal Stem Cell Marker	Keratin (K3-K13)

Limbal Epithelial Stem Cells (LESCs)

- At the **corneoscleral junction** in an area known as the **limbus,** there is a population of **limbal epithelial stem cells (LESCs).**
- **LESCs** share common features with other adult somatic stem cells including **small size** and **high nuclear to cytoplasmic ratio**. They also **lack expression of differentiation markers** such as cytokeratins 3 and 12.
- Many types of organ-specific stem cells, including **LESC** have been recently shown to exhibit a **side population (SP) phenotype**.
- The **SP cells** are able to **efflux Hoechst 33342 dye** through the **ATPbinding cassette transporter Bcrpl/ ABCG2.**

  - **ABCG2** has therefore been proposed to be a **universal marker for stem cells**.
  - **In putative LESCs**, this protein has been **immunolocalised to the cell membrane** and **cytoplasm of a population of limbal basal cells** and a few suprabasal cells.
  - Furthermore, ABCG2 positive cells produce higher colony forming efficiency values in vitro than their negative counterparts.

166. **Ans. d. Masson trichrome** *(Ref: Kanski 7/e p212-224; Parson's 22/e p212-214, 21/e p207-209; Yanoff and Duker 4/e p261)*

Masson trichrome stain is used for diagnosis of granular dystrophy of cornea.

Granular dystrophy:
- Inheritance is **AD** with the **gene locus on 5q31**
- Onset: **First decade with recurrent erosions**
- Signs (in chronological order):
  - **Small, white, sharply demarcated deposits resembling crumbs** or **snowflakes in the central anterior stroma**
  - Increase in number of lesions with deeper and outward spread but not reaching the limbus
  - Gradual confluence causing **impairment of visual acuity**
- **Histology shows amorphous hyaline deposits,** which **stain bright red with Masson trichrome**.

AIIMS May 2015

Corneal Dystrophies

- Group of **progressive**, usually **bilateral,** mostly **genetically determined**, **non-inflammatory, opacifying** disorders
- Manifest usually during **1st or 2nd decade**
- Types of Corneal Dystrophies

Anterior Corneal Dystrophies

Epithelial Dystrophies	Bowman layer Dystrophies

- **Epithelial basement membrane dystrophy (Cogan microcystic** or **map-dot-fingerprint Dystrophy):**
  – **MC type of dystrophy** seen in clinical practice[Q]
  – Neither familial nor progressive
  – Characterized by **recurrent corneal erosions**
  – **Signs: Dot-like opacities, Epithelial microcysts, Subepithelial map-like patterns and Whorled fingerprint-like lines[Q].**
  – **Meesmann dystrophy: Tiny epithelial cysts in interpalpebral area**
  – Lisch dystrophy
  – Stocker Holt dystrophy
	- **Reis Buckler dystrophy** (AD): Characterized by **recurrent corneal erosions**
	- Honey comb dystrophy (AD)
	- Central Schnyder dystrophy (AD)

Stromal Dystrophies

Feature	Granular (AD)	Lattice (AD)	Macular (AR)
Age of onset	1st decade	1st decade	1st decade
Diminished vision	By 4th or 5th decade	By 2nd or 3rd decade	1st or 2nd decade
Corneal Erosions	Uncommon	Frequent	Common
Opacities	**Small, white, sharply demarcated deposits resembling crumbs** or **snowflakes in the central anterior stroma**	**Early refractile tiny lines** and **dots** **Subepithelial spots** Diffuse central haze Limbal zone clear except in extreme cases	**Indistinct margins** **Hazy intervening stroma** **Extends to limbus** Endothelium affected Central lesions more anterior Peripheral lesions more posterior
Corneal thickness	Normal	Normal	**Thinned**
Material accumulated	**Hyaline[Q]**	**Amyloid[Q]**	**Mucopolysaccharides[Q]**
Stains	**Masson trichrome[Q]**	**Congo red[Q]**	**Alcian blue[Q]**
Distinguishing clinical features	Clear limbal zone	Lattice lines	Opacities reach limbus, Most severe

Posterior (Endothelial) Dystrophies

Cornea Guttata	Fuchs Endothelial Dystrophy (AD)	Posterior Polymorphous Dystrophy (AD)

- **Focal accumulations of collagen** on the **posterior surface of Descemet membrane**
- The lesions appear as **warts** or **excrescences** and are **secreted by abnormal endothelial cells.**
- Signs:
  – **Tiny dark spots[Q]**
  – **'Beaten metal' appearance[Q]**
  – **Hassall-Henle bodies[Q]**
	- More common in **women, slowly progressive** disease, occurs in **old age.**
	- **Signs:**
	  – **'Beaten-metal' appearance**
	  – **Central stromal edema** and blurred vision
	  – Persistent epithelial edema results in bullae (**bullous keratopathy**)
		- Vesicular, geographical band like opacities on posterior corneal surface with **endothelial dysfunction**
		- **Signs: Stromal and epithelial edema**
		- Associated with **open angle glaucoma, angle closure glaucoma** due to iridocorneal adhesions

167. Ans. b. Right head tilt *(Ref: Yanoff and Duker 4/e p1228)*

Right trochlear nerve palsy is accompanied by compensatory contralateral head tilt (left head tilt), not the right head tilt.

*"The classical sign of unilateral fourth nerve palsy is a contralateral head tilt (an 'ocular' torticollis). It is **exhibited by most patients** and is **usually the sole presenting sign in children**, although non-ophthalmological causes must also be considered."-Yanoff and Duker 4/e p1228*

*"**Fourth nerve palsy** present with **vertical diplopia** and is commonly **accompanied by compensatory contralateral head tilt**. **Torsional diplopia**, which **results from ocular cyclotorsion**, **often accompanies vertical diplopia** in acquired fourth nerve palsy."*

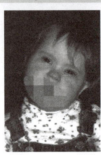

Congenital right trochlear nerve palsy with compensatory left head tilt.

Trochlear Nerve Palsy

- **Fourth nerve palsy** present with **vertical diplopia** and is commonly **accompanied by compensatory contralateral head tilt.**
- **Weakness of the superior oblique muscle allows unopposed action of its direct antagonist**, which results in an **ipsilateral hypertropia** and **excyclotorsion**. **Vertical diplopia** or vague reports of 'eyestrain' or **other difficulty reading in down gaze** are the **most common complaints vocalized in fourth nerve palsy**.
  - The **classical sign of unilateral fourth nerve palsy is a contralateral head tilt (an 'ocular' torticollis)**. It is **exhibited by most patients** and is **usually the sole presenting sign in children**, although non-ophthalmological causes must also be considered^Q.
- **Torsional diplopia**, which **results from ocular cyclotorsion**, **often accompanies vertical diplopia** in acquired fourth nerve palsy.
- **Excyclotorsion of the hypertropic eye** suggests **fourth nerve palsy because of weakened intorsion**
- **Esotropia greatest in down gaze** (so called **V-pattern esotropia** with >15 prism diopter difference between upgaze and downgaze) because of weakened abduction in depression (the superior oblique acts as an abductor). **Esotropia is more evident in bilateral trochlear nerve palsy.**
- Hypertropia is greatest in the vertical field of action of the superior oblique muscle.
  - MC cause of trochlear nerve palsy: Idiopathic^Q
  - MC cause of vertical strabismus: Trochlear nerve palsy^Q
  - **Nuclear or fascicular lesion** causes **partial or complete paralysis of the contralateral superior oblique muscle**. So in case of **nuclear lesion, ipsilateral head tilt occurs**^{Q}.

168. Ans. a. Malignancy   *(Ref: Yanoff and Duker 4/e p1339)*

Evisceration of eye is not done in malignancy

*"**Evisceration** is the surgical technique that **removes the entire intraocular contents of the eye** while **leaving the scleral shell** and **extraocular muscle attachments intact**. Evisceration surgery is a simpler procedure than enucleation surgery and offers better preservation of the orbital anatomy and natural motility of the ophthalmic socket tissues.*

In cases of documented or suspected intraocular malignant tumors, evisceration is contraindicated."-Yanoff and Duker 4/e p1339

Enucleation	Evisceration	Exenteration
• **Removal of eyeball with a portion of optic nerve** from the orbit while **preserving all other orbital structures.**	• **Removal of the eye with its inner two coats, leaving behind the sclera** and **extraocular muscles.** • **Frill evisceration** is **preferred** over simple evisceration.	• **Most radical** • Involves **removal of the eye, adnexa** and **part of the bony orbit**

Contd...

Contd...

Enucleation		Evisceration	Exenteration
Indications		**Indications**	**Indications**
Absolute	Relative	• Panophthalmits[Q] • Expulsive choroidal hemorrhage[Q] • Bleeding anterior staphyloma[Q] • Endophthalmitis not responding to antibiotics[Q]	• Large orbital tumors[Q] • Orbital extension of intraocular tumor
• Retinoblastoma[Q] • Malignant melanoma[Q]	• Phthisis bulbi[Q] • Endophthalmitis[Q] • Painful blind eye • Mutilating ocular • Anterior staphyloma[Q] • Congenital anophthalmia • Severe microphthamia		

169. **Ans. b. Macular cones** *(Ref: Yanoff and Duker 4/e p460)*
Multifocal ERG is useful to assess the function of macular cones.

Multifocal ERG (mfERG)
• The multifocal ERG (mfERG) has supplanted focal ERG testing and records multiple local ERG responses elicited from the central 40–50 degrees of the retina under light-adapted conditions.   • These responses are then displayed individually so that **abnormal spatial variations** can be **localized to their corresponding areas in the macula, perimacula, or remaining posterior pole.**
• Clinically, **mfERG testing is most useful to assess macular function** in patients with **unexplained or central loss of vision** who may have a normal full-field ERG.
• The **mfERG can aid in the diagnosis of macular diseases including Stargardt's dystrophy, cone dystrophy, occult macular dystrophy**, and **hydroxychloroquine toxicity.**   • **Ring ratio analysis of mfERGs** provides a quantitative measure that can be helpful in early detection of diseases that cause **dysfunction in the pericentral macula**, such as in **hydroxychloroquine toxicity.**

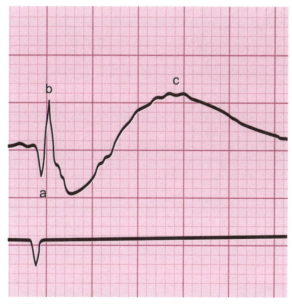

Fig. 21: Typical electroretinogram showing a, b and c waves. The dip in the lower line indicates the point of stimulation.

AIIMS ESSENCE

Electroretinogram (ERG)

- In **ERG**, changes in the resting potential of the eye, induced by the stimulation of the eye with a light stimulus, are measured.

In the normal dark-adapted eye, after a fleeting early receptor potential, three components are seen:	
Negative a-wave	• Possibly **representing the activity of the rods and cones**[Q]
Positive (composite) b-wave	• Arising in the **inner retinal layers; and, with strong stimuli,** a secondary rise in potential[Q]
c-wave	• **Related not to visual processes** but **to retinal metabolism, associated particularly with the pigmentary epithelium[Q].**

- The **ERG measures a global response** and essentially **gives an indication of the activity of the entire retina**, that is, of the **rods and cones** and **their immediate connections**.
- The **rod response** is selectively tested in the dark-adapted state with a blue light stimulus (**scotopic ERG**).
- The **cones** are tested in bright light (**photopic ERG**) or with a flickering light stimulus of >20 Hz, which is higher than the critical fusion frequency of rods.
- The **pattern ERG** indicates the **activity of the central macular region** and its corresponding nerve connections; it is **used to diagnose early glaucomatous damage**.

ERG (Normal ERG is biphasic)	
Extinguished ERG	• Advanced retinitis pigmentosa, CRAO, complete old retinal detachment, advanced siderosis
Subnormal ERG	• **Early retinitis pigmentosa,** large area of retina is not functioning
Negative ERG	• Gross disturbances of retinal circulation
Pattern ERG	• Indicates activity of central macular region
Multifocal ERG	• For disorders of **central retina/fovea**

170. **Ans. d. Ascorbate** *(Ref: Yanoff and Duker 4/e p353)*

As compared to blood, vitreous humor has high concentration of ascorbate.

Ingredient	Human Aqueous Humor	Human Vitreous Humor	Balanced Salt Solution
Sodium	**162.9**	144	155.7
Potassium	2.2-3.9	5.5	**10.1**
Calcium	1.8	1.6	3.3
Magnesium	1.1	1.3	**1.5**
Chloride	131.6	**177**	128.9
Bicarbonate	**20.15**	15	-
Phosphate	**0.62**	0.4	-
Lactate	2.5	**7.8**	-
Glucose	2.7-3.7	3.4	-
Ascorbate	1.06	**2**	-
Glutathione	0.0019	-	-
Citrate	-	-	5.8
Acetate	-	-	28.6
pH	7.38	-	7.6
Osmolality	304	-	298

171. **Ans. c. Magnification is 5 times** *(Ref: Parson's 22/e p137-139, 20/e p126-133; Yanoff and Duker 4/e p69)*

Magnification is direct ophthalmoscopy is 15 times. In indirect ophthalmoscopy, magnification is 4-5 times.

Direct ophthalmoscopy:
- Image is **virtual, erect**[Q]
- **Magnification: About 15 times**[Q]
- **Area of field in focus: About 2 disc diopters**[Q]
- **Illumination: Not so bright, so not useful in hazy media**

Features	Direct ophthalmoscopy	Indirect Ophthalmoscopy
Condensing lens	Not required	Required (Convex lens)
Examination distance	As close to patient's eye as possible	At an arm's length
Image	Virtual, erect[Q]	Real, inverted[Q]
Magnification	About 15 times[Q]	4-5 times[Q]
Illumination	Not so bright, so not useful in hazy media	Bright, so useful for hazy media[Q]
Area of field in focus	About 2 disc diopters[Q]	About 8 disc diopters[Q]
Stereopsis	Absent	Present
Accessible fundus view	Slightly beyond equator	Up to Ora serrata i.e. Peripheral retina[Q]
Examination through hazy media	Not possible	Possible[Q]
Patient position	Sitting	Supine
Ease	Easy procedure for visualization of posterior pole of retina	Difficult, require training

ENT

172. **Ans. b. Bilateral vocal cord palsy**   *(Ref: Dhingra 7/e p339, 6/e p300)*

Transverse cordotomy or Kashima operation is done for bilateral vocal cord palsy.

Bilateral Recurrent Laryngeal Nerve Paralysis (Bilateral Abductor Paralysis)
• **Neuritis or surgical trauma (thyroidectomy)** are the **most important causes**. • **Position of cords:** As **all the intrinsic muscles of larynx are paralyzed**, the **vocal cords lie in median or paramedian[Q] position** due to **unopposed action of cricothyroid muscles**
Clinical Features:
• As both the cords lie in median or paramedian position, so there is **dyspnea and stridor** but **voice is good[Q]**
Treatment:
• **Emergency tracheostomy** or **widening the respiratory airway** without a permanent tracheostomy by arytenoidectomy with suture, arytenoidopexy (fixing the arytenoid in lateral position), lateralization of vocal cord and laser cordectomy (**replaced by less invasive techniques**)

Less Invasive Techniques for Bilateral RLN Paralysis	
1. **Transverse cordotomy (Kashima operation)**	• **Soft tissue at the junction of membranous cord** and **vocal process of arytenoid** is **excised laterally with laser.** • This provides good airway. In case airway is still insufficient more tissue can be removed at subsequent operation.
2. **Partial arytenoidectomy**	• **Medial part of arytenoid is excised with laser**. • Sometimes only the vocal process of arytenoids is ablated.
3. **Reinnervation procedures**	• These have been **used to innervate paralyzed posterior cricoarytenoid muscle by implanting a nerve-muscle pedicle of sternohyoid** or **omohyoid muscle with its nerve supply from ansa hypoglossi.** • These procedures have not been very successful.
4. **Thyroplasty type II**	• It creates **lateral expansion of larynx** and is similar to vocal cord lateralization. Quality of voice may not be good.

173. **Ans. a. Tympanometry**   *(Ref: Dhingra 7/e p62-63, 6/e p59)*

Eustachian tube function is assessed by both tympanometry and Politzer test. Tympanometry is better than Politzer test.

Rhinomanometry	• **Rhinomanometry** is a standard diagnostic tool aiming to **objectively evaluate the respiratory function of the nose.**
	• It **measures pressure and flow during normal inspiration and expiration through the nose.**
	• Increased pressure during respiration is a result of increased resistance to airflow through nasal passages (nasal blockage), while increased flow, which means the speed of airstream, is related to better patency.
	• **Nasal obstruction leads to increased values of nasal resistance.**
	• Rhinomanometry may be used to measure **only one nostril at a time (anterior rhinomanometry)** or **both nostrils simultaneously (posterior rhinomanometry).**
Vestibular Evoked Myogenic Potential (VEMP)	• It is a **neurophysiological assessment technique** used to **determine the function of the otolithic organs (utricle and saccule) of the inner ear.**
	• It complements the information provided by caloric testing and other forms of inner ear (vestibular apparatus) testing.

Eustachian Tube Function Tests

1. Valsalva test:

- **Principle: Build positive pressure in the nasopharynx so that air enters the eustachian tube**
- If air enters the middle ear, tympanic membrane will move outwards which can be **verified by otoscope or microscope.**
- **Failure of this test does not prove blockage of the tube** because only about 65% of persons can successfully perform this test.
- **It should be avoided in the presence of: Atrophic scar of tympanic membrane** which can rupture, and **infections of nose and nasopharynx** (infected secretions are likely to be pushed into the middle ear causing otitis media)

2. Politzer test:

- **Done in children** who are **unable to perform Valsalva test.**
- In this test, olive-shaped tip of Politzer's bag is introduced into the patient's nostril on the side of which the tubal function is desired to be tested.
- Other nostril is closed and the bag compressed while at the same time the patient swallows (he can be given sips of water).
- By means of an auscultation tube, connecting the patient's ear under test to that of the examiner, a hissing sound is heard if tube is patent.
- Compressed air can also be used instead of Politzer's bag. The test is also used therapeutically to ventilate the middle ear.

  • **Both Valsalva and Politzer tests are outdated** and **rarely used clinically for assessment of Eustachian tube function.**

3. Eustachian tube catheterization:

- Nose is first anesthetized by topical spray of lignocaine and then a **eustachian tube catheter**, the tip of which is bent, is **passed along the floor of the nose till it reaches the nasopharynx**. Here it is rotated 90° medially and gradually on the posterior border of nasal septum.
- It is then rotated 180° laterally so that the tip lies against the tubal opening
- A politzer bag is now connected to the catheter and air is insufflated.
- **Entry of air into middle ear is verified by an auscultation tube**. The procedure of catheterization should be gentle as, it is known to cause complications (injury to eustachian tube, bleeding from nose).

4. Toynbee test:

- While the above three tests use a positive pressure, **Toynbee's maneuver causes negative pressure**.
- It is more physiological test.
- It is performed by asking the patient to swallow while nose has been pinched.
- This draws air into middle ear into the nasopharynx and **causes inward movement of tympanic membrane**, which is verified by the examiner otoscopically or with a microscope.

5. Tympanometry:

- In this test, **positive and negative pressures are created in the external ear canal** and the patient swallows repeatedly.
- **The ability of the tube to equilibrate positive and negative pressures to the ambient pressure indicates normal tubal function.**
- The test can be done both in patients with perforated or intact tympanic membrane.

Contd...

Eustachian Tube Function Tests

6. Radiological Test:
- A radio-opaque dye, e.g. hypaque or lipoidal instilled into the middle ear through a pre-existing perforation and X-rays taken should delineate the tube and any obstruction.
- **The time taken by the dye to reach the nasopharynx also indicates its clearance function.**

7. Saccharine or methylene blue test:
- Saccharine solution is placed into the middle ear through a pre-existing perforation. The time taken by it to reach the pharynx and impart a sweet test is also a measure of clearance function.
- Similarly, methylene blue dye can be instilled into the middle ear and the time taken by it to stain the pharyngeal secretions can be noted.
- **Indirect evidence of drainage/clearance function** is established when **ear-drops instilled into the ear with tympanic membrane perforation causes bad taste in the throat.**

8. Sonotubometry:
- A tone is presented to the nose and it's recording taken from the external canal.
- The tone is heard louder when the tube is patent.
- It also tells the duration for which the tube remains open.
- It is a **non-invasive technique** and provides **information on active tubal opening**.
- Accessory sounds produced in the nasopharynx during swallowing, may interfere with the test results.

---

174. Ans. b. Cidofovir *(Ref: Dhingra 7/e p346, 6/e p305)*

Topical treatment for recurrent respiratory papillomatosis includes cidofovir.

*"**Many antiviral drugs like cidofovir have been used to treat laryngeal papillomatosis**, but none completely stops the tumors from growing. Most antivirals are injected to control the frequency of tumor growth."*

See Q. No. 178 AIIMS May 2016.

175. Ans. c. Internal maxillary artery *(Ref: Dhingra 7/e p281-282, 5/261-263)*

***The** main vessel involved in bleeding from Juvenile nasopharyngeal angiofibroma is Internal maxillary artery.*

*"**Juvenile Nasopharyngeal Angiofibroma:** The **main feeding vessel** in most of the cases is **internal maxillary artery**, branch of external carotid artery."*

Juvenile Nasopharyngeal Angiofibroma

- **MC benign tumor of nasopharynx[Q]** (but overall angiofibroma is rare).
- **MC site: Posterior part of nasal cavity** close to the margin of sphenopalatine foramen.
- Seen almost **exclusively in males** of **10–20 years[Q]**
- **Testosterone dependent** tumor, seen in **pre-pubertal to adolescent males[Q]**
- **Locally invasive vasoformative** tumor consisting of **endothelium lined vessels** with **no muscle coat.**
- **Major blood supply:** From **internal maxillary artery[Q]**

Clinical Features:
- **MC symptom: Spontaneous profuse and recurrent epistaxis[Q].**
- **Progressive nasal obstruction**, denasal speech, hyposmia or anosmia, **broadening of nasal bridge[Q]**.
- **Otalgia, conductive hearing loss, serous otitis media** due to **eustachian tube obstruction[Q].**

> - **Tumor in the orbit** causes **proptosis** and **frog-face deformity[Q]**; diplopia and diminished vision.

- **Tumor in infratemporal fossa** can cause **trismus** and **bulge of parotid.**
- II, III, IV, V, VI cranial nerve can be involved.

1578 **AIIMS ESSENCE**

Contd...

Juvenile Nasopharyngeal Angiofibroma
• **Signs:** Splaying of nasal bones, **pink or purplish mass** obstructing one or both choanae in nasopharynx, **swelling of cheek** and fullness of face.
• In an **adolescent male, profuse recurrent episodes of nosebleed** suggests **juvenile nasopharyngeal angiofibroma** until proven otherwise[Q]

Diagnosis:
- **IOC: CT scan of head** with **contrast enhancement**

    • CT shows **extent, bony destruction** or **displacements** and **anterior bowing of the posterior wall of maxilla** due to tumor enlarging in pterygopalatine fossa
    • **Antral sign** or **Holman Miller sign**[Q]:
        – **Pathognomic of angiofibroma.**
        – **Anterior bowing of the posterior wall of maxilla** due to tumor enlarging in pterygopalatine fossa

- **MRI:** To view the **soft tissue extension** and is complementary to CT scan.
- **Carotid angiography:** Shows **extent of the tumor**, its **vascularity** and **feeding vessel**[Q]

    • Biopsy is **contraindicated in juvenile nasopharyngeal angiofibroma**[Q]

Treatment:
- **Surgical excision is treatment of choice**[Q].
- **Preoperative embolization and estrogen therapy** or **cryotherapy** or **radiotherapy reduce blood loss** in surgery.
- **Preoperative embolization of the tumour reduces its blood supply** and **causes less bleeding**, if tumour removal is performed within 24–48 hour of embolization before collaterals have time to develop.

Surgical approach for Nasopharyngeal Angiofibroma
• **Surgical approach of choice: Midfacial degloving approach** to nasopharynx.
• **Wilson approach**[Q]: **Transpalatal approach** is for **tumor confined to nasopharynx.**
• **Lateral rhinotomy: For larger tumors** involving nasal cavity, paranasal sinuses.
• Other Approaches:
– **Sardana's approach**[Q]: **Transpalatine + Sublabial**
– **Extended Denker's approach**[Q].

Recurrence:
- **Recurrence rate after surgery: 30-50%**
- Recurrences usually become evident **within 2–3 years of initial resection.**

SKIN

176. Ans. c. Lichen nitidus *(Ref: Mark Lebwohl 2/e p345; Fitzpatrick 6/e p2157)*

Grouped pinhead lesions on elbow, abdomen, penis and dorsum of hand in a child as shown in the picture is highly suggestive of lichen nitidus.

"Lichen scrofulosorum is an uncommon asymptomatic lichenoid eruption of minute papule occurring in children and adolescents with strongly positive tuberculin reaction. It mainly involves perifollicular distribution on abdomen, chest, back and proximal limbs. A hallmark is that superficial epitheloid dermal granuloma surround hair follicles and sweat ducts and may occupy several dermal papillae."

Lichen Nitidus
• Lesion and etiology are similar, but size is smaller 1.2 mm (**pinhead size**[Q])
• Occurs as **grouped lesions** on **elbow, abdomen, penis** and **dorsum of hand**[Q]
• Mucosal or nail changes are rare
• **Self-limiting, non-itchy**[Q]

Contd...

Contd...

Lichen Nitidus

Histopathology:
- Dense, **circumscribed** and distinctive **infiltrate** of **histio-lymphocytic cells** situated directly beneath **thinned epidermis** results in widening of papillary dermis with **elongation and the appearance of embracement by neighboring rete ridges (Ball in clutch appearance^Q)**.
- Thinned epidermis demonstrates **central parakeratosis^Q**, variable /focal hyper keratosis **without hypergranulosis**, minimal hydropic degeneration and few dyskeratotic cells

Treatment:
- Antihistaminics particularly **Astemazole^Q** is effective.

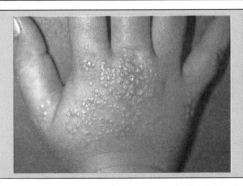 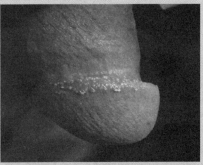

Lichen Scrofulosorum

- Lichen scrofulosorum is a **lichenoid eruption of minute papules^Q**
- Occurs in **children and adolescents with tuberculosis**.

Pathogenesis:
- Usually associated with **chronic tuberculous disease of the LNs and bones^Q**

Clinical Features:
- **Eruption is asymptomatic** and is **usually confined to the trunk^Q**.
- Lesions consist of **symptomless, small, firm, follicular or parafollicular papules** of a yellowish or pink color with **flat-top** or bear a minute horny spine or fine scales on their surface^Q.
- It mainly **involves perifollicular distribution on abdomen, chest, back and proximal limbs^Q**.

Histopathology:
- A hallmark is that **superficial epitheloid dermal granuloma surround hair follicles and sweat ducts** and may occupy several dermal papillae^Q.

Treatment:
- **Antituberculous therapy** results in **complete resolution** within a matter of weeks^Q.

Feature	Lichen Nitidus	Lichen planus
Symptoms	Asymptomatic	Itchy (marked)
Cutaneous lesion	• Multiple, discrete (or closely grouped), minute, pinpoint to pinhead sized^Q (1-2 mm), flat/ round or dome shaped papule with a glistening (shiny surface)^Q. • Papules are flesh colored or pink or shiny hypopigmented^Q (in blacks)	• Larger, plain (flat) topped, polygonal, pruritic, pink/purple (violaceous) papule^Q
Wickham's striae	Absent	Present^Q
Grouping	Present^Q	Usually not
Mucous membrane involvement	Uncommon	Common^Q (Variably present)

Contd...

Contd...

Site	• Most frequently on **flexural surfaces of upper extremities i.e. arm, forearm, wrist and dorsal surface of hands,** lower abdomen, breast, the **glans** and **shaft of penis** and other areas of **genital region**[Q]	• **Flexures** (wrist), **extremities** (shin), **lower back and genitals**[Q]

177. Ans. c. Post Kala Azar dermal leishmaniasis   *(Ref: Harrison 19/e p1391)*

A 26-year-old man from Bihar comes with juicy looking papules over face and back of neck, which were hypopigmented and normoaesthetic. History revealed an episode of prolonged fever in childhood. Diagnosis is Post Kala-Azar dermal Leishmaniasis.

*"Post Kala-Azar Dermal Leishmaniasis: On the **Indian subcontinent** and in **Sudan** and other **East African countries**, 2–50% of patients develop **skin lesions concurrent with or after the cure of visceral leishmaniasis.** Most common are **hypopigmented macules, papules,** and/or **nodules or diffuse infiltration of the skin** and sometimes of the oral mucosa."*
-Harrison 19/e p1391

Diagnosis of Post Kala-Azar Dermal Leishmaniasis (PKDL) is based on:

- **History of kala-azar** in the past (1-5 years ago) or **living in endemic area**.
- Presence of **"juicy" erythematous nodules on the central part of the face**[Q]
- **Hypopigmented macules** on the central part of the trunk.
- **No nerve involvement**

Post Kala-Azar Dermal Leishmaniasis (PKDL)
• **Endemic in Bihar (India), Sudan (Africa)**
• On the **Indian subcontinent** and in **Sudan** and other **East African countries**, 2–50% of patients develop **skin lesions concurrent with or after the cure of visceral leishmaniasis**[Q].
Characteristic Features:
• **Most common are hypopigmented macules, papules,** and/or **nodules or diffuse infiltration of the skin** and sometimes of the oral mucosa[Q].

Characterized by presence of three types of Skin Lesions
• **Erythematous juicy nodules on the central part (peri-orificial area) face**[Q]
• **Hypopigmented macules on the trunk**[Q]
• **Photosensitivity**[Q]

Diagnosis:

- In PKDL, **parasites are scanty in hypopigmented macules** but may be seen and **cultured more easily from nodular lesions**[Q].
- **Diagnosis is based on history and clinical findings,** but **rK39** and other serologic tests are positive in most cases[Q].

Demonstration of Organisms
• **Specimen taken using a tissue smear,** preferably a **nodule/plaque**[Q].
• **Stained with Giemsa stain or acridine orange**[Q]
• **Serology-Antibodies to RK 39**[Q]

Treatment:

- **Indian PKDL is treated with pentavalent antimonials for 60–120 days**[Q]
- Alternative: **Amphotericin-B**
- **Oral miltefosine for 12 weeks**[Q], in the usual daily doses, cures most patients with Indian PKDL.

> • In **East Africa**, a **majority of patients experience spontaneous healing.** In those with **persistent lesions**, the response to 60 days of treatment with a **pentavalent antimonial** is good.

178. Ans. c. Drugs *(Ref: Neena Khanna 4/e p83)*

The above picture shows forearm with extensive reddish bullae involving >30% body surface area and description are typical of the spectrum of Steven-Johnson syndrome and toxic epidermal necrolysis. Toxic epidermal necrolysis (TEN), also known as Lyell's syndrome, is a rare, life-threatening skin condition that is usually caused by a reaction to drugs.

See Q. No. 181 AIIMS November 2015.

AIIMS May 2015

179. Ans. b. Cyclosporine *(Ref: Roxburgh's 18/e p148-150; Harrison 19/e p348, 18/e p399; Fitzpatrick's 7/e p192, 959-960)*

The given picture shows multiple small pustules over the skin. This is a case of pustular psoriasis of pregnancy. Among the given drugs, only cyclosporine is used in pregnancy.

"Pustular Psoriasis of Pregnancy (Impetigo Herpetiformis): Systemic steroids are the mainstay of therapy during pregnancy. Cyclosporine may be used to treat cases refractory to high-dose systemic steroid."

Pustular Psoriasis of Pregnancy (Impetigo Herpetiformis)
• **Variant of pustular psoriasis** attributable to **hormonal changes in pregnancy.**

Clinical features
• Generally seen in **third trimester**
• Characterized by **erythematous patches** with margins studded with subcorneal pustules.
• **Eruption typically originates in flexural areas**, rash may be **pruritic or painful**[Q].
 	
      • Subungual lesions may result in **onycholysis.**
      • **Face, palms and soles** are **commonly spared**[Q].

Laboratory investigations: • **Leukocytosis with neutrophilia, raised ESR** • **Iron deficiency anemia, hypoalbuminemia**

Treatment:
• **Resolution after delivery is the norm.**
• However, given its consistently progressive course, **treatment is indicated to reduce the risk of fetal and maternal complications.**
 	
      • **Systemic steroids** are the **mainstay of therapy during pregnancy**[Q]
      • **Cyclosporine** may be used to treat cases refractory to high-dose systemic steroid

180. Ans. b. Acne rosacea *(Ref: Rooks 8/e p43.1-43.10; Fitzpatrick 7/e p704-708; Roxburgh 18/e p172-178; Harrison 19/e p352, 18/e p404, 444)*

The most likely diagnosis of this 25-year-old girl with erythematous papules on the face as seen in the picture with exacerbated of the lesions on excessive sweating, sun exposure and emotional disturbance is acne rosacea.

Acne rosacea
• It is characterized by **erythema of central face persisting for months or more**[Q]. • **Convex areas of nose, cheeks, chin** and **forehead are characteristically involved**, whereas **perioral and periorbital areas are spared**[Q]. • **Vascular abnormalities:** May be associated with an abnormal **vascular reactivity (exaggerated flushing response to heat, spicy food, alcohol and stress)** but no pharmacological defect has been found.
Epidemiology: • **Peak incidence:** 4th and 5th decades. • **Gender:** More frequent in **females**
Clinical Features: • **Factors, which trigger flushing:** Emotional stress, hot drinks, spicy foods, alcohol, and **withdrawal of steroids.**

Primary Features	Secondary Features
• **Intermittent flushing** followed by **more perma-nent telangiectasia, papules, pustules**[Q]	• Facial burning or stinging, edema, plaques, a dry appearance, peripheral flushing, and ocular manifestations

• The primary **differentiating feature** between acne vulgaris and rosacea **is presence of open and closed comedones in acne**[Q]. Both conditions may coexist, although **rosacea most often begins** and **reaches its peak incidence in the decades after acne declines.**

AIIMS ESSENCE

181. Ans. a. Nevus of ota   *(Ref: Neena Khanna 4/e p355)*

The given picture shows irregular bluish lesion in left superior conjunctiva in a female patient. Most probable diagnosis is Nevus of Ota.

Nevus of Ota
• **Nevus of Ota** is **more common in females**[Q,] Asian and African-American patients • **Present at birth** or **appears in infancy**.
Characteristic Features:
• **Macular pigmentation**: More prominent **slate grey hyperpigmentation** due to dermal melanocytes and **brownish epidermal pigmentation**. • **Distribution along the maxillary division of the trigeminal nerve**. • **Pigmentation of sclera** (slate gray) and **conjunctiva** (brown) often present • Patchy involvement of the conjunctiva, hard palate, pharynx, nasal mucosa, buccal mucosa, or tympanic membrane occurs in some patients.
Diagnosis:
• **Nevus of Ota** differs from a more common dermal melanocytosis patch, not only by its **distribution** but also by having a **speckled** rather than a uniform **appearance**. • Nevus of Ota also has a **greater concentration of elongated, dendritic dermal melanocytes located in the upper** rather than the lower **portion of the dermis**.
Treatment:
• **Laser therapy** may effectively decrease the pigmentation but can be unpredictable.

Nevus of Ito	• It is localized to the **supraclavicular, scapular** and **deltoid regions**. • **More diffuse in its distribution** and less mottled than nevus of Ota. • It is also a **form of mid-dermal melanocytosis**[Q] • The only available treatments are **masking with cosmetics and laser therapy**[Q]	
Mongolian spots	• Seen commonly in **Mongoloid**[Q] and **Negroid infants** • Bluish ill-defined macules • **Seen in lumbosacral**[Q] **region** • **Regress by 4 years**[Q] **of age**	
Becker's Nevus	• **More common in men**[Q] • **Begins shortly before, at or after puberty**[Q] • Appears as a **hyperpigmented patch**, which has a **characteristic splashed appearance**. Over period of time, coarse dark hairs appear on the lesion and sometimes skin texture is altered. • Seen over chest and shoulders, becomes thickened and often hairy	

AIIMS May 2015

1583

182. Ans. d. BB *(Ref: Rooks 7/e p29.1-29.19, Fitzpatrick 6/e p1962-1969)*

Inverted saucer-shaped lesions are characteristic feature of borderline leprosy.

"Often a single lesion is present surrounded by several smaller ones. Skin and nerves are the only directly affected tissues in BL (Borderline Lepromatous). The skin lesions consist of erythematous macules or plaques. Inverted saucer-shaped annular lesions are characteristic."

See Q. No. 186 AIIMS May 2016.

183. Ans. b. Segmental vitiligo *(Ref: Fitzpatrick 7/e p624-625, Rooks 8/e p58.39-58.51; Harrison 19/e p357-359, 18/e p409-412)*

A lady came with unilateral white skin lesions with leukotrichia as shown in the picture. Most likely diagnosis is segmental vitiligo.

Segmental Vitiligo:

- **Occurs along a nerve segment**
- **Common on face** along the branches of **trigeminal nerve**[Q]
- **Stable course**, i.e., lesions increase initially (6-12 months) and then remain static.
- **Leukotrichia** on the depigmented areas as well as away from vitiliginous areas frequently seen. **Margins are feathery**.

Piebaldism	<ul><li>Rare autosomal dominant condition</li><li>Present at birth, usually remain unchanged throughout life</li><li>Characterized by stable areas of vitiligo-like amelanotic skin associated with a white forelock[Q]</li><li>Most common is frontal median or paramedian patch, associated with a mesh of white hair (white forelock)[Q]</li><li>Often white patches occur on the upper chest, abdomen and limbs bilaterally, but not necessarily symmetrically[Q]</li></ul>

Waardenburg syndrome	<ul><li>Autosomal dominant</li><li>Characterized by:
	  – Sensorineural hearing loss[Q]
	  – Pigment abnormalities (heterochromia iridis, white forelock, patchy skin depigmentation)[Q]
	  – Craniofacial abnormalities (synophrys, flat nasal root)</li></ul>

See Q. No. 177 AIIMS November 2015.

184. Ans. b. Bullous pemphigoid *(Ref: Fitzpatrick 7/e p432-441; Rooks 8/e p40.27, 13.19, 10.12-10.28)*

The most likely diagnosis in this patient with tens blisters on normal looking skin associated urticarial plaques as seen in the figure are bullous pemphigoid.

Immunologically Mediated Blistering Disease				
Disease	**Pemphigus vulgaris**	**Bullous Pemphigoid**	**Linear IgA Disease**	**Dermatitis Herpetiformis**
Auto antigen	Desmoglein 3[Q]	BP230 > BP180	BPAG 2	Epidermal and tissue transglutaminase
Histology	Epidermal **Acantholytic** blister in **suprabasal spinous cell layer**	**Subepidermal** blister with **eosinophil rich infiltrate**[Q] in perivascular and vesicular sites.	**Subepidermal** blister with **neutrophils in dermal papillae**[Q]	**Subepidermal blister with neutrophils in Dermal papillae**[Q]
Direct Immuno-fluorescence Microscopy	Cells surface **deposits of IgG on keratinocytes in fishnet pattern**	**Linear band of IgG** and/or C3 in epidermal **BMZ**	**Linear band of IgA, in epidermal BMZ**	**Granular deposits of IgA in dermal papillae**[Q]
Associations	**HLA-DR4 and DRW6**[Q]	HLA-DQ β1 * 0301	– HLA-B8 (+) – TNF2 allele	**Subclinical gluten sensitive enteropathy (100%)** HLA-B8 (60%)/ DRW3 (95%) and HLA-DQW2 haplotype (95-100%)

Contd...

Contd...

Disease	Pemphigus vulgaris	Bullous Pemphigoid	Linear IgA Disease	Dermatitis Herpetiformis
Clinical features	Flaccid blisters, denuded skin, oro-mucosal lesions[Q]	Large tense blisters on flexor surfaces and trunk[Q]	Pruritic small papules on extensor surfaces occasionally larger, acneiform blisters in adults	Extremely pruritic small vesicles on elbows, knees, buttocks and posterior neck[Q]

Pemphigoid

- **Large, tense blisters on flexor surface** located over **lower part of body**[Q] (limbs >trunk)
- **Non-itchy** and **painless**[Q]
- Mainly seen in patients **over 60 years**[Q]
- **Mucosa** is **not involved**[Q]

Pathology:

- **Subepidermal blisters without acantholysis**[Q]
- Subepidermal collection of **IgG, C3-complement**, eosinophils, polymorphs[Q]

Diagnosis:

- **Direct immunofluorescence: Linear band of IgG** and/or **C3 in** epidermal basement membrane zone[Q]

Treatment:

- Systemic steroids, immunosuppressants

---

185. Ans. b. Varicella zoster *(Ref: Fitzpatrick 7/e p490-493, 1873-1898; Rooks 8/e p33.14-33.22; Roxburgh 18/52-54)*

Vesicles on shin and giant cell on Tzanck smear suggest the diagnosis of Herpes Zoster.

Tzanck Smear

- **Cytological examination of skin blisters**
- After rupturing roof of the blister, the floor is scraped with a surgical blade and material is transferred on to a microscopic slide and fixed.
- **Slides are stained with Giemsa stain, Wright's stain** or **toluidine blue** and examined under the microscope.

Disorder	Finding
Pemphigus	Acantholytic cells[Q]
Bullous pemphigoid	Predominantly **eosinophil**[Q]
Chronic bullous disease of childhood	Predominantly **neutrophils**[Q]
Varicella zoster	**Multinucleated giant cells**[Q]
Herpes simplex infection	**Multinucleated giant cells**[Q]
Toxic epidermal necrolysis	Necrotic cells

Herpes Zoster

- Caused by **Varicella Zoster (chicken pox) virus**[Q], one attack gives life long immunity
- **Thoracic nerves (intercostal nerves)**[Q], **ophthalmic division of trigeminal nerve** and other **spinal nerves** are **most commonly affected**[Q]

Pathology:

- **Ballooning** is **characteristic**[Q]
- **Tzanck smear: Multinucleated giant cells**[Q]

Clinical Features:

- Prodrome of segmental **pain** begins **1-4 days before the eruption**[Q], erythema and edema is rapidly followed by appearance of **grouped vesicles unilateral and in a segmental distribution (MC thoracic dermatome)**[Q], mucous membrane within the affected dermatome may be involved
- Unilateral vesicular eruption within a dermatome associated with severe pain
- The dermatome from T3 to L3 are most frequently involve

Contd...

Contd...

Herpes Zoster
Complications:
• **Post-herpetic neuralgia**[Q] (persistent neuralgic pain)
• Corneal ulcer and scarring (zoster of ophthalmic division of trigeminal nerve), eye involvement is indicated when **vesicles are present on the side of nose- Hutchinson's sign**[Q]
Variants:
A.Ramsay Hunt Syndrome: H. zoster involving sensory branch of **facial nerve**[Q]
B.Zoster opthalmicus: H. zoster involving ophthalmic division of **trigeminal nerve.**[Q]

ANAESTHESIA

186.   r . **a. Ramifentanyl, midazolam, propofol** *(Ref: Miller's 8/e p726; Lee 13/e p158-160; Morgan 3/e p173, 884)*

Drug combination, which can be used for day care surgery are ramifentanyl, midazolam and propofol.

"Any induction agents used in day-case anesthesia should ensure a smooth induction, good immediate recovery and a rapid return to street fitness. Propofol is now used widely as the primary induction agent, which has advantage of rapid recovery and low incidence of post-operative nausea and vomiting."

Preferable agents in Day Care Anaesthesia
• **Mivacurium**[Q] (muscle relaxant of choice, shortest duration of action)
• **Succinylcholine**[Q] (for Ultra short period of profound **muscle relaxation; Disadvantage: Post-operative myalgia**)
• **Isoflurane**[Q] (volatile inhalational agent)
• **Alfentanyl**[Q]
• **Propofol**[Q] (inducing agent of choice)
• **Midazolam**[Q] (for initial anaxiolysis and sedation)
• Mnemonic: **Manmohan Singh Is A Prime Minister**

Anesthetic Agent of Choice	
• **Day care**	**Propofol**[Q]
• **Ischemic heart disease**	**Etomidate**[Q]
• **Congenital heart disease (left to right shunt): ASD, VSD, PDA**	**Sevoflurane**[Q]
• **Congenital heart disease (right to left shunt)** • **Congestive heart failure** • **Shock** • **Asthma and COPD**	**Ketamine**[Q]
• **For producing deliberate hypotension** • **Cardiac surgery** • **Neurosurgery**	**Isoflurane**[Q]
• **Epilepsy** • **Thyrotoxicosis**	**Thiopentone**[Q]
• **For electroconvulsive therapy**	**Methohexitone**[Q]

187. **Ans. b. Propofol** *(Ref: Miller 6/e p318-320; Morgan 4/e p200-202; Lee 13/e p158-160)*

Propofol causes pain on IV administration.

*"**Propofol** is **oil-based** preparation containing **soyabean oil, egg lecithin** and **glycerol**. As it **contains oil** so **injection is painful** and should be **preceded or mixed with lignocaine.**"*

Contd...

Propofol
• Consists of a phenol ring with isopropyl group attached (**2, 6 di-isopropylphenol**[Q]).
• Available as **milky white** solution in **1%** and **2%** concentration.
• It is **oil-based** preparation containing **soyabean oil, egg lecithin** and **glycerol**[Q].

• As it **contains oil** so **injection is painful** and should be **preceded or mixed with lignocaine.**
     • **Fospropofol** is a **water based preparation** approved for use but not widely available.
     • It is **mandatory to use propofol within 6 hours after opening the vial** (As **egg** is a **good media for bacterial growth** and it **does not have preservative** therefore **once opened**, there are **chances of bacterial contamination**)

Mechanism of Action:

- Similar to thiopentone (action is mediated **through GABA-A subtype**)

Anaesthetic Properties

- **Induction** is achieved in one arm brain circulation time i.e., **15 seconds.**
- **Consciousness** is regained **after 2-8 minutes due to redistribution**[Q].
- **Elimination half-life: 2-4 hours; Rapid recovery**[Q]
- **No antanalgesic property; Not a muscle relaxant**[Q]

Dose: 2 mg/kg

Metabolism

- **Mainly metabolized in liver** but significant **30% extrahepatic metabolism** also occurs in **lungs** and **excreted via kidneys**[Q].
- **Clearance rate is 10 times more rapid than thiopentone** so recovery is rapid.
- **All metabolic products** of propofol are **inactive.**

Systemic Effects of Propofol	
CVS	• **Myocardial depression**[Q] • Systemic vascular resistance is reduced **without compensatory tachycardia**[Q]. • **Hypotension** produced is significant
Respiratory system	• **Incidence of apnea is higher** (25-30%) than thiopentone. • **Respiratory depression** is more severe and prolonged than thiopentone • Induces **bronchodilatation in COPD patients**[Q]. • **Depression of upper airway reflexes** is more than thiopentone and therefore **most preferred for surgeries done under laryngeal mask airway without muscle relaxants**[Q].
CNS	• Effective like thiopentone for **brain protection**. It is **reliable amnestic**. • It is **not an anticonvulsant** rather it can produce **muscle twitching** and **myoclonic activity**[Q].
Eye	• **Reduces IOP**[Q]
GIT	• **Antipruritic**[Q]

Uses of Propofol:

- **IV agent of choice for day care surgery** (Because of **early induction, rapid and smooth recovery, inactive metabolites** and **antiemetic effects**)[Q]
- **Agent of choice for total intravenous anaesthesia** (TIVA) along with opioids (**alfentanil** or **remifentanil**)[Q]
- **Propofol infusion** is used to **produce sedation in ICU**[Q].
- **Agent of choice for induction** in susceptible individuals for **malignant hyperthermia**[Q].
- **Most preferred for surgeries associated with high incidence of nausea and vomiting** like **laparoscopic** or **middle ear surgeries** because of it's **antiemetic property**[Q]

Contd...

Contd...

Propofol	
Disadvantages of Propofol	**Contraindications of Propofol**
1. **Apnea is more profound** and **longer**[Q] 2. **Hypotension** is **more severe**[Q] 3. **Injection is painful**[Q] 4. **Solution** is **less stable (6 hours)**[Q] 5. **Chances of sepsis with contaminated solution** are high[Q] 6. **Myoclonic activity** can be produced. 7. Sexual fantasies and hallucinations are additional side effects. 8. **Increased chances of aspiration in high risk cases**[Q] (Because of **maximum inhibition of airway reflexes**)	1. **Increased chances of aspiration** it is **contra-indicated throughout the pregnancy** (except abortion) including cesarean section. 2. **Avoid propofol during breast feeding** 3. **Children <3 years** 4. Patients at **high risk of aspiration** like **full stomach** patients.
Propofol infusion syndrome	**Egg allergy is not a contraindication**
• **Rare but lethal** complication • Seen if **propofol infusion** is **continued for >48 hours**[Q] • Common in **children** • Occurs because of **failure of free fatty acid metabolism** caused by propofol. • **Associated with severe metabolic acidosis**, acute cardiac failure, cardiomyopathy, skeletal myopathy, hyperkalemia lipemia and hepatomegaly.	• **Egg allergy** is almost always **from egg white (albumin) not from lecithin** (which is prepared from yoke)[Q] • **History of egg allergy is not a contraindication for propofol**[Q].

188. Ans. d. Dexmedetomidine *(Ref: KDT 7/e p384; Katzung 13/e p145, 12/e p445)*

This patient is having bradycardia and hypotension. Dexmedetomidine *is contraindicated in* hypovolemia, hypotension, heart block *and* congestive heart failure.

*"Side effects of dexmedetomidine are similar to those with clonidine (**hypotension, bradycardia and dry mouth**). Contraindications to the use of Dexmedetomidine include **hypovolemia, hypotension, heart block** and **congestive heart failure** prior to administration."*

Fentanyl	• **Decreases heart rate** but **fall in BP is slight**
Etomidate	• **Most cardiovascular stable agent** among all IV inducing agents
Ketamine	• **Increases oxygen demand, heart rate, cardiac output and BP** • **Avoided** in patients with **ischemic heart disease or vascular aneurysm** • **IV inducing agent of choice for shock**

Dexmedetomidine
• **Dexmedetomidine** is a **centrally active selective alpha-2 agonist** with **strong sedative properties**[Q]   • **Introduced for sedating critically ill/ventilated patients in intensive care units.** It is **also being used as an adjunct to anaesthesia**[Q].   • **Analgesia and sedation** are produced with **little respiratory depression**.   • Sympathetic response to stress and noxious stimulus is blunted.
Pharmacokinetics: • Administered by **IV infusion; Half-life: 2–3 hours**   • **Metabolized in the liver and excreted,** mainly as metabolites, **in the urine.**
Properties: • **Sedation, hypnosis;** at high doses **anxiolysis, sympatholysis and analgesia**
Side effects: • **Side effects** are similar to those with clonidine (**hypotension, bradycardia and dry mouth**).

Contd...

Contd...

Dexmedetomidine
Uses:
• As premedication **(anxiolysis)** • Adjuvant to reduce the dose of analgesics **(Analgesic property)** • Adjuvant to reduce the dose of IV and inhalational anesthetics **(Sedative property)** • **To attenuate cardiovascular response to intubation (it causes hypotension and bradycardia)**
Contraindications:
• **Hypovolemia, hypotension, heart block** and **congestive heart failure**

189. **Ans. a. Atracurium** *(Ref: Goodman Gilman 12/e p264; Morgan 4/e p221; Lee 13/e p191,192)*

Muscle relaxant that can be used in a patient with high serum bilirubin of 6.0 and serum creatinine of 4.5 mg/dL is Atracurium because of unique metabolism independent of hepatic and renal functions and ensured degradation.

See Q. No. 188 AIIMS May 2016.

RADIOLOGY

190. **Ans. a. FDG-18 PET CT** *(Ref: Harrison 19/e p270 e4, 18/e p1846)*

Best noninvasive investigation to check for viability of myocardium is FDG-18 PET CT.

*"Viable myocardium is myocardium which due to ischemia does not contract normally at rest but **has the potential to recover its function, either by itself over time or after revascularization**. PET is generally regarded as the gold standard for the assessment of myocardium viability. PET identifies ischemic or hibernating myocardium in 10-20% of the regions that would be classified as fibrotic or infracted by thallium and technetium labelled compounds."*

*"For the **evaluation of myocardial viability** in patients with ischemic cardiomyopathy, **myocardial perfusion imaging (with SPECT or PET) is usually combined with metabolic imaging** (i.e., fluorodeoxyglucose [FDG] PET). In hospital settings lacking access to PET scanning, thallium-201 SPECT imaging is an excellent alternative."-Harrison 19/e p270 e4*

*"PET has traditionally been regarded as the **gold standard technique for the assessment of myocardial viability**. The positron-emitting tracer F-18 fluorodeoxyglucose (FDG) assesses myocardial glucose metabolism and is an indicator of myocardial viability. Because uptake is heterogeneous in normal myocardium in the fasting state, **oral glucose loading or a combination of insulin and glucose infusions is used to enhance myocardial uptake**. With reduced myocardial blood flow and ischemia, substrate utilization switches from fatty acids and lactate toward glucose, leading to enhanced myocardial FDG uptake. This pattern of **enhanced FDG uptake in regions of decreased perfusion** (termed flow/ metabolism "mismatch") **identifies areas of ischemic or hibernating myocardium** that are **likely to improve in function after revascularization**."*

Radiopharmaceutical	Imaging Technique	Physical Half-Life	Application
Technetium-99m sestamibi	**SPECT**	6 hour	Myocardial perfusion imaging
Technetium-99m tetrofosmin	**SPECT**	6 hour	Myocardial perfusion imaging
Thalium-201	**SPECT**	72 hour	Myocardial perfusion imaging
Iodine-123 metaiodobenzylguanidine (MIBG)	**SPECT**	13 hour	**Cardiac sympathetic innervation[Q]**
Rubidium-82	**PET**	76 seconds	Myocardial perfusion imaging
13N-ammonia	**PET**	10 minutes	Myocardial perfusion imaging
18F-fluorodeoxyglucose	**PET**	110 minutes	**Myocardial viability and inflammation imaging[Q]**

*"For the **evaluation of myocardial viability** in patients with ischemic cardiomyopathy, **myocardial perfusion imaging (with SPECT or PET)** is usually combined with metabolic imaging (i.e., fluorodeoxyglucose [FDG] PET). In hospital settings lacking access to PET scanning, thallium-201 SPECT imaging is an excellent alternative."* -Harrison 19/e p270 e4

191. **Ans. d. Plain radiograph**   *(Ref: Hurst's The Heart 13/e p1050)*

    Best method to know the position and integrity of ICD is plain radiograph.

    *"**ICD Insertion Procedure:** The procedure takes about 30 to 60 minutes to complete. A chest x-ray is performed after the procedure to be sure the leads are in the proper position."*

    *"**Lead dislodgement** may be **radiographically visible** or it may be a **microdislodgement**, where there is **no radiographic change** in **position**, but there is significant increase in pacing threshold and/or decline in electrogram amplitude."*
    -Hurst's The Heart 13/e p1050

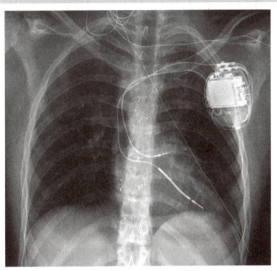

ICD Insertion Procedure

- An ICD is inserted after the person is given a sedative and a local anesthetic is injected into the skin.
- The surgery involves making an **incision below one of the collarbones**.
- The leads will be placed into the heart through the vein that runs next to the collarbone.
- **Up to two leads** will be **placed inside the heart**. **One lead** will be placed **in the ventricle** and **one may be placed in the atrium**, on the **right side of heart**.
- During the operation, **routine electrical measurements of the heart** will be made **to be sure that the leads are positioned correctly**.
- After the leads are in place, they are **connected to the ICD**. The **device** will be **placed under the skin in the upper chest**.
- The clinician may trigger the heart to beat rapidly, and then use the ICD to deliver a shock to the heart and stop the rapid beating; this is usually done one to five times to make sure the ICD functions properly.

> - The procedure takes about 30 to 60 minutes to complete. A chest X-ray is performed after the procedure to be sure the leads are in the proper position[Q].

192. **Ans. b. Intradural extramedullary tumor**   *(Ref: Sutton 6/e p254; Neurology in Clinical Practice 4/e Vol I p579)*

    Expansion of the contrast filled space in myelography is seen in intradural extramedullary tumor.

    *"The **expansion of contrast filled space**, i.e. **the subarachnoid space**, is seen in any intramedullary extradural lesion like meningioma. Sometimes a filling defect causing a meniscus sign may also be demonstrable."*

Findings in Intradural Extramedullary Spinal Tumors	Findings in Spinal Dysraphism
• Deviation of the spinal cord away from mass[Q] • Ipsilateral subarachnoid space enlargement[Q] • Contralateral subarachnoid space effacement • Intradural filling defect **outlined by sharp meniscus of contrast** (**Meniscus sign**) • The subarachnoid space is blocked and **CSF above the block remains unopacified**.	• **Contrast filling** and **associated meningocele** in addition to **dural ectasia** and **low-lying conus**. • **Tethered spinal cord** to be posteriorly located, sometimes tenting the dorsal thecal sac. • **Filum is thickened** with **lack of cord movement** in various positions.

Classification of spinal lesions

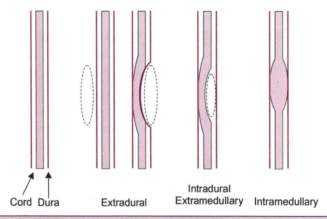

Cord Dura   Extradural   Intradural Extramedullary   Intramedullary

Myelography

- Myelography is the **radiographic investigation of the spinal canal for the diagnosis of space occupying** and **obstructive lesion**.
- It requires **contrast agent** to be **injected into subarachnoid space**.
- **MRI has replaced myelography**, because it is invasive and less informative[Q].

Intraspinal Masses

- Spinal cord has a covering called duramater. The space between dura and spinal cord is called subarachnoid space.

Intramedullary Mass (Within spinal cord)	Extramedullary Mass (Outside spinal cord)	
	Intradural (In subarachnoid space)	**Extradural** (Outside dura)
• **Ependymoma**[Q] • **Astrocytoma**[Q] • Teratoma • Infarct • Hematoma	• **Meningioma**[Q] • **Metastases**[Q] • Subdural empyema	• Prolapsed intervertebral disc • **Metastases, myeloma**[Q] • **Neurofibroma**[Q] • **Neuroblastoma**[Q] • Ganglioneuroma, lymphoma • Hematoma, abscess • Arachnoid cyst

Levels of Block in Myelography

Site	Typical Appearance
Extradural block	• Feathered appearance[Q]
Intradural Extramedullary block	• Meniscus sign[Q] • Widening of ipsilateral subarachnoid space[Q]
Intramedullary block	• Widening of the cord[Q] • Trouser leg appearance[Q]

AIIMS May 2015

PSYCHIATRY

193. Ans. a. Akathisia *(Ref: Kaplan and Sadock 11/e p329, 871; Niraj Ahuja 7/e p59)*

Akathisia is not a part of catatonia.

*"Akathisia is characterized by a **subjective and objective sense of restlessness, anxiety, and agitation**. Although a trial of anticholinergics for the treatment of neuroleptic-induced acute akathisia is reasonable, these drugs are not generally considered as effective as the **β-adrenergic receptor antagonists, the benzodiazepines, and clonidine.**"-Kaplan and Sadock 11/e p871*

Ambitendency is an example of negativism. It can be considered as a form of ambivalence. Ambivalence is a sign of Schizophrenia.

Catatonia
• Catatonia is a clinical syndrome characterized by **striking behavioral abnormalities** that may include **motoric immobility or excitement**, **profound negativism**, or **echolalia** (mimicry of speech) or **echopraxia** (mimicry of movement).   • **MC cause of catatonia** is **schizophrenia**[Q].
Epidemiology:
• Uncommon condition **mostly seen in advanced primary mood** or **psychotic illnesses**.   • Among inpatients with catatonia, **25-50% are related to mood disorders** (e.g., major depressive episode, recurrent, with catatonic features), and **10%** are associated with **schizophrenia.**
Etiology:
• **Medical conditions: Neurological disorders** (e.g., nonconvulsive status epilepticus and head trauma), **infections** (e.g., encephalitis), and **metabolic disturbances** (e.g., hepatic encephalopathy, hyponatremia and hypercalcemia).   • **Medications: Corticosteroids, immunosuppressants and antipsychotics**
<table><tr><td>**According to DSM-5, Catatonia associated with Another Mental Disorder is diagnosed if the clinical picture is dominated by at least three of the following:** 1. **Catalepsy** (i.e., passive induction of a posture held against gravity) 2. **Waxy flexibility** (i.e., slight and even resistance to positioning by examiner) 3. **Stupor** (no psychomotor activity; not actively relating to environment) 4. **Agitation**, not influenced by external stimuli 5. **Mutism** (i.e., no, or very little, verbal response (Note: not applicable if there is an established aphasia) 6. **Negativism** (i.e., opposing or not responding to instructions or external stimuli) 7. **Posturing** (i.e., spontaneous and active maintenance of a posture against gravity) 8. **Mannerisms** (i.e., odd caricature of normal actions) 9. **Stereotypies** (i.e., repetitive, abnormally frequent, non-goal movements) 10. **Grimacing** 11. **Echolalia** (i.e., mimicking another's speech) 12. **Echopraxia** (i.e., mimicking another's movements)</td></tr></table>
Treatment:
• **Primary treatment modality**: Identify and correct the underlying medical or pharmacological cause.   • **Benzodiazepines** can provide **temporary improvement in symptoms**   • **ECT is appropriate for catatonia due to a general medical condition**, especially if the **catatonia is life threatening** (e.g., inability to eat) or has developed into **lethal (malignant) catatonia.**

Schizophrenia
• **Dementia praecox** was coined by **Emil Kraepelin**[Q].   • **Schizophrenia** was coined by Eugen **Bleuler**[Q].

Schizophrenia	
Schneider's first rank symptoms	**Bleuler's "4A"**

1. Hallucinations
    a. Audible thoughts
    b. Voices heard arguing
    c. **Voices commenting on ones action**[Q]
 2. **Delusional perception**
	1. **Ambivalence**[Q] (confusion)
	 2. **Autism**[Q] (withdrawal into self)
	 3. **Affect disturbances**[Q]
	 4. **Association disturbance**[Q]

Contd...

Contd...

Schneider's first rank symptoms	Bleuler's "4A"

3. **Thought alienation phenomenon**
   a. Thought withdrawal
   b. Thought insertion
   c. Thought diffusion/broadcasting
 4. **Passivity phenomenon**
   a. **Made feeling (affect)[Q]**
   b. Made impulses
   c. Made volition or acts
   d. **Somatic passivity**	

Schizophrenia	
Type	**Feature**
1. Catatonic	• **Best prognosis**, late onset • **Mutism, rigidity, waxy flexibility, negativism, echolalia, echopraxia,** mannerism, grimacing, automatic obedience, ambitendency, verbigeration, Lethal **catatonia** or Pernicious catatonia
2. Paranoid	• **Most common** type • **Later age of onset, better prognosis than others** • Characterized by **presence of delusions and hallucinations of persecution, reference, grandeur, control or infidelity.** • **Personality is well reserved** • **Amphetamine** causes similar syndrome
3. Simple	• **Worst prognosis** • **Most difficult diagnosis**
4. Ptropf	• **Schizophrenia in presence of mental retardation**
5. Hebephrenic	• **Early onset and bad prognosis** • Senseless giggling and mirror gazing
6. Undifferentiated	

- The delusions included in 1st rank symptoms of schizophrenia are **primary delusions[Q]** also known as **autoconthous delusions[Q]**. These are **characteristic of schizophrenia.**

194. **Ans. a. Obsessive compulsive disorder** *(Ref: Kaplan and Sadock 11/e p390; Niraj Ahuja 7/e p90)*

Pathological doubts (feeling of uncertainty) and excessive sense or responsibility are both symptoms of OCD. (See explanation of question number 200)

Generalized Anxiety disorder
• **Characterized by a pattern of frequent, persistent worry and anxiety** that is **out of proportion to the impact of the event or circumstance** that is the focus of the worry.
Clinical Features:
• **Essential characteristics** are **sustained and excessive anxiety** and **worry accompanied by either motor tension or restlessness[Q].**   • The **anxiety is excessive** and **interferes with other aspects of a person's life.** This pattern must occur more days than not for at least 3 months.   • **Motor tension** is most commonly manifested as **shakiness, restlessness and headaches[Q].**
Treatment:
• **Most effective treatment** is probably one that **combines psychotherapeutic, pharmacotherapeutic and supportive approaches.**   • Major psychotherapeutic approaches are **cognitive-behavioral, supportive, and insight oriented.**

AIIMS May 2015

195. Ans. a. Self-exemption *(Ref: http://www.ncbi.nlm.nih.gov/pubmed/10170434; Kaplan and Sadock 11/e p590)*

There are many psychological barriers that need to be overcome in order to successfully quit smoking. Self-exempting belief is one of them.

"Self-exempting beliefs: A large majority of smokers have the belief that 'it will never happen to me'. For example, someone who runs everyday and doesn't drink alcohol may think that they have less chances of developing lung cancer than the next smoker because their lifestyle 'balances out' the cigarettes. This is not true. Every smoker has the same risk of negative health outcomes associated with smoking as the next smoker."

Prochaska and DiClemente's Stages of Change Model		
Stage of Change	**Characteristics**	**Techniques**
Precontemplation	**Not currently considering change:** "Ignorance is bliss"	• Validate lack of readiness Clarify: decision is theirs • Encourage re-evaluation of current behavior • Encourage self-exploration, not action • Explain and personalize the risk
Contemplation	**Ambivalent about change:** "Sitting on the fence" Not considering change within the next month	• Validate lack of readiness • Clarify: decision is theirs • Encourage evaluation of pros and cons of behavior change • Identify and promote new, positive outcome expectations
Preparation	**Some experience with change and are trying to change:** "Testing the waters" Planning to act within 1 month	• Identify and assist in problem solving re: obstacles • Help patient identify social support • Verify that patient has underlying skills for behavior change • Encourage small initial steps
Action	**Practicing new behavior for 3-6 months**	• Focus on restructuring cues and social support • Bolster self-efficacy for dealing with obstacles • Combat feelings of loss and reiterate long-term benefits
Maintenance	**Continued commitment to sustaining new behavior** Post-6 months to 5 years	• Plan for follow-up support • Reinforce internal rewards • Discuss coping with relapse
Relapse	**Resumption of old behaviors:** "Fall from grace"	• Evaluate trigger for relapse

196. Ans. c. *(Ref: Niraj Ahuja 7/e p113)*

A person with histrionic, shy, anxious avoidant personality comes under cluster C.

Cluster	Disorders
Cluster A (Odd and eccentric)	• Paranoid PD • Schizoid PD • Schizotypal PD
Cluster B (Dramatic, emotional and erratic)	• Antisocial PD • **Histrionic PD** • Narcissistic PD • Borderline PD
Cluster C (Anxious and fearful)	• **Anxious (avoidant) PD** • Dependent PD • Anankastic (Obsessive and compulsive) PD

197. Ans. a. Resperidone *(Ref: Kaplan and Sadock 11/e p1091; Niraj Ahuja 7/e p168)*

The given clinical scenario suggests motor and vocal tics associated with Tourette's disorder. Antipsychotics (haloperidol, resperidone) are used in this condition.

Tic Disorders
• In **DSM-IV-TR**, a **tic** is defined as a **sudden, rapid, recurrent, non-rhythmic, stereotyped motor movement** or **vocalization** that is experienced as **irresistible**, but **can be suppressed** for varying lengths of time. • **Usually markedly diminished during sleep.**

Contd...

AIIMS ESSENCE

Contd...

Tic Disorders		
Types of Tic Disorders		
Tourette's disorder	**Chronic motor or vocal tic disorder**	**Transient tic disorder**
• Characterized by **multiple motor** and **one or more vocal tics** that have been present at some time in the illness, although not necessarily concurrently. • **Ticks occur many times a day** nearly every day for **>1 year** with **no more 3 consecutive tic-free months.**	• Chronic motor or vocal tic disorder is similar, but each does not include both kinds of tics.	• Transient tic disorder involves motor and/or vocal tics that have been present for at least 2 weeks, but less than 1 year.

Treatment:

• **Pharmacotherapy is the treatment of choice**
• **Behavior therapy** maybe **used as an adjunct**.

> • **Drug of Choice for tic disorder: Haloperidol**[Q]
> • Other useful drugs: **Resperidone, Olanzapine, Aripiprazole** etc[Q].

• **SSRIs** like **fluoxetine** for co-morbid **obsessive-compulsive symptoms**.
• **Methylphenidate** and **Imipramine** are used in **ADHD** (attention Deficit hyperactivity disorder), usually seen in children

198. **Ans. c. Promethazine**   *(Ref: Harrison 19/e p2624, 18/e p3544; Katzung 13/e p500-501, 12/e p495)*

Rigidity and inability to move eyes after haloperidol use in a patient of Schizophrenia is highly suggestive of acute muscular dystonia. Treatment with IM anticholinergic (benztropine) or IV/IM antihistaminic (diphenhydramine hydrochloride)[Q] almost always relieves the symptoms. Promethazine, 25-50 mg IV or IM, has been used less frequently but readily available.

Acute Muscular Dystonia:

• **Bizarre muscle spasms, mostly involving linguo-facial muscles-grimacing, torticollis, locked jaw**[Q]
• Occurs **within few hours of single dose** or at the **most in the first week of therapy**[Q]
• **More common in children below 10 years and in girls, particularly after parenteral administration**[Q]
• **Treatment: Central anticholinergic**[Q]**, promethazine**[Q] **or hydroxyzine**

Neuroleptic Induced Acute Dystonia
• About 10% of all patients experience **dystonia as an adverse effect of dopamine receptor antagonist**, usually **in the first few hours or days of treatment**[Q] **(early onset during the course of treatment with neuroleptics).**
• **Most common in young men** (< 40 years old) • **Most common with high doses of high potency dopamine receptor antagonist**[Q] especially via IM route (haloperidol is high potency drug and 20 mg/day is high dose)**, shortly after starting the drug or increasing its dose**[Q].
• It results from **dopaminergic hyperactivity in the basal ganglia,** that occurs when the CNS levels of dopamine receptor antagonist drug begin to fall between doses.

Clinical Features:

Dystonic movements result from a slow, sustained muscular contraction or spasm that can result in an involuntary movement. It can involve the:	
• **Face (grimacing)**[Q] • **Neck (spasmodic torticollis**[Q] or retrocollis) • Jaw (forced opening resulting in dislocation of jaw or **trismus**[Q]) • **Tongue (protrusions, twisting)**[Q] • **Eye (oculogyric crisis**[Q] characterized by eyes' upward lateral movement)	• **Dystonic posture of limb and trunk**[Q]. • Spinal muscles **(opisthotonos)**[Q], • Blepharospasm, **glossopharyngeal and laryngo-pharyngeal dystonia**, which can result in dysarthria, dysphagia, and even trouble breathing, which can cause cyanosis

• Unlike other types of dystonia, an **oculogyric crisis may occur late in treatment**.
• **Children are particularly likely to exhibit opisthotonos, scoliosis, lordosis, and writhing movements**.

Contd...

AIIMS May 2015

Contd...

Neuroleptic Induced Acute Dystonia
Treatment:
• Treatment with **IM anticholinergic (benztropine) or IV/IM antihistaminic (diphenhydramine hydrochloride)**[Q] **almost always relieves the symptoms.**
• **Promethazine,** 25-50 mg IV or IM, has been **used less frequently but readily available**

Extrapyramidal Disturbances of anti-Psychotic drugs
• These are the **major dose limiting side effects**[Q]
• **More prominent with high potency drugs like fluphenazine, haloperidol, pimozide etc**[Q].
• **Least with thioridazine, clozapine, olanzapine,** and **low doses of resperidone**[Q].
• These are of following types:
A. Parkinsonism:
• With typical manifestations-**rigidity, tremor, hypokinesia, mask like facies, shuffling gait**[Q]
• Appears **between 1-4 weeks of therapy**[Q]
• **Treatment: Central anticholinergic drugs**[Q]

Rabbit syndrome
• A rare form of extrapyramidal side effect is **perioral tremors "rabbit syndrome"**
• Occurs years after of therapy
• **Treatment: Central anticholinergic drugs**[Q]

B. Acute muscular dystonia:
• **Bizarre muscle spasms, mostly involving linguo-facial muscles-grimacing, torticollis, locked jaw**[Q]
• Occurs **within few hours of single dose** or at the **most in the first week of therapy**[Q]
• **More common in children below 10 years and in girls, particularly after parenteral administration**[Q]
• **Treatment: Central anticholinergic**[Q], **promethazine**[Q] or hydroxyzine

C. Akathisia:
• Restlessness, feeling of discomfort, apparent agitation manifested as **compelling desire to move about but without anxiety**[Q]
• **Between 1-8 weeks of therapy**[Q]
• No specific antidote is available
• **Treatment: Propranolol**[Q]

D. Malignant neuroleptic syndrome:
• **Occurs rarely with high doses of potent agents**[Q]
• Marked rigidity, immobility, tremor, fever, semi-consciousness, fluctuating BP and heart rate, myoglobin may be present in blood-lasts 5-10 days after drug withdrawal and may be fatal[Q].
• **Treatment: Stop neuroleptic, Bromocriptine**[Q]

E. Tardive dyskinesia:
• **Occurs late in therapy (Chronic therapy), sometimes even after withdrawal of neuroleptic**[Q]
• Manifests as purposeless involuntary facial and limb movements like constant chewing, pouting, puffing of cheeks, lip licking, choreoathetoid movements[Q]
• **More common in elderly women**[Q]
• Probably a manifestation of progressive neuronal degeneration along with supersensitivity to DA
• **Accentuated by anticholinergics and temporarily suppressed by high doses of neuroleptics**[Q]

199. **Ans. c. Tremors**   *(Ref: Kaplan and Sadock 11/e p596; Niraj Ahuja 7/e p38)*

Key symptom in alcohol withdrawal syndrome is tremors.

AIIMS ESSENCE

*"The **classic sign of alcohol withdrawal is tremulousness**, although the **spectrum of symptoms can expand to include psychotic and perceptual symptoms** (e.g., delusions and hallucinations), seizures, and the symptoms of delirium tremens (DTs), called alcohol delirium in DSM-5. **Tremulousness (commonly called the "shakes" or the "jitters") develops 6 to 8 hours after the cessation of drinking, the psychotic and perceptual symptoms begin in 8 to 12 hours, seizures in 12 to 24 hours, and DTs anytime during the first 72 hours,** although physicians should watch for the development of DTs for the first week of withdrawal. The syndrome of withdrawal sometimes skips the usual progression and, for example, goes directly to DTs."-Kaplan and Sadock 11/e p596*

Withdrawal Syndromes	
Substance	**Features**
Opioid	• **Yawning[Q]**, Insomnia, Dysphoric mood • Water loss from different orifices[Q] **(Lacrimation[Q], sweating[Q], diarrhea[Q], vomiting, rhinorrhea[Q])** • **Increased vitals[Q]** (BP, Pulse, RR, Temperature)[Q] • Pupillary dilation, **piloerection[Q]**

Alcohol	• **Hang over (MC)[Q]**
	• **Hallucinations[Q] (usually auditory) and illusions[Q]**
	• **Insomnia[Q]**
	• **Tremors/Seizures (Alcoholic seizures/Rum fits): Classic sign**
	• **Delirium tremens:**
	  – Occurs **within 5 days[Q]** of complete or **significant abstinence[Q]** from heavy alcohol drinking
	  – Recovery occurs within 7 days
	  – Characteristic features are **clouding of consciousness[Q], disorientation[Q], hallucinations (mostly visual and auditory)[Q], illusion[Q], autonomic disturbances[Q], agitation[Q] and insomnia[Q].**

Cocaine	• Increased or decreased
	  – **Sleep (hypersomnia[Q] or insomnia)**
	  – Psychomotor activity
	• **Vivid unpleasant dreams[Q]**
	• Increased apetite and fatigue

200. **Ans. b. Exposure and response prevention**   *(Ref: Kaplan and Sadock 11/e p406)*

From the above description it is clear that this patient is suffering from OCD. Treatment of choice for OCD is behaviour therapy. Exposure and response prevention is the preferred and principal approach. It is most effective in compulsions.

*"**Behavior Therapy:** Although few head-to-head comparisons have been made, **behavior therapy is as effective as pharmacotherapies in OCD,** and some data indicate that the **beneficial effects are longer lasting with behavior therapy.***

*Many clinicians, therefore, consider **behavior therapy the treatment of choice for OCD.** Behavior therapy can be conducted in both outpatient and inpatient settings. **The principal behavioral approaches in OCD are exposure and response prevention.** Desensitization, thought stopping, flooding, implosion therapy, and aversive conditioning have also been used in patients with OCD. In behavior therapy, patients must be truly committed to improvement."-Kaplan and Sadock 11/e p406*

See Q. No. 197 AIIMS November 2016.